ORAL RADIOLOGY
Principles and Interpretation

ORAL RADIOLOGY
Principles and Interpretation

STUART C. WHITE, DDS, PhD
Professor, Section of Oral and Maxillofacial Radiology
School of Dentistry
University of California, Los Angeles
Los Angeles, California

MICHAEL J. PHAROAH, DDS, MSc, FRCD(C)
Professor, Department of Radiology
Faculty of Dentistry
University of Toronto
Toronto, Ontario
Canada

FIFTH EDITION

Selected illustrations by Donald O'Connor

with 1325 *illustrations*

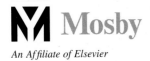
Mosby
An Affiliate of Elsevier

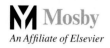

Mosby

An Affiliate of Elsevier

11830 Westline Industrial Drive
St. Louis, Missouri 63146

ORAL RADIOLOGY: PRINCIPLES AND INTERPRETATION   ISBN 0-323-02001-1

Previous editions copyrighted 1982, 1987, 1994, and 2000

Publishing Director: Linda L. Duncan
Executive Editor: Penny Rudolph
Senior Developmental Editor: Kimberly Alvis
Publishing Services Manager: Pat Joiner
Project Manager: Karen M. Rehwinkel
Senior Designer: Gail Morey Hudson
Cover Design: M-W Design, Inc.

Printed in China

Last digit is the print number: 9   8   7   6   5   4   3   2

Contributors

Kathryn A. Atchison, DDS, MPH
Professor and Associate Dean for
  Research and Knowledge Management
University of California, School of Dentistry
Los Angeles, California

Byron W. Benson, DDS, MS
Professor, Department of Diagnostic Sciences
Baylor College of Dentistry, Texas A&M University System
Dallas, Texas

Sharon L. Brooks, DDS, MS
Professor
Department of Oral Medicine/Pathology/Oncology;
Associate Professor, Department of Radiology
University of Michigan School of Medicine
Ann Arbor, Michigan

Laurie C. Carter, DDS, MA, PhD
Associate Professor and Director
Oral and Maxillofacial Radiology
Department of Oral Pathology
Virginia Commonwealth University, School of Dentistry
Richmond, Virginia

Neil L. Frederiksen, DDS, PhD
Professor and Director, Oral and Maxillofacial Radiology
Department of Diagnostic Sciences
Baylor College of Dentistry
Texas A&M University System Health Science Center
Dallas, Texas

Mel L. Kantor, DDS, MPH
Professor
Division of Oral and Maxillofacial Radiology
Department of Diagnostic Sciences
UMDNJ New Jersey Dental School
Newark, New Jersey

Ernest W.N. Lam, DMD, PhD, FRCD(C)
Associate Professor and Chair
Division of Oral and Maxillofacial Radiology;
Adjunct Associate Professor of Oncology
Department of Dentistry, University of Alberta
Edmonton, Alberta
Canada

Linda Lee, DDS, MSc, Dipl ABOP, FRCD(C)
Assistant Professor
Department of Biological and Diagnostic Sciences
Faculty of Dentistry, University of Toronto;
Staff Dentist, Department of Dental Oncology
Princess Margaret Hospital, University Health Network
Toronto, Ontario
Canada

John B. Ludlow, DDS, MS
Associate Professor
Department of Diagnostic Sciences and General
  Dentistry
University of North Carolina, School of Dentistry
Chapel Hill, North Carolina

Alan G. Lurie, DDS, PhD
Professor and Head, Oral and Maxillofacial Radiology;
Professor, Diagnostic Imaging and Therapeutics
Division of Oral and Maxillofacial Radiology
University of Connecticut, School of Dental Medicine
Farmington, Connecticut

André Mol, DDS, MS, PhD
Assistant Professor
Department of Diagnostic Sciences and General
  Dentistry
University of North Carolina
Chapel Hill, North Carolina

Carol Anne Murdoch-Kinch, DDS, PhD
Clinical Associate Professor
Department of Oral Medicine, Pathology, and
  Oncology
University of Michigan, School of Dentistry;
Attending Physician
Oral and Maxillofacial Surgery and Hospital Dentistry
University of Michigan Health System
Ann Arbor, Michigan

C. Grace Petrikowski, DDS, MSc, Dip. Oral Rad, FRCD(C)
Associate Professor, Department of Radiology
Faculty of Dentistry, University of Toronto
Toronto, Ontario
Canada

Axel Ruprecht, DDS, MScD, FRCD(C)
Professor and Director, Oral and Maxillofacial Radiology
Department of Oral Pathology, Radiology, and Medicine
College of Dentistry;
Professor, Department of Radiology
College of Medicine, University of Iowa
Iowa City, Iowa

Vivek Shetty, DDS, Dr Med Dent
Associate Professor
Department of Oral and Maxillofacial Surgery
University of California, School of Dentistry
Los Angeles, California

Sotirios Tetradis, DDS, PhD
Associate Professor
Department of Oral and Maxillofacial Radiology
University of California, School of Dentistry
Los Angeles, California

Ann Wenzel, PhD, DrOdont
Professor and Head
Department of Oral Radiology, Royal Dental College
Faculty of Health Sciences, University of Aarhus
Aarhus, Denmark

Robert E. Wood, DDS, PhD, FRCD(C)
Associate Professor
Department of Oral Radiology
Faculty of Dentistry, University of Toronto;
Active Staff, Department of Dental Oncology
Princess Margaret Hospital, University Health Network
Toronto, Ontario
Canada

To our wives and children
Liza
Heather and **Kelly**

Linda
Jayson, Edward, and **Lian**

Preface

Each new edition of this textbook provides the opportunity to include recent progress in the rapidly changing field of diagnostic imaging. We note with particular satisfaction the recent recognition by the American Dental Association of Oral and Maxillofacial Radiology as their ninth specialty. The ADA's definition of *oral and maxillofacial radiology* is: the specialty of dentistry and discipline of radiology concerned with the production and interpretation of images and data produced by all modalities of radiant energy that are used for the diagnosis and management of diseases, disorders, and conditions of the oral and maxillofacial region. It is the continuing goal of our text to present the underlying science of diagnostic imaging as well as describe the core principles of image production and interpretation for the dental student.

In this edition the chapters on panoramic imaging and extraoral radiographic examinations have been extensively rewritten and expanded beyond radiographic technique and anatomy to provide new emphasis on radiographic interpretation. These chapters now lead the reader through systematic approaches to evaluate the complex anatomic relationships displayed on panoramic and skull radiographs for evidence of abnormalities. In recent years there has been a major move to digital imaging in dentistry. We added a new chapter, *Digital Imaging*, that explains the various types of digital imaging available in dentistry, the underlying concepts of how the different methods work, and their comparative strengths and weaknesses in clinical usage. Just within the last two years cone-beam tomography has become available in dentistry. The chapter on specialized radiographic techniques now explains how this technology works and how it is best used in dentistry. The chapter on dental caries has also been expanded and updated. The chapters on radiographic manifestations of disease in the orofacial region have been updated to include the latest information on etiology and diagnosis. The chapter on orofacial implants has been expanded and updated to keep abreast of this rapidly changing field. We improved the images throughout the book and added examples of advanced imaging where appropriate.

Stuart C. White
Michael J. Pharoah

Preface

Acknowledgments

We have drawn upon the special talents of many of our colleagues as authors of chapters, some for the first time and others for return visits. We thank all for sharing their knowledge and skills. In particular we welcome the first timers: Dr. Alan G. Lurie—*Panoramic Imaging,* Drs. Sotirios Tetradis and Mel L. Kantor—*Extraoral Radiographic Examinations,* Drs. John B. Ludlow and André Mol—*Digital Imaging,* Dr. Ann Wenzel—*Dental Caries,* Dr. Ernest W.N. Lam—*Paranasal Sinuses,* Dr. Laurie C. Carter—*Soft Tissue Calcification and Ossification,* and Dr. Carol Anne Murdoch-Kinch—*Developmental Disturbances of the Face and Jaws.* We also wish to acknowledge the insightful thoughts of Mr. Charlie Brayer and Ms. Ruth K. Arbuckle related to x-ray film and intensifying screens. The immense knowledge and experience of all these individuals adds immeasurably to this text. We are most grateful for the skillful and generous support from the staff at Elsevier for their energy and creativity in the presentation of the content. And finally, we thank our students whose sharp eyes and minds constantly discover new ways for us to improve this book.

Stuart C. White
Michael J. Pharoah

Contents

PART I
THE PHYSICS OF IONIZING RADIATION
1   Radiation Physics, 3
    In collaboration with
    ALBERT G. RICHARDS

PART II
BIOLOGIC EFFECTS OF RADIATION
2   Radiation Biology, 25

PART III
RADIATION SAFETY AND PROTECTION
3   Health Physics, 47
    NEIL L. FREDERIKSEN

PART IV
IMAGING PRINCIPLES AND TECHNIQUES
4   X-Ray Film, Intensifying Screens, and Grids, 71

5   Projection Geometry, 86

6   Processing X-Ray Film, 94

7   Radiographic Quality Assurance and Infection
    Control, 110

8   Intraoral Radiographic Examinations, 121

9   Normal Radiographic Anatomy, 166

10 Panoramic Imaging, 191
    ALAN G. LURIE

11 Extraoral Radiographic Examinations, 210
    SOTIRIOS TETRADIS ■ MEL L. KANTOR

12 Digital Imaging, 225
    JOHN B. LUDLOW ■ ANDRÉ MOL

13 Specialized Radiographic Techniques, 245
    NEIL L. FREDERIKSEN

14 Guidelines for Prescribing Dental
    Radiographs, 265
    SHARON L. BROOKS ■ KATHRYN A. ATCHISON

PART V
RADIOGRAPHIC INTERPRETATION OF PATHOLOGY
15 Principles of Radiographic Interpretation, 281

16 Dental Caries, 297
    ANN WENZEL

17 Periodontal Diseases, 314

18 Dental Anomalies, 330

19 Inflammatory Lesions of the Jaws, 366
    LINDA LEE

20 Cysts of the Jaws, 384

21 Benign Tumors of the Jaws, 410

22 Malignant Diseases of the Jaws, 458
    ROBERT E. WOOD

23 Diseases of Bone Manifested in the Jaws, 485

24 Systemic Diseases Manifested in the
    Jaws, 516

25 Diagnostic Imaging of the
    Temporomandibular Joint, 538
    C. GRACE PETRIKOWSKI

26 Paranasal Sinuses, 576
    AXEL RUPRECHT ■ ERNEST W.N. LAM

27 Soft Tissue Calcification and Ossification, 597
    LAURIE C. CARTER

28 Trauma to Teeth and Facial Structures, 615

29 Developmental Disturbances of the Face and
    Jaws, 639
    CAROL ANNE MURDOCH-KINCH

30 Salivary Gland Radiology, 658
    BYRON W. BENSON

31 Orofacial Implants, 677
    VIVEK SHETTY ■ BYRON W. BENSON

ORAL RADIOLOGY
Principles and Interpretation

PART ONE

The Physics of Ionizing Radiation

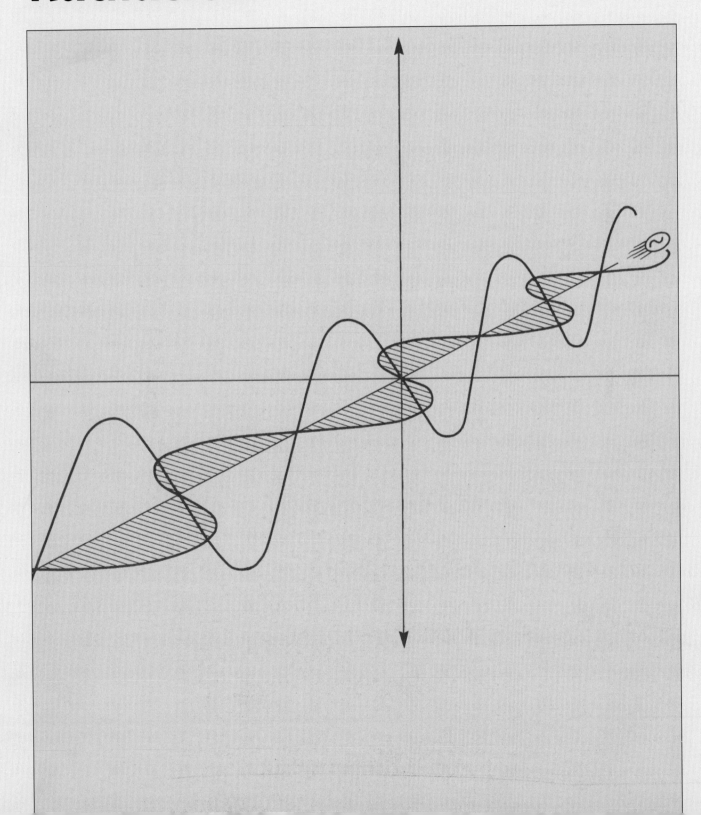

1

Radiation Physics

In collaboration with

ALBERT G. RICHARDS

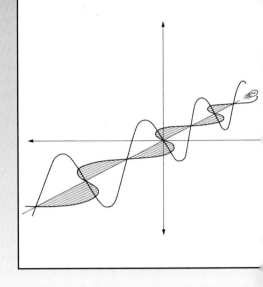

Composition of Matter

Matter is anything that occupies space and has inertia. It has mass and can exert force or be acted on by a force. Matter occurs in three states—solid, liquid, and gas—and may be divided into elements and compounds. Atoms, the fundamental units of elements, cannot be subdivided by ordinary chemical methods but may be broken down into smaller (subatomic) particles by special high-energy techniques. More than 100 subatomic particles have been described*; the so-called *fundamental* particles (electrons, protons, and neutrons) are of greatest interest in radiology because the generation, emission, and absorption of radiation occur at the subatomic level.

ATOMIC STRUCTURE

Because the atom cannot be directly observed, various models are used to describe its structure, each of which is capable of explaining observable actions. The phenomena associated with radiology employ the quantum mechanical model proposed by Niels Bohr in 1913. Bohr conceived the atom as a miniature solar system, at the center of which is the nucleus, analogous to the sun. Electrons revolve around this nucleus at high speeds, analogous to the planets orbiting the sun. In all atoms except hydrogen, the nucleus consists of two primary subatomic particles: protons and neutrons. A single proton constitutes the nucleus of the hydrogen atom.

*The Particle Adventure: the fundamentals of matter and force: http://www.particleadventure.org.

Electrons orbit the nucleus of all atoms. All electrons are alike, as are all protons and neutrons.

Figure 1-1, *A,* illustrates Bohr's model, using a stylized rendering of three atoms. The paths of the electrons are drawn as sharply defined orbits to facilitate graphic representation of the generation of x rays and their interaction with matter. In reality the orbit should be represented by broad parameters defining a space in which the electron is most likely to be found. The orbits, or shells, lie at defined distances from the nucleus and are identified by a letter (Fig. 1-1, *B*). The innermost shell is the K shell, and the next in order are the L, M, N, O, P, and Q shells. The shells also have numbers for identification: 1 for the K shell, 2 for the L shell, and so on. These are the principal quantum numbers, represented by the letter *n*. No known atom has more than seven shells. Only two electrons may occupy the K shell, with increasingly larger numbers of electrons occupying the outer shells. The maximal number of electrons in a given shell is $2(n^2)$, where *n* is the principal quantum number.

Electrons, protons, and neutrons have unique characteristics. The electron carries an electrical charge of −1, the proton a charge of +1, and the neutron no charge at all. The mass of an electron at rest is about 9.1×10^{-28} g. In contrast, the mass of a proton is 1.67×10^{-24} g, which is 1836 times the mass of an electron. The mass of a neutron is 1.68×10^{-24} g, making it 1852 times heavier than an electron and slightly heavier than a proton. Most of the mass of an atom consists of protons and neutrons concentrated in the nucleus. The nucleus contributes only a small fraction (about $^1/_{100,000}$) of the total size of an atom; most of the size of an atom consists of the cloud of orbiting electrons.

3

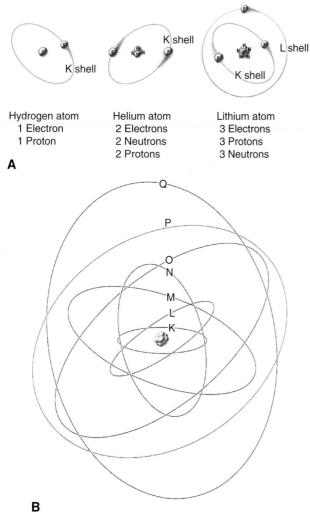

A

Hydrogen atom
1 Electron
1 Proton

Helium atom
2 Electrons
2 Neutrons
2 Protons

Lithium atom
3 Electrons
3 Protons
3 Neutrons

B

FIG. **1-1**   **A,** Atomic structures of hydrogen, helium, and lithium showing orbiting electrons surrounding neutrons and protons in the nucleus. **B,** Atom showing the structure and identification of electron shells around the nucleus.

The number of protons contained in the nucleus determines the positive charge. Because any atom in its ground state is electrically neutral, the total number of protons and electrons it carries must be the same. The number of protons in the nucleus also determines the identity of an element. This is its atomic number *(Z)*. Consequently, each of the more than 100 elements has a definitive atomic number, a corresponding number of orbital electrons, and unique chemical and physical properties. Nearly the entire mass of the atom consists of the protons and neutrons in the nucleus. The total number of protons and neutrons in the nucleus of an atom is its atomic mass *(A)*.

The electrostatic attraction between a positively charged nucleus and its negatively charged electrons balances the centrifugal force of the rapidly revolving electrons and maintains them in their orbits. Consequently, the amount of energy required to remove an electron from a given shell must exceed the electrostatic force of attraction between it and the nucleus. This is called the *electron binding energy* of the electron (or *ionization energy*) and is specific for each shell of each element. Electrons in the K shell of a given element have the greatest binding energy because they are closest to the nucleus. The binding energy of the electrons in each successive shell decreases. For an electron to move from a specific orbit to another orbit farther from the nucleus, energy must be supplied in an amount equal to the difference in binding energies between the two orbits. In contrast, in moving an electron from an outer orbit to one closer to the nucleus, energy is lost and given up in the form of electromagnetic radiation (see "Characteristic Radiation," p. 13). The K-shell electrons or any other electrons of large (high-Z) atoms have greater binding energies than those in comparable shells of smaller (low-Z) atoms. This is because large atoms have more protons and thus bind the orbital electrons more tightly to the nucleus than do small atoms.

IONIZATION

When the number of orbiting electrons in an atom is equal to the number of protons in its nucleus, the atom is electrically neutral. If an electrically neutral atom loses an electron, it becomes a positive ion and the free electron is a negative ion. This process of forming an ion pair is termed *ionization.* Electrons can be lost from an atom by heating or by interactions (collisions) with high-energy x rays or particles such as protons. Such ionization requires sufficient energy to overcome the electrostatic force binding the electrons to the nucleus. The electrons in the inner shells (K, L, and M) are so tightly bound to the nucleus that only x rays, gamma rays, and high-energy particles can remove them. In contrast, the electrons in the outer shells have such low binding energies that they can be easily displaced by photons of lower energy (e.g., ultraviolet or visible light).

Nature of Radiation

Radiation is the transmission of energy through space and matter. It may occur in two forms: particulate and electromagnetic.

PARTICULATE RADIATION

Particulate radiation consists of atomic nuclei or subatomic particles moving at high velocity. Alpha particles, beta particles, and cathode rays are examples of particulate radiation. Alpha particles are helium nuclei consisting of two protons and two neutrons. They result from the radioactive decay of many elements. Because of their double charge and heavy mass, alpha particles densely ionize matter through which they pass. Accordingly, they quickly give up their energy and penetrate only a few microns of body tissue. (An ordinary sheet of paper absorbs them.) After stopping, alpha particles acquire two electrons and become neutral helium atoms.

Beta particles are electrons emitted by radioactive nuclei. High-speed beta particles are able to penetrate matter to a greater depth than alpha particles, to a maximum of 1.5 cm in tissue. This deeper penetration occurs because beta particles are smaller and lighter and carry a single negative charge; therefore they have a much lower probability of interacting with matter than do alpha particles. Accordingly, they ionize matter much less densely than alpha particles. Beta particles are used in radiation therapy for treatment of skin lesions. Cathode rays are also high-speed electrons but are produced by manufactured devices (e.g., x-ray tubes).

The capacity of particulate radiation to ionize atoms depends on its mass, velocity, and charge. The rate of loss of energy from a particle as it moves along its track through matter (tissue) is its *linear energy transfer* (LET). A particle loses kinetic energy each time it ionizes adjacent matter; the greater its physical size and charge and the lower its velocity, the greater is its LET. For example, alpha particles, with their high charge and low velocity, lose kinetic energy rapidly and have short path lengths (are densely ionizing); thus they have a high LET. Beta particles are much less densely ionizing because of their lighter mass and lower charge and thus have a lower LET. They penetrate through tissue more readily than do alpha particles.

ELECTROMAGNETIC RADIATION

Electromagnetic radiation is the movement of energy through space as a combination of electric and magnetic fields (Fig. 1-2). It is generated when the velocity of an electrically charged particle is altered. Gamma rays, x rays, ultraviolet rays, visible light, infrared radiation (heat), microwaves, and radio waves are all examples of electromagnetic radiation (Fig. 1-3). Gamma rays are photons that originate in the nuclei of radioactive atoms. They typically have greater energy than x rays. X rays, in contrast, are produced extranuclearly from the interaction of electrons with nuclei in x-ray machines. The types of radiation in this spectrum are ionizing or nonionizing, depending on their energy. If

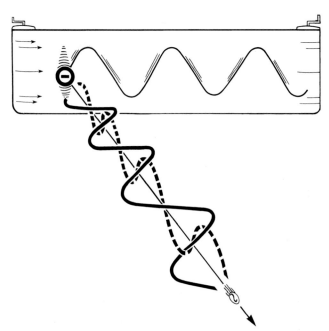

FIG. **1-2** A vibrating negatively charged particle generates electromagnetic radiation. Oscillations of the particle are traced on a strip recorder; they are equal in frequency to the electromagnetic waves produced.

sufficient energy is associated with the radiation to remove orbital electrons from atoms in the irradiated matter, the radiation is ionizing.

Some of the properties of electromagnetic radiation are best expressed by wave theory, whereas others are most successfully described by quantum theory. The wave theory of electromagnetic radiation maintains that radiation is propagated in the form of waves, not unlike the waves resulting from a disturbance in water. Such waves consist of electric and magnetic fields oriented in planes at right angles to one another that oscillate perpendicular to the direction of motion (Fig. 1-4). All electromagnetic waves travel at the velocity of light (3.0×10^8 m per sec; the velocity of light is represented by the letter c) in a vacuum. Waves of all kinds exhibit the properties of wavelength (λ) and frequency (ν). Wavelength and frequency of electromagnetic radiation are related as follows:

$$\lambda \times \nu = c = 3 \times 10^8 \text{ meters/second}$$

where λ is in meters and ν is in cycles per second (hertz). Wave theory is more useful for considering radiation in bulk when millions of quanta are being examined, as in experiments dealing with refraction, reflection, diffraction, interference, and polarization.

Quantum theory considers electromagnetic radiation as small bundles of energy called *photons*. Each photon travels at the speed of light and contains a

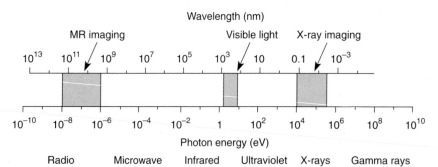

FIG. **1-3** Electromagnetic spectrum showing the relationship among wavelength, photon energy, and physical properties of various portions of the spectrum. Photons with shorter wavelengths have higher energy. Photons used in dental radiography have a wavelength of 0.1 to 0.001 nm.

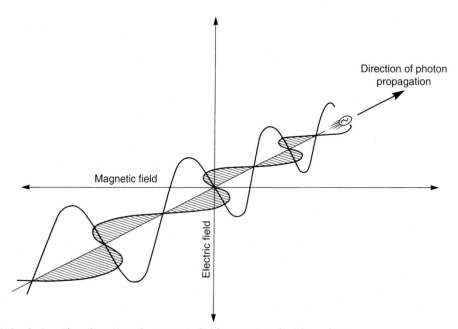

FIG. **1-4** The electric and magnetic fields associated with a photon.

specific amount of energy. The unit of photon energy is the *electron volt* (eV) (Fig. 1-5). The relationship between wavelength and photon energy is as follows:

$$E = h \times c/\lambda$$

where E is energy in kiloelectron volts (keV), h is Planck's constant (6.626×10^{-34} joule-seconds, or 4.3×10^{-18} keV), c is the velocity of light, and λ is wavelength in nanometers. This expression may be simplified as follows:

$$E = 1.24/\lambda$$

The quantum theory of radiation has been successful in correlating experimental data on the interaction of radiation with atoms, the photoelectric effect, and the production of x rays.

Typically, high-energy photons such as x rays and gamma rays are characterized by their energy, whereas lower-energy photons (ultraviolet through radio waves) are characterized by their wavelength.

The X-Ray Machine

The heart of an x-ray machine is the x-ray tube and its power supply. The x-ray tube is positioned within the tube head, along with some components of the power supply (Fig. 1-6). Often the tube is recessed within the

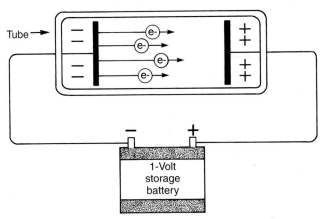

FIG. **1-5** An electron volt is the amount of energy acquired by one electron accelerating through a potential difference of 1 volt (1.602×10^{-19} joules).

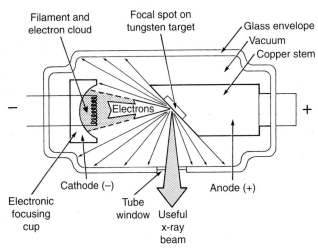

FIG. **1-7** X-ray tube with the major components labeled.

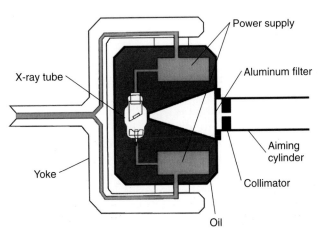

FIG. **1-6** Tube head (including the recessed x-ray tube), components of the power supply, and the oil that conducts heat away from the x-ray tube.

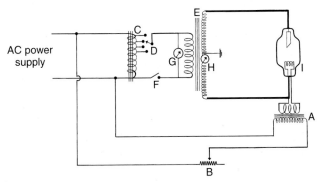

FIG. **1-8** Dental x-ray machine circuitry with the major components labeled. *A,* Filament step-down transformer; *B,* filament current control (mA switch); *C,* autotransformer; *D,* kVp selector dial (switch); *E,* high-voltage transformer; *F,* x-ray timer (switch); *G,* tube voltage indicator (volt-meter); *H,* tube current indicator (ammeter); *I,* x-ray tube.

tube head to improve the quality of the radiographic image (see Chapter 5). The tube head is supported by an arm that is usually mounted on a wall. A control panel allows the operator to adjust the time of exposure and often the energy and exposure rate of the x-ray beam.

X-RAY TUBE

All dental and medical x-ray tubes are called *Coolidge tubes* because they follow the original design of W. C. Coolidge introduced in 1913. The basic apparatus for generating x rays, the x-ray tube, is composed of a cathode and an anode (Fig. 1-7). The cathode serves as the source of electrons that flow to the anode. The cathode and anode lie within an evacuated glass envelope or tube. When electrons from the cathode

strike the target in the anode, they produce x rays. For the x-ray tube to function, a power supply is necessary to (1) heat the filament to generate electrons, and (2) establish a high-voltage potential between the anode and cathode to accelerate the electrons (Fig. 1-8).

Cathode

The cathode (see Fig. 1-7) in an x-ray tube consists of a filament and a focusing cup. The *filament* is the source of electrons within the x-ray tube. It is a coil of tungsten wire about 2 mm in diameter and 1 cm or less in length. It is mounted on two stiff wires that support it and carry the electric current. These two mounting wires lead through the glass envelope and connect to both the high- and low-voltage electrical sources. The filament is heated to incandescence by the flow of current from

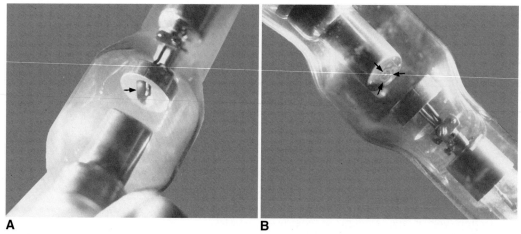

FIG. **1-9** **A,** Focusing cup *(arrow)* containing a filament in the cathode of the tube from a dental x-ray machine. **B,** Focal spot area *(arrows)* on the target of the tube. The size and shape of the focal area approximate those of the focusing cup.

the low-voltage source and emits electrons at a rate proportional to the temperature of the filament.

The filament lies in a *focusing cup* (Fig. 1-9, *A;* see also Fig. 1-7), a negatively charged concave reflector made of molybdenum. The focusing cup electrostatically focuses the electrons emitted by the incandescent filament into a narrow beam directed at a small rectangular area on the anode called the *focal spot* (Fig. 1-9, *B;* see also Fig. 1-7). The electrons move in this direction because they are repelled by the negatively charged cathode and attracted to the positively charged anode. The x-ray tube is evacuated to prevent collision of the moving electrons with gas molecules, which would significantly reduce their speed. This also prevents oxidation and "burnout" of the filament.

Anode

The anode consists of a tungsten target embedded in a copper stem (see Fig. 1-7). The purpose of the *target* in an x-ray tube is to convert the kinetic energy of the electrons generated from the filament into x-ray photons. This is an inefficient process with more than 99% of the electron kinetic energy converted to heat. The target is made of tungsten, a material that has several characteristics of an ideal target material. It has a high atomic number (74), high melting point, high thermal conductivity, and low vapor pressure at the working temperatures of an x-ray tube. A target made of a *high atomic number* material is best because it is most efficient in producing x rays. Because heat is generated at the anode, the requirement for a target with a *high melting point* is clear. Tungsten also has *high thermal conductivity,* thus dissipating heat into the copper stem. Finally, the

low vapor pressure of tungsten at high temperatures also helps maintain the vacuum in the tube at high operating temperatures.

The tungsten target is typically embedded in a large block of copper to dissipate heat. Copper, a good *thermal conductor,* dissipates heat from the tungsten, thus reducing the risk of the target melting. In addition, insulating oil between the glass envelope and the housing of the tube head carries heat away from the copper stem. This type of anode is a *stationary anode.*

The *focal spot* is the area on the target to which the focusing cup directs the electrons from the filament. The sharpness of the radiographic image increases as the size of the focal spot—the radiation source—decreases (see Chapter 5). The heat generated per unit target area, however, becomes greater as the focal spot decreases in size. To take advantage of a small focal spot while distributing the electrons over a larger area of the target, the target is placed at an angle to the electron beam (Fig. 1-10). The projection of the focal spot perpendicular to the electron beam (the *effective focal spot*) is smaller than the actual size of the focal spot. Typically, the target is inclined about 20 degrees to the central ray of the x-ray beam. This causes the effective focal spot to be almost 1×1 mm, as opposed to the actual focal spot, which is about 1×3 mm. The effect is a small apparent source of x rays and an increase in sharpness of the image (see Fig. 5-2) with a larger actual focal spot for heat dissipation.

Another method of dissipating the heat from a small focal spot is to use a *rotating anode.* In this case the tungsten target is in the form of a beveled disk that rotates when the tube is in operation (Fig. 1-11). As a result, the

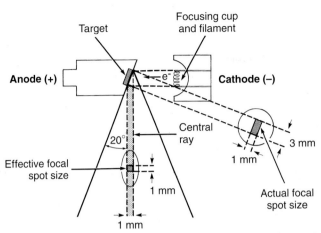

FIG. **1-10** The angle of the target to the central ray of the x-ray beam has a strong influence on the apparent size of the focal spot. The projected effective focal spot is much smaller than the actual focal spot size.

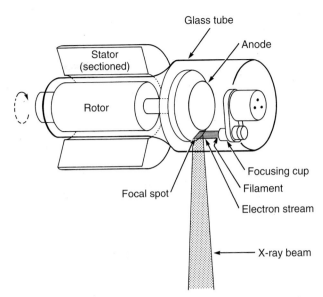

FIG. **1-11** X-ray tube with a rotating anode, which allows heat at the focal spot to spread out over a large surface area.

electrons strike successive areas of the target, widening the focal spot by an amount corresponding to the circumference of the beveled disk and distributing the heat over this expanded area. As a consequence, small focal spots can be used with tube currents of 100 to 500 milliamperes (mA), 10 to 50 times that possible with stationary targets. The target and rotor (armature) of the motor lie within the x-ray tube, and the stator coils (which drive the rotor at about 3000 revolutions per minute) lie outside the tube. Such rotating anodes are not used in intraoral dental x-ray machines but may be used in tomographic or cephalometric units and in medical x-ray machines requiring higher radiation output.

POWER SUPPLY

A brief review of some aspects of an electric circuit may be useful in understanding the power supply in an x-ray machine. An electric current is the movement of electrons in a conductor, for example, a wire. The rate of the current flow—the number of electrons moving past a point in a second—is measured in *amperes*. It depends on two factors: the pressure, or voltage, of the current, measured in volts, and the resistance of the conductor to the flow of electricity, measured in ohms. Ohm's law relates these units:

$$V = I \times R$$

where *V* is the electric potential in volts, *I* is the current flow in amperes, and *R* is the resistance of the conductor in ohms. Such an electric circuit is often compared to a simple water supply system in which the rate of water flow through a pipe (amperes) depends both on the water pressure (volts) and the pipe resistance or diameter (ohms).

The primary functions of the power supply of an x-ray machine are to (1) provide a low-voltage current to heat the x-ray tube filament by use of a step-down transformer and (2) generate a high potential difference between the anode and cathode by use of a high-voltage transformer. These transformers and the x-ray tube lie within an electrically grounded metal housing called the *head* of the x-ray machine. An electrical insulating material, usually oil, surrounds the transformers.

Tube Current

The *filament step-down transformer* (see Fig. 1-8, *A*) reduces the voltage of the incoming alternating current (AC) to about 10 volts. Its operation is regulated by the filament current control (mA switch) (see Fig. 1-8, *B*), which adjusts the resistance and thus the current flow through the low-voltage circuit, including the filament. This in turn regulates the temperature of the filament and thus the number of electrons emitted. The *tube current* is the flow of electrons through the tube, that is, from the filament to the anode and then back to the filament through the wiring of the power supply. The mA setting on the filament current control refers to the tube current, which is measured by the ammeter (see Fig. 1-8, *H*).

Tube Voltage

A high voltage is required between the anode and cathode to generate x rays. An *autotransformer* (see

Fig. 1-8, *C*) converts the primary voltage from the input source into the secondary voltage. The secondary voltage is regulated by the kilovolts peak (kVp) selector dial (see Fig. 1-8, *D*). The kVp dial selects a voltage from different levels on the autotransformer and applies it across the primary winding of the *high-voltage transformer*. The kVp dial therefore controls the voltage between the anode and cathode of the x-ray tube. The high-voltage transformer (see Fig. 1-8, *E*) provides the high voltage required by the x-ray tube to accelerate the electrons from the cathode to the anode and generate x rays. It accomplishes this by boosting the peak voltage of the incoming line current to as high as 60 to

100 kV, thus boosting the peak energy of the electrons passing through the tube to as high as 60 to 100 keV. The kVp selector dial setting thus determines the peak kilovoltage across the tube (see Fig. 1-8, *I*).

Because the line current is AC (60 cycles per second), the polarity of the x-ray tube alternates at the same frequency (Fig. 1-12, *A*). When the polarity of the voltage applied across the tube causes the target anode to be positive and the filament to be negative, the electrons around the filament accelerate toward the positive target and current flows through the tube (Fig. 1-12, *B*). Because the line voltage is variable, the voltage potential between the anode and cathode varies. As the

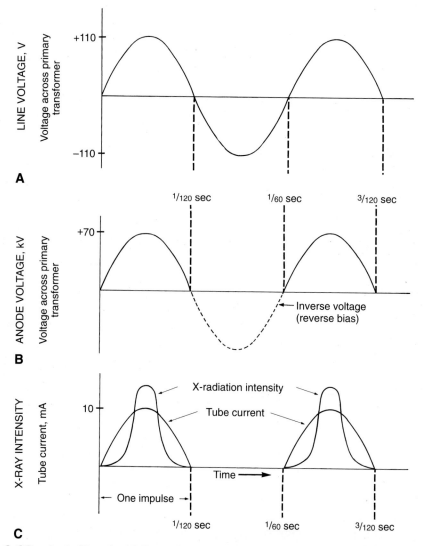

FIG. 1-12 **A,** A 60-cycle AC line voltage at a primary transformer. **B,** Voltage at the anode varies up to the kVp setting (70 in this case). **C,** The intensity of radiation produced at the anode increases as the anode voltage increases. (Modified from Johns HE, Cunningham JR: The physics of radiology, ed 3, Springfield, Ill, 1969, Charles C Thomas.)

tube voltage is increased, the speed of the electrons toward the anode increases. When the electrons strike the focal spot of the target, some of their energy converts to x-ray photons. X rays are produced at the target with greatest efficiency when the voltage applied across the tube is high. Therefore the intensity of x-ray pulses tends to be sharply peaked at the center of each cycle (Fig. 1-12, *C*). During the following half (or negative half) of the cycle, the polarity of the AC reverses, and the filament becomes positive and the target negative (see Fig. 1-12, *B*). At these times the electrons stay in the vicinity of the filament and do not flow across the gap between the two elements of the tube. This half of the cycle is called *inverse voltage* or *reverse bias* (see Fig. 1-12, *B*). No x rays are generated during this half of the voltage cycle (see Fig. 1-12, *C*). Therefore when an x-ray tube is powered with 60-cycle AC, 60 pulses of x rays are generated each second, each having a duration of $^1/_{120}$ second. This type of power supply circuitry, in which the alternating high voltage is applied directly across the x-ray tube, limits x-ray production to half the AC cycle and is called *self-rectified* or *half-wave rectified*. Almost all conventional dental x-ray machines are self-rectified.

A tube energized with a self-rectifying power supply must not be operated for extended periods. With overuse the target may get so hot that it emits electrons, and during the negative half cycle, the inverse voltage may drive electrons from the target to the filament, causing the filament to overheat and melt. The glass envelope also may be damaged if the electrons are driven in the wrong direction by the reverse bias on the tube.

Some dental x-ray manufacturers produce machines that replace the conventional 60-cycle AC high-voltage current of the x-ray tube with a high-frequency power supply. This effect is an essentially constant potential between the anode and cathode. The result is that the mean energy of the x-ray beam produced by these x-ray machines is higher than that from a conventional half-wave rectified machine operated at the same voltage. This is because the number of lower-energy (nondiagnostic) x rays is reduced. These photons are produced as the voltage across the x-ray tube rises from zero to its peak and then decreases back again to zero during the voltage cycle in the half-wave rectified machine. For a given voltage setting and radiographic density, the images resulting from these constant-potential machines have a longer contrast scale and lower patient dose compared with conventional x-ray machines.

TIMER

A timer is built into the high-voltage circuit to control the duration of the x-ray exposure (see Fig. 1-8, *F*). The timer controls the length of time that high voltage is applied to the tube and therefore the time during which tube current flows and x rays are produced. Before the high voltage is applied across the tube, however, the filament must be brought to operating temperature to ensure an adequate rate of electron emission. Subjecting the filament to continuous heating at normal operating current is not practical because maintaining the filament at a high temperature for a long period shortens its life. Failure of the filament is a common source of malfunction of x-ray tubes. To minimize filament burnout, the timing circuit first sends a current through the filament for about half a second to bring it to the proper operating temperature. After the filament is heated, the timer then applies power to the high-voltage circuit. In some circuit designs, a continuous low-level current passing through the filament maintains it at a safe low temperature. In this case the delay to preheat the filament before each exposure is even shorter. Accordingly, the machine should be left on continuously during working hours.

Some x-ray machine timers are calibrated in fractions and whole numbers of seconds. The time intervals on other timers are expressed as number of impulses per exposure (e.g., 3, 6, 9, 15). Such numbers represent the number of impulses of radiation emitted during the exposure; thus the number of impulses divided by 60 (the frequency of the power source) gives the exposure time in seconds. Therefore a setting of 30 impulses means that there will be 30 impulses of radiation and is equivalent to a half-second exposure.

TUBE RATING AND DUTY CYCLE

Each x-ray machine comes with *tube rating* specifications that describe the maximal exposure time the tube can be energized without risk of damage to the target from overheating. These specifications describe in graph form the maximal safe intervals (seconds) that the tube can be used for a range of voltages (kVp) and filament current (mA) values. These tube ratings generally do not impose any restrictions on tube use for daily intraoral radiography. If a dental x-ray unit is to be used for extraoral exposures, however, the tube-rating chart should be mounted by the machine for easy reference.

Duty cycle relates to the frequency with which successive exposures can be made. The heat buildup at the anode is measured in heat units defined by the following equation: heat units (HU) = kVp × mA × seconds. The heat storage capacity for anodes of dental diagnostic tubes is approximately 20 kHU. Because of heat generated at the anode, the interval between successive exposures must be long enough for its dissipation. This characteristic is a function of the size of the anode and the method used to cool it. The cooling characteristics of anodes are described by the maximal number of heat units it can store without damage and the heat dissipation rate, which can be determined from the cooling curves provided by the manufacturer of each tube.

Production of X Rays

Electrons traveling from the filament to the target convert some of their kinetic energy into x-ray photons by the formation of bremsstrahlung and characteristic radiation.

BREMSSTRAHLUNG

Bremsstrahlung interactions, the primary source of x-ray photons from an x-ray tube, are produced by the sudden stopping or slowing of high-speed electrons at the target. (*Bremsstrahlung* means "braking radiation" in German.) When electrons from the filament strike the tungsten target, x-ray photons are created if the electrons hit a target nucleus directly or if their path takes them close to a nucleus. If a high-speed electron directly hits the nucleus of a target atom, all its kinetic energy is transformed into a single x-ray photon (Fig. 1-13, *A*). The energy of the resultant photon (in keV) is numerically equal to the energy of the electron. This in turn is equal to the kilovoltage applied across the x-ray tube at the instant of its passage.

Most high-speed electrons, however, have near or wide misses with atomic nuclei (Fig. 1-13, *B*). In these interactions, a negatively charged high-speed electron is attracted toward the positively charged nuclei and loses some of its velocity. This deceleration causes the electron to lose some kinetic energy, which is given off in the form of many new photons. The closer the high-speed electron approaches the nuclei, the greater is the electrostatic attraction on the electron, the braking effect, and the energy of the resulting bremsstrahlung photons.

Bremsstrahlung interactions generate x-ray photons with a continuous spectrum of energy. The energy of an x-ray beam may be described by identifying the peak operating voltage (in kVp). A dental x-ray machine operating at a peak voltage of 70,000 volts (70 kVp), for example, applies a fluctuating voltage of as much as 70 kVp across the tube. This tube therefore produces x-ray photons with energies ranging to a maximum of 70,000 eV (70 keV). Fig. 1-14 demonstrates the continuous spectrum of photon energies produced by an x-ray machine operating at 100 kVp. The reasons for this continuous spectrum are as follows:

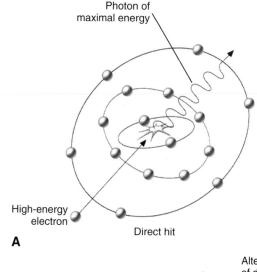

A

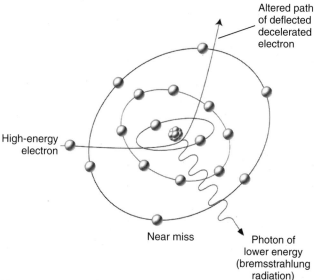

B

FIG. **1-13**   Bremsstrahlung radiation is produced by the direct hit of electrons on the nucleus in the target **(A)** or by the passage of electrons near the nucleus, which results in electrons being deflected and decelerated **(B)**.

1. The continuously varying voltage difference between the target and filament, which is characteristic of half-wave rectification, causes the electrons striking the target to have varying levels of kinetic energy.
2. The bombarding electrons pass at varying distances around tungsten nuclei and are thus deflected to varying extents. As a result, they give up varying amounts of energy in the form of bremsstrahlung photons.
3. Most electrons participate in many bremsstrahlung interactions in the target before losing all their kinetic energy. As a consequence, an electron carries differing amounts of energy at the time of each interaction with a tungsten nucleus that results in the generation of an x-ray photon.

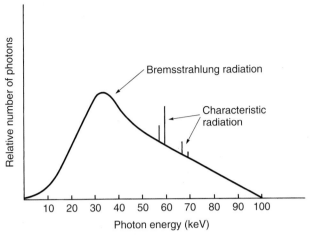

FIG. **1-14** Spectrum of photons emitted from an x-ray beam generated at 100 kVp. The vast preponderance of radiation is bremsstrahlung, with a minor addition of characteristic radiation.

CHARACTERISTIC RADIATION

Characteristic radiation occurs when an electron from the filament displaces an electron from a shell of a tungsten target atom, thereby ionizing the atom. When this happens, a higher energy electron in an outer shell of the tungsten atom is quickly attracted to the void in the deficient inner shell (Fig. 1-15). When the outer-shell electron replaces the displaced electron, a photon is emitted with an energy equivalent to the difference in the two orbital binding energies. Characteristic radiation from the K shell occurs only above 70 kVp with a tungsten target and occurs as discrete increments compared with bremsstrahlung radiation (see Fig. 1-14). The energies of characteristic photons are a function of the energy levels of various electron orbital levels and

hence are characteristic of the target atoms. Characteristic radiation is only a minor source of radiation from an x-ray tube.

Factors Controlling the X-Ray Beam

The x-ray beam emitted from an x-ray tube may be modified by altering the beam exposure length (timer), exposure rate (mA), beam energy (kVp and filtration), beam shape (collimation), and target-patient distance.

EXPOSURE TIME

Figure 1-16 portrays the changes in the x-ray spectrum that result when the exposure time is increased while the tube current (mA) and voltage (kVp) remain constant. When the exposure time is doubled, the number of photons generated at all energies in the x-ray emission spectrum is doubled, but the range of photon energies is unchanged. Therefore changing the time simply controls the *quantity* of the exposure, the number of photons generated.

TUBE CURRENT (mA)

Figure 1-17 illustrates the changes in the spectrum of photons that result from increasing tube current (mA) while maintaining constant tube voltage (kVp) and exposure time. As the mA setting is increased, more power is applied to the filament, which heats up and releases more electrons that collide with the target to produce radiation. Therefore the quantity of radiation produced by an x-ray tube (i.e., the number of photons that reach the patient and film) is directly proportional

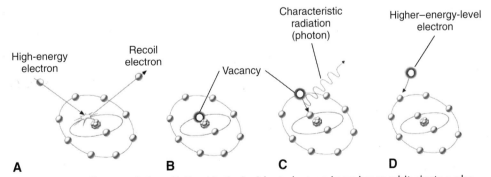

FIG. **1-15** Characteristic radiation. **A,** An incident electron in an inner orbit ejects a photoelectron, creating a vacancy. **B,** This vacancy is filled by an electron from an outer orbit. **C,** A photon is emitted with energy equal to the difference in energy levels between the two orbits. **D,** Electrons from various orbits may be involved, giving rise to other photons. The energies of the photons thus created are characteristic of the target atom.

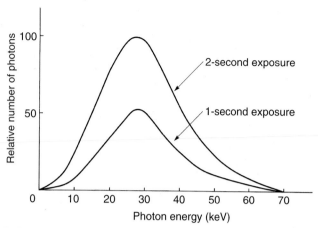

FIG. 1-16 Spectrum of photon energies showing that as exposure time increases (kVp and tube voltage held constant), so does the total number of photons. The mean energy and maximal energy of the beams are unchanged.

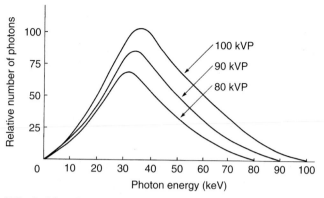

FIG. 1-18 Spectrum of photon energies showing that as the kVp is increased (tube current and exposure time held constant), there is a corresponding increase in the mean energy of the beam, the total number of photons emitted, and the maximal energy of the photons.

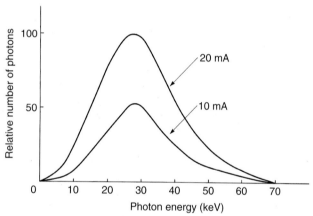

FIG. 1-17 Spectrum of photon energies showing that as tube current (mA) increases (kVp and exposure time held constant), so does the total number of photons. The mean energy and maximal energy of the beams are unchanged. Compare with Fig. 1-16.

to the tube current (mA) and the time the tube is operated. The quantity of radiation produced is expressed as the product of time and tube current. The quantity of radiation remains constant regardless of variations in mA and time as long as their product remains constant. For instance, a machine operating at 10 mA for 1 second (10 mAs) produces the same quantity of radiation when operated at 20 mA for 0.5 second (10 mAs), although in practice some dental x-ray machines fall slightly short of this ideal constancy.

TUBE VOLTAGE (kVp)

Figure 1-18 shows the influence of changing tube voltage (kVp) on the spectrum of photon energies in

an x-ray beam. Increasing the kVp increases the potential difference between the cathode and anode, thus increasing the energy of each electron when it strikes the target. This results in an increased efficiency of conversion of electron energy into x-ray photons, and thus an increase in (1) the number of photons generated, (2) their mean energy, and (3) their maximal energy. The increased number of photons produced per unit time by use of higher kVp results from the greater efficiency in the production of bremsstrahlung photons that occurs when increased numbers of higher-energy electrons interact with the target.

The ability of x-ray photons to penetrate matter depends on their energy. High-energy x-ray photons have a greater probability of penetrating matter, whereas relatively low-energy photons have a greater probability of being absorbed. Therefore the higher the kVp and mean energy of the x-ray beam, the greater the penetrability of the beam through matter. A useful way to characterize the penetrating quality of an x-ray beam (its energy) is by its half-value layer (HVL). The HVL is the thickness of an absorber, such as aluminum, required to reduce by one half the number of x-ray photons passing through it. As the average energy of an x-ray beam increases, so does its HVL. The term *beam quality* refers to the mean energy of an x-ray beam.

FILTRATION

Although an x-ray beam consists of a spectrum of x-ray photons of different energies, only photons with sufficient energy to penetrate through anatomic structures and reach the image receptor (usually film) are useful for diagnostic radiology. Those that are of low energy (long wavelength) contribute to patient exposure (and

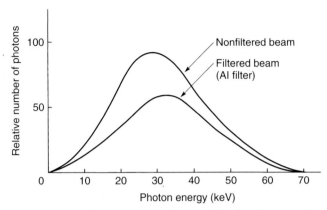

FIG. **1-19** Filtering an x-ray beam with aluminum preferentially removes low-energy photons, thereby reducing the beam intensity and increasing its mean energy.

risk) but do not have enough energy to reach the film. Consequently, to reduce patient dose, the less-penetrating photons should be removed. This can be accomplished, in part, by placing an aluminum filter in the path of the beam. Fig. 1-19 illustrates how the addition of an aluminum filter alters the energy distribution of the unfiltered beam. The aluminum preferentially removes many of the lower-energy photons with lesser effect on the higher-energy photons that are able to penetrate to the film.

In determinations of the amount of filtration required for a particular x-ray machine, kVp and inherent filtration of the tube and its housing must be considered. *Inherent filtration* consists of the materials that x-ray photons encounter as they travel from the focal spot on the target to form the usable beam outside the tube enclosure. These materials include the glass wall of the x-ray tube, the insulating oil that surrounds many dental tubes, and the barrier material that prevents the oil from escaping through the x-ray port. The inherent filtration of most x-ray machines ranges from the equivalent of 0.5 to 2 mm of aluminum. *Total filtration* is the sum of the inherent filtration plus any added *external filtration* supplied in the form of aluminum disks placed over the port in the head of the x-ray machine. Governmental regulations require the total filtration in the path of a dental x-ray beam to be equal to the equivalent of 1.5 mm of aluminum to 70 kVp, and 2.5 mm of aluminum for all higher voltages (see Chapter 3).

COLLIMATION

A collimator is a metallic barrier with an aperture in the middle used to reduce the size of the x-ray beam (Fig. 1-20) and therefore the volume of irradiated tissue within the patient. Round and rectangular collimators are most frequently used in dentistry. Dental x-ray beams are usually collimated to a circle 2$\frac{3}{4}$ inches (7 cm) in diameter. A round collimator (see Fig. 1-20, *A*) is a thick plate of radiopaque material (usually lead) with a circular opening centered over the port in the x-ray head through which the x-ray beam emerges. Typically, round collimators are built into open-ended aiming cylinders. Rectangular collimators (see Fig. 1-20, *B*) further limit the size of the beam to just larger than the x-ray film. It is important to reduce the beam to the size of the film to reduce further unnecessary patient exposure. Some types of film-holding instruments also provide rectangular collimation of the x-ray beam (see Chapters 3 and 8).

Use of collimation also improves image quality. When an x-ray beam is directed at a patient, the tissues

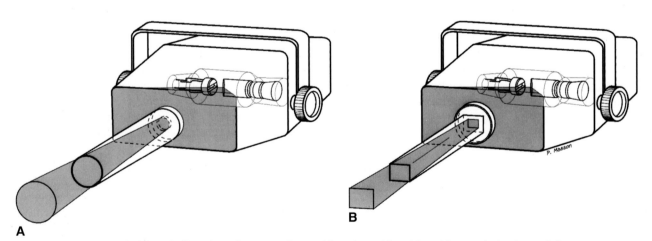

FIG. **1-20** Collimation of an x-ray beam *(dotted area)* is achieved by restricting its useful size. **A,** Circular collimator. **B,** Rectangular collimator restricts area of exposure to just larger than the detector size.

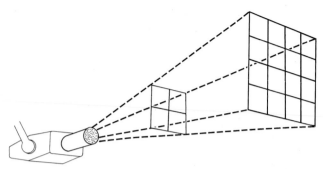

FIG. **1-21**   The intensity of an x-ray beam is inversely proportional to the square of the distance between the source and the point of measure.

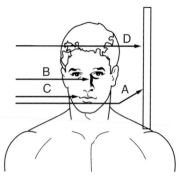

FIG. **1-22**   Photons in an x-ray beam interact with the object primarily by Compton scattering *(A)*, in which case the scattered photon may strike the film and degrade the radiographic image by causing film fog, or photoelectric absorption *(B)*. Relatively few photons undergo coherent scattering within the object *(C)* or pass through the object without interacting and expose the film *(D)*.

absorb about 90% of the x-ray photons and 10% of the photons pass through the patient and reach the film. Many of the absorbed photons generate scattered radiation within the exposed tissues by a process called *Compton scattering* (see below). These scattered photons travel in all directions, and some reach the film and degrade image quality. Collimating the beam to reduce the exposure area and thus the number of scattered photons reaching the film can minimize the detrimental effect of scattered radiation on the images.

INVERSE SQUARE LAW

The intensity of an x-ray beam at a given point (number of photons per cross-sectional area per unit exposure time) depends on the distance of the measuring device from the focal spot. For a given beam the intensity is inversely proportional to the square of the distance from the source (Fig. 1-21). The reason for this decrease in intensity is that the x-ray beam spreads out as it moves from the source. The relationship is as follows:

$$\frac{I_1}{I_2} = \frac{(D_2)^2}{(D_1)^2}$$

where *I* is intensity and *D* is distance. Therefore if a dose of 1 gray (Gy) is measured at a distance of 2 m, a dose of 4 Gy will be found at 1 m, and 0.25 Gy at 4 m.

Therefore changing the distance between the x-ray tube and patient has a marked effect on beam intensity. Such a change requires a corresponding modification of the kVp or mAs if the exposure of the film is to be kept constant.

Interactions of X Rays With Matter

The intensity of an x-ray beam is reduced by interaction with the matter it encounters. This attenuation results from interactions of individual photons in the beam with atoms in the absorber. The x-ray photons are either absorbed or scattered out of the beam. In absorption, photons ionize absorber atoms and convert their energy into kinetic energy of the absorber electrons. In scattering, photons are ejected out of the primary beam as a result of interactions with the orbital electrons of absorber atoms. In a dental x-ray beam there are three means of beam attenuation: (1) coherent scattering, (2) photoelectric absorption, and (3) Compton scattering (Fig. 1-22). In addition, about 9% of the primary photons pass through the patient without interaction (Table 1-1).

COHERENT SCATTERING

Coherent scattering (also known as *classical, elastic,* or *Thompson scattering*) may occur when a low-energy incident photon (less than 10 keV) passes near an outer electron of an atom (which has a low binding energy). The incident photon interacts with the electron by causing it to become momentarily excited at the same frequency as the incoming photon (Fig. 1-23). The incident photon ceases to exist. The excited electron then returns to the ground state and generates another x-ray photon with the same frequency and energy as in the incident beam. Usually the secondary photon is emitted at an angle to the path of the incident photon. In effect, the direction of the incident x-ray photon is altered. This interaction accounts for only about 8% of the total number of interactions (per exposure) in a dental examination (see Table 1-1). Coherent scattering contributes very little to film fog because the total quantity

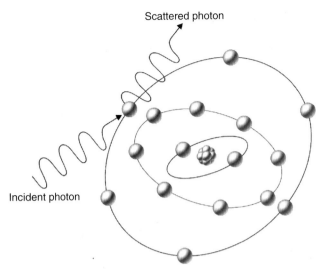

FIG. **1-23** Coherent scattering resulting from the interaction of a low-energy incident photon with an outer electron, causing the outer electron to vibrate momentarily. After this, a scattered photon of the same energy is emitted at a different angle from the path of the incident photon.

TABLE **1-1** *Fate of 2,000,000 Incident Photons in Bitewing Projections*			
INTERACTION	PRIMARY PHOTONS	SCATTERED PHOTONS*	TOTAL†
Coherent scattering	148,905	156,234	305,139
Photoelectric absorption	536,208	522,082	1,058,290
Compton scattering	1,131,878	1,098,720	2,230,598
Exit	183,009	758,701	941,710
TOTAL	2,000,000	2,535,737	4,535,737

From Gibbs SJ: Personal communication, 1986.
*Scattered photons result from primary, Compton, and coherent interactions.
†Note that the sum of the total number of photoelectric interactions and photons that exit the patient equals the total number of incident photons.

of scattered photons is small and its energy level is too low for much of it to reach the film.

PHOTOELECTRIC ABSORPTION

Photoelectric absorption is critical in diagnostic imaging. This process occurs when an incident photon collides with a bound electron in an atom of the absorb-ing medium. At this point the incident photon ceases to exist. The electron is ejected from its shell and becomes a recoil electron (photoelectron) (Fig. 1-24). The kinetic energy imparted to the recoil electron is equal to the energy of the incident photon minus that used to overcome the binding energy of the electron. The absorbing atom is now ionized because it has lost an electron. In the case of atoms with low atomic numbers (e.g., those in most biologic molecules), the binding energy is small. As a result the recoil electron acquires most of the energy of the incident photon. Most photoelectric interactions occur in the K shell because the density of the electron cloud is greater in this region and a higher probability of interaction exists. About 30% of photons absorbed from a dental x-ray beam are absorbed by the photoelectric process.

An atom that has participated in a photoelectric interaction is ionized as a result of the loss of an electron. This electron deficiency (usually in the K shell) is instantly filled, usually by an L-shell electron, with the release of characteristic radiation (see Fig. 1-15). Whatever the orbit of the replacement electron, the characteristic photons generated are of such low energy that they are absorbed within the patient and do not fog the film.

Recoil electrons ejected during photoelectric absorption travel only short distances in the absorber before they give up their energy through secondary ionizations. As a consequence, all the energy of incident photons that undergo photoelectric interaction is deposited in the patient. Although this is beneficial in producing high-quality radiographs, because no scattered radiation fogs the film, it is potentially deleterious for patients because of increased radiation absorption.

The frequency of photoelectric interaction varies directly with the *third power of the atomic number* of the absorber. For example, because the effective atomic number of compact bone (Z = 13.8) is greater than that of soft tissue (Z = 7.4), the probability that a photon will be absorbed by a photoelectric interaction in bone is approximately 6.5 times greater than in an equal thickness of soft tissue. This difference is readily seen on dental radiographs as a difference in optical density of the image. It is this difference in the absorption that makes the production of a radiographic image possible.

COMPTON SCATTERING

Compton scattering occurs when a photon interacts with an outer orbital electron (Fig. 1-25). About 62% of the photons that are absorbed from a dental x-ray beam are absorbed by this process. In this interaction the incident photon collides with an outer electron, which

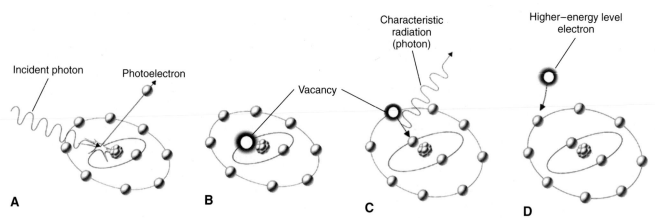

FIG. **1-24**   Photoelectric absorption. **A,** Photoelectric absorption occurs when an incident photon gives up all its energy to an inner electron ejected from the atom (a photoelectron). **B,** An electron vacancy in the inner orbit results in ionization of the atom. **C,** An electron from a higher energy level fills the vacancy and emits characteristic radiation. **D,** All orbits are subsequently filled, completing the energy exchange.

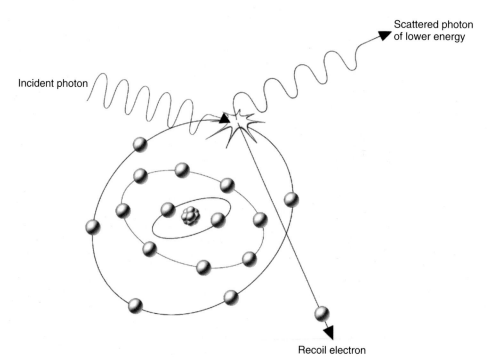

FIG. **1-25**   Compton absorption occurs when an incident photon interacts with an outer electron, producing a scattered photon of lower energy than the incident photon and a recoil electron ejected from the target atom.

receives kinetic energy and recoils from the point of impact. The path of the incident photon is deflected by its interaction and is scattered from the site of the collision. The energy of the scattered photon equals the energy of the incident photon minus the sum of the kinetic energy gained by the recoil electron and its binding energy. As with photoelectric absorption,

Compton scattering results in the loss of an electron and ionization of the absorbing atom. Scattered photons continue on their new paths, causing further ionizations. Similarly, the recoil electrons also give up their energy by ionizing other atoms.

The probability of a Compton interaction is directly proportional to the *electron density* of the absorber. The number of electrons in bone (5.55×10^{23}/cc) is greater than in soft tissue (3.34×10^{23}/cc); therefore the probability of Compton scattering is correspondingly greater in bone than in tissue. In a dental x-ray beam, approximately 62% of the photons undergo Compton scattering.

Scattered photons travel in all directions. The higher the energy of the incident photon, however, the greater the probability that the angle of scatter of the secondary photon will be small and its direction will be forward. Approximately 30% of the scattered photons formed during a dental x-ray exposure (primarily from Compton scattering) exit through the patient's head. This is advantageous to the patient because some of the energy of the incident x-ray beam escapes the tissue, but it is disadvantageous because it causes nonspecific film darkening. Scattered photons darken the film while carrying no useful information because their paths are altered.

DIFFERENTIAL ABSORPTION

The importance of photoelectric absorption and Compton scattering in diagnostic radiography relates to differences in the way photons are absorbed by various anatomic structures. The number of photoelectric and Compton interactions is greater in hard tissues than in soft tissues. As a consequence, more photons in the beam exit the patient after passing through soft tissue than through hard tissue. Thus while the *incident beam,* the beam striking the patient, is spatially homogenous, the *remnant beam,* the beam that exits the patient, is spatially heterogeneous. This remnant beam strikes the image receptor (film), resulting in greater exposure of the film behind soft tissue than behind hard tissues. It is this differential exposure of the film that allows a radiograph to reveal the morphology of enamel, dentin, bone, and soft tissues.

SECONDARY ELECTRONS

In both photoelectric absorption and Compton scattering, electrons are ejected from their orbits in the absorbing material after interaction with x-ray photons. These secondary electrons give up their energy in the absorber by either of two processes: (1) collisional interaction with other electrons, resulting in ionization or excitation of the affected atom, and (2) radiative interactions, which produce bremsstrahlung radiation, resulting in the emission of low-energy x-ray photons. Secondary electrons eventually dissipate all their energy, mostly as heat by collisional interactions, and come to rest.

BEAM ATTENUATION

As an x-ray beam travels through matter, its intensity is reduced (attenuated). This results from loss of individual photons, primarily through photoelectric absorption and Compton scattering interactions. The reduction of beam intensity is predictable because it depends on physical characteristics of the beam and absorber. A monochromatic beam of photons, a beam in which all the photons have the same energy, provides a good example. When only the primary (not scattered) photons are considered, a constant fraction of the beam is attenuated as the beam moves through each unit thickness of an absorber. Therefore 1.5 cm of water may reduce a beam intensity by 50%, the next 1.5 cm by another 50% (to 25% of the original intensity), and so on. This is an exponential pattern of absorption (Fig. 1-26). The HVL described earlier in this chapter is a measure of beam energy describing the amount of an absorber that reduces the beam intensity by half; in the

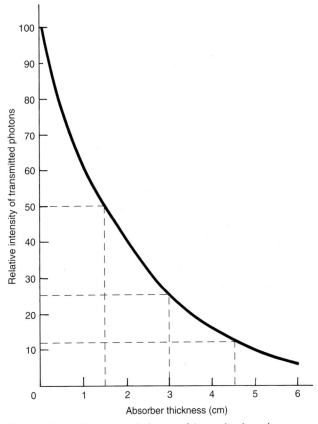

FIG. **1-26** Exponential decay of intensity in a homogeneous photon beam through the absorber, where the HVL is 1.5 cm of absorber. The curve for a heterogeneous x-ray beam does not drop quite as precipitously because of the preferential removal of low-energy photons and the increased mean energy of the resulting beam.

TABLE 1-2
Summary of Radiation Quantities and Units

QUANTITY	SI UNIT	TRADITIONAL UNIT	CONVERSION
Exposure	Air kerma (Gy)	Roentgen (R)	1 Gy = 100 rad 1 rad = 0.01 Gy (1 cGy)
Absorbed dose	Gray (Gy)	Rad	1 Gy = 100 rad 1 rad = 0.01 Gy (1 cGy)
Equivalent dose	Sievert (Sv)	Rem	1 Sv = 100 rem 1 rem = 0.01 Sv (1 cSv)
Effective dose	Sievert (Sv)	—	—
Radioactivity	Becquerel (Bq)	Curie (Ci)	1 Bq = 2.7×10^{-11} Ci 1 Ci = 3.7×10^{10} Bq

Data from The NIST Reference on Constants, Units, and Uncertainty: http://physics.nist.gov/cuu/Units/units.html.

preceding example, the HVL is 1.5 cm. The absorption of the beam depends primarily on the thickness and mass of the absorber and the energy of the beam.

The range of photon energies in an x-ray beam is wide. Low-energy photons are much more likely than high-energy photons to be absorbed. As a consequence the superficial layers of an absorber tend to remove the low-energy photons and transmit the higher-energy photons. Therefore as an x-ray beam passes through matter, the intensity of the beam decreases, but the mean energy of the resultant beam increases. In contrast to the absorption of a monochromatic beam, an x-ray beam is absorbed less and less by each succeeding unit of absorber thickness. For example, the first 1.5 cm of water might absorb about 40% of the photons in an x-ray beam with a mean energy of 50 kVp. The mean energy of the remnant beam might increase 20% as a result of the loss of lower-energy photons. The next 1.5 cm of water removes only about 30% of the photons as the average energy of the beam increases another 10%. If the water test object is thick enough, the mean energy of the remnant beam approaches the peak voltage applied across the tube and absorption becomes similar to that of a monochromatic beam.

The attenuation of a beam depends on both the energy of the incident beam and the composition of the absorber. In general, as the energy of the beam increases, so does the transmission of the beam through the absorber. When the energy of the incident photon is raised to the binding energy of the K-shell electrons of the absorber, however, the probability of photoelectric absorption increases sharply and the number of transmitted photons is greatly decreased. This is called *K-edge absorption*. (The probability that a photon will interact with an orbital electron is greatest when the energy of the photon equals the binding energy of the electron; it decreases as the photon energy increases.) Photons with energy less than the binding energy of K-shell electrons interact photoelectrically only with electrons in the L shell and in shells even farther from the nucleus. Rare earth elements are sometimes used as filters because their K edges (50.2 keV for gadolinium) greatly increase the absorption of high-energy photons. This is desirable because these high-energy photons are not as likely to contribute to a radiographic image as mid-energy photons.

Dosimetry

Determining the quantity of radiation exposure or dose is termed *dosimetry*. The term *dose* is used to describe the amount of energy absorbed per unit mass at a site of interest. *Exposure* is a measure of radiation based on its ability to produce ionization in air under standard conditions of temperature and pressure (STP).

UNITS OF MEASUREMENT

Table 1-2 presents some of the more frequently used units for measuring quantities of radiation. In recent years a move has occurred to use a modernized version of the metric system called the *SI system* (Système International d'Unités)*. This book uses SI units. The SI system uses *base units* including the kilogram (mass), the meter (length), the second (time), the amphere

---

*The NIST Reference on Constants, Units, and Uncertainty: http://physics.nist.gov/cuu/Units/units.html.

(electric current), and the mole (amount of substance). SI derived units, including newton (force) and joule (energy), evolve from these base units. The units below are SI derived units with special names.

Exposure

Exposure is a measure of radiation quantity, the capacity of radiation to ionize air. The SI unit of exposure is air kerma, an acronym for *kinetic energy released in matter*. Kerma measures the kinetic energy transferred from photons to electrons and is expressed in units of dose (Gy), where 1 Gy equals 1 joule/kg. Kerma is the sum of the initial kinetic energies of all the charged particles liberated by uncharged ionizing radiation (neutrons and photons) in a sample of matter, divided by the mass of the sample. It has replaced the roentgen (R), the traditional unit of radiation exposure measured in air.

Absorbed Dose

Absorbed dose is a measure of the energy absorbed by any type of ionizing radiation per unit mass of any type of matter. The SI unit is the gray (Gy), where 1 Gy equals 1 joule/kg. The traditional unit of absorbed dose is the rad (*radiation absorbed dose*), where 1 rad is equivalent to 100 ergs/g of absorber. One gray equals 100 rads.

Equivalent Dose

The equivalent dose (H_T) is used to compare the biologic effects of different types of radiation to a tissue or organ. It is the sum of the products of the absorbed dose (D_T) averaged over a tissue or organ and the radiation weighting factor (W_R):

$$H_T = \sum W_R \times D_T$$

Equivalent dose is expressed as a sum to allow for the possibility that the tissue or organ is exposed to more than one type of radiation. The radiation weighting factor is chosen for the type and energy of the radiation involved. Thus high-LET radiations (which are more damaging to tissue than low-LET radiations) have a correspondingly higher W_R. For example, the W_R of photons is 1; of 5 keV neutrons and high-energy protons, 5; and of alpha particles, 20. The unit of equivalent dose is the sievert (Sv). For diagnostic x-ray examinations 1 Sv equals 1 Gy. The traditional unit of equivalent dose is the rem (*roentgen equivalent man*). One sievert equals 100 rem.

Effective Dose

The effective dose (E) is used to estimate the risk in humans. It is the sum of the products of the equivalent dose to each organ or tissue (H_T) and the tissue weighting factor (W_T):

$$E = \sum W_T \times H_T$$

The tissue weighting factors include gonads, 0.20; red bone marrow, 0.12; esophagus, 0.05; thyroid, 0.05; skin, 0.01; and bone surface, 0.01. The unit of effective dose is the sievert (Sv). The use of this term is described more fully in Chapter 3.

Radioactivity

The measurement of radioactivity (A) describes the decay rate of a sample of radioactive material. The SI unit is the becquerel (Bq); 1 Bq equals 1 disintegration/second. The traditional unit is the curie (Ci), which corresponds to the activity of 1 g of radium (3.7×10^{10} disintegrations/second). Accordingly, 1 mCi equals 37 megaBq; and 1 Bq equals 2.7×10^{-11} Ci.

BIBLIOGRAPHY

Bushberg JT: The essential physics of medical imaging, ed 2. Baltimore, 2001, Lippincott Williams & Wilkins.

Bushong SC: Radiologic science for technologists: physics, biology, and protection, ed 7. St Louis, 2001, Mosby.

Curry TS, Dowdey JE, Murry RC: Christensen's introduction to the physics of diagnostic radiology, ed 4. Philadelphia, 1990, Lea & Febiger.

International Commission on Radiological Protection: Radiation protection; Radiological Protection and Safety in Medicine; ICRP Publication 73, 1996, Elsevier Science.

PART ■ TWO
Biologic Effects of Radiation

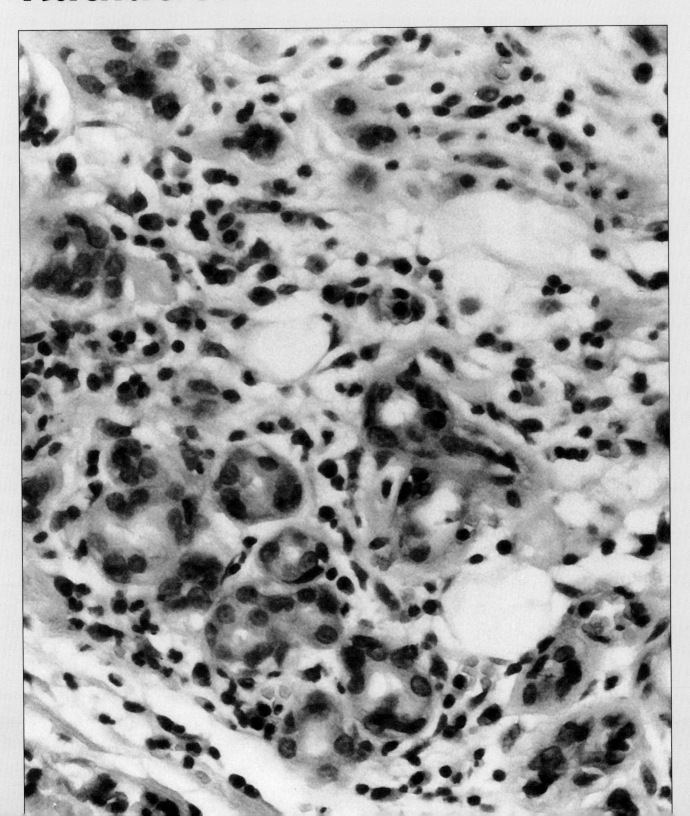

CHAPTER 2

Radiation Biology

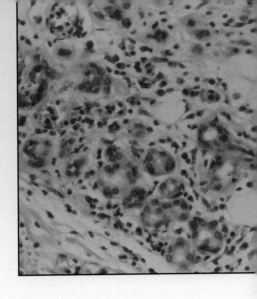

Radiation biology is the study of the effects of ionizing radiation on living systems. This discipline requires studying many levels of organization within biologic systems spanning broad ranges in size and temporal scale. The initial interaction between ionizing radiation and matter occurs at the level of the electron within the first 10^{-13} second after exposure. These changes result in modification of biologic molecules within the ensuing seconds to hours. In turn, the molecular changes may lead to alterations in cells and organisms that persist for hours, decades, and possibly even generations. If enough cells are killed in an individual, it may cause injury or death. If cells are modified, such changes may lead to cancer or disorders in the descendents of the exposed individual.

Biologic effects of ionizing radiation may be divided into two broad categories: deterministic effects and stochastic effects. *Deterministic effects* are those effects in which the severity of response is proportional to the dose. These effects, usually cell killing, occur in all people when the dose is large enough. Deterministic effects have a dose threshold below which the response is not seen. Examples of deterministic effects include oral changes after radiation therapy. In contrast, *stochastic effects* are those for which the probability of the occurrence of a change, rather than its severity, is dose-dependent. Stochastic effects are all-or-none: a person either has or does not have the condition. For example, radiation-induced cancer is a stochastic effect because greater exposure of a person or population to radiation increases the probability of cancer but not its severity. Stochastic effects are believed not to have dose thresholds.

Radiation Chemistry

Radiation acts on living systems through direct and indirect effects. When the energy of a photon or secondary electron ionizes biologic macromolecules, the effect is termed *direct*. Alternatively, the photon may be absorbed by water in an organism, ionizing the water molecules. The resulting ions form free radicals (radiolysis of water) that in turn interact with and produce changes in the biologic molecules. Because intermediate changes involving water molecules are required, this series of events is termed *indirect*.

DIRECT EFFECT

Direct alteration of biologic molecules (RH, where R is the molecule and H is a hydrogen atom) by ionizing radiation begins with absorption of energy by the biologic molecule and formation of unstable free radicals (atoms or molecules having an unpaired electron in the valence shell). The generation of free radicals occurs in less than 10^{-10} second after the passage of a photon. They are extremely reactive and have very short lives, quickly reforming into stable configurations by dissociation (breaking apart) or cross-linking (joining of two molecules). Free radicals play a dominant role in producing molecular changes in biologic molecules.

Free radical production:

$$\text{RH} + \text{x-radiation} \rightarrow R^{\bullet} + H^{+} + e^{-}$$

Free radical fates:
Dissociation:

$$R^{\bullet} \rightarrow X + Y^{\bullet}$$

Cross-linking:

$$R^\bullet + S^\bullet \rightarrow RS$$

Because the altered molecules differ structurally and functionally from the original molecules, the consequence is a biologic change in the irradiated organism. *Approximately one third of the biologic effects of x-ray exposure result from direct effects.*

RADIOLYSIS OF WATER

Because water is the predominant molecule in biologic systems (about 70% by weight), it frequently participates in the interactions between x-ray photons and the biologic molecules of an organism. A complex series of chemical changes occurs in water after exposure to ionizing radiation. Collectively these reactions result in the radiolysis of water. The first step is ionization of water resulting from the absorption of a photon or interaction with a photoelectron or Compton electron. Displacement of an electron from the water molecule results in an ion pair, a positively charged water molecule (H_2O^+) and the displaced electron:

$$\text{photon} + H_2O \rightarrow e^- + H_2O^+$$

$$\text{photoelectron } e^- + H_2O \rightarrow 2e^- + H_2O^+$$

The displaced electron is usually captured by a water molecule to form a negatively charged water molecule (H_2O^-):

$$e^- + H_2O \rightarrow H_2O^-$$

These molecules are not stable and dissociate rapidly to form a hydroxyl ion and hydrogen free radical:

$$H_2O^- \rightarrow OH^- + H^\bullet$$

The positively charged water molecule reacts with another water molecule to form a hydroxyl free radical:

$$H_2O^+ + H_2O \rightarrow H_3O^+ + OH^\bullet$$

Water may also be excited and dissociate directly into hydrogen and hydroxyl free radicals:

$$\text{Photon} + H_2O \rightarrow H_2O^* \rightarrow OH^\bullet + H^\bullet$$

Although the radiolysis of water is extremely complex, on balance water is largely converted to hydrogen and hydroxyl free radicals.

When dissolved molecular oxygen (O_2) is present in irradiated water, hydroperoxyl free radicals may also be formed:

$$H^\bullet + O_2 \rightarrow HO_2^\bullet$$

Hydroperoxyl free radicals also may contribute to the formation of hydrogen peroxide in tissues:

$$HO_2^\bullet + H^\bullet \rightarrow H_2O_2$$

$$HO_2^\bullet + HO_2^\bullet \rightarrow O_2 + H_2O_2$$

Both peroxyl radicals and hydrogen peroxide are oxidizing agents that can significantly alter biologic molecules and cause cell destruction. They are considered to be major toxins produced in the tissues by ionizing radiation.

INDIRECT EFFECTS

Indirect effects are those in which hydrogen and hydroxyl free radicals, produced by the action of radiation on water, interact with organic molecules. The interaction of hydrogen and hydroxyl free radicals with organic molecules can result in the formation of organic free radicals. About two thirds of radiation-induced biologic damage results from indirect effects. Such reactions may involve the removal of hydrogen:

$$RH + OH^\bullet \rightarrow R^\bullet + HO_2$$

$$RH + H^\bullet \rightarrow R^\bullet + H_2$$

The $OH^\bullet$ free radical is more important in causing such damage.

Organic free radicals are unstable and transform into stable altered molecules as described in the earlier section in this chapter on direct effects (p. 25). These altered molecules have different chemical and biologic properties from the original molecules. The important role of water radiolysis and the indirect action of radiation may be seen by comparing the radiation dose required to inactivate enzymes when dry or in solution. The dose required to inactivate 37% of dry yeast invertase is 110 kGy but only 60 kGy when the enzyme is irradiated in solution.

CHANGES IN BIOLOGIC MOLECULES

Nucleic Acids

The last few decades have seen a growing appreciation for the crucial role of nucleic acids in determining cellular functions. It is clear that damage to the deoxyribonucleic acid (DNA) molecule is the primary mechanism for radiation-induced cell death, mutation, and carcinogenesis. Radiation produces a number of different types of alterations in DNA, including the following:
- Breakage of one or both DNA strands
- Cross-linking of DNA strands within the helix, to other DNA strands, or to proteins
- Change or loss of a base
- Disruption of hydrogen bonds between DNA strands

The most important types of damage are single- and double-strand breakage. Most single-strand breakage is of little biologic consequence as the broken stand is repaired using the intact second strand as a template. However, misrepair of a strand can result in a mutation and consequent biologic effect. Double-strand breakage occurs when both strands of a DNA molecule are damaged at the same location or within a few base pairs. In this instance repair is greatly complicated by the lack of an intact template strand and misrepair is common. Double-strand breakage is believed to be responsible for most cell killing and carcinogenesis as well as mutation.

Proteins

Irradiation of proteins in solution usually leads to changes in their secondary and tertiary structures through disruption of side chains or the breakage of hydrogen or disulfide bonds. Such changes lead to denaturation. The primary structure of the protein is usually not significantly altered. Irradiation may also induce intermolecular and intramolecular cross-linking. When an enzyme is irradiated, the biologic effect of the radiation may become amplified. For example, inactivation of an enzyme molecule results in its failure to convert many substrate molecules to their products. Thus many molecules become subsequently affected, although only a small number were initially damaged. The dose of radiation required to induce significant amounts of protein denaturation (or enzyme inactivation) is much higher than that required to induce gross cellular changes or cell death. Such data suggest that radiation-induced changes in protein structure and function are not the major cause of radiation effects after absorption of moderate doses (2 to 4 Gy) of radiation.

Radiation Effects at the Cellular Level

EFFECTS ON INTRACELLULAR STRUCTURES

The effects of radiation on intracellular structures result from radiation-induced changes in their macromolecules. Although the initial molecular changes are produced within a fraction of a second after exposure, cellular changes resulting from moderate exposures usually require a minimum of hours to become apparent. These changes are manifest initially as structural and functional changes in cellular organelles. Later, cell death may occur.

Nucleus

A wide variety of radiobiologic data indicate that the nucleus is more radiosensitive (in terms of lethality) than the cytoplasm, especially in dividing cells. *The sensitive site in the nucleus is the DNA within chromosomes.*

Chromosome Aberrations

Chromosomes serve as useful markers for radiation injury. They may be easily visualized and quantified,

and the extent of their damage is related to cell survival. Chromosome aberrations are observed in irradiated cells at the time of mitosis when the DNA condenses to form chromosomes. The type of damage that may be observed depends on the stage of the cell in the cell cycle at the time of irradiation.

Fig. 2-1 shows the stages of the cell cycle. If radiation exposure occurs after DNA synthesis (i.e., in G_2 or mid- and late S), only one arm of the affected chromosome is broken (chromatid aberration) (Fig. 2-2, *A*). If the radiation-induced break occurs before the DNA has replicated (i.e., in G_1 or early S), the damage manifests as a break in both arms (chromosome aberration) at the next mitosis (Fig. 2-2, *B*). Most simple breaks are repaired by biologic processes and go unrecognized. Fig. 2-3 illustrates several common forms of

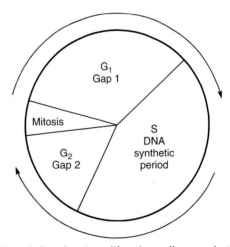

FIG. **2-1** Cell cycle. A proliferating cell moves in the cycle from mitosis to gap 1 (G_1) to the period of DNA synthesis (*S*) to gap 2 (G_2) to the next mitosis.

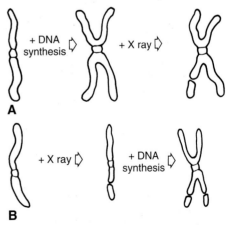

FIG. **2-2** Chromosome aberrations. **A**, Irradiation of the cell after DNA synthesis results in a single-arm (chromatid) aberration. **B**, Irradiation before DNA synthesis results in a double-arm (chromosome) aberration.

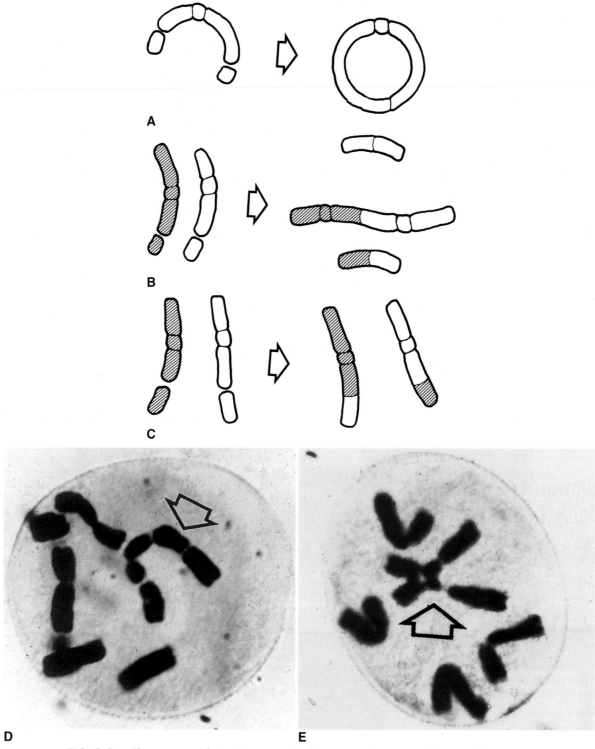

FIG. **2-3**   Chromosome aberrations. **A,** Ring formation plus acentric fragment; **B,** dicentric formation; **C,** translocation. In **D** and **E** the arrows point to tetracentric exchange and chromatid exchange taking place in *Trandescantia,* an herb. (**D** and **E,** Courtesy Dr. M. Miller, Rochester, NY.)

chromosome aberrations resulting from incorrect repair. Such radiation-induced aberrations may result in unequal distribution of chromatin material to daughter cells or prevent completion of a subsequent mitosis. Chromosome aberrations have been detected in peripheral blood lymphocytes of patients exposed to medical diagnostic procedures. Moreover, the survivors of the atomic bombings of Hiroshima and Nagasaki have demonstrated chromosome aberrations in circulating lymphocytes more than 2 decades after the radiation exposure. The frequency of aberrations is generally proportional to the radiation dose received.

Cytoplasm

Radiation effects occur in cellular structures other than nuclei and chromosomes. After relatively large doses of radiation (30 to 50 Gy), mitochondria demonstrate increased permeability, swelling, and disorganization of the internal cristae. Such permeability and structural changes probably play only a minor role in the cellular changes seen in rapidly dividing cells after exposure to moderate doses of radiation (2 to 4 Gy).

EFFECTS ON CELL KINETICS

The effects of radiation on the kinetics (turnover rate) of a cell population have been studied in rapidly dividing cell systems, such as skin and intestinal mucosa, and in cell culture systems. Irradiation of such cell populations will cause a reduction in size of the irradiated tissue as a result of mitotic delay (inhibition of progression of the cells through the cell cycle) and cell death (usually during mitosis).

Mitotic Delay

Mitotic delay occurs after irradiation of a population of dividing cells. Fig. 2-4 illustrates the effect of radiation on mitotic activity. A low dose of radiation induces mild mitotic delay in G_2 cells. The delayed cells subsequently pass through mitosis with other (nondelayed) cells, giving rise to an elevated mitotic index. A moderate dose results in a longer mitotic delay (G_2 block) and some cell death. The area under the curve of the following supranormal mitotic index is smaller than that of the preceding mitotic delay, indicating some cell death. Larger doses may cause a profound mitotic delay with incomplete recovery.

Cell Death

Mitosis-linked death in a cell population is loss of the capacity for mitotic division. Cell death is caused by damage to the nucleus that results in chromosome aberrations. This damage causes the cell to die, usually during attempt to complete the first few mitoses after

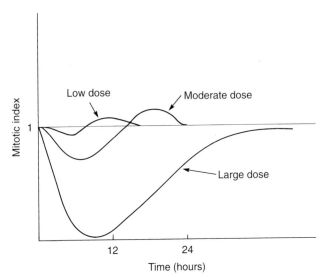

FIG. **2-4** Radiation-induced mitotic delay. The degree of delay in a replicating cell population depends on the amount of exposure. The larger the dose, the greater the reduction in mitotic activity and the more prolonged the recovery.

irradiation. Reproductive death occurs in a dividing cell population after exposure to a moderate dose of radiation, which accounts for the radiosensitivity of tissues. When a population of nondividing cells is irradiated, much larger doses and longer time intervals are required for induction of interphase death.

Survival curves are used to study the response of replicating cells exposed in culture. Single cells grown in tissue culture are dispersed onto plates, where they form colonies. The plates are irradiated before colony growth, and the effect of the irradiation on the reproductivity of the cells is studied.

Survival curves have helped researchers understand the response of cells to irradiation under various conditions. Fig. 2-5 shows typical survival curves for cells exposed to x radiation in which the fraction of surviving cells is compared with the absorbed dose. The value n is the extrapolation number and measures the size of the shoulder. The shoulder in the survival curve represents either the accumulation of sublethal damage before cells die or a measure of the repair process active early in the period of irradiation. D_0 indicates the slope of the straight portion of the curve. It measures the amount of radiation required to reduce the number of colony-forming cells to 37% and thus is the dose required to deliver an average of one cell-killing event per cell.

Recovery

Cell recovery involves enzymatic repair of single-strand breaks of DNA. Because of this repair, a higher total

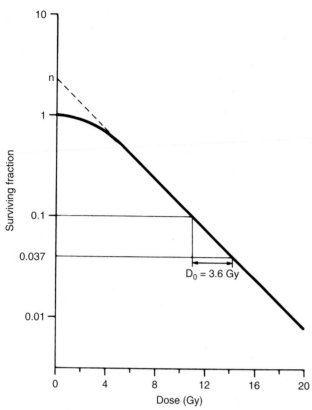

FIG. **2-5**   Survival curve for mammalian cells grown in culture after irradiation. In this case the cells have an extrapolation number (*n*) of about 2 and a D_0 of about 3.6 Gy. The n value is a measure of the size of the shoulder; D_0 is the amount of radiation required to reduce the surviving population to 37% of its former size.

dose is required to achieve a given degree of cell killing when multiple fractions are used (e.g., in radiation therapy) than when the same total dose is given in a single brief exposure. Damage to both strands of DNA at the same site (usually caused by particulate radiation) is usually lethal to the cell.

RADIOSENSITIVITY AND CELL TYPE

Different cells from various organs of the same individual may respond to irradiation quite differently. This variation was recognized as early as 1906 by the French radiobiologists Bergonié and Tribondeau. They observed that the most radiosensitive cells are those that (1) have a high mitotic rate, (2) undergo many future mitoses, and (3) are most primitive in differentiation. These findings are still true except for lymphocytes and oocytes, which are very radiosensitive even though they are highly differentiated and nondividing.

Mammalian cells may be divided into five categories of radiosensitivity on the basis of histologic observations of early cell death:

1. *Vegetative intermitotic cells* are the most radiosensitive. They divide regularly, have long mitotic futures, and do not undergo differentiation between mitoses. These are stem cells that retain their primitive properties and whose function is to replace themselves. Examples include early precursor cells, such as those in the spermatogenic or erythroblastic series, and basal cells of the oral mucous membrane.
2. *Differentiating intermitotic cells* are somewhat less radiosensitive than vegetative intermitotic cells because they divide less often. They divide regularly, although they undergo some differentiation between divisions. Examples of this class include intermediate dividing and replicating cells of the inner enamel epithelium of developing teeth, cells of the hematopoietic series that are in the intermediate stages of differentiation, spermatocytes, and oocytes.
3. *Multipotential connective tissue cells* have intermediate radiosensitivity. They divide irregularly, usually in response to a demand for more cells, and are also capable of limited differentiation. Examples are vascular endothelial cells, fibroblasts, and mesenchymal cells.
4. *Reverting postmitotic cells* are generally radioresistant because they divide infrequently. They also are generally specialized in function. Examples include the acinar and ductal cells of the salivary glands and pancreas as well as parenchymal cells of the liver, kidney, and thyroid.
5. *Fixed postmitotic cells* are most resistant to the direct action of radiation. They are the most highly differentiated cells and, once mature, are incapable of division. Examples of these cells include neurons, striated muscle cells, squamous epithelial cells that have differentiated and are close to the surface of oral mucous membrane, and erythrocytes.

Radiation Effects at the Tissue and Organ Level

The radiosensitivity of a tissue or organ is measured by its response to irradiation. Loss of moderate numbers of cells does not affect the function of most organs. However, with loss of large numbers of cells, all affected organisms display a clinical result. The severity of this change depends on the dose and thus the amount of cell loss. The following discussion pertains to the effect of irradiation of tissues and organs when the exposure is restricted to a small area. Moderate doses to a localized area may lead to repairable damage. Comparable doses to a whole organism may result in death from damage to the most sensitive systems in the body.

SHORT-TERM EFFECTS

The short-term effects of radiation on a tissue are determined primarily by the sensitivity of its parenchymal cells. If continuously proliferating tissues (e.g., bone marrow, oral mucous membranes) are irradiated with a moderate dose, cells are lost primarily by mitosis-linked death. The extent of cell loss depends on damage to the stem cell pools and the proliferative rate of the cell population. The effects of irradiation of such tissues become apparent relatively quickly as a reduction in the number of mature cells in the series. Tissues composed of cells that rarely or never divide (e.g., muscle) demonstrate little or no radiation-induced hypoplasia over the short term. The relative radiosensitivity of various tissues and organs is shown in Box 2-1.

LONG-TERM EFFECTS

The long-term deterministic effects of radiation on tissues and organs depend primarily on the extent of damage to the fine vasculature. The relative radiosensitivity of capillaries and connective tissue is intermediate between that of differentiating intermitotic cells and reverting postmitotic cells. Irradiation of capillaries causes swelling, degeneration, and necrosis. These changes increase capillary permeability and initiate a slow progressive fibrosis around the vessels. As a result, deposition of fibrous scar tissue is increased around the

vessels, leading to premature narrowing and eventual obliteration of vascular lumens. This impairs the transport of oxygen, nutrients, and waste products and results in death of all cell types. The net result is progressive fibroatrophy of the irradiated tissue.

Such progressive atrophic changes lead to a loss of cell function and a reduced resistance of irradiated tissue to infection and trauma. These cellular changes are the basis for long-term radiation-induced atrophy of tissues and organs. Death of parenchymal cells after moderate exposure is thus the result of (1) mitotic-linked death of rapidly dividing cells in the short term and (2) the consequences of progressive fibroatrophy on all cell types over time.

MODIFYING FACTORS

The response of cells to irradiation depends on variations in exposure parameters and the environment of the cell.

Dose

The severity of deterministic damage seen in irradiated tissues or organs depends on the amount of radiation received. Very often a clinical threshold dose exists below which no adverse effects are seen. All individuals receiving doses above the threshold level show damage in proportion to the dose.

Dose Rate

The term *dose rate* indicates the rate of exposure. For example, a total dose of 5 Gy may be given at a high dose rate (5 Gy/min) or a low dose rate (5 mGy/min). Exposure of biologic systems to a given dose at a high dose rate causes more damage than exposure to the same total dose given at a lower dose rate. When organisms are exposed at lower dose rates, a greater opportunity exists for repair of damage, thereby resulting in less net damage. Fig. 2-6 illustrates the effects of dose rate schematically.

Oxygen

The radioresistance of many biologic systems increases by a factor of 2 or 3 when irradiation is conducted with reduced oxygen (hypoxia). The greater cell damage sustained in the presence of oxygen is related to the increased amounts of hydrogen peroxide and hydroperoxyl free radicals formed. The oxygen enhancement ratio measures the extent of this damage. It is the dose required to achieve a given endpoint (e.g., 50% survival of a cell population) under anoxic conditions divided by the dose required to produce the same endpoint under fully oxygenated conditions. Fig. 2-7 demonstrates the influence of oxygen on cell survival

---

BOX 2-1
Relative Radiosensitivity of Various Organs

HIGH	INTERMEDIATE	LOW
Lymphoid organs	Fine vasculature	Optic lens
Bone marrow	Growing cartilage	Mature
Testes	Growing bone	erythrocytes
Intestines	Salivary glands	Muscle cells
Mucous	Lungs	Neurons
membranes	Kidney	
	Liver	

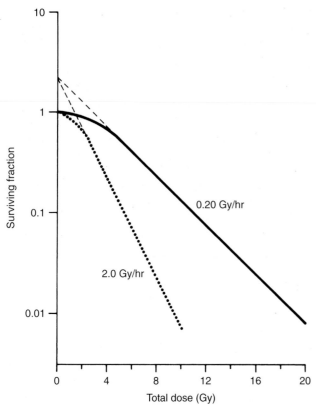

FIG. **2-6**   Survival curve for mammalian cells grown in culture after irradiation at low and high dose rates. Exposure at a high dose rate kills more cells per unit dose because less time exists for repair of sublethal damage.

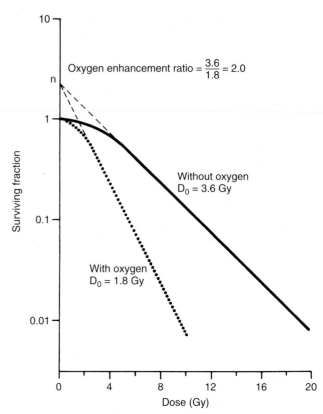

FIG. **2-7**   Survival curve for mammalian cells grown in culture after irradiation with and without oxygen. The presence of oxygen increases the cells' sensitivity to radiation. In this example the D_0 value is reduced from 3.6 Gy when irradiated without oxygen to 1.8 Gy in the presence of oxygen. The oxygen enhancement ratio measures the influence of oxygen.

curves. This is important clinically because hyperbaric oxygen therapy may be used during radiation therapy of tumors having hypoxic cells.

Linear Energy Transfer

In general, the dose required to produce a certain biologic effect is reduced as the linear energy transfer (LET) of the radiation is increased. Thus higher-LET radiations (e.g., alpha particles) are more efficient in damaging biologic systems because their high ionization density is more likely than x rays to induce double-strand breakage in DNA. Low-LET radiations such as x rays deposit their energy uniformly in the absorber and thus are more likely to cause single-strand breakage and less biologic damage. When the biologic response to different types of radiation is compared, it is common to use the term *relative biologic effectiveness* (RBE), where x rays are used as a reference. For instance, if the dose of x rays required to kill 50% of the cells in a culture was 5 Gy and the dose of neutrons required to achieve the same end point was 2 Gy, then the RBE of neutrons would be 2.5 (5 Gy ÷ 2 Gy).

Radiation Effects on the Oral Cavity

RATIONALE OF RADIOTHERAPY

The oral cavity is irradiated during the course of treating radiosensitive oral malignant tumors, usually squamous cell carcinomas. The specific treatment of choice for a lesion depends on many tumor variables such as radiosensitivity, histology, size, location, invasion into adjacent structures, and duration of symptoms. Radiation therapy for malignant lesions in the oral cavity is usually indicated when the lesion is radiosensitive, advanced, or deeply invasive and cannot be approached surgically. Combined surgical and radiotherapeutic treatment often provides optimal treatment. Increasingly, chemotherapy is being combined with radiation therapy and surgery.

Fractionation of the total x-ray dose into multiple small doses provides greater tumor destruction than is possible with a large single dose. Fractionation characteristically also allows increased cellular repair of normal tissues, which are believed to have an inherently greater capacity for recovery than tumor cells. Fractionation also increases the mean oxygen tension in an irradiated tumor, rendering the tumor cells more radiosensitive. This results from rapid killing of tumor cells and shrinkage of the tumor mass after the first few fractions, reducing the distance that oxygen must diffuse from the fine vasculature through the tumor to reach the remaining viable tumor cells. The fractionation schedules currently in use have been established empirically.

RADIATION EFFECT ON ORAL TISSUES

The following sections describe the deterministic effects of a course of radiotherapy on the normal tissue of the oral cavity. This discussion assumes that 2 Gy is delivered daily, bilaterally through 8- × 10-cm fields over the oropharynx, for a weekly exposure of 10 Gy. This continues typically until a total of 50 Gy is administered.

Cobalt is often the source of gamma radiation; however, on occasion small implants containing radon or iodine-125 are placed directly in a tumor mass. Such implants deliver a high dose of radiation to a relatively small volume of tissue in a short time.

Oral Mucous Membrane

The oral mucous membrane contains a basal layer composed of radiosensitive vegetative and differentiating intermitotic cells. Near the end of the second week of therapy, as some of these cells die, the mucous membranes begin to show areas of redness and inflammation (mucositis). As the therapy continues, the irradiated mucous membrane begins to break down, with the formation of a white to yellow pseudomembrane (the desquamated epithelial layer). At the end of therapy the mucositis is usually most severe, discomfort is at a maximum, and food intake is difficult. Good oral hygiene minimizes infection. Topical anesthetics may be required at mealtimes. Secondary yeast infection by *Candida albicans* is a common complication and may require treatment.

After irradiation is completed, the mucosa begins to heal rapidly. Healing is usually complete by about 2 months. At later intervals (months to years) the mucous membrane tends to become atrophic, thin, and relatively avascular. This long-term atrophy results from progressive obliteration of the fine vasculature and fibrosis of the underlying connective tissue. These atrophic changes complicate denture wearing because they may cause oral ulcerations of the compromised tissue. Ulcers can result from a denture sore, radiation necrosis, or tumor recurrence. A biopsy may be required to make the differentiation.

Taste Buds

Taste buds are sensitive to radiation. Doses in the therapeutic range cause extensive degeneration of the normal histologic architecture of taste buds. Patients often notice a loss of taste acuity during the second or third week of radiotherapy. Bitter and acid flavors are more severely affected when the posterior two thirds of the tongue is irradiated, and salt and sweet when the anterior third of the tongue is irradiated. Taste acuity usually decreases by a factor of 1,000 to 10,000 during the course of radiotherapy. Alterations in the saliva may account partly for this reduction, which may proceed to a state of virtual insensitivity, with recovery to near-normal levels some 60 to 120 days after irradiation.

Salivary Glands

The major salivary glands are at times unavoidably exposed to 20 to 30 Gy during radiotherapy for cancer in the oral cavity or oropharynx. The parenchymal component of the salivary glands is rather radiosensitive (parotid glands more so than submandibular or sublingual glands). A marked and progressive loss of salivary secretion is usually seen in the first few weeks after initiation of radiotherapy, The extent of reduced flow is dose-dependent and reaches essentially zero at 60 Gy. The mouth becomes dry (xerostomia) and tender, and swallowing is difficult and painful because the residual saliva also loses its normal lubricating properties.

Patients with irradiation of both parotid glands are more likely to complain of dry mouth than are those with unilateral irradiation. The small volume of viscous saliva that is secreted usually has a pH value 1 unit below normal (i.e., an average of 5.5 in irradiated patients compared with 6.5 in unexposed individuals). This pH is low enough to initiate decalcification of normal enamel. In addition, the buffering capacity of saliva falls as much as 44% during radiation therapy. If some portions of the major salivary glands have been spared, dryness of the mouth usually subsides in 6 to 12 months because of compensatory hypertrophy of residual salivary gland tissue. Reduced salivary flow that persists beyond a year is unlikely to show significant recovery.

Histologically an acute inflammatory response may occur soon after the initiation of therapy, particularly involving the serous acini. In the months after irradiation the inflammatory response becomes more chronic and the glands demonstrate progressive fibrosis, adiposis, loss of fine vasculature, and concomitant parenchymal degeneration (Fig. 2-8), thus accounting for the xerostomia.

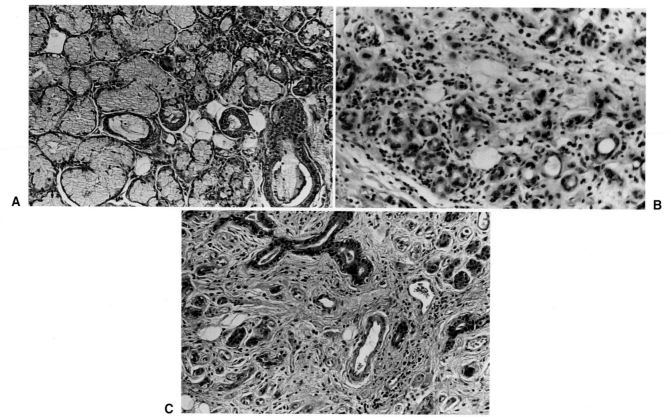

FIG. **2-8**   Radiation effects on human submandibular salivary glands. **A,** Normal gland. **B,** A gland 6 months after exposure to radiotherapy. Note the loss of acini and presence of chronic inflammatory cells. **C,** A gland 1 year after exposure to radiotherapy. Note the loss of acini and extensive fibrosis.

Salivary changes have a profound influence on the oral microflora and secondarily on the dentition, often leading to radiation caries. After radiotherapy that includes the major salivary glands, the microflora undergo a pronounced change, rendering them acidogenic in the saliva and plaque. Patients receiving radiation therapy to oral structures have increases in *Streptococcus mutans*, *Lactobacillus*, and *Candida*. Because of their small volume of thick, viscous, acidic saliva, such patients are quite prone to radiation caries.

Teeth

Irradiation of teeth with therapeutic doses during their development severely retards their growth. Such irradiation may be for local disease (e.g., eosinophilic granuloma) or a generalized condition (leukemia being treated with whole-body irradiation followed by bone marrow transplantation). If it precedes calcification, irradiation may destroy the tooth bud. Irradiation after calcification has begun may inhibit cellular differentiation, causing malformations and arresting general

growth. Children receiving radiation therapy to the jaws may show defects in the permanent dentition such as retarded root development, dwarfed teeth, or failure to form one or more teeth (Fig. 2-9). Teeth irradiated during development may complete calcification and erupt prematurely. In general, the severity of the damage is dose-dependent. Irradiation of teeth may retard or abort root formation, but the eruptive mechanism of teeth is relatively radiation-resistant. Irradiated teeth with altered root formation still erupt.

Adult teeth are very resistant to the direct effects of radiation exposure. Pulpal tissue, which consists primarily of reverting and fixed postmitotic cells, demonstrates long-term fibroatrophy after irradiation. Radiation has no discernible effect on the crystalline structure of enamel, dentin, or cementum, and radiation does not increase their solubility.

Radiation Caries

Radiation caries is a rampant form of dental decay that may occur in individuals who receive a course of radio-

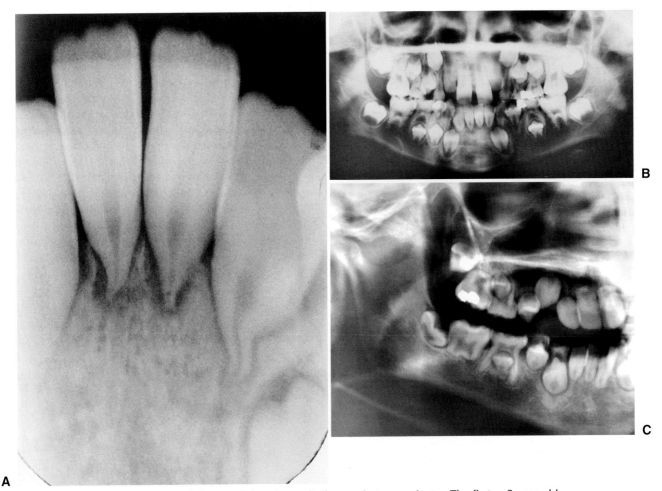

FIG. **2-9** Dental abnormalities after radiotherapy in two patients. The first, a 9-year-old girl who received 35 Gy at the age of 4 years because of Hodgkin's disease, had severe stunting of the incisor roots with premature closure of the apices at 8 years **(A)** and retarded development of the mandibular second premolar crowns with stunting of the mandibular incisor, canine, and premolar roots at 9 years **(B)**. The other patient **(C)** a 10-year-old boy who received 41 Gy to the jaws at age 4 years, had severely stunted root development of all permanent teeth with a normal primary molar. (**A** and **B**, Courtesy Mr. P.N. Hirschmann, Leeds, England; **C**, Courtesy Dr. James Eischen, San Diego, Calif.)

therapy that includes exposure of the salivary glands. The carious lesions result from changes in the salivary glands and saliva, including reduced flow, decreased pH, reduced buffering capacity, and increased viscosity. Because of the reduced or absent cleansing action of normal saliva, debris accumulates quickly. Irradiation of the teeth by itself does not influence the course of radiation caries.

Clinically, three types of radiation caries exist. The most common is widespread superficial lesions attacking buccal, occlusal, incisal, and palatal surfaces. Another type involves primarily the cementum and dentin in the cervical region. These lesions may progress around the teeth circumferentially and result in loss of the crown. A final type appears as a dark pig-

mentation of the entire crown. The incisal edges may be markedly worn. Some patients develop combinations of all these lesions (Fig. 2-10). The histologic features of the lesions are similar to those of typical carious lesions. It is the rapid course and widespread attack that distinguish radiation caries.

The best method of reducing radiation caries is daily application for 5 minutes of a viscous topical 1% neutral sodium fluoride gel in custom-made applicator trays. Use of topical fluoride causes a 6-month delay in the irradiation-induced elevation of *Streptococcus mutans*. Avoidance of dietary sucrose, in addition to the use of a topical fluoride, further reduces the concentrations of *S. mutans* and *Lactobacillus*. The best result is achieved from a combination of restorative dental procedures,

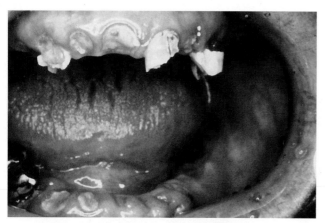

FIG. **2-10**   Radiation caries. Note the extensive loss of tooth structure in both jaws resulting from radiation-induced xerostomia.

excellent oral hygiene, and topical applications of sodium fluoride. Patient cooperation in maintaining oral hygiene is extremely important. Teeth with gross caries or periodontal involvement are often extracted before irradiation.

Bone

Treatment of cancers in the oral region often includes irradiation of the mandible. The primary damage to mature bone results from radiation-induced damage to the vasculature of the periosteum and cortical bone, which are normally already sparse. Radiation also acts by destroying osteoblasts and, to a lesser extent, osteoclasts. Subsequent to irradiation, normal marrow may be replaced with fatty marrow and fibrous connective tissue. The marrow tissue becomes hypovascular, hypoxic, and hypocellular. In addition, the endosteum becomes atrophic, showing a lack of osteoblastic and osteoclastic activity, and some lacunae of the compact bone are empty, an indication of necrosis. The degree of mineralization may be reduced, leading to brittleness, or little altered from normal bone. When these changes are so severe that bone death results, the condition is termed *osteoradionecrosis.*

Osteoradionecrosis is the most serious clinical complication that occurs in bone after irradiation. The decreased vascularity of the mandible renders it easily infected by microorganisms from the oral cavity. This bone infection may result from radiation-induced breakdown of the oral mucous membrane, by mechanical damage to the weakened oral mucous membrane such as from a denture sore or tooth extraction, through a periodontal lesion, or from radiation caries. This infection may cause a nonhealing wound in irradiated bone that is difficult to treat (Fig. 2-11). It is more common in the mandible than in the maxilla, probably

because of the richer vascular supply to the maxilla and the fact that the mandible is more frequently irradiated. The higher the radiation dose absorbed by the bone, the greater the risk for osteoradionecrosis.

Patients must be referred for dental care before undergoing a course of radiation therapy to reduce the severity of or prevent radiation caries and osteoradionecrosis. Radiation caries can be minimized by restoring all carious lesions before radiation therapy and initiating preventive techniques of good oral hygiene and daily topical fluoride. The risk for osteoradionecrosis and infection can be minimized by removing all poorly supported teeth, allowing sufficient time for the extraction wounds to heal before beginning radiation therapy, and adjusting dentures to minimize the risk for denture sores. When teeth must be

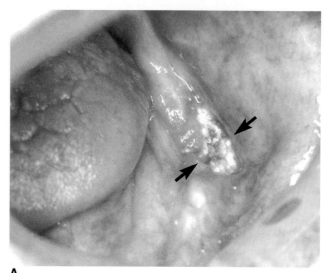

A

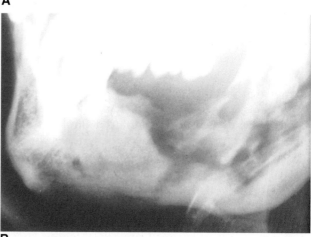

B

FIG. **2-11** Osteoradionecrosis. **A,** Area of exposed mandible after radiotherapy. Note the loss of oral mucosa. **B,** Destruction of irradiated bone resulting from the spread of infection.

removed from irradiated jaws, the dentist should use atraumatic surgical technique to avoid elevating the periosteum, provide antibiotic coverage, and use low-concentration epinephrine-containing local anesthetics that do not contain lidocaine.

Often patients require a radiographic examination to supplement the clinical examination. These radiographs are especially important because untreated caries leading to periapical infection can be quite severe with the compromised vascular supply to bone. The amount of added radiation is negligible compared with the amount received during therapy and should not serve as a reason to defer radiographs. Whenever possible, however, it is desirable to avoid taking radiographs during the first 6 months after completion of radiotherapy to allow time for the mucous membrane to heal.

Effects of Whole-Body Irradiation

When the whole body is exposed to low or moderate doses of radiation, characteristic changes (called the *acute radiation syndrome*) develop. The clinical picture after whole-body exposure is quite different from that seen when a relatively small volume of tissue is exposed.

ACUTE RADIATION SYNDROME

The acute radiation syndrome is a collection of signs and symptoms experienced by persons after acute whole-body exposure to radiation. Information about this syndrome comes from animal experiments and human exposures in the course of medical radiotherapy, atom bomb blasts, and radiation accidents. Individually the clinical symptoms are not unique to radiation exposure, but taken as a whole, the pattern constitutes a distinct entity (Table 2-1). The following

TABLE **2-1** *Acute Radiation Syndrome*	
DOSE (GY)	MANIFESTATION
1 to 2	Prodromal symptoms
2 to 4	Mild hematopoietic symptoms
4 to 7	Severe hematopoietic symptoms
7 to 15	Gastrointestinal symptoms
50	Cardiovascular and central nervous system symptoms

discussion pertains to whole-body exposure at a relatively high dose rate.

Prodromal Period
Within the first minutes to hours after exposure to whole-body irradiation of about 1.5 Gy, symptoms characteristic of gastrointestinal tract disturbances may occur. The individual may develop anorexia, nausea, vomiting, diarrhea, weakness, and fatigue. These early symptoms constitute the prodromal period of the acute radiation syndrome. Their cause is not clear but probably involves the autonomic nervous system. The severity and time of onset may be of significant prognostic value because they are dose-related: the higher the dose, the more rapid the onset and the greater the severity of symptoms.

Latent Period
After this prodromal reaction comes a latent period of apparent well-being, during which no signs or symptoms of radiation sickness occur. The extent of the latent period is also dose-related. It extends from hours or days at supralethal exposures (greater than approximately 5 Gy) to a few weeks at sublethal exposures (less than 2 Gy). Symptoms follow the latent period when individuals are exposed in the lethal range (approximately 2 to 5 Gy) or supralethal range.

Hematopoietic Syndrome
Whole-body exposures of 2 to 7 Gy cause injury to the hematopoietic stem cells of the bone marrow and spleen. The high mitotic activity of these cells and the presence of many differentiating cells make the bone marrow a highly radiosensitive tissue. As a consequence, doses in this range cause a rapid and profound fall in the numbers of circulating granulocytes, platelets, and finally erythrocytes. The mature circulating granulocytes, platelets, and erythrocytes themselves are very radioresistant, however, because they are non-replicating cells. Their paucity in the peripheral blood after irradiation reflects the radiosensitivity of their precursors.

The differential changes in the blood count do not all appear at the same time (Fig. 2-12). Rather, the rate of fall in the circulating levels of a cell depends on the life span of that cell in the peripheral blood. Granulocytes, with short lives in circulation, fall off in a matter of days, whereas red blood cells, with their long lives in circulation, fall off only slowly.

The clinical consequences of the depression of these cellular elements become evident as the circulating levels decline. Hence, in the weeks after radiation injury, infection appears first, followed later by anemia. The clinical signs of the hematopoietic syndrome

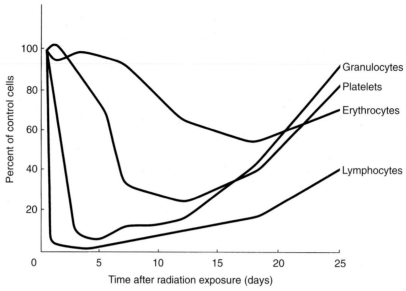

FIG. **2-12**   Radiation effects on blood cells. When whole-body exposure inhibits the replacement of circulating cells by stem cell proliferation, the duration of the circulating cells' survival is largely determined by their life span.

include infection (in part from the lymphopenia and granulocytopenia), hemorrhage (from the thrombocytopenia), and anemia (from the erythrocyte depletion). Individuals may survive exposure in this range if the bone marrow and spleen recover before the patient dies of one or more clinical complications. The probability of death is low after exposures at the low end of this range but much higher at the high end. When death results from the hematopoietic syndrome, it usually occurs 10 to 30 days after irradiation.

Because periodontitis results in a likely source of entry for microorganisms into the bloodstream, the role of the dentist is important in preventing infection in hematopoietic syndrome. After moderate injury, about 7 to 10 days pass before clinically significant leukopenia develops. During this time the dentist should remove all sites of infection from the mouth. The removal of sources of infection, the vigorous administration of antibiotics, and in some cases the transplantation of bone marrow have saved individuals suffering from the acute radiation syndrome.

Gastrointestinal Syndrome

Whole-body exposures in the range of 7 to 15 Gy cause extensive damage to the gastrointestinal system. This damage, in addition to the hematopoietic damage described previously, causes signs and symptoms called the *gastrointestinal syndrome.* Individuals exposed in this range may experience the prodromal stage within a few hours of exposure. Typically from the second through about the fifth day, no symptoms are present (latent

period) and the patient feels well. Such exposure, however, causes considerable injury to the rapidly proliferating basal epithelial cells of the intestinal villi and leads to a loss of the epithelial layer of the intestinal mucosa. The turnover time for cells lining the small intestine is normally 3 to 5 days. Because of the denuded mucosal surface, plasma and electrolytes are lost; efficient intestinal absorption cannot occur. Ulceration also occurs, with hemorrhaging of the intestines. All these changes are responsible for the diarrhea, dehydration, and loss of weight that are observed. Endogenous intestinal bacteria readily invade the denuded surface, producing septicemia.

The level of radiation required to produce the gastrointestinal syndrome (more than 7 Gy) is much greater than that causing sterilization of the blood-forming tissues. However, death (from destruction of the rapidly self-renewing cells in the intestines) occurs before the full effect of the radiation on hematopoietic systems can be evidenced. At about the time that developing damage to the gastrointestinal system reaches a maximum, the effect of bone marrow depression is just beginning to be manifested. By the end of 24 hours, the number of circulating lymphocytes falls to a very low level. This is followed by decreases in the number of granulocytes and then of platelets (see Fig. 2-12). The result is a marked lowering of the body's defense against bacterial infection and a decrease in effectiveness of the clotting mechanism. The combined effects on these stem cell systems cause death within 2 weeks from a combination of factors that include fluid and electrolyte loss, infection, and possibly nutritional impairment. Thirty of the firefighters at the accident site at Chernobyl, Ukraine, died in the first few months of the hematopoietic syndrome or gastrointestinal syndrome.

Cardiovascular and Central Nervous System Syndrome

Exposures in excess of 50 Gy usually cause death in 1 to 2 days. The few human beings who have been exposed at this level showed collapse of the circulatory system with a precipitous fall in blood pressure in the hours preceding death. Autopsy revealed necrosis of cardiac muscle. Victims also may show intermittent stupor, incoordination, disorientation, and convulsions suggestive of extensive damage to the nervous system. Although the precise mechanism is not fully understood, these latter symptoms most likely result from radiation-induced damage to the neurons and fine vasculature of the brain.

The syndrome is irreversible, and the clinical course may run from only a few minutes to about 48 hours before death occurs. The cardiovascular and central nervous system syndromes have such a rapid course that the irradiated individual dies before the effects of damage to the bone marrow and gastrointestinal system can develop.

The initial clinical problems govern the management of different forms of the acute radiation syndrome. Antibiotics are indicated when infection threatens or the granulocyte count falls. Fluid and electrolyte replacement is used as necessary. Whole blood transfusions are used to treat anemia, and platelets may be administered to arrest thrombocytopenia. Bone marrow grafts are indicated between identical twins because there is no risk for graft-versus-host disease. Patients also receive such grafts when exposed to 8 to 10 Gy for treatment of leukemia.

RADIATION EFFECTS ON EMBRYOS AND FETUSES

Embryos and fetuses are considerably more radiosensitive than adults because most embryonic cells are relatively undifferentiated and rapidly mitotic. Prenatal irradiation may lead to death or specific developmental abnormalities depending on the stage of development at the time of irradiation. The description below of abnormalities resulting from embryo or fetal irradiation pertains to exposures far higher than those received during the course of dental radiography. The fetus of a patient exposed to dental radiography receives less than 0.25 µGy from a full-mouth examination when a leaded apron is used.

The effects of radiation on human embryos and fetuses have been studied in women exposed to diagnostic or therapeutic radiation during pregnancy and in women exposed to radiation from the atomic bombs dropped at Hiroshima and Nagasaki. These embryos received exposures of 0.5 to 3 Gy (well more than one million times the exposure from a dental examination). Exposures during the first few days after conception are thought to cause undetectable death of the conceptus.

The most sensitive period for inducing developmental abnormalities is during the period of organogenesis, between 18 and 45 days of gestation. These effects are deterministic in nature. The most common abnormality among the Japanese children exposed early in gestation was reduced growth and reduced head circumference (microcephaly), often associated with mental retardation. Other abnormalities included small birth size, cataracts, genital and skeletal malformations, and microphthalmia. The period of maximal sensitivity of the brain is 8 to 15 weeks postconception. The frequency of severe mental retardation after exposure to 1 Gy during this period is about 43%.

Irradiation during the fetal period (more than 50 days after conception) does not cause gross malformations. However, general retardation of growth persists through life. Evidence also exists for an increased risk for childhood cancer, both leukemia and solid tumors, after irradiation in utero. However, the risks to the embryo and fetus from exposure to radiation are less than from other sources. Table 2-2 shows that maternal smoking and alcohol consumption pose a greater risk than low-level radiation exposure.

Late Somatic Effects

Somatic effects are those seen in the irradiated individual. The most important are radiation-induced cancers. Such lesions are a stochastic effect of radiation in that the probability of an individual's getting cancer depends on the amount of radiation exposure but the severity of the disease is not related to the dose.

CARCINOGENESIS

Radiation causes cancer by modifying the DNA. Although most such damage is repaired, imperfect repair may be transmitted to daughter cells and result in cancer. Data on radiation-induced cancers come primarily from populations of people that have been exposed to high levels of radiation; however, in principle even low doses of radiation may initiate cancer formation in a single cell. By far, the group of individuals most intensively studied for estimating the cancer risk

TABLE 2-2
Comparative Risks During Pregnancy

RISK FACTOR	RESULT	RATE OF RISK
Irradiation during gestation 10 mGy	Death from childhood leukemia	1 in 3,333
	Death from other childhood cancer	1 in 3,571
Maternal smoking 1 pack or more per day	Infant death	1 in 3
Maternal alcohol consumption 2 to 4 drinks per day	Signs of fetal alcohol syndrome	1 in 10
	Major malformation at delivery	3 in 100

Modified from Mettler F, Moseley R: Medical effects of ionizing radiation, Orlando, Fla, 1985, Grune & Stratton.

from radiation are the Japanese atomic bomb survivors. The cases of more than 120,000 individuals have been followed since 1950, of whom 91,000 were exposed. An estimated 7,827 deaths from cancer of all types had been observed in this group by 1990, most resulting from natural causes, with only 87 leukemias and 334 solid cancers attributed to radiation exposure.

British patients treated with spinal irradiation for ankylosing spondylitis have also demonstrated leukemia and other cancers. Several studies of patients receiving many fluoroscopic examinations in the course of treatment for tuberculosis, as well as women treated with radiation for postpartum mastitis, have helped researchers understand the risk for inducing breast cancer. The effects of thyroid gland exposure have also been studied in irradiated patients. Some Israeli children received radiation treatments to the scalp to aid in treatment for ringworm, whereas infants in Rochester, New York, were irradiated to reduce the size of their thymus glands. Many other studies on smaller groups of patients have provided useful information.

Estimation of the number of cancers induced by radiation is difficult. Most of the individuals in the studies mentioned above received exposure in excess of the diagnostic range. Thus the probability that a cancer will result from a small dose can be estimated only by interpolation from the rates observed after exposure to larger doses. Furthermore, radiation-induced cancers are not distinguishable from cancers produced by other causes. This means that the number of cancers can be estimated only as the number of excess cases found in exposed groups compared with the number in unexposed groups of people.

BOX 2-2
Susceptibility of Different Tissues to Radiation-Induced Cancer

HIGH	MODERATE	LOW
Colon	Breast (women)	Bladder
Stomach	Esophagus	Liver
Lung		Thyroid
Bone marrow (leukemia)		Skin
		Bone surface
		Brain
		Salivary glands

In the United States, cancer accounts for nearly 20% of all deaths. Accordingly, the estimated number of deaths attributable to low-level radiation exposure is a small fraction of the total number that occur spontaneously. Estimates indicate that a single, brief whole-body exposure of 100 mGy (about 30 times the average annual exposure) to 100,000 people would result in about 500 additional cancer deaths over the lifetime of the exposed individuals. This would be in addition to the 20,000 that would occur spontaneously. Such a calculation assumes a linear dose-response relationship and no threshold dose below which no risk exists. These assumptions may be in error and, if so, most likely overestimate the actual risk. Tissues vary in their susceptibility to radiation-induced cancer (Box 2-2). Estimation of the risks associated with dental radiography are considered in Chapter 3, Health Physics.

The mechanism of induction of cancer by ionizing radiation is not well understood. Most likely the basis is radiation-induced gene mutation. Most investigators believe that radiation acts as an initiator, that is, it induces a change in the cell so that it no longer undergoes terminal differentiation. Evidence also exists that radiation acts as a promoter, stimulating cells to multiply. Finally, it may also convert premalignant cells into malignant ones.

The following brief discussion of somatic effects of exposure to radiation pertains primarily to those organs exposed in the course of dental radiography. All radiation-induced cancers, other than leukemia, generally show the following:

1. Most cancers appear approximately 10 years after exposure, and the elevated risk remains for as long as most exposed populations are followed, presumably for the lifetime of the exposed individuals.
2. The risk from exposure during childhood is estimated to be about twice as great as the risk during adulthood.
3. The number of excess cancers induced by radiation is considered to be a multiple of the spontaneous rate rather than independent of the spontaneous rate.

Thyroid Cancer

The incidence of thyroid carcinomas (arising from the follicular epithelium) increases in human beings after exposure. Only about 10% of individuals with such cancers die from their disease. The best-studied groups are Israeli children irradiated to the scalp for ringworm; children in Rochester, New York, irradiated to the thymus gland; and survivors of the atomic bomb in Japan. Susceptibility to radiation-induced thyroid cancer is greater early in childhood than at any time later in life, and children are more susceptible than adults. Females are 2 to 3 times more susceptible than males to radiogenic and spontaneous thyroid cancers. The fallout from the accident at the Chernobyl nuclear power plant, primarily iodine-131, is believed to have caused about 1,800 cases of thyroid cancer in children.

Esophageal Cancer

The data pertaining to esophageal cancer are relatively sparse. Excess cancers are found in the Japanese atomic bomb survivors and in patients treated with x radiation for ankylosing spondylitis.

Brain and Nervous System Cancers

Patients exposed to diagnostic x-ray examinations in utero and to therapeutic doses in childhood or as adults (average midbrain dose of about 1 Gy) show excess numbers of malignant and benign brain tumors. Additionally, a case-control study has shown an association between intracranial meningiomas and previous medical or dental radiography. The strongest association was with a history of exposure to full-mouth dental radiographs when less than 20 years of age. Because of their age it is likely that these patients received substantially more exposure than is the case today with contemporary techniques.

Salivary Gland Cancer

The incidence of salivary gland tumors is increased in patients treated with irradiation for diseases of the head and neck, in Japanese atomic bomb survivors, and in persons exposed to diagnostic x radiation. An association between tumors of the salivary glands and dental radiography has been shown, the risk being highest in persons receiving full-mouth examinations before the age of 20 years. Only individuals who received an estimated cumulative parotid dose of 500 mGy or more showed a significant correlation between dental radiography and salivary gland tumors.

Cancer of Other Organs

Other organs such as the skin, paranasal sinuses, and bone marrow (with respect to multiple myeloma) also show excess neoplasia after exposure. However, the mortality and morbidity rates expected after head and neck exposure are much lower than for the organs described previously.

Leukemia

The incidence of leukemia (other than chronic lymphocytic leukemia) rises after exposure of the bone marrow to radiation. Atomic bomb survivors and patients irradiated for ankylosing spondylitis show a wave of leukemias beginning soon after exposure, peaking at around 7 years, and returning nearly to baseline rates within 40 years. Leukemias appear sooner than solid tumors because of the higher rate of cell division and differentiation of hematopoietic stem cells compared with the other tissues. Persons younger than 20 years are more at risk than adults.

OTHER LATE SOMATIC EFFECTS

A number of late somatic effects other than carcinogenesis have been found in the survivors of the atomic bombing of Hiroshima and Nagasaki.

Growth and Development

Children exposed in the bombings showed impairment of growth and development. They have reduced height, weight, and skeletal development. The younger the individual was at the time of exposure, the more pronounced the effects.

Mental Retardation

Studies of individuals exposed in utero have shown that the developing human brain is radiosensitive. An estimated 4% chance of mental retardation per 100 mSv exists at 8 to 15 weeks of gestational age, with less risk occurring from exposure at other gestational ages. During this period, rapid production of neurons and migration of these immature neurons to the cerebral cortex occur. The exposure to the embryo from a full set of dental radiographs, using a leaded apron, is less than 3 μSv.

Cataracts

The threshold for induction of cataracts (opacities in the lens of the eye) ranges from about 2 Gy when the dose is received in a single exposure to more than 5 Gy when the dose is received in multiple exposures over a period of weeks. These doses are far in excess of those received with contemporary dental radiographic techniques. Most affected individuals are unaware of their presence.

Radiation Genetics

GENE MUTATION

Radiation may induce damage in the genetic material of reproductive cells, and the offspring of irradiated parents may experience the effects of such damage. In his pioneering work in this field, Muller (1927) reported radiation-induced mutations in *Drosophila* (fruit flies). Later the husband-and-wife team of Russell and Russell studied radiation-induced mutations in over 7 million mice. Intensive work in this field established a number of basic principles of radiation genetics. In general, radiation causes increased frequency of spontaneous mutations rather than inducing new mutations. Furthermore, the frequency of mutations increases in direct proportion to the dose, even at very low doses, with no evidence of a threshold. The vast majority of mutations are deleterious to the organism. Dose rate is important in that at low dose rates the frequency of induced mutations is greatly reduced. Males are much more radiosensitive than females. The rate of mutations is reduced as the time between exposure and conception increases.

Effects on Humans

Current knowledge of genetic effects (those effects seen in the progeny of irradiated persons) after radiation exposure comes largely from the atomic bomb survivors. To date, no such radiation-related genetic damage has been demonstrated. No increase has occurred in adverse pregnancy outcome, leukemia or other cancers, or impairment of growth and development in the children of atomic bomb survivors. These findings do not exclude the possibility that such damage occurs but do show that it must be at a very low frequency.

Doubling Dose

One way to measure the risk from genetic exposure is by determining the *doubling dose*. This is the amount of radiation a population requires to produce in the next generation as many additional mutations as arise spontaneously. In human beings the genetic doubling dose for mutations resulting in death is approximately 2 Sv. Because the average person receives far less gonadal radiation, radiation contributes relatively little to genetic damage in populations.

For comparison, the gonadal dose to males from a full-mouth radiographic examination is very low, about 1 μSv or less. This exposure is contributed largely by the maxillary views, which are angled caudally. The dose to the ovaries is about 50 times less, in the range of 0.02 μSv. Table 2-3 shows the estimated genetic effects resulting from 10 mSv per generation (10,000 times the dose from a full-mouth radiographic examination).

TABLE 2-3
Estimated Genetic Effects of 10 mSv per Generation

DISORDER	CURRENT INCIDENCE/10^6 LIVEBORN	ADDITIONAL FIRST-GENERATION CASES/10^6 LIVEBORN
Autosomal dominant		
Severe	2,500	5 to 20
Mild	7,500	1 to 15
X-linked	400	<1
Recessive	2,500	<1
Congenital abnormalities	20,000 to 30,000	10

Modified from Committee on the Biological Effects of Ionizing Radiations: Health effects of exposure to low levels of ionizing radiation, BEIR V, Washington, DC, 1990, National Academy Press.

BIBLIOGRAPHY

Bushong SC: Radiologic science for technologists: physics, biology, and protection, 7th ed, St. Louis, 2001, Mosby.

Dowd SB, Tilson, ER: Practical radiation protection and applied radiobiology, 2nd ed, Philadelphia, 1999, WB Saunders.

Hall EJ: Radiobiology for the radiologist, 5th ed, Philadelphia, 2002, Lippincott Williams & Wilkins.

Mettler F, Kelsey C, Ricks R: Medical management of radiation accidents, Boca Raton, Fla., 1990, CRC Press.

Prasad KN: Handbook of radiobiology, 2nd ed, Boca Raton, Fla., 1995, CRC Press.

Steel GG: Basic clinical radiobiology, 3rd ed, London, 2002, Hodder Arnold.

SUGGESTED READINGS

GENETIC EFFECTS

United Nations Scientific Committee on the Effects of Atomic Radiation: HEREDITARY EFFECTS OF RADIATION, UNSCEAR 2001, http://www.unscear.org/reports/2001.html.

ODONTOGENESIS

Dahllof G: Craniofacial growth in children treated for malignant diseases, Acta Odontol Scand 56:378, 1998.

Kaste SC, Hopkins KP, Jenkins JJ III: Abnormal odontogenesis in children treated with radiation and chemotherapy: imaging findings, AJR Am J Roentgenol 162:1407, 1994.

Kimeldorf DJ: Radiation-induced alterations in odontogenesis and formed teeth. In Berdgis CC, editor: Pathology of irradiation, Baltimore, 1971, Williams & Wilkins.

Maguire A, Welbury RR: Long-term effects of antineoplastic chemotherapy and radiotherapy on dental development, Dent Update 23:188, 1996.

Nasman M, Forsberg CM, Dahllof G: Long-term dental development in children after treatment for malignant disease, Eur J Orthod 19:151, 1997.

OSTEORADIONECROSIS

Cronje FJ: A review of the Marx protocols: prevention and management of osteoradionecrosis by combining surgery and hyperbaric oxygen therapy, Sadj 53:469, 1998.

Hao SP, Chen HC, Wei FC, Chen CY, Yeh AR, Su JL: Systematic management of osteoradionecrosis in the head and neck, Laryngoscope 109:1324, 1999.

Mealey BL, Semba SE, Hallmon WW: The head and neck radiotherapy patient: part 2—management of oral complications, Compendium 15:442, 1994.

Semba SE, Mealey BL, Hallmon WW: The head and neck radiotherapy patient: part 1—oral manifestations of radiation therapy, Compendium 15:250, 1994.

Thorn JJ, Hansen HS, Specht L, Bastholt L: Osteoradionecrosis of the jaws: clinical characteristics and relation to the field of irradiation, J Oral Maxillofac Surg 58:1088, 2000.

Vanderpuye V, Goldson A: Osteoradionecrosis of the mandible, J Natl Med Assoc 92:579, 2000.

Vudiniabola S, Pirone C, Williamson J, Goss AN: Hyperbaric oxygen in the therapeutic management of osteoradionecrosis of the facial bones, Int J Oral Maxillofac Surg 29:435, 2000.

RADIATION CARIES

Brown RS, Martin RE, Keene H: Cariogenic infection control in the management of post-irradiation caries, J Gt Houst Dent Soc 68:19, 1996.

Carl W: Oral complications of local and systemic cancer treatment, Curr Opin Oncol 7:320, 1995.

Epstein JB, van der Meij EH, Lunn R, Stevenson-Moore P: Effects of compliance with fluoride gel application on caries and caries risk in patients after radiation therapy for head and neck cancer, Oral Surg Oral Med Oral Pathol Oral Radiol Endod 82:268, 1996

Epstein JB, van der Meij EH, Emerton SM, Le ND, Stevenson-Moore P: Compliance with fluoride gel use in irradiated patients, Spec Care Dentist 15:218, 1995.

Garg AK, Malo M: Manifestations and treatment of xerostomia and associated oral effects secondary to head and neck radiation therapy, J Am Dent Assoc 128:1128, 1997.

Greenspan D: Xerostomia: diagnosis and management, Oncology (Huntingt) 10:7, 1996.

Jansma J et al: The effect of x-ray irradiation on the demineralization of bovine dental enamel, Caries Res 22:199, 1988.

Lacatusu S, Francu D, Francu L: The patients with cariogenic high-risk after the cervico-facial radiotherapy and their management, Rev Med Chir Soc Med Nat Iasi 100:193, 1996.

Lacatusu S, Francu L, Francu D: Clinical and therapeutical aspects of rampant caries in cervico-facial irradiated patients, Rev Med Chir Soc Med Nat Iasi 100:198, 1996.

Pankhurst CL, Smith EC, Rogers JO, Dunne SM, Jackson SH, Proctor G: Diagnosis and management of the dry mouth: Part 1, Dent Update 23:56, 1996.

Papas A et al: Double blind clinical trial of a remineralizing dentifrice in the prevention of caries in a radiation therapy population, Gerodontology 16:2, 1999.

SALIVA AND SALIVARY GLANDS

Blom M, Lundeberg T: Long-term follow-up of patients treated with acupuncture for xerostomia and the influence of additional treatment, Oral Dis 6:15, 2000.

Eisbruch A, Kim HM, Terrell JE, Marsh LH, Dawson LA, Ship JA: Xerostomia and its predictors following parotid-sparing irradiation of head-and-neck cancer, Int J Radiat Oncol Biol Phys 50:695, 2001.

Eisbruch A, Ship JA, Kim HM, Ten Haken RK: Partial irradiation of the parotid gland, Semin Radiat Oncol 11:234, 2001.

Eisbruch A, Ten Haken RK, Kim HM, Marsh LH, Ship JA: Dose, volume, and function relationships in parotid salivary glands following conformal and intensity-modulated irradiation of head and neck cancer, Int J Radiat Oncol Biol Phys 45:577, 1999.

Garg AK, Malo M: Manifestations and treatment of xerostomia and associated oral effects secondary to head and neck radiation therapy, J Am Dent Assoc 128:1128, 1997.

Guchelaar HJ, Vermes A, Meerwaldt JH: Radiation-induced xerostomia: pathophysiology, clinical course and supportive treatment, Support Care Cancer 5:281, 1997.

Horiot JC et al: Post-radiation severe xerostomia relieved by pilocarpine: a prospective French cooperative study, Radiother Oncol 55:233, 2000.

Land CE et al: Incidence of salivary gland tumors among atomic bomb survivors, 1950-1987: evaluation of radiation-related risk, Radiat Res 146:28, 1996.

Niedermeier W, Matthaeus C, Meyer C, Staar S, Muller RP, Schulze HJ: Radiation-induced hyposalivation and its treatment with oral pilocarpine, Oral Surg Oral Med Oral Pathol Oral Radiol Endod 86:541, 1998.

Reddy SP, Leman CR, Marks JE, Emami B: Parotid-sparing irradiation for cancer of the oral cavity: maintenance of oral nutrition and body weight by preserving parotid function, Am J Clin Oncol 24:341, 2001.

Silverman, S: Oral cancer: Complications of therapy, Oral Surg Oral Med Oral Pathol Oral Radiol Endod 88:122, 1999.

Thakkar SS: Researchers make slow headway in managing dry mouth, J Natl Cancer Inst 89:1337, 1997.

SOMATIC EFFECTS

1990 Recommendations of the International Commission on Radiological Protection, ICRP Publ. 60, Annals of the ICRP 21, 1990.

Committee on the Biological Effects of Ionizing Radiations: Health effects of exposure to low levels of ionizing radiation, BEIR V, Washington, D.C., 1990, National Academies Press.

Committee on Health Effects of Exposure to Radon (BEIR VI): Health Effects of Exposure to Radon: Time for Reassessment?, Washington, DC, 1994, National Academies Press.

Putnam FW: Hiroshima and Nagasaki revisited: the Atomic Bomb Casualty Commission and the Radiation Effects Research Foundation, Perspect Biol Med 37:515, 1994.

Schull WJ: Effects of atomic radiation: a half-century of studies from Hiroshima and Nagasaki, New York, 1995, Wiley-Liss.

United Nations Scientific Committee on the Effects of Atomic Radiation: Sources and Effects of Ionizing Radiation, UNSCEAR 2000 Report to the General Assembly, with scientific annexes, volume I: sources, http://www.unscear.org/reports/2000_1.html.

United Nations Scientific Committee on the Effects of Atomic Radiation: Sources and Effects of Ionizing Radiation, UNSCEAR 2000 Report to the General Assembly, with scientific annexes, volume II: effects, http://www.unscear.org/reports/2000_2.html.

TASTE

Bartoshuk LM: Chemosensory alterations and cancer therapies, NCI Monogr 9:179, 1990.

Epstein JB, Stevenson-Moore P: A clinical comparative trial of saliva substitutes in radiation-induced salivary gland hypofunction, Spec Care Dentist 12:21, 1992.

Fernando IN et al: The effect of head and neck irradiation on taste dysfunction: a prospective study, Clin Oncol (R Coll Radiol) 7:173, 1995.

Mossman KL: Frequent short-term oral complications of head and neck radiotherapy, Ear Nose Throat J 73:316, 1994.

Schwartz LK, Weiffenbach JM, Valdez IH, Fox PC: Taste intensity performance in patients irradiated to the head and neck, Physiol Behav 53:671, 1993.

PART THREE

Radiation Safety and Protection

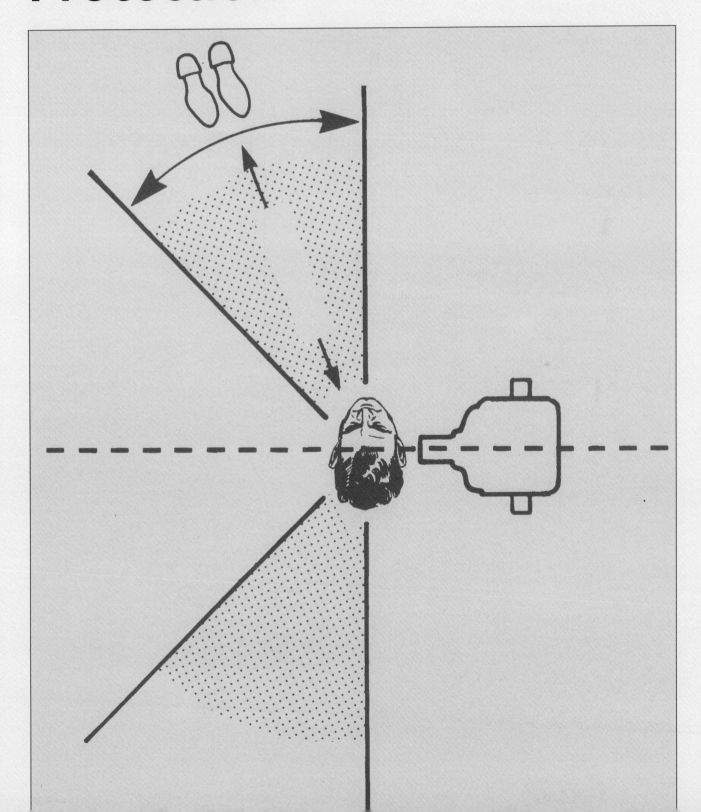

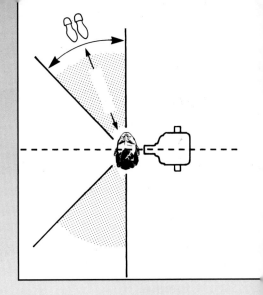

CHAPTER 3

Health Physics

NEIL L. FREDERIKSEN

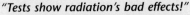

"Tests show radiation's bad effects!"
"Radiation cloud over medicine!"
"Single dose of 'safe' radiation found harmful!"
"Diagnostic x rays deserve that negative reaction!"

These headlines have appeared in newspapers across the U.S. over the years. Before an appointment with their dentist, a patient may read one of these articles and understandably form a negative opinion concerning the use of x rays for diagnostic purposes. Practitioners must be prepared to discuss intelligently the benefits and possible hazards involved with the use of x rays and be able to describe the steps taken to reduce the hazard.

Practitioners who administer ionizing radiation must become familiar with the magnitude of radiation exposure encountered in medicine and dentistry, the possible risk that such exposure entails, and the methods used to affect exposure and reduce dose. This information provides the necessary background for explaining to concerned patients the benefits and possible hazards involved with the use of x rays. This chapter is dedicated to the application of radiation protection principles, collectively known as *health physics*.

Sources of Radiation Exposure

A wide variety of conditions and circumstances, some that are controllable and others that are not, result in radiation exposure from a multitude of sources. Although the sources of radiation exposure are many and varied, they are categorized as being derived from two sources: natural and artificial (Table 3-1). The radi-

ation from these sources results in an average annual effective dose of 3.6 mSv to a person living in the U.S.

The effective dose, the dosimetric quantity used to relate radiation exposure to risk, is derived as follows: the equivalent dose (H_T), a quantity that expresses all kinds of radiation on a common scale, is defined as the sum of the products of the absorbed dose in grays (D) and the radiation weighting factor (w_R). The unit of equivalent dose is the Sievert. The effective dose (E) is the sum of the equivalent doses to each tissue (H_T), multiplied by each tissue's weighting factor (w_T):

$$E = \Sigma H_T \times w_T$$

The International Commission on Radiological Protection (ICRP) defines tissue weighting factors. These factors allow practitioners to obtain a value for E that is estimated to be a measure of the somatic and genetic radiation-induced risks, even if the body is not uniformly exposed. The quantities of dose listed in Table 3-1 are an average for the total population. The contribution to the radiation exposure of an individual from each component may vary by one or more orders of magnitude depending on factors discussed later in this chapter.

NATURAL RADIATION

An appreciation of the magnitude of radiation doses from natural sources is necessary to put radiation expo-

TABLE 3-1
Average Annual Effective Dose of Ionizing Radiation (mSv) to a Member of the U.S. Population

SOURCE	DOSE
Natural	
EXTERNAL	
Cosmic	0.27
Terrestrial	0.28
INTERNAL	
Radon	2.00
Other	0.40
NATURAL TOTAL	3.00
Artificial	
MEDICAL	
X-ray diagnosis	0.39
Nuclear medicine	0.14
CONSUMER PRODUCTS	**0.10**
OTHER	
Occupational	<0.01
Nuclear fuel cycle	<0.01
Fallout	<0.01
Miscellaneous	<0.01
ARTIFICIAL TOTAL	0.60
NATURAL PLUS ARTIFICIAL	3.60

From National Council on Radiation Protection and Measurements: NCRP Reports 93, 1987; 94, 1987; 95, 1987; 100, 1989.

sure into perspective. All life on earth has evolved over time in a continuous exposure to natural radiation. Still today natural or background radiation is the largest contributor (83%) to the radiation exposure of people living in the U.S. (Fig. 3-1; see also Table 3-1). Background radiation from external and internal sources yields an average annual E of about 3 mSv.

External Sources

External exposure results from cosmic and terrestrial radiation, both of which originate from the environment. These sources contribute about 16% of the radiation exposure to the population.

Cosmic radiation. Cosmic radiation includes energetic subatomic particles, photons of extraterrestrial origin that reach the earth (primary cosmic radiation) and to a lesser extent the particles and photons (secondary cosmic radiation) generated by the interactions of

primary cosmic radiation with atoms and molecules of the earth's atmosphere. In the lower atmosphere the EE from cosmic radiation is primarily a function of altitude, almost doubling with each 2000-meter increase in elevation, because less atmosphere is present to attenuate the radiation. Therefore at sea level the exposure from cosmic radiation is about 0.24 mSv per year; at an elevation of 1600 m (approximately 1 mile, or the elevation of Denver, CO), it is about 0.50 mSv per year; and at an elevation of 3200 m (approximately 2 miles, or the elevation of Leadville, CO), it is about 1.25 mSv per year. Cosmic radiation is also greater at higher latitudes because charged particles from space are deflected toward the poles by the earth's magnetic field. In addition to causing an increase in cosmic-ray dose at the poles, the interaction of these charged particles results in light being emitted by the earth's upper atmosphere. This visual display in the northern hemisphere is called the *aurora borealis,* or "northern lights." Considering the altitude and latitude distribution of the U.S. population and a 20% reduction in exposure because of structural shielding during time spent indoors, the average cosmic radiation E rate is about 0.26 mSv per year.

Cosmic radiation also includes exposure resulting from airline travel. As more people travel frequently above the protection of the earth's atmosphere, cosmic radiation becomes a more significant contributor to exposure. An airline flight of 5 hours in the middle latitudes at an altitude of 12 km may result in a dose equivalent of about 25 μSv. Airline flight crews on northern routes at high altitudes from the U.S. to Europe may also receive significant exposures. Crews originating in Europe are currently classified as radiation workers and subjected to occupational dose limits (Table 3-2). This classification has yet to be adopted in the U.S.

Thus in total, cosmic radiation, including that occurring during airline travel, contributes an exposure of 0.27 mSv, or about 8% of the average annual E.

Terrestrial radiation. Exposure from terrestrial sources comes from radioactive nuclides in the soil. The extent of exposure varies with the type of soil and its content of the naturally occurring radionuclides potassium-40 and the radioactive decay products of uranium-238 and thorium-232. Most of the gamma radiation from these sources comes from the top 20 cm of soil, with only a small contribution by airborne radon and its decay products. Indoor exposure from radionuclides is very close to that occurring outdoors. This results from a balance between the shielding provided by structural materials and the exposure from radioactive nuclides contained within these shielding materials.

It is estimated that the average terrestrial exposure rate is about 0.28 mSv per year, or approximately 8% of

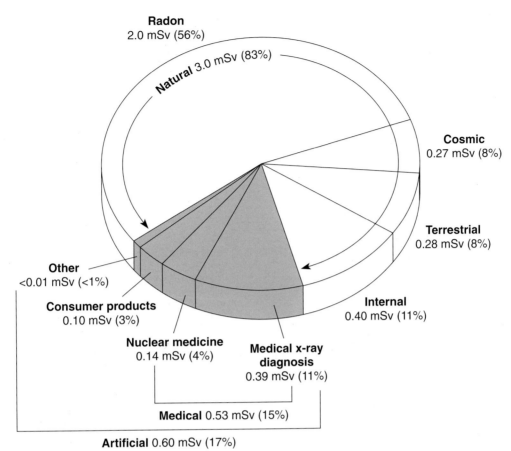

Radon
2.0 mSv (56%)

Natural 3.0 mSv (83%)

Cosmic
0.27 mSv (8%)

Terrestrial
0.28 mSv (8%)

Internal
0.40 mSv (11%)

Medical x-ray diagnosis
0.39 mSv (11%)

Nuclear medicine
0.14 mSv (4%)

Consumer products
0.10 mSv (3%)

Other
<0.01 mSv (<1%)

Medical 0.53 mSv (15%)

Artificial 0.60 mSv (17%)

FIG. **3-1**   The distribution of natural and artificial radiation. Natural radiation contributes more exposure than artificial radiation; x-ray diagnosis is the largest component of artificial radiation.

the average annual E to a person living in the U.S. This quantity of radiation exposure appears minimal compared with that received by individuals living in certain towns and villages of coastal Brazil and Kerala, India, where the gamma radiation dose levels can be as high as 13 mSv per year. These unusually high terrestrial radiation levels are caused by a high content of thorium-232 in the soil.

Internal Sources

The sources of internal radiation are radionuclides that are taken up from the external environment by inhalation and ingestion. Because an organism cannot discriminate between isotopes of a chemical element, all isotopes, radioactive or not, have an equal chance, modified by frequency of occurrence, of being incorporated into the body. This source, which results in about 67% (2.4 mSv) of the radiation exposure of the population, includes radon and its short-lived decay products.

Radon. Radon, a decay product in the uranium series, is estimated to be responsible for approximately 56% of

the radiation exposure of the U.S. population. As such, it is the largest single contributor to natural radiation (2.0 mSv). The ubiquitous noble gas radon (radon-222) is transported in the water and air that enter our homes and buildings and by itself does little harm. However, radon decays to form solid products that emit α-particles (^{218}Po, ^{214}Po, ^{214}Pb, and ^{214}Bi). These decay products become attached to dust particles that can be deposited in the respiratory tract, contributing an average annual equivalent dose to the bronchial epithelium in the U.S. population of 24 mSv. Exposure to this quantity of radiation may cause as many as 10,000 to 20,000 lung cancer deaths per year in the U.S., mostly in smokers.

Other internal sources. The second largest source (11%) of natural radiation results from the ingestion of food and water that contain radionuclides. The average annual E due to the presence of uranium and thorium and their decay products (primarily potassium-40, but also rubidium-87, carbon-14, tritium, and a dozen or more extraterrestrially produced radionuclides) is estimated at 0.4 mSv per year in the U.S. An interesting

TABLE 3-2
Recommendations on Annual Limits for Human Exposure to Ionizing Radiation

RECOMMENDATION	NCRP	ICRP
Occupational Dose Limits		
Relative to stochastic effects	50 mSv annual effective dose limit and [10 mSv][age (yr)] cumulative effective dose limit	50 mSv annual effective dose limit and 100 mSv in 5 yr cumulative effective dose limit
Relative to deterministic effects	150 mSv annual equivalent dose limit to lens of eye and 500 mSv annual equivalent dose limit to skin and extremities	150 mSv equivalent dose limit to lens of eye and 500 mSv annual equivalent dose limit to skin and extremities
Nonoccupational (Public) Dose Limits		
Relative to stochastic effects	5 mSv annual effective dose limit for infrequent exposure and 1 mSv annual effective dose limit for continuous exposure	1 mSv annual effective dose limit and, if higher, not to exceed annual average of 1 mSv over 5 yr
Relative to deterministic effects	50 mSv annual equivalent dose limit to lens of eye, skin, and extremities	15 mSv annual equivalent dose limit to lens of eye and 50 mSv annual equivalent dose limit to lens of eye, skin, and extremities
Embryo-fetus	0.5 mSv equivalent dose limit per month after after pregnancy is known	2 mSv equivalent dose limit after the pregnancy has been declared
Negligible individual dose*	0.01 mSv annual effective dose	None established

From National Council on Radiation Protection and Measurements: NCRP Report 116, 1993, and International Commission on Radiological Protection: Radiation protection, ICRP Publication 60, 1990.
*That dose below which any effort to reduce the radiation exposure cannot be justified.

source of internal exposure is the Brazil nut. This nut has relatively high concentrations of radioactive nuclides. A person consuming 100 g of Brazil nuts per week (not an unreasonable amount in Brazil) would receive an annual dose of 0.2 mSv.

ARTIFICIAL RADIATION

Human beings, with all their technologic advances, have contributed a number of sources of radiation to the environment. These may be categorized into three major groups—medical diagnosis and treatment, consumer and industrial products and sources, and other minor sources—which, in total, contribute an average annual E of about 0.6 mSv, or 17% of the annual radiation exposure to the U.S. population.

Medical Diagnosis and Treatment

In 1993 it was estimated that more than 1 billion medical x-ray examinations and 300 million dental examinations are performed annually worldwide. Radiation used in the healing arts is the single largest component (0.53 mSv) of artificial radiation to which the

U.S. population is exposed and second only to radon as a source. Although sources in this group include radiation therapy and diagnosis, diagnostic x-ray exposure is the largest contributor, with an average annual E of about 0.39 mSv. The contribution made by oral radiography has been excluded from this calculated total because dental examinations are responsible for an average annual E of less than the negligible individual dose (0.01 mSv; see Table 3-2). Dental x-ray examinations are responsible for only 2.5% of the average annual E resulting from x-ray diagnosis and 0.3% of the total average annual E.

Consumer and Industrial Products and Sources

Although only a minor contributor to the average annual E (3%), consumer and industrial products and sources contain some of the most interesting and unsuspected sources. In total, this group, which includes the domestic water supply (10 to 60 µSv), combustible fuels (1.0 to 6.0 µSv), dental porcelain (0.1 µSv), television receivers (less than 10 µSv), pocket watches (1.0 to 5.0 $\times$ 10^{-2} µSv), smoke alarms (less than 1.0 $\times$ 10^{-2} µSv), and airport inspection systems (less than 1.0×10^{-2} µSv), contributes about 0.10 mSv to the average annual E.

The contribution resulting from use of tobacco products is also included in this category. Estimating the average annual E to the population from this source is difficult with current information. Nevertheless, by making several assumptions, the E for the average smoker can be calculated. The annual average dose to a small area of the bronchial epithelium may be estimated to be 8.0 mGy as a result of the ^{210}Pb and ^{210}Po contained within tobacco. Applying a radiation quality factor (w_R) of 20 for alpha particles (^{210}Pb and ^{210}Po are alpha emitters) yields an annual equivalent dose (H_T) to the lungs of 160 mSv. Using a tissue-weighting factor (w_T) of 0.08 for the portion of lungs exposed results in a calculation of an effective dose of approximately 13 mSv for the average smoker, by far the largest source of exposure from consumer products.

Other Artificial Sources

Other artificial radionuclides are a product of modern times. After periods of nuclear weapons testing in the 1950s and early 1960s, the fission products cesium-137, strontium-90, and iodine-131 were discovered in humans. Released into the environment by aboveground nuclear explosions, 90 of which occurred at the Nevada Test Site, these radiation sources reached the body through normal food chains.

Of these sources, strontium-90 and iodine-131 are perhaps the most important. Because of its chemical similarity to calcium, strontium-90, a beta emitter, is readily assimilated in the bones and teeth of children and young adults. Concentration in these areas is a reason for concern because of its long half-life (28.8 years) and slow turnover rate (the effective half-life in bone is 17.5 years). Iodine-131 (a gamma emitter) accumulates in the thyroid gland. It has been estimated that the average cumulative dose to the thyroid of approximately 160 million people in the U.S. resulting from the Nevada tests was 0.02 Gy, or about 21 times that delivered by a complete mouth survey (see Thyroid Dose, p. ••). The late effects of these exposures have yet to be determined. Currently, fallout is no longer considered a significant source of exposure to the public because of the cessation of atmospheric testing of nuclear weapons.

Nuclear power (which may contribute in total only about 0.01 mSv to the average annual E) is another artificial source that is of particular concern to the public. However, nuclear power and support facilities, in normal operation, add only about 0.6 µSv to the average annual E, a quantity up to 10 times less than that contributed by the release of naturally occurring radionuclides from the combustion of coal, natural gas, and oil.

In spite of this relatively low contribution to the average annual E made by nuclear power, accidents do happen that result in significant exposure to certain segments of the population. Between 1945 and 1987, 284 nuclear reactor accidents, excluding Chernobyl, were reported in several countries, resulting in the exposure of more than 1300 people, with 33 fatalities. In the majority of these accidents, the public was not directly affected. This was not the case, however, in the Three Mile Island incident in the U.S. and at Chernobyl in the Ukraine. After the Three Mile Island nuclear plant incident in 1979, studies showed that the maximum individual dose was less than 1.0 mSv and individuals living within a 16-km radius of the plant received an average dose of only 0.08 mSv, an added exposure equal to some 2.7% of their natural background radiation exposure. From 1982 to 1984, a temporary increase occurred in the incidence of cancer among those living near the nuclear plant. This finding was not expected in view of the relatively long latent period for radiation-induced malignancy. Instead it was believed to be a result not of exposure to radiation, but of early detection as a result of increased surveillance of cancer prompted by postaccident concern.

The nuclear accident at Chernobyl in 1986 made clear that the use of nuclear power facilities carries the real potential of causing considerable harm if not properly controlled. In that event, 29 persons in the immediate vicinity of the plant died of acute radiation injury in the first months after exposure. The long-term risk to the general population is not known.

Exposure and Dose in Radiography

The goal of health physics is to prevent the occurrence of deterministic effects and reduce the likelihood of stochastic effects by minimizing the exposure of office personnel and patients during radiographic examinations. A *deterministic effect* is defined as any somatic effect that increases in severity as a function of radiation dose after a threshold has been reached. These effects, resulting from relatively large doses of radiation not generally encountered in diagnostic radiology, may occur soon after exposure or months to years after exposure. Examples of deterministic effects include cataracts, skin erythema, fibrosis, and abnormal growth and development following exposure in utero. A *stochastic effect* is defined as one whose probability rather than severity is a function of radiation dose without a threshold. Stochastic effects represent an all-or-none response, modified by individual risk factors. These effects may occur after exposure to relatively low doses of radiation such as those that may be encountered in diagnostic radiology. Cancers and genetic effects are examples of stochastic effects.

DOSE LIMITS

Recognition of the harmful effects of radiation and the risks involved with its use led the National Council on Radiation Protection and Measurements (NCRP) and the International Commission on Radiological Protection (ICRP) to establish guidelines for limitations on the amount of radiation received by both occupationally exposed individuals and the public. Since their establishment in the 1930s, these dose limits have been revised downward several times. These revisions reflect the increased knowledge gained over the years concerning the harmful effects of radiation and the increased ability to use radiation more efficiently. The current occupational exposure limits have been established to ensure that the probability for stochastic effects is as low as reasonably and economically feasible (see Table 3-2).

Compliance with these limits should ensure that the risk for individual radiation workers being afflicted with fatal cancer as a result of their occupational exposure is no greater than the risk for fatal accidents in nonradiation occupations. Nonoccupational dose limits for members of the public have been established at 10% of that of occupationally exposed individuals. This lower dose limit was set because of uncertainties associated with risk estimates, the wider variation in mortality risks and levels of exposure to natural radiation, and the wider range of sensitivities to radiation found among the general public. The negligible individual dose, established by the NCRP, is considered to be the dose below which any effort to reduce the radiation exposure may not be cost-effective. In spite of the Council's endorsement of the nonthreshold hypothesis for purposes of radiation safety, it is believed that the impact on society of radiation exposure of this magnitude is negligible.

Although receiving 50 mSv of whole-body radiation exposure in 1 year as a result of performing one's occupation may be considered to present minimal risk, every effort should be made to keep the dose to all individuals as low as practical. All unnecessary radiation exposure should be avoided. This is a philosophy of radiation protection everyone should recognize. It is based on the principle of ALARA (*As Low As Reasonably Achievable*), which recognizes the possibility that no matter how small the dose, some stochastic effect may result. Industrial workers in radiation industries appear to be acting in accordance with this philosophy,

insofar as their average annual individual effective dose is 1.56 mSv, 3% of the annual limit. The dosage for individuals occupationally exposed in the operation of dental x-ray equipment is even less: 0.2 mSv, or 0.4% of the allowable limit.

It is important to realize that these dose limits were formulated by the NCRP and ICRP, private nonprofit organizations, and as such have no force of law. Although the federal government and most state governments accept these recommendations, all those who administer ionizing radiation should consult with their state's bureau of radiation control or safety to obtain information on applicable and current laws. In addition, these dose limits apply only to exposure from manmade sources and do not apply to either natural radiation or radiation exposure that patients receive in the course of dental and medical treatment.

PATIENT EXPOSURE AND DOSE

Patient dose from dental radiography is usually reported as the amount of radiation received by a target organ. One of the most common measurements is skin or surface exposure. The surface exposure, obtained by direct measurement, is the simplest way to record a patient's exposure to x rays. Of little significance in itself, it is used in the calculation of doses received by organs that lie at or near the point of measurement. Radiosensitive target organs commonly reported include bone marrow, thyroid gland, and gonads. The mean active bone marrow dose is an important measurement because bone marrow is the target organ believed responsible for radiation-induced leukemia. Particular concern has been expressed over exposure of the thyroid because this gland has one of the highest radiation-induced cancer rates. The gonad dose is important because of suspected genetic responses to diagnostic x-ray exposure.

Patient dose has also been reported as the effective dose, E. This method of reporting resulted from an inability to make direct comparisons between radiographic techniques themselves and background radiation exposure in terms of dose because of the limited area of the body exposed during diagnostic radiology. It is only through the E that possible adverse effects from irradiation to a limited portion of the body can be compared with possible adverse effects from irradiation of the whole body.

Mean Active Bone Marrow Dose

The mean active bone marrow dose was derived as a specific tissue dose relevant to a particular stochastic effect, leukemia. The mean active bone marrow dose is that dose of radiation averaged over the entire active bone marrow. The mean active bone marrow dose resulting from an intraoral full-mouth survey of 21 films exposed with round collimation is 0.142 mSv; the same survey exposed with rectangular collimation results in a dose of only 0.06 mSv. Panoramic radiography may contribute a mean active bone marrow dose of about 0.01 mSv per film. For comparison, the mean active bone marrow dose from one chest film is 0.03 mSv.

Thyroid Dose

The proximity of the thyroid gland to the x-ray beam is of crucial importance in determining the magnitude of dose received. For example, a radiographic examination of the cervical spine may consist of four separate exposures that in total are responsible for a dose to the thyroid of about 5.5 mGy. During this examination, the thyroid gland is almost directly in the center of the radiation field. On the other hand, a radiograph of the chest may result in a thyroid dose of only 0.01 mGy, mainly from scatter radiation. The dose to the thyroid from oral radiography is fairly low. A 21-film complete mouth examination results in a thyroid dose of 0.94 mGy, one sixth that resulting from a radiographic examination of the cervical spine. Likewise, the thyroid dose from panoramic radiography is about 0.074 mGy, 1% that from a cervical spinal examination.

Gonad Dose

Radiographs of the abdomen result in the highest dose to the gonads; those involving the head, neck, and extremities result in the lowest. For example, a radiograph of the kidneys, ureters, and bladder (retrograde pyelogram) delivers a gonad dose of 1.07 mGy to women and 0.08 mGy to men, whereas a radiograph of the skull delivers a gonadal dose of less than 0.005 mGy in both sexes. Dental x-ray examinations result in a genetically insignificant dose of only 0.001 mGy. This contribution is only 0.003% of the average annual background exposure.

Comparative Exposure

It is tempting to make a direct comparison of the previously discussed values for purposes of risk estimation. However, the statement that a single dental periapical radiograph delivers more than 10 times the radiation of a chest film (in terms of surface exposure, that is, 217 versus 16 mR) is not entirely true because of differences in the area and critical organs exposed. These differences may be compensated for by a calculation of the E, which is an estimate of the uniform whole-body exposure carrying the same probability of radiation effect as a partial-body exposure. By this method of calculation, a complete mouth survey of 20 films made by

methods that were optimized for dose (i.e., E-speed film, rectangular collimation) has been found to deliver less than half the amount of radiation of a single chest film and less than 1% of the amount of a barium study of the intestines (Table 3-3).

ESTIMATES OF RISK

The degree of risk that may be associated with exposure to ionizing radiation may be expressed in two ways: equivalent natural exposure and probability of stochastic effects. Equivalent natural exposure is calculated as the product of the E resulting from a specific radiographic examination and the average daily E (8 μSv) delivered by natural sources (see Table 3-3). Dentists may use this expression of exposure to discuss potential risk with patients from a perspective that may be more easily understood. The dentist may point out to the patient that by optimizing the intraoral radiographic technique (E-speed film, rectangular collimation), the days of equivalent exposure may be reduced from about $2\frac{1}{2}$ weeks (18.8 days) to only about 2 days. This time is quite low when compared with over $1\frac{1}{2}$ years, which is equivalent to that delivered by a barium examination of the lower intestinal tract. For another example, the dependence of physical location within the U.S. on exposure to natural radiation may be used. The E resulting from cosmic radiation in Denver is 0.24 mSv (240 μSv) higher than the average of the U.S. because of its high elevation and reduced atmospheric protection. This means that a person living in an average location in the U.S. who had one complete mouth survey and one panoramic film made by optimized techniques every year (total E for these examinations = 43 μSv; see Table 3-3) would incur less than one fifth the risk for a person living in Denver who was not exposed to dental radiography. Put another way, if a person living in an average location in the U.S. had 14 complete mouth surveys (238 μSv) made by optimized techniques every year, he or she would incur only the same risk as a person living in Denver who was not exposed to dental radiography.

The primary risk from dental radiography is radiation-induced cancer. The risk for cancer being induced in humans as a result of exposure to low doses of radiation is difficult to estimate for a number of reasons. First, the number of known radiation-induced cases is small and the doses too high to allow for interpolation to low doses with any degree of certainty. Second, cancer is a prevalent disease. It is estimated that in the U.S. in 2002 almost 1,300,000 new cases of cancer were diagnosed and over 550,000 people died from cancer. This makes the low incidence resulting from radiation exposure difficult to detect. Third, radiation-induced

TABLE **3-3**

Effective Dose, Equivalent Natural Exposure, and Probability of Stochastic Effects From Diagnostic X-ray Examinations

SURVEY	E (μSv)	DAYS OF EQUIVALENT NATURAL EXPOSURE	PROBABILITY OF STOCHASTIC EFFECTS ($\times 10^{-6}$)
Intraoral			
Round collimation, D-speed film*			
Periapical—15 films	111	13.9	8.1
Interproximal—4 films	38	4.8	2.8
Complete mouth survey—19 films	150	18.8	11.0
Rectangular collimation, E-speed film†			
Complete mouth survey—20 films	33	4.1	2.4
Extraoral			
Panoramic‡	26	3.3	1.9
Computed tomography			
Maxilla	104§ to 1,202‖	13.0 to 150.3	7.6 to 87.7
Mandible	761§ to 3,324‖	95.1 to 415.5	55.6 to 242.7
Lower gastrointestinal (GI)¶	4060	507.5	55.6 to 242.7
Upper GI¶	2440	305.0	178.1
Abdomen¶	560	70.0	40.9
Skull¶	220	27.5	16.1
Chest¶	80	10.0	5.8

*Avendanio B et al: Effective dose and risk assessment from detailed narrow beam radiography, Oral Surg Oral Med Pathol Radiol Endod 82:713, 1996.
†White SC: 1992 assessment of radiation risks from dental radiography, Dentomaxillofac Radiol 21:118, 1992.
‡Frederikson NL, Benson BS, Sokolowski TW: Effective dose and risk assessment from film tomography used for dental implant diagnostics, Dentomaxillofac Radiol 23:123, 1994.
§Frederiksen NL, Benson BW, Sokolowski TW: Effective dose and risk assessment from computed tomography of the maxillofacial complex, Dentomaxillofac Radiol 24:55, 1995.
‖Scaf G et al: Dosimetry and cost of imaging osseointegrated implants with film-based and computed tomography, Oral Surg Oral Med Pathol Oral Radiol Endod 83:41, 1997.
¶National Council on Radiation Protection and Measurements: Exposure of the U.S. population from diagnostic medical radiation, NCRP Report 100, Bethesda, Md, 1989.

cancers are clinically indistinguishable from cancers induced by other causes. Finally, the time between radiation exposure and the development of cancer may be years to decades, during which time individuals may be subjected to other carcinogens.

In spite of these difficulties, the ICRP has developed an estimate that includes the probability for the induction of both fatal and nonfatal cancer and hereditary effects in an exposed population. The probability coefficient for these stochastic effects resulting from exposure to low doses of radiation is $7.3 \times 10^{-2} \, \text{Sv}^{-1}$. The product of this probability coefficient and the E resulting from a specific radiographic examination, which yields a probability of occurrence per million exposed people, is shown in Table 3-3. These data show that the risk for developing cancer or some heritable effect from radiation received as a result of intraoral radiography is estimated to be at most 11 per million examinations. If the contribution made by hereditary effects were ignored (assuming these 11 cases per million examinations to be cancers), then exposure of everyone in the population would increase the number of new cases of invasive cancer by only 0.2%.

Everyone is subject to risks in everyday life. Newspapers and news magazines occasionally publish articles dealing with the level of such risks. In consideration of the potential risk associated with dental radiography, it might be good to keep in mind that the average person's risk for death as a result of an accident while a patient in hospital is about 230 per million; choking to death, 13 per million; and dying in a boating accident, 4.6 per million. The risk from these events is greater than the risk from intraoral radiographic procedures.

In addition, people needlessly expose themselves to x radiation. There is a current trend for having body CT scans in hopes of detecting early signs of cancer, coronary artery disease, and other abnormalities. What most people do not realize is that a combined CT scan of the chest and abdomen delivers an E dose equal to almost 1000 radiographs of the chest! Furthermore, this increased exposure is often incurred for what is considered to be an unnecessary test: there is insufficient scientific evidence to justify CT screening for patients with no symptoms or family history suggesting disease.

Although the risk involved with dental radiography is certainly small in comparison with many other risks that are a common part of everyday life such as smoking or consumption of fatty foods, no basis exists to assume that it is zero. Despite the fact that diagnostic radiation appears to be a weak carcinogen, the risk is increased because of the large number of people exposed. Practitioners must conclude that it is their responsibility to ensure that patients avoid even the smallest unnecessary dose of radiation.

Methods of Exposure and Dose Reduction

> "The guiding principle for use of diagnostic radiology in dentistry is to enhance the diagnostic benefits of dental radiographs and minimize the associated radiation risks to patients and staff."*

In this section, methods of exposure and dose reduction are described that can be used in oral radiography. Each subsection begins with a recommendation of either the American Dental Association (ADA) Council on Dental Materials, Instruments, and Equipment or the Council on Scientific Affairs based on optimal use of the radiologic process. This is followed by a discussion of ways in which these recommendations can be satisfied. Included in the text are NCRP recommendations and federal regulations concerning the use of ionizing radiation.

In addition to federal regulations, states have their own laws dealing with ionizing radiation. Although most of them closely follow the recommendations of the ADA and the NCRP, all practitioners should consult their local bureau of radiation control or safety to obtain information on current and applicable laws.

PATIENT SELECTION

> ... dentists (should) exercise professional judgment when prescribing diagnostic radiographs for dental patients. Diagnostic radiography should be used only after clinical examination, consideration of the patient's history and consideration of both the dental and the general health needs of the patient.†

No question exists about the diagnostic utility of radiographs; almost half of all carious teeth can be found only by radiographic examination. In spite of this usefulness, the potential exists for misapplication, resulting in increased patient exposure. In three out of four cases, orthodontists were found to be confident in their diagnosis before evaluating any existing radiographic evidence. In some instances, less than 1% of all radiographs made were found to have any influence on

---

*From ADA Council on Scientific Affairs: An Update on Radiographic Practices: Information and Recommendations, J Am Dent Assoc 132:234, 2001.
†From ADA Council on Dental Materials, Instruments, and Equipment: Recommendations on radiographic practices: an update, 1988, J Am Dent Assoc 118:115, 1989.

patient care. These findings may cast some doubt on the reliability of "professional judgment" as the sole criterion for patient selection. Realization of this prompted two national conferences to conclude that a need exists for the development and implementation of more specific radiographic selection criteria to guide the practitioner's professional judgment. Such criteria could serve as more definitive guidelines for patient selection, which in turn might reduce the number of unproductive radiographic examinations and patient exposure to x rays.

Radiographic selection criteria, also known as high-yield or referral criteria, are clinical or historical findings that identify patients for whom a high probability exists that a radiographic examination will provide information affecting their treatment or prognosis. The Dental Patient Selection Criteria Panel, established by the Center for Devices and Radiological Health of the Food and Drug Administration, was assigned the responsibility of formulating selection criteria for oral radiography (see Chapter 14). When used in ordering radiographs for caries detection, these guidelines have been found to result in 43% fewer radiographs being made while missing what was felt to be an insignificant number of lesions (3.3%). Additionally, when these guidelines were used, the number of missed intraosseous and other dental conditions was considered inconsequential, given the range of variability among clinicians in diagnosis and treatment. In spite of these findings, only a little more than a third of dentists chose to prescribe selectively according to the patient's needs.

CONDUCT OF THE EXAMINATION

When the decision has been made that a radiographic examination is justified (patient selection), the way in which the examination is conducted greatly influences patient exposure to x radiation. The conduct of the examination may be divided into choice of equipment, choice of technique, operation of equipment, and processing and interpretation of the radiographic image.

Choice of Equipment

The choice of equipment includes selection of the image receptor, focal spot-to-film distance, x-ray beam collimation, filtration, and the type of leaded apron and collar.

Receptor selection.   **The ADA has taken the following position:**

> The basis for selecting film types, film-intensifying screen combinations and other image receptors is to obtain the

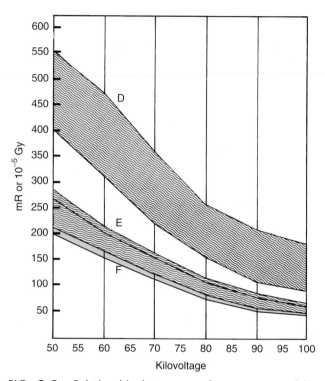

Acceptable X-Ray Exposure Ranges
Speed Groups D, E, and F Film

FIG. 3-2   Relationship between surface exposures delivered to a patient by exposure of group D, E, and F (in light gray) intraoral films and diagnostic density at various kilovoltages. (Modified from HHS Pub [FDA] 85-8245, 1985.)

maximum sensitivity (speed) consistent with the image quality required for the diagnostic task.*

Intraoral image receptors.   In 1920, the Eastman Kodak Company introduced what it referred to as *regular dental x-ray film.* The images produced by this film were excellent for that time, but the speed was so slow that a radiograph of the maxillary molar area of an adult required 9 seconds of exposure. Since that time, progressively faster films have been developed. Beginning with the letter designation "A," film speed has almost doubled with the introduction of each new speed group. Currently, intraoral dental x-ray film is available in three speed groups—D, E, and F. Clinically, film of speed group E is almost twice as fast (sensitive) as film of group D and about 50 times as fast as regular dental x-ray film (Fig. 3-2). F-speed film requires about 75% the exposure of E-speed film and only about 40% that of D-speed.† In

---

*From ADA Council on Scientific Affairs: An Update on Radiographic Practices: Information and Recommendations, J Am Dent Assoc 132:234, 2001.

†Because speed groups include a range of exposures, clinically there is not an exact doubling of speed when going from speed groups D to E or E to F.

TABLE 3-4
Factors Affecting the Radiographic Quality of a Diagnostic Film

IMAGE FACTORS	CLARITY	IMAGE SIZE	SHAPE DISTORTION	FILM DENSITY	RADIOGRAPHIC CONTRAST
kVp*				X	X
mAs*	X			X	X
Collimation*		X		X	X
Filtration*				X	X
Focal spot size†	X	X			
Object-to-film distance†	X	X			
Focal spot-to-film distance†	X	X		X	
Motion	X	X			
Alignment‡			X		
Subject density§	X			X	X
Subject shape§	X			X	X
Film speed§	X			X	X
Developing time‖				X	X
Technique‡	X	X	X		
Screen speed§	X	X		X	X

*See Chapter 1.
†See Chapter 5.
‡See Chapter 8.
§See Chapter 4.
‖See Chapter 6.

practice, this means that the 9-second exposure required for regular film in 1920 has been reduced to about 0.2 second with the use of E-speed film and 0.15 second with F-speed film.

Faster films are desirable from the standpoint of exposure reduction. However, the possible decrease in image quality associated with increased speed, obtained in part by increasing the size or shape of silver halide crystals in the film's emulsion, must also be considered (Table 3-4). If shorter exposure times are realized at the expense of image quality, it is not beneficial to use faster film. Shortly after the introduction of F-speed film (Insight, Eastman Kodak Company) in 2000, studies were undertaken to compare film of speed group F with that of speed groups D and E in terms of the diagnostic quality of the image. It was found that F-speed film had the same useful density range, latitude, contrast, and image quality as D- and E-speed films when processed in a roller-transport type automatic processor. Studies of the comparative diagnostic value of D-, E-, and F-speed film suggest that the faster F-speed film can be used in routine intraoral radiographic examinations without sacrifice of diagnostic information. In spite of the reported benefits of using intraoral film of faster speed groups, the majority of dentists in the U.S. continue to use D-speed film.

Patient dose reductions of 75% compared with D-speed film, 50% compared with E-speed film, and about 40% compared with F-speed film may be achieved using digital intraoral radiography. This significant reduction in patient dose must be balanced against the decreased image resolution associated with digital imaging.

Intensifying screens. Contemporary intensifying screens used in extraoral radiography use the rare earth elements gadolinium and lanthanum. These rare earth phosphors emit green light on interaction with x rays. Compared with the older calcium tungstate screens, rare earth screens decrease patient exposure by as much as 55% in panoramic and cephalometric radiography.

A further reduction in patient exposure during extraoral radiography may be achieved with the use of T-grain film. Introduced as T-Mat by the Eastman Kodak Company in 1983, this film contains silver halide grains that are tabular or flat rather than pebblelike in shape. With their flat surface oriented toward the x-ray source, these grains present a greater cross-section, which increases their ability to gather light from intensifying screens. T-grain film used with rare earth screens is twice as fast as calcium tungstate screen-film combinations and $1^1/_3$ times as fast as conventional rare earth screen-film combinations with no loss in image quality. This same T-grain technology was incorporated into intraoral film by Kodak to achieve the faster speeds of E and F films.

Extraoral films exposed by intensifying screens achieve a level of image resolution that is about half that of direct exposure intraoral film. One reason for image degradation in extraoral imaging systems is *crossover*, which refers to the loss of image sharpness and resolution resulting from light emitted by one screen passing through the film to expose the emulsion on the opposite side of the double emulsion film. The Ultra-Vision (DuPont) and Ektavision (Kodak) screen film systems were designed to minimize crossover by using phosphors that emit ultraviolet light, which is less able to pass through the film base to expose the opposite emulsion. Results have shown that images produced by these systems have higher resolution than corresponding rare earth screen-film systems. This allows for the use of a screen one speed class higher and a 50% reduction in patient exposure.

Unlike digital intraoral imaging, there is no significant dose reduction to be gained by replacing extraoral screen-film systems with digital imaging. Image resolution with digital systems appears to approach that obtained with rare earth regular-speed screens matched with T-Mat film (see Chapter 12, Digital Imaging).

Focal spot-to-film distance. The ADA states the following:

> The combination of proper collimation and extended source-patient distance (focal spot-to-film distance) will reduce the amount of radiation to the patient.*

Two standard focal spot-to-film distances (FSFDs) have evolved over the years for use in intraoral radiography, one 20 cm (8 inches) and the other 41 cm (16 inches). When the x-ray tube is operated above 50 kVp, each of these distances satisfies the federal regulation that the x-ray source–skin distance must not be less than 18 cm

(7 inches) (assuming a 2.5-cm [1-inch] distance from the skin surface to the film). Inasmuch as both distances comply with federal law, the decision as to which should be used may then be based on which FSFD results in less patient exposure and the best diagnostic image.

Use of an FSFD longer distance results in a 32% reduction in exposed tissue volume. This is because at the greater distance, the x-ray beam is less divergent (Fig. 3-3). A reduction in exposed tissue volume should be reflected in a reduction in the E. This finding was confirmed by a study that reported a 30% decrease in the E resulting from the use of a 30-cm FSFD instead of a 20-cm FSFD for a simulated 19-film complete mouth survey using D-speed film. Indeed, a study of patient exposures from intraoral radiographic examinations compared a 40-cm FSFD with a 20-cm FSFD in terms of organ doses and found a 38% to 45% decrease in thyroid exposure.

The use of a longer FSFD also results in a smaller apparent focal spot size and thereby theoretically increases the resolution of the radiograph (see Chapter 5). The clinical significance of the effect of focal spot size on image resolution, however, has been questioned.

Collimation. The ADA recommends the following:

> The tissue area (and volume) exposed to the primary x-ray beam should not exceed the minimum coverage consistent with meeting diagnostic requirements and clinical feasibility.†

The federal government requires that the x-ray beam used in intraoral radiography be collimated so that the field of radiation at the patient's skin surface is "contained in a circle having a diameter of no more than 7 cm ($2^3/_4$ inches)" when the x-ray tube is operated above 50 kVp. In view of the dimensions of no. 2 intraoral film (3.2×4.1 cm), a field size of this magnitude is almost three times that necessary to expose the film. Consequently, limiting the size of the x-ray beam even more than required by law may significantly reduce patient exposure. This results in not only decreased patient exposure but also increased image quality (see Table 3-4 and Fig. 3-3). Additionally, the amount of radiation scatter generated is proportional to the area exposed. If scatter radiation is decreased, film fog is decreased and image quality is increased.

There are several means to limit of the size of the x-ray beam. First, a rectangular position-indicating device (PID) may be attached to the radiographic tube

---

*From ADA Council on Scientific Affairs: An Update on Radiographic Practices: Information and Recommendations, J Am Dent Assoc 132:234, 2001.

†From ADA Council on Scientific Affairs: An Update on Radiographic Practices: Information and Recommendations, J Am Dent Assoc 132:234, 2001.

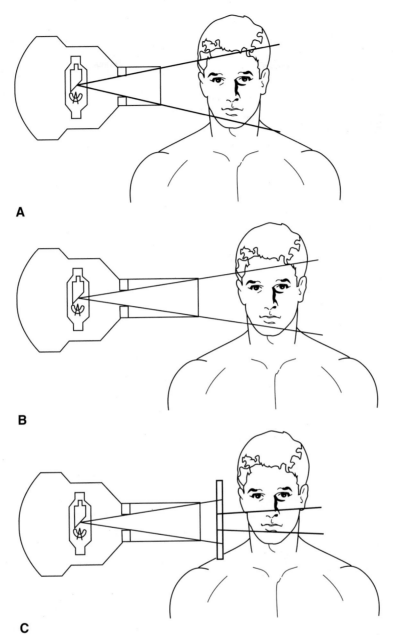

FIG. **3-3** Effect of FSFD and collimation on the volume of tissue irradiated. A larger volume of irradiated tissue results from **A** (with shorter FSFD) than from **B** (in which the longer FSFD produces a less divergent beam). In **C** the collimator between the round PID and the patient produces the effect of a rectangular PID on the tube housing or a rectangular collimating face shield on the film-holding instrument. This rectangular collimator (close to the patient in **C**) results in a smaller, less divergent beam and a smaller volume of tissue irradiated than in **A** or **B**.

housing (Fig. 3-4). Use of a rectangular PID having an exit opening of 3.5×4.4 cm (1.38×1.34 inches) reduces the area of the patient's skin surface exposed by 60% over that of a round (7 cm) PID (see Fig. 3-3, C). Depending on the FSFD, use of rectangular collimation may result in a 71% to 80% decrease in the E, a significant reduction. This reduction in beam size, however, may make aiming the beam difficult. To avoid

the possibility of unsatisfactory radiographs (cone cutting), a film-holding instrument that centers the beam over the film is recommended (Fig. 3-5).

Second, film holders with rectangular collimators may be used with round PIDs (Fig. 3-6); these holders reduce patient exposure to the same degree as rectangular PIDs. In a study reviewing the E delivered during complete mouth examinations made with film holders

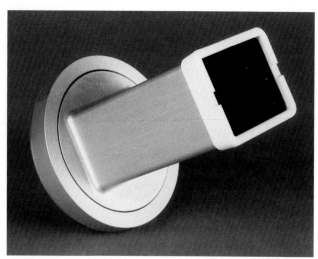

FIG. **3-4**   A rectangular PID, which may be used to reduce the area of patient skin exposed. (Courtesy Dentsply Rinn, Elgin, Ill.)

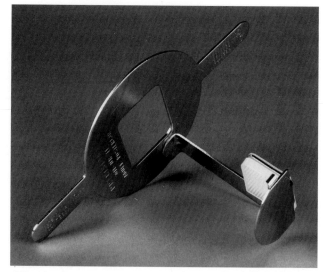

FIG. **3-6**   Precision film-holding instrument. The face shield of the instrument absorbs radiation except for that required to expose the film. (Courtesy Masel Enterprises, Bristol, Penn.)

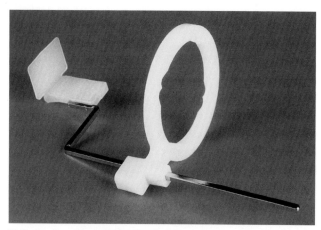

FIG. **3-5**   Rinn XCP film-holding instrument. (Courtesy Dentsply Rinn, Elgin, Ill.)

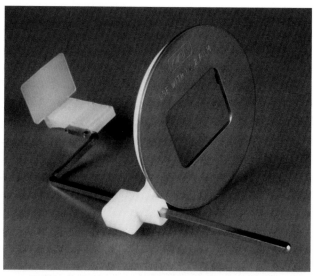

FIG. **3-7**   Rinn XCP instrument with a rectangular collimator clipped to the aiming ring. As with the Precision instrument (see Fig. 3-6), the collimator of this instrument absorbs radiation except for that required to expose the film. (Courtesy Dentsply Rinn, Elgin, Ill.)

using round and rectangular collimation, rectangular collimation reduced the patient dose from intraoral examinations by about 60% (see Table 3-4). Both the Precision instrument (Masel Enterprises, Bristol, PA) and the XCP instrument (Dentsply/Rinn, Elgin, IL) with a rectangular collimator clipped to the aiming ring (Fig. 3-7) may be expected to produce similar results.

The benefits of rectangular collimation relative to image quality and patient exposure do not appear to be realized in clinical practice. Less than 10% of dentists surveyed use rectangular collimation.

Filtration.   The ADA recommends the following:

> Beam filtration should comply with federal and state regulations. The most judicious use of filtration involves selective filtration of excessively high-energy as well as excessively low-energy radiation.*

The x-ray beam emitted from the radiographic tube consists of not only high-energy x-ray photons, but also many photons with relatively lower energy (see Chapter

---

*From ADA Council on Scientific Affairs: An Update on Radiographic Practices: Information and Recommendations, J Am Dent Assoc 132:234, 2001.

1). Low-energy photons, which have little penetrating power, are absorbed mainly by the patient and contribute nothing to the information on the film. The purpose of filtration is to remove these low-energy x-ray photons selectively from the x-ray beam. This results in decreased patient exposure with no loss of radiologic information (see Table 3-4).

When an x-ray beam is filtered with 3 mm of aluminum, the surface exposure is reduced to about 20% of that with no filtration. In light of this and other information, the federal government has designated the specific amount of filtration required for dental x-ray machines operating at various kilovoltages. These quantities, expressed as beam quality (half-value layer [HVL]), are listed in Table 3-5.

Patient exposure may be reduced even further by removing both low- and high-energy x-ray photons from the beam, leaving the mid-range energy photons to expose the film. This suggestion resulted from the finding that the x-ray energies most effective in producing the image are between 35 and 55 keV. Selective filtration of both low- and high-energy photons has been demonstrated with the rare earth elements samarium, erbium, yttrium, niobium, gadolinium, terbium-activated gadolinium oxysulfide (Lanex, Eastman Kodak), and thulium-activated lanthanum oxybromide (Quanta III, DuPont). The use of these materials in combination with aluminum filtration may reduce patient exposure by 20% to 80% compared with conventional aluminum filtration alone, which attenuates few high-energy photons. However, exposure reduction achieved with rare earth filtration has costs. Use of these filters requires a significant increase in exposure time (as much as 50%), increasing both x-ray tube loading and the possibility of patient movement during exposure. Additionally, image quality may suffer because of a decrease in contrast, sharpness, and resolution.

Leaded aprons and collars. The ADA recommends the following:

> Leaded thyroid collars are strongly recommended. Although scatter radiation to the patient's abdomen is extremely low, leaded aprons should be used to minimize patient's exposure to radiation.*

The gonad dose resulting from oral radiography is minimal (see Gonad Dose, p. 53). The philosophy of radiation protection currently in practice, however, is based on the principles of ALARA. This philosophy recognizes the possibility that, no matter how small the dose, some adverse effect may result. Consequently, any dose that can be reduced without difficulty, great expense, or inconvenience should be reduced. Current data show that the mean exposure at skin entrance for a single dental periapical film is 217 mR. If the gonad dose is equal to 1/10,000 of the total beam exposure, as it has been estimated, the dose from one dental periapical film can be calculated to be 0.02 mR. In spite of the fact that this quantity is 50 times less than the negligible dose (see Table 3-2), according to ALARA it should be reduced if possible. Leaded aprons are useful because they attenuate as much as 98% of the scatter radiation to the gonads (Fig. 3-8). Similarly, thyroid shields reduce the exposure of this gland by as much as 92% (Fig. 3-9). No difficulty, great expense, or inconvenience is encountered with their use; instead, using them demonstrates a real concern for the welfare of the patient. However, use of fast film and rectangular collimation are far more important means of protecting the patient.

This and other information regarding the dose to the fetus during oral radiographic procedures and NCRP recommendations concerning embryo-fetus exposure resulted in the decision by the Dental Patient Selection Criteria Panel to propose that oral radiographic examinations were not contraindicated because of pregnancy. However, the decision of whether to use x rays when the patient is pregnant is an individual one. The patient should be made aware of both the need for radiographs and the relative magnitude of exposure before any films are made.

TABLE 3-5
Minimum Half-Value Layer

MEASURED X-RAY TUBE VOLTAGE	MINIMUM HALF-VALUE LAYER
(kVp)	(mm Al)
30 to 70	1.5
71	2.1
80	2.3
90	2.5
100	2.7

From Code of Federal Regulations 21, Subchapter J: Radiological health, part 1000, Washington, D.C., 1994, Office of the Federal Register, General Services Administration.

*From ADA Council on Scientific Affairs: An Update on Radiographic Practices: Information and Recommendations, J Am Dent Assoc 132:234, 2001.

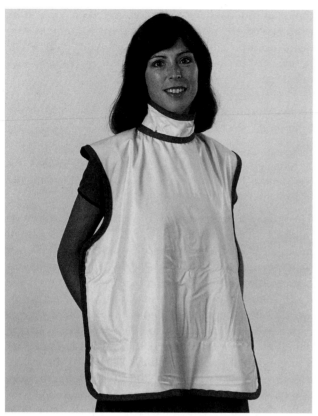

FIG. **3-8**   Leaded apron with a thyroid collar attached.

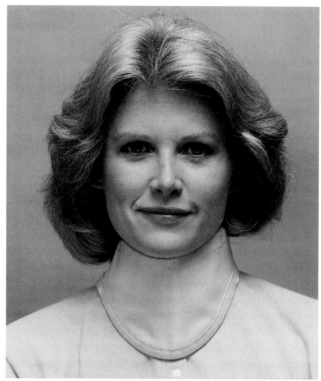

FIG. **3-9**   Thyroid collar for use when one is not attached to the leaded apron.

CHOICE OF INTRAORAL TECHNIQUE

Receptor/film holders that position the receptor to coincide with the collimated x-ray beam should be used. . . . radiographic film (or any image receptor) should not be held in the oral cavity by the patient or the dental professional.*

Currently no recommendations or regulations deal specifically with intraoral radiographic techniques. Consequently, the choice of technique (bisection of the angle or paralleling long cone) is left to the practitioner. Regardless of the technique chosen, a film holder should be used. A significant reduction in the number of unacceptable periapical films was found when film holders were used instead of patient manual support.

The decision as to which technique is used should be based on the diagnostic quality of the resultant radiographs, the efficiency of using radiation, and the convenience of the technique (see Table 3-4). The more efficient the technique, the fewer radiograph retakes

will be required, along with less patient exposure. A study of comparative efficiencies of the bisection and parallel techniques found that the number of undiagnostic radiographs was reduced by more than half when intraoral complete mouth examinations were made with the paralleling technique. If it is assumed that all undiagnostic radiographs are remade, use of the bisection technique leads to a significant increase in patient exposure. This study used the Rinn XCP instrument for parallel film placement (see Fig. 3-5), but similar reports on efficiency have appeared using the Precision instrument (see Fig. 3-6). The Precision instrument with rectangular field collimation reduces patient exposure even more, although similar results might be obtained with the Rinn XCP instrument and a rectangular PID (see Figs. 3-4 and 3-5) or with a rectangular collimator clipped to the aiming ring (see Fig. 3-7; see also Collimation, p. 58).

Operating the Equipment

Exposure settings should be established for optimal image quality.*

---

*From ADA Council on Scientific Affairs: An Update on Radiographic Practices: Information and Recommendations, J Am Dent Assoc 132:234, 2001.

*From ADA Council on Scientific Affairs: An Update on Radiographic Practices: Information and Recommendations, J Am Dent Assoc 132:234, 2001.

TABLE 3-6
Milliampere-Seconds Required to Expose Speed Group D and E Intraoral Radiographic Film to Diagnostic Density at a Focal Spot-to-Film Distance (FSFD) of 16 Inches

OPERATING KILOVOLTAGE*	MILLIAMPERE-SECONDS†					
	D			E		
	LOW	HIGH	MEAN	LOW	HIGH	MEAN
70	6.7	10.9	8.8	3.6	4.8	4.2
90	3.1	6.0	4.6	1.7	2.6	2.2

*Using a half wave–rectified x-ray machine with minimal HVL, as shown in Table 3-5.
†For an 8-inch FSFD, divide by 4.

Kilovoltage. The recommendation for selection of operating kilovoltage is stated in very general terms:

> A kilovoltage best suited to the diagnostic purpose should be used. The range of 70 to 100 kilovolt peak is suitable for most purposes.*

Kilovoltage is the exposure factor that controls the energy of the x-ray beam (see Chapter 1). As the kilovoltage is decreased, the effective energy of the x-ray beam is decreased and radiographic image contrast increases (see Table 3-4). In theory, an image of high contrast should be better suited for visualizing large differences in density within an object such as caries or soft tissue calcifications. However, the effect of kilovoltage on the accuracy of caries diagnosis has been reported to be negligible. As the kilovoltage is increased, the effective energy of the x-ray beam is increased and radiographic image contrast decreases. An image of low contrast allows for the visualization of smaller differences in density within an object. This type of image contrast may be more useful for periodontal diagnosis, where minute changes in bone must be detected. High-kilovoltage techniques, which produce images of low contrast, also reduce the effective dose delivered per intraoral examination. It was found that the *E* resulting from the production of comparable-density radiographs was reduced by as much as 23% in one study, with an increase in kilovoltage from 70 to 90.

The introduction of constant-potential (fully rectified), high-frequency or direct current (DC) dental x-ray units has made possible the production of diagnostic-quality radiographs with lower kilovoltage and at reduced levels of radiation. The surface exposure required to produce a comparable radiographic density using a constant-potential unit is approximately 25% less than that of a conventional self-rectified unit operating at the same kilovoltage. Currently several manufacturers produce DC units.

Milliampere-seconds. Of the three technical conditions (tube voltage, filtration, and exposure time), exposure time has been shown to be the most crucial factor in influencing diagnostic quality. In terms of exposure, optimal image quality means that the radiograph is of diagnostic density, neither overexposed (too dark) nor underexposed (too light). Both overexposed and underexposed radiographs result in repeat exposures, thereby leading to needless additional patient exposure. Image density is controlled by the quantity of x rays produced, which in turn is best controlled by the combination of milliamperage and exposure time, termed *milliampere-seconds (mAs)* (see Table 3-4 and Chapter 1). Diagnostic density is, for the most part, a matter of personal preference subject to certain guidelines. Patient exposure is directly related to mAs. Table 3-6 lists average mAs values needed to expose an intraoral film to proper density. Typically a radiograph of correct density will demonstrate very faint soft tissue outlines. Enamel and dentin will have an optical density of about 1.0. Optimal image density can be obtained by using values listed, after considering the age and physical stature of the patient. For example, 3.5 mAs is suggested for an average adult when F-speed film and an operating kilovoltage of 70 are used. This value may be arrived at by using a milliamperage of 10 and an exposure time of 0.35 second. If the kilovoltage is increased to reduce image contrast, the mAs must be decreased or the radiograph will be overexposed.

Phototiming is routinely employed in some medical radiographic procedures. This technique uses a phototimer to measure the quantity of radiation

*From ADA Council on Dental Materials, Instruments, and Equipment: Recommendations on radiographic practices: an update, 1988, J Am Dent Assoc 118:115, 1989.

reaching the film and automatically terminates the exposure when enough radiation has reached the film to provide the required density. A form of this technology is currently available with some panoramic machines.

PROCESSING THE FILM

Film processing should be performed under the manufacturer-recommended conditions with proper processing equipment and a darkroom with safelights. Alternatively, an automatic processor with an appropriate safelight hood may be used.*

A major cause of unnecessary patient exposure is the deliberate overexposure of films compensated by underdevelopment of the film. Not only does this procedure result in needless exposure of the patient but it also results in films that are of inferior diagnostic quality (because of incomplete development). On the other hand, a properly exposed radiograph is of no value if all its diagnostic information is lost as a result of poor processing procedures (see Table 3-4). One dental insurance carrier reported that some 6% of the dental radiographs it received were not readable because of improper processing. Another study of 500 panoramic radiographs found that the average film contained at least one processing error. Time-temperature processing, in an adequately equipped and maintained darkroom, is the best way to ensure optimal film quality (see Chapter 6). For optimizing image quality, care must be exercised in the selection of processing solutions. Processing solutions have been found to affect film speed, contrast, and latitude even when the solution manufacturer's directions have been strictly followed. To help ensure optimal image quality, the technician should follow the film manufacturer's recommendation for processing solutions, not the solution manufacturer's directions.

The use of machines to process dental x-ray film has become widespread. Over 90% of dentists surveyed have reported using dental film processors. Film processors, however, can actually increase patient exposure if not correctly maintained. Approximately 30% of all films retaken because of incorrect film density were directly related to processor variability. The introduction of a comprehensive maintenance program was found to reduce this retake rate significantly, resulting in a substantial savings in both patient exposure and operating costs.

---

*From ADA Council on Scientific Affairs: An Update on Radiographic Practices: Information and Recommendations, J Am Dent Assoc 132:234, 2001.

Interpretation of the Image

Radiographic images should be viewed under proper conditions with an illuminated viewer to obtain maximum available information.*

Radiographs are best viewed in a semidarkened room with light transmitted through the films; all extraneous light should be eliminated. In addition, radiographs should be studied with the aid of a magnifying glass to detect even the smallest change in image density. A variable-intensity light source should also be available. This may compensate for overexposed or underexposed radiographs or radiographs with processing artifacts. Many radiographs can be saved in this way, precluding the necessity of remaking the film and subjecting the patient to additional radiation exposure.

At the beginning of this section it was stated that optimizing the radiologic process is the best way to ensure maximal patient benefit with minimal patient and operator exposure. Although the importance of this cannot be overemphasized, in spite of everything that can be done to optimize the radiologic process, the diagnostic accuracy of radiographic caries diagnosis is only about 70%. This fact should stimulate individuals to place a greater emphasis on accurate radiographic interpretation. Currently, failure to diagnose problems is an increasing source of liability claims.

PROTECTION OF PERSONNEL

Unless protective shielding is provided for the operator, the installation (operatory) should be so arranged so that the operator can stand at least six feet from the patient and in a location that is not in the path of the x-ray beam during exposure.†

The methods of dose reduction discussed thus far have emphasized the effect on patient exposure. It should be apparent, however, that any procedure or technique that reduces radiation exposure to the patient also reduces the possibility of operator or office personnel exposure. In addition to those mentioned, several other steps can be taken to reduce the chance of occupational exposure.

Perhaps the single most effective way of limiting occupational exposure is the establishment of radiation

---

*From ADA Council on Scientific Affairs: An Update on Radiographic Practices: Information and Recommendations, J Am Dent Assoc 132:234, 2001.
†From ADA Council on Scientific Affairs: An Update on Radiographic Practices: Information and Recommendations, J Am Dent Assoc 132:234, 2001.

safety procedures that are understood and followed by all personnel. Such written procedures are currently mandated by several states. The procedures described below are based on a number of important facts concerning x rays:

- They travel in straight lines from their source.
- The intensity of the radiation beam diminishes fairly rapidly as the distance from the source increases (inverse square law).
- They can be scattered or deflected in their path of travel.

First, every effort should be made so that the operator can leave the room or take a position behind a suitable barrier or wall during exposure of the film. Dental operatories should be designed and constructed to meet the minimal shielding requirement of the NCRP. This recommendation states that walls must be of sufficient density or thickness that the exposure to nonoccupationally exposed individuals (e.g., someone occupying an adjacent office) is no greater than $100\,\mu Gy$ per week. In most instances, it is not necessary to line the walls with lead to meet this requirement. Walls constructed of gypsum wallboard (drywall or sheet rock) have been found to be adequate for the average dental office. The following factors are considered in calculating specific barrier thickness required: (1) workload, an expression of the amount of radiation emitted at a given kilovoltage in milliamperes per week; (2) use, the fraction of time an x-ray beam is directed toward the barrier; (3) occupancy, an estima-

tion of the amount of time the area behind the barrier is occupied; and (4) maximum permissible E. Examples of the way these parameters are used in calculating required barrier thickness can be found in NCRP Report 35.

If leaving the room or making use of some other barrier is impossible, strict adherence to what has been termed the *position-and-distance rule* is required: The operator should stand at least 6 feet from the patient, at an angle of 90 to 135 degrees to the central ray of the x-ray beam (Fig. 3-10). When applied, this rule not only takes advantage of the inverse square law to reduce x-ray intensity but also considers that in this position most scatter radiation is absorbed by the patient's head. All practitioners should check their state's regulations for use of ionizing radiation regarding operator position during x-ray exposures. At least one state (New Mexico) requires that the operator leave the room during the exposure. Thus the position-and-distance rule is in violation of that state's regulations.

Second, the operator should never hold films in place. Ideally, film-holding instruments should be used (see Collimation, p. 58). If correct film placement and retention are still not possible, a parent or other individual responsible for the patient should be asked to hold the film in place and, of course, be afforded adequate protection with a leaded apron. Under no circumstances should this person be one of the office staff.

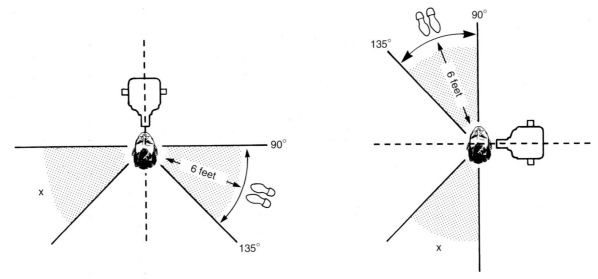

FIG. **3-10** Position-and-distance rule. If no barrier is available, the operator should stand at least 6 feet from the patient, at an angle of 90 to 135 degrees to the central ray of the x-ray beam when the exposure is made.

LANDAUER®

Landauer, Inc. 2 Science Road   Glenwood, Illinois 60425-1586
Telephone: (708) 755-7000   Facsimile: (708) 755-7016
www.landauerinc.com

SAMPLE ORGANIZATION
RADIATION SAFETY OFFICER
2 SCIENCE ROAD
GLENWOOD, IL 60425

RADIATION DOSIMETRY REPORT

luXel®

ACCOUNT NO.	SERIES CODE	ANALYTICAL WORK ORDER	REPORT DATE	DOSIMETER RECEIVED	REPORT TIME IN WORK DAYS	PAGE NO.
103702	RAD	992150087	06/13/03	06/09/03	4	1

PARTICIPANT NUMBER	NAME (ID NUMBER / BIRTH DATE / SEX)	DOSIMETER	USE	RADIATION QUALITY	DOSE EQUIVALENT (MREM) FOR PERIODS SHOWN BELOW			YEAR TO DATE DOSE EQUIVALENT (MREM)			LIFETIME DOSE EQUIVALENT (MREM)			RECORDS FOR YEAR	INCEPTION DATE (MM/YY)
					DEEP DDE	EYE LDE	SHALLOW SDE	DEEP DDE	EYE LDE	SHALLOW SDE	DEEP DDE	EYE LDE	SHALLOW SDE		
FOR MONITORING PERIOD:					05/01/03 - 05/31/03			2003							
0000H	CONTROL CONTROL CONTROL	J P U	CNTRL CNTRL CNTRL		M M	M M	M M M							5	07/97 07/97 07/97
00189	ADAMS, HEATHER 336235619 08/31/1968 F	P	WHBODY		M	M	M	9	10	12	29	31	42	5	07/01
00191	ADDISON, JOHN 471563287 10/04/1968 M	J	WHBODY	PN P NF	90 60 30	90 60 30	90 60 30	100 70 30	100 70 30	100 70 30	200 170 30	200 170 30	200 170 30	5	07/01
00202	HARRIS, KATHY 587582144 06/09/1960 F	P U	WHBODY RFINGR		M	M	M M	M	M	M 30	M	M	M 30	5	02/02 02/02
00005	MEYER, STEVE 982778955 07/15/1964 M	P P U	COLLAR WAIST ASSIGN NOTE RFINGR	PL P	119 10 19	119 11 119	113 11 113	33	185	174	1387	2308	2320	5	08/97 08/97 08/97
			ASSIGNED DOSE BASED ON EDE 1 CALCULATION				140						690		2180	
00203	STEVENS, LEE 335478977 08/25/1951 M	P U	WHBODY RFINGR		ABSENT ABSENT			M	M	M M	M	M	M M	4	07/02 07/02
00204	WALKER, JANE 416995421 03/21/1947 F	P	WHBODY		3	3	3	12	11	11	22	21	21	5	11/02
00188	WEBSTER, ROBERT 355381469 05/15/1972 M	P	WHBODY NOTE		40 CALCULATED	40	40	200	200	200	240	240	240	5	07/01

M: MINIMAL REPORTING SERVICE OF 1 MREM
ELECTRONIC MEDIA TO FOLLOW THIS REPORT

QUALITY CONTROL RELEASE: LMR   1 - PR   6774 - PT131 - N1   -21587

NVLAP®
NVLAP LAB CODE 100518-0**

FIG. 3-11 Sample radiation dosimetry report showing that George Smith received an exposure of 0.60 mSv (60 mrem) during the month reported. The report also shows totals for the calendar quarter, year to date, and permanent or lifetime exposure. (Courtesy Landauer, Inc., Glenwood, IL.)

Third, neither the operator nor patient should hold the radiographic tube housing during the exposure. Suspension arms should be adequately maintained to prevent housing movement and drift.

The best way to ensure that personnel are following office safety rules such as those described previously is with personnel-monitoring devices. Commonly referred to as *film badges*, these devices provide a useful record of occupational exposure. Their use is not only recommended but also required by law in certain states. Several companies in the U.S. offer film badge services. For a reasonable charge, these services provide badges that contain either a piece of sensitive film or a radiosensitive crystal (thermoluminescent dosimeter) and a printed report of accumulated exposure at regular intervals (Fig. 3-11). These reports indicate any undesirable change in work habits and help remove any apprehension office staff members may have about the possibility of exposure to x rays.

QUALITY ASSURANCE

A quality assurance program should be established to ensure high-quality radiographic images.*

Quality assurance may be defined as any planned activity to ensure that a dental office will consistently produce high-quality images with minimum exposure to patients and personnel (see Chapter 7). Studies have indicated that dentists may be needlessly exposing their patients to compensate for improper exposure techniques, film processing practices, and darkroom procedures. One study reported that only 33% of panoramic radiographs that accompanied biopsy specimens were of acceptable diagnostic quality. However, when

*From ADA Council on Scientific Affairs: An Update on Radiographic Practices: Information and Recommendations, J Am Dent Assoc 132:234, 2001.

Following should be inspected at suitable intervals:
X-ray unit
- Leakage radiation
- Verification of FSFD
- Stability of radiographic tube housing
- X-ray beam
  - Alignment
  - Collimation
  - Quality
- Timer accuracy
- Integrity of exposure switch
Darkroom
- Light leaks
- Adequacy of safe lighting
- Cleanliness
Ancillary equipment
- Leaded aprons and collars
- The brightness and color of view boxes
Procedures should be established for the following:
- Use of a reference film
- Proper handling and storage of film, cassettes, screens, grids, and chemicals
- X-ray exposure factors (posted by control console)
- Film processing techniques (posted in darkroom)
- Maintenance of processing systems

From National Council on Radiation Protection and Measurements: NCRP Report 99, Washington, D.C., 1988, NCRP Publications.

demands were placed on dentists to improve their techniques, the number of unsatisfactory radiographs was significantly reduced. Two studies by a dental insurance carrier demonstrated that after claims were rejected for unsatisfactory radiographs and the dentist was made aware of the errors and ways in which they could be corrected, the number of satisfactory radiographs submitted doubled. This suggests that when the dentist is presented with guidelines for quality assurance, along with proper motivation, patient exposure can be dramatically reduced.

Currently some states require dental offices to establish written guidelines for quality assurance and maintain written records of quality assurance tests. Regardless of requirements, each dental office should establish maintenance and monitoring procedures as outlined in Box 3-1 according to the NCRP. The frequency of these inspections varies according to state regulations and manufacturers' directions.

CONTINUING EDUCATION

Practitioners should stay informed of new information on radiation safety issues, as well as developments in equipment, materials and techniques and adopt appropriate items to improve radiographic practices.*

Those who administer ionizing radiation must become familiar with the magnitude of exposure encountered in medicine, dentistry, and everyday life; the possible risks associated with such exposure; and the methods used to affect exposure and dose reduction. Although this chapter presents some of this information, acquiring knowledge and developing and maintaining skills is an ongoing process.

BIBLIOGRAPHY

ADA Council on Dental Materials, Instruments, and Equipment: Recommendations on radiographic practices: an update, 1988, J Am Dent Assoc 118:115, 1989.

ADA Council on Scientific Affairs: An Update on Radiographic Practices: Information and Recommendations, J Am Dent Assoc 132:234, 2001.

Bushberg JT, Seibert JA, Leidholdt EM, Boone JM: The Essential Physics of Medical Imaging, ed 2, Baltimore, 2001, Lippincott Williams and Wilkins.

Bushong SC: Radiologic Science for Technologists: Physics, Biology, and Protection, ed 7, St. Louis, 2001, Mosby.

Code of Federal Regulations 21, Subchapter J: Radiological health, part 1000, Office of the Federal Register, General Services Administration, Washington, D.C., 1994.

Committee on the Biological Effects of Ionizing Radiations: Health effects of exposure to low levels of ionizing radiation. BEIR V, National Academy Press, Washington, D.C., 1990.

Curry TS, Dowdey JE, Murry RC: Christensen's Physics of Diagnostic Radiology, ed 4, Philadelphia, 1990, Lea and Febiger.

International Commission on Radiological Protection: Radiation protection, ICRP Publ. 60, Oxford, England, 1990.

Hall EJ: Radiobiology for the Radiologist, ed 5, Baltimore, 2000, Lippincott Williams and Wilkins.

National Council on Radiation Protection and Measurements: Control of radon in houses, NCRP Report 103, Bethesda, Md, 1989.

National Council on Radiation Protection and Measurements: Dental x-ray protection, NCRP Report 35, Bethesda, Md, 1970.

National Council on Radiation Protection and Measurements: Exposure of the population in the U.S. and Canada from natural background radiation, NCRP Report 94, Bethesda, Md, 1987.

*From ADA Council on Scientific Affairs: An Update on Radiographic Practices: Information and Recommendations, J Am Dent Assoc 132:234, 2001.

National Council on Radiation Protection and Measurements: Exposure of the U.S. population from diagnostic medical radiation, NCRP Report 100, Bethesda, Md, 1989.

National Council on Radiation Protection and Measurements: Exposure of the U.S. population from occupational radiation, NCRP Report 101, Bethesda, Md, 1989.

National Council on Radiation Protection and Measurements: Ionizing radiation exposure of the population of the U.S., NCRP Report 93, Bethesda, Md, 1987.

National Council on Radiation Protection and Measurements: Limitation of exposure to ionizing radiation, NCRP Report 116, Bethesda, Md, 1993.

National Council on Radiation Protection and Measurements: Quality assurance for diagnostic imaging, NCRP Report 99, Bethesda, Md, 1990.

National Council on Radiation Protection and Measurements: Radiation exposure of the U.S. population from consumer products and miscellaneous sources, NCRP Report 95, Bethesda, Md, 1987.

Nationwide Evaluation of X-Ray Trends (NEXT): 1993 Dental x-ray data, Washington, D.C., 1993, HHS Publication (FDA).

U.S. Department of Health and Human Services, FDA: Guidelines for prescribing dental radiographs, Rockville, Md., 1987, HHS Publication FDA 88-8273.

PART ■ FOUR
Imaging Principles and Techniques

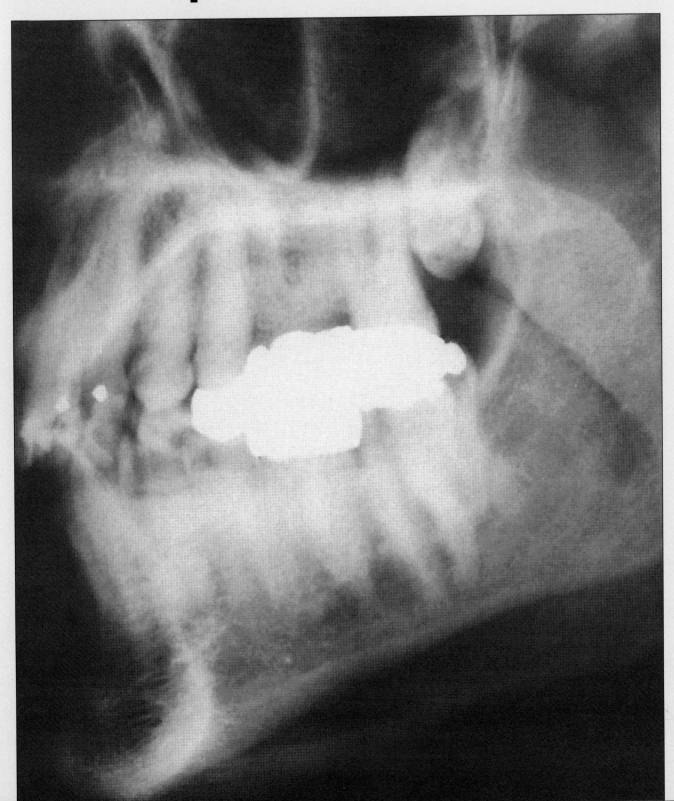

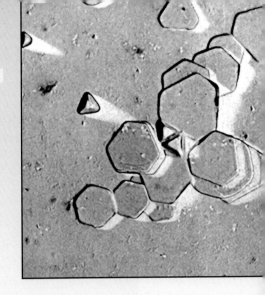

CHAPTER 4

X-Ray Film, Intensifying Screens, and Grids

A beam of x-ray photons that passes through the dental arches is reduced in intensity (attenuated) by absorption and scattering of photons out of the primary beam. The pattern of the photons that exits the subject, the remnant beam, conveys information about the structure and composition of the absorber. For this information to be useful diagnostically, the remnant beam must be recorded on an image receptor. The image receptor most often used in dental radiography is x-ray film. This chapter describes x-ray film and its properties, as well as the use of intensifying screens and grids to modify radiographic images. Digital radiographic systems, which also may be used to make radiographs, are described in Chapter 12.

X-Ray Film

COMPOSITION

X-ray film has two principal components: emulsion and base. The emulsion, which is sensitive to x rays and visible light, records the radiographic image. The base is a plastic supporting material onto which the emulsion is coated (Fig. 4-1).

Emulsion

The two principal components of emulsion are silver halide grains, which are sensitive to x radiation and visible light, and a vehicle matrix in which the crystals are suspended. The *silver halide grains* are composed primarily of crystals of silver bromide. The composition of a dental film emulsion is shown in Table 4-1. Iodide is added to Ultra-Speed film because its large diameter (compared with bromine) disrupts the regularity of the silver bromide crystal structure, thereby increasing its sensitivity to x radiation. Iodide is not used in InSight film. The photosensitivity of the silver halide crystals also depends on the presence of trace amounts of a sulfur-containing compound. In addition, trace amounts of gold are sometimes added to silver halide crystals to improve their sensitivity.

The silver halide grains in InSight film are flat, tabular crystals with a mean diameter of about 1.8 μm (Fig. 4-2). Ultra-Speed film is composed of globular-shaped crystals about 1 μm in diameter. The tabular grains of the InSight film are oriented parallel with the film surface to offer a large cross-sectional area to the x-ray beam (Fig. 4-3). As a result, InSight film requires only about half the exposure of Ultra-Speed film.

In the manufacture of film, the silver halide grains are suspended in a surrounding *vehicle* that is applied to both sides of the supporting base. The vehicle, composed of gelatinous and nongelatinous materials, keeps the silver halide grains evenly dispersed. To ensure good adhesion of the emulsion to the film base, a thin layer of adhesive material is added to the base before the emulsion is applied. During film processing, the vehicle absorbs the processing solutions, allowing the chemicals to reach and react with the silver halide grains. An additional layer of vehicle is added to the film emulsion as an overcoat; this barrier helps protect the film from damage by scratching, contamination, or pressure from rollers when an automatic processor is used.

Film emulsions are sensitive to both x-ray photons and visible light. Film intended to be exposed by x rays is called *direct exposure film*. All intraoral dental film is direct exposure film. *Screen film*, which is sensitive to visible light, is used with intensifying screens that emit

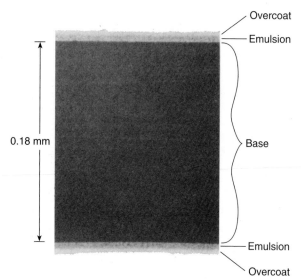

FIG. **4-1** Scanning electron micrograph of Kodak InSight dental x-ray film (300×). Note the overcoat, emulsion, and base on this double-emulsion film. (Courtesy Eastman Kodak, Rochester, N.Y.)

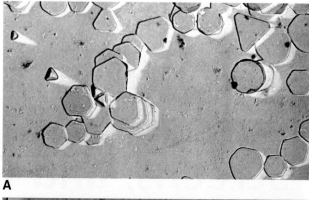

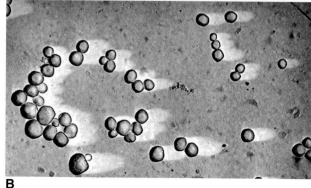

FIG. **4-2** Scanning electron micrographs of emulsion comparing flat tabular silver bromide crystals of InSight film (**A**) with globular silver halide crystals of Ultra-Speed film (**B**). (Courtesy Eastman Kodak, Rochester, N.Y.)

visible light. Screen film and intensifying screens are used for extraoral projections such as panoramic and skull radiographs. Intensifying screens are described later in this chapter.

Base

The function of the film base is to support the emulsion. The base must have the proper degree of flexibility to allow easy handling of the film. The base for dental x-ray film is 0.18 mm thick and is made of polyester polyethylene terephthalate. The film base is uniformly translucent and casts no pattern on the resultant radiograph. Some believe that a base with a slight blue tint improves viewing of diagnostic detail. The film base must also withstand exposure to processing solutions without becoming distorted.

INTRAORAL X-RAY FILM

A number of manufacturers around the world make intraoral dental x-ray film. In each case the film is made as a double-emulsion film, that is, coated with an emulsion on each side of the base. With a double layer of emulsion, less radiation can be used to produce an image. Direct exposure film is used for intraoral examinations because it provides higher-resolution images than screen-film combinations. Some diagnostic tasks, such as detection of incipient caries or early periapical disease, require this higher resolution.

One corner of each dental film has a small, raised dot that is used for film orientation. When the film is placed in the patient's mouth, the side of the film with the raised dot is always positioned facing the x-ray tube. The side of the film with the depression is thus oriented

TABLE **4-1** *Coating Weight Per Film Side (mg/cm²)*					
FILM TYPE	SILVER	BROMIDE	IODIDE	EMULSION VEHICLE	OVERCOAT VEHICLE
InSight	0.81-1.03	0.63-0.71	0	0.70-0.80	0.07-0.11
Ultra-Speed	0.92	0.67	0.02	0.59	0.16

Courtesy Eastman Kodak, Rochester, N.Y.

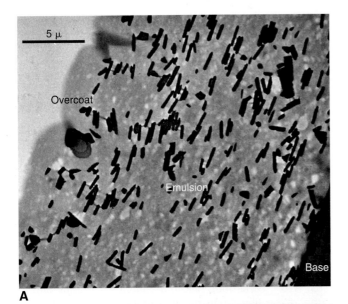

A

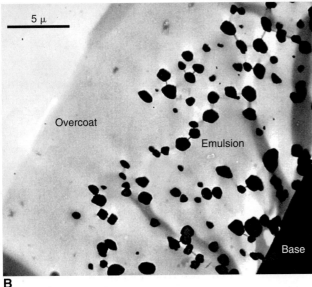

B

FIG. **4-3** Cross-sectional electron microscopic image of emulsion of InSight film **(A)** and Ultra-Speed film **(B).** Note that the orientation of the tabular crystals in the InSight film is essentially parallel to the film surface to increase the exposure surface area of the crystals to the x-ray beam. (Courtesy Eastman Kodak, Rochester N.Y.)

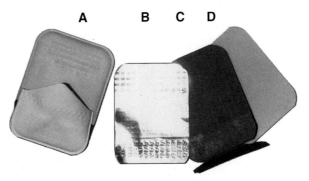

FIG. **4-4** Moisture- and light-proof packet **(A)** contains an opening tab on the side opposite the tube. Inside is a sheet of lead foil **(B)** and a black, lightproof, interleaf paper wrapper **(C)** that is folded around the film **(D).** Film is packaged with one or two sheets of film.

toward the patient's tongue. After the film has been processed, the dot is used to identify the image as being the patient's right or left side (see Fig. 6-22).

Intraoral x-ray film packets contain either one or two sheets of film (Fig. 4-4). When double-film packs are used, the second film serves as a duplicate record that can be sent to insurance companies or to a colleague. The film is encased in a protective black paper wrapper and then in an outer white paper or plastic wrapping, which is resistant to moisture. The outer wrapping clearly indicates the location of the raised dot and

identifies which side of the film should be directed toward the x-ray tube.

Between the wrappers in the film packet is a thin lead foil backing with an embossed pattern. The foil is positioned in the film packet behind the film, away from the tube. This lead foil serves several purposes. It shields the film from backscatter (secondary) radiation, which fogs the film and reduces subject contrast (image quality). It also reduces patient exposure by absorbing some of the residual x-ray beam. Perhaps most important, however, is the fact that if the film packet is placed backwards in the patient's mouth so that the tube side of the film is facing away from the x-ray machine, the lead foil will be positioned between the subject and the film. In this circumstance most of the radiation is absorbed by the lead foil and the resulting radiograph is light and shows the embossed pattern in the lead foil. This combination of a light film with the characteristic pattern indicates that the film packet was put in the patient's mouth backwards and that the patient's right side–left side designation indicated by the film dot was reversed.

Because intraoral direct exposure film packets have several uses and are used in large adults as well as small children, the film packets are made in a variety of sizes. The composition of the film is identical in each case.

Periapical View

Periapical views are used to record the crowns, roots, and surrounding bone. Film packs come in three sizes: 0 for small children ($22 \times 35\,mm$); 1, which is relatively narrow and used for views of the anterior teeth ($24 \times 40\,mm$); and 2, the standard film size used for adults ($31 \times 41\,mm$) (Fig. 4-5).

Bitewing View

Bitewing (interproximal) views are used to record the coronal portions of the maxillary and mandibular teeth in one image. They are useful for detecting

FIG. **4-5** Dental x-ray film is commonly supplied in various sizes. *Left,* Occlusal film; *top right,* adult posterior film; *middle right,* adult anterior film; *bottom right,* child-size film (in vinyl wrapping).

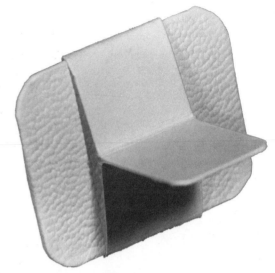

FIG. **4-6** Paper loop placed around a size 2 adult film to support the film when the patient bites on the tab for a bitewing projection. This projection reveals the tooth crowns and alveolar crests.

interproximal caries and evaluating the height of alveolar bone. Size 2 film normally is used in adults; the smaller size 1 is preferred in children. In small children, size 0 may be used. A relatively long size 3 also is available.

Bitewing films often have a paper tab projecting from the middle of the film, on which the patient bites to support the film (Fig. 4-6). This tab is rarely visualized and does not interfere with the diagnostic quality of the image. Film-holding instruments for bitewing projections also are available.

Occlusal View

Occlusal film is more than three times larger than size 2 film (57 × 76 mm) (see Fig. 4-5). It is used to show larger areas of the maxilla or mandible than may be seen on a periapical film. These films also are used to obtain right-angle views to the usual periapical view. The name derives from the fact that the film usually is held in position by having the patient bite lightly on it to support it between the occlusal surfaces of the teeth (see Chapter 8).

SCREEN FILM

The extraoral projections used most frequently in dentistry are the panoramic, cephalometric, and other skull views. For these projections and for virtually all other extraoral radiography, screen film is used with intensifying screens (described later in this chapter) to reduce patient exposure. Screen film is different from dental intraoral film. It is designed to be sensitive to visible light because it is placed between two intensifying screens when an exposure is made. The intensifying screens absorb x rays and emit visible light, which exposes the screen film. Silver halide crystals are inherently sensitive to ultraviolet (UV) and blue light (300 to 500 nm) and thus are sensitive to screens that emit UV and blue light. When film is used with screens that emit green light, the silver halide crystals are coated with sensitizing dyes to increase absorption. Because the properties of intensifying screens vary, the dentist should use the appropriate screen-film combination recommended by the screen and film manufacturer so that the emission characteristics of the screen match the absorption characteristics of the film.

Several general types of screen film are suitable for extraoral radiography. Several manufacturers supply high-contrast, medium-speed film suitable for skull radiography. Other films are available that are faster (i.e., they require less radiation exposure), but these provide less image detail. Such films should be considered for panoramic radiography when fine image detail is not available because of movement of the x-ray tube head during the exposure.

Another type of film provides less contrast and a wider latitude. This type reveals a wide range of densities and is most suitable for cephalometric radiography, when both bony and soft tissue details are desired.

The design of screen films changes constantly to optimize imaging characteristics. Kodak, for example, has introduced T-Mat films, which have tabular-shaped (flat) grains of silver halide (Fig. 4-7). The tabular (T) grains are oriented with their relatively large, flat sur-

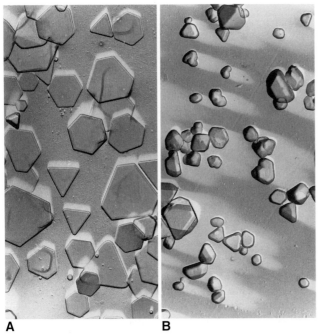

A   **B**

FIG. **4-7**   T grains of silver halide in an emulsion of T-Mat film **(A)** are larger and flatter than the smaller, thicker crystals in an emulsion of conventional film **(B)**. Note that the flat surfaces of the T grains are oriented parallel with the film surface, facing the radiation source. (Courtesy Eastman Kodak, Rochester, N.Y.)

FUNCTION

The presence of intensifying screens creates an image receptor system that is 10 to 60 times more sensitive to x rays than the film alone. Consequently, use of intensifying screens means a substantial reduction in the dose of x radiation to which the patient is exposed. Intensifying screens are used with films for virtually all extraoral radiography, including panoramic, cephalometric, and skull projections. In general, the resolving power of screens is related to their speed: the slower the speed of a screen, the greater its resolving power and vice versa. Intensifying screens are not used intraorally with periapical or occlusal films because their use would reduce the resolution of the resulting image below that necessary for diagnosis of much dental disease.

COMPOSITION

Intensifying screens are made of a base supporting material, a phosphor layer, and a protective polymeric coat (Fig. 4-8). In all dental applications, intensifying screens are used in pairs, one on each side of the film, and they are positioned inside a cassette (Fig. 4-9). The purpose of a cassette is to hold each intensifying screen in contact with the x-ray film to maximize the sharpness of the image. Most cassettes are rigid, but they may be flexible.

faces facing the radiation source, providing a larger cross-section (target) and resulting in increased speed without loss of sharpness. In addition, green-sensitizing dyes are added to the surface of the tabular grains, increasing their light-gathering capability and reducing the crossover of light from the phosphor layer on one side of the intensifying screen to the film emulsion on the other. Kodak's new Ektavision system includes an absorbing dye in the emulsion to prevent crossover of light from one screen to the other emulsion. This increases the sharpness of the image.

Intensifying Screens

Early in the history of radiography, scientists discovered that various inorganic salts or phosphors fluoresce (emit visible light) when exposed to an x-ray beam. The intensity of this fluorescence is proportional to the x-ray energy absorbed. These phosphors have been incorporated into intensifying screens for use with screen film. The sum of the effects of the x rays and the visible light emitted by the screen phosphors exposes the film in an intensifying cassette.

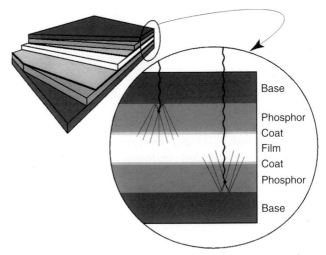

Base
Phosphor
Coat
Film
Coat
Phosphor
Base

FIG. **4-8**   The image on the left shows a schematic of two intensifying screens (shades of gray) enclosing a film (white). The detailed view on the right shows x-ray photons entering at the top, traveling through the base, and striking phosphors in the base. The phosphors emit visible light, exposing the film. Some visible light photons may reflect off the reflecting layer of the base.

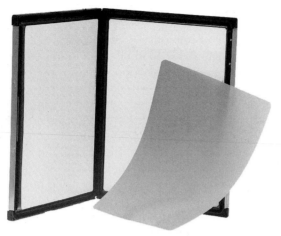

FIG. **4-9**   *Cassette for 8- × 10-inch film.* When the cassette is closed, the film is supported in close contact between two intensifying screens.

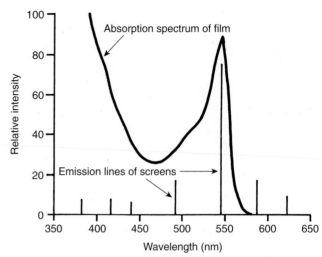

FIG. **4-10**   Relative sensitivity of Kodak T-Mat film (continuous line) and emission lines of a Kodak Lanex and Ektavision screens (gadolinium oxysulfide, terbium activated). Intensifying screens emit light as a series of relatively narrow line emissions. The maximal emission of the screen at 545 nm corresponds well to a high-sensitivity region of the film. (Data courtesy Eastman Kodak, Rochester, N.Y.)

Base

The base material of most intensifying screens is some form of polyester plastic that is about 0.25 mm thick. The base provides mechanical support for the other layers. In some intensifying screens the base also is reflective; thus it reflects light emitted from the phosphor layer back toward the x-ray film. This has the effect of increasing the light emission of the intensifying screen. However, it also results in some image "unsharpness" because of the divergence of light rays reflected back to the film. Some fine detail intensifying screens omit *the reflecting layer* to improve image sharpness. In other intensifying screens the base is not reflective, and a separate coating of titanium dioxide is applied to the base material to serve as a reflecting layer.

Phosphor Layer

The phosphor layer is composed of phosphorescent crystals suspended in a polymeric binder. When the crystals absorb x-ray photons, they fluoresce (see Fig. 4-8). The phosphor crystals often contain rare earth elements, most commonly lanthanum and gadolinium. Their fluorescence can be increased by the addition of small amounts of elements such as thulium, niobium, or terbium. Common phosphor combinations used in intensifying screens are shown in Table 4-2.

Some rare earth compounds are efficient phosphors. In the energy range typically used in dental radiography, a pair of rare earth intensifying screens absorbs about 60% of the photons that reach the cassette after passing through a patient. These phosphors are about 18% efficient in converting this x-ray energy to visible light. Rare earth screens convert each absorbed x-ray photon into about 4,000 lower-energy, visible light (green or blue) photons. These visible photons then expose the film.

Different phosphors fluoresce in different portions of the spectrum. For example, light emission from Kodak Lanex (Fig. 4-10) rare earth intensifying screens ranges from 375 to 600 nm and peaks sharply at 545 nm (green). Figure 4-10 shows the spectral emission of a rare earth screen and the spectral sensitivity of an appropriate film. Other intensifying screens have a major peak at 350 nm (UV) and another at 450 nm (blue). It is important to match green-emitting screens with green-sensitive films and blue-emitting screens with blue-sensitive films.

The speed and resolution of a screen depends on many factors including:
- Phosphor type and phosphor conversion efficiency
- Thickness of phosphor layer and coating weight (amount of phosphor/unit volume)

TABLE **4-2** *Rare Earth Elements Used in Intensifying Screens*	
EMISSION	PHOSPHOR
Green	Gadolinium oxysulfide, terbium activated
Blue and UV	Yttrium tantalate, niobium activated

TABLE **4-3** *Speeds of Selected Rare-Earth Screens*						
SPEED CLASS	AGFA	FUJI	KODAK	KONICA	STERLING/DUPONT	3M
Green Emitting Screens						
100	Curix Ortho Fine	HR Fine	Lanex Fine	KF	—	Trimax 2
200	Curix Ortho Medium	HR Medium	Lanex Medium	KM	—	Trimax 4
400	Curix Ortho Regular	HR Regular	Lanex Regular	KR Ektavision	Quanta V	Trimax 8
600	Curix Ortho Fast	HR Fast	Lanex Fast	KS	—	Trimax 12
Blue Emitting Screens						
100	—	—	—	—	Quanta Detail	—
400	MR 400	—	—	RD	Quanta Fast Detail	—
800	MR 800	—	—	RB	Quanta Rapid	Trilight 8

- Presence of reflective layer
- Presence of light-absorbing dye in phosphor binder or protective coating
- Phosphor grain size

Fast screens have large phosphor crystals and efficiently convert x-ray photons to visible light but produce images with lower resolution. As the size of the crystals or the thickness of the screen decreases, the speed of the screen also declines but image sharpness increases. Fast screens also have a thicker phosphor layer and a reflective layer, but these properties also decrease sharpness. In deciding on the combination to use, the practitioner must consider the resolution requirements of the task for which the image will be used. Table 4-3 shows several contemporary screens and their speed class. Most dental extraoral diagnostic tasks can be accomplished with screen-film combinations that have a speed of 400 or faster.

Protective Coat

A protective polymer coat (up to 15 μm thick) is placed over the phosphor layer to protect the phosphor and provide a surface that can be cleaned. The intensifying screens should be kept clean because any debris, spots, or scratches may cause light spots on the resultant radiograph.

Image Characteristics

Processing an exposed x-ray film causes it to become dark in the exposed area. The degree and pattern of film darkening depend on numerous factors, including the energy and intensity of the x-ray beam, composition of the subject imaged, film emulsion used, and characteristics of film processing. This section describes the major imaging characteristics of x-ray film.

RADIOGRAPHIC DENSITY

When a film is exposed by an x-ray beam (or by light, in the case of screen-film combinations) and then processed, the silver halide crystals in the emulsion that were struck by the photons are converted to grains of metallic silver. These silver grains block the transmission of light from a viewbox and give the film its dark appearance. The overall degree of darkening of an exposed film is referred to as *radiographic density*. This density can be measured as the optical density of an area of an x-ray film where:

$$\text{Optical density} = \text{Log}_{10}\frac{I_o}{I_t}$$

where I_o is the intensity of incident light (e.g., from a viewbox) and I_t is the intensity of the light transmitted through the film. Thus the measurement of film density also is a measure of the opacity of the film. With an optical density of 0, 100% of the light is transmitted; with a density of 1, 10% of the light is transmitted; with a density of 2, 1% of the light is transmitted, and so on.

A plot of the relationship between film optical density and exposure is called a *characteristic curve* (Fig.

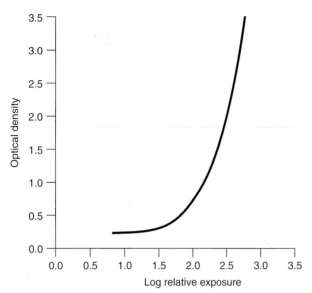

FIG. **4-11** *Characteristic curve of direct exposure film.* The contrast (slope of the curve) is greater in the high-density region than in the low-density region.

4-11). It usually is shown as the relation between the optical density of the film and the logarithm of the corresponding exposure. As exposure of the film increases, its optical density increases. A film is of greatest diagnostic value when the structures of interest are imaged on the relatively straight portion of the graph, between 0.6 and 3.0 optical density units. The characteristic curves of films reveal much information about film contrast, speed, and latitude.

An unexposed film, when processed, shows some density. This is caused by the inherent density of the base and added tint, as well as the development of unexposed silver halide crystals. This minimal density is called *gross fog,* or *base plus fog.* The optical density of gross fog typically is 0.2 to 0.3.

Radiographic density is influenced by exposure and the thickness and density of the subject.

Exposure

The overall film density depends on the number of photons absorbed by the film emulsion. Increasing the milliamperage (mA), peak kilovoltage (kVp), or exposure time increases the number of photons reaching the film and thus increases the density of the radiograph. Reducing the distance between the focal spot and film also increases film density.

Subject Thickness

The thicker the subject, the more the beam is attenuated and the lighter the resultant image (Fig. 4-12). If exposure factors intended for adults are used on

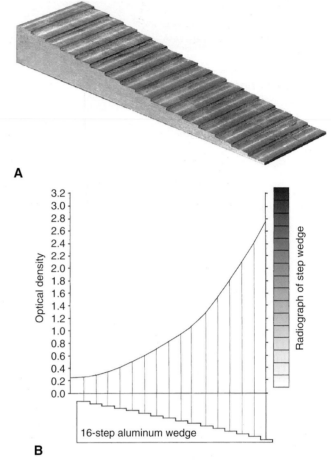

FIG. **4-12**   **A,** Aluminum step wedge. **B,** Graph of the optical density of a radiograph made by exposing the step wedge. Note that as the thickness of the aluminum decreases, more photons are available to expose the film and the image becomes progressively darker.

children or edentulous patients, the resultant films are dark because a smaller amount of absorbing tissue is in the path of the x-ray beam. The dentist should vary exposure (either kVp or time) according to the patient's size to produce radiographs of optimal density.

Subject Density

Variations in the density of the subject exert a profound influence on the image. The greater the density of a structure within the subject, the greater the attenuation of the x-ray beam directed through that subject or area. In the oral cavity the relative densities of various natural structures, in order of decreasing density, are enamel, dentin and cementum, bone, muscle, fat, and air. Metallic objects (e.g., restorations) are far denser than enamel and hence better absorbers. Because an x-ray beam is differentially attenuated by these absorbers, the resultant beam carries information that is recorded on the radiographic film as light and dark areas. Dense objects (which are strong absorbers) cause the radiographic image to be light and are said to be *radiopaque*. Objects with low densities are weak absorbers. They allow most photons to pass through, and they cast a dark area on the film that corresponds to the *radiolucent* object.

RADIOGRAPHIC CONTRAST

Radiographic contrast is a general term that describes the range of densities on a radiograph. It is defined as the difference in densities between light and dark regions on a radiograph. Thus an image that shows both light areas and dark areas has *high contrast*. This also is referred to as a *short gray scale of contrast* because few shades of gray are present between the black and white images on the film. A radiographic image composed only of light gray and dark gray zones has *low contrast,* also referred to as having a *long gray scale of contrast* (Fig. 4-13). The radiographic contrast of an image is the result of the interplay of subject contrast, film contrast, and scattered radiation.

Subject Contrast

Subject contrast is the range of characteristics of the subject that influences radiographic contrast. It is influenced largely by the subject's thickness, density, and atomic number. The subject contrast of a patient's head and neck exposed in a lateral cephalometric view is high. The dense regions of the bone and teeth absorb most of the incident radiation, whereas the less dense soft tissue facial profile transmits most of the radiation.

Subject contrast also is influenced by beam energy and intensity. The energy of the x-ray beam, selected by the kVp, influences image contrast. Fig. 4-14 shows an aluminum step wedge exposed to x-ray beams of differing energies. Because increasing the kVp increases the overall density of the image, the exposure time has been adjusted so that the density of the middle step in each case is comparable. As the kVp of the x-ray beam increases, subject contrast decreases. Similarly, when relatively low kVp energies are used, subject contrast increases. Most clinicians select a kVp in the range of 70 to 80. At higher values the exposure time is reduced, but the loss of contrast may be objectionable because subtle changes may be obscured.

Changing the time or mA of the exposure (and holding the kVp constant) also influences subject contrast. If the film is excessively light or dark, contrast of anatomic structures is diminished. Subtle changes in the mA may also slightly change subject contrast by changing the location of the radiographed structures on the characteristic curve, as described previously.

Film Contrast

Film contrast describes the capacity of radiographic films to display differences in subject contrast, that is, variations in the intensity of the remnant beam. A high-contrast film reveals areas of small difference in subject contrast more clearly than does a low-contrast film. Film contrast usually is measured as the average slope of the diagnostically useful portion of the characteristic curve (Fig. 4-15): the greater the slope of the curve in this region, the greater the film contrast. In this illustration, film A has a higher contrast than film B. When the slope of the curve in the useful range is greater than 1, the film exaggerates subject contrast. This desirable feature, which is found in most diagnostic film, allows

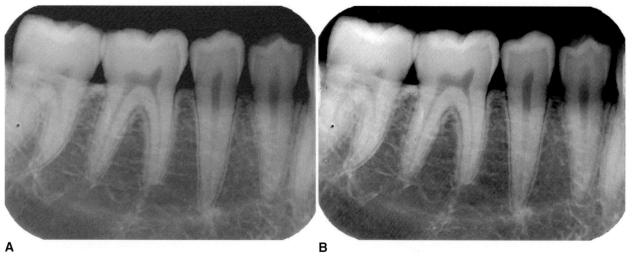

A   **B**

FIG. **4-13** Radiograph of a dried mandible revealing low contrast **(A)** and high contrast **(B)**.

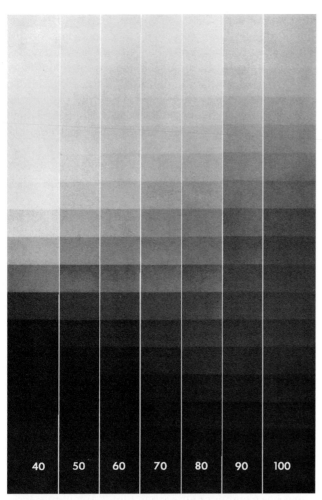

FIG. **4-14**   Radiographs of a step wedge made at 40 to 100 kVp. As the kVp increases, the mA is reduced to maintain the uniform middle-step density. Note the long gray scale (low contrast) with high kVp. (Courtesy Eastman Kodak, Rochester, N.Y.)

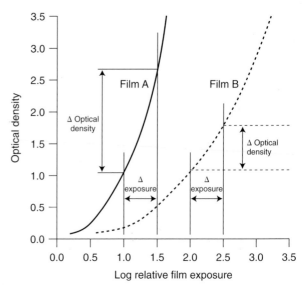

FIG. **4-15**   Characteristic curves of two films demonstrating the greater inherent contrast of film *A* compared with film *B*. The slope of film *A* is greater than that of film *B;* thus film *A* shows a greater change in optical density than film *B* for a constant change in exposure. The fact that film *A* is faster than film *B* in this figure is unrelated to film contrast.

visualization of structures that differ only slightly in density. For example, the remnant beam in the region of a tooth pulp chamber will be more intense (greater exposure) than the beam from the surrounding enamel crown. A high-contrast film will show a greater contrast (difference in optical density) between these structures than a low-contrast film. Films used with intensifying screens typically have a slope in the range of 2 to 3.

As can be seen in Fig. 4-11, film contrast also depends on the density range being examined. With dental direct-exposure film, the slope of the curve continually increases with increasing exposure. As a result, properly exposed films have more contrast than underexposed (light) films.

Film processing is another factor that influences film contrast. Film contrast is maximized by optimal film processing conditions. Mishandling of the film through incomplete or excessive development diminishes contrast of anatomic structures. Improper handling of film, such as storage at too high a temperature, exposure to excessively bright safelights, or light leaks in the darkroom, also degrades film contrast.

Fog on an x-ray film results in increased film density arising from causes other than exposure to the remnant beam. Film contrast is reduced by the addition of this undesirable density. Common causes of film fog are improper safelighting, storage of film at too high a temperature, and development of film at an excessive temperature or for a prolonged period. Film fog can be reduced by proper film processing and storage.

Scattered Radiation

Scattered radiation results from photons that have interacted with the subject by Compton or coherent interactions. These interactions cause the emission of photons that travel in directions other than that of the primary beam. The consequent scattered radiation causes fogging of a radiograph, an overall darkening of the image that results in loss of radiographic contrast. In most dental applications the best means of reducing scattered radiation are to (1) use a relatively low kVp, (2) collimate the beam to the size of the film to prevent scatter from an area outside the region of the image, and (3) use grids in extraoral radiography.

TABLE 4-4
Intraoral Film Speed Classification

FILM SPEED GROUP	SPEED RANGE (RECIPROCAL ROENTGENS*)
C	6-12
D	12-24
E	24-48
F	48-96

From Council on Dental Materials and Devices: Dentist's desk reference: materials, instruments, and equipment, ed 2, Chicago, 1983, American Dental Association.
*Reciprocal Roentgens are the reciprocal of the exposure in Roentgens required to obtain a film with an optical density of 1.0 above base plus fog after processing.

RADIOGRAPHIC SPEED

Radiographic speed refers to the amount of radiation required to produce an image of a standard density. Film speed frequently is expressed as the reciprocal of the exposure (in roentgens) required to produce an optical density of 1 above gross fog. A fast film requires a relatively low exposure to produce a density of 1, whereas a slower film requires a longer exposure for the processed film to have the same density. Film speed is controlled largely by the size of the silver halide grains and their silver content.

The speed of dental intraoral x-ray film is indicated by a letter designating a particular group (Table 4-4). The fastest dental film currently available has a speed rating of F. Only films with a D or faster speed rating are appropriate for intraoral radiography. Currently the types of film used most often in the U.S. are Kodak Ultra-Speed (group D) and Kodak InSight (group E or F, depending on processing conditions). InSight film is preferred because it requires only about half the exposure of Ultra-Speed film and offers comparable contrast and resolution. F-speed film is faster than the D-speed type because tabular crystal grains are used in the emulsion of F-speed film. The characteristic curves in Fig. 4-16 show that InSight film (curve on the left) is faster than Ultra-Speed film (curve on the right) because less exposure is required to produce the same level of density even though the two films have similar contrast.

Although film speed can be increased slightly by processing the film at a higher temperature, this is achieved at the expense of increased film fog and graininess. Processing in depleted solutions can lower the effective speed. It is always preferable to use fresh processing solutions and follow the recommended processing time and temperature.

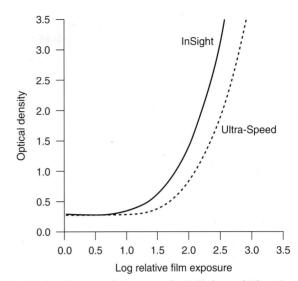

FIG. **4-16** *Characteristic curves for InSight and Ultra-Speed film.* InSight film is faster and has essentially the same contrast as Ultra-Speed film. (Courtesy Eastman Kodak, Rochester, N.Y.)

FILM LATITUDE

Film latitude is a measure of the range of exposures that can be recorded as distinguishable densities on a film. A film optimized to display a wide latitude can record a subject with a wide range of subject contrast. A film with a characteristic curve that has a long straight-line portion and a shallow slope has a wide latitude (Fig. 4-17). As a consequence, wide variations in the amount of radiation exiting the subject can be recorded. Films with a wide latitude have lower contrast (i.e., a long gray scale) than do films with a narrow latitude. Wide-latitude films are useful when both the osseous structures of the skull and the soft tissues of the facial region must be recorded.

To some extent the operator can modify the latitude of an image. A high kVp produces images with a wide latitude and low contrast. Reduced exposure produces a somewhat lighter image and shows a slightly wider range of anatomic structures with lower contrast. Wide-latitude film is recommended for imaging structures with a wide range of subject densities.

RADIOGRAPHIC NOISE

Radiographic noise is the appearance of uneven density of a uniformly exposed radiographic film. It is seen on a small area of film as localized variations in density. The primary causes of noise are radiographic mottle and radiographic artifact. Radiographic mottle is uneven density resulting from the physical structure of

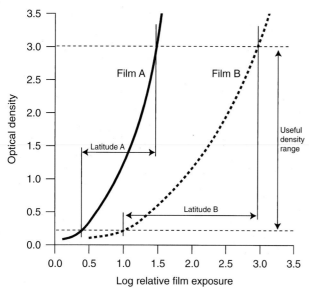

FIG. **4-17** Characteristic curves for two films demonstrating greater inherent latitude of film *B* compared with film *A*. The slope of film *B* is less steep than that of film *A;* therefore film *B* records a greater range of exposures within the useful density range than does film *A.*

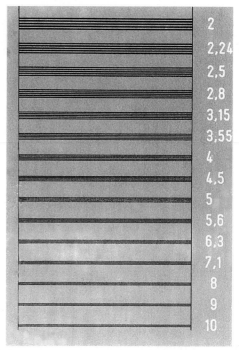

FIG. **4-18** Radiograph of a resolving power target consisting of groups of radiopaque lines and radiolucent spaces. Numbers at each group indicate the line pairs per millimeter represented by the group.

the film or intensifying screens. Radiographic artifacts are defects caused by errors in film handling, such as fingerprints or bends in the film, or errors in film processing, such as splashing developer or fixer on a film or marks or scratches from rough handling.

On intraoral dental film, mottle may be seen as *film graininess,* which is caused by the visibility of silver grains in the film emulsion, especially when magnification is used to examine an image. Film graininess is most evident when high-temperature processing is used.

Radiographic mottle is also evident when the film is used with fast intensifying screens. Two important causes of the phenomenon are *quantum mottle* and *screen structure mottle.* Quantum mottle is caused by a fluctuation in the number of photons per unit of the beam cross-sectional area absorbed by the intensifying screen. Quantum mottle is most evident when fast film-screen combinations are used. Under these conditions the relative nonuniformity of the beam is highest. The longer exposures required by slower film-screen combinations tend to average out the beam pattern and thereby reduce quantum mottle. Screen structure mottle is graininess caused by screen phosphors. It is most evident when fast screens with large crystals are used.

RADIOGRAPHIC BLURRING

Sharpness is the ability of a radiograph to *define an edge precisely* (e.g., the dentinoenamel junction, a thin tra-

becular plate). *Resolution,* or resolving power, is the ability of a radiograph to record *separate structures* that are close together. It usually is measured by radiographing an object made up of a series of thin lead strips with alternating radiolucent spaces of the same thickness. The groups of lines and spaces are arranged in the test target in order of increasing numbers of lines and spaces per millimeter (Fig. 4-18). The resolving power is measured as the highest number of line pairs (a line pair being the image of an absorber and the adjacent lucent space) per millimeter that can be distinguished on the resultant radiograph when examined with low-power magnification. Typically, panoramic film-screen combinations can resolve about five line pairs per millimeter; periapical film, which has better resolving power, can delineate clearly more than 20 line pairs per millimeter.

Radiographic blur is caused by image receptor (film and screen) blurring, motion blurring, and geometric blurring.

Image Receptor Blurring

With intraoral dental x-ray film, the *size and number of the silver grains* in the film emulsion determines image sharpness: the finer the grain size, the finer the

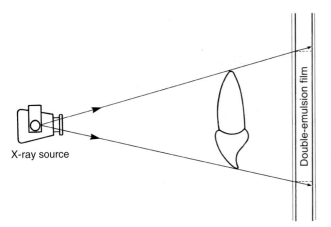

FIG. **4-19**   Parallax unsharpness results when double-emulsion film is used because of the slightly greater magnification on the side of the film away from the x-ray source. Parallax unsharpness is a minor problem in clinical practice.

sharpness. In general, slow-speed films have fine grains and faster films have larger grains.

Use of *intensifying screens* in extraoral radiography has an adverse effect on image sharpness. Some degree of sharpness is lost because visible light and ultraviolet radiation emitted by the screen spread out beyond the point of origin and expose a film area larger than the phosphor crystal (see Fig. 4-8). The spreading light causes a blurring of fine detail on the radiograph. Intensifying screens with large crystals are relatively fast, but image sharpness is diminished. Furthermore, fast intensifying screens have a relatively thick phosphor layer, which contributes to dispersion of light and loss of image sharpness. Diffusion of light from a screen can be minimized and image sharpness maximized by ensuring as close contact as possible between the intensifying screen and film.

The presence of an image on each side of a double-emulsion film also causes a loss of image sharpness through *parallax* (Fig. 4-19). Parallax results from the apparent change in position or size of a subject when it is viewed from different perspectives. Because dental film has a double coating of emulsion and the x-ray beam is divergent, the images recorded on each emulsion vary slightly in size. In intraoral images, the effect of parallax on image sharpness is unimportant but is most apparent when wet films are viewed. Under these conditions the emulsion is swollen with water and the loss of image sharpness caused by parallax is more evident. When intensifying screens are used, parallax distortion contributes to image unsharpness because light from one screen may cross the film base and reach the emulsion on the opposite side. This problem can

be solved by incorporating dyes into the base that absorb the light emitted by the screens.

Motion Blurring

Image sharpness also can be lost through movement of the film, subject, or x-ray source during exposure. Movement of the x-ray source in effect enlarges the focal spot and diminishes image sharpness. Patient movement can be minimized by stabilizing the patient's head with the chair headrest during exposure. Using a higher mA and kVp and correspondingly shorter exposure times also helps resolve this problem.

Geometric Blurring

Several geometric factors influence image sharpness. Loss of image sharpness results in part because photons are not emitted from a point source (focal spot) on the target in the x-ray tube. The larger the focal spot, the greater the loss of image sharpness. Also, image sharpness is improved by increasing the distance between the focal spot and the object and reducing the distance between the object and the image receptor. Various means of optimizing projection geometry are discussed in Chapter 5.

IMAGE QUALITY

Image quality describes the subjective judgment by the clinician of the overall appearance of a radiograph. It combines the features of density, contrast, latitude, sharpness, resolution, and perhaps other parameters. Various mathematic approaches have been used to evaluate these parameters further, but a thorough discussion of them is beyond the scope of this text. The *detective quantum efficiency (DQE)* is a basic measure of the efficiency of an imaging system. It encompasses image contrast, blur, speed, and noise. Often a system can be optimized for one of these parameters, but this usually is achieved at the expense of others. For instance, a fast system typically has a high level of noise. Even with these and other sophisticated approaches, however, more information is needed for complete understanding of all the factors responsible for the subjective impression of image quality.

Grids

When an x-ray beam strikes a patient, many of the incident photons undergo Compton interactions and produce scattered photons. Typically the number of scattered photons in the remnant beam that reach the film is two to four times the number of primary photons that do not undergo absorption. The amount of scattered radiation increases with increasing subject thickness, field size, and kVp (energy of the x-ray beam).

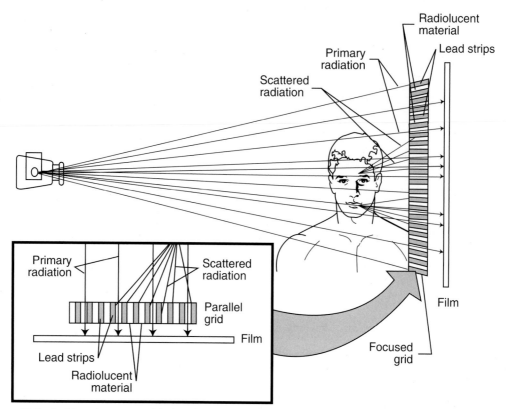

FIG. **4-20**   An x-ray grid absorbs scattered x-ray photons from the primary beam and prevents them from fogging the film. In a focused grid the absorber plates are angled toward the anode; in a parallel grid the absorber plates are parallel.

These scattered photons produce fog on the film and reduce the subject contrast.

FUNCTION

The function of a grid is to reduce the amount of scattered radiation exiting a subject that reaches the film. The grid, which is placed between the subject and the film, preferentially removes the scattered radiation and spares primary photons; this reduces nonimaging exposure and increases subject contrast.

COMPOSITION

A grid is composed of alternating strips of a radiopaque material (usually lead) and strips of radiolucent material (often plastic). The diagram in Fig. 4-20 shows the interaction between a grid and an x-ray beam. When secondary photons generated in the subject are scattered toward the film, they usually are absorbed by the radiopaque material in the grid. This occurs because the direction of the scattered photons deviates from that of the primary beam, and consequently they cannot pass through the parallel plates of the grid.

Focused grids are used most often. In a focused grid the strips of radiopaque material are all directed toward a common point, the focal spot of the x-ray tube, some distance away. Because the lead strips are angled toward the focal spot, their direction coincides with the paths of diverging photons in the primary x-ray beam. The lead strips absorb the scattered photons as their paths diverge from those of the primary photons. A focused grid can be used only within a range of distances from the focal spot where the alignment of lead strips closely coincides with the path of the diverging x-ray beam. The range of distances is specified on the grid.

Grids are manufactured with a varying number of line pairs of absorbers and radiolucent spaces per inch. Grids with 80 or more line pairs per inch do not show objectionable grid lines on the image. The ratio of grid thickness to the width of the radiolucent spacer is known as the *grid ratio.* The higher the grid ratio, the more effectively scattered radiation is removed from the x-ray beam. Grids with a ratio of 8 or 10 are preferred.

The image of the radiolucent grid lines on the film can be deleted by moving the grid perpendicular to the direction of the grid lines (but not moving the subject or the film) during exposure. This has the effect of blurring out the radiolucent lines and allowing a more uniform exposure. This movement does not interfere with the absorption of scattered photons. The apparatus for moving a grid is called a *Bucky*.

To compensate for the absorbing materials in the grid, the exposure required when a grid is used is approximately double that needed without a grid. Therefore grids should be used only when the improvement in diagnostic image quality is sufficient to justify the added exposure. For example, with lateral cephalometric examinations made for assessing the growth and development of the facial region (Chapter 11), use of a grid usually is not indicated because the improved contrast does not aid in identification of anatomic landmarks.

BIBLIOGRAPHY

Bushberg JT: The essential physics of medical imaging, ed 2, Baltimore, 2001, Lippincott Williams & Wilkins.

Bushong SC: Radiologic science for technologists: physics, biology, and protection, ed 7, St. Louis, 2001, Mosby.

Council on Dental Materials and Devices: Revised American Dental Association specification no. 22 for intraoral dental radiographic film adapted, JADA 80:1066, 1970.

Curry TS III et al: Christensen's physics of diagnostic radiology, ed 4, Philadelphia, 1990, Lea & Febiger.

Haus AG: The AAPM/RSNA physics tutorial for residents: measures of screen-film performance, Radiographics 16:1165, 1996.

Ludlow JB, Platin E, Mol A: Characteristics of Kodak InSight, an F-speed intraoral film, Oral Surg Oral Med Oral Pathol Oral Radiol Endod 91:120-9, 2001.

Nair MK, Nair UP: An in-vitro evaluation of Kodak InSight and Ektaspeed Plus film with a CMOS detector for natural proximal caries: ROC analysis. Caries Res 35:354-9, 2001.

Thunthy KH, Ireland EJ. A comparison of the visibility of caries on Kodak F-speed (InSight) and D-speed (Ultraspeed) films. LDA J 60:31-2, 2001.

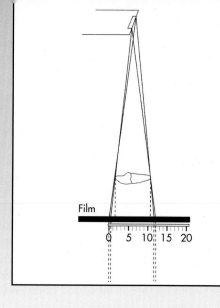

CHAPTER 5

Projection Geometry

A *radiograph is a two-dimensional representation* of a three-dimensional object. To obtain the maximal value from a radiograph, a clinician must have a clear understanding of normal anatomy and then mentally reconstruct a three-dimensional image of the anatomic structures of interest from one or more of these two-dimensional views. Using high-quality radiographs greatly facilitates this task. The principles of projection geometry describe the effect of focal spot size and position (relative to the object and the film) on image clarity, magnification, and distortion. Clinicians use these principles to maximize image clarity, minimize distortion, and localize objects in the image field.

Image Sharpness and Resolution

Several geometric considerations contribute to image clarity, particularly image sharpness and resolution. *Sharpness* measures how well a boundary between two areas of differing radiodensity is revealed. Image *spatial resolution* measures how well a radiograph is able to reveal small objects that are close together. Although sharpness and resolution are two distinct features, they are interdependent, being influenced by the same geometric variables. For clinical diagnosis it is desirable to optimize conditions that will result in images with high sharpness and resolution.

When x rays are produced at the target in an x-ray tube, they originate from all points within the area of the focal spot. Because these rays originate from different points and travel in straight lines, their projections of a feature of an object do not occur at exactly the same location on a film. As a result, the image of the edge of an object is slightly blurred rather than

sharp and distinct. Fig. 5-1 shows the path of photons that originate at the margins of the focal spot and provide an image of the edges of an object. The resulting blurred zone of unsharpness on an image causes a loss in image clarity by reducing sharpness and resolution. The larger the focal spot area, the greater the loss of clarity.

Three methods exist for minimizing this loss of image clarity and improving the quality of radiographs:
1. *Use as small an effective focal spot as practical.* Dental x-ray machines should have a nominal focal spot size of 1.0 mm or less. Some tubes used in extraoral radiography have effective focal spots measuring 0.3 mm, which greatly adds to image clarity. X-ray tube manufacturers use as small an effective focal spot size as is consistent with the requirements for heat dissipation. As described in Chapter 1, the size of the effective focal spot is a function of the angle of the target with respect to the long axis of the electron beam. A large angle distributes the electron beam over a larger surface and decreases the heat generated per unit of target area, thus prolonging tube life. However, this results in a larger effective focal spot and loss of image clarity (Fig. 5-2). A small angle has a greater wearing effect on the target but results in a smaller effective focal spot, decreased unsharpness, and increased image sharpness and resolution. This angle of the face of the target to the central x-ray beam is usually between 10 and 20 degrees.
2. *Increase the distance between the focal spot and the object by using a long, open-ended cylinder.* Fig. 5-3 shows how increasing the focal spot–to–object distance reduces image blurring by reducing the divergence of the x-ray beam. The longer focal spot–to–object distance minimizes blurring by using photons whose paths

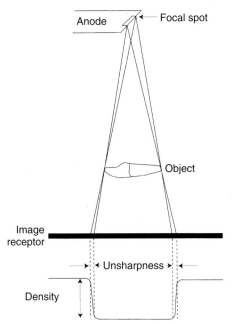

FIG. 5-1 Photons originating at different places on the focal spot result in a zone of unsharpness on the radiograph. The density of the image changes from a high background value to a low value in the area of an edge of enamel, dentin, or bone.

are almost parallel. The benefits of using a long focal spot–to-object distance support the use of long, open-ended cylinders as aiming devices on dental x-ray machines.

3. *Minimize the distance between the object and the film.* Fig. 5-4 shows that as the object-to-film distance is reduced, the unsharpness decreases, resulting in enhanced image clarity. This is the result of minimizing the divergence of the x-ray photons.

Image Size Distortion

Image size distortion (magnification) is the increase in size of the image on the radiograph compared with the actual size of the object. The divergent paths of photons in an x-ray beam cause enlargement of the image on a radiograph. Image size distortion results from the relative distances of the focal spot–to-film and object-to-film (see Figs. 5-3 and 5-4). Accordingly, increasing the focal spot–to-film distance and decreasing the object-to-film distance minimizes image magnification. The use of a long, open-ended cylinder as an

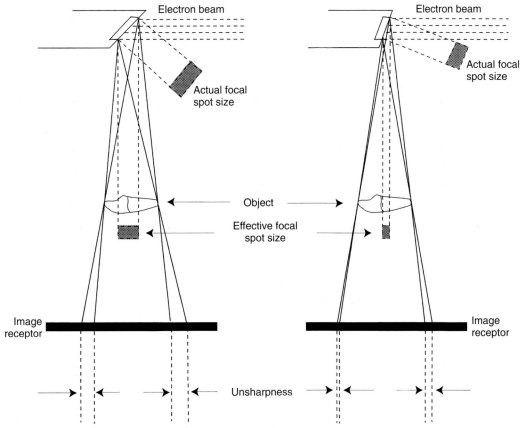

FIG. 5-2 Decreasing the angle of the target perpendicular to the long axis of the electron beam decreases the actual focal spot size and decreases heat dissipation and thereby tube life. It also decreases the effective focal spot size, thus increasing the sharpness of the image.

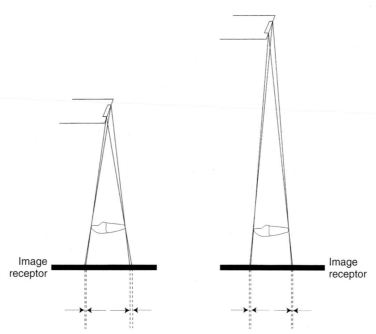

FIG. **5-3**   Increasing the distance between the focal spot and the object results in an image with increased sharpness and less magnification of the object.

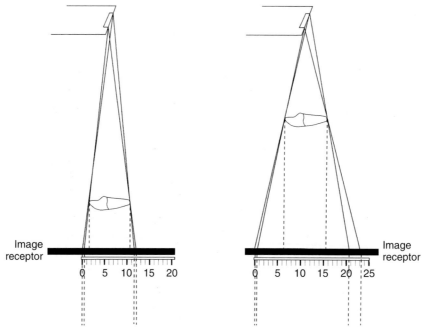

FIG. **5-4**   Decreasing the distance between the object and the film increases the sharpness and results in less magnification of the object.

aiming device on an x-ray machine thus reduces the magnification of images on a periapical view. Furthermore, as mentioned above, this technique also improves image clarity by increasing the distance between the focal spot and object.

Image Shape Distortion

Image shape distortion is the result of unequal magnification of different parts of the same object. This situation arises when not all the parts of an object are at the same focal spot–to-object distance. The physical shape of the object may often prevent its optimal orientation, resulting in some shape distortion. Such a phenomenon is seen by the differences in appearance of the image on a radiograph compared with the true shape. To minimize shape distortion, the practitioner should make an effort to align the tube, object, and film carefully, using the following guidelines:

1. *Position the film parallel to the long axis of the object.* Image shape distortion is minimized when the long axes of the film and tooth are parallel. Fig. 5-5 shows that the central ray of the x-ray beam is perpendicular to the film, but the object is not parallel to the film. The resultant image is distorted because of the unequal distances of the various parts of the object from the film. This type of shape distortion is called *foreshortening* because it causes the radiographic image to be shorter than the object. Fig. 5-6 shows

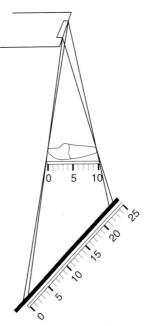

FIG. **5-6** Elongation of a radiographic image results when the central ray is perpendicular to the object but not to the film.

the situation when the x-ray beam is oriented at right angles to the object but not to the film. This results in *elongation,* with the object appearing longer on the film than its actual length.

2. *Orient the central ray perpendicular to the object and film.* Image shape distortion occurs if the object and film are parallel but the central ray is not directed at right angles to each. This is most evident on maxillary molar projections (Fig. 5-7). If the central ray is oriented with an excessive vertical angulation, the palatal roots appear disproportionately longer than the buccal roots.

The practitioner can prevent distortion errors by aligning the object and film parallel with each other and the central ray perpendicular to both.

Paralleling and Bisecting-Angle Techniques

From the earliest days of dental radiography, a clinical objective has been to produce accurate images of dental structures that are normally visually obscured. An early method for aligning the x-ray beam and film with the teeth and jaws was the *bisecting-angle technique* (Fig. 5-8). In this method the film is placed as close to the teeth as possible without deforming it. However, when the film is in this position, it is not parallel to the long axes of the teeth. This arrangement inherently causes

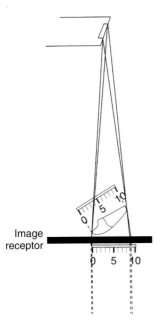

Image receptor

FIG. **5-5** Foreshortening of a radiographic image results when the central ray is perpendicular to the film but the object is not parallel with the film.

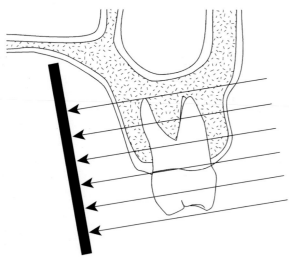

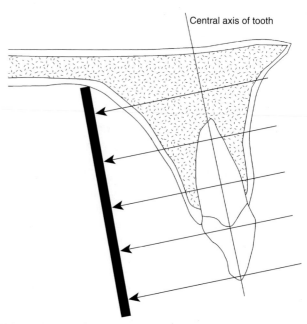

FIG. **5-7**   The central ray should be perpendicular to the long axes of both the tooth and the film. When the direction of the x-ray beam is not at right angles to the long axis of the tooth, the appearance of the tooth is distorted, as seen by apparent elongation of the length of the palatal roots. Additionally, distortion of the relationship of the height of the alveolar crest relative to the cementoenamel junction (CEJ) occurs. In this case the buccal alveolar crest appears to lie superior to the palatal CEJ.

FIG. **5-9**   In the paralleling technique the central ray is directed at a right angle to the central axes of the object and the film.

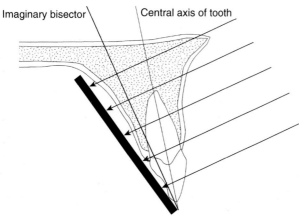

FIG. **5-8**   In the bisecting-angle technique the central ray is directed at a right angle to the imaginary plane that bisects the angle formed by the film and the central axis of the object. This method results in an image that is the same length as the object.

distortion. Nevertheless, by directing the central ray perpendicular to an imaginary plane that bisects the angle between the teeth and the film, the practitioner can make the length of the tooth's image on the film correspond to the actual length of the tooth. This angle between a tooth and the film is especially apparent when teeth are radiographed in the maxilla or anterior

mandible. Even though the projected length of a tooth is correct, the image is still distorted because the film and object are not parallel and the x-ray beam is not directed at right angles to them. This distortion tends to increase along the image toward the apex.

When the central ray is not perpendicular to the bisector plane, the length of the image of a projected tooth changes. If the central ray is directed at an angle that is more positive than perpendicular to the bisector, the image of the tooth is *foreshortened*. Likewise, if it is inclined with more negative angulation to the bisector, the image is *elongated*. In recent years, the bisecting-angle technique has been used less frequently for general periapical radiography as use of the paralleling technique has increased.

The *paralleling technique* is the preferred method for making intraoral radiographs. It derives its name as the result of placing the film parallel with the long axis of the tooth (Fig. 5-9). This procedure minimizes image distortion and best incorporates the imaging principles described in the first three sections of this chapter.

To achieve this parallel orientation, the practitioner often must position the film toward the middle of the oral cavity, away from the teeth. Although this allows the teeth and film to be parallel, it results in some image magnification and loss of definition by increasing unsharpness. As a consequence, the paralleling technique also uses a relatively long open-ended aiming cylinder ("cone") to increase the focal spot-to-object distance. This directs only the most central and parallel rays of the beam to the film and teeth and reduces image magnification while increasing image sharpness and resolution. The paralleling technique has benefited from the development of fast-speed film emulsions, which allow relatively short exposure times in spite of an increased target-to-object distance.

Because it is desirable to position the film near the middle of the oral cavity with the paralleling technique, film holders should be used to support the film in the patient's mouth. Chapter 8 discusses film-holding instruments and techniques for intraoral radiography using the paralleling technique.

Object Localization

In clinical practice, the dentist must often derive from a radiograph three-dimensional information concerning patients. The dentist may wish to use radiographs, for example, to determine the location of a foreign object or an impacted tooth within the jaw. Two methods are frequently used to obtain such three-dimensional information. The first is to examine two films projected at right angles to each other. The second method is to employ the so-called tube shift technique.

Fig. 5-10 shows the first method, in which *two projections taken at right angles to one another* localize an object in or about the maxilla in three dimensions. In clinical practice the position of an object on each radiograph is noted relative to the anatomic landmarks. This allows the observer to determine the position of the object or area of interest. For example, if a radiopacity is found near the apex of the first molar on a periapical

radiograph, the dentist may take an occlusal projection to identify its mediolateral position. The occlusal film may reveal a calcification in the soft tissues located laterally or medially to the body of the mandible. This information is important in determining the treatment required. The right-angle (or cross-section) technique is best for the mandible. On a maxillary occlusal projection the superimposition of features in the anterior part of the skull may frequently obscure the area of interest.

The second method used to identify the spatial position of an object is the *tube shift technique.* Other names for this procedure are the *buccal object rule* and *Clark's rule* (Clark described it in 1910). The rationale for this procedure derives from the manner in which the relative positions of radiographic images of two separate objects change when the projection angle at which the images were made is changed.

Fig. 5-11 shows two radiographs of an object exposed at different angles. Compare the position of the object in question on each radiograph with the reference structures. If the tube is shifted and directed at the reference object (e.g., the apex of a tooth) from a more mesial angulation and the object in question also moves mesially with respect to the reference object, the object lies lingual to the reference object.

Alternatively, if the tube is shifted mesially and the object in question appears to move distally, it lies on the

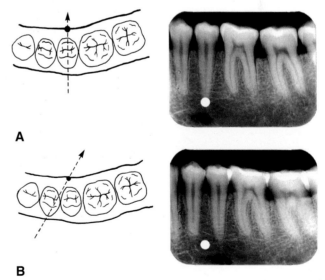

FIG. **5-11** The position of an object may be determined with respect to reference structures using the tube shift technique. In **A**, an object on the lingual surface of the mandible may appear apical to the second premolar. When another radiograph is made of this region angulated from the mesial, **B**, the object appears to have moved mesially with respect to the second premolar apex ("same lingual" in the acronym *SLOB*).

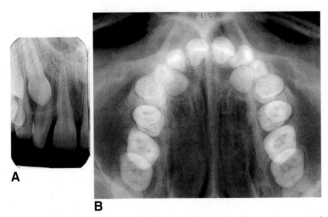

FIG. **5-10** **A**, The periapical radiograph shows impacted canine lying apical to roots of lateral incisor and first premolar. **B**, The vertex occlusal view shows that the canine lies palatal to the roots of the lateral incisor and first premolar.

buccal aspect of the reference object (Fig. 5-12). These relations can be easily remembered by the acronym *SLOB: Same Lingual, Opposite Buccal.* Thus if the object in question appears to move in the same direction with respect to the reference structures as does the x-ray tube, it is on the lingual aspect of the reference object; if it appears to move in the opposite direction as the x-ray tube, it is on the buccal aspect. If it does not move with respect to the reference object, it lies at the same depth (in the same vertical plane) as the reference object.

Examination of a conventional set of full-mouth films with this rule in mind demonstrates that the incisive foramen is indeed located lingual (palatal) to the roots of the central incisors and that the mental foramen lies buccal to the roots of the premolars. This technique assists in determining the position of impacted teeth, presence of foreign objects, and other abnormal conditions. It works just as well when the x-ray machine is moved vertically as horizontally.

The dentist may have two radiographs of a region of the dentition that were made at different angles, but no record exists of the orientation of the x-ray machine. Comparison of the anatomy displayed on the images helps distinguish changes in horizontal or vertical angulation. The relative positions of osseous landmarks with respect to the teeth helps identify changes in horizontal or vertical angulation. Fig. 5-13 shows the inferior border of the zygomatic process of the maxilla over the molars. This structure lies buccal to the teeth and appears to move mesially as the x-ray beam is oriented more from the distal. Similarly, as the angulation of the beam is increased vertically, the zygomatic process is projected occlusally over the teeth.

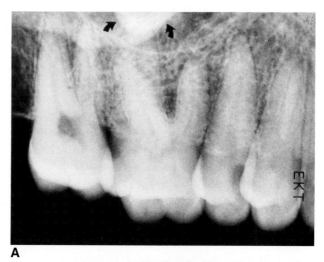

A

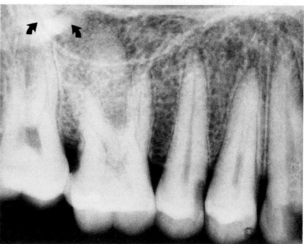

B

FIG. **5-13** The position of the maxillary zygomatic process in relation to the roots of the molars can help in identifying the orientation of projections. In **A**, the inferior border of the process lies over the palatal root of the first molar, whereas in **B**, it lies posterior to the palatal root of the first molar. This indicates that when **A** was made, the beam was oriented more from the posterior than when **B** was made. The same conclusion can be reached independently by examining the roots of the first molar. In **A**, the palatal root lies behind the distobuccal root, but in **B**, it lies between the two buccal roots.

A

B

FIG. **5-12** The position of an object can be determined with respect to reference structures using the tube shift technique. In **A**, an object on the buccal surface of the mandible may appear apical to the second premolar. When another radiograph is made of this region angulated from the mesial, **B**, the object appears to have moved distally with respect to the second premolar apex ("opposite buccal" in the acronym *SLOB*).

BIBLIOGRAPHY

BUCCAL OBJECT RULE

Chenail B, Aurelio JA, Gerstein H: A model for teaching the Buccal Object Moves Most Rule, J Endod 9:452-3, 1983.

Clark CA: A method of ascertaining the relative position of unerupted teeth by means of film radiographs, Proc R Soc Med Odontol Sect 3:87, 1910.

Goerig AC, Neaverth EJ: A simplified look at the buccal object rule in endodontics, J Endod 13:570, 1987.

Jacobs SG: Radiographic localization of unerupted teeth: further findings about the vertical tube shift method and other localization techniques, Am J Orthod Dentofacial Orthop 118:439-47, 2000.

Jacobs SG: Radiographic localization of unerupted maxillary anterior teeth using the vertical tube shift technique: the history and application of the method with some case reports, Am J Orthod Dentofacial Orthop 116:415-23, 1999.

Khabbaz MG, Serefoglou MH: The application of the buccal object rule for the determination of calcified root canals, Int Endod J 29:284-7, 1996.

Ludlow JB: The Buccal Object Rule, Dentomaxillofac Radiol 28:258, 1999.

Reader A: A teaching model for the buccal object rule, J Dent Educ 48:469-72, 1984.

PARALLELING TECHNIQUE

Forsberg J, Halse A: Radiographic simulation of a periapical lesion comparing the paralleling and the bisecting-angle techniques, Int Endod J 27:133-8, 1994.

Forsberg J: A comparison of the paralleling and bisecting-angle radiographic techniques in endodontics, Int Endod J 20:177-82, 1987.

Schulze RK, d'Hoedt B: A method to calculate angular disparities between object and receptor in "paralleling technique," Dentomaxillofac Radiol 31:32-8, 2002.

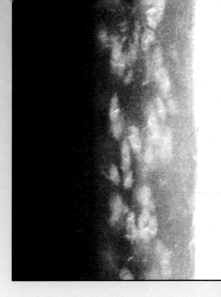

CHAPTER **6**

Processing X-Ray Film

T**he recording medium (image receptor)** most frequently used in dental radiography is radiographic film. When a beam of photons exits an object and exposes an x-ray film, it chemically changes the photosensitive silver halide crystals in the film emulsion. These chemically altered silver bromide crystals constitute the latent (invisible) image on the film. The developing process converts the latent image into the visible radiographic image.

Formation of the Latent Image

Film emulsion consists of photosensitive crystals containing primarily silver bromide suspended in a vehicle and layered on a thin sheet of transparent plastic base. Some cystals also contain small amounts of silver iodide. These silver halide crystals also contain a few free silver ions (interstitial silver ions) in the spaces between the crystalline lattice atoms (Fig. 6-1, *A*). The crystals are chemically sensitized by the addition of trace amounts of sulfur compounds, which bind to the surface of the crystals. The sulfur compounds play a crucial role in image formation. Along with physical irregularities in the crystal produced by iodide ions, sulfur compounds create *sensitivity sites,* the sites in the crystals that are sensitive to radiation. Each crystal has many sensitivity sites, which begin the process of image formation by trapping the electrons generated when the emulsion is irradiated. Exposure to radiation chemically alters the photosensitive silver halide crystals to produce the latent image. Processing the exposed film in developer and fixer converts the latent image into the visible radiographic image.

When the silver halide crystals are irradiated, x-ray photons interact primarily with the bromide ions by Compton and photoelectric interactions (Fig. 6-1, *B*). These interactions result in the removal of an electron from the bromide ions. By the loss of an electron, a bromide ion is converted into a neutral bromine atom. The free electrons move through the crystal until they reach a sensitivity site, where they become trapped and impart a negative charge to the site. The negatively charged sensitivity site then attracts positively charged free interstitial silver ions (Fig. 6-1, *C*). When a silver ion reaches the negatively charged sensitivity site, it is reduced and forms a neutral atom of metallic silver (Fig. 6-1, *D*). The sites containing these neutral silver atoms are now called *latent image sites.* This process occurs numerous times within a crystal. The overall distribution of latent image sites in a film after exposure constitutes the latent image.

Film processing converts the latent image into one that can be visualized (Fig. 6-2). The neutral silver atoms at each latent image site (see Fig. 6-2, *B*) render the crystals sensitive to development and image formation. The larger the aggregate of neutral silver atoms, the more sensitive the crystal is to the effects of the developer. Most latent image sites that are capable of being developed in an optimally exposed film have at least four or five silver atoms. Developer converts silver bromide crystals with neutral silver atoms deposited at the latent image sites into black, solid silver metallic grains (see Fig. 6-2, *C*). These solid silver grains block light from a viewbox. Fixer removes unexposed, undeveloped silver bromide crystals (those without latent image sites), leaving the film clear in unexposed areas (see Fig. 6-2, *D*). Thus the radiographic image is composed of the light (radiopaque) areas, where few photons reached the film, and dark (radiolucent) areas of the film that were struck by many photons.

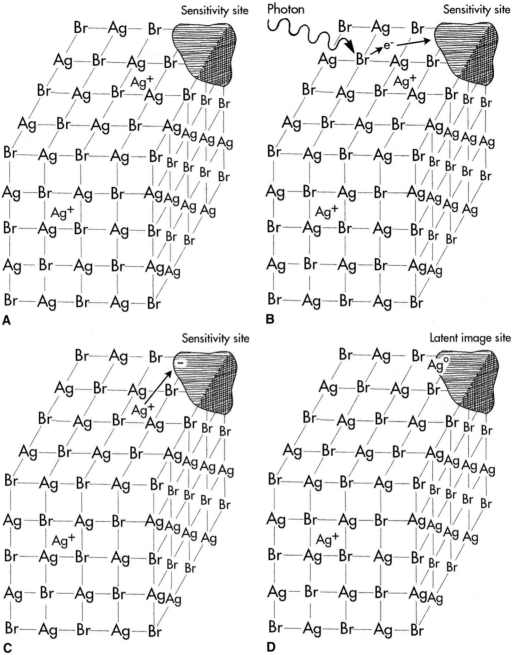

FIG. **6-1** **A,** A silver bromide crystal in the emulsion of an x-ray film contains mostly silver and bromide ions in a crystal lattice. There are also free interstitial silver ions and areas of trace chemicals that form sensitivity sites. **B,** Exposure of the crystal to photons in an x-ray beam results in the release of electrons, usually by interaction of the photon with a bromide ion. Bromide ions are converted to bromine atoms, and the recoil electrons have sufficient kinetic energy to move about in the crystal. When electrons reach a sensitivity site, they impart a negative charge to this region. **C,** Free interstitial silver ions (with a positive charge) are attracted to the negatively charged sensitivity site. **D,** When the silver ions reach the sensitivity site, they acquire an electron and become neutral silver atoms. These silver atoms now constitute a latent image site. The collection of latent image sites over the entire film constitutes the latent image. Developer causes the neutral silver atoms at the latent image sites to initiate the conversion of silver ions in the crystal into one large grain of metallic silver.

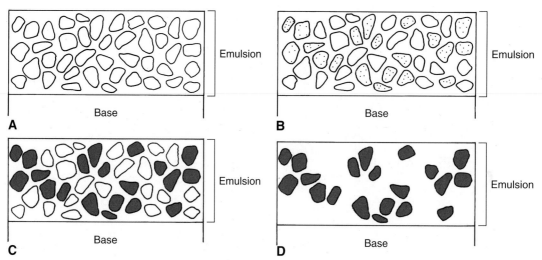

FIG. **6-2** *Emulsion changes during film processing.* **A,** Before exposure, many silver bromide crystals are present in the emulsion. **B,** After exposure, the exposed crystals containing neutral silver atoms at latent image sites constitute the latent image (shaded areas in the crystals). **C,** The developer converts the exposed crystals containing neutral silver atoms at the latent image sites into solid grains of metallic silver. **D,** The fixer dissolves the unexposed, undeveloped silver bromide crystals leaving only the solid silver grains. (Courtesy C.L. Crabtree, DDS, Bureau of Radiological Health, Rockville, Md.)

Processing Solutions

Film processing involves the following procedures:
1. Immerse exposed film in developer.
2. Rinse film in a water bath.
3. Immerse film in fixer.
4. Wash film in water bath.
5. Dry film and mount for viewing.

This chapter first describes the function of developer and fixer. Procedures for each of these steps are described later.

DEVELOPER SOLUTION

The developer reduces all silver ions in the exposed crystals of silver halide (those with a latent image) to metallic silver grains (see Fig. 6-2). To produce a diagnostic image, this reduction process must be restricted to crystals containing latent image sites. To accomplish this, the reducing agents used as developers are catalyzed by the neutral silver atoms at the latent image sites (see Fig. 6-2, *B*). The silver atoms act as a bridge by which electrons from the reducing agents reach silver ions in the crystal and convert them to solid grains of metallic silver. Individual crystals are developed completely or not at all during the recommended developing times (see Fig. 6-2, *C*). Variations in density on the processed radiographs are the result of different ratios of developed (exposed) and undeveloped (unexposed)

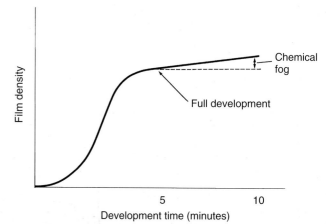

FIG. **6-3** Relationship between film density and development time. The density of film rises quickly initially and then levels off, increasing more slowly because of chemical fogging.

crystals. Areas with many exposed crystals are denser because of their higher concentration of black metallic silver grains after development. If the developer remains too long in contact with silver bromide halide crystals that do not contain a latent image, it slowly reduces these crystals also, thereby overdeveloping the image.

When an exposed film is developed, the developer initially has no visible effect (Fig. 6-3). After this initial phase, the density increases, very rapidly at first and then more slowly. Eventually all the exposed crystals develop (become reduced to black metallic silver), and the developing agent starts to reduce the unexposed crystals. The development of unexposed crystals results in chemical fog on the film. The interval between maximal density and fogging explains why a properly exposed film does not become overdeveloped even though it may be in contact with the developer longer than the recommended interval. Thus dark films usually are the result of overexposure rather than overdevelopment.

The developing solution contains four components, all dissolved in water: (1) developer, (2) activator, (3) preservative, and (4) restrainer.

Developer

The primary function of the developing solution is to convert the exposed silver halide crystals into metallic silver grains. This process begins at the latent image sites, where electrons from the developing agents are conducted into the silver halide crystal and reduce the constituent silver ions (approximately 1 billion to 10 billion) to solid grains of metallic silver. Two developing agents are used in dental radiology: a pyrazolidone-type compound, usually Phenidone (1-phenyl-3-pyrazolidone), and hydroquinone (paradihydroxy benzene). Phenidone serves as the first electron donor that converts silver ions to metallic silver at the latent image site. This electron transfer generates the oxidized form of Phenidone. Hydroquinone provides an electron to reduce the oxidized Phenidone back to its original active state so that it can continue to reduce silver halide grains to metallic silver. Unexposed crystals, those without latent images, are unaffected during the time required for reduction of the exposed crystals.

Activator

The developers are active only at alkaline pH values, usually around 10. This is achieved with the addition of alkali compounds (activators) such as sodium or potassium hydrozide. Buffers are used to maintain this condition—usually sodium bicarbonate. The activators also cause the gelatin to swell so that the developing agents can diffuse more rapidly into the emulsion and reach the suspended silver bromide crystals.

Preservative

The developing solution contains an antioxidant or preservative, usually sodium sulfite. The preservative protects the developers from oxidation by atmospheric oxygen and thus extends their useful life. The preservative also combines with the brown oxidized developer to produce a colorless soluble compound. If not removed, oxidation products interfere with the developing reaction and stain the film.

Restrainer

Bromide, usually as potassium bromide, and benzotriazole are added to the developing solution to restrain development of unexposed silver halide crystals. Although bromide and benzotriazole depress the reduction of both exposed and unexposed crystals, they are much more effective in depressing the reduction of unexposed crystals. Consequently, the restrainers act as antifog agents and increase contrast.

DEVELOPER REPLENISHER

In the normal course of film processing, Phenidone and hydroquinone are consumed, and bromide ions and other by-products are released into solution. Developer also becomes inactivated by exposure to oxygen. These actions produce a "seasoned" solution, and the film speed and contrast stabilize. The developing solution of both manual and automatic developers should be replenished with fresh solution each morning to prolong the life of the seasoned developer. The recommended amount to be added daily is 8 ounces of fresh developer (replenisher) per gallon of developing solution. This assumes the development of an average of 30 periapical or five panoramic films per day. Some of the used solution may need to be removed to make room for the replenisher.

RINSING

After development the film emulsion swells and becomes saturated with developer. At this point the films are rinsed in water for 30 seconds with continuous, gentle agitation before they are placed in the fixer. Rinsing dilutes the developer, slowing the development process. It also removes the alkali activator, preventing neutralization of the acid fixer. This rinsing process is typical for manual processing but is not used with automatic processing.

FIXING SOLUTION

The primary function of fixing solution is to dissolve and remove the undeveloped silver halide crystals from the emulsion (see Fig. 6-2, *D*). The presence of unexposed crystals causes film to be opaque. If these crystals are not removed, the image on the resultant radiograph is dark and nondiagnostic. Fig. 6-4 is a photomicrograph of film emulsion showing the solid silver grains after fixer has removed the unexposed

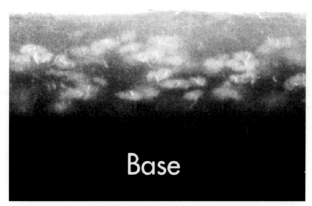

FIG. **6-4** Scanning electron micrograph of a processed emulsion of Kodak Ultra-Speed dental x-ray film (5000 ×). Note the white-appearing solid silver grains above the base. (Courtesy Eastman Kodak, Rochester, N.Y.)

silver bromide crystals. (Compare it with Fig. 4-2, *A*, which shows the unprocessed emulsion.) A second function of fixing solution is to harden and shrink the film emulsion. As with developer, fixer should be replenished daily at the rate of 8 ounces per gallon.

Fixing solution also contains four components, all dissolved in water: (1) clearing agent, (2) acidifier, (3) preservative, and (4) hardener.

Clearing Agent
After development the film emulsion must be cleared by dissolving and removing the unexposed silver halide. An aqueous solution of ammonium thiosulfate ("hypo") dissolves the silver halide grains. It forms stable, water-soluble complexes with silver ions, which then diffuse from the emulsion. The clearing agent does not have a rapid effect on the metallic silver grains in the film emulsion, but excessive fixation results in a gradual loss of film density because the grains of silver slowly dissolve in the acetic acid of the fixing solution.

Acidifier
The fixing solution contains an acetic acid buffer system (pH 4 to 4.5) to keep the fixer pH constant. The acidic pH is required to promote good diffusion of thiosulfate into the emulsion and of silver thiosulfate complex out of the emulsion. The acid fixing solution also inactivates any carryover developing agents in the film emulsion, blocking continued development of any unexposed crystals while the film is in the fixing tank.

Preservative
Ammonium sulfite is the preservative in the fixing solution, as it is in the developer. It prevents oxidation of the thiosulfate clearing agent, which is unstable in the acid environment of the fixing solution. It also binds with any colored oxidized developer carried over into the fixing solution and effectively removes it from the solution, which prevents oxidized developer from staining the film.

Hardener
The hardening agent most often used is aluminum sulfate. Aluminum complexes with the gelatin during fixing and prevents damage to the gelatin during subsequent handling. The hardeners also reduce swelling of the emulsion during the final wash. This lessens mechanical damage to the emulsion and limits water absorption, thus shortening drying time.

WASHING

After fixing, the processed film is washed in a sufficient flow of water for an adequate time to ensure removal of all thiosulfate ions and silver thiosulfate complexes. Washing efficiency declines rapidly when the water temperature falls below 60° F. Any silver compound or thiosulfate that remains because of improper washing discolors and causes stains, which are most apparent in the radiopaque (light) areas. This discoloration results from the thiosulfate reacting with silver to form brown silver sulfide, which can obscure diagnostic information.

Darkroom Equipment

The darkroom should be convenient to the x-ray machines and dental operatories and should be at least 4×5 feet (1.2×1.5 m) (Fig. 6-5). One of the most important requirements is that it be lightproof. To accomplish this, a light-tight door or doorless maze (if space permits) is used. The door should have a lock to prevent accidental opening, which might allow an unexpected flood of light that can ruin opened films. The room must be well ventilated for the comfort of those working in the area and to exhaust the heat from the dryer and moisture from the drying films. Also, a comfortable room temperature helps maintain optimal conditions for developing, fixing, and washing solutions. If supplies (including unexposed x-ray film) are to be stored in the darkroom, ventilation is doubly important because temperatures of 90° F or higher can cause a generalized increase in density (film fog) on the film.

SAFELIGHTING
Equipment
The processing room should have both white illumination and safelighting. Safelighting is low-intensity illu-

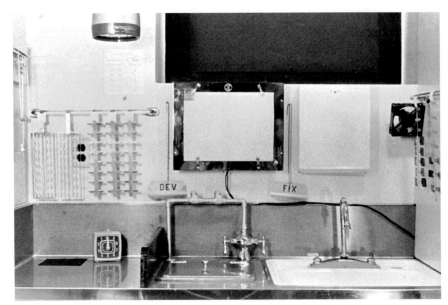

FIG. **6-5** Darkroom work area. *Left*, Film mounting area, timer, film racks, and safelight above. *Middle*, Developing and fixing tanks below the viewbox and stirring paddles. *Right*, Sink and drying racks with fan. (Courtesy C.L. Crabtree, M.D., Bureau of Radiological Health, Rockville, Md.)

mination of relatively long wavelength (red) that does not rapidly affect open film but permits one to see well enough to work in the area. It is best to place one safelight (Fig. 6-6) above the work area on the wall behind the processing tanks and somewhat to the right of the fixing tank. To minimize the fogging effect of prolonged exposure, the safelight should have a 15-watt bulb and should be mounted at least 4 feet above the surface where opened films are handled.

X-ray films are very sensitive to the blue-green region of the spectrum and less sensitive to yellow and red wavelengths. Accordingly, the red GBX-2 filter is recommended as a safelight in darkrooms where either intraoral or extraoral films are handled, because this filter transmits light only at the red end of the spectrum (Fig. 6-7). Film handling under a safelight should be limited to about 5 minutes because film emulsion shows some sensitivity to light from a safelight with prolonged exposure. The older ML-2 filters (yellow light) are not appropriate for fast intraoral dental film or extraoral panoramic or cephalometric film.

MANUAL PROCESSING TANKS

All dental offices should have the capability to develop film by tank processing, if only as a backup for an automatic processor or digital imaging system. The tank must have hot and cold running water and a means of maintaining the temperature between 60° and 75° F. A practical size for a dental office is a master tank about 20×25 cm (8×10 inches) that can serve as a water

jacket for two removable inserts that fit inside (Fig. 6-8). The insert tanks usually hold 3.8 L (1 gallon) of developer or fixer and are placed within the outer, larger master tank. The outer tank holds the running water for maintaining the temperature of the developer and fixer in the insert tanks and for washing films. The developer customarily is placed in the insert tank on the left side of the master tank and the fixer in the insert tank on the right. All three tanks should be made of stainless steel, which does not react with the processing solutions and is easy to clean. The master tank should have a cover to reduce oxidation of the processing solutions, protect the developing film from accidental exposure to light, and minimize evaporation of the processing solutions.

THERMOMETER

The temperature of the developing, fixing, and washing solutions should be closely controlled. A thermometer can be left in the water circulating through the master tank to monitor its temperature. The most desirable thermometers clip onto the side of the tank. Thermometers may contain alcohol or metal, but they should not contain mercury because they could break and contaminate the processor or solutions.

TIMER

The x-ray film must be exposed to the processing chemicals for specific intervals. An interval timer is

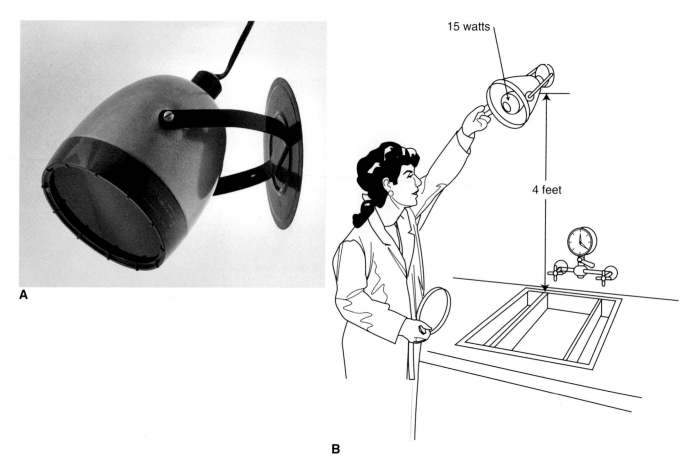

A   B

FIG. **6-6** **A,** A safelight may be mounted on the wall or ceiling in the darkroom and should be at least 4 feet from the work surface. **B,** The safelight uses a GBX-2 filter and 15-watt bulb.

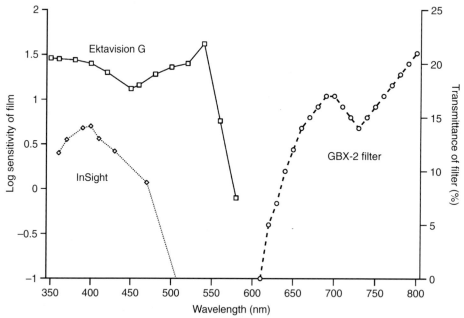

FIG. **6-7** Spectral sensitivities of Ektavision G film *(heavy line with squares)* and InSight film *(thin line with diamonds)* shown with the transmission characteristics of a GBX-2 filter *(broken line with circles)*. Note that the films are more sensitive in the blue-green portion of the spectrum (shorter than 600 nm); the GBX-2 filter transmits primarily red light (longer than 600 nm).

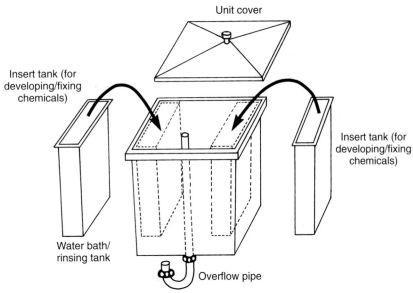

FIG. **6-8** *Processing tank.* The developing and fixing tanks are inserted into a bath of running water with an overflow drain.

indispensable for controlling development and fixation times.

DRYING RACKS

Two or three drying racks can be mounted on a convenient wall for film hangers. Drip trays are placed underneath the racks to catch water that may run off the wet films. An electric fan can be used to circulate the air and speed the drying of films, but it should not be pointed directly at the films. Also, cabinet dryers are available that circulate warm air around the film and accelerate drying. Excessive heat must be avoided because it may damage the emulsion. If dryers are installed in the darkroom, they should be ventilated outside the darkroom to preclude high humidity and heat, which are detrimental to any unexposed film stored in the room.

Manual Processing Procedures

Manual processing of film requires the following eight steps:

1. *Replenish solutions*—The first step in manual tank processing is to replenish the developer and fixer. Add fresh developer (replenisher) and fixer (8 ounces per gallon) to maintain the proper strength of each solution. Check the solution levels to ensure that the developer and fixer cover the films on the top clips of the film hangers.

2. *Stir solutions*—Next, stir the developer and fixing solution to mix the chemicals and equalize the temperature throughout the tanks. To prevent cross-contamination, use a separate paddle for each solution. It is best to label one paddle for the developer and the other for the fixer. Because proper developing time varies with the temperature of the solution, check the temperature of the developer after stirring.

3. *Mount films on hangers*—Using only safelight illumination in the darkroom, remove the exposed film from its lightproof packet or cassette. Hold the films only by their edges to avoid damage to the film surface. Clip the bare film onto a film hanger, one film to a clip (Fig. 6-9). To avoid any possible confusion later, label the film racks with the patient's name and the exposure date.

4. *Set timer*—Check the temperature of the developer and set the interval timer to the time indicated by the manufacturer for the solution temperature. For intraoral film processing in conventional solutions, use the following development times:

TEMPERATURE	DEVELOPMENT TIME
68° F	5 minutes
70° F	$4^1/_2$ minutes
72° F	4 minutes
76° F	3 minutes
80° F	$2^1/_2$ minutes

Processing films at either higher or lower temperatures and for longer or shorter times than recommended by the manufacturer reduces the contrast of

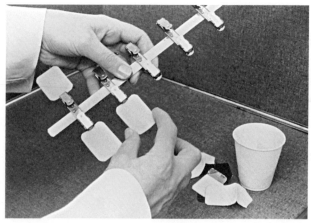

FIG. **6-9**   Films are mounted securely on film clips. Film is always held by its edges to avoid fingerprints on the image. (Courtesy C.L. Crabtree, DDS, Bureau of Radiological Health, Rockville, Md.)

the processed film. Also, processing too long or at temperatures higher than those recommended can result in film fog, which may diminish film contrast and diagnostic information.

5. *Develop*—Start the timer mechanism and immerse the hanger and films immediately in the developer. Agitate the hanger mildly for 5 seconds to sweep air bubbles off the film. Leave the films in the developer for the predetermined time without further agitation. When removing the films, drain the excess developer into the wash bath.

6. *Rinse*—After development, remove the film hanger from the developer and place in the running water bath for 30 seconds. Agitate the films continuously in the rinse water to remove excess developer, thus slowing development and minimizing contamination of the fixer.

7. *Fix*—Place the hanger and film in the fixer solution for 10 minutes and agitate for 5 of every 30 seconds. This eliminates bubbles and brings fresh fixer into contact with the emulsion. Excess fixation (several hours) removes some of the metallic silver grains, diminishing the density of the film. When the films are removed, drain the excess fixer into the wash bath.

8. *Wash and dry*—After fixation of the films is complete, place the hanger in running water for at least 10 minutes to remove residual processing solutions. After the films have been washed, remove surface moisture by gently shaking excess water from the films and hanger. Dry the films in circulating, moderately warm air. If the films dry rapidly with small drops of water clinging to their surface, the areas under the drops dry more slowly than the surrounding areas. This uneven drying causes distor-

tion of the gelatin, leaving a drying artifact in some cases. The result is spots that frequently are visible and detract from the usefulness of the finished radiograph. After drying, the films are ready to mount.

Rapid-Processing Chemicals

In recent years a number of manufacturers have produced rapid-processing solutions. These solutions typically develop films in 15 seconds and fix them in 15 seconds at room temperature. They have the same general formulation as conventional processing solutions but often contain a higher concentration of hydroquinone. They also have a more alkaline pH than conventional solutions, which causes the emulsion to swell more, thus providing greater access to developer. These solutions are especially advantageous in endodontics and in emergency situations, when short processing time is essential. Although the resultant images may be satisfactory, they often do not achieve the same degree of contrast as films processed conventionally, and they may discolor over time if not fully washed. After viewing, rapidly processed films are placed in conventional fixing solution for 4 minutes and washed for 10 minutes. This improves the contrast and helps keep them stable in storage. Conventional solutions are preferred for most routine use.

Changing Solutions

All processing solutions deteriorate as a result of continued use and exposure to air. Although regular replenishment of the developer and fixer prolongs their useful life, the buildup of reaction products eventually causes these solutions to cease functioning properly. Exhaustion of the developer results from oxidation of the developing agents, depletion of the hydroquinone, and buildup of bromide. Use of exhausted developer results in films that show reduced density and contrast. When fixer becomes exhausted, silver thiosulfate complexes form and halide ions build up. The increased concentration of silver thiosulfate complexes slows the rate of diffusion of these complexes from the emulsion. The halide ions slow the rate of clearing of unexposed silver halide crystals. These changes result in films with incomplete clearing that turn brown with age. With regular replenishment, solutions may last 3 or 4 weeks before they must be changed. When the developer and fixer are replaced, the solutions must be prepared according to the directions on the containers.

A simple procedure can help determine when solutions should be changed. A double film packet instead of a single film packet is exposed on one projection for the first patient radiographed after new solutions have been prepared. One film is placed in the patient's chart, and the other is mounted on a corner of a viewbox in the darkroom. As successive films are processed, they are compared with this reference film. Loss of image contrast and density become evident as the solutions deteriorate, indicating when the time has come to change them. The fixer is changed when the developer is changed.

Automatic Film Processing

Equipment is available that automates all processing steps (Fig. 6-10). Although automatic processing has a number of advantages, the most important is the time saved. Depending on the equipment and the temperature of operation, an automatic processor requires only 4 to 6 minutes to develop, fix, wash, and dry a film. Many dental automatic processors have a light-shielded (daylight loading) compartment in which the operator can unwrap films and feed them into the machine without working in a darkroom. This is desirable because the individual doing the developing does not have to work in the dark. However, special care must be taken to maintain infection control when using these daylight-loading compartments (see Chapter 7).

When extraoral films are processed, the light-shielded compartment is removed to provide room for feeding the larger film into the processor. Another

attractive feature of the automatic system is that the density and contrast of the radiographs tend to be consistent. However, because of the higher temperature of the developer and the artifacts caused by rollers, the quality of films processed automatically often is not as high as that of those carefully developed manually. With automatically processed films, more grain usually is evident in the final image.

Whether automatic processing equipment is appropriate for a specific practice depends on the dentist and the nature and volume of the practice. The equipment is expensive and must be cleaned frequently. Also, the automated equipment may break down, and conventional darkroom equipment may still be needed as a backup system.

MECHANISM

Automatic processors have an in-line arrangement. Typically, this consists of a transport mechanism that picks up the unwrapped film and passes it through the developing, fixing, washing, and drying sections (Fig. 6-11). The transport system most often used is a series of rollers driven by a constant-speed motor that operates through gears, belts, or chains. The rollers often consist of independent assemblies of multiple rollers in a rack, with one rack for each step in the operation. Although these assemblies are designed and positioned so that the film crosses over from one roller to the next, the operator may remove them independently for soaking, cleaning, and repairing.

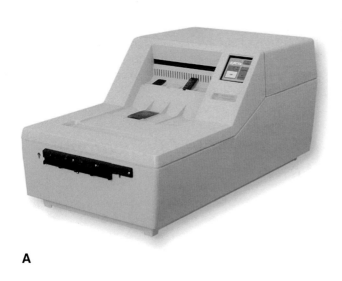

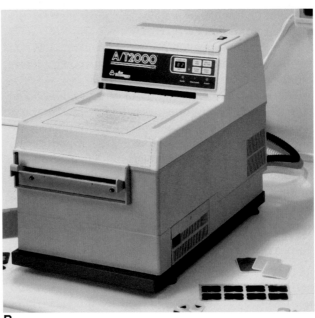

A

B

FIG. **6-10** *Automatic film processors.* **A,** Excel. **B,** A/T 2000XR. (**A,** Courtesy Dent-X, Elmsford, N.Y.; **B,** courtesy Air Techniques, Inc., Hicksville, N.Y.)

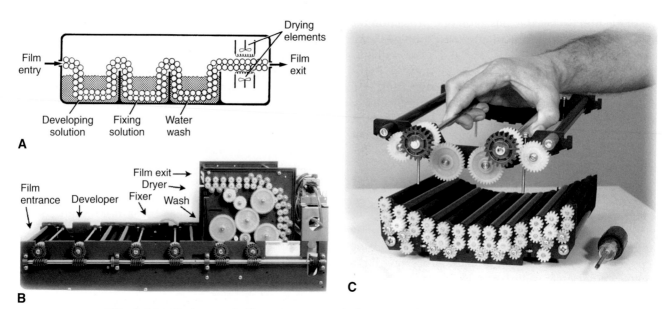

FIG. **6-11**   **A,** Automatic film processors typically consist of a roller assembly that transports the film through developing, fixing, washing, and drying stations. **B,** Internal assembly demonstrating series of developer, fixer, and wash stations with dryer unit above wash station. **C,** Detail of one of the roller units that advances the film through the processing solutions. (**B** and **C,** Courtesy Dent-X, Elmsford, N.Y.)

The primary function of the rollers is to move the film through the developing solutions, but they also serve at least three other purposes. First, their motion helps keep the solutions agitated, which contributes to the uniformity of processing. Second, in the developer, fixer, and water tanks the rollers press on the film emulsion, forcing some solution out of the emulsion. The emulsions rapidly fill again with solution, thus promoting solution exchange. Finally, the top rollers at the crossover point between the developer and fixer tanks remove developing solution, minimizing carryover of developer into the fixer tank. This feature helps maintain the uniformity of processing chemicals.

The chemical compositions of the developer and fixer are modified to operate at higher temperatures than those used for manual processing and to meet the more rapid development, fixing, washing, and drying requirements of automatic processing. The fixer has an additional hardener that helps the emulsion withstand the rigors of the transport system.

REPLENISHMENT

It is important to maintain the constituents of the developer and fixer carefully to preserve the optimal sensitometric and physical properties of the film emulsion within the narrow limits imposed by the speed and temperature of automatic processing. As the activity of the developing and fixing solutions lessens, its effect on the film diminishes. To compensate for this loss of activity, some automatic processors include an automatic replenishment system, which adds fresh developer to the developer tank and fresh fixer to the fixer tank. As with manual processing, 8 ounces of fresh developer and fixer should be added per gallon of solution per day. This assumes an average workload of 30 intraoral or 5 extraoral films per day. Insufficient replenishment of the developer results in a loss of image contrast. Exhaustion of the fixing solution causes poor clearing of the film, insufficient hardening of the emulsion, and unreliable transport from the fixer assembly through the drying operation.

Management of Radiographic Wastes

To prevent environmental damage, many communities and states have passed laws governing the disposal of wastes. Such laws often derive from the federal Resource Conservation and Recovery Act of 1976. Although dental radiographic waste constitutes only a small potential hazard, it should be discarded properly. The primary ingredient of concern in processing solutions is the dissolved silver found in used fixer. Another material of concern is the lead foil found in film packets.

Several means are available for properly disposing of the silver and lead. Silver may be recovered from the fixer by using either metallic replacement or electroplating methods. Metallic replacement uses cartridges through which waste solutions are poured. In this process, iron goes into the solution and the silver precipitates as a sludge. In the electroplating method, the waste solutions come in contact with two electrodes, through which a current passes. The cathode captures the silver. In either case, the scrap silver can be sold to silver refiners and buyers.

The lead foil is separated from the packet and collected until enough has been accumulated to sell to a scrap metal dealer. Dental offices also should consider using companies licensed to pick up waste materials.

The names of such companies can be found in the telephone directory or obtained from the state hazardous waste management agency.

Common Causes of Faulty Radiographs

Although film processing can produce radiographs of excellent quality, inattention to detail may lead to many problems and images that are diagnostically suboptimal. Poor radiographs contribute to a loss of diagnostic information and loss of professional and patient time. Box 6-1 presents a list of common causes of faulty radiographs. The steps necessary for correction are self-evident.

BOX **6-1**
Common Problems in Film Exposure and Development

Light Radiographs (Fig. 6-12)
- Processing errors
  Underdevelopment (temperature too low; time too short; thermometer inaccurate)
  Depleted developer solution
  Diluted or contaminated developer
  Excessive fixation
- Underexposure
  Insufficient milliamperage
  Insufficient peak kilovoltages
  Insufficient time
  Film-source distance too great
  Film packet reversed in mouth (Fig. 6-13)

Dark Radiographs (Fig. 6-14)
- Processing errors
  Overdevelopment (temperature too high; time too long)
  Developer concentration too high
  Inadequate fixation
  Accidental exposure to light
  Improper safelighting
- Overexposure
  Excessive milliamperage
  Excessive peak kilovoltage
  Excessive time
  Film-source distance too short

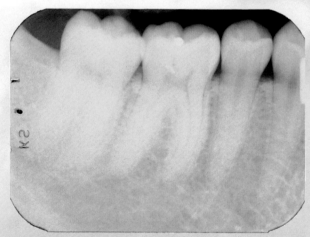

FIG. **6-12**   A radiograph that is too light because of inadequate processing or insufficient exposure.

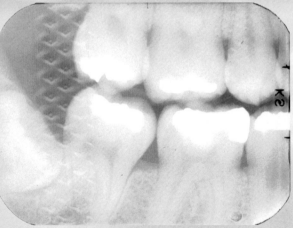

FIG. **6-13**   A radiograph that is too light because the film packet was placed backward in the patient's mouth. Note the characteristic markings caused by exposure through the lead foil in the film packaging.

Continued

BOX **6-1**
Common Problems in Film Exposure and Development—cont'd.

Insufficient Contrast (Fig. 6-15)
- Underdevelopment
- Underexposure
- Excessive peak kilovoltage
- Excessive film fog

Film Fog (Fig. 6-16)
- Improper safelighting (improper filter; excessive bulb wattage; inadequate distance between safelight and work surface; prolonged exposure to safelight)
- Light leaks (cracked safelight filter; light from doors, vents, or other sources)
- Overdevelopment
- Contaminated solutions
- Deteriorated film (stored at high temperature; stored at high humidity; exposed to radiation; outdated)

Dark Spots or Lines (Fig. 6-17)
- Fingerprint contamination
- Black wrapping paper sticking to film surface
- Film in contact with tank or another film during fixation

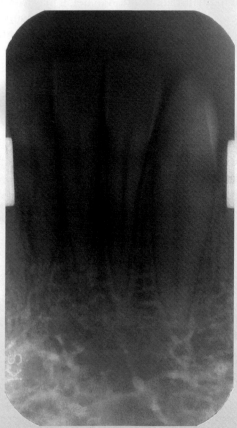

FIG. **6-14** A radiograph that is too dark because of overdevelopment or overexposure.

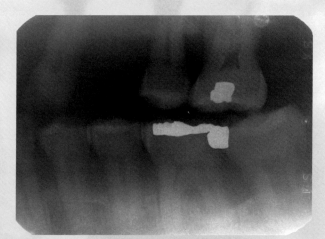

FIG. **6-16** Fogged radiograph marked by lack of image detail.

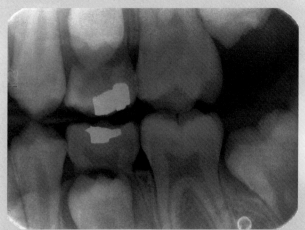

FIG. **6-15** A radiograph with insufficient contrast, showing gray enamel and gray pulp chambers.

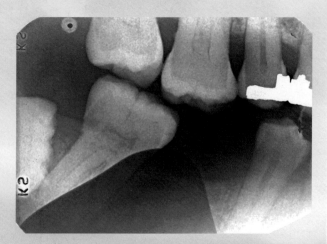

FIG. **6-17** Dark spot on an x-ray film caused by film contact with the tank wall during fixation.

BOX 6-1
Common Problems in Film Exposure and Development—cont'd.

- Film contaminated with developer before processing
- Excessive bending of film
- Static discharge to film before processing
- Excessive roller pressure during automatic processing
- Dirty rollers in automatic processing

Light Spots (Fig. 6-18)
- Film contaminated with fixer before processing
- Film in contact with tank or another film during development
- Excessive bending of film

Yellow or Brown Stains
- Depleted developer
- Depleted fixer
- Insufficient washing
- Contaminated solutions

Blurring (Fig. 6-19)
- Movement of patient
- Movement of x-ray tube head
- Double exposure

Partial Images (Fig. 6-20)
- Top of film not immersed in developing solution
- Misalignment of x-ray tube head ("cone cut")

Emulsion Peel
- Abrasion of image during processing
- Excessive time in wash water

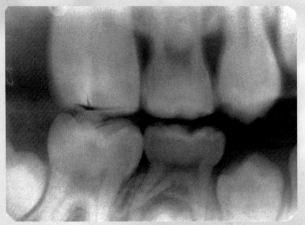

FIG. **6-19** Blurred radiograph caused by movement of the patient during exposure.

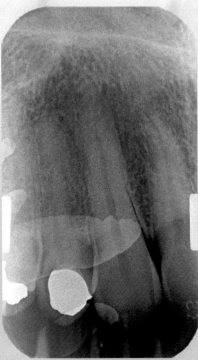

FIG. **6-18** Light spots on an x-ray film caused by film contact with drops of fixer before processing.

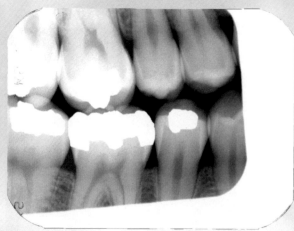

FIG. **6-20** Partial image caused by poor alignment of the tube head with the film rectangular collimator.

Mounting Radiographs

Radiographs must be preserved and maintained in the most satisfactory and useful condition. Periapical, interproximal, and occlusal films are best handled and stored in a film mount (Fig. 6-21). The operator can handle them with greater ease, and there is less chance of damaging the emulsion. Mounts are made of plastic or cardboard and may have a clear plastic window that covers and protects the film. However, the window may have scratches or imperfections that interfere with radiographic interpretation. The operator can arrange several films from the same individual in a film mount in the proper anatomic relationship. This facilitates correlation of the clinical and radiographic examinations. Opaque mounts are best because they prevent stray light from the viewbox from reaching the viewer's eyes.

The preferred method of positioning periapical and occlusal films in the film mount is to arrange them so that the images of the teeth are in the anatomic position and have the same relationship to the viewer as when the viewer faces the patient. The radiographs of the teeth in the right quadrants should be placed in the left side of the mount and those of the left quadrants in the right side. This system, advocated by the American Dental Association, allows the examiner's gaze to shift from radiograph to tooth without crossing the midline. The alternative arrangement, with the images of the right quadrants on the right side of the mount and those of the left quadrant on the left, is not recommended.

Identification Dot

A round impression in a corner of each film, the "dot," allows rapid and proper film orientation (Fig. 6-22). The manufacturer orients the film in the packet so that the convex side of the dot is toward the front of the packet and faces the source of radiation. Consequently, to mount the films with the images of the teeth in the anatomic position as described above, each film is first oriented with the convex side of the dot toward the viewer. Then, on the basis of the features of the teeth and anatomic landmarks in the adjacent bone, the films are arranged in their normal sequential relationship in the mount.

Duplicating Radiographs

Occasionally radiographs must be duplicated; this is best accomplished with duplicating film. The film to be duplicated is placed against the emulsion side of the duplicating film, and the two films are held in position by a glass-topped cassette or photographic printing frame. The films are exposed to light, which passes through the clear areas of the original radiograph and exposes the duplicating film. The duplicating film is then processed in conventional x-ray processing solutions.

Unlike conventional x-ray film, duplicating film gives a positive image. Thus areas exposed to light come out clear, as on the original radiograph. Duplication typically results in images with less resolution and more

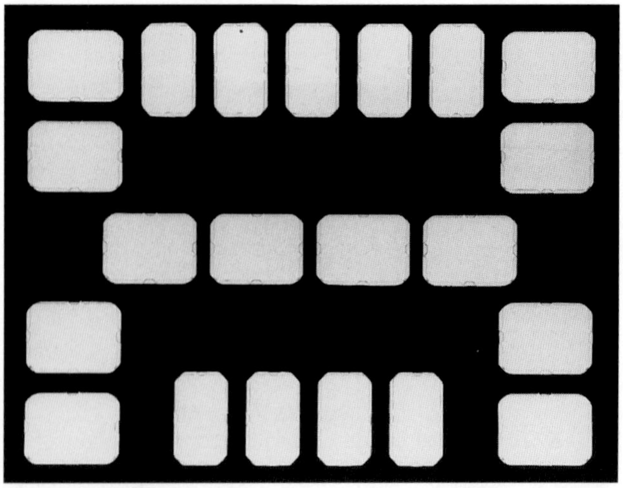

FIG. **6-21** Film mount for holding nine narrow anterior periapical views, eight posterior periapical view, and four bitewing views.

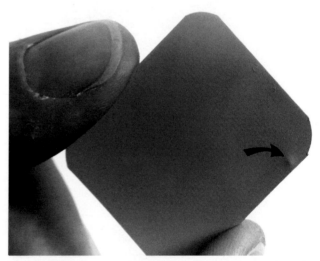

FIG. **6-22** The raised film dot (arrow) indicates the tube side of the film and identifies the patient's right and left sides.

contrast than the original radiograph. The best images are obtained when a circular, ultraviolet light source is used. In contrast to the usual negative film, images on duplicating film that are too dark or too light are underexposed or overexposed, respectively.

BIBLIOGRAPHY

Akdeniz BG, Lomcali G: Densitometric evaluation of four radiographic processing solutions, Dentomaxillofac Radiol 27:102-6, 1998.

Eikenberg S, Vandre R: Comparison of digital dental X-ray systems with self-developing film and manual processing for endodontic file length determination, J Endod 26:65-7, 2000.

Farman TT, Farman AG: Evaluation of a new F speed dental X-ray film. The effect of processing solutions and a comparison with D and E speed films, Dentomaxillofac Radiol 29:41-5, 2000.

Fitterman AS et al: Processing chemistry for medical imaging, Technical and Scientific Monograph No 5, N-327, Rochester, N.Y., 1995, Eastman Kodak.

Geist JR, Gleason MJ: Densitometric properties of rapid manual processing solutions: abbreviated versus complete rapid processing, J Endod 21:180-4, 1995.

Haist G: Modern photographic processing, vol 1, New York, 1979, Wiley & Sons.

Kitts EL: The AAPM/RSNA physics tutorial for residents: physics and chemistry of film and processing, Radiographics 16:1467, 1996.

Lindequist S, Madsen JE, Christensen I, Nielsen B: Film processing and the environment. Reducing pollution, water consumption, and costs, Acta Radiol 39:332-6, 1998.

Ludlow JB, Platin E, Delano EO, Clifton L: The efficacy of caries detection using three intraoral films under different processing conditions, J Am Dent Assoc 128:1401-8, 1997.

Mees DEK, James TH: The theory of the photographic process, New York, 1977, Macmillan.

Rout PG, Rogers SN, Chapman M, Rippin JW: A comparison of manual and automatic processing in general dental practice, Br Dent J 181:99-101, 1996.

Syriopoulos K, Velders XL, Sanderink GC, van Ginkel FC, van der Stelt PF: Sensitometric evaluation of four dental x-ray films using five processing solutions, Dentomaxillofac Radiol 28:73-9, 1999.

Stanczyk DA, Paunovich ED, Broome JC, Fatone MA: Microbiologic contamination during dental radiographic film processing, Oral Surg Oral Med Oral Pathol 76:112-9, 1993.

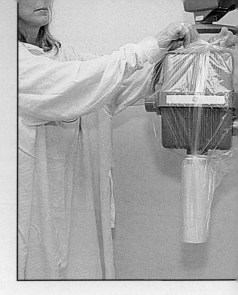

CHAPTER 7

Radiographic Quality Assurance and Infection Control

A *quality assurance program in radiology* is a series of procedures made to ensure optimal and consistent operation of each component in the imaging chain. When all components are functioning properly, the result is consistently high-quality radiographs made with low exposure to patients and office personnel.

The goal of an infection control program is to avoid cross-contamination among patients and between patients and operators.

Radiographic Quality Assurance

Because radiographs are indispensable for patient diagnosis, the dentist must ensure that optimal exposure and film processing conditions are maintained. To reach this goal, a quality assurance program includes evaluation of the performance of x-ray machines, manual and automatic processing procedures, image receptors, and viewing conditions. Optimization of these components results in the most diagnostic images and the lowest exposure for patients. It is best if one individual is given the responsibility for implementing the quality assurance program and to take corrective action when indicated. Most of these steps are quickly accomplished yet can have a significant influence on radiographic quality (Box 7-1).

DAILY TASKS

Several tasks should be performed daily to ensure excellent radiographs.

Compare Radiographs With Reference Film

A simple and effective means for constant monitoring of the quality of images produced in an office is to check daily films against a reference film. Soon after film-processing solutions are replaced, mount a patient film that has been properly exposed and processed with exact time-temperature technique on a corner of the viewbox. This image, with optimal density and contrast, serves as a reference for the radiographs made in the following days and weeks (Fig. 7-1). All subsequent images should be compared with this reference film.

Comparison of daily images with the reference film may reveal problems before they interfere with the diagnostic quality of the images. When a problem is identified, it is important to determine the probable source and take corrective action. For instance, if the processing solutions have become depleted, the resultant radiographs are light and have reduced contrast. Both developer and fixer should be changed when degradation of the image quality is evident. Light images may also result from cold solutions or insufficient developing time. Dark images may be caused by excessive developing time, developer that is too warm, or light leaks.

Enter Findings in Retake Log

Another simple and effective means of reducing the number of faulty radiographs is to keep a retake log. Record all errors for films that must be reexposed.

Replenish Processing Solutions

At the beginning of each workday, check the levels of the processing solutions and replenish if necessary. Replenish the developer with fresh developing solution and the fixer with fresh fixing solution.

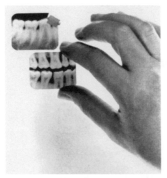

FIG. **7-1** Check radiographs daily against a reference film made with fresh solutions. As processing solutions become exhausted, the daily images become increasingly light and lose contrast. When these changes are clear, change both the developer and the fixer. (Courtesy C.L. Crabtree, DDS, Bureau of Radiological Health, Rockville, Md.)

BOX 7-1
Schedule of Radiographic Quality Assurance Procedures

Daily
- Compare radiographs with reference film
- Enter findings in retake log
- Replenish processing solutions
- Check temperature of processing solutions
- Make step-wedge test of processing system

Weekly
- Replace processing solutions
- Clean processing equipment
- Clean viewboxes
- Review retake log

Monthly
- Check darkroom safelighting
- Clean intensifying screens
- Rotate film stock
- Check exposure charts

Yearly
- Calibrate x-ray machine

Check Temperature of Processing Solutions

At the beginning of each workday, check the temperature of the processing solutions. The solutions must reach the optimal temperature before use—68° F (20° C) for manual processing and 82° F (28° C) for heated automatic processors. The instructions accompanying the film and processor verify the optimal temperature. Unheated automatic processors should be located away from windows or heaters that may cause their temperature to vary during the day. Proper temperature regulation is required for accurate time-temperature processing.

Make Step-Wedge Test of Processing System

Quality control of manual and automatic film processing is important because deficiencies in this process are the most common cause of faulty radiographs. A step-wedge test provides accurate monitoring of day-to-day processing conditions. It measures the speed of the imaging system and image contrast. Both are sensitive measures of the processing environment. A step wedge is readily made with the lead foil from film packets. Stack five sheets together and staple at one end (Fig. 7-2). Cut off 4/5 of the top layer, 3/5 of the second layer, 2/5 of the third layer, and 1/5 of the fourth layer to create a five-step wedge. Lay the wedge on top of a film packet and expose using the usual setting for an adult bitewing view. The resultant image should show five steps from dark to light. Save the first film after changing to fresh processing solution for comparison with images made on subsequent days.

Monitor the processing solutions at the beginning of each day with a step-wedge image to ensure that the processing system is operational for patient care. If a step-wedge image is too light, it is most likely that the processing solutions are depleted or too cold. If the solutions are at the proper temperature, the developer has become depleted and should be changed. Solutions that are excessively warm cause a dark image.

WEEKLY TASKS

Replace Processing Solutions

The replacement frequency of processing solutions depends primarily on the rate of use of the solutions but also on the size of tanks, whether a cover is used, and the temperature of the solutions. In most offices the solutions should be changed weekly or every other week. The results of the step-wedge test will help determine the proper frequency.

Clean Processing Equipment

Regular cleaning of the processing equipment is necessary for optimal operation. Clean the solution tanks of manual and automatic processing equipment when the solutions are changed. Clean the rollers of automatic film processors weekly according to the manufacturer's instructions. After cleaning, rinse the tanks and rollers twice as long as the manufacturer recommends to prevent the cleaner from interfering with the action of the film-processing solutions.

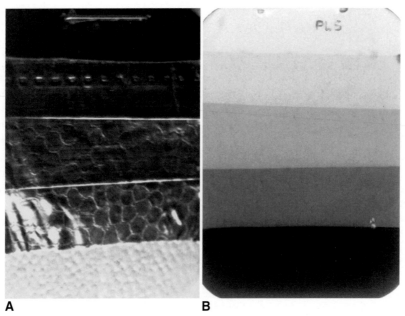

FIG. **7-2**   **A,** Step wedge made of strips of lead foil from film packets. This step wedge is positioned over a film, and an exposure is made. **B,** Processed radiograph showing each step. Such an image should be made daily after replenishing processing solutions and compared with an image made with fresh solutions. When the step wedge has become one full step lighter, it is time to change both the developer and the fixer.

Clean Viewboxes

Clean viewboxes weekly to remove any particles or defects that may interfere with film interpretation.

Review Retake Log

Review the retake record weekly and identify any recurring problems with film processing conditions or operator technique. Use this information to educate staff or to initiate corrective actions.

MONTHLY TASKS

Check Darkroom Safelighting

Film becomes fogged in the darkroom because of inappropriate safelight filters, excessive exposure to safelights, and stray light from other sources. Such films are dark, show low contrast, and have a muddy gray appearance. Inspect the darkroom monthly to assess the integrity of the safelights (preferably GBX-2 filters with 15-watt bulbs). The glass filter should be intact, with no cracks. To check for light leaks in a darkroom, turn off all lights, allow your vision to accommodate to the dark, and check for light leaks, especially around doors and vents. Mark light leaks with chalk or masking tape. Weather stripping is useful for sealing light leaks under doors.

The following simple penny test can be used monthly to evaluate for fogging caused by inappropriate safe-lighting conditions (Fig. 7-3):

1. Open the packet of an exposed film and place the test film in the area where the films are usually unwrapped and clipped on the film hanger.
2. Place a penny on the film and leave it in this position for the approximate time required to unwrap and mount a full-mouth set of films, usually about 5 minutes.
3. Develop the test film as usual. If the image of the penny is visible on the resultant film, the room is not light-safe for the particular film tested. Each type of film used in the office should be tested to measure the integrity of the darkroom.

Clean Intensifying Screens

Clean all intensifying screens in panoramic and cephalometric film cassettes monthly. The presence of scratches or debris results in recurring light areas on the resultant images. The foam supporting the screens must be intact and capable of holding both screens closely against the film. If close contact between the film and screens is not maintained, the image loses sharpness.

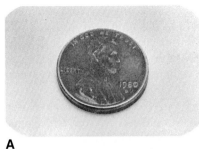

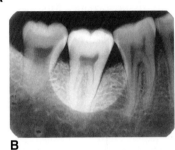

FIG. **7-3** *Penny test for unsafe illumination.* **A,** Leave a penny on the exposed duplicate film from the double-film pack on the working surface during the time that any film would be opened (usually about 5 minutes). **B,** If the processed radiograph shows an outline of the penny, the film is being fogged by inappropriate safelighting conditions.

X-ray machine: brand name		
Location: room		
mA: 15		
kVp: 70		
E-speed film: brand name		

	Exposure time	
Projection	Seconds	Impulses
Adult periapicals		
Incisors	0.25	15
Premolars	0.30	18
Molars	0.35	21
Occlusal	0.40	24
Adult bitewings		
Premolar	0.30	18
Molar	0.35	21
Edentulous periapicals		
Incisors	0.20	12
Premolars	0.25	15
Molars	0.30	18
Occlusal	0.35	21
Children		
Anterior periapicals	0.25	15
Posterior periapicals	0.25	15
Bitewing	0.25	15
Occlusal	0.30	18

FIG. **7-4** Sample wall chart showing identification information for x-ray machine, film type, mA and kVp settings, and appropriate exposure times for various anatomic locations and patient sizes. Note that the optimal exposure times must be determined empirically in each office because they vary with the machine settings used, source-to-skin distance, and other factors.

Rotate Film Stock

Dental x-ray film is quite stable when properly handled. Store it in a cool, dry facility away from a radiation source. Rotate stock when new film is received so that old film does not accumulate in storage. Always use the oldest film first—but never after its expiration date has passed.

Check Exposure Charts

Each month inspect exposure tables listing the proper peak kilovoltage (kVp), milliamperes (mA), and exposure times for making radiographs of each region of the oral cavity posted by each x-ray machine (Fig. 7-4). Verify that the information is legible and accurate. These tables help ensure that all operators use the appropriate exposure factors. Typically the mA is fixed at its highest setting; the kVp is fixed, usually at 70 kVp; and the exposure time is varied to account for patient size and location of the area of interest in the mouth. Exposure times are initially determined empirically. Careful time-temperature processing (described in Chapter 6) must be used with fresh solutions during this initial determination of exposure times.

YEARLY TASKS

Calibrate X-Ray Machine

X-ray machines are generally quite stable and only rarely is a malfunction of the machine the cause of poor radiographs. Accordingly, machines need to be calibrated only annually unless a specific problem is identified or substantive repair is necessary that may affect operation. Usually dental service companies or health physicists should make these machine measurements because of the specialized equipment required. The following parameters should be measured:

1. X-ray output—Use a radiation dosimeter to measure the intensity and reproducibility of radiation output (Fig. 7-5). Acceptable values are shown in Fig. 3-2.
2. Collimation and beam alignment—The field diameter for dental intraoral x-ray machines should be no greater than $2\frac{3}{4}$ inches. The tip of the position-indicating device (PID, aiming cylinder) should be

closely aligned with the x-ray beam. This may be evaluated by making a star pattern with dental films, marking them with pinholes, and centering the aiming cylinder over the pattern (Fig. 7-6). Expose the films using usual bitewing values, process the films, and reconstitute the star pattern. The size and alignment of the beam can then be determined.

For panoramic machines the beam exiting the patient should not be larger than the film slit holding the film cassette. This may be tested by taping dental films in front of and behind the slit. A pin stick should be made through both films to allow subsequent

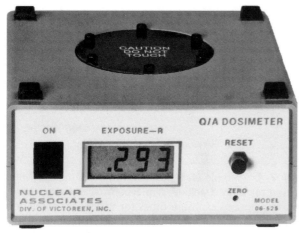

FIG. **7-5** *Device for measuring exposure output of an x-ray machine.* The aiming cylinder of the x-ray machine is positioned on the center of the top and an exposure made. The display on the front gives the output in Roentgens.

realignment. Expose, process, and realign both films. The exposure to the film in front of the slit should be comparable in size to the film exposure behind the slit. Service is required if the front film exposure is larger than or not well oriented with the film exposure behind the slit.

3. Beam energy—The kVp or half-value layer (HVL) of the beam should be measured to ensure that the beam has sufficient energy for film exposure without excessive soft tissue dosage. Measurement of kVp requires specialized equipment. It should be accurate within 5 kVp. Measurement of HVL requires a dosimeter. The HVL should be at least 1.5 mm aluminum (Al) at 70 kVp and 2.5 mm Al at 90 kVp.

4. Timer—Electric pulse counters count the number of pulses generated by an x-ray machine during a preset time interval. The timer should be accurate and reproducible.

5. mA—Verify the linearity of the mA control if two or more mA settings are available on the machine. Make an exposure using the usual adult bitewing setting. Then reduce the mA to the lower value and select another exposure time, ensuring that the product of the mA and time in seconds (impulses) is the same as for the adult bitewing. For example, if the machine has 10- and 15-mA settings, and 15 mA and 24 impulses are used for adult bitewings, select 15 mA and 24 impulses for the first exposure and measure the dose. Make a second exposure at 10 mA and 36 impulses and measure the dose. The dose at each exposure combination should be the same ($15 \times 24 = 10 \times 36$). A discrepancy implies nonlinearity in the mA control or a fault in the timer.

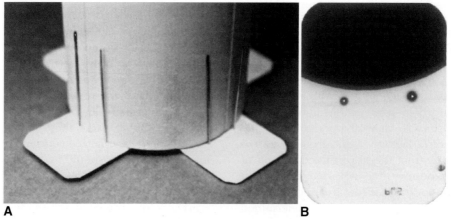

A   **B**

FIG. **7-6** **A,** The alignment of the collimation of the x-ray beam and the end of the aiming cylinder can be checked by making a cross pattern of film, centering the aiming cylinder, marking the periphery with needles, and making an exposure. **B,** One of the processed radiographs showing the dark exposed area just inside the holes. If this pattern is seen on all films, then good alignment is demonstrated.

The step wedge described above may also be used in place of the dosimeter. In this case the density of each step of each image should be the same.

6. Tube head stability—The tube head should be stable when placed around the patient's head, and it should not drift during the exposure. When the tube head is not stable, service is necessary to adjust the suspension mechanism.

7. Focal spot size—Measure the size of the focal spot because it may become enlarged with excessive heat buildup within an x-ray machine. An enlarged focal spot contributes to geometric fuzziness in the resultant image. A specialized piece of equipment is required for this test.

Infection Control

Dental personnel and patients are at increased risk for acquiring tuberculosis, herpes viruses, upper respiratory infections, and hepatitis strains A through E. After the recognition of acquired immunodeficiency syndrome (AIDS) in the 1980s, rigorous hygienic procedures were introduced in dental offices. The primary goal of infection-control procedures is to prevent cross-contamination between patients as well as between patients and health care providers. The potential for cross-contamination in dental radiography is great. An operator's hands may become contaminated by contact with a patient's mouth and saliva-contaminated films and film holders. The operator then must adjust the x-ray tube head and PID, as well as the x-ray machine control panel, to make the exposure. Cross-contamination also may occur when operators open film packets to process the films in the darkroom. The procedures described in the following sections minimize or eliminate cross-contamination (Box 7-2). Each dental office or practice should have a written policy describing its infection control practices. It is best if one individual in

a practice, usually the dentist, assumes responsibility for implementing these procedures. This person also educates other members of the practice.

APPLY UNIVERSAL PRECAUTIONS

Universal precautions are infection control guidelines designed to protect workers from exposure to diseases spread by blood and certain body fluids. Under universal precautions, all human blood and saliva are treated as if known to be infectious for human immunodeficiency virus (HIV) and hepatitis B virus. Accordingly, the means used to protect against cross-contamination are used universally, that is, for all individuals. The American Dental Association and the Centers for Disease Control and Prevention stress the use of universal precautions because many patients are unaware that they are carriers of infectious disease or choose not to reveal this information.

Wear Gloves During All Radiographic Procedures

Always wear gloves when making radiographs or handling contaminated film packets or associated materials such as cotton rolls and film-holding instruments, or when removing barrier protections from surfaces and radiographic equipment. After seating the patient, wash your hands and put on disposable gloves in sight of the patient if the operatory arrangement permits.

Keep charts away from sources of contamination and do not handle them during the radiographic examination. Make chair adjustments in advance, or make adjustments on control surfaces that are covered, such as the headrest control.

Disinfect and Cover X-Ray Machine, Working Surfaces, Chair, and Apron

The goal of preventing cross-contamination is addressed in part by disinfecting all surfaces and by using barriers to isolate equipment from direct contact. Although barriers greatly aid infection control, they do not replace the need for effective surface cleaning and disinfection. Experience has demonstrated that, during the daily activity of treatment, failure of mechanical barriers is common. It is advantageous and reassuring to the operator to know that whenever this happens, the surfaces that may become accidentally exposed are clean and disinfected. Any surface that may be contaminated should be surface-disinfected. This includes the x-ray machine control panel, tube head, and beam alignment device, dental chair and headrest, surfaces on which film is placed, leaded apron and thyroid collar, and doorknob of operatory. Operators should avoid touching walls and other surfaces with contami-

---

> **BOX 7-2**
> ## Key Steps in Radiographic Infection Control
>
> - Apply Universal Precautions
> - Wear Gloves During All Radiographic Procedures
> - Disinfect and Cover X-Ray Machine, Working Surfaces, Chair, and Apron
> - Sterilize Nondisposable Instruments
> - Use Barrier-Protected Film (Sensor) or Disposable Container
> - Prevent Contamination of Processing Equipment

nated gloves. Good surface disinfectants include iodophors, chlorines, and synthetic phenolic compounds. Although the American Dental Association does not recommend specific chemical disinfectants and sterilants, it does suggest that when dentists use a chemical agent for disinfection or sterilization, the agent should carry Environmental Protection Agency (EPA) registration. The agent should also be tuberculocidal—an effective killer of tuberculosis—and capable of preventing other infectious diseases, including hepatitis B and HIV.

Use barriers to cover working surfaces that were previously cleaned and disinfected. Barriers protect the underlying surface from becoming contaminated. An effective barrier for the countertops and x-ray control console is plastic wrap, which may be conveniently stored in a butcher's paper dispenser mounted on a wall (Fig. 7-7). When covering the x-ray control console, be sure to include the exposure switch and the expo-

sure time control if they are integral parts of the unit (Fig. 7-8). The application of plastic wrap over the kVp meter may cause electrostatic deflection of the meter needle and result in an erroneous voltage reading. Experiment with your equipment to determine whether the application of plastic wrap influences the meter reading. Cover an x-ray exposure switch that is independent of the console with a sandwich bag or food storage bag, or wrap it with plastic wrap.

The dental chair headrest, headrest adjustments, and chair back may be easily covered with a plastic bag (Fig. 7-9). Cover the x-ray tube head, PID, and yoke while they are still wet with disinfectant with a barrier to stop any dripping (Fig. 7-10). Secure the bag by tying a knot in the open end or by placing a heavy rubber band over the x-ray tube head just proximal to the swivel. Also clean, disinfect, and cover the leaded apron between patients because it is frequently contaminated with saliva as the result of handling (readjusting its position) during a radiographic procedure. Suspend the apron on a heavy coat hanger to permit turning front to back. Spray it with a detergent containing disinfectant; then wipe and cover with the same type of plastic garment bag used for the x-ray head and chair back (Fig. 7-11). The operatory is now prepared for radiography.

Panoramic and cephalometric equipment should receive the same maintenance for decontamination and disinfection as other equipment. Clean the panoramic bite blocks, chin rest, and patient handgrips with detergent-iodine disinfectant and cover with a plastic bag. Disposable bite blocks may be used. Carefully wipe the head-positioning guides, control panel, and exposure

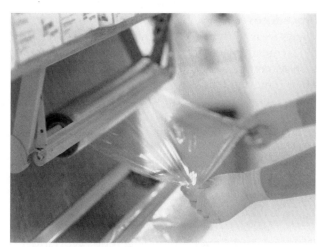

FIG. **7-7** Obtain plastic wrap from dispenser to cover countertops and x-ray machine console.

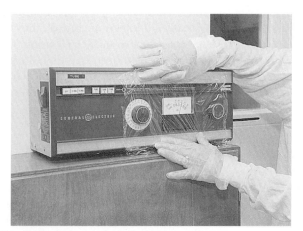

FIG. **7-8** Cover console with plastic wrap on parts that are touched during the radiographic examination.

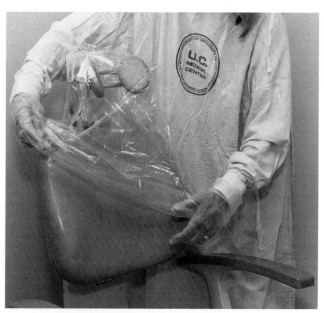

FIG. **7-9** Place a new garment bag over chair and headrest for each patient.

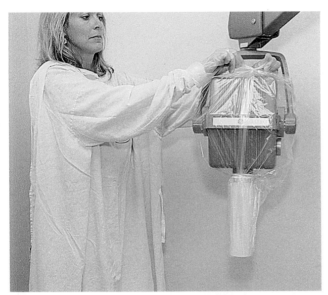

FIG. **7-10** Slip a plastic garment bag over x-ray tube head. Place a large rubber band just proximal to the swivel or tie ends, as shown here. Pull the plastic tight over the PID and secure with a light rubber band slipped over the PID and placed next to the head.

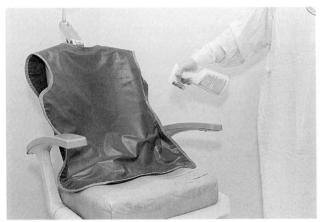

FIG. **7-11** Spray hanging apron with disinfectant; then dry and cover with a garment bag.

switch with a paper towel that is well moistened with disinfectant. The radiographer should wear disposable gloves while positioning and exposing the patient. Remove gloves before removing the cassette from the machine for processing because the cassette and film remain extraoral and should not be handled while wearing contaminated disposable gloves. Clean and disinfect cephalostat ear posts, ear post brackets, and forehead support or nasion pointer with iodine-detergent disinfectant. These may then also be covered in plastic.

After completing patient exposures, remove the barriers, spray contaminated working surfaces (includ-ing those in the darkroom) and the apron with disinfectant, and wipe them as described previously. Then replace the barriers in preparation for the next patient.

Sterilize Nondisposable Instruments

The film-holding instruments described in Chapter 8 can be sterilized with steam under pressure (auto-claved) or with exposure to ethylene oxide gas. The Precision instrument can also be dry-heat sterilized, but the plastic XCP instruments cannot. Both should be mechanically cleaned in soapy water and well rinsed to remove saliva before sterilizing. The instruments may now be placed in sterilization bags. The bite blocks used with the Precision instruments are disposable and should be discarded after use. After sterilization, keep the instruments in bags for storage and subsequent transport to the radiography area. When the instruments are taken to the radiography area, it is good technique to remove them from the bag immediately before use. After use, replace instruments in the bag to reinforce cleanliness in the area. Use the same sterilization bag to transport the contaminated instruments back to the cleaning and sterilizing room.

Use Barrier-Protected Film (Sensor) or Disposable Container

Film should be obtained in advance from a central source. To prevent contamination of bulk supplies of film, dispense them in procedure quantities. Prepackage the required number of films for a full-mouth or interproximal series in coin envelopes or paper cups in the central preparation room. Dispense these envelopes of films with the film-holding instruments. For unanticipated occasions in which an unusual number of films are required, a small container of films can be on hand in the central preparation and steriliz-ing room. No one wearing contaminated gloves should retrieve a film from this supply. Films should be dis-pensed only by staff members with clean hands or wearing clean gloves.

Film packets may be packaged in a plastic envelope (Fig. 7-12), which protects the film from contact with saliva and blood during exposure. Barrier-protected film fits in the Precision and XCP film-holding instru-ments (Fig. 7-13). An attractive feature of the protec-tive envelopes is the ease with which they may be opened and the film extracted. For best results, immerse the packet in a disinfectant after the films have been exposed in the patient's mouth. Then dry the packet and open, allowing the film to drop out. The barrier envelopes can be conveniently opened in a lighted area, the film dropped onto a clean work area or into a clean paper or plastic cup, and the film transferred to the daylight loader or darkroom for processing.

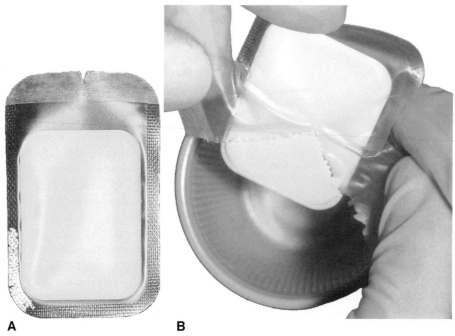

FIG. **7-12** *Dental film with a plastic barrier to protect film from contact with saliva.* **A**, Note notch on side of plastic envelope for opening. **B**, During opening, the plastic is removed and the clean film allowed to drop into a container.

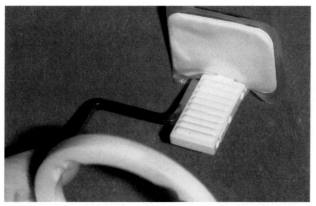

FIG. **7-13** Film-holding instrument with barrier envelope protecting film from saliva.

If barrier-protected film is not used, the exposed film should be placed in a disposable container for later transport to the darkroom for processing. Paper film packets are exposed to saliva and possibly blood during exposure in the patient's mouth. To prevent saliva from seeping into a paper film packet, place a paper towel beside the container for exposed films. Use this towel to wipe each film as you remove it from the patient's mouth and before placing it with the other exposed films. This problem may also be avoided by using film packaged in vinyl.

Sensors for digital imaging are not sterilizable; thus it is important to use a barrier to protect them from contamination when placed in the patient's mouth. Typically the manufacturers of these sensors recommend use of plastic barrier sheaths. However, experience has shown that these plastic barrier sheaths often tear or leak and thus cannot be relied on for protection of the sensor. The supplemental use of latex finger cots provides significant added protection and is recommended for routine use when using digital sensors.

Prevent Contamination of Processing Equipment

After making all exposures, remove your gloves and take the container of contaminated films to the darkroom. The goal in the darkroom is to break the infection chain so that only clean films are placed into processing solutions. Lay out two towels on the darkroom working surface. Place the container of contaminated films on one of these towels. After removing the exposed film from its packet, place it on the second towel. The film packaging is discarded on the first towel with the container.

Removing film from a packet without touching (contaminating) it is a relatively simple procedure. Fig. 7-14 illustrates the method for opening a contaminated film packet while wearing contaminated gloves without touching the film. Put on a clean pair of gloves, pick up the film packet by the color-coded end, and pull the tab

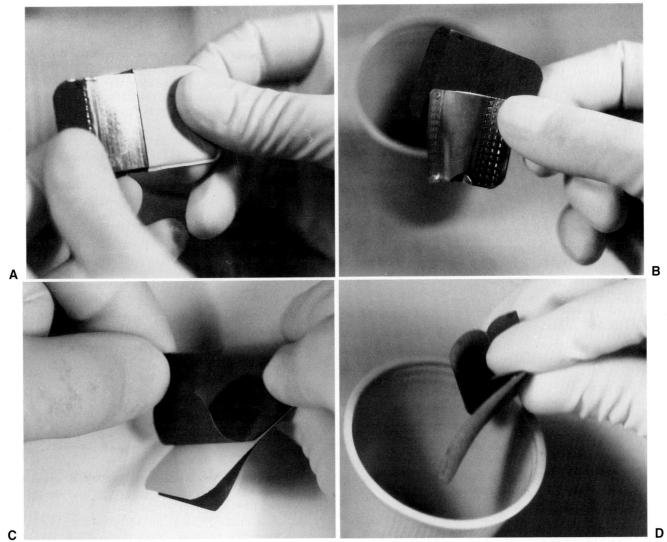

FIG. **7-14** *Method for removing films from packet without touching them with contam-inated gloves.* **A,** Open packet tab and slide lead foil and black interleaf paper from wrapping. **B,** Rotate foil away from black paper and discard. **C,** Open paper wrapping. **D,** Allow film to fall into a clean cup.

upward and away from the packet to reveal the black paper tab wrapped over the end of the film. Now, holding the film over the second towel, carefully grasp the black paper tab that wraps the film and pull the film from the packet. When the film is pulled from the packet, it will fall from the paper wrapping onto the clean towel. The paper wrapper may need to be shaken lightly to cause the film to fall free. Place the packaging materials on the first paper towel. After opening all films, gather the contaminated packaging and container and discard them along with the contaminated gloves. Process the clean films in the usual manner. It

is not necessary to wear gloves when handling processed films, film mounts, or patient charts.

An alternate procedure when exposing films in vinyl packaging is to place the exposed film, still in the protective plastic envelope, in an approved disinfecting solution when it is removed from the mouth and after wiping it with a paper towel. It should remain in the disinfectant after the exposure of the last film for the recommended time. Immersion for 30 seconds in a 5.25% solution of sodium hypochlorite is effective.

Automatic film processors with daylight loaders offer a special problem because of the risk for contaminating the sleeves with contaminated gloves or film packets. One approach is to clean the films by immersion in a disinfectant, with or without a plastic envelope, as described above. With this method the operator cleans the films, puts on clean gloves, and then takes only cleaned film packets into the daylight loader. An alternate approach is to open the top of the loader, place a clean barrier on the bottom, and insert the cup of exposed film packets and a clean cup. The operator then closes the top, puts on clean gloves, pushes his or her hands through the sleeve, and opens the film packets, allowing the film to drop into the clean cup. After all film packets have been opened, remove the contaminated gloves, load the films into the developer, and remove hands. Then the top of the loader may be removed and the contaminated materials removed.

BIBLIOGRAPHY

QUALITY ASSURANCE

ADA Council on Scientific Affairs: An update on radiographic practices: information and recommendations, J Am Dent Assoc 132:234-8, 2001.

American Academy of Dental Radiology Quality Assurance Committee: Recommendations for quality assurance in dental radiography, Oral Surg Oral Med Oral Pathol 55:421, 1983.

Goren AD et al: Updated quality assurance self-assessment exercise in intraoral and panoramic radiography, American Academy of Oral and Maxillofacial Radiology, Radiology Practice Committee, Oral Surg Oral Med Oral Pathol Oral Radiol Endod 89:369-74, 2000.

Michel R, Zimmerman TL: Basic radiation protection considerations in dental practice, Health Phys 77:S81-3, 1999.

National Radiological Protection Board: Guidance Notes for Dental Practitioners on the Safe Use of X-Ray Equipment, June 2001 (www.nrpb.org.uk).

Platin E, Janhom A, Tyndall D: A quantitative analysis of dental radiography quality assurance practices among North Carolina dentists, Oral Surg Oral Med Oral Pathol Oral Radiol Endod 1998;86:115-20.

Kodak Dental Radiography Series: Quality assurance in dental radiography, N-416, Rochester, NY, 1995, Eastman Kodak.

Whaites E, Brown J: An update on dental imaging, Br Dent J 185:166-72, 1998.

X-Ray Inspection Service: Quality assurance for dental facilities, Ontario, Canada, 1990, Ministry of Health.

Yoshiura K et al: Assessment of image quality in dental radiography, part 1: phantom validity, Oral Surg Oral Med Oral Pathol Oral Radiol Endod 87:115-22, 1999.

INFECTION CONTROL

American Academy of Oral and Maxillofacial Radiology infection control guidelines for dental radiographic procedures, Oral Surg Oral Med Oral Pathol 73:248, 1992.

American Dental Association: Infection control recommendations for the dental office and dental laboratory, JADA 127:672, 1996.

American Dental Association Council on Scientific Affairs and American Dental Association Council on Dental Practice: Infection control recommendations for the dental office and the dental laboratory, JADA 127:672, 1996.

Anderson K: Staying healthy in the dental office, CDS Rev 90:16-23, 1997.

Bachman CE et al: Bacterial adherence and contamination during radiographic processing, Oral Surg Oral Med Oral Pathol 70:669, 1990.

Centers for Disease Control and Prevention: Guidelines for Infection Control in Dental Health-Care Settings, MMWR 52(RR-17), 2003.

Cottone JA, Terezhalmy GT, Molinari JA: Practical infection control in dentistry, Baltimore, 1996, Williams & Wilkins.

Glass BJ: Infection control in dental radiology, NY State Dent J 60:42, 1994.

Hokett SD, Honey JR, Ruiz F, Baisden MK, Hoen MM: Assessing the effectiveness of direct digital radiography barrier sheaths and finger cots, J Am Dent Assoc 131:463-7, 2000.

Hubar JS, Gardiner DM: Infection control procedures used in conjunction with computed dental radiography, Int J Comput Dent 3:259-67, 2000.

Hubar JS, Oeschger MP: Optimizing efficiency of radiograph disinfection, Gen Dent 43:360-2, 1995.

Katz JO et al: Infection control protocol for dental radiology, Gen Dent 38:261, 1990.

Miller CH, Palenik CJ: Infection control and management of hazardous materials for the dental team, ed 2, St. Louis, 1998, Mosby.

Packota GV, Komiyama K: Surface disinfection of saliva-contaminated dental X-ray film packets, J Can Dent Assoc 58:747-51, 1992.

Puttaiah R, Langlais RP, Katz JO, Langland OE: Infection control in dental radiology, CDA J 23:21-2, 1995.

Rahmatulla M, Almas K, al-Bagieh N: Cross infection in the high-touch areas of dental radiology clinics, Indian J Dent Res 7:97-102, 1996.

Reams GJ, Baumgartner JC, Kulild JC: Practical application of infection control in endodontics, J Endod 21:281-4, 1995.

Stanczyk DA, Paunovich ED: Microbiologic contamination during dental radiographic film processing, Oral Surg Oral Med Oral Pathol 76:112, 1993.

Thomas LP, Abramovitch K: Aseptic techniques for dental radiography, J Greater Houston Dent Soc 63:21, 1992.

Tullner JB, Zeller G, Hartwell G, Burton J: A practical barrier technique for infection control in dental radiology, Compendium 13:1054-6, 1992.

U.S. Department of Labor, Occupational Safety and Health Administration: Occupational exposure to bloodborne pathogens, final rule, Federal Register 56(235):64004, 1991.

Wolfgang L: Analysis of a new barrier infection control system for dental radiographic film, Compend Cont Ed Dent 13:68, 1993.

Wyche CJ: Infection control protocols for exposing and processing radiographs, J Dent Hyg 70:122-6, 1996.

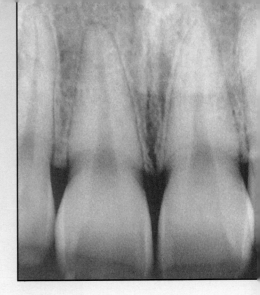

CHAPTER 8

Intraoral Radiographic Examinations

Intraoral radiographic examinations are the backbone of imaging for the general dentist. Intraoral radiographs can be divided into three categories: periapical projections, bitewing projections, and occlusal projections. Periapical radiographs should show all of a tooth, including the surrounding bone. Bitewing radiographs show only the crowns of teeth and the adjacent alveolar crests. Occlusal radiographs show an area of teeth and bone larger than periapical radiographs. When intraoral digital image receptors are used, the radiographic principles are the same as those for radiographic film.

A full-mouth set of radiographs consists of periapical and bitewing projections (Fig. 8-1). These projections, when well exposed and properly processed, can provide considerable diagnostic information to complement the clinical examination. As with any clinical procedure, the operator must clearly understand the goals of dental radiography and the criteria for evaluating the quality of performance.

Radiographs should be made only when a clear diagnostic need exists for the information the radiograph may provide. Accordingly, the frequency of such examinations varies with the individual circumstances of each patient (see Chapter 14).

Criteria of Quality

Every radiographic examination should produce radiographs of optimal diagnostic quality, incorporating the following features:

- Radiographs should record the complete areas of interest on the image. In the case of intraoral periapical radiographs, the full length of the roots and at least 2 mm of the periapical bone must be visible. If evidence of a pathologic condition is present, the area of the entire lesion plus some surrounding normal bone should show on one radiograph. Sometimes, however, this is not possible to achieve on a periapical radiograph; in such an instance an occlusal projection may be required as well as an extraoral projection. Bitewing examinations should demonstrate each posterior proximal surface at least once.
- Radiographs should have the least possible amount of distortion. Most distortion is caused by improper angulation of the x-ray beam rather than by curvature of the structures being examined or inappropriate positioning of the film. Close attention to proper positioning of the film and x-ray tube results in diagnostically useful images.
- Radiographs should have optimal density and contrast to facilitate interpretation. Although mA, kVp, and exposure time are crucial parameters influencing density and contrast, faulty processing can adversely affect the quality of a properly exposed radiograph.

When evaluating radiographs and considering whether to retake a view, the practitioner should consider the initial reason for making the image. When a full-mouth set is indicated, it is not necessary to retake a view that fails to open a contact or show a periapical region if the missing information is available on another view. If a single view or only a few views are needed, they should be repeated only if they fail to reveal the desired information.

Periapical Radiography

Two intraoral projection techniques are commonly used for periapical radiography: the paralleling tech-

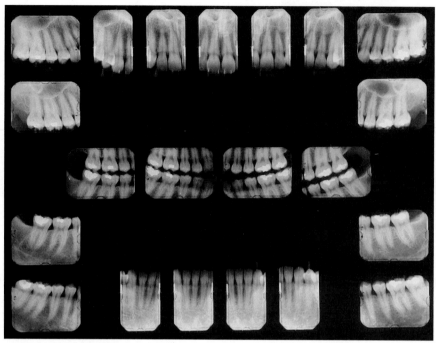

FIG. **8-1**   Mounted full-mouth set of radiographs consisting of 17 periapical views and four bitewing views.

nique and the bisecting-angle technique. Although each technique has evolved as the result of efforts to minimize image distortion, most clinicians prefer the paralleling technique because it provides a less distorted view of the dentition. The following discussion describes the principles and uses of the paralleling technique to obtain a full-mouth set of radiographs. When anatomic configuration (e.g., palate and floor of the mouth) precludes strict adherence to the paralleling concept, slight modifications may have to be made. If the anatomic constraints are extreme, some of the principles of the bisecting-angle technique may be used to accomplish the required film placement and determine the vertical angulation of the tube. The bisecting-angle technique is described later in the chapter.

GENERAL STEPS FOR MAKING AN EXPOSURE

- *Greet and seat the patient*—Position the patient upright in the chair with the back and head well supported and briefly describe the procedures that are to be performed. Position the dental chair low for maxillary projections and elevated for mandibular projections. Ask the patient to remove eyeglasses and all removable appliances. Drape the patient with a lead apron regardless of whether a single film or a full series is to be made. Do not comment on any discomfort the patient may experience during the

procedure. If it seems necessary to apologize for any discomfort, do it after the examination.
- *Adjust the x-ray unit setting*—Set the x-ray machine for the proper kVp, mA, and exposure time according to the recommendations of the film manufacturer or guidelines that experience has demonstrated produce the highest-quality films with the least radiation exposure to the patient.
- *Position the tube head*—Bring the tube head to the side to be examined so that it is readily available after the film has been positioned.
- *Wash hands thoroughly*—Wash your hands with soap and water, preferably in front of the patient or at least in an area where the patient can observe or be aware of the washing. Put on disposable gloves.
- *Examine the oral cavity*—Before placing the film in the mouth, examine the teeth to estimate their axial inclination, which influences the placement of the film. Also note tori or other obstructions that modify film placement.
- *Position the film*—Insert the film into the film-holding device, and position the film in the region of the patient's mouth to be examined. Leading with the apical end of the film, rotate the film into the oral cavity. Place the film as far from the teeth as possible. This provides the maximal space available in the midline of the palate and the greatest depth toward the center of the floor of the mouth. The added space allows the film to be oriented parallel with the

long axis of the teeth. First rest the film gently on the palate or floor of the mouth. Next, rotate the instrument either up or down until the bite-block rests on the teeth to be radiographed. Place a cotton roll between the bite-block and the teeth opposite those being radiographed. This helps stabilize the instrument and in many cases contributes to the patient's comfort. Then ask the patient to close his or her mouth gently, holding the instrument and film in place. If the bite-block is not on the teeth when the patient closes, the film moves into the palate or floor of the mouth and may cause discomfort.

- *Position the x-ray tube*—Adjust the vertical and horizontal angulation of the tube head to correspond to the beam-guiding instrument. The end of the aiming cylinder of the x-ray machine must be flush or parallel with the face shield of the Precision instrument or the guide ring of the XCP instrument. The aiming cylinder does not have to be centered on the face shield. Alignment is satisfactory when the aiming cylinder covers the port and is within the limits of the face shield. When a beam-guiding instrument is not used, aim the central ray at the appropriate entry point on the skin (identified later in this chapter). Caution the patient not to move.
- *Make the exposure*—Make the exposure using the preset exposure parameters. After exposure, remove the film from the patient's mouth, dry it with a paper towel, and place it in an appropriate receptacle outside the exposure area. Encourage the patient along the way.

A typical full-mouth set of radiographs consists of 21 films (Box 8-1; see also Fig. 8-1). Establish a regular sequence when making exposures to avoid overlooking individual projections. Make the anterior projections before the posterior projections because the former causes less discomfort for the patient. The following description of procedures pertains to the paralleling technique. When using this technique, use film-holding instruments that also guide the position of the x-ray tube. Position each film-holding instrument to locate the film in the position described. Using a film-holding device with an external guide for film positioning automatically establishes the point of entry.

PARALLELING TECHNIQUE

The essence of the paralleling technique (also called the *right-angle* or *long-cone technique*) is that the x-ray film is supported parallel to the long axis of the teeth and the central ray of the x-ray beam is directed at right angles to the teeth and film (Fig. 8-2). This orientation of the film, teeth, and central ray minimizes geometric distortion. To reduce geometric distortion further, the x-ray source should be located relatively distant from the teeth. The use of a long source-to-object distance reduces the apparent size of the focal spot. These factors result in images with less magnification and increased definition.

Film-Holding Instruments

Use film-holding instruments to position the film properly in the patient's mouth and maintain the film in position. To position the film parallel to the teeth and project the periapical areas onto the film, position the film away from the teeth and toward the center of the

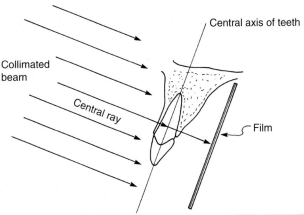

FIG. **8-2** Paralleling technique illustrates the parallelism between the long axis of the tooth and the film. The central ray is directed perpendicular to each.

BOX **8-1**
Projections

Anterior Periapical (use no. 1 film)
- Maxillary central incisors: one projection
- Maxillary lateral incisors: two projections
- Maxillary canines: two projections
- Mandibular centrolateral incisors: two projections
- Mandibular canines: two projections

Posterior Periapical (use no. 2 film)
- Maxillary premolars: two projections
- Maxillary molars: two projections
- Maxillary distomolar (as needed): two projections
- Mandibular premolars: two projections
- Mandibular molars: two projections
- Mandibular distomolar (as needed): two projections

Bitewing (use no. 2 film)
- Premolars: two projections
- Molars: two projections

mouth to use the maximal height of the palate. The long source-to-object distance used in the paralleling technique minimizes the disadvantages imposed by the increased object-to-film distance. For maxillary projections, the superior border of the film generally rests at the height of the palatal vault in the midline. Similarly, for mandibular projections, use the film to displace the tongue toward the midline to allow the inferior border of the film to rest on the floor of the mouth away from the mucosa on the lingual surface of the mandible.

A number of available commercial devices can hold the film parallel and at varying distances from the teeth (Fig. 8-3). The Precision instrument (Masel, Bristol, PA) and the XCP instrument used with a rectangular aiming device (Rinn Corp., Elgin, IL) are recom-

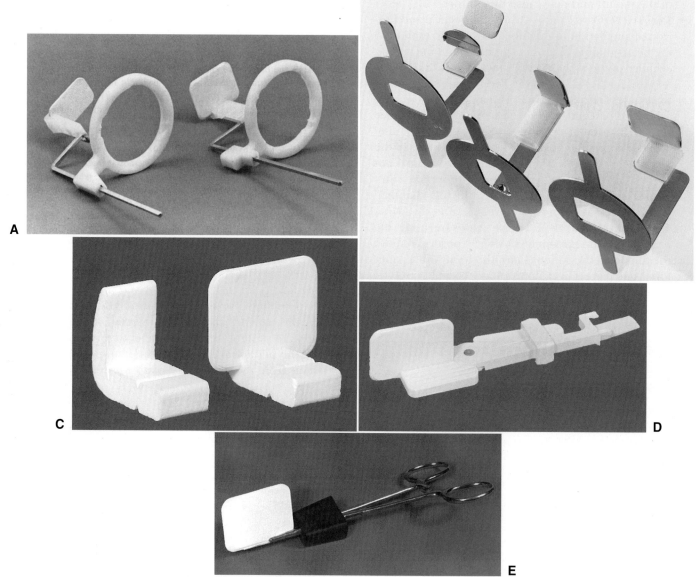

FIG. **8-3**   *Film-holding instruments.*   **A,** XCP instruments: *left,* instrument for anterior views; *right,* instrument for posterior views. During use, the aiming cylinder on the x-ray tube head is positioned against the localizing ring. **B,** Precision x-ray film holders show instruments for posterior projections *(left and right)* and anterior projections *(middle).* During use, the cylinder on the x-ray tube head is positioned against the face shield. **C,** Stabe bite-blocks. **D,** Snap-A-Ray intraoral film holder. **E,** Hemostat and rubber bite-block. (**A, C,** and **D,** Courtesy Dentsply Rinn, Elgin, Ill.)

mended because they significantly reduce patient exposure by limiting the field of exposure to the size of the film.

Angulation of the Tube Head

Adjust the position of the x-ray machine's tube head in the vertical and horizontal planes such that the central ray is oriented perpendicular to the long axis of the teeth and film. Vertical angulation usually is described in positive or negative degrees, established by the dial on the side of the tube head. The horizontal direction of the beam primarily influences the degree of overlapping of the images of the crowns at the interproximal spaces (Fig. 8-4). Control the third dimension by bringing the end of the aiming cylinder up to the film-holding instrument or within 2 cm of the patient's face.

BISECTING-ANGLE TECHNIQUE

The bisecting-angle technique is based on a simple geometric theorem, Cieszynski's rule of isometry, which states that two triangles are equal when they share one complete side and have two equal angles. Dental radiography applies the theorem as follows: Position the film as close as possible to the lingual surface of the teeth, resting in the palate or in the floor of the mouth (Fig. 8-5). The plane of the film and the long axis of the teeth form an angle with its apex at the point where the film is in contact with the teeth. Construct an imaginary line that bisects this angle and direct the central ray of the beam at right angles to this bisector. This forms two triangles with two equal angles and a common side (the imaginary bisector). Consequently, when these conditions are satisfied, the images cast on the film theoretically are the same length as the projected object. To reproduce the length of each root of a multirooted tooth accurately, the central beam must be angled differently for each root. Another limitation of this technique is that the alveolar ridge often projects more coronally than its true position.

Film-Holding Instruments

Several methods can be used to support films intraorally for bisecting-angle projections. The preferred method is to use a film-holding instrument (e.g., the Snap-A-Ray) or bisecting-angle instrument. Both provide an external device for localizing the x-ray beam. The bisecting-angle instrument uses a fixed average bisecting angle. The method most often used is to have the patient support the film from the lingual surface with his or her forefinger. However, this method has several drawbacks. Patients often use excessive force and bend the film, causing distortion of the image. Also, the film might slip without the operator's expertise, resulting in an improper image field. Finally, without an external guide to the position of the film, the x-ray beam may miss part of the film, resulting in a partial image (*cone cut*).

Positioning of the Patient

To radiograph the maxillary arch, the patient's head should be positioned upright with the sagittal plane vertical and the occlusal plane horizontal. When the mandibular teeth are to be radiographed, the head is tilted back slightly to compensate for the changed occlusal plane when the mouth is opened.

Film Placement

The projections described for the paralleling technique may also be used for the bisecting-angle technique.

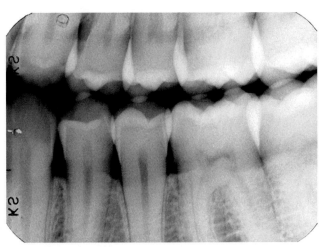

FIG. **8-4**   Horizontal overlapping of crowns is the result of misdirection of the central ray.

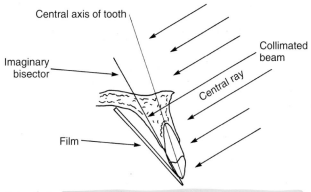

FIG. **8-5**   Bisecting-angle technique shows the central ray directed at a right angle to the plane that bisects the angle between the long axis of the tooth and the film.

PARALLELING TECHNIQUE
Maxillary Central Incisor Projection

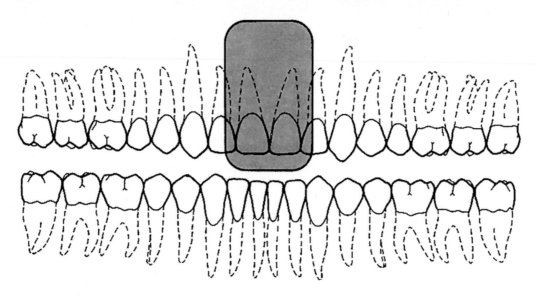

Image field. The field of view on these radiographs *(shaded area)* should include both central incisors and their periapical areas.

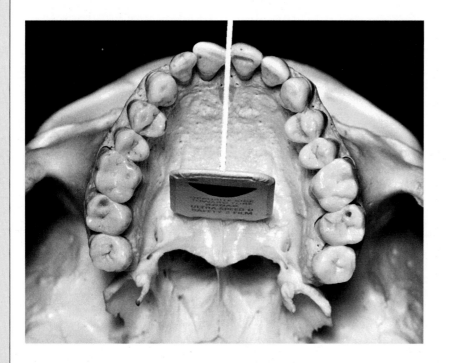

Film placement. Place a no. 1 film at about the level of the second premolars or first molars to take advantage of the maximal palatal height so that the entire length of the teeth can be projected on it. Have the film resting on the palate with its midline centered with the midline of the arch. Position the packet's long axis parallel to the long axis of the maxillary central incisors.

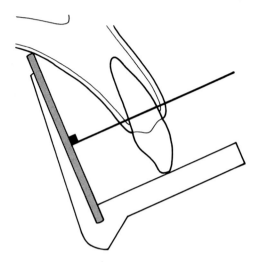

Projection of central ray.* Direct the central ray through the contact point of the central incisors and perpendicular to the plane of the films and roots of the teeth. Because the axial inclination of the maxillary incisors is about 15 to 20 degrees, the vertical angulation of the tube should be at the same positive angle. The tube should have 0 horizontal angulation.

---

* Projection of the central ray and point of entry are described in the discussion of the paralleling technique for instances when a film-holding device without a tube-alignment ring or face shield is used. When using a film-holding device with a tube-alignment ring or face shield, position the device in the mouth to give the appropriate horizontal and vertical angulation.

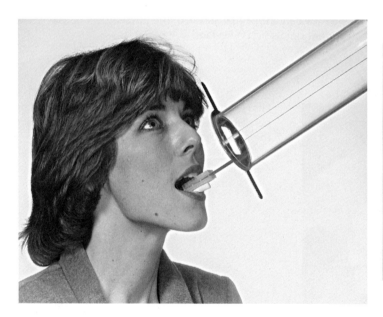

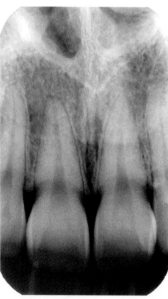

Point of entry. Direct the point of entry of the central ray high on the lip, in the midline, just below the septum of the nostril. If the palatal vault is unusually low or a palatal torus is present, it may be necessary to tilt the film holder positively and compromise a completely parallel relationship between the film and the teeth to ensure that the periapical region is included on the image.

PARALLELING TECHNIQUE
Maxillary Lateral Projection

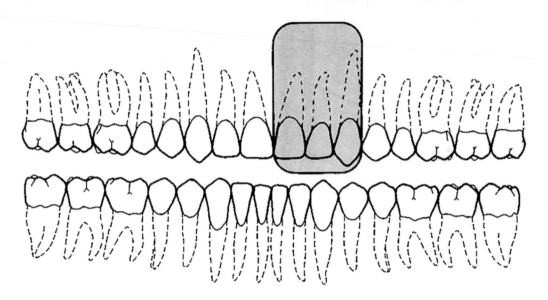

Image field. This projection should show the lateral incisor and its periapical field centered on the radiograph. Include the mesial interproximal area with the distal aspect of the central incisor on the radiograph so that no overlap is evident.

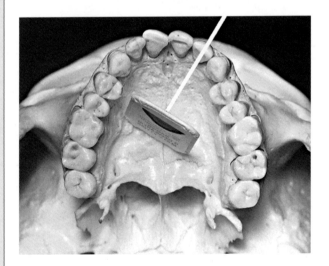

Film placement. Place a no. 1 film deep in the oral cavity parallel with the long axis and the mesiodistal plane of the maxillary lateral incisor.

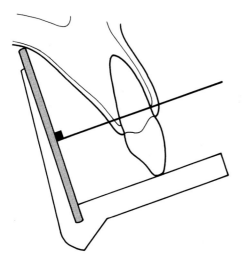

Projection of central ray. Direct the central ray through the middle of the lateral incisor, with no overlapping of the margins of the crowns at the interproximal space on its mesial aspect. Do not attempt to visualize the distal contact with the canine.

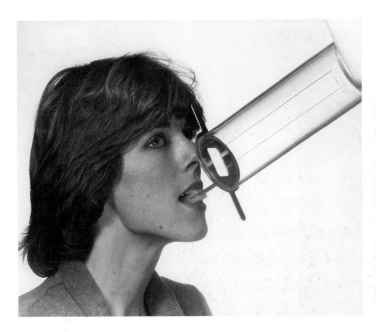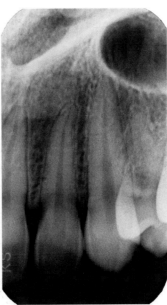

Point of entry. Orient the central ray to enter high on the lip about 1 cm from the midline.

PARALLELING TECHNIQUE
Maxillary Canine Projection

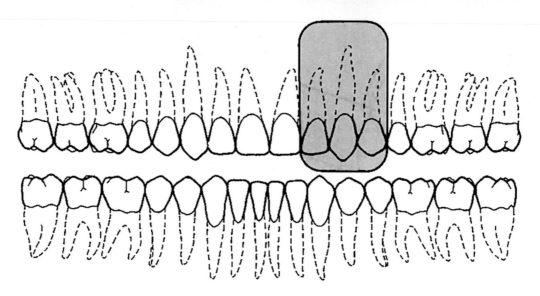

Image field. This projection should demonstrate the entire canine, with its periapical area, in the midline of the radiograph. Open the mesial contact area. Ignore the distal contact because it will be visualized on other projections.

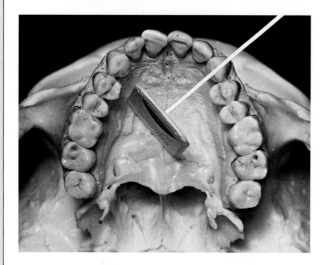

Film placement. Place a no. 1 film against the palate, well away from the palatal surface of the teeth. Orient the film packet with its anterior edge at about the middle of the lateral incisor and its long axis parallel with the long axis of the canine.

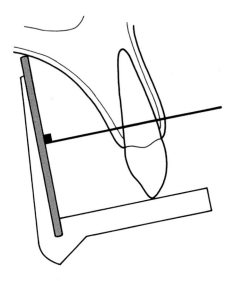

Projection of central ray. Position the holding instrument so that it directs the beam through the mesial contact of the canine. Do not attempt to open the distal contact.

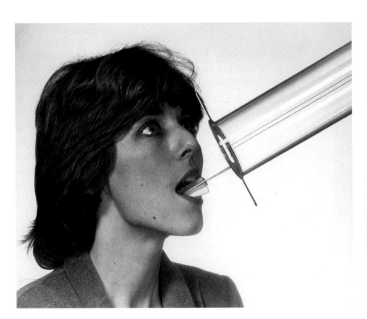

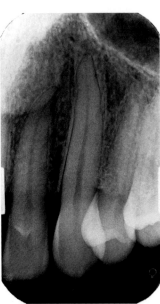

Point of entry. Direct the central ray through the canine eminence. The point of entry will be at about the intersection of the distal and inferior borders of the ala of the nose.

PARALLELING TECHNIQUE
Maxillary Premolar Projection

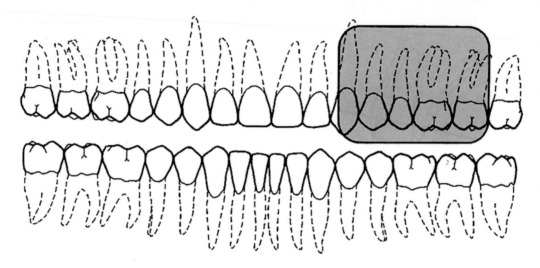

Image field. The radiograph of this region should include the images of the distal half of the canine and the premolars, with room for at least the first molar.

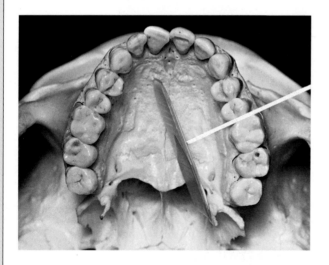

Film placement. Place a no. 2 film in the mouth with the long dimension parallel with the occlusal plane and in the midline. The packet should cover the distal half of the canine, the premolars, and the first molar; it probably will reach to the mesial portion of the second molar. Orient the Precision posterior instrument so that the tip of the canine is in the anterior groove of the bite-block. This ensures that the image includes the distal half of the canine. The exact position of the canine tip in this groove depends on the size of the mouth. The plane of the film should be nearly vertical to correspond with the long axis of the premolar teeth. Position the film-holding device so that the long axis of the film is parallel with the mean buccal plane of the premolars. This establishes the proper horizontal angulation.

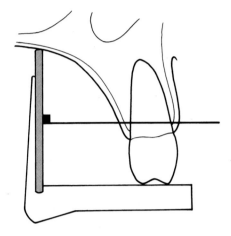

Projection of central ray. Direct the central ray perpendicular to the film. The horizontal angulation of the holding instrument should be adjusted to permit the beam to pass through the interproximal area between the first and second premolars.

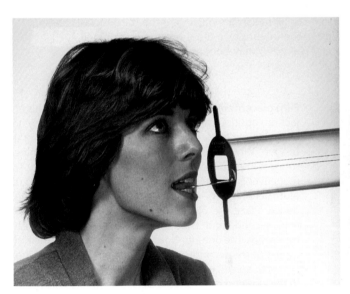

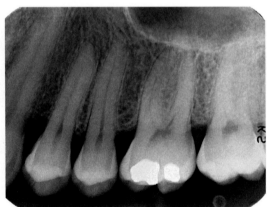

Point of entry. Place the holding instrument so that the central ray passes through the center of the second premolar root. This point usually is below the pupil of the eye.

PARALLELING TECHNIQUE
Maxillary Molar Projection

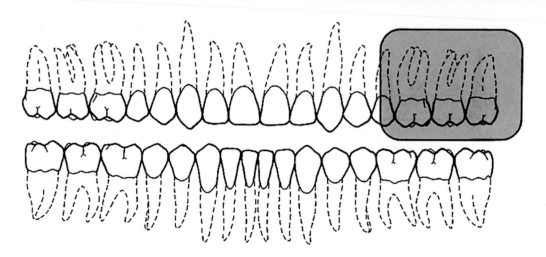

Image field. The radiograph of this region should show the images of the distal half of the second premolar, the three maxillary permanent molars, and some of the tuberosity. Include the same area on the film even if some or all molars are missing. If the third molar is impacted in an area other than the region of the tuberosity, a distal oblique or extraoral projection (e.g., panoramic or oblique lateral jaw view) may be required.

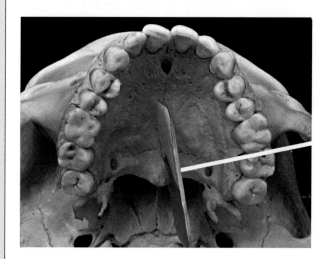

Film placement. When placing the no. 2 film for this projection, position the wide dimension of the film nearly horizontal to minimize brushing the palate and dorsum of the tongue. When the film is in the region to be examined, rotate it into position with a firm and definite motion. This maneuver is important in avoiding the gag reflex, and resolute action by the operator enhances the patient's confidence. Place the film far enough posterior to cover the first, second, and third molar areas and some of the tuberosity. The anterior border should just cover the distal aspect of the second premolar. To cover the molars from crown to apices, place the film at the midline of the palate. In this position room should be available to orient the film parallel with the molar teeth. The mesial or distal rotation of the film-holding device should ensure that the long axis of the film is parallel with the mean buccal plane of the molars (to establish the proper horizontal angulation). A shallow palate may require slight tipping of the holding instrument to avoid bending the film.

NOTE: In some cases the size of the mouth (length of the arch) does not allow positioning of the film (holding device) as far posterior as recommended for the molar projection. However, by placing the film-holding device so that half the tube alignment ring or face shield is behind the outer canthus of the eye, the molars and part of the tuberosity usually can be included in the image of the molar projection.

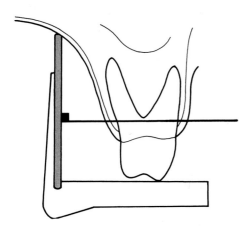

Projection of central ray. Direct the central ray perpendicular to the film. Adjust the horizontal angulation of the film-holding instrument to direct the beam at right angles to the buccal surfaces of the molar teeth. Orient the horizontal angulation of the Precision instrument so that the lateral groove on the bite-block is parallel with the mean buccal plane of the molars.

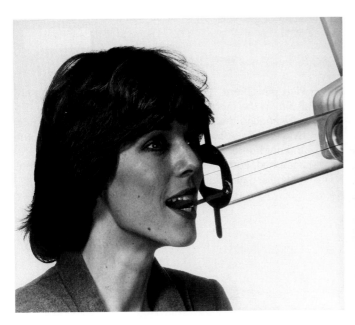

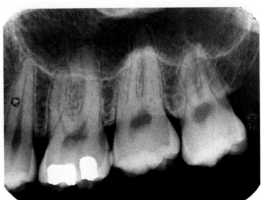

Point of entry. The point of entry of the central ray should be on the cheek below the outer canthus of the eye and the zygoma at the position of the maxillary second molar.

PARALLELING TECHNIQUE
Maxillary Distal Oblique Molar Projection

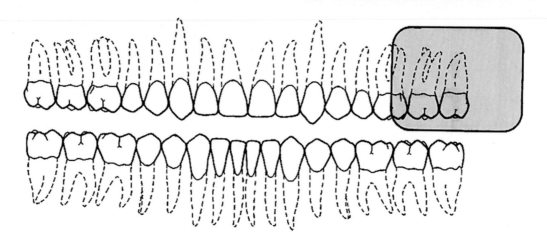

Image field. This projection provides a view of the maxillary tuberosity region more posterior than usually is seen in the molar projection. It allows detection or evaluation of impacted teeth or pathologic conditions in the bone of this area.

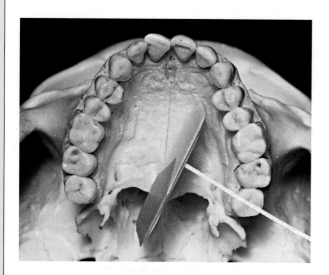

Film placement. Position the holding device with a no. 2 film in the molar region of the maxilla and rotate distally, angling the film across the midline so that the posterior border is away from the teeth of interest and the anterior border is near the molars on the side being radiographed. Position this film with a definite movement to minimize patient discomfort.

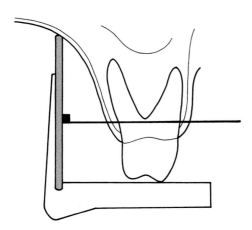

Projection of central ray. Direct the central ray from the posterior aspect through the third molar region and perpendicular to the angled film, projecting the more posterior objects anteriorly onto the film.

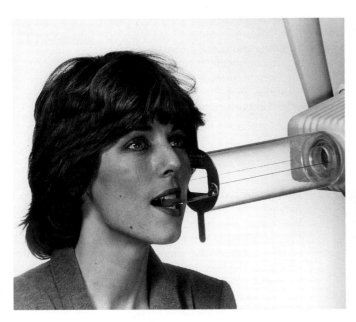

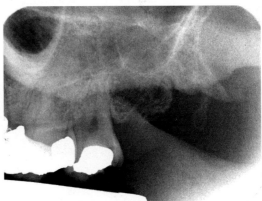

Point of entry. The central ray enters the maxillary third molar region just below the middle of the zygomatic arch, distal to the lateral canthus of the eye.

NOTE: Occasionally a hypersensitive patient gags when a film is placed for the usual maxillary molar projection. However, if a modified distal oblique projection is used, moving the posterior border of the film more medially frequently is less irritating to the patient, and the image is obtained with comfort. The patient's reaction of relief indicates when a sufficient rotation has been achieved. Although this maneuver may result in some overlapping of the molar contact areas, these surfaces will be apparent on the bitewing projection. Slight overlapping of contact areas is preferable to no radiograph of the region.

PARALLELING TECHNIQUE
Mandibular Centrolateral Projection

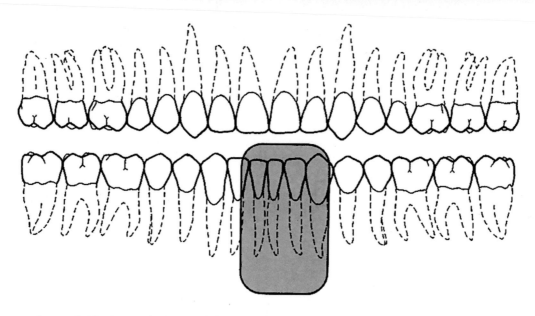

Image field. Center the image of the mandibular central and lateral incisors and their periapical areas on the film. Because the space in this area frequently is restricted, use two of the narrower anterior periapical films for the incisors to provide good coverage with minimal discomfort. In addition, the incisor contact areas are better visualized on two narrower anterior films because the angulation of the central ray can be adjusted for the contact area on each side.

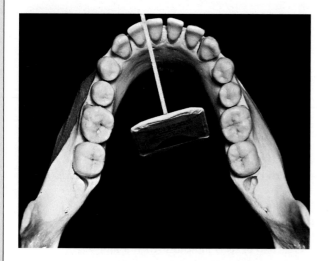

Film placement. Place the long dimension of the no. 1 film vertically behind the central and lateral incisors with the contact area centered and the lower border below the tongue. Position the film posteriorly as far as possible, usually between the premolars. With the film resting gently on the floor of the mouth as the fulcrum, tip the instrument downward until the film-holder bite-block is resting on the incisors. Instruct the patient to close the mouth slowly. As the patient is closing slowly and the floor of the mouth is relaxing, rotate the instrument with the teeth as the fulcrum to align the film to be more parallel with the teeth.

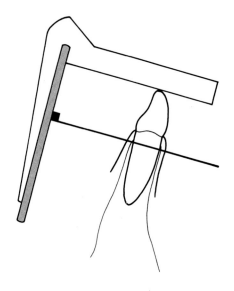

Projection of central ray.   Orient the central ray through the interproximal space between the central and lateral incisors.

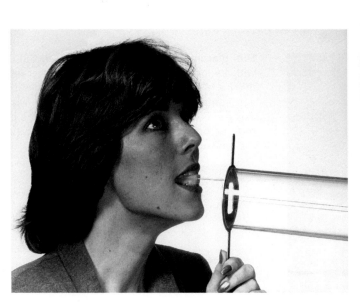

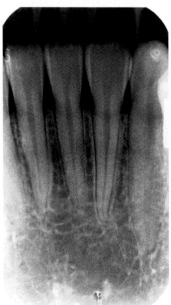

Point of entry.   The central ray enters below the lower lip and about 1 cm lateral to the midline.

PARALLELING TECHNIQUE
Mandibular Canine Projection

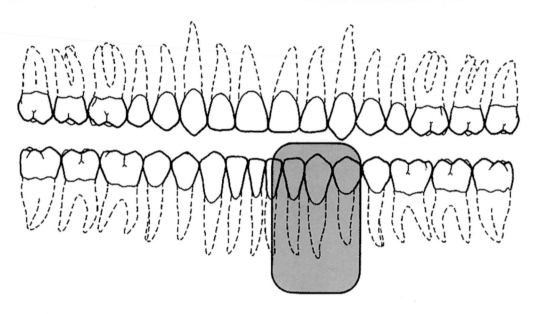

Image field. This image should show the entire mandibular canine and its periapical area. Open its mesial contact area. The distal contact is included on other projections.

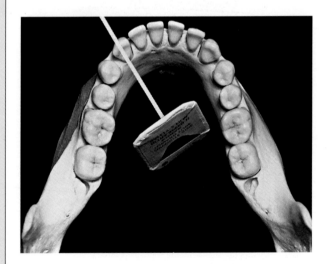

Film placement. Place a no. 1 film packet in the mouth with its long dimension vertical and the canine in the midline of the film. Position it as far lingual as the tongue and contralateral alveolar process permit, with its long axis parallel and in line with the canine. The instrument must be tipped with the bite-block on the canine before the patient is asked to close.

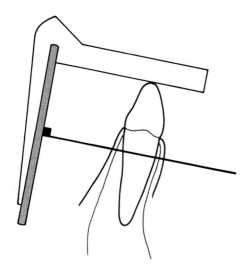

Projection of central ray. Direct the central ray through the mesial contact of the canine without regard to the distal contact.

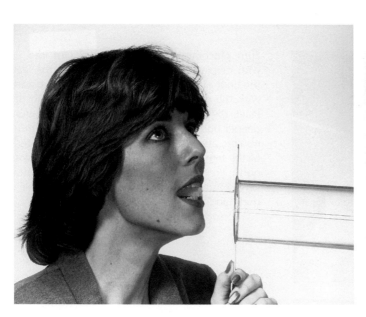

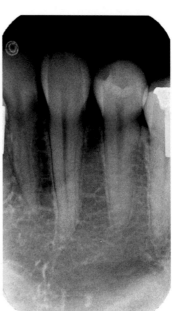

Point of entry. The point of entry is nearly perpendicular to the ala of the nose, over the position of the canine, and about 3 cm above the inferior border of the mandible.

PARALLELING TECHNIQUE
Mandibular Premolar Projection

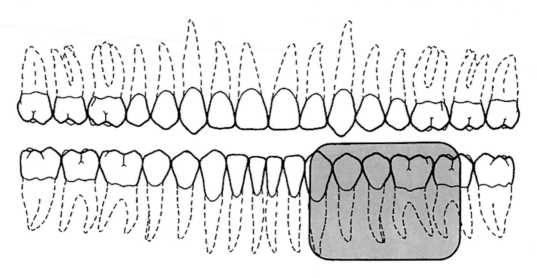

Image field. The radiograph of this area should show the distal half of the canine, the two premolars, and the first molar.

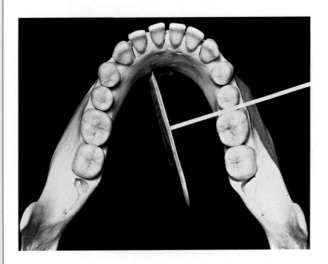

Film placement. Bring the no. 2 film into the mouth with its plane nearly horizontal. Rotate the lead edge to the floor of the mouth between the tongue and the teeth with the anterior border near the midline of the canine. Place the film away from the teeth to position it in the deeper portion of the mouth. Placing the film toward the midline also provides more room for the anterior border of the film in the curvature of the jaw as it sweeps anteriorly. Prevent the anterior border from contacting the very sensitive attached gingiva on the lingual surface of the mandible.

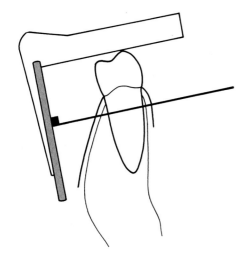

Projection of central ray. Position the film-holding instrument to project the central ray through the second premolar-molar area. The vertical angulation should be small, nearly parallel with the occlusal plane, to keep the film as nearly parallel with the long axis of the teeth as possible. Adjust the horizontal angulation and the placement of the film-holding device to direct the beam through the premolar contact points.

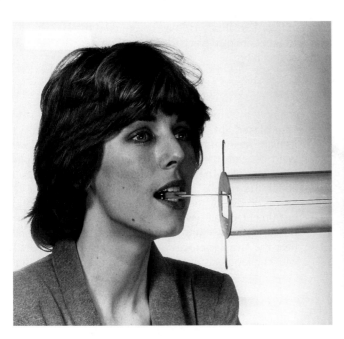

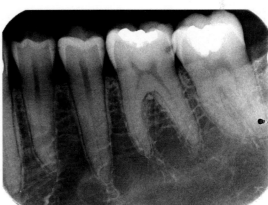

Point of entry. The point of entry of the central ray is below the pupil of the eye and about 3 cm above the inferior border of the mandible.

PARALLELING TECHNIQUE
Mandibular Molar Projection

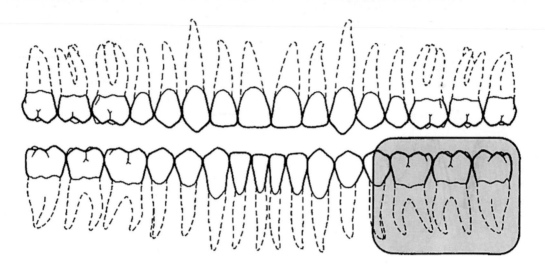

Image field. The radiograph of this region should include the distal half of the second premolar and the three mandibular permanent molars. In the case of an impacted third molar or a pathologic condition distal to the third molar, a distal oblique molar projection or even additional extraoral projections (panoramic or lateral ramus) may be required to demonstrate the area adequately. If the molar area is edentulous, place the film far enough posterior to include the retromolar area in the examination.

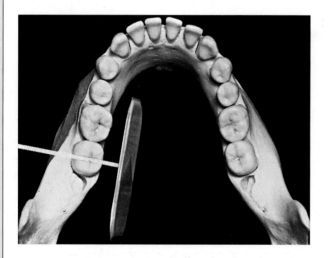

Film placement. Place the no. 2 film in the mouth with its plane nearly horizontal. Rotate the inferior edge downward beneath the lateral border of the tongue, displacing it medially. The anterior edge of the film should be at about the middle of the second premolar. Orient the lateral groove of the bite-block used with the Precision instrument parallel with the mean plane of the molars' buccal surfaces. In most cases the tongue forces the film near the alveolar process and molars, aligning it parallel with the long axis of the teeth and the line of occlusion.

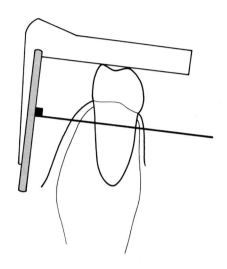

Projection of central ray. Proper placement of the holding instrument directs the central ray through the second molar. Adjust the horizontal angulation to project the beam through the contact areas. Because of the slight lingual inclination of the molars, the central ray may have some slight positive angulation (approximately 8 degrees).

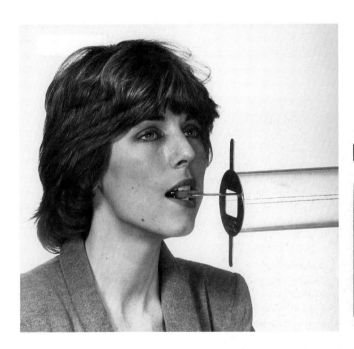

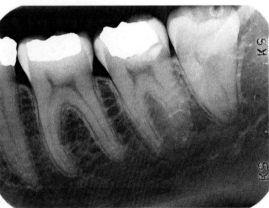

Point of entry. Direct the point of entry of the central ray below the outer canthus of the eye about 3 cm above the inferior border of the mandible.

PARALLELING TECHNIQUE
Mandibular Distal Oblique Molar Projection

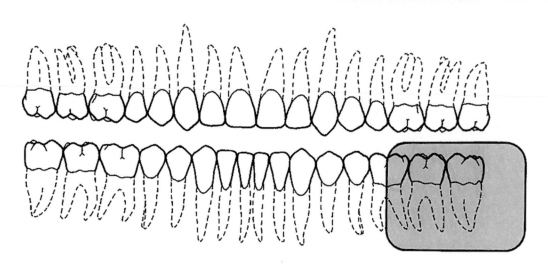

Image field. The distal oblique projection provides a view of the third molar and the retromolar area of the mandible that usually is not included in the molar radiograph. It is intended primarily for detection or examination of impacted teeth and pathologic conditions in the bone in this area rather than for the teeth themselves; the images of the teeth are distorted and overlap because of the oblique path of the x-ray beam. This projection may eliminate the requirement for an extraoral radiograph of the area.

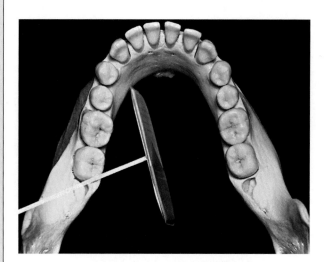

Film placement. Place the film holder in the floor of the mouth between the tongue and alveolar process and parallel with the long axis of the molars. Position the instrument as far posteriorly as possible and then rotate the film-holding device distally, moving the posterior margin of the film toward the midline. The beam is directed posteroanteriorly, and more distal objects are projected anteriorly onto the film.

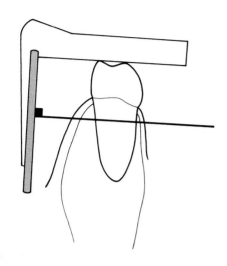

Projection of central ray. The position of the holding instrument projects the central ray from a more posterior aspect through the third molar area to the film.

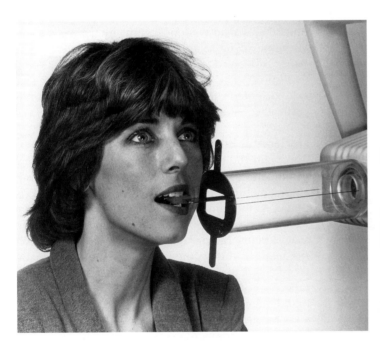

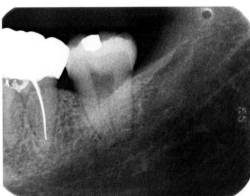

Point of entry. Orient the point of entry about 3 cm above the antegonial notch on the inferior border of the mandible, in line with the anterior border of the ramus.

Alternatively, the anterior region is often covered by using a no. 2 film behind the central incisors in the midline and one lingual to each canine. The film is positioned behind the area of interest, with the apical end against the mucosa on the lingual or palatal surface. The occlusal or incisal edge is oriented against the teeth with an edge of the film extending just beyond the teeth. If necessary for the patient's comfort, the anterior corner of the film can be softened by bending it before it is placed against the mucosa. Care must be taken not to bend the film excessively because this may result in considerable image distortion and pressure defects in the emulsion that are apparent on the processed film.

Angulation of the Tube Head

Horizontal angulation. When a film-holding device with a beam-localizing ring is used, the instrument is positioned horizontally so that when the tube is aligned with the ring, the central ray is directed through the contacts in the region being examined. If the film-holding device does not have a beam-localizing feature, the tube is pointed so as to direct the central ray through the contacts. In this situation the radiation beam is also centered on the film. This angulation usually is at right angles (in the horizontal projection) to the buccal or facial surfaces of the teeth in each region.

Vertical angulation. In practice, the clinician's goal is to aim the central ray of the x-ray beam at right angles to a plane bisecting the angle between the film and the long axis of the tooth. This principle works well with flat, two-dimensional structures, but teeth that have depth or are multirooted show evidence of distortion. Excessive vertical angulation results in foreshortening of the image, whereas insufficient vertical angulation results in image elongation. The angle that

directs the central ray perpendicular to the bisecting plane varies with the individual's anatomy. Several measurements can be used as a general guide when the occlusal plane is oriented parallel with the floor (Box 8-2).

BITEWING EXAMINATIONS

Bitewing (also called *interproximal*) radiographs include the crowns of the maxillary and mandibular teeth and the alveolar crest on the same film. Bitewing films are particularly valuable for detecting interproximal caries in the early stages of development before it becomes clinically apparent. Because of the horizontal angle of the x-ray beam, these radiographs also may reveal secondary caries below restorations that may escape recognition in the periapical views. Bitewing projections are also useful for evaluating the periodontal condition. They provide a good perspective of the alveolar bone crest, and changes in bone height can be assessed accurately through comparison with the adjacent teeth. In addition, because of the angle of projection directly through the interproximal spaces, the bitewing film is especially effective and useful for detecting calculus deposits in interproximal areas. (Because of its relatively low radiodensity, calculus is better visualized on radiographs made with reduced exposure.) The long axis of bitewing films usually are oriented horizontally but may be oriented vertically.

Horizontal Bitewing Films

To obtain the desirable characteristics of the bitewing examination described above, the beam is carefully aligned between the teeth and parallel with the occlusal plane. As the film or film-holding instrument is placed in the mouth, the portion of the mandibular quadrant that is being radiographed is in view. The position of the teeth in this segment of the mandibular quadrant is evaluated, and the beam is directed through the contacts. Some difference may exist in the curvature of the mandibular and maxillary arches. However, when the x-ray beam is accurately directed through the mandibular premolar contacts, overlapping is minimal or absent in the maxillary premolar segment. A few degrees of tolerance are available in the horizontal angulation before overlapping becomes critical. The contact between the maxillary first and second molars often is angled a few degrees more anteriorly than between the mandibular first and second molars. The aiming cylinder is positioned about +10 degrees to project the beam parallel with the occlusal plane (occlusal dentinoenamel junction [DEJ]). This minimizes overlapping of the opposing cusps onto the occlusal surface and thus improves

---

BOX 8-2
*Angulation Guidelines for Bisecting-Angle Projections**

PROJECTION	MAXILLA	MANDIBLE
Incisors	+40 degrees	−15 degrees
Canines	+45 degrees	−20 degrees
Premolars	+30 degrees	−10 degrees
Molars	+20 degrees	−5 degrees

*When the occlusal plane is oriented parallel with the floor.
NOTE: With a positive (+) angulation the aiming tube is pointed downward, and with a negative (−) angulation it is pointed upward.

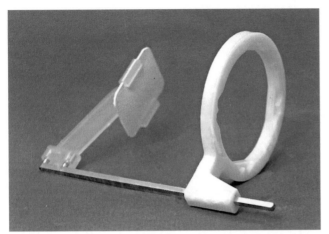

FIG. **8-6** Film-holding device for bitewing radiographs. Note the external localizing ring, which is used to position the aiming tube of the x-ray machine to ensure that the entire film is in the x-ray beam.

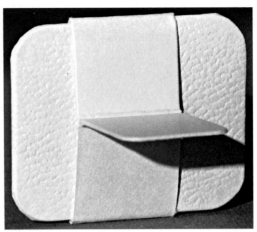

FIG. **8-7** Bitewing loop, showing the tab that the patient bites on to support the film during exposure.

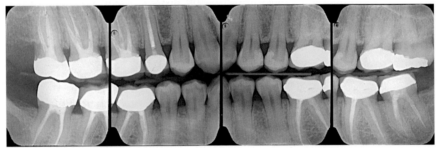

FIG. **8-8** *A set of vertical bitewings.* Orienting the length of the film vertically increases the likelihood that even in patients with extensive alveolar bone loss, the residual alveolar crests in the maxilla and the mandible will be recorded on the radiograph.

the probability of detecting early occlusal lesions at the DEJ.

The XCP bitewing instrument has an external guide ring for positioning the tube head. This reduces the possibility of cone cutting the film (Fig. 8-6). To position the XCP instrument properly, the guide bar is placed parallel with the direction of the beam that opens the contacts of the dentition being examined.

A film fitted with a bitewing tab or loop may be used instead of a holding device (Fig. 8-7). The film is placed in a comfortable position lingual to the teeth to be examined. The aiming cylinder is oriented in the predetermined direction that passes the x-ray beam through the interproximal spaces. To help prevent cone cutting, the central ray is directed toward the center of the bitewing tab, which protrudes to the buccal side. The beam is angulated +7 to +10 degrees vertically to preclude overlap of the cusps onto the occlusal surface.

Two posterior bitewing views, a premolar and a molar, are recommended for each quadrant. However, for children 12 years old or younger, one bitewing film (no. 2 film) usually suffices. The premolar projection should include the distal half of the canines and the crowns of the premolars. Because the mandibular canines usually are more mesial than the maxillary canines, the mandibular canine is used as the guide for placement of the premolar bitewing film. The molar bitewing film is placed 1 or 2 mm beyond the most distally erupted molar (maxillary or mandibular).

Vertical Bitewing Films

Vertical bitewing films usually are used when the patient has moderate to extensive alveolar bone loss. Orienting the length of the film vertically increases the likelihood that the residual alveolar crests in the maxilla and the mandible will be recorded on the radiograph (Fig. 8-8). The principles for positioning the film and orienting the x-ray beam are otherwise the same as for horizontal bitewing projections.

PREMOLAR BITEWING PROJECTION

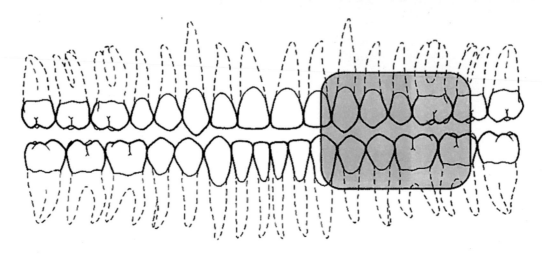

Image field. This projection should cover the distal portion of the mandibular canine anteriorly and show equally the crowns of the maxillary and mandibular premolar teeth.

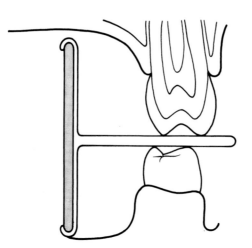

Film placement. Place the film between the tongue and the teeth, far enough from the lingual surface of the teeth to prevent interference by the palate on closing and parallel to the long axes of the teeth. The anterior border of the film should extend beyond the contact area between the mandibular canine and first premolar. Hold the film in place until the patient's mouth is completely closed. Holding the film while closing prevents it from being displaced distally.

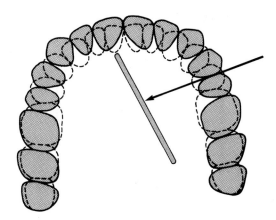

Projection of central ray. Adjust the horizontal angulation of the cone to project the central ray to the center of the film through the premolar contact areas. To compensate for the slight inclination of the film against the palatal mucosa, the vertical angulation should be about +5 degrees. (In the drawing, the mandibular teeth are in *dashed lines*.)

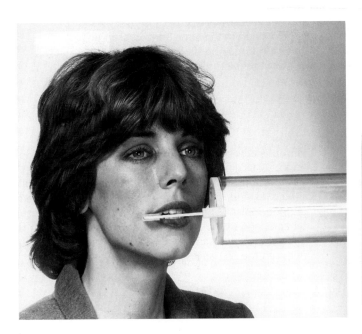

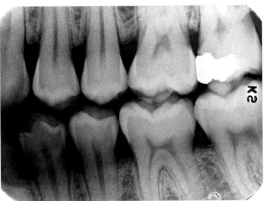

Point of entry. Identify the point of entry by retracting the cheek and determining that the central ray will enter the line of occlusion at the point of contact between the second premolar and first molar.

MOLAR BITEWING PROJECTION

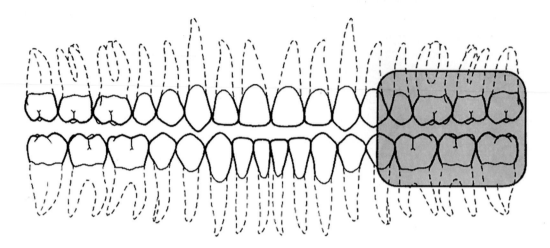

Image field. This projection should show the distal surface of the most posterior erupted molar and equally the crowns of the maxillary and mandibular molars. Because the maxillary and mandibular molar contact areas may not be open from the same horizontal angulation, they may not be visible on one film. In this case it may be desirable to open the maxillary molar contacts because the mandibular molar contacts usually are open on the periapical films.

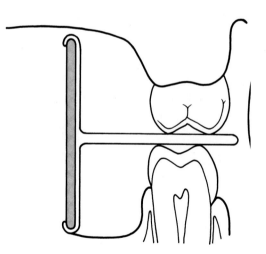

Film placement. Place the film between the tongue and teeth, as far lingual as practical to avoid contacting the sensitive attached gingiva. The distal margin of the film should extend 1 to 2 mm beyond the most posterior erupted molar. When using the XCP, adjust the horizontal angulation by placing the guide bar parallel with the direction of the central ray to open the contact area between the first and second molars.

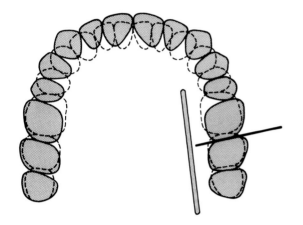

Projection of central ray. Project the central ray to the center of the film and through the contact of the first and second maxillary molars. Angle the central ray slightly from the anterior because the molar contacts usually are not oriented at right angles to the buccal surfaces of these teeth. A vertical angulation of +10 degrees is recommended. (In the drawing, the mandibular teeth are in *dashed lines.*)

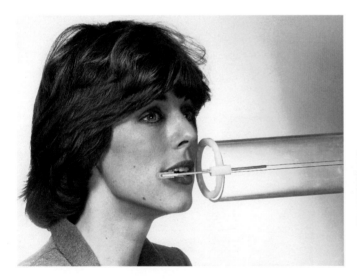

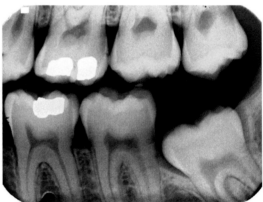

Point of entry. The central ray should enter the cheek below the lateral canthus of the eye at the level of the occlusal plane.

ANTERIOR MAXILLARY OCCLUSAL PROJECTION

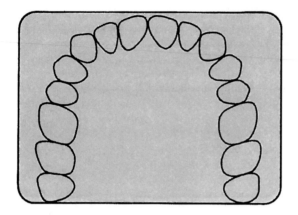

Image field. The primary field of this projection includes the anterior maxilla and its dentition, as well as the anterior floor of the nasal fossa and teeth from canine to canine.

Film placement. Adjust the patient's head so that the sagittal plane is perpendicular and the occlusal plane is horizontal to the floor. Place the film in the mouth with the exposure side toward the maxilla, the posterior border touching the rami, and the long dimension of the film perpendicular to the sagittal plane. The patient stabilizes the film by gently closing the mouth or using gentle bilateral thumb pressure.

Projection of central ray. Orient the central ray through the tip of the nose toward the middle of the film with approximately +45 degrees vertical angulation and 0 degrees horizontal angulation.

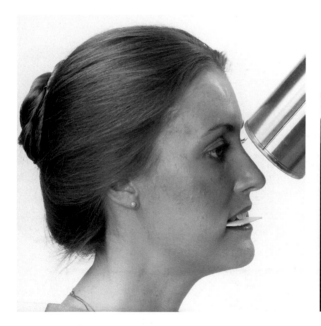

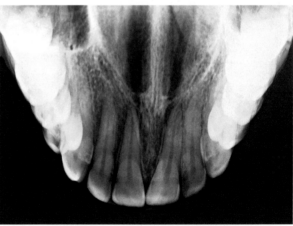

Point of entry. The central ray enters the patient's face approximately through the tip of the nose.

CROSS-SECTIONAL MAXILLARY OCCLUSAL PROJECTION

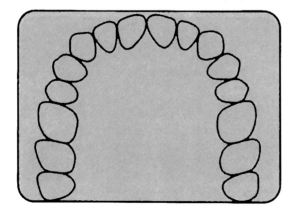

Image field. This projection shows the palate, zygomatic processes of the maxilla, anteroinferior aspects of each antrum, nasolacrimal canals, teeth from second molar to second molar, and nasal septum.

Film placement. Seat the patient upright with the sagittal plane perpendicular to the floor and the occlusal plane horizontal. Place the film, with its long dimension perpendicular to the sagittal plane, crosswise in the mouth. Gently push the film in backward until it contacts the anterior border of the mandibular rami. The patient stabilizes the film by gently closing the mouth.

Projection of central ray. Direct the central ray at a vertical angulation of +65 degrees and a horizontal angulation of 0 degrees, to the bridge of the nose just below the nasion, toward the middle of the film.

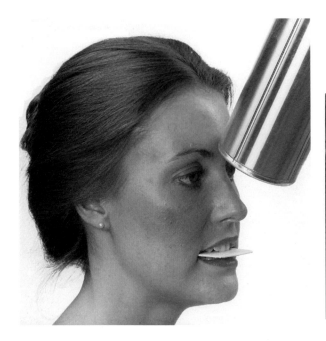

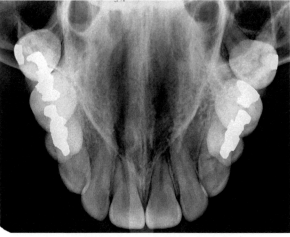

Point of entry. Generally, the central ray enters the patient's face through the bridge of the nose.

LATERAL MAXILLARY OCCLUSAL PROJECTION

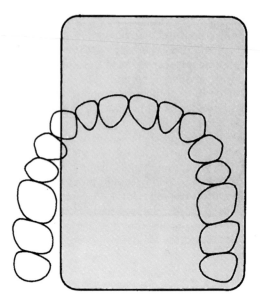

Image field. This projection shows a quadrant of the alveolar ridge of the maxilla, inferolateral aspect of the antrum, tuberosity, and teeth from the lateral incisor to the contralateral third molar. In addition, the zygomatic process of the maxilla superimposes over the roots of the molar teeth.

Film placement. Place the film with its long axis parallel with the sagittal plane and on the side of interest, with the tube side toward the side of the maxilla in question. Push the film posteriorly until it touches the ramus. Position the lateral border parallel with the buccal surfaces of the posterior teeth, extending laterally approximately 1 cm past the buccal cusps. Ask the patient to close gently to hold the film in position.

Projection of central ray. Orient the central ray with a vertical angulation of +60 degrees, to a point 2 cm below the lateral canthus of the eye, directed toward the center of the film.

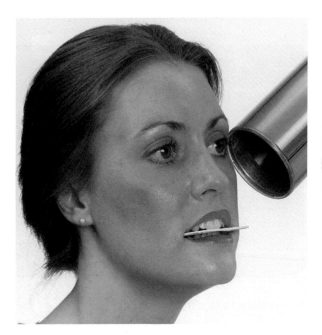
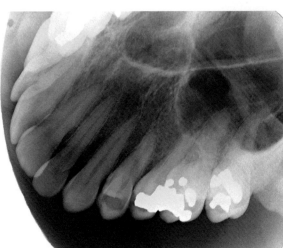

Point of entry. The central ray enters at a point approximately 2 cm below the lateral canthus of the eye.

ANTERIOR MANDIBULAR OCCLUSAL PROJECTION

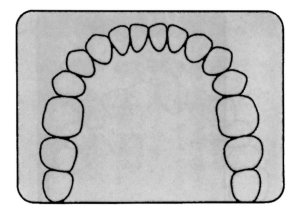

Image field. This projection includes the anterior portion of the mandible, dentition from canine to canine, and inferior cortical border of the mandible.

Film placement. Seat the patient tilted back so that the occlusal plane is 45 degrees above horizontal. Place the film in the mouth with the long axis perpendicular to the sagittal plane and push it posteriorly until it touches the rami. Center the film with the pebbled side (tube side) down and ask the patient to bite lightly to hold the film in position.

Projection of central ray. Orient the central ray with −10 degrees angulation through the point of the chin toward the middle of the film; this gives the ray −55 degrees of angulation to the plane of the film.

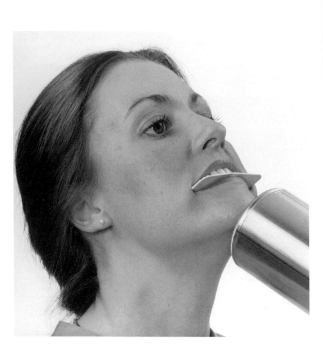

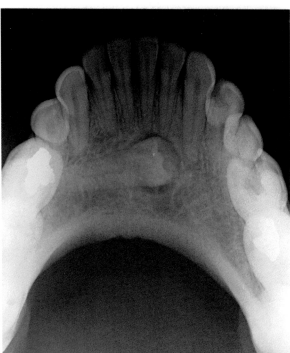

Point of entry. The point of entry of the central ray is in the midline and through the tip of the chin.

CROSS-SECTIONAL MANDIBULAR OCCLUSAL PROJECTION

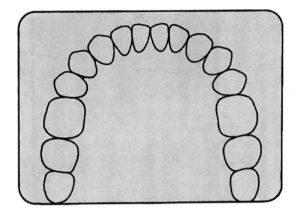

Image field. This projection includes the soft tissue of the floor of the mouth and reveals the lingual and buccal plates of the mandible from second molar to second molar. When this view is made to examine the floor of the mouth (e.g., for sialoliths), the exposure time should be reduced to one half the time used to create an image of the mandible.

Film placement. Seat the patient in a semireclining position with the head tilted back so that the ala-tragus line is almost perpendicular to the floor. Place the film in the mouth with its long axis perpendicular to the sagittal plane and with the tube side toward the mandible. The anterior border of the film should be approximately 1 cm beyond the mandibular central incisors. Ask the patient to bite gently on the film to hold it in position.

Projection of central ray. Direct the central ray at the midline through the floor of the mouth approximately 3 cm below the chin, at right angles to the center of the film.

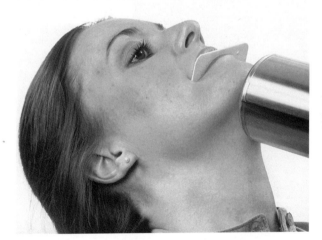

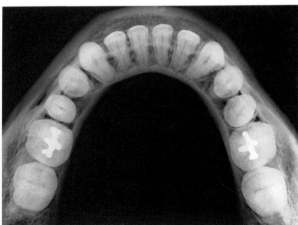

Point of entry. The point of entry of the central ray is in the midline through the floor of the mouth approximately 3 cm below the chin.

LATERAL MANDIBULAR OCCLUSAL PROJECTION

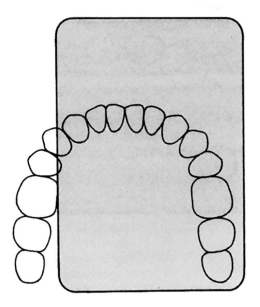

Image field. This projection covers the soft tissue of half the floor of the mouth, the buccal and lingual cortical plates of half of the mandible, and the teeth from the lateral incisor to the contralateral third molar. When this view is used to provide an image of the floor of the mouth, the exposure time should be reduced to one half that used to provide an image of the mandible.

Film placement. Seat the patient in a semireclining position with the head tilted back so that the ala-tragus line is almost perpendicular to the floor. Place the film in the mouth with its long axis initially parallel with the sagittal plane and with the pebbled side down toward the mandible. Place the film as far posterior as possible, then shift the long axis buccally (right or left) so that the lateral border of the film is parallel with the buccal surfaces of the posterior teeth and extends laterally approximately 1 cm.

Projection of central ray. Direct the central ray perpendicular to the center of the film through a point beneath the chin, approximately 3 cm posterior to the point of the chin and 3 cm lateral to the midline.

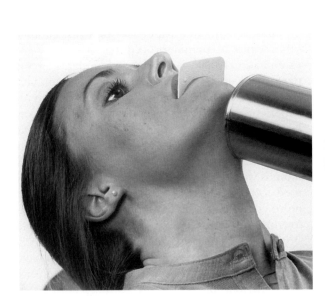

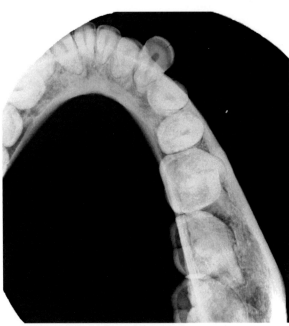

Point of entry. The point of entry of the central ray is beneath the chin, approximately 3 cm posterior to the chin and approximately 3 cm lateral to the midline.

Occlusal Radiography

An occlusal radiograph displays a relatively large segment of a dental arch. It may include the palate or floor of the mouth and a reasonable extent of the contiguous lateral structures. Occlusal radiographs also are useful when patients are unable to open wide enough for periapical radiographs or for other reasons cannot accept periapical radiography. Because occlusal radiographs are exposed at a steep angulation, they may be used with conventional periapical radiographs to determine the location of objects in all three dimensions. Typically, the occlusal radiograph is especially useful in the following cases:

- To precisely locate roots and supernumerary, unerupted, and impacted teeth (this technique is especially useful for impacted canines and third molars)
- To localize foreign bodies in the jaws and stones in the ducts of sublingual and submandibular glands
- To demonstrate and evaluate the integrity of the anterior, medial, and lateral outlines of the maxillary sinus
- To aid in the examination of patients with trismus, who can open their mouths only a few millimeters; this condition precludes intraoral radiography, which may be impossible or at least extremely painful for the patient
- To obtain information about the location, nature, extent, and displacement of fractures of the mandible and maxilla
- To determine the medial and lateral extent of disease (e.g., cysts, osteomyelitis, malignancies) and to detect disease in the palate or floor of the mouth

To make an occlusal radiograph, a relatively large film ($7.7 \times 5.8\,cm$ [3×2.3 inches]) is inserted between the occlusal surfaces of the teeth. As its name implies, the film lies in the plane of occlusion. The "tube" side of this film is positioned toward the jaw to be examined, and the x-ray beam is directed through the jaw to the film. Because of its size, the film allows examination of relatively large portions of the jaw. Standardized projections are used, which stipulate a desired relationship between the central ray, film, and region being examined. However, the clinician should feel free to modify these relationships to meet a specific clinical requirement.

Radiographic Examination of Children

Concern about radiation protection is most important for children because of their greater sensitivity to irradiation. The best way to reduce unnecessary exposure is for the dentist to make the minimal number of films required for the individual patient. These judgments are based on a careful clinical examination and consideration of the patient's age, medical history, growth considerations, and general oral health, as well as whether caries is present and the time elapsed since previous examinations. Prudence suggests making bitewing examinations for caries assessment at periodic intervals after the patient's contacts have closed. The frequency should be determined partly by the patient's caries rate. A periapical survey often is recommended for children early in the mixed dentition stage. Special attention should be paid to procedures that reduce exposure (see Chapter 3) including use of fast film, proper processing, beam-limiting devices, and leaded aprons and thyroid shields.

Radiography in a child can be an interesting and challenging experience. Although the principles of periapical radiography for children are the same as for adults, in practice children present special considerations because of their small anatomic structures and possible behavioral problems. The smaller size of the arches and dentition requires the use of smaller periapical film. The relatively shallow palate and floor of the mouth may require further modification of film placement. Special radiographic examinations using occlusal film for extraoral projections have been suggested.

PATIENT MANAGEMENT

Children often are apprehensive about the radiographic examination, much as they are about many other types of dental procedures. The radiographic examination usually is the first manipulative procedure performed on a young patient. If this examination is nonthreatening and comfortable, subsequent dental experiences usually are accepted with little or no apprehension. This apprehension is best allayed by familiarizing children with the procedure, which is done by explaining it in a manner they can comprehend. It often is wise to describe the x-ray machine as a camera used to take pictures of teeth. The child can become more comfortable with the film and x-ray machine by touching them before the examination. The operator should carry on a conversation with children to distract them and gain their confidence. It may be advantageous for the child to watch an older brother or sister being radiographed or to have the parent or dental assistant serve as a model. For children who experience a gagging sensation, the clinician can have them breathe through their nose, curl their toes, make a fist, or follow other such devices to distract their attention from the radiographic procedure. However, if the procedure is postponed until the next appointment, the gag reflex may not be encountered or often is much easier for the patient to control. It is especially important to explain to the patient that the procedure will be much easier the next time—plant the positive thought.

EXAMINATION COVERAGE

When a complete radiographic survey is necessary, it should show the periapical region of all teeth, the proximal surfaces of all posterior teeth, and the crypts of the developing permanent teeth. The number of projections required depends on the child's size. Also, an exposure appropriate to the child's size should be used. For example, a 50% reduction in the mA used for the usual young adult gives the proper density for patients under 10 years of age. Exposure is reduced about 25% for those between 10 and 15 years of age.

Primary Dentition (3 to 6 Years)

A combination of projections can be used to provide adequate coverage for the pedodontic patient. This examination may consist of two anterior occlusal films, two posterior bitewing films, and up to four posterior periapical films as indicated (Fig. 8-9). For the maxillary and interproximal projections, the child is seated upright with the sagittal plane perpendicular to and the occlusal plane parallel with the floor (horizontal plane). For mandibular projections, except the occlusal, the child is seated upright with the sagittal plane perpendicular. The tragus corner of the mouth line is oriented parallel to the floor. Some find that a panoramic film, rather than the four periapical films, is more informative and results in less exposure to the child (see Chapter 3).

Maxillary anterior occlusal projection. Place a no. 2 film in the mouth with its long axis perpendicular to the sagittal plane and the pebbled surface toward the maxillary teeth. Center the film on the midline with the anterior border extending just beyond the incisal edges of the anterior teeth. Direct the central ray at a vertical angulation of +60 degrees through the tip of the nose toward the center of the film.

Mandibular anterior occlusal projection. Seat the child with the head tipped back so that the occlusal plane is about 25 degrees above the plane of the floor. Place a no. 2 film with the long axis perpendicular to the sagittal plane and the pebbled surface toward the mandibular teeth. Orient the central ray at −30 degrees vertical angulation and through the tip of the chin toward the film.

Bitewing projection. Use a no. 0 film with a paper loop film holder. Place the film in the child's mouth as in the adult premolar bitewing projection. The image field should include the distal half of the canine and the deciduous molars. Use a positive vertical angulation of +5 to +10 degrees. Orient the horizontal angle to direct the beam through the interproximal spaces.

Deciduous maxillary molar periapical projection. Use a no. 0 film in a modified XCP or BAI bite-block, either with or without the aiming ring and indicator bar. Position the film in the midline of the palate with the anterior border extending to the maxillary primary canine. The image field of this projection should include the distal half of the primary canine and both primary molars.

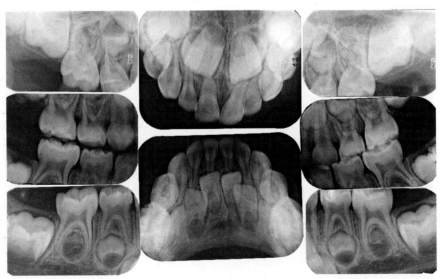

FIG. **8-9** Radiographic examination of primary dentition consists of two anterior occlusal views, four posterior periapical views, and two bitewing views.

Deciduous mandibular molar projection. Position a no. 0 film in a modified XCP or BAI bite-block, with or without the aiming ring and indicator bar, between the posterior teeth and tongue. The exposed radiograph should show the distal half of the mandibular primary canine and the primary molar teeth.

Mixed Dentition (7 to 12 Years)

A complete examination of the mixed dentition, if indicated, consists of two incisor periapical films, four canine periapical films, four posterior periapical films, and two or four posterior bitewing films (Fig. 8-10). For the maxillary and interproximal projections, seat the child upright with the sagittal plane perpendicular and the occlusal plane parallel to the floor. For the mandibular projections, seat the child upright with the sagittal plane perpendicular and the ala-tragus line parallel to the floor. Use the Precision Pedodontic or XCP instruments for larger children. The BAI bite-blocks may be more comfortable for smaller individuals.

Maxillary anterior periapical projection. Center a no. 1 film on the embrasure between the central incisors in the mouth behind the maxillary central and lateral incisors. Center the film on the midline.

Mandibular anterior periapical projection. Position a no. 1 film behind the mandibular central and lateral incisors.

Canine periapical projection. Position a no. 1 film behind each of the canines.

Deciduous and permanent molar periapical projection. Position a no. 1 or no. 2 film (if the child is large enough) with the anterior edge behind the canine.

Posterior bitewing projection. Expose bitewing projections in the premolar region with no. 1 or no. 2 film as previously described, using either bitewing tabs or the Rinn bitewing instrument. Expose four bitewing projections when the second permanent molars have erupted.

Special Considerations

The radiographic procedures that have been described in this chapter are for the "well" patient. These procedures may need to be modified for patients who have unusual difficulties. Specific modifications depend on the patient's physical and emotional characteristics. As with any dental procedure, however, the dental assistant begins the examination by showing appreciation of the patient's condition and sympathy for any problems that might occur for either of them. If the assistant is kind but firm, the patient's confidence increases, which helps the patient relax and cooperate. Following are a few conditions and circumstances that may be encountered, with some recommendations and suggestions that may help the clinician achieve an adequate radiographic examination.

INFECTION

Infection in the orofacial structures may result in edema and lead to trismus of some of the muscles of mastication. As a result, intraoral radiography may be painful to the patient and difficult for both the patient and radiologist. Under such circumstances extraoral or occlusal techniques may offer the only possibility of an examination. The choice of a specific extraoral projec-

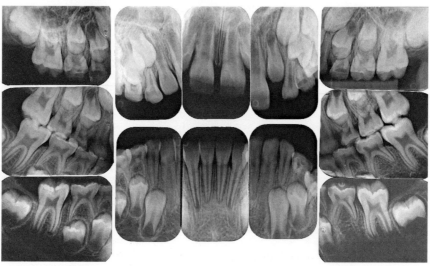

FIG. **8-10**   Radiographic examination of mixed dentition consists of two incisor views, four canine views, four posterior views, and two bitewing views.

tion depends on the condition and the areas to be examined. Although the resulting radiograph may not be ideal in many respects, it usually provides more useful information than the diagnostician would have without it. In the case of edema in an area to be examined, increase exposure time to compensate for the tissue swelling.

TRAUMA

A patient who has suffered trauma may have a dental or facial fracture. Dental fractures are best appreciated using periapical or occlusal radiographs. Special care must be taken when making these views because of the condition of the patient. Skeletal fractures are usually best seen with panoramic or other extraoral views, or a CT examination. In some cases patients with fractures of the facial skeleton may be bedridden because of involvement of other injuries. Consequently, an extraoral radiographic examination with the patient in the supine position is necessary. However, the circumstances need not compromise the techniques, and satisfactory intraoral radiographs can be produced if the proper relative positions of the tube, patient, and film are observed.

MENTALLY DISABLED PATIENTS

Patients with mental disabilities may cause some difficulty for the radiologist who is attempting an examination. The difficulty usually is the result of the patient's lack of coordination or inability to comprehend what is expected. However, by performing the radiographic examination speedily, unpredictable moves by the patient can be minimized. In some cases sedation may be required.

PHYSICALLY DISABLED PATIENTS

Patients with physical disabilities (e.g., loss of vision, loss of hearing, loss of the use of any or all extremities, congenital defects such as cleft palate) may require special handling during a radiographic examination. These patients usually are cooperative and eager to assist. They may be accustomed to so much discomfort and inconvenience that their tolerance level is high, and they are not challenged by the relatively slight irritation represented by the x-ray procedures. Generally, intraoral and extraoral radiographic examinations may be performed for these patients if a good rapport between the patient and radiology technician is established and maintained. Members of the patient's family often are very helpful in assisting the patient into and out of the examination chair and in film positioning and holding, inasmuch as they usually are familiar with the patient's condition and accustomed to coping with it.

GAG REFLEX

Occasionally, patients who need a radiographic examination manifest a gag reflex at the slightest provocation. These patients usually are very apprehensive and frightened by unknown procedures; others simply seem to have very sensitive tissue that precipitates a gag reflex when stimulated. This sensitivity is manifested when the film is placed in the oral cavity. To overcome this disability, the radiologist should make an effort to relax and reassure the patient. The radiologist can describe and explain the procedures. Often gagging can be controlled if the operator bolsters the patient's confidence by demonstrating technical competence and showing authority tempered with compassion. The gag reflex often is worse when a patient is tired; therefore it is advisable to perform the examination in the morning, when the individual is well rested, especially in the case of children.

Stimulating the posterior dorsum of the tongue or the soft palate usually initiates the gag reflex. Consequently, during the placement of the film, the tongue should be very relaxed and positioned well to the floor of the mouth. This can be accomplished by asking the patient to swallow deeply just before opening the mouth for placement of the film. (The dentist should never mention the tongue, nor ask patients to relax the tongue; this usually makes them more conscious of it and precipitates involuntary movements.) The film is carried into the mouth parallel to the occlusal plane. When the desired area is reached, the film is rotated with a decisive motion, bringing it into contact with the palate or the floor of the mouth. Sliding it along the palate or tongue is likely to stimulate the gag reflex. Also, the dentist must keep in mind that the longer the film stays in the mouth, the greater the possibility that the patient will start to gag. The patient should be advised to breathe rapidly through the nose because mouth breathing usually aggravates this condition.

Any little exercise that can be devised that does not interfere with the x-ray examination but shifts the patient's attention from the film and the mouth is likely to relieve the gag reaction. Asking patients to hold their breath often can create such a distraction or to keep a foot or arm suspended during film placement and exposure. In extreme cases, topical anesthetic agents in mouthwashes or spray can be administered to produce temporary numbness of the tongue and palate to reduce gagging. However, in our experience this procedure gives limited results. The most effective approach is to reduce apprehension, minimize tissue irritation, and encourage rapid breathing through the nose. If all measures fail, an extraoral examination may be the only means, short of administering general anesthesia, to examine the patient radiographically.

RADIOGRAPHIC TECHNIQUES FOR ENDODONTICS

Radiographs are essential to the practice of endodontics. Not only are they indispensable for determining the diagnosis and prognosis of pulp treatment, they also are the most reliable method of managing endodontic treatment. The presence of a rubber dam, rubber dam clamp, and root canal instruments may complicate an intraoral periapical examination by impairing pro-per film positioning and aiming cylinder angulation. Despite these obstacles, certain requirements must be observed:

1. The tooth being treated must be centered in the image.
2. The film must be positioned as far from the tooth and apex as the region permits to ensure that the apex of the tooth and some periapical bone are apparent on the radiograph.

Projection Technique

For maxillary projections, the patient is seated so that the sagittal plane is perpendicular and the occlusal plane is parallel to the floor. For mandibular projections, the patient is seated upright with the sagittal plane perpendicular and the tragus corner of the mouth line parallel to the floor. A hemostat is used as a film holder because it occupies minimal space and is easy for the operator and patient to manage (see Fig. 8-3, *E*); specially designed instruments for endodontic use also may be used (Fig. 8-11).

A no. 2 periapical film is used for all projections. For anterior projections, the film is grasped along the edge of the short dimension of the film. For posterior projections, the long side of the film is engaged. The film in the hemostat is inserted into the mouth with the film parallel to the occlusal plane. The film is placed in the

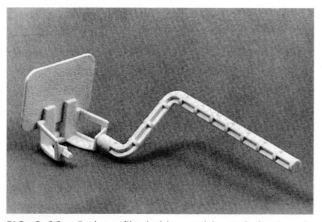

FIG. 8-11 Endoray film holder used for endodontic radiographs. (Courtesy Dentsply Rinn, Elgin, Ill.)

proper position by rotating the hemostat and film into a position as near parallel as possible to the long axis of the tooth to be radiographed.

The aiming cylinder is aligned so as to direct the central ray perpendicular to the center of the film. The plane of the end of the aiming cylinder should be parallel with the hemostat handle. After the film is positioned, the patient's hand is guided, with instructions, to hold and stabilize the hemostat against the teeth in the same arch during exposure. As an alternative, the hemostat can be inserted through a bite-block onto which the patient can bite, providing stabilization of the instrument and film.

Often a single radiograph of a multirooted tooth made at the normal vertical and horizontal projection does not display all the roots. In these cases, when it is prudent to separate the roots on multirooted teeth, a second projection may be made. The horizontal angulation is altered 20 degrees mesially to the hemostat handle for the maxillary premolars, 20 degrees mesially or distally for the maxillary molars, or 20 degrees distally for an oblique projection of the mandibular molar roots.

If a sinus tract is encountered, its course is tracked by threading a no. 40 gutta-percha cone through the tract before the radiograph is made. It also is possible to localize and determine the depth of periodontal defects with this gutta-percha tracking technique.

A final radiograph of the treated tooth is made to demonstrate the quality of the root canal filling and the condition of the periapical tissues after removal of the clamp and rubber dam.

PREGNANCY

Although a fetus is sensitive to ionizing radiation, the amount of exposure received by an embryo or fetus during dental radiography is extremely low. No incidences have been reported of damage to a fetus from dental radiography. Regardless, prudence suggests that such radiographic examinations be kept to a minimum consistent with the mother's dental needs. As with any patient, radiographic examination is limited during pregnancy to cases with a specific diagnostic indication. With the low patient dose afforded by use of optimal radiation safety techniques (see Chapter 3), an intraoral or extraoral examination can be performed whenever a reasonable diagnostic requirement exists.

EDENTULOUS PATIENTS

Radiographic examination of edentulous patients is important, whether the area of interest is one tooth or an entire arch. These areas may contain roots, residual infection, impacted teeth, cysts, or other pathologic entities that may adversely affect the usefulness of prosthetic appliances or the patient's health. After a determination has been made that these entities are not present, repeated examinations to detect them are not warranted. Edentulous patients typically represent an older age group, and their potential for developing malignant tumors is higher. However, the low probability of developing a malignancy does not constitute a continuing indication for periodic radiographic examination in the absence of other clinical signs or symptoms. After a determination has been made that the jaws are free of disease, periodic radiographs are not warranted in the absence of symptoms.

Radiographic Techniques for Edentulous Patients

If available, a panoramic examination of the edentulous jaws is most convenient. If abnormalities of the alveolar ridges are identified, the higher resolution of periapical film is used to make intraoral projections to supplement the panoramic examination.

In a completely or partly edentulous patient, a film-holding device is used for intraoral radiography of the alveolar ridges. Placement of the film-holding instrument may be complicated by its tipping into the voids normally occupied by the crowns of the missing teeth. To manage this difficulty, cotton rolls are placed between the ridge and the film holder, supporting the holder in a horizontal position. An orthodontic elastic to hold cotton rolls to the bite-block on the film holder often is useful when several such projections must be exposed. With elastics, it is simple to maneuver the cotton rolls into the areas that require support. The patient may steady the film-holding instrument with a hand or an opposing denture.

If panoramic equipment is not available, an examination consisting of 14 intraoral films provides an excellent survey. The exposure required for an edentulous ridge is approximately 25% less than that for a dentulous ridge. This examination consists of seven projections in each jaw (adult no. 2 film) as follows:

Central incisors (midline)	1 projection
Lateral-canine	2 projections
Premolar	2 projections
Molar	2 projections

BIBLIOGRAPHY

Adriaens PA, De Boever J, Vande Velde F: Comparison of intra-oral long-cone paralleling radiographic surveys and orthopantomographs with special reference to the bone height, J Oral Rehabil 9:355-65, 1982.

Biggerstaff RH, Phillips JR: A quantitative comparison of paralleling long-cone and bisection-of-angle periapical radiography, Oral Surg Oral Med Oral Pathol 62:673-7, 1976.

Dubrez B, Jacot-Descombes S, Cimasoni G: Reliability of a paralleling instrument for dental radiographs, Oral Surg Oral Med Oral Pathol Oral Radiol Endod 80:358-64, 1995.

Forsberg J, Halse A: Radiographic simulation of a periapical lesion comparing the paralleling and the bisecting-angle techniques, Int Endod J 27:133-8, 1994.

Graf JM, Mounir A, Payot P, Cimasoni G: A simple paralleling instrument for superimposing radiographs of the molar regions, Oral Surg Oral Med Oral Pathol 66:502-6, 1988.

Medwedeff FM, Elcan PD: A precision technique to minimize radiation, Dent Surv 43:45, 1967.

Scandrett FR et al: Radiographic examination of the edentulous patient. 1. Review of the literature and preliminary report comparing three methods, Oral Surg 35:266, 1973.

Schulze RK, d'Hoedt B: A method to calculate angular disparities between object and receptor in "paralleling technique," Dentomaxillofac Radiol 31:32-8, 2002.

Updegrave WJ: Right angle (paralleling) dental radiography with the conventional short (8 inch) tube, Gen Dent 29:220-4, 1981.

Weclew TV: Comparing the paralleling extension cone technique and the bisecting angle technique, J Acad Gen Dent 22:18-20, 1974.

Weissman DD, Longhurst GE: Clinical evaluation of a rectangular field collimating device for periapical radiography, JADA 82:580, 1971.

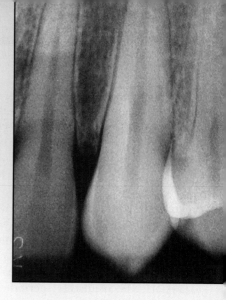

CHAPTER 9

Normal Radiographic Anatomy

The *radiographic recognition of disease* requires a sound knowledge of the radiographic appearance of normal structures. Intelligent diagnosis mandates an appreciation of the wide range of variation in the appearance of normal anatomic structures. Similarly, most patients demonstrate many of the normal radiographic landmarks, but it is a rare patient who shows them all. Accordingly, the absence of one or even several such landmarks in any individual should not necessarily be considered abnormal.

Teeth

Teeth are composed primarily of dentin, with an enamel cap over the coronal portion and a thin layer of cementum over the root surface (Fig. 9-1). The enamel cap characteristically appears more radiopaque than the other tissues because it is the most dense naturally occurring substance in the body. Being 90% mineral, it causes the greatest attenuation of x-ray photons. The dentin is about 75% mineralized, and because of its lower mineral content its radiographic appearance is roughly comparable to that of bone. Dentin is smooth and homogeneous on radiographs because of its uniform morphology. The enamelo-dentinal junction, between enamel and dentin, appears as a distinct interface that separates these two structures. The thin layer of cementum on the root surface has a mineral content (50%) comparable to that of dentin. Cementum is not usually apparent radiographically because the contrast between it and dentin is so low and the cementum layer is so thin.

Diffuse radiolucent areas with ill-defined borders may be apparent radiographically on the mesial or distal aspects of teeth in the cervical regions between the edge of the enamel cap and the crest of the alveolar ridge (Fig. 9-2). This phenomenon, called *cervical burnout,* is caused by the normal configuration of the affected teeth, which results in decreased x-ray absorption in the areas in question. Close inspection will reveal intact edges of the proximal surfaces. Furthermore, the perception of these radiolucent areas results from the contrast with the adjacent, relatively opaque enamel and alveolar bone. Such radiolucencies should be anticipated in almost all teeth and not be confused with root surface caries, which frequently have a similar appearance.

The pulp of normal teeth is composed of soft tissue and consequently appears radiolucent. The chambers and root canals containing the pulp extend from the interior of the crown to the apices of the roots. Although the shape of most pulp chambers is fairly uniform within tooth groups, great variations exist among individuals in the size of the pulp chambers and the extent of pulp horns. The practitioner must anticipate such variations in the proportions and distribution of the pulp and verify them radiographically when planning restorative procedures.

In normal, fully formed teeth the root canal may be apparent, extending from the pulp chamber to the apex of the root. An apical foramen is usually recognizable (Fig. 9-3). In other normal teeth the canal may appear constricted in the region of the apex and not discernible in the last millimeter or so of its length (Fig. 9-4). In this case the canal may occasionally exit on the side of the tooth, just short of the radiographic apex. Lateral canals may occur as branches of an otherwise normal root canal. They may extend to the apex and end in a normal, discernible foramen or may exit the

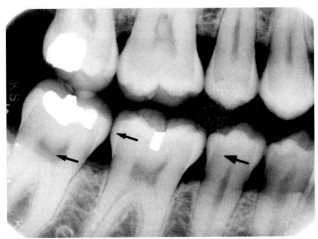

FIG. **9-1** Teeth are composed of pulp (*arrow* on the second molar), enamel (*arrow* on the first molar), dentin (*arrow* on the second premolar), and cementum (usually not visible radiographically).

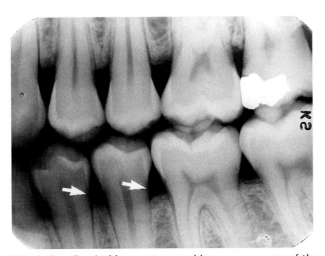

FIG. **9-2** Cervical burnout caused by overexposure of the lateral portion of teeth between the enamel and alveolar crest (*arrows*).

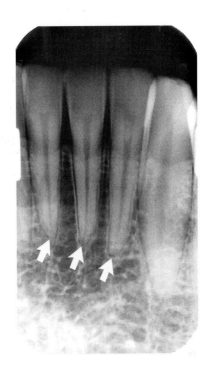

FIG. **9-3** Root canals open at the apices of adult incisors (*arrows*).

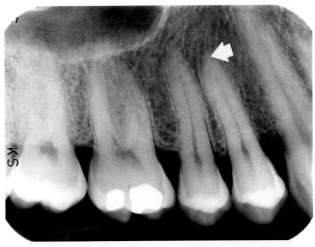

FIG. **9-4** Although the root canal is not radiographically visible in the apical 2 mm of a tooth, anatomically it is present (*arrow*).

side of the root. In either case, two or more terminal foramina might cause endodontic treatment to fail if they are not identified.

At the end of a developing tooth root the pulp canal diverges and the walls of the root rapidly taper to a knife edge (Fig. 9-5). In the recess formed by the root walls and extending a short distance beyond is a small, rounded, radiolucent area in the trabecular bone, surrounded by a thin layer of hyperostotic bone. This is the dental papilla bounded by its bony crypt. The papilla forms the dentin and the primordium of the pulp. When the tooth reaches maturity, the pulpal walls in the apical region begin to constrict and finally come into close apposition. Awareness of this sequence and

its radiographic pattern is often useful in evaluating the stage of maturation of the developing tooth; it also helps avoid misidentifying the apical radiolucency as a periapical lesion.

In a mature tooth, the shape of the pulp chamber and canal may change. With aging occurs a gradual deposition of secondary dentin. This process begins apically, proceeds coronally, and may lead to pulp obliteration. Trauma to the tooth (e.g., from caries, a blow, restorations, attrition, or erosion) also may stimulate dentin production, leading to a reduction in size of the pulp chamber and canals. Such cases usually include evidence of the source of the pathologic stimulus. In the case of a blow to the teeth, however, only the patient's recollection may suggest the true reason for the reduced pulp chamber size.

Supporting Structures

LAMINA DURA

A radiograph of sound teeth in a normal dental arch demonstrates that the tooth sockets are bounded by a

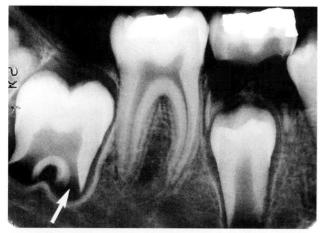

FIG. **9-5**   A developing root shown by a divergent apex around the dental papilla *(arrow)*, which is enclosed by an opaque bony crypt.

thin radiopaque layer of dense bone (Fig. 9-6). Its name, *lamina dura* ("hard layer"), is derived from its radiographic appearance. This layer is continuous with the shadow of the cortical bone at the alveolar crest. It is only slightly thicker and no more highly mineralized than the trabeculae of cancellous bone in the area. Its radiographic appearance is caused by the fact that the x-ray beam passes tangentially through many times the thickness of the thin bony wall, which results in its observed attenuation. Developmentally the lamina dura is an extension of the lining of the bony crypt that surrounds each tooth during development.

The appearance of the lamina dura on radiographs may vary. When the x-ray beam is directed through a relatively long expanse of the structure, the lamina dura appears radiopaque and well defined. When the beam is directed more obliquely, however, the lamina dura appears more diffuse and may not be discernible. In fact, even if the supporting bone in a healthy arch is intact, identification of a lamina dura completely surrounding every root on each film is frequently difficult, although it usually is evident to some extent about the roots on each film (Fig. 9-7). In addition, small variations and disruptions in the continuity of the lamina dura may result from superimpositions of cancellous bone and small nutrient canals passing from the marrow spaces to the periodontal ligament.

The thickness and density of the lamina dura on the radiograph vary with the amount of occlusal stress to which the tooth is subjected. The lamina dura is wider and more dense around the roots of teeth in heavy occlusion, and thinner and less dense around teeth not subjected to occlusal function.

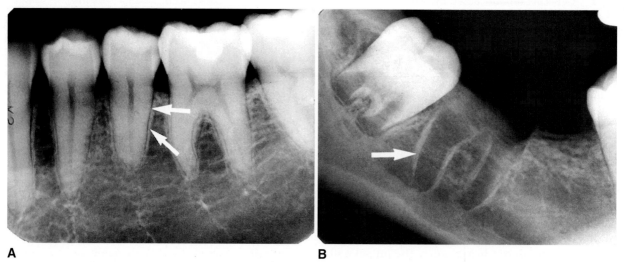

A   **B**

FIG. **9-6**   The lamina dura *(arrows)* appears as a thin opaque layer of bone around teeth, **A,** and around a recent extraction socket, **B.**

The image of a double lamina dura is not uncommon if the mesial or distal surfaces of roots present two elevations in the path of the x-ray beam. A common example of this is seen on the buccal and lingual eminences on the mesial surface of mandibular first molar roots (Fig. 9-8).

The appearance of the lamina dura is a valuable diagnostic feature. The presence of an intact lamina dura around the apex of a tooth strongly suggests a vital pulp. Because of the variable appearance of the lamina dura, however, the absence of its image around an apex on a radiograph may be normal. Rarely, in the absence of disease the lamina dura may be absent from a molar root extending into the maxillary sinus. The clinician is therefore advised to consider other signs and symptoms, as well as the integrity of the lamina dura, when establishing a diagnosis and treatment.

ALVEOLAR CREST

The gingival margin of the alveolar process that extends between the teeth is apparent on radiographs as a radiopaque line, the alveolar crest (Fig. 9-9). The level of this bony crest is considered normal when it is not more than 1.5 mm from the cementoenamel junction of the adjacent teeth. The alveolar crest may recede apically with age and show marked resorption with periodontal disease. Radiographs can demonstrate only the position of the crest; determining the significance of its level is primarily a clinical problem (see Chapter 17).

The length of the normal alveolar crest in a particular region depends on the distance between the teeth in question. In the anterior region the crest is reduced to only a point of bone between the close-set incisors. Posteriorly it is flat, aligned parallel with and slightly below a line connecting the cementoenamel junctions of the adjacent teeth. The crest of the bone is continuous with the lamina dura and forms a sharp angle with it. Rounding of these sharp junctions is indicative of periodontal disease.

The image of the crest varies from a dense layer of cortical bone to a smooth surface without cortical bone.

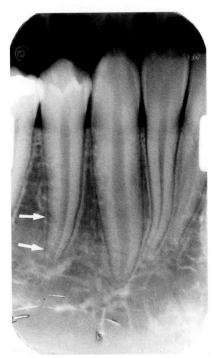

FIG. 9-7 The lamina dura is poorly visualized on the distal surface of this premolar *(arrows)* but is clearly seen on the mesial surface.

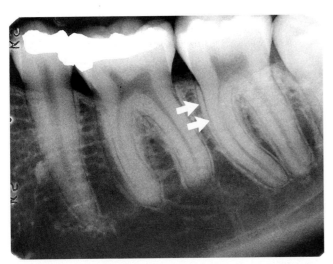

FIG. 9-8 A double periodontal ligament space and lamina dura *(arrows)* may be seen when there is a convexity of the proximal surface of the root.

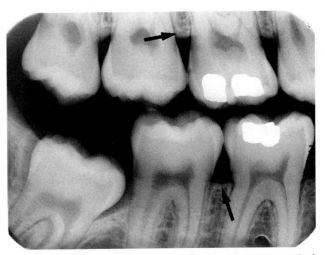

FIG. 9-9 The alveolar crests *(arrows)* are seen as cortical borders of the alveolar bone.

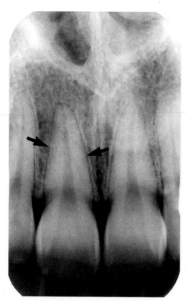

FIG. **9-10**   The periodontal ligament space *(arrows)* is seen as a narrow radiolucency between the tooth root and lamina dura.

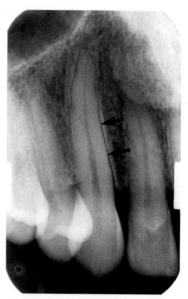

FIG. **9-11**   The periodontal ligament space appears wide on the mesial surface of this canine *(arrows)* and thin on the distal surface.

In the latter case the trabeculae at the surface are of normal size and density. In the posterior regions this range of radiodensity of the crest is presumed to be normal if the bone is at a proper level in relation to the teeth. The absence of an image of cortex between the incisors, however, is considered by many to be an indication of incipient disease, even if the level of the bone is not abnormal.

PERIODONTAL LIGAMENT SPACE

Because the periodontal ligament (PDL) is composed primarily of collagen, it appears as a radiolucent space between the tooth root and the lamina dura. This space begins at the alveolar crest, extends around the portions of the tooth roots within the alveolus, and returns to the alveolar crest on the opposite side of the tooth (Fig. 9-10).

The PDL varies in width from patient to patient, from tooth to tooth in the individual, and even from location to location around one tooth (Fig. 9-11). Usually it is thinner in the middle of the root and slightly wider near the alveolar crest and root apex, suggesting that the fulcrum of physiologic movement is in the region where the PDL is thinnest. The thickness of the ligament relates to the degree of function because the PDL is thinnest around the roots of embedded teeth and those that have lost their antagonists. The reverse is not necessarily true, however, because an appreciably wider space is not regularly observed in persons with especially heavy occlusion or bruxism.

The shape of the tooth creates the appearance of a double PDL space. When the x-ray beam is directed so that two convexities of a root surface appear on a film, the double PDL space is seen (see Fig. 9-8).

CANCELLOUS BONE

The cancellous bone (also called *trabecular bone* or *spongiosa*) lies between the cortical plates in both jaws. It is composed of thin radiopaque plates and rods (trabeculae) surrounding many small radiolucent pockets of marrow. The radiographic pattern of the trabeculae shows considerable intrapatient and interpatient variability, which is normal and not a manifestation of disease. To evaluate the trabecular pattern in a specific area, the practitioner should examine the trabecular distribution, size, and density and compare them throughout both jaws. This frequently demonstrates that a particularly suspect region is characteristic for the individual.

The trabeculae in the anterior maxilla are typically thin and numerous, forming a fine, granular, dense pattern (Fig. 9-12), and the marrow spaces are consequently small and relatively numerous. In the posterior maxilla the trabecular pattern is usually quite similar to that in the anterior maxilla, although the marrow spaces may be slightly larger.

In the anterior mandible the trabeculae are somewhat thicker than in the maxilla, resulting in a coarser pattern (Fig. 9-13), with trabecular plates that are oriented more horizontally. The trabecular plates are also

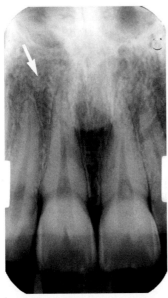

FIG. **9-12** The trabecular pattern in the anterior maxilla is characterized by fine trabecular plates and multiple small trabecular spaces *(arrow).*

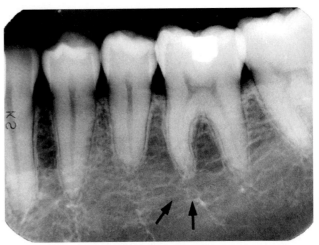

FIG. **9-14** The trabecular pattern in the posterior mandible is quite variable, generally showing large marrow spaces and sparse trabeculation, especially inferiorly *(arrows).*

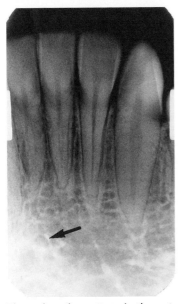

FIG. **9-13** The trabecular pattern in the anterior mandible is characterized by coarser trabecular plates and larger marrow spaces *(arrow)* than in the anterior maxilla.

fewer than in the maxilla, and the marrow spaces are correspondingly larger. In the posterior mandible the periradicular trabeculae and marrow spaces may be comparable to those in the anterior mandible but are usually somewhat larger (Fig. 9-14). The trabecular plates are oriented mainly horizontally in this region also. Below the apices of the mandibular molars the

number of trabeculae dwindles still more. In some cases the area from just below the molar roots to the inferior border of the mandible may appear to be almost devoid of trabeculae. The distribution and size of the trabeculae throughout both jaws show a relationship to the thickness (and strength) of the adjacent cortical plates. It may be speculated that where the cortical plates are thick (e.g., in the posterior region of the mandibular body), internal bracing by the trabeculae is not required, so there are relatively few except where required to support the alveoli. By contrast, in the maxilla and anterior region of the mandible, where the cortical plates are relatively thin and less rigid, trabeculae are more numerous and lend internal bolstering to the jaw. Occasionally the trabecular spaces in this region are very irregular, with some so large that they mimic pathologic lesions.

If trabeculae are apparently absent, suggesting the presence of disease, it is often revealing to examine previous radiographs of the region in question. This helps determine whether the current appearance represents a change from a prior condition. An abnormality is more likely when the comparison indicates a change in the trabecular pattern. If prior films are not available, it is frequently useful to repeat the radiographic examination at a reduced exposure because this often demonstrates the presence of an expected but sparse trabecular pattern that was overexposed and burned out in the initial projection. Finally, if prior films are not available and reduced exposure does not allay the examiner's apprehension, it may be appropriate to expose another radiograph at a later time to monitor for ominous changes. Again, considerable variation may exist in trabecular pattern among patients, so examining all regions of the jaws is important in evaluating a trabecular pattern for any individual. This enables the dentist to determine the general nature of the particular pattern and whether any areas deviate appreciably from that norm.

The buccal and lingual cortical plates of the mandible and maxilla do not cast a discernible image on periapical radiographs.

MAXILLA

Intermaxillary Suture

The intermaxillary suture (also called the *median suture*) appears on intraoral periapical radiographs as a thin radiolucent line in the midline between the two portions of the premaxilla (Fig. 9-15). It extends from the alveolar crest between the central incisors superiorly through the anterior nasal spine and continues posteriorly between the maxillary palatine processes to the posterior aspect of the hard palate. It is not unusual for this narrow radiolucent suture to terminate at the alveolar crest in a small rounded or V-shaped enlargement (Fig. 9-16). The suture is limited by two parallel radiopaque borders of thin cortical bone on each side of the maxilla. The radiolucent region is usually of uniform width. The adjacent cortical margins may be either smooth or slightly irregular. The appearance of the intermaxillary suture depends on both anatomic variability and the angulation of the x-ray beam through the suture.

Anterior Nasal Spine

The anterior nasal spine is most frequently demonstrated on periapical radiographs of the maxillary central incisors (Fig. 9-17). Located in the midline, it lies some 1.5 to 2 cm above the alveolar crest, usually at or just below the junction of the inferior end of the nasal septum and the inferior outline of the nasal fossa. It is radiopaque because of its bony composition and is usually V-shaped.

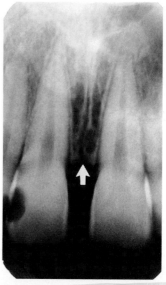

FIG. **9-16**   The intermaxillary suture may terminate in a V-shaped widening *(arrow)* at the alveolar crest.

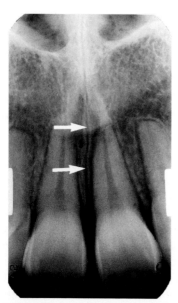

FIG. **9-15**   The intermaxillary suture *(arrows)* appears as a curving radiolucency in the midline of the maxilla.

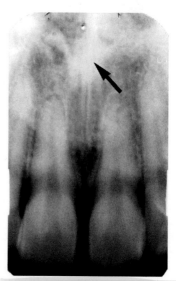

FIG. **9-17**   The anterior nasal spine is seen as an opaque V-shaped projection from the floor of the nasal fossa in the midline *(arrow)*.

Nasal Fossa

Because the air-filled nasal fossa (cavity) lies just above the oral cavity, its radiolucent image may be apparent on intraoral radiographs of the maxillary teeth, especially in central incisor projections. On periapical radiographs of the incisors the inferior border of the fossa appears as a radiopaque line extending bilaterally away from the base of the anterior nasal spine (Fig. 9-18). Above this line is the radiolucent space of the inferior portion of the fossa. If the radiograph was made with the x-ray beam directed in the sagittal plane, the relatively radiopaque nasal septum is seen arising in the midline from the anterior nasal spine (Fig. 9-19). The shadow of the septum may appear wider than anticipated and not sharply defined because the image is a superimposition of septal cartilage and vomer bone. Also the septum frequently deviates slightly from the midline, and its plate of bone (the vomer) is somewhat curved.

The nasal cavity contains the hazy shadows of the inferior conchae extending from the right and left lateral walls for varying distances toward the septum. These conchae fill varying amounts of the lateral portions of the fossa (Fig. 9-20). The floor of the nasal fossa and a small segment of the nasal cavity not uncommonly are projected high onto a maxillary canine radiograph (Fig. 9-21). Also, in the posterior maxillary region, the floor of the nasal cavity and a portion of the fossa above it may be seen in the region of the maxillary sinus. (It is not possible from a single radiograph to determine which of two superimposed structures is

in front of or behind the other unless the conclusion is based on an awareness of the anatomic features and relationships.) It may falsely convey the impression of a septum in the sinus or a limiting superior sinus wall (Fig. 9-22).

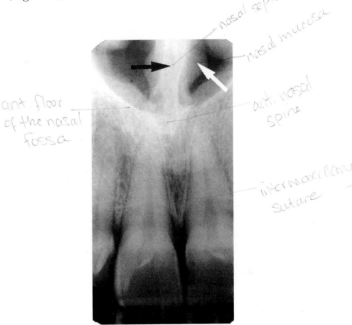

FIG. **9-19** The nasal septum *(black arrow)* arises directly above the anterior nasal spine and is covered on each side by nasal mucosa *(white arrow)*.

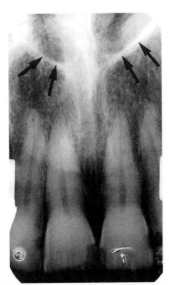

FIG. **9-18** The anterior floor of the nasal fossa *(arrows)* appears as opaque lines extending laterally from the anterior nasal spine.

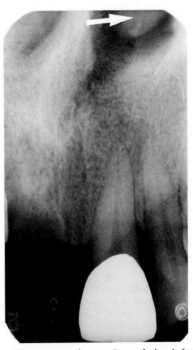

FIG. **9-20** The mucosal covering of the inferior concha *(arrow)* is occasionally visualized in the nasal fossa.

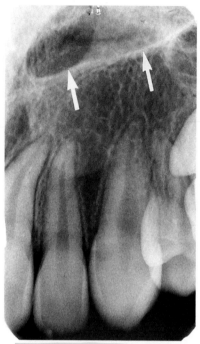

FIG. **9-21**   The floor of the nasal fossa *(arrows)* may often be seen extending above the maxillary lateral incisor and canine.

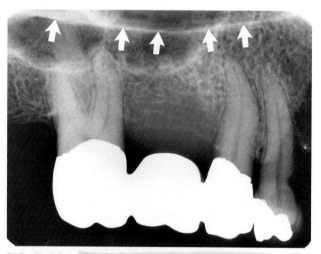

FIG. **9-22**   The floor of the nasal fossa *(arrows)* extends posteriorly, superimposed with the maxillary sinus.

Incisive Foramen

The incisive foramen (also called the *nasopalatine or anterior palatine foramen*) in the maxilla is the oral terminus of the nasopalatine canal. It transmits the nasopalatine vessels and nerves (which may participate in the innervation of the maxillary central incisors) and lies in the midline of the palate behind the central incisors at approximately the junction of the median palatine and

incisive sutures. Its radiographic image is usually projected between the roots and in the region of the middle and apical thirds of the central incisors (Fig. 9-23). The foramen varies markedly in its radiographic shape, size, and sharpness. It may appear smoothly symmetric, with numerous forms, or very irregular, with a well-demarcated or ill-defined border. The position of the foramen is also variable and may be recognized at the apices of the central incisor roots, near the alveolar crest, anywhere in between, or extending over the entire distance. The great variability of its radiographic image is primarily the result of (1) the differing angles at which the x-ray beam is directed for the maxillary central incisors and (2) some variability in its anatomic size.

Familiarity with the incisive foramen is important because it is a potential site of cyst formation. An incisive canal cyst is radiographically discernible: it frequently causes a readily perceived enlargement of the foramen and canal. The presence of a cyst is presumed if the width of the foramen exceeds 1 cm or if enlargement can be demonstrated on successive radiographs. Also, if the radiolucency of the normal foramen is projected over the apex of one central incisor, it may suggest a pathologic periapical condition. The absence of pathosis is indicated by a lack of clinical symptoms and an intact lamina dura around the central incisor in question.

The lateral walls of the nasopalatine canal are not usually seen but on occasion can be visualized on a projection of the central incisors as a pair of radiopaque lines running vertically from the superior foramina of the nasopalatine canal to the incisive foramen (Fig. 9-24).

Superior Foramina of the Nasopalatine Canal

The nasopalatine canal originates at two foramina in the floor of the nasal cavity. The openings are on each side of the nasal septum, close to the anteroinferior border of the nasal cavity, and each branch passes downward somewhat anteriorly and medially to unite with the canal from the other side in a common opening, the incisive (nasopalatine) foramen. The superior foramina of the canal occasionally appear in projections of the maxillary incisors, especially when an exaggerated vertical angle is used. When apparent radiographically, they can be recognized as two radiolucent areas above the apices of the central incisors in the floor of the nasal cavity near its anterior border and on both sides of the septum (Fig. 9-25). They are usually round or oval, although they make take a variety of outlines depending on the angle of projection.

Lateral Fossa

The lateral fossa (also called *incisive fossa*) is a gentle depression in the maxilla near the apex of the lateral

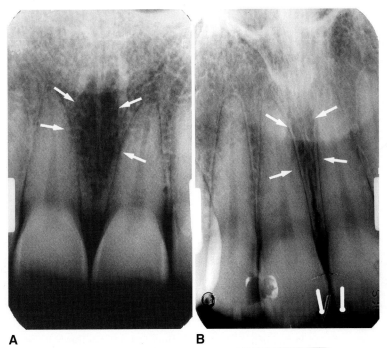

A   **B**

FIG. **9-23**   **A,** The incisive foramen appears as an ovoid radiolucency *(arrows)* between the roots of the central incisors. **B,** Note its borders, which are diffuse but within normal limits.

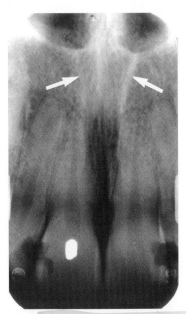

FIG. **9-24**   The lateral walls of the nasopalatine canal *(arrows)* extend from the incisive foramen to the floor of the nasal fossa.

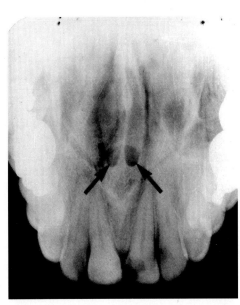

FIG. **9-25**   The superior foramina of the nasopalatine canal *(arrows)* appear just lateral to the nasal septum and posterior to the anterior nasal spine.

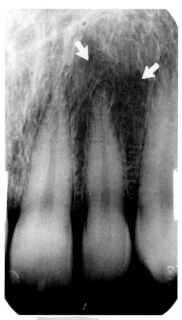

FIG. **9-26**   The lateral fossa is a diffuse radiolucency *(arrows)* in the region of the apex of the lateral incisor. It is formed by a depression in the maxilla at this location.

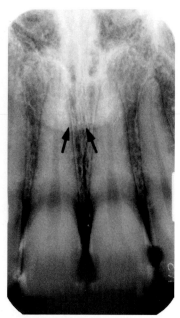

FIG. **9-27**   The soft tissue outline of the nose *(arrows)* is superimposed on the anterior maxilla.

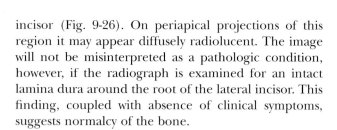

incisor (Fig. 9-26). On periapical projections of this region it may appear diffusely radiolucent. The image will not be misinterpreted as a pathologic condition, however, if the radiograph is examined for an intact lamina dura around the root of the lateral incisor. This finding, coupled with absence of clinical symptoms, suggests normalcy of the bone.

Nose

The soft tissue of the tip of the nose is frequently seen in projections of the maxillary central and lateral incisors, superimposed over the roots of these teeth. The image of the nose has a uniform, slightly opaque appearance with a sharp border (Fig. 9-27). Occasionally the radiolucent nares can be identified, especially when a steep vertical angle is used.

Nasolacrimal Canal

The nasal and maxillary bones form the nasolacrimal canal. It runs from the medial aspect of the anteroinferior border of the orbit inferiorly, to drain under the inferior concha into the nasal cavity. Occasionally it can be visualized on periapical radiographs in the region above the apex of the canine, especially when steep vertical angulation is used (Fig. 9-28). The nasolacrimal canals are routinely seen on maxillary occlusal projections (see Chapter 8) in the region of the molars (Fig. 9-29).

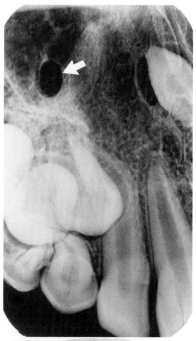

FIG. **9-28**   The nasolacrimal canal *(arrow)* is occasionally seen near the apex of the canine when steep vertical angulation is used. Note the mesiodens (supernumerary tooth) superior to the central incisor.

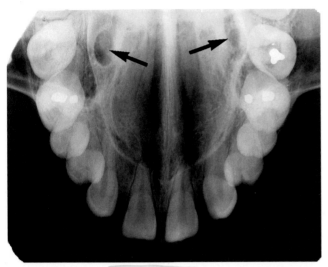

FIG. **9-29** The nasolacrimal canals are commonly seen as ovoid radiolucencies *(arrows)* on maxillary occlusal projections.

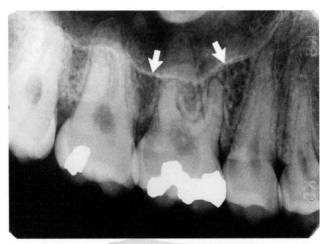

FIG. **9-30** The inferior border of the maxillary sinus *(arrows)* appears as a thin radiopaque line near the apices of the maxillary premolars and molars.

Maxillary Sinus

The maxillary sinus, like the other paranasal sinuses, is an air-containing cavity lined with mucous membrane. It develops by the invagination of mucous membrane from the nasal cavity. Being the largest of the paranasal sinuses, it normally occupies virtually the entire body of the maxilla. Its function is unknown.

The sinus may be considered as a three-sided pyramid, with its base the medial wall adjacent to the nasal cavity and its apex extending laterally into the zygomatic process of the maxilla. Its three sides are (1) the superior wall forming the floor of the orbit, (2) the anterior wall extending above the premolars, and (3) the posterior wall bulging above the molar teeth and maxillary tuberosity. The sinus communicates with the nasal cavity via the ostium some 3 to 6 mm in diameter positioned under the posterior aspect of the middle turbinate.

The borders of the maxillary sinus appear on periapical radiographs as a thin, delicate, tenuous radiopaque line (actually a thin layer of cortical bone) (Fig. 9-30). In the absence of disease it appears continuous, but on close examination it can be seen to have small interruptions in its smoothness or density. These discontinuities are probably illusions caused by superimposition of small marrow spaces. In adults the sinuses are usually seen to extend from the distal aspect of the canine to the posterior wall of the maxilla above the tuberosity.

The maxillary sinuses show considerable variation in size. They enlarge during childhood, achieving mature size by the age of 15 to 18 years. They may change during adult life in response to environmental factors. The right and left sinuses usually appear similar in shape and size, although marked asymmetry is occasionally present. The floors of the maxillary sinus and nasal cavity are seen on dental radiographs at approximately the same level around the age of puberty. In older individuals the sinus may extend farther into the alveolar process, and in the posterior region of the maxilla its floor may appear considerably below the level of the floor of the nasal cavity. Anteriorly each sinus is restricted by the canine fossa and is usually seen to sweep superiorly, crossing the level of the floor of the nasal cavity in the premolar or canine region. Consequently, on periapical radiographs of the canine, the floors of the sinus and nasal cavity are often superimposed and may be seen crossing one another, forming an inverted Y in the area (Fig. 9-31).

The outline of the nasal fossa is usually heavier and more diffuse than that of the thin, delicate cortical bone denoting the sinus. The degree of extension of the maxillary sinus into the alveolar process is extremely variable. In some projections the floor of the sinus will be well above the apices of the posterior teeth; in others it may extend well beyond the apices toward the alveolar ridge. In response to a loss of function (associated with the loss of posterior teeth) the sinus may expand farther into the alveolar bone, occasionally extending to the alveolar ridge (Fig. 9-32).

The roots of the molars usually lie in close apposition to the maxillary sinus. Root apices may project anatomically into the floor of the sinus, causing small elevations or prominences. The thin layer of bone covering the root is seen as a fusion of the lamina dura and

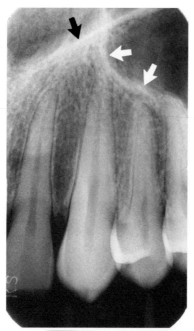

FIG. **9-31**   The anterior border of the maxillary sinus *(white arrows)* crosses the floor of the nasal fossa *(black arrow)*.

the floor of the sinus. Rarely, defects may be present in the bony covering of the root apices in the sinus floor, and a periapical radiograph will fail to show lamina dura covering the apex.

When the rounded sinus floor dips between the buccal and palatal molar roots and is medial to the premolar roots, the projection of the apices is superior to the floor. This appearance conveys the impression that the roots project into the sinus cavity, which is an illusion. As the positive vertical angle of the projection is increased, the roots medial to the sinus appear to project farther into the sinus cavity. In contrast, the roots lateral to the sinus appear to move either out of the sinus or farther away from it as the angle is increased.

The intimate relationship between sinus and teeth leads to the possibility that clinical symptoms originating in the sinus may be perceived in the teeth, and vice versa. This proximity of sinus and teeth is in part a consequence of the gradual developmental expansion of the maxillary sinus, which thins the sinus walls and opens the canals that traverse the anterolateral and posterolateral walls and carry the superior alveolar nerves. The nerves are then in intimate contact with the membrane lining the sinus. As a result, an acute inflammation of the sinus is frequently accompanied by pain in the maxillary teeth innervated by that portion of the nerve proximal to the insult. Subjective symptoms in the area of the maxillary posterior teeth may require careful analysis to differentiate tooth pain from sinus pain.

Frequently, thin radiolucent lines of uniform width are found within the image of the maxillary sinus (Fig. 9-33). These are the shadows of neurovascular canals or grooves in the lateral sinus walls that accommodate the posterior superior alveolar vessels, their branches, and the accompanying superior alveolar nerves. Although they may be found coursing in any direction (including vertically), they are usually seen running a curved posteroanterior course that is convex toward the alveolar process. On occasion they may be found to branch, and rarely also to extend outside the image of the sinus and continue as an interradicular channel. Because such

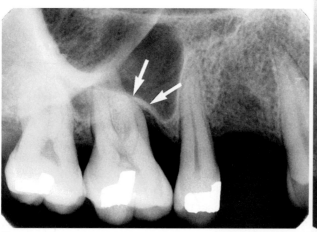

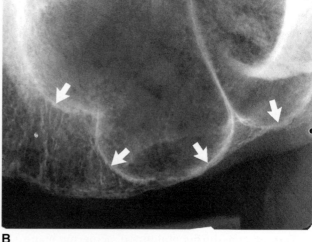

A   **B**

FIG. **9-32**   The floor of the maxillary sinus *(arrows)* extends toward the crest of the alveolar ridge in response to missing teeth.

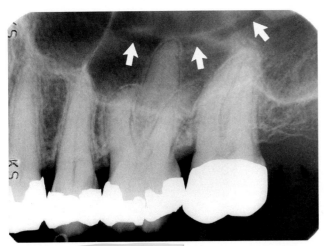

FIG. **9-33** Neurovascular canals *(arrows)* in the lateral wall of the maxillary sinus.

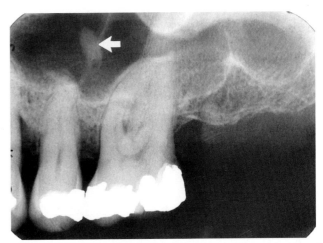

FIG. **9-35** This bony nodule *(arrow)* is a normal variant of the floor of the maxillary sinus.

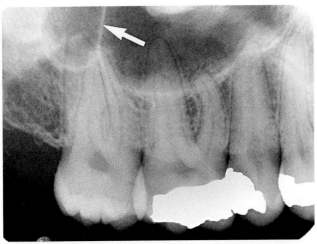

FIG. **9-34** A septum *(arrow)* in the maxillary sinus formed by a low ridge of bone on the sinus wall. (See also Fig. 9-32, *B*).

vascular markings are not seen in the walls of cysts, they may serve to distinguish a normal sinus from a cyst.

Often one or several radiopaque lines traverse the image of the maxillary sinus (Fig. 9-34). These septa represent folds of cortical bone projecting a few millimeters away from the floor and wall of the antrum. They are usually oriented vertically, although horizontal bony ridges also occur, and it is not uncommon for them to vary in number, thickness, and length. Septa are believed by some to have been formed through the uneven resorption of bone as the sinus was pneumatized, but others hold that they are remnants of incompletely fused cavities from which the sinus formed. They appear on many periapical intraoral radiographs, although seldom in extraoral projections because for this view the x-ray beam is rarely directed tangential to them. Although septa appear to separate the sinuses into distinct compartments, this is seldom the case because the septa are usually of limited extent. It has been reported, however, that in 1% to 10% of examined skulls, complete septa did in fact divide the sinus into individual compartments, each compartment with separate ostia for drainage. Septa deserve attention because they sometimes mimic periapical pathoses, and the chambers they create in the alveolar recess may complicate the search for a root fragment displaced into the sinus.

The floor of the maxillary sinus occasionally shows small radiopaque projections, which are nodules of bone (Fig. 9-35). These must be differentiated from root tips, which they resemble in shape. In contrast to a root fragment, which is quite homogeneous in appearance, the bony nodules often show trabeculation; and although they may be quite well defined, at certain points on their surface they blend with the trabecular pattern of adjacent bone. A root fragment may also be recognized by the presence of a root canal. It is not uncommon to see the floor of the nasal fossa in periapical views of the posterior teeth superimposed on the maxillary sinus (see Fig. 9-22). The floor of the nasal fossa is usually oriented more or less horizontally, depending on film placement, and is superimposed high on maxillary views. The image, a solid opaque line, frequently appears somewhat thicker than the adjacent sinus walls and septa.

Zygomatic Process and Zygomatic Bone

The zygomatic process of the maxilla is an extension of the lateral maxillary surface that arises in the region of the apices of the first and second molars and serves

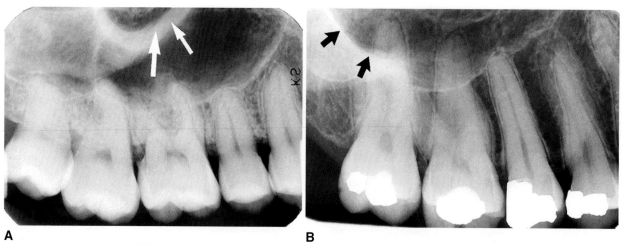

A   **B**

FIG. **9-36**   The zygomatic process of the maxilla *(arrows)* protrudes laterally from the maxillary wall. Its size may be quite variable: small with thick borders (**A**) or large with thin borders (**B**).

as the articulation for the zygomatic bone. On periapical radiographs the zygomatic process appears as a U-shaped radiopaque line with its open end directed superiorly. The enclosed rounded end is projected in the apical region of the first and second molars (Fig. 9-36). The size, width, and definition of the zygomatic process are quite variable, and its image may be large, depending on the angle at which the beam was projected. The maxillary antrum may expand laterally into the zygomatic process of the maxilla (and even into the zygomatic bone after the maxillozygomatic suture has fused), thereby resulting in a relatively increased radiolucent region within the U-shaped image of the process.

When the sinus is recessed deep within the process (and perhaps into the zygomatic bone), the image of the air space within the process is dark and typically the walls of the process are rather thin and well defined (in contrast to the very dark radiolucent air space). When the sinus exhibits relatively little penetration of the maxillary process (usually in younger individuals or those who have maintained their posterior teeth and vigorous masticatory function), the image of the walls of the zygomatic process tends to be somewhat thicker, and the appearance of the sinus in this region is somewhat smaller and more opaque.

The inferior portion of the zygomatic bone may be seen extending posteriorly from the inferior border of the zygomatic process of the maxilla (thereby completing the zygomatic arch between the zygomatic processes of the maxillary and temporal bones). It can be identified as a uniform gray or white radiopacity over the apices of the molars (Fig. 9-37). The prominence of the molar apices superimposed on the shadow of the

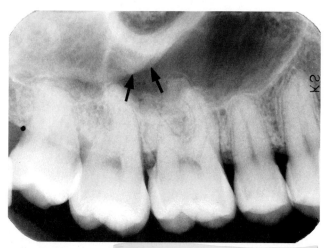

FIG. **9-37**   The inferior border of the zygomatic arch *(arrows)* extends posteriorly from the inferior portion of the zygomatic process of the maxilla.

zygomatic bone, and the amount of detail supplied by the radiograph, depends in part on the degree of aeration (pneumatization) of the zygomatic bone that has occurred, on the bony structure, and on the orientation of the x-ray beam.

Nasolabial Fold

An oblique line demarcating a region that appears to be covered by a veil of slight radiopacity frequently traverses periapical radiographs of the premolar region (Fig. 9-38). The line of contrast is sharp, and the area of increased radiopacity is posterior to the line. The line is the nasolabial fold, and the opaque veil is the thick cheek tissue superimposed on the teeth and the

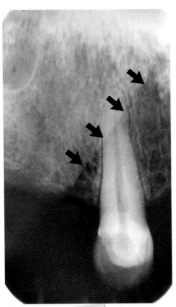

FIG. **9-38** The nasolabial fold *(arrows)* extends across the canine-premolar region.

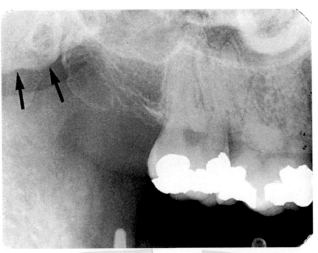

FIG. **9-39** Pterygoid plates *(arrows)* located posterior to the maxillary tuberosity.

alveolar process. The image of the fold becomes more evident with age, as the repeated creasing of the skin along the line (where the elevator of the lip, zygomatic head, and orbicularis all insert into the skin) and the degeneration of the elastic fibers finally lead to the formation and deepening of permanent folds. This radiographic feature frequently proves useful in identifying the side of the maxilla represented by a film of the area if it is edentulous and few other anatomic features are demonstrated.

Pterygoid Plates

The medial and lateral pterygoid plates lie immediately posterior to the tuberosity of the maxilla. The image of these two plates is extremely variable, and on many intraoral radiographs of the third molar area they do not appear at all. When they are apparent, they almost always cast a single radiopaque homogeneous shadow without any evidence of trabeculation (Fig. 9-39). Extending inferiorly from the medial pterygoid plate may be seen the hamular process (Fig. 9-40), which on close inspection can show trabeculae.

MANDIBLE

Symphysis

Radiographs of the region of the mandibular symphysis in infants demonstrate a radiolucent line through the midline of the jaw between the images of the forming deciduous central incisors (Fig. 9-41). This suture usually fuses by the end of the first year of life, after

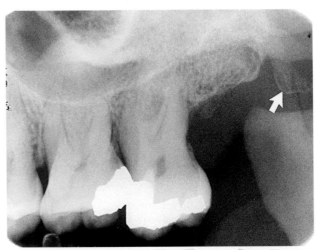

FIG. **9-40** The hamular process *(arrow)* extends downward from the medial pterygoid plate.

which it is no longer radiographically apparent. It is not frequently encountered on dental radiographs because few young patients have cause to be examined radiographically. If this radiolucency is found in older individuals, it is abnormal and may suggest a fracture or a cleft.

Genial Tubercles

The genial tubercles (also called the *mental spine*) are located on the lingual surface of the mandible slightly above the inferior border and in the midline. They are bony protuberances, more or less spine-shaped, that often are divided into a right and left prominence and a superior and inferior prominence. They serve to attach the genioglossus muscles (at the superior

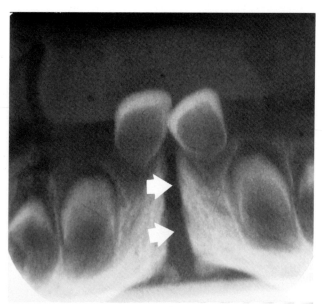

FIG. **9-41**   Mandibular symphysis *(arrows)* in a newborn infant. Note the bilateral supernumerary primary incisors adjacent to it.

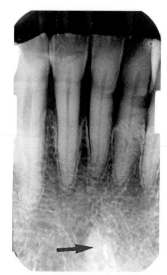

FIG. **9-43**   The genial tubercles *(arrow)* appear as a radiopaque mass, in this case without evidence of the lingual foramen.

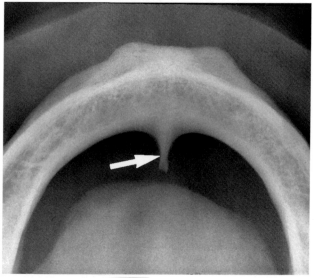

FIG. **9-42**   Genial tubercles *(arrow)* on the lingual surface of the mandible in this cross-sectional mandibular occlusal view.

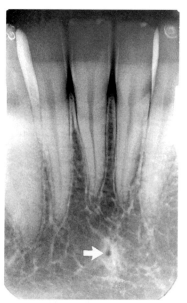

FIG. **9-44**   Lingual foramen *(arrow)*, with a sclerotic border, in the symphyseal region of the mandible.

tubercles) and the geniohyoid muscles (at the inferior tubercles) to the mandible. They are well visualized on mandibular occlusal radiographs as one or more small projections (Fig. 9-42). Their appearance on periapical radiographs of the mandibular incisor region is variable: often they appear as a radiopaque mass (up to 3 to 4 mm in diameter) in the midline below the incisor roots (Fig. 9-43). They also may not be apparent at

all. When the genial tubercles are seen on periapical films, it is often possible to see the lingual foramen (Fig. 9-44). This foramen contains an artery carrying blood from the sublingual arteries into the bony chin.

Mental Ridge

On periapical radiographs of the mandibular central incisors, the mental ridge (protuberance) may occasionally be seen as two radiopaque lines sweeping

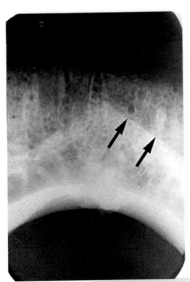

FIG. **9-45** Mental ridge *(arrows)* on the anterior surface of the mandible, seen as a radiopaque ridge.

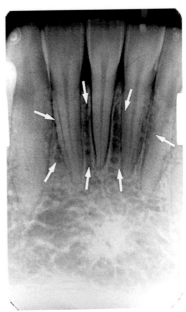

FIG. **9-46** The mental fossa is a radiolucent depression on the anterior surface of the mandible *(arrows)* between the alveolar ridge and mental ridge.

bilaterally forward and upward toward the midline (Fig. 9-45). They are of variable width and density and may be found to extend from low in the premolar area on each side up to the midline, where they lie just inferior to or are superimposed on the mandibular incisor tooth roots. The image of the mental ridge is most prominent when the beam is directed parallel with the surface of the mental tubercle (as when using the bisecting-angle technique).

Mental Fossa

The mental fossa is a depression on the labial aspect of the mandible extending laterally from the midline and above the mental ridge. Because of the resulting thinness of jawbone in this area, the image of this depression may be similar to that of the submandibular fossa (see below) and may, likewise, be mistaken for periapical disease involving the incisors (Fig. 9-46).

Mental Foramen

The mental foramen is usually the anterior limit of the inferior dental canal that is apparent on radiographs (Fig. 9-47). Its image is quite variable, and it may be identified only about half the time because the opening of the mental canal is directed superiorly and posteriorly. As a result, the usual view of the premolars is not projected through the long axis of the canal opening. This circumstance is responsible for the variable appearance of the mental foramen. Although the wall of the foramen is of cortical bone, the density of the foramen's image varies, as does the shape and definition of its border. It may be round, oblong, slitlike, or

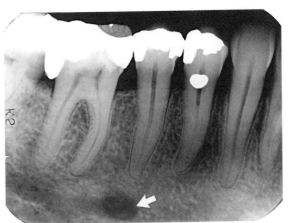

FIG. **9-47** The mental foramen *(arrow)* appears as an oval radiolucency near the apex of the second premolar.

very irregular and partially or completely corticated. The foramen is seen about halfway between the lower border of the mandible and the crest of the alveolar process, usually in the region of the apex of the second premolar. Also, because it lies on the surface of the mandible, the position of its image in relation to the tooth roots is influenced by projection angulation. It may be projected anywhere from just mesial of the permanent first molar roots to as far anterior as mesial of the first premolar root. The image of two mental foramina, one above the other, has also been observed.

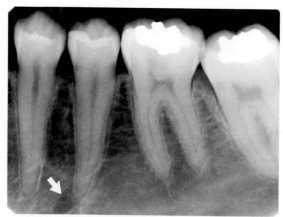

FIG. **9-48**   The mental foramen *(arrow)* (over the apex of the second premolar) may simulate periapical disease. Continuity of the lamina dura around the apex, however, indicates the absence of periapical abnormality.

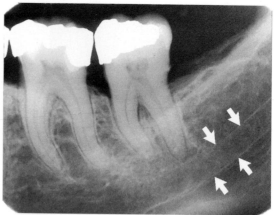

FIG.   **9-49**   Mandibular   canal.   Arrows   denote   its radiopaque superior and inferior cortical borders.

When the mental foramen is projected over one of the premolar apices, it may mimic periapical disease (Fig. 9-48). In such cases, evidence of the inferior dental canal extending to the suspect radiolucency or a detectable lamina dura in the area would suggest the true nature of the dark shadow. It is well to point out, however, that the relative thinness of the lamina dura superimposed with the radiolucent foramen may result in considerable "burnout" of the lamina dura image, which will complicate its recognition. Nevertheless, a second radiograph from another angle is likely to show the lamina dura clearly, as well as some shift in position of the radiolucent foramen relative to the apex.

Mandibular Canal

The radiographic image of the mandibular canal is a dark linear shadow with thin radiopaque superior and inferior borders cast by the lamella of bone that bounds the canal (Fig. 9-49). Sometimes the borders are seen only partially or not at all. The width of the canal shows some interpatient variability but is usually rather constant anterior to the third molar region. The canal's course may be apparent between the mandibular foramen and the mental foramen. Only rarely is the image of its anterior continuation toward the midline discernible on the radiograph.

The relationship of the mandibular dental canal to the roots of the lower teeth may vary, from one in which there is close contact with all molars and the second premolar to one in which the canal has no intimate relation to any of the posterior teeth. In the usual picture, however, the canal is in contact with the apex of the third molar, and the distance between it and the other roots increases as it progresses anteriorly. When the apices of the molars are projected over the canal,

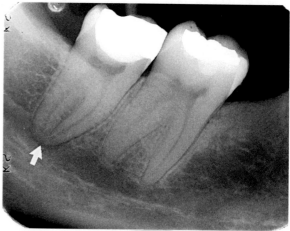

FIG. **9-50**   The mandibular canal superimposed over the apex of a molar causes the image of the periodontal ligament space to appear wider *(arrow)*. The presence of an intact lamina dura, however, indicates that there is no periapical disease.

the lamina dura may be overexposed, conveying the impression of a missing lamina or a thickened PDL space that is more radiolucent than apparently normal for the patient (Fig. 9-50). To ensure the soundness of such a tooth, other clinical testing procedures must be employed (e.g., vitality testing). Because the canal is usually located just inferior to the apices of the posterior teeth, altering the vertical angle for a second film of the area is not likely to separate the images of the apices and canal.

Nutrient Canals

Nutrient canals carry a neurovascular bundle and appear as radiolucent lines of fairly uniform width. They are most often seen on mandibular periapical radiographs running vertically from the inferior dental canal directly to the apex of a tooth (Fig. 9-51) or into the interdental space between the mandibular incisors (Fig. 9-52). They are visible in about 5% of all patients and are more frequent in blacks, males, older persons, and individuals with high blood pressure or advanced periodontal disease. They also indicate a thin ridge, useful in implant assessment. Because they are anatomic spaces with walls of cortical bone, their images occasionally have hyperostotic borders. At times

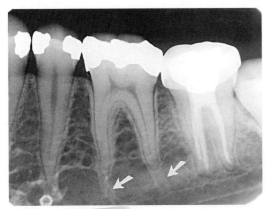

FIG. **9-51** Nutrient canals *(arrows),* demonstrated by radiopaque cortical borders, descend from the mandibular first molar.

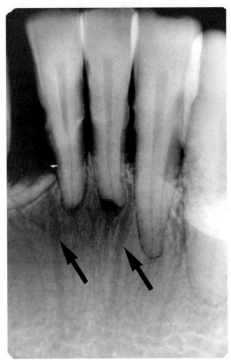

FIG. **9-52** Nutrient canals demonstrated by radiolucencies *(arrows)* in the anterior mandible of a patient with severe periodontal disease.

a nutrient canal will be oriented perpendicular to the cortex and appear as a small round radiolucency simulating a pathologic radiolucency.

Mylohyoid Ridge

The mylohyoid ridge is a slightly irregular crest of bone on the lingual surface of the mandibular body. Extending from the area of the third molars to the lower border of the mandible in the region of the chin, it serves as an attachment for the mylohyoid muscle. Its radiographic image runs diagonally downward and forward from the area of the third molars to the premolar region, at approximately the level of the apices of the posterior teeth (Fig. 9-53). Sometimes this image is superimposed on the images of the molar roots. The margins of the image are not usually well defined but appear quite diffuse and of variable width. The contrary is also observed, however, where the ridge is relatively dense with sharply demarcated borders (Fig. 9-54). It will be more evident on periapical radiographs when the beam is positioned with excessive negative angulation. In general, as the ridge becomes less defined, its anterior and posterior limits blend gradually with the surrounding bone.

Submandibular Gland Fossa

On the lingual surface of the mandibular body, immediately below the mylohyoid ridge in the molar area, there is frequently a depression in the bone. This concavity accommodates the submandibular gland and often appears as a radiolucent area with the sparse trabecular pattern characteristic of the region (Fig. 9-55). This trabecular pattern is even less defined on radiographs of the area because it is superimposed on the relatively reduced mass of the concavity. The

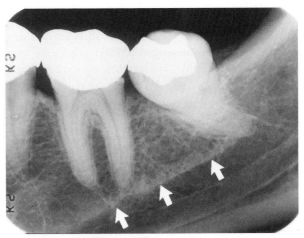

FIG. **9-53** Mylohyoid ridge *(arrows)* running at the level of the molar apices and above the mandibular canal.

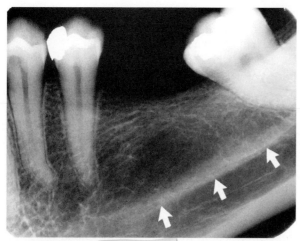

FIG. **9-54**   The mylohyoid ridge *(arrows)* may be dense, especially when a radiograph is exposed with excessive negative angulation.

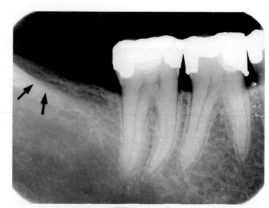

FIG. **9-56**   External oblique ridge *(arrows)*, seen as a radiopaque line near the alveolar crest in the mandibular third molar region.

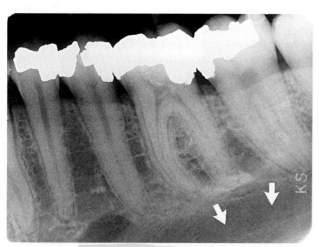

FIG. **9-55**   Submandibular gland fossa *(arrows)*, indicated by a poorly defined radiolucency and sparse trabecular bone below the mandibular molars.

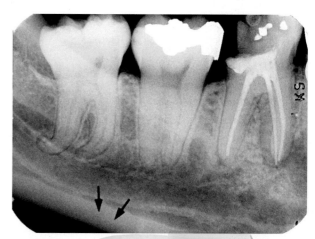

FIG. **9-57**   The inferior border of the mandible *(arrows)* is seen as a dense, broad radiopaque band.

radiographic image of the fossa is sharply limited superiorly by the mylohyoid ridge and inferiorly by the lower border of the mandible, but is poorly defined anteriorly (in the premolar region) and posteriorly (at about the ascending ramus). Although the image may appear strikingly radiolucent, accentuated as it is by the dense mylohyoid ridge and inferior border of the mandible, awareness of its possible presence should preclude its being confused with a bony lesion by the inexperienced clinician.

External Oblique Ridge

The external oblique ridge is a continuation of the anterior border of the mandibular ramus. It follows an anteroinferior course lateral to the alveolar process, being relatively prominent in its upper part and jutting

considerably on the outer surface of the mandible in the region of the third molar (Fig. 9-56). This bony elevation gradually flattens, and usually disappears, at about where the alveolar process and mandible join below the first molar. The ridge is a line of attachment of the buccinator muscle. Characteristically, it is projected onto posterior periapical radiographs superior to the mylohyoid ridge, with which it runs an almost parallel course. It appears as a radiopaque line of varying width, density, and length, blending at its anterior end with the shadow of the alveolar bone.

Inferior Border of the Mandible

Occasionally the inferior mandibular border will be seen on periapical projections (Fig. 9-57) as a characteristically dense, broad radiopaque band of bone.

Coronoid Process

The image of the coronoid process of the mandible is frequently apparent on periapical radiographs of the

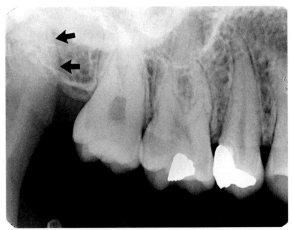

FIG. **9-58** Coronoid process of the mandible *(arrows)* superimposed on the maxillary tuberosity.

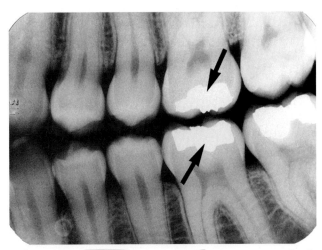

FIG. **9-59** Amalgam restorations appear completely radiopaque *(arrows)*.

maxillary molar region as a triangular radiopacity, with its apex directed superiorly and somewhat anteriorly, superimposed on the region of the third molar (Fig. 9-58). In some cases it may appear as far forward as the second molar and be projected above, over, or below these molars, depending on the position of the jaw and the projection of the x-ray beam. Usually the shadow of the coronoid process is homogeneous, although internal trabeculation can be seen in some cases. Its appearance on maxillary molar radiographs results from the downward and forward movement of the mandible when the mouth is open. Consequently, if the opacity reduces the diagnostic value of a film and the film must be remade, the second view should be acquired with the mouth minimally open. (This contingency must be considered whenever this area is radiographically examined.) On occasion, and especially when its shadow is dense and homogeneous, the coronoid process is mistaken for a root fragment by the neophyte clinician. The true nature of the shadow can be easily demonstrated by obtaining two radiographs with the mouth in different positions and noting the change in position of the suspect shadow.

Restorative Materials

Restorative materials vary in their radiographic appearance, depending primarily on their thickness, density, and atomic number. Of these, the atomic number is most influential.

A variety of restorative materials may be recognized on intraoral radiographs. The most common, silver amalgam, is completely radiopaque (Fig. 9-59). Gold is equally opaque to x rays, whether cast as a crown or inlay (Fig. 9-60) or condensed as gold foil. Stainless

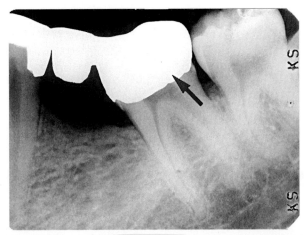

FIG. **9-60** A cast gold crown, appearing completely radiopaque *(arrow)*, serves as the terminal abutment of a bridge.

steel pins also appear radiopaque (Fig. 9-61). Often a calcium hydroxide base is placed in a deep cavity to protect the pulp. Although such base material may be radiolucent, most is radiopaque (Fig. 9-62). Another material of comparable radiopacity is gutta-percha, a rubberlike substance used to fill tooth canals during endodontic therapy (Fig. 9-63). Silver points were previously used to obliterate canals during endodontic therapy (Fig. 9-64). Other restorative materials that appear rather radiolucent on intraoral films include silicates, usually in combination with a base but now seldom used (Fig. 9-65), composite, usually in anterior teeth (Fig. 9-66), and porcelain, now usually fused to a metallic coping (Fig. 9-67). Composite restorative materials may also be opaque (Fig. 9-68). In addition, stainless steel crowns (Fig. 9-69) and orthodontic appliances around teeth (Fig. 9-70) are relatively radiopaque.

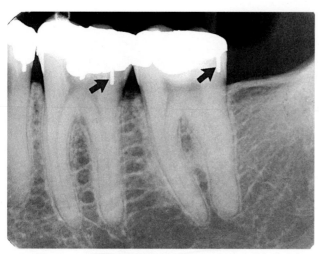

FIG. **9-61**   Stainless steel pins *(arrows)* provide retention for amalgam restorations.

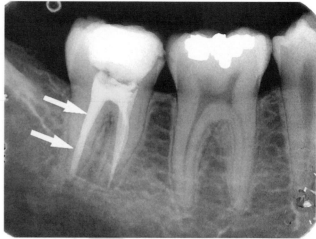

FIG. **9-63**   Gutta-percha *(arrows)* is a radiopaque rubber-like material used in endodontic therapy.

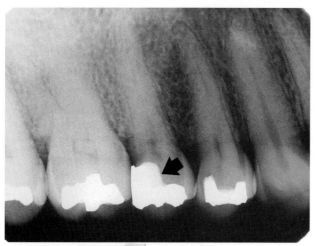

FIG. **9-62**   Base material *(arrow)* is usually radiopaque but less opaque than the amalgam restoration.

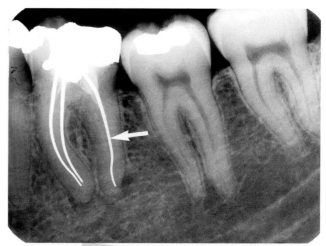

FIG. **9-64**   Silver points *(arrow)* were used to fill the root canals in this patient.

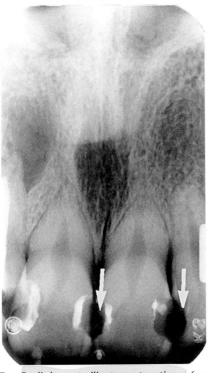

FIG. **9-65**   Radiolucent silicate restorations *(arrows)* were placed over a base to protect the pulp in this patient.

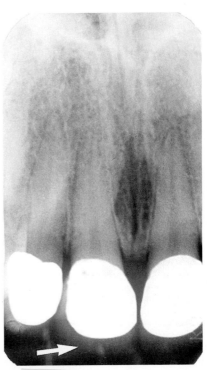

FIG. **9-67**   Porcelain appears radiolucent *(arrow)* over a metal coping.

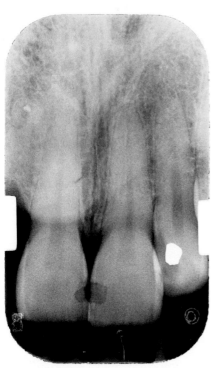

FIG. **9-66**   Composite restorations may be radiolucent and may suggest caries but can be recognized by their well-demarcated border with dentin.

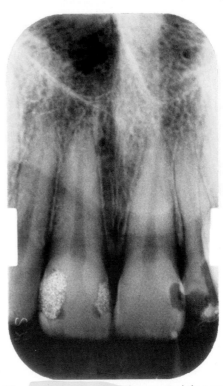

FIG. **9-68**   Composite restorations containing particles of barium glass are radiopaque and not likely to be confused with caries.

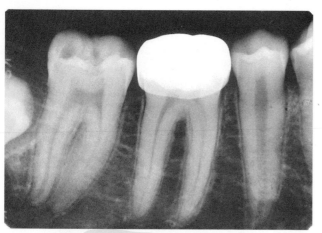

FIG. **9-69** Stainless steel crowns appear mostly radiopaque.

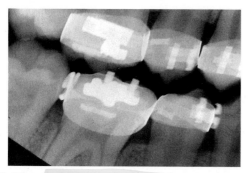

FIG. **9-70** Orthodontic appliances have a characteristic radiopaque appearance.

BIBLIOGRAPHY

Berkovitz BKB, Holland GR, Moxham BL: Oral Anatomy, Histology & Embryology, ed 3, London, 2002, Mosby.

Kasle MJ: An Atlas of Dental Radiographic Anatomy, ed 4, Philadelphia, 1994, WB Saunders.

Lusting JP, London D, Dor BL, Yanko R: Ultrasound identification and quantitative measurement of blood supply to the anterior part of the mandible. Oral Surg Oral Med Oral Pathol Oral Radiol Endod 96(5): 625-9, 2003.

CHAPTER 10

Panoramic Imaging

ALAN G. LURIE

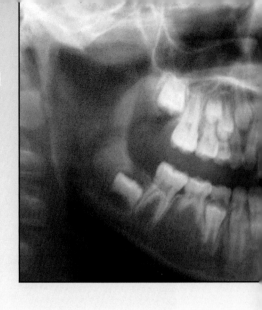

Panoramic imaging (also called **pantomography**) is a technique for producing a single tomographic image of the facial structures that includes both the maxillary and mandibular dental arches and their supporting structures (Fig. 10-1). This is a curvilinear variant of conventional tomography and is also based on the principle of the reciprocal movement of an x-ray source and an image receptor around a central point or plane, called the *image layer,* in which the object of interest is located. Objects in front of or behind this image layer are not clearly captured because of their movement relative to the center of rotation of the receptor and x-ray source.

The principal advantages of panoramic images include the following:

- Broad coverage of the facial bones and teeth
- Low patient radiation dose
- Convenience of the examination for the patient
- Ability to be used in patients unable to open their mouths
- Short time required to make a panoramic image, usually in the range of 3 to 4 minutes (includes the time necessary for positioning the patient and the actual exposure cycle)
- Patient's ready understandability of panoramic films, making them a useful visual aid in patient education and case presentation

Panoramic images are most useful clinically for diagnostic problems requiring broad coverage of the jaws. Common examples include evaluation of trauma, location of third molars, extensive disease, known or suspected large lesions, tooth development (especially in the mixed dentition), retained teeth or root tips (in edentulous patients), and developmental anomalies. These tasks do not require the high resolution and sharp detail available on intraoral images. Panoramic imaging is often used as the initial evaluation image that can provide the required insight or assist in determining the need for other projections. Panoramic images are also useful for patients who do not tolerate intraoral procedures well. However, when a full-mouth series of radiographs is available for a patient receiving general dental care, typically little or no additional useful information is gained from a simultaneous panoramic examination.

The main disadvantage of panoramic radiography is that the images do not display the fine anatomic detail available on intraoral periapical radiographs. Thus panoramic imaging is not as useful as periapical radiography for detecting small carious lesions, fine structure of the marginal periodontium, or periapical disease. The proximal surfaces of premolars also typically overlap. Accordingly, the availability of a panoramic radiograph for an adult patient often does not preclude the need for intraoral films for the diagnoses of most commonly encountered dental diseases. Other problems associated with panoramic radiography include unequal magnification and geometric distortion across the image. Occasionally the presence of overlapping structures, such as the cervical spine, can hide odontogenic lesions, particularly in the incisor region. Furthermore, clinically important objects may be situated outside the plane of focus (image layer) and may appear distorted or not present at all.

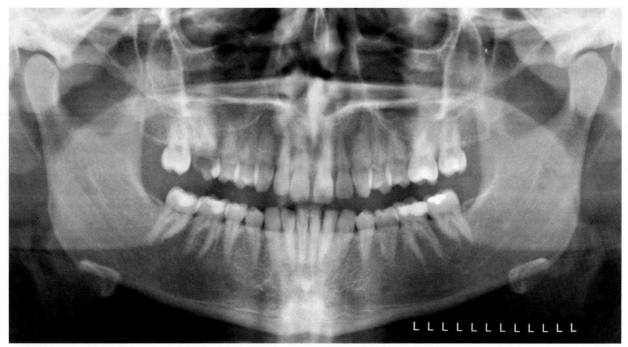

FIG. **10-1**   Maxilla, mandible, and dentition in a 12-year-old child (panoramic view).

Principles of Panoramic Image Formation

The first to describe the principles of panoramic radiography were Paatero and, working independently, Numata. The illustrations in this section explain the operation of a panoramic machine. Two adjacent disks rotate at the same speed in opposite directions as an x-ray beam passes through their centers of rotation (Fig. 10-2). Lead collimators in the shape of a slit, located at the x-ray source and at the image receptor, limit the central ray to a narrow vertical beam. Radiopaque objects *A, B, C,* and *D* stand upright on disk 1 and rotate

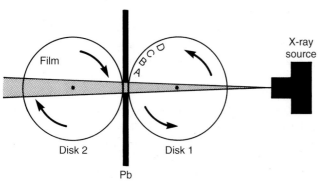

FIG. **10-2**   Movement of the film and objects (*A, B, C,* and *D*) about two fixed centers of rotation. *Pb,* Lead collimator.

past the slit. Their images are recorded on the receptor, which also moves past the slit at the same time. The objects are displayed sharply on the receptor because they are moving past the slit at the same rate and in the same direction as the receptor. This causes their moving shadows to appear stationary in relation to the moving receptor. Other objects between the letters and the center of rotation of disk 1 rotate with a slower velocity and are blurred on the receptor. Any objects between the x-ray source and the center of rotation of disk 1 move in the opposite direction of the receptor, and their shadows are also blurred on the receptor.

Fig. 10-3 shows that the same relationship of moving film to image is achieved if disk 1 is held stationary and the x-ray source is rotated so that the central ray constantly passes through the center of rotation of disk 1 and, simultaneously, both disk 2 and the lead collimator (Pb) rotate around the center of disk 1. Note that although disk 2 moves, the receptor on this disk also rotates past the slit. In this situation, as before, the objects *A* through *D* move through the x-ray beam in the same direction and at the same rate as the receptor. To obtain optimal image definition, it is crucial that the speed of the receptor passing the collimator slit (Pb) be maintained equal to the speed at which the x-ray beam sweeps through the objects of interest.

In the case where the receptor is a charge-coupled device (CCD) array, the image is electronically transmitted to the controlling computer as the x-ray beam

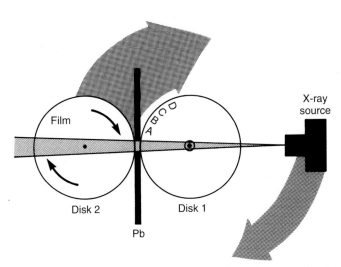

FIG. **10-3** Movement of the film and x-ray source about one fixed center of rotation. *Pb*, Lead collimator.

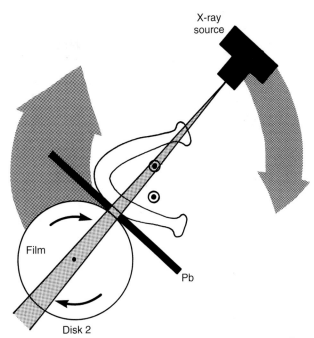

FIG. **10-4** Movement of the film and x-ray source about a shifting center of rotation. *Pb*, Lead collimator.

hits it, and this transmission is continuous as the x-ray source and receptor travel around the patient. The resulting geometric projection characteristics are the same as if film or a photostimulable phosphor plate (PSP) had been used. This holds true for geometric distortions such as magnification and elongation, the presence of ghost images, superimposition of the c-spine over midline structures, overlap of teeth, and left-right size variations from lack of proper positioning of the patient sagittal plane in the instrument.

Fig. 10-4 shows a patient in the place of disk 1, and objects *A* through *D* represent teeth and surrounding bone. In practice, the center of rotation is located off to the side, away from the objects being imaged. During the exposure cycle, the machine automatically shifts to one or more additional rotation centers. The rate of movement of the receptor behind the slit is regulated to be the same as that of the central ray sweeping through the dental structures on the side of the patient nearest the receptor. Structures on the opposite side of the patient (near the x-ray tube) are distorted and appear out of focus because the x-ray beam sweeps through them in the direction opposite that in which the image receptor is moving. In addition, structures near the x-ray source are so magnified (and their borders so blurred) that they are not seen as discrete images on the resultant image. These structures appear only as diffuse phantom or ghost images. Because of both these circumstances, only structures near the receptor are usefully captured on the resultant image. Structures located more centrally in the body relative to the jaws, such as the hyoid bone and epiglottis, appear on the right, left, and sometimes central areas of the final image.

Most panoramic machines now use a continuously moving center of rotation rather than multiple fixed locations. Fig. 10-5 shows a continually moving center of rotation. This feature optimizes the shape of the image layer to reveal the teeth and supporting bone. This center of rotation is initially near the lingual surface of the right body of the mandible when the left temporomandibular joint (TMJ) is imaged. The rotation center moves forward along an arc that ends just lingual to the symphysis of the mandible when the midline is imaged. The arc is reversed as the opposite side of the face is imaged. In some contemporary panoramic machines, the shape of the image layer can be adjusted to better conform to the shape of the patients' mandibulofacial anatomy or to better show specific anatomic areas such as the temporomandibular joints or the maxillary sinuses. This is accomplished through varying the shape of the moving center of rotation and allows better representation of children, unusually configured patients, and specific anatomic sites of interest.

The Image Layer

The image layer is a three-dimensional curved zone (or *focal trough*) in which the structures lying within the layer are reasonably well defined on final panoramic image. The structures seen on a panoramic image are primarily those located within the image layer. Objects

X-ray
source

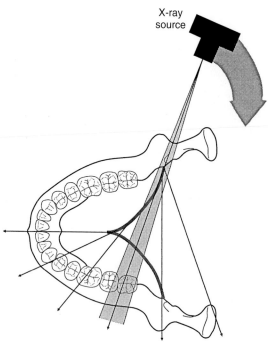

FIG. **10-5** *Movement of the x-ray source and beam.* The dark line shows a continuously moving center of rotation. As the source moves behind the patient's neck and the anterior teeth are imaged, the center of rotation moves forward along the arc *(dark line)* toward the sagittal plane. The x-ray source continues to move around the patient to image the opposite side.

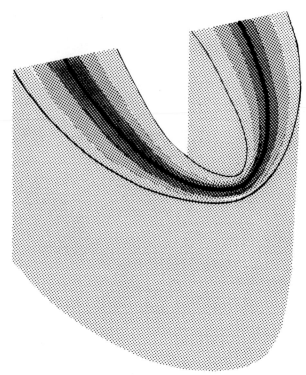

FIG. **10-6** *Focal trough.* The closer to the center of the trough *(dark zone)* an anatomic structure is positioned, the more clearly it is imaged on the resulting radiograph.

outside the image layer are blurred, magnified, or reduced in size and are sometimes distorted to the extent of not being recognizable. The shape of the image layer varies with the brand of equipment used. Fig. 10-6 shows the general shape of the image layer used in panoramic machines. The factors that affect its size are variables that influence image definition: arc path, velocity of the receptor and x-ray tube head, alignment of the x-ray beam, and collimator width. The location of the image layer can change with extensive machine use, so recalibration may be necessary if consistently suboptimal images are produced.

As the position of an object is moved within the image layer, the size and shape of the resultant image change. Fig. 10-7 illustrates the influence of patient positioning on image size and shape. Fig. 10-7, *A* and *B*, shows a mandible supporting a brass ring properly aligned in the middle of the image layer. Note the even magnification of the ring and the images of the anterior teeth in proper proportion. Fig. 10-7, *C* and *D*, shows the same mandible positioned 5 mm anterior to the middle of the center of the image layer. This position causes distortion of the ring in the horizontal dimension, with the ring appearing thinner, and a commensurate decreased width

of the images of the teeth. Fig. 10-7, *E* and *F*, shows the same mandible positioned 5 mm posterior to the middle of the focal trough. Now the horizontal distortion results in the ring appearing wider and a commensurate increased width of the projected teeth. On these images the vertical dimension, in contrast to the horizontal dimension, is little altered, even though it appears to be. These distortions result from the reciprocal horizontal movements of the receptor and x-ray source. Thus, as a general rule, when the structure of interest, in this case the mandible, is displaced to the lingual side of its optimal position in the image layer, toward the x-ray source, the beam passes more slowly through it than the speed at which the receptor moves. Consequently, the images of the structures in this region are elongated horizontally on the image and they appear wider. Alternatively, when the mandible is displaced toward the buccal aspect of the image layer, the beam passes at a rate faster than normal through the structures. In the example shown, because the receptor is moving at the proper rate, the representations of the anterior teeth are compressed horizontally on the image and they appear thinner. Special attention must be paid to these considerations in following the progress of a bony lesion, especially in the anterior region. As a result of improper

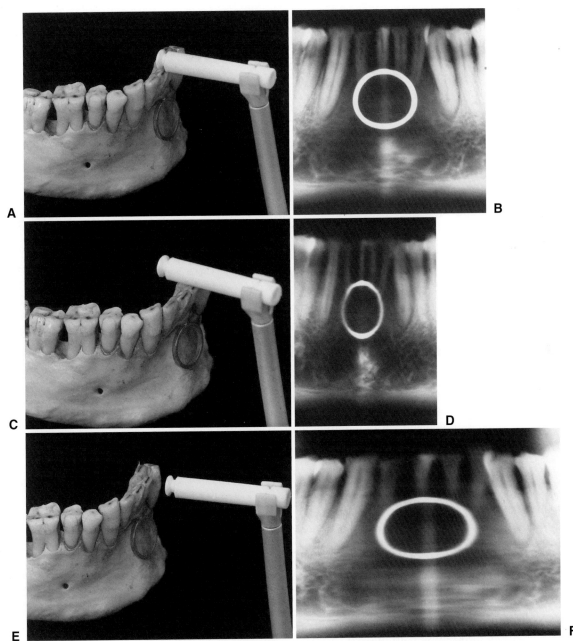

FIG. **10-7**   **A**, Mandible supporting a metal ring positioned at the center of the focal trough. The incisal edges of the mandibular teeth are indexed by a bite rod–positioning device. The mandible is positioned at the center of the trough. **B**, Resultant panoramic radiograph. **C**, Mandible and ring positioned 5 mm anterior to the focal trough. The incisal edges of the teeth are anterior to the trough. **D**, Resultant panoramic radiograph demonstrating the horizontal minification of both ring and mandibular teeth. **E**, Mandible and ring positioned 5 mm posterior to the focal trough. The incisal edges of the teeth are also posterior to the trough. **F**, Resultant panoramic radiograph demonstrating the horizontal magnification of both ring and mandibular teeth.

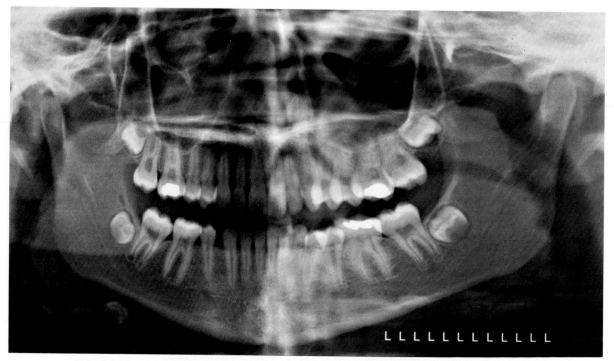

FIG. **10-8**   Panoramic image showing positioning error—rotation of the sagittal plane. The patient's head was rotated to the left, moving the right side closer to the receptor and the left side farther from the receptor. Note the relative magnification of the left-sided molar teeth, mandibular ramus, and condyle. It is important to recognize this fairly common distortion and not to mistake it for a skeletal asymmetry.

patient positioning, the lesion may appear greater (enlarging) (see Fig. 10-7, *F*) or reduced (healing) (see Fig. 10-7, *D*) on successive images. Thus the importance of careful alignment and positioning of the patient's dental arches within the area of the image layer is apparent.

The same principle applies to the patient's sagittal plane being rotated in the image layer. The posterior structures on the side to which the patient's head is rotated are magnified in horizontal dimension, as they are moved away from the image receptor, whereas posterior structures on the opposite side are moved closer to the image receptor and are reduced in horizontal dimension. The resulting image will show horizontally large molar teeth and mandibular ramus on one side and horizontally smaller molar teeth and mandibular ramus on the other side. This must not be confused with a congenital or developmental facial asymmetry. This positioning artifact is demonstrated in Fig. 10-8.

Panoramic Machines

A number of companies manufacture high-quality film-based and digital panoramic machines. The Orthopantomograph 100 (Instrumentarium) (Fig. 10-9), the Orthophos Plus (Sirona), the Orthoralix S (Gendex

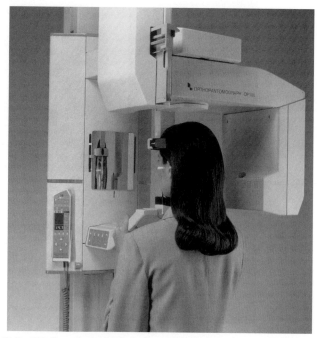

FIG. **10-9**   Orthopantomograph OP100 panoramic machine. (Courtesy Instrumentarium Imaging Inc., Milwaukee, WI.)

Division, Dentsply International), and the ProMax (PLANMECA) Panoramic machine (Fig. 10-10) are all highly versatile. In addition to producing standard panoramic images of the jaws, they have the capability of adjusting to patients of various sizes as well as making frontal and lateral images of the TMJs. These machines also are capable of producing tomographic views through the sinuses and cross-sectional views of the maxilla and mandible. The ProMax (PLANMECA) Panoramic machine acquires these views by using a linear tomography program designed to use SCARA (Selectively Compliant Articulated Robotic Arm) movements with ProMax software and pivoting cassette movements. Each machine also has the capability for adding a cephalometric attachment to allow exposure of standardized skull views. Some machines further have the capability of automated exposure control. This is accomplished by measuring the amount of radiation passing through the patient's mandible during the initial part of the exposure and adjusting the imaging factors (kVp, mA, and speed of imaging movements) to obtain a correctly exposed image.

There are now computer-controlled multimodality machines in which the direction and speed of movement of the tube head and film are highly variable, in some cases including multidirectional tomography. This allows the machines to be programmed to make tomographic views through many areas of the head. For instance, they can be programmed to image frontal or lateral views of the TMJs, coronal or sagittal sections

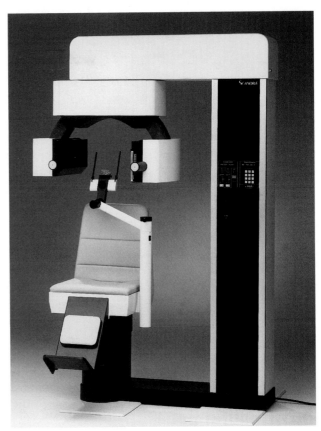

FIG. **10-11** Scanora multimodality machine. (Courtesy Soredex Inc., Milwaukee, WI.)

through the maxillary sinuses, and cross-sectional cuts through a predetermined portion of the maxilla or mandible. These machines have much greater versatility than the conventional panoramic machines, and they are more expensive. The Scanora (Soredex) (Fig. 10-11) and CommCAT (Imaging Sciences International) (Fig. 10-12), for example, have the capability of making conventional panoramic images as well as many special-purpose examinations of the facial skeleton. Most of the special examinations made on these machines use circular or hypocycloidal tomography (see Chapter 13).

Patient Positioning and Head Alignment

To obtain diagnostically useful panoramic radiographs, the technologist must properly prepare patients and position their heads carefully in the image layer. Remove dental appliances, earrings, necklaces, hairpins, and any other metallic objects in the head and neck region. It may also be wise to demonstrate the machine to the patient by cycling it while explaining

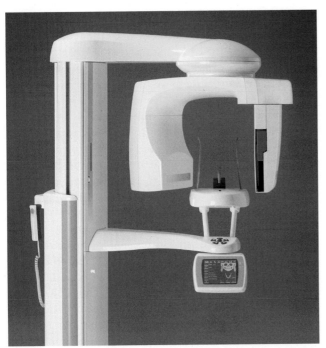

FIG. **10-10** ProMax (PLANMECA) Panoramic machine. (Courtesy Planmeca Inc., Roselle, IL.)

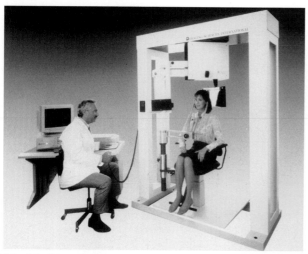

FIG. **10-12**   The CommCAT Imaging System is capable of panoramic radiography as well as complex motion tomography of the TMJ and jaws. (Courtesy Imaging Sciences International, Hatfield, PA.)

the need to remain still during the procedure. This is particularly true for children, who may be anxious. Instruct children to look forward and not follow the tube head with their eyes.

The anteroposterior position radiograph of the patient is typically achieved by having patients place the incisal edges of their maxillary and mandibular incisors into a notched positioning device (the bite block). Be sure patients do not shift their mandible to either side when making this protrusive movement. The midsagittal plane must be centered within the image layer of the particular x-ray unit. Failure to position the midsagittal plane in the rotational midline of the machine results in a radiograph showing right and left sides that are unequally magnified in the horizontal dimension (see Fig. 10-8). Poor midline positioning is a common error, causing horizontal distortion in the posterior regions and, on occasion, nondiagnostic, clinically unacceptable images. A simple method for evaluating the degree of horizontal distortion of the image is to compare the apparent width of the mandibular first molars bilaterally. The smaller side is too close to the receptor, and the larger side is too close to the x-ray source.

The patient's chin and occlusal plane must be properly positioned to avoid distortion. The occlusal plane is aligned so that it is lower anteriorly, angled 20 to 30 degrees below the horizontal plane. A general guide for chin positioning is to place the patient so that a line from the tragus of the ear to the outer canthus of the eye is parallel with the floor. If the chin is tipped too high, the occlusal plane on the radiograph appears flat or inverted and the image of the mandible is distorted

(Fig. 10-13, *A*). In addition, a radiopaque shadow of the hard palate is superimposed on the roots of the maxillary teeth. If the chin is tipped too low, the teeth become severely overlapped, the symphyseal region of the mandible may be cut off the film, and both mandibular condyles may be projected off the superior edge of the film (Fig. 10-13, *B*). Patients are positioned with their backs and spines as erect as possible and their necks extended. Having patients place their feet on a foot support and using a cushion for back support may facilitate proper back positioning in seated units. These devices help straighten the spine, minimizing the artifact produced by a shadow of the spine.

Proper neck extension is best accomplished by using a gentle upward force on the mastoid eminences when positioning the head in a manner similar to applying cervical traction. Allowing patients to slump their heads and necks forward causes a large opaque artifact in the midline created by the superimposition of an increased mass of cervical spine. This shadow obscures the entire symphyseal region of the mandible and may require that the radiograph be retaken (Fig. 10-14). Finally, after patients are positioned in the machine, instruct them to swallow and hold the tongue on the roof of the mouth. This raises the dorsum of the tongue to the hard palate, eliminating the air space and providing optimal visualization of the apices of the maxillary teeth.

Image Receptors

Intensifying screens (see Chapter 4) are routinely used in panoramic radiography because they significantly reduce the amount of radiation required for properly exposing a radiograph. Fast films combined with high-speed (rare earth) screens are indicated for most examinations. In most cases, the manufacturer provides panoramic machines with intensifying screens. The type of screen (manufacturer and model) is printed in black letters on each screen and clearly projected onto the radiograph. With rare earth screens and fast films, the patient's skin exposure from panoramic radiography is approximately equivalent to four bitewing views taken using E-speed film.

Several manufacturers have developed direct digital acquisition panoramic machines. The receptor on such a machine is either an array of charge-coupled devices (CCD) or a film-sized photostimulable storage phosphor plate (PSP) rather than film. The CCD array transmits an electronic signal to the controlling computer, which displays the image on the viewscreen as it is being acquired. The software of the unit makes internal adjustments to the acquired data to render an

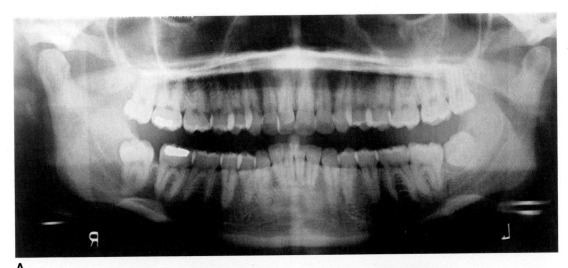

A

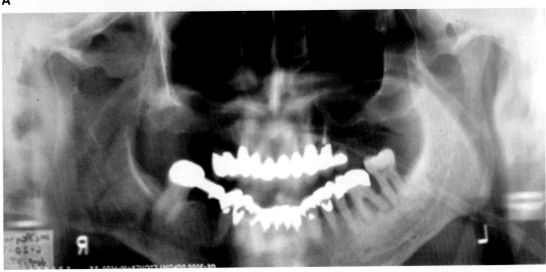

B

FIG. **10-13** *Panoramic radiographs demonstrating poor patient head alignment.* **A,** The chin and occlusal plane are rotated upward, resulting in overlapping images of the teeth and an opaque shadow (the hard palate) obscuring the roots of the maxillary teeth. **B,** The chin and occlusal plane are rotated downward, cutting off the symphyseal region on the radiograph and distorting the anterior teeth.

interpretable image on the screen. The PSP plate is processed in the same manner as intraoral PSPs, and a similar image characteristic adjustmentis automatically performed by the software package. Both of these digital modalities allow the user to perform postprocessing modifications on the image, including linear contrast and density adjustments, black/white reversal, area of interest magnification, edge enhancement, and color rendering. Most units acquire and store their electronic data in DICOM format (*D*igital *I*maging and *CO*mmunication in *M*edicine); this allows for rapid telecommunication of images worldwide to all DICOM–compliant workstations. DICOM is the

international standard language for the electronic communication of digital images, whether they are radiographs, photographs, histopathologic slides, or any other type of "picture image." The American Dental Association has recommended that all digital x-ray units manufactured after 2004 be DICOM–compliant. These units are becoming more widely used as dentistry increases its use of direct digital imaging and electronic patient records. All panoramic images should have some mechanism for automatically marking the patient's left and/or right sides on the image. Also, the patient's name, age, and the date the image was acquired should be indicated with markers,

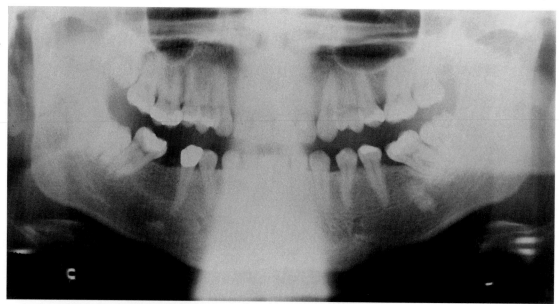

FIG. **10-14**   *Panoramic radiograph of an improperly positioned patient.* Note the large radiopaque region in the middle. This artifact (called a "spine-shadow ghost") can be prevented by having the patient sit straight and align or stretch the neck.

photographic imprinting, or glued labels. The dentist's name must be on the image. No significant anatomic structures should be obscured by any of these labels or markings. Also, no parts of the image should be trimmed to make the film fit the patient's chart.

Panoramic Film Darkroom Techniques

Special darkroom procedures are needed when panoramic film is being processed. These films are far more light-sensitive than intraoral films, especially after they have been exposed. Thus a reduction in darkroom lighting from that used for conventional intraoral film is necessary. A Kodak GBX-2 filter can be installed with a 15-watt bulb at least 4 feet from the working surface. A ML-2 filter should not be used because it fogs panoramic film. Panoramic film should be developed either manually or in automatic film processors using the manufacturer's recommendations. Obtaining optimal results relies on the same care to develop, rinse, fix, and wash panoramic films as is taken with intraoral films.

Interpreting the Panoramic Image

As with all image interpretation, the starting points are the systematic approach to analyzing the image and a

thorough understanding of the appearances of the normal anatomic structures on the image. Panoramic images are quite different from intraoral images and demand a disciplined and focused approach to their interpretation. Recognizing normal anatomic structures on panoramic radiographs is challenging because of the complex anatomy of the midface, the superimposition of various anatomic structures, and the changing projection orientation. The many potential artifacts associated with machine and patient movement, patient positioning, and unusual patient anatomy must be identified and understood. *The absence of a normal anatomic structure may be the most important finding on the image.* Thus it is essential to identify the presence and integrity of all of the major anatomic structures.

Most images in dentistry are two-dimensional representations of three-dimensional structures. Thus on a posterior-anterior (PA) skull film, orbital rims, nasal conchae, teeth, cervical vertebrae, and petrous ridges are all in sharp focus on the image, even though they may be as much as a foot apart from each other. Although this presents less of an interpretation problem when viewing panoramic images, which are curved image "slices" of the mandibulofacial tissues, there is still a thickness to the tomogram that must be considered and the interpreter must relate the structures on the image to their relative positions in the midfacial skeleton. An example of this three-dimensionality is the relative positioning of the external oblique and mylohyoid ridges in the mandible: on the panoramic image, they generally both appear sharp, whereas physically the external oblique ridge is on the mandibular buccal surface and the mylohyoid ridge is on the mandibular lingual surface, separated by several millimeters. When viewing panoramic images, it is important to remember this principle and to attempt visualization of the structures three-dimensionally in your mind.

It is helpful to view the image as if you were looking at the patient, with the structures on the patient's right side positioned on your left (Fig. 10-15). Thus the image is presented to you in the same orientation as that of periapical and bitewing images, making the interpretation more comfortable. It is extremely important to recognize the planes of the patient that are represented in different parts of the panoramic image. The panoramic image is actually three images in one: left and right lateral images posterior to the canines and a posterior-anterior image anterior to the canines. The anterior sextants are subject to the most dimensional distortion, and to superimposition artifacts due to the cervical vertebrae. Thus a useful mental approach to the panoramic image is to consider it as two lateral views surrounding a PA view in the middle, a sort of Mercator projection of the mid- and lower face. This mental approach to viewing the panoramic image

is illustrated by the panoramic and lateral and PA cephalometric images in Fig. 10-16.

As with all image viewing, mask out extraneous light from around the image, dim the room lights, and when possible, work seated in a quiet room. This applies equally to viewing digital images on a computer display and traditional film radiographs on a viewbox.

APPEARANCES OF IMPORTANT ANATOMIC STRUCTURES ON THE PANORAMIC IMAGE

The Mandible

Studying the mandible (Figs. 10-17 and 10-18) can be compartmentalized into the major anatomic areas of this curved bone:
- Condylar process and temporomandibular joint
- Coronoid process
- Ramus
- Body and angle
- Anterior sextant
- Teeth and supporting structures

You should be able to follow a cortical border around the entire bone, with the exception of the dentate

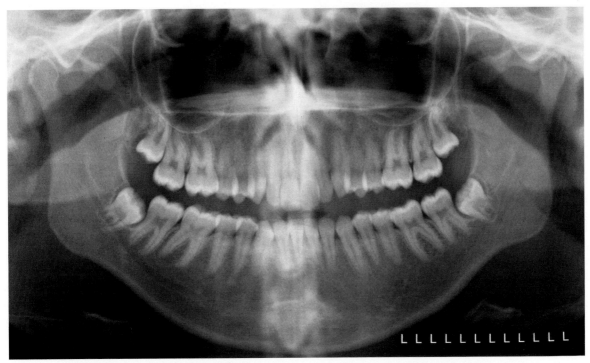

FIG. **10-15** *Properly acquired and displayed panoramic image of an adult patient.* Note that the patient's left side is indicated on the image and that the image is oriented as if you were facing the patient. This is the same orientation used with a full mouth series, making it easier to orient yourself and interpret the image.

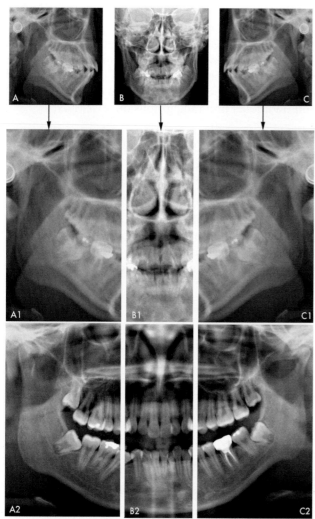

FIG. **10-16   Intellectual segmentation of the panoramic image.** The panoramic image is composed of right and left lateral images connected in the middle by a PA image; it looks similar to a Mercator projection of the globe. This is appreciated by comparing the segmented panoramic image and the labeled structures with the matching cephalometric films acquired on the same patient. **A-C** show left lateral, PA, and right lateral cephalometric images. These images are cropped and aligned to produce **A1-C1. A2-C2** show a segmented panoramic image on the same patient. Note the similarities between the lateral cephalometric images and the panoramic image posterior to the canines and between the PA cephalometric image and the panoramic image between the canines. Thus, when interpreting a panoramic image, you should think of viewing left and right lateral projections of the midface, connected in the middle by a PA projection.

areas. This border should be smooth, without interruptions (step deformities), and have symmetrical thicknesses in comparable anatomic areas (e.g., angles, inferior borders of bodies, posterior borders of rami) The trabeculation of the mandible tends to be more plentiful in the anterior regions, whereas the marrow compartment increases toward the angle and into the ramus; however, these trabecular patterns and densities should be relatively symmetrical. This is especially true in children, who have very sparse trabeculation throughout the deciduous and mixed dentition stages.

The mandibular condyle is generally positioned slightly anteroinferior to its normal closed position as the patient has to slightly open and protrude the mandible to engage the positioning device in most panoramic machines. Remember that you can assess the TMJ for gross anatomic changes of the condylar head and glenoid fossa; you cannot evaluate the soft tissues, such as the articular disc and posterior ligamentous attachment. Also keep in mind the fact that the glenoid fossa is part of the temporal bone and as such it can be pneumatized by the mastoid air cells. This can result in the appearance of a multilocular radiolucency in the articular eminence and the roof of the glenoid fossa, a variant of normal. More definitive osseous assessment of the TMJ is accomplished using complex motion tomography, and magnetic resonance imaging (MRI) is the examination of choice for evaluation of the disc and pericondylar soft tissues (Brooks, 1997).

Shadows of other structures that can be superimposed over the mandibular ramal area include the following:

- Pharyngeal airway shadow—especially when the patient was unable to expel the air and place the tongue in the palate during the exposure
- Posterior wall of the nasopharynx
- Cervical vertebrae—especially in patients with pronounced anterior lordosis, typically seen in severely osteoporotic individuals
- Ear lobe and ear decorations
- Soft palate and uvula
- Dorsum of the tongue
- Ghost shadow of the opposite side of the mandible

From the angle of the mandible, continue viewing anteriorly toward the symphyseal region. A fracture often manifests as a discontinuity (step deformity) in the inferior border; a sharp change in the level of the occlusal plane indicates that the fracture passes through the tooth-bearing area, whereas a cant in the entire occlusal table without a step deformity in the occlusal plane indicates that the fracture is posterior to the tooth-bearing area. The width of the cortical bone

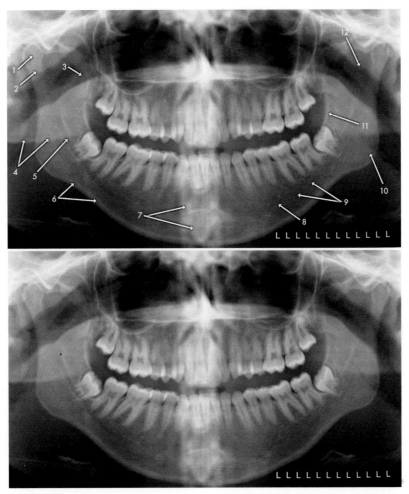

FIG. **10-17** **Mandibular bony anatomic structures on the panoramic image.** The labeled *(top)* and unlabeled *(bottom)* images are duplicates of the same patient. *1,* Mandibular condyle. *2,* Neck of mandibular condyle. *3,* Coronoid process of mandible. *4,* Ghost image—posterior aspect of inferior border of left side of mandible. *5,* Inferior alveolar (mandibular) canal. *6,* Inferior border of mandible. *7,* Superimposed shadow of cervical vertebrae. *8,* Mental foramen. *9,* Submandibular fossa (lingual salivary gland depression)—see also Fig. 10-19. *10,* Mandibular angle. *11,* External oblique ridge. *12,* Sigmoid notch.

at the inferior border of the mandible should be at least 3 mm in adults and of uniform density. The bone may be thinned locally by an expansile lesion such as a cyst or thinned generally by systemic diseases such as hyperparathyroidism and osteoporosis. Compare the outlines of both sides of the mandible for symmetry, noting any changes. Asymmetry of size may result from improper patient positioning or conditions such as hemifacial hyperplasia or hypoplasia. The hyoid bone may be projected below or onto the inferior border of the mandible.

Trabeculation is most evident within the alveolar process. The mandibular canals and mental foramina are usually clearly visualized in the ramus and body

regions of the body of the mandible. Typically the canals exhibit uniform width or gentle tapering from the mandibular foramina to the mental foramina. They may be less well seen in the first molar and premolar regions. They usually rise to meet the mental foramina, often looping several millimeters anterior of the mental foramina. This is termed the *anterior loop* of the mandibular canal, and its position and extent are considerations when planning dental implants in the mandibular canine regions. A bulging of the canal suggests a neural tumor; however, it should be noted that slight widening at the point that the canal bends to enter the body of the mandible from the ramus is a variation of normal. Examine the mandible for

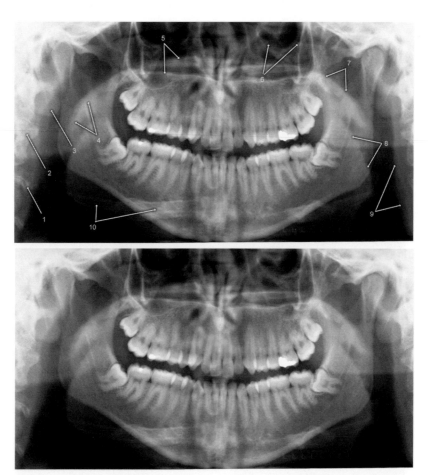

FIG. **10-18**   **Spinal, neck, and soft tissue anatomic structures on the panoramic image.** The labeled *(top)* and unlabeled *(bottom)* images are duplicates of the same patient. *1,* Schwall's node (variant of normal anatomy of the vertebral body). *2,* Cervical vertebra. *3,* Ear lobe. *4,* Soft palate and uvula. *5,* Hard palate (the lower line is the palatal surface; the upper line is the floor of the nasal cavity). *6,* Orbital rim. *7,* Floor of nasopharynx (upper surface of soft palate). *8,* Posterior surface of tongue. *9,* Posterior pharyngeal wall. *10,* Hyoid bone.

radiolucencies or opacities. The midline is more opaque because of the mental protuberance, increased trabecular numbers, and attenuation of the beam as it passes through the cervical spine. Many modern panoramic machines automatically increase the exposure factors as they pass across the cervical spine region in an attempt to minimize this opacity; nevertheless, some opacity is generally seen in the anterior regions of the image. There are often depressions on the lingual surfaces of the mandible that are occupied by the sub-mandibular and sublingual glands: these depressions are termed the *lingual salivary gland depressions,* or *fossae,* and are often more radiolucent. This anatomic feature is shown on a panoramic image, a periapical image, a coronal CT image, and a dry skull in Fig. 10-19.

The Midfacial Region

The midface (Fig. 10-20; see also Fig. 10-18) is a complex mixture of bones, air cavities, and soft tissues, all of which appear on panoramic images. Individual bones that may appear on the panoramic image of the midfacial include temporal, zygoma, mandible, frontal, maxilla, sphenoid, ethmoid, vomer, nasal, turbinate, and palate; thus it is somewhat of a misnomer to refer to the midfacial region on the panoramic image as the *maxilla.* Maintaining the discipline and focus of a systemic examination of all aspects of the midfacial images is difficult and critical in the overall examination of the panoramic image.

As with the mandible, the maxilla can be compartmentalized into major sites for examination:

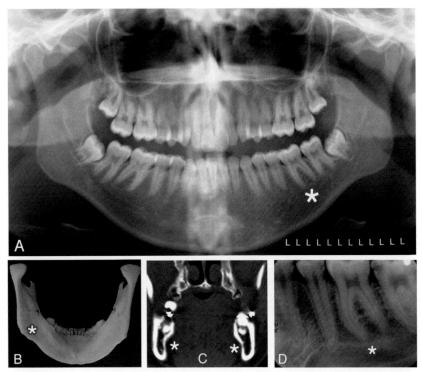

FIG. **10-19**   The submandibular fossa (lingual salivary gland depression), a concavity often found on the posterior lingual surface of the mandible. This triangularly shaped area is bounded anatomically by the mylohyoid ridge, the inferior border of the mandibular body, and the posterior border of the mandibular ramus. Asterisk (*) indicates the area of the submandibular fossa on the various images. **A,** Panoramic image. **B,** Photograph of the lingual side of a dried mandible. **C,** Coronal CT scan through the molar region of the mandible. **D,** Mandibular molar periapical image.

- Cortical boundary of the maxilla, including the posterior border and the alveolar ridge
- Pterygomaxillary fissure
- Maxillary sinuses
- Zygomatic complex, including inferior and lateral orbital rims, zygomatic process of maxilla, and anterior portion of zygomatic arch
- Nasal cavity and conchae
- Temporomandibular joint (already viewed in the mandible, but revisiting important structures is always a good idea in image interpretation)
- Maxillary dentition and supporting alveolus

Examining the cortical outline of the maxilla is a good way to center your examination of the midface. The posterior border of the maxilla extends from the superior portion of the pterygomaxillary fissure down to the tuberosity region and around to the other side. The posterior border of the pterygomaxillary fissure is the pterygoid spine of the sphenoid bone (the anterior border of the pterygoid plates). Occasionally, the sphenoid sinus may extend into this structure. The pterygomaxillary fissure itself has an inverted teardrop appearance; it is very important to identify this area on both sides of the image, because maxillary sinus mucoceles and carcinomas will characteristically destroy the posterior maxillary border, which is then manifested as loss of the pterygomaxillary fissure. Also, LeFort fractures of the maxilla always involve the pterygoid plate(s), and this will often be initially diagnosed by disturbances of the integrity of the pterygomaxillary fissure on the panoramic image. In fact, this may be the only evidence for such a fracture on the panoramic image. To clarify the three-dimensional anatomy of the pterygomaxillary fissure, Fig. 10-21 shows this structure in a dried skull, in an axial CT image, and in the panoramic image.

The maxillary sinuses are usually well visualized on panoramic images. Identify each of the borders and then note whether they are entirely outlined with cortical bone, roughly symmetric, and comparable in radiographic density. The borders should be present and intact. The medial border of the maxillary sinus is the

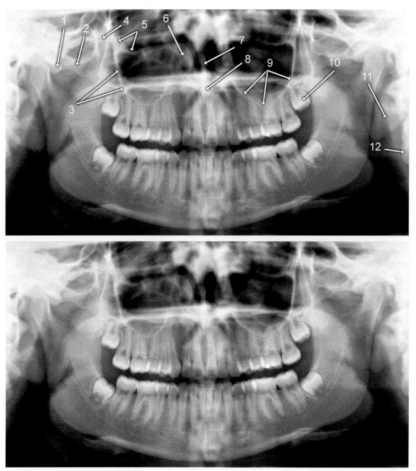

FIG. **10-20**   **Maxillary, or mid-facial, bony anatomic structures on the panoramic image.** The labeled *(top)* and unlabeled *(bottom)* images are duplicates of the same patient. *1,* Articular tubercle of the temporal bone (articular eminence of the temporomandibular joint). *2,* Zygomatic arch. *3,* Zygomatic process of the maxilla. *4,* Pterygomaxillary fissure (see also Fig. 10-21). *5,* Orbital rim. *6,* Inferior nasal concha. *7,* Nasal septum. *8,* Anterior nasal spine. *9,* Floor of the maxillary sinus. *10,* Developing third molar. *11,* Ear lobe. *12,* Cervical vertebra.

lateral border of the nasal cavity, however this interface is not demonstrated on the panoramic image. The superior border, or roof, of the maxillary sinus is the floor of the orbit; this interface is demonstrated on the panoramic image in its most anterior aspect. Although it is useful to compare right and left maxillary sinuses when looking for abnormalities, it is important to remember that the sinuses are frequently nonpathologically asymmetric relative to size, shape, and presence and numbers of septae. The posterior aspect of the sinus is more opaque because of superimposition of the zygoma. Examine each sinus for evidence of a mucous retention cyst, mucoperiosteal thickening, and other sinus abnormalities.

The zygomatic complex, or "buttress" of the midface, is a very complex anatomic area, with contributions from the frontal, zygomatic, and maxillary bones. It includes the lateral and inferior orbital rims, the zygomatic process of the maxilla, and the zygomatic arch. The zygomatic process of the maxilla arises over the maxillary first and second molar. The maxillary sinus can pneumatize the zygomatic process of the maxilla up to the zygomaticomaxillary suture. This can result in the appearance of an elliptical, corticated radiolucency in the maxillary sinus, possibly superimposed over the roots of a molar tooth, on a panoramic image. The inferior border of the zygomatic arch extends posteriorly from the inferior portion of the zygomatic process of the maxilla and extends posteriorly to the articular tubercle and glenoid fossa of the temporal bone. Note also the superior border of the zygomatic arch, which curves superiorly to form the lateral aspect of the lateral

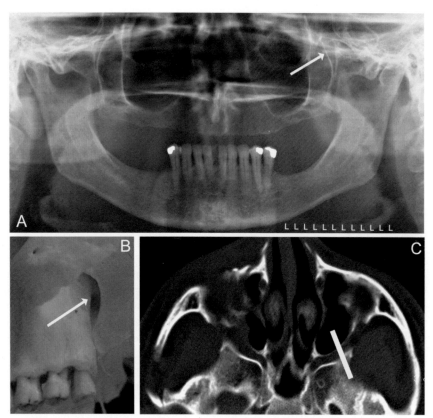

FIG. **10-21**   The pterygomaxillary fissure, a space between the posterior surface of the maxilla and the anterior border of the pterygoid plates. **A** shows the inverted teardrop shape of the fissure on a panoramic image. **B** shows the fissure on a dried skull. **C** shows the approximate section of the panoramic image layer through the pterygomaxillary fissure on an axial CT section *(white bar)*.

orbital rim. The zygomaticotemporal suture lies in the middle of the zygomatic arch and may simulate a fracture if visualized. Additionally, the mastoid air cells occasionally pneumatize the temporal bone all the way to the zygomaticotemporal suture, giving the glenoid fossa of the TMJ the appearance of having a multilocular, or "soap-bubbly," radiolucency that is, in fact, a variant of normal.

The nasal fossa may show the nasal septum and inferior concha, including both the bone and its mucosal covering. The conchae, composed of an internal bone, the turbinate, and covering cartilage and mucosa, are seen in a coronal manner in the anterior portion of the image and in a sagittal manner in the posterior portions of the panoramic image. These structures can appear as very large, homogeneous, soft tissue densities superimposed over the maxillary sinuses and occasionally the anterior nasopharynx.

Soft Tissues

A number of opaque soft tissue structures (Fig. 10-22; see also Fig. 10-18) may be identified on panoramic radiographs, including the tongue arching across the film under the hard palate (roughly from the region of the right angle of the mandible to the left angle), lip markings (in the middle of the film), the soft palate extending posteriorly from the hard palate (see Fig. 10-15, *6*) over each ramus, the posterior wall of the oral and nasal pharynx, the nasal septum, ear lobes, nose, and nasolabial folds. Radiolucent airway shadows superimpose on normal anatomic structures and may be demonstrated by the borders of adjacent soft tissues. These include the nasal fossa, nasal pharynx, oral cavity, and oral pharynx. The epiglottis and thyroid cartilage are often seen in panoramic images. Occasionally the air space between the dorsum of the tongue and the soft palate simulates a fracture through the angle of the mandible.

Superimpositions and Ghost Images

Many radiopaque objects out of the image layer superimpose on the image of normal anatomic structures. This results when the x-ray beam projects through a dense object (e.g., an earring, the spinal column, the

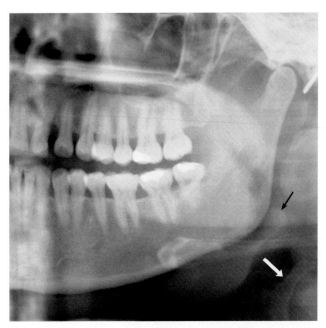

FIG. 10-22   Normal structures occasionally seen in the neck area on panoramic images. The *white arrow* indicates the superior aspect of the thyroid cartilage, which can be mistaken for a vascular calcification. The *black arrow* indicates the epiglottis. Also note the ear decoration posterior to the condylar head.

mandibular ramus, or the hard palate) that is in the path of the x-ray beam but out of the portion of the focal trough being imaged. The object typically appears blurred and projects either over the midline structures, as with the cervical vertebrae, or onto the opposite side of the radiograph in reversed configuration and more cranially positioned than the real structure (see Fig. 10-17). These contralateral images are termed *ghost images*, and they may obscure normal anatomy or be mistaken for pathology.

Dentition

Finally, evaluate the teeth and supporting alveolar bone. If the anterior teeth are excessively wide or narrow, this suggests malposition of the patient. Similarly, if the teeth are wider on one side than the other, this suggests that the patient's sagittal plane was rotated. Although gross caries and periapical and periodontal disease may be evident, subtle disease requires intraoral images for diagnosis. The proximal surfaces of the premolar teeth often overlap, which further interferes with caries interpretation.

One of the strengths of the panoramic image is the demonstration of the complete dentition. Although

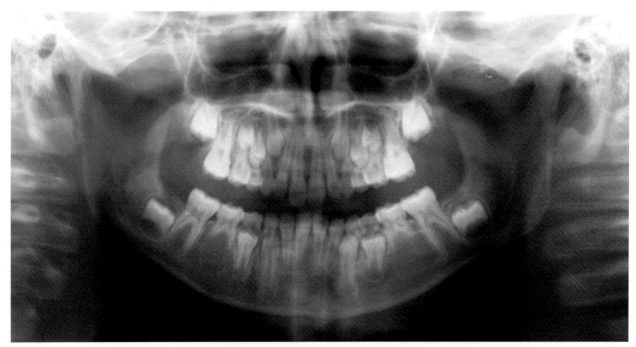

FIG. 10-23 Panoramic image showing late mixed dentition of an 11-year-old patient. The panoramic image can be useful in identifying the presence or absence, as well as developmental status, of the permanent dentition. In this patient, the mandibular second premolars are congenitally absent, and the mandibular deciduous second molars are not undergoing root resorption, indicating that they will be retained. The permanent canines, second molars, and first and second premolars are in various stages of mineralization, with most of them beginning to erupt.

rare situations occur in which positioning of the patient and of an ectopic tooth place the tooth out of the image layer, all of the teeth are generally seen on the image. Thus the interpretation must always include identification of all erupted and developing teeth (Fig. 10-23). The teeth should be examined for gross abnormalities of number, position, and anatomy. Existing dentistry, including endodontic obturations, crowns, and other fixed restorations, should be noted.

It is particularly important to examine impacted third molars closely. Their orientation, the numbers and configurations of the roots, the relationships of the tooth components to critical anatomic structures such as the mandibular canal, the floor and posterior wall of the maxillary sinus, the maxillary tuberosity, and adjacent teeth, as well as the presence of abnormalities in the pericoronal and/or periradicular bone, must be carefully studied. Suspected abnormalities of the dentition seen on panoramic images generally requires intraoral imaging for a more definitive demonstration of the area.

BIBLIOGRAPHY

Brooks SL, et al: Imaging of the temporomandibular joint. A position paper of the American Academy of Oral and Maxillofacial Radiology, Oral Surg Oral Med Oral Pathol Oral Radiol Endod 83:609-618, 1997.

Chomenko AG: Atlas for maxillofacial pantomographic interpretation, Chicago, 1985, Quintessence Publishing.

Langland OE, et al: Panoramic radiology, ed 2, Philadelphia, 1989, Lea & Febiger.

Moore WE (ed): Successful Panoramic Radiography. KODAK Dental Radiography Series, http://www.kodak.com/global/en/health/dental/publications/proEdDental.jhtml, 2001.

Numata H: Consideration of the parabolic radiography of the dental arch, J Shimazu Stud 10:13, 1933.

Paatero YV: A new tomographic method for radiographing curved outer surfaces, Acta Radiol 32:177, 1949.

Paatero YV: The use of a mobile source of light in radiography, Acta Radiol 29:221, 1948.

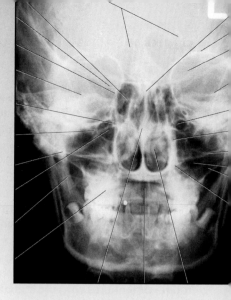

CHAPTER 11

Extraoral Radiographic Examinations

SOTIRIOS TETRADIS ■ MEL L. KANTOR

In extraoral radiographic examinations both the x-ray source and image receptor (film or electronic sensor) are placed outside the patient's mouth. This chapter describes the most common extraoral radiographic examinations in which the source and sensor remain static. These include the *lateral cephalometric* projection of the sagittal or median plane; the *submentovertex* projection of the transverse or horizontal plane; the *Waters, posteroanterior cephalometric,* and *reverse-Towne* projections of the coronal or frontal plane; and the *oblique lateral* projections of the mandibular body and ramus. Panoramic radiography is described in Chapter 10, and other more complex imaging modalities are described in Chapter 13.

Technique

The first step in obtaining a radiograph is the selection of the appropriate projection for the pertinent diagnostic task. However, for pedagogical reasons, this chapter begins with the technical facets of obtaining the extraoral views to make the reader familiar with the various projections.

Extraoral radiographs are produced with conventional dental x-ray machines, certain models of panoramic machines, or higher-capacity medical x-ray units. Cephalometric and skull views require at least a 20×25 cm (8×10 inch) image receptor, whereas oblique lateral projections of the mandible can be obtained with a 13×18 cm (5×7 inch) image receptor. It is critical to correctly and clearly label the right and

left side of the image. This usually is done by placing a metal marker (an *R* or an *L*) on the outside of the cassette in a corner in which the marker does not obstruct diagnostic information.

The proper exposure parameters depend on the patient's size, anatomy, and head orientation; image receptor speed; x-ray source-to-receptor distance; and whether or not grids are used. In cases of known or suspected disease, medium- or high-speed rare-earth screen-film combinations provide optimal balance between diagnostic information and patient exposure. For orthodontic purposes, high-speed combinations reduce patient exposure without compromising the identification of anatomic landmarks necessary for cephalometric analysis. Although radiographic grids reduce scattered radiation and improve contrast and resolution, they result in higher patient exposure. Cephalometry does not require the use of grids. However, grids could improve the radiographic appearance of fine structures, such as trabecular architecture, and aid in the diagnosis of disease.

Proper positioning of the x-ray source, patient, and image receptor requires patience, attention to detail, and experience. The main anatomic landmark used in patient positioning during extraoral radiography is the canthomeatal line, which joins the central point of the external auditory canal to the outer canthus of the eye. The canthomeatal line forms approximately a 10-degree angle with the Frankfort plane, the line that connects the superior border of the external auditory canal with the infraorbital rim. The image receptor and patient placement, central beam direction, and resultant image for the lateral, submentovertex, Waters, posteroanterior, reverse-Towne, and mandibular oblique lateral projections are summarized in Table 11-1 and are described in detail below.

LATERAL CEPHALOMETRIC PROJECTION (LATERAL SKULL PROJECTION)

Image Receptor and Patient Placement

The image receptor is positioned parallel to the patient's midsagittal plane. The site of interest is placed toward the image receptor to minimize distortion. In cephalometric radiography, the patient is placed with the left side toward the image receptor (USA standards), and a wedge filter at the tube head is positioned over the anterior aspect of the beam to absorb some of the radiation and allow visualization of soft tissues of the face.

Position of the Central X-Ray Beam

The central beam is perpendicular to the midsagittal plane of the patient and the plane of the image receptor and is centered over the external auditory meatus.

Resultant Image (Fig. 11-1)

Exact superimposition of right and left sides is impossible because structures on the side near to the image receptor are magnified less than the same structures on the side far from the image receptor. Bilateral structures close to the midsagittal plane demonstrate less discrepancy in size when compared with bilateral structures farther away from the midsagittal plane.

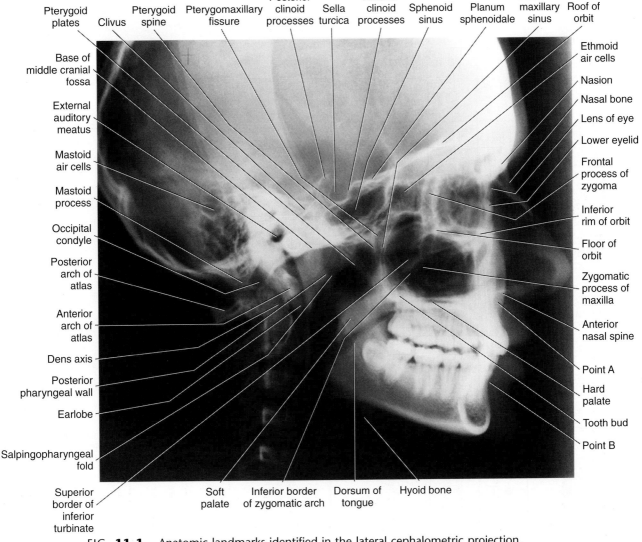

FIG. **11-1** Anatomic landmarks identified in the lateral cephalometric projection.

TABLE 11-1
Technical Aspects of Extraoral Radiographic Projections and Resultant Images

	Lateral Ceph	SMV	Waters	PA Ceph	Reverse Towne	Oblique Lateral Body	Oblique Lateral Ramus
Patient placement	Film parallel to midsagittal plane	Canthomeatal line parallel to film	Canthomeatal line at 37° with film	Canthomeatal line at 10° with film	Canthomeatal line at −30° with film	Film in contact with cheek at molar area	Film in contact with cheek at ramus area
Central beam	Beam perpendicular to film	Beam perpendicular to film	Beam perpendicular to film	Beam perpendicular to film	Beam perpendicular to film	Beam aims at the molar-premolar area	Beam aims at the ramus area
Diagram of patient placement							
Illustration of patient placement							
Skull view							
Resultant image							

Structures close to the midsagittal plane (e.g., the clinoid processes and inferior turbinates) should be nearly superimposed.

SUBMENTOVERTEX (BASE) PROJECTION

Image Receptor and Patient Placement
The image receptor is positioned parallel to patient's transverse plane and perpendicular to the midsagittal and coronal planes. To achieve this, the patient's neck is extended as far backwards as possible, with the canthomeatal line forming a 10-degree angle with the image receptor.

Position of the Central X-Ray Beam
The central beam is perpendicular to the image receptor, directed from below the mandible towards the vertex of the skull (hence the name *submentovertex*, or *SMV*), and centered about 2 cm anterior to a line connecting the right and left condyles.

Resultant Image (Fig. 11-2)
The midsagittal plane (represented by an imaginary line extending from the interproximal space of the maxillary central incisors through the nasal septum, to the middle of the anterior arch of the atlas, and to the dens) should divide the skull image in two symmetric halves. The buccal and lingual cortical plates of the mandible should be projected as uniform opaque lines. An underexposed view is required for the evaluation of the zygomatic arches as they will be overexposed or "burned out" on radiographs obtained with normal exposure factors.

WATERS PROJECTION

Image Receptor and Patient Placement
The image receptor is placed in front of the patient and perpendicular to the midsagittal plane. The patient's head is tilted upward so that the canthomeatal line forms a 37-degree angle with the image receptor. If the patient's mouth is open, the sphenoid sinus will be seen superimposed over the palate.

Position of the Central X-Ray Beam
The central beam is perpendicular to the image receptor and centered in the area of the maxillary sinuses.

Resultant Image (Fig. 11-3)
The midsagittal plane (represented by an imaginary line extending from the interproximal space of the maxillary central incisors through the nasal septum and the middle of the bridge of the nose) should divide the

skull image in two symmetric halves. The petrous ridge of the temporal bone should be projected below the floor of the maxillary sinus.

POSTEROANTERIOR CEPHALOMETRIC PROJECTION (POSTEROANTERIOR SKULL PROJECTION)

Image Receptor and Patient Placement
The image receptor is placed in front of the patient, perpendicular to the midsagittal plane and parallel to the coronal plane. The patient is placed so that the canthomeatal line forms a 10-degree angle with the horizontal plane and the Frankfurt plane is perpendicular to the image receptor. In the posteroanterior skull projection, the canthomeatal line is perpendicular to the image receptor.

Position of the Central X-Ray Beam
The central beam is perpendicular to the image receptor, directed from the posterior to the anterior (hence the name *posteroanterior*, or *PA*), parallel to patient's midsagittal plane, and is centered at the level of the bridge of the nose.

Resultant Image (Fig. 11-4)
The midsagittal plane (represented by an imaginary line extending from the interproximal space of the central incisors through the nasal septum and the middle of the bridge of the nose) should divide the skull image in two symmetric halves. The superior border of the petrous ridge should lie in the lower third of the orbit.

REVERSE-TOWNE PROJECTION (OPEN-MOUTH)

Image Receptor and Patient Placement
The image receptor is placed in front of the patient, perpendicular to the midsagittal and parallel to the coronal plane. The patient's head is tilted downward so that the canthomeatal line forms a 25- to 30-degree angle with the image receptor. To improve the visualization of the condyles, the patient's mouth is opened so that the condylar heads are located inferior to the articular eminence. When requesting this image to evaluate the condyles, it is necessary to specify "open-mouth, reverse-Towne" otherwise a standard Towne view of the occiput may result.

Position of the Central X-Ray Beam
The central beam is perpendicular to the image receptor and parallel to patient's midsagittal plane and is centered at the level of the condyles.

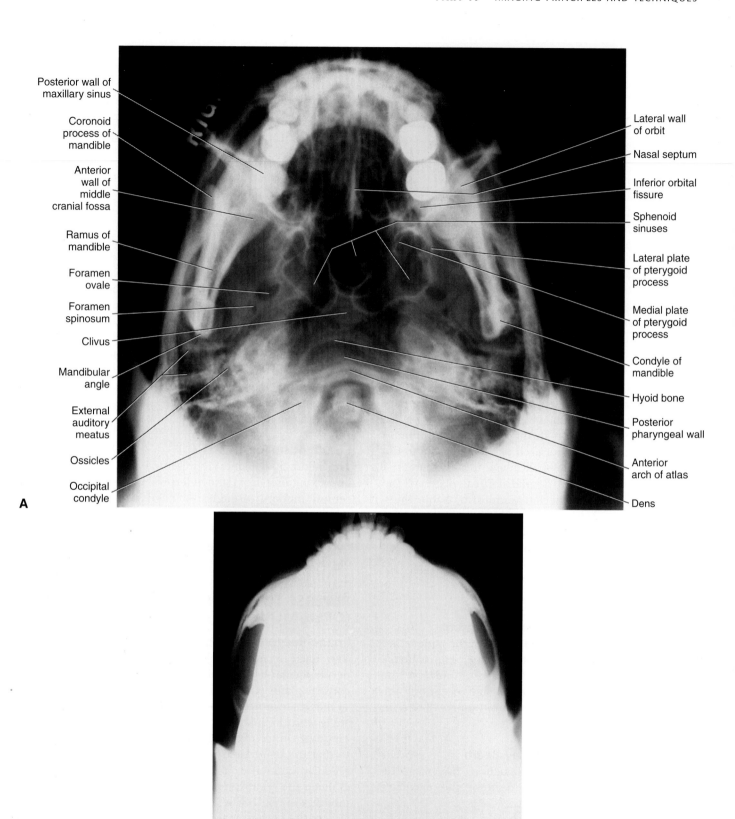

Posterior wall of
maxillary sinus

Coronoid
process of
mandible

Anterior
wall of
middle
cranial fossa

Ramus of
mandible

Foramen
ovale

Foramen
spinosum

Clivus

Mandibular
angle

External
auditory
meatus

Ossicles

Occipital
condyle

Lateral wall
of orbit

Nasal septum

Inferior orbital
fissure

Sphenoid
sinuses

Lateral plate
of pterygoid
process

Medial plate
of pterygoid
process

Condyle of
mandible

Hyoid bone

Posterior
pharyngeal wall

Anterior
arch of atlas

Dens

A

B

FIG. **11-2**   **A,** Anatomic landmarks identified in the submentovertex projection. **B,** An underexposed submentovertex view reveals the zygomatic arches.

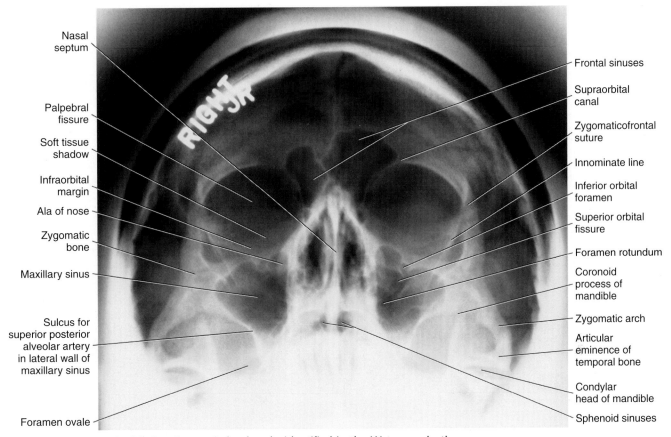

Nasal septum
Palpebral fissure
Soft tissue shadow
Infraorbital margin
Ala of nose
Zygomatic bone
Maxillary sinus
Sulcus for superior posterior alveolar artery in lateral wall of maxillary sinus
Foramen ovale

Frontal sinuses
Supraorbital canal
Zygomaticofrontal suture
Innominate line
Inferior orbital foramen
Superior orbital fissure
Foramen rotundum
Coronoid process of mandible
Zygomatic arch
Articular eminence of temporal bone
Condylar head of mandible
Sphenoid sinuses

FIG. **11-3** Anatomic landmarks identified in the Waters projection.

Resultant Image (Fig. 11-5)

The midsagittal plane (represented by an imaginary line extending from the middle of the foramen magnum and the posterior arch of the atlas through the middle of the bridge of the nose and the nasal septum) should divide the skull image in two symmetric halves. The petrous ridge of the temporal bone should be superimposed at the inferior part of the occipital bone, and the condylar heads should be projected inferior to the articular eminence.

MANDIBULAR OBLIQUE LATERAL PROJECTIONS

MANDIBULAR BODY PROJECTION

Image Receptor and Patient Placement

The image receptor is placed against the patient's cheek on the side of interest and centered in the molar-premolar area. The lower border of the cassette is parallel and at least 2 cm below the inferior border of the mandible. The head is tilted towards the side being examined, and the mandible is protruded.

Position of the Central X-Ray Beam

The central beam is directed toward the molar-premolar region from a point 2 cm below the angle of the opposite side of the mandible.

Resultant Image (Fig. 11-6)

A clear image of the teeth, the alveolar ridge, and the body of the mandible should be obtained. If significant distortion is present, the head was tilted excessively. If the contralateral side of the mandible is superimposed over the area of interest, the head was not tilted sufficiently.

MANDIBULAR RAMUS PROJECTION

Image Receptor and Patient Placement

The image receptor is placed over the ramus and far enough posteriorly to include the condyle. The lower border of the cassette is parallel and at least 2 cm below the inferior border of the mandible. The head is tilted towards the side being examined such that the condyle of the area of interest and the contralateral angle of the

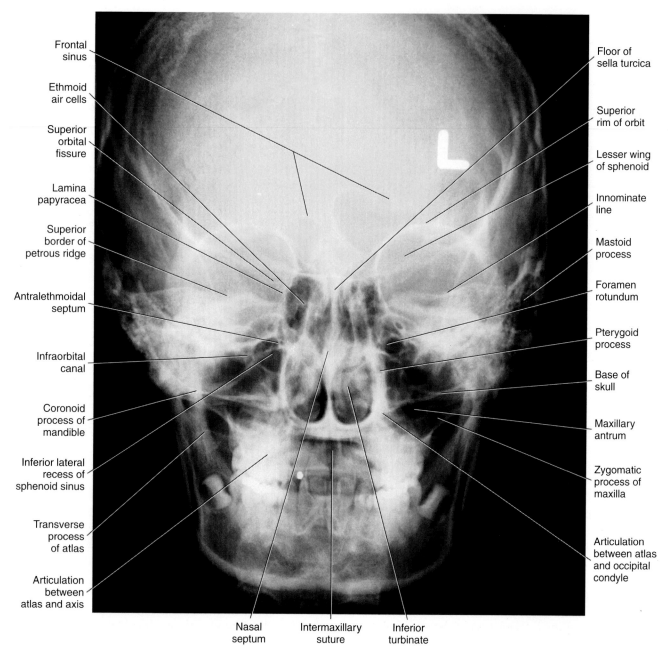

FIG. **11-4** Anatomic landmarks identified in the posteroanterior cephalometric projection.

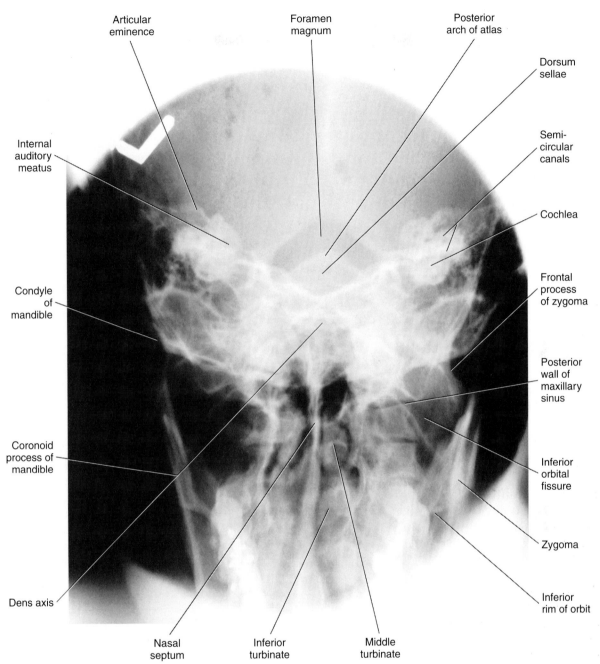

FIG. **11-5** Anatomic landmarks identified in the open-mouth reverse-Towne projection.

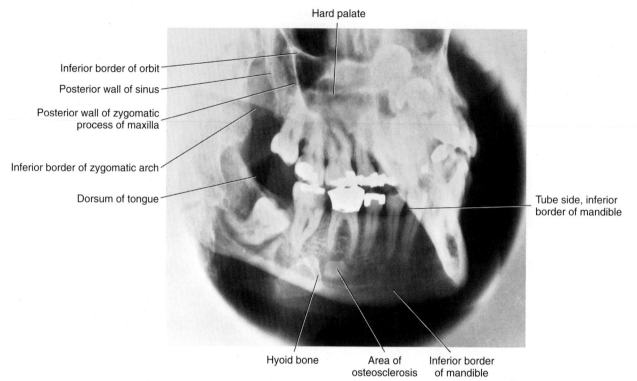

Hard palate

Inferior border of orbit

Posterior wall of sinus

Posterior wall of zygomatic process of maxilla

Inferior border of zygomatic arch

Dorsum of tongue

Tube side, inferior border of mandible

Hyoid bone   Area of osteosclerosis   Inferior border of mandible

FIG. **11-6**   Anatomic landmarks identified in the oblique lateral projection of the mandibular body.

mandible form a horizontal line. The mandible is protruded.

Position of the Central X-Ray Beam

The central beam is directed toward the center of the imaged ramus, from 2 cm below the inferior border of the opposite side of the mandible at the area of the first molar.

Resultant Image (Fig. 11-7)

A clear image of the third molar-retromolar area, angle of the mandible, ramus, and condyle head should be obtained. If significant distortion is present, the head was tilted excessively. If the contralateral side of the mandible is superimposed over the area of interest, the head was not tilted sufficiently.

Evaluation of the Image

Extraoral images should first be evaluated for overall quality. Proper exposure and processing will result in an image with good contrast and density. Proper patient positioning prevents unwanted superimpositions and distortions and facilitates identification of anatomic landmarks. Interpreting poor-quality images can lead to diagnostic errors and subsequent treatment errors.

The first step in the interpretation of radiographic images is the identification of anatomy. A thorough knowledge of normal radiographic anatomy and the appearance of normal variants is critical for the identification of pathology. Abnormalities cause disruptions of normal anatomy. Detecting the altered anatomy precedes classifying the type of change and developing a differential diagnosis. What is not detected cannot be interpreted. Figs. 11-1 through 11-7 present the major anatomic landmarks that can be identified in the various extraoral projections.

Interpretation of extraoral radiographs should be thorough, careful, and meticulous. Images should be interpreted in a room with reduced ambient light, and peripheral light from the viewbox or monitor should be masked. A systematic, methodical approach should be used for the visual exploration or interrogation of the diagnostic image. A method for the visual interrogation of extraoral projections is presented below. This method is not the only approach to examining radiographic images. Any technique that reliably ensures that the entire image will be examined is equally appropriate.

- LATERAL PROJECTION (Fig. 11-8)

  Step 1. Evaluate the base of the skull and calvarium. Identify the mastoid air cells, clivus, clinoid processes, sella turcica, sphenoid sinuses, and roof of the orbit.

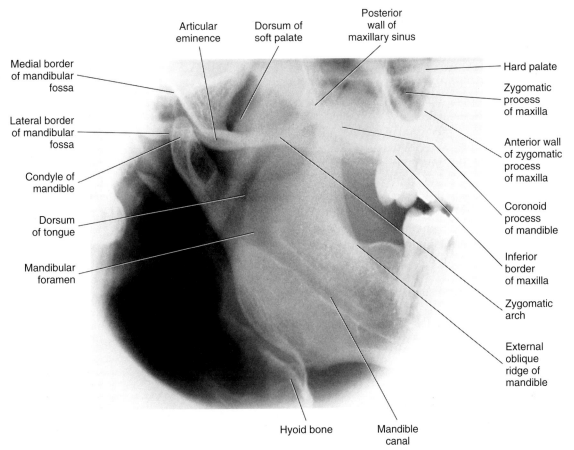

Medial border
of mandibular
fossa

Lateral border
of mandibular
fossa

Condyle of
mandible

Dorsum
of tongue

Mandibular
foramen

Articular
eminence

Dorsum of
soft palate

Posterior
wall of
maxillary sinus

Hard palate

Zygomatic
process
of maxilla

Anterior wall
of zygomatic
process
of maxilla

Coronoid
process
of mandible

Inferior
border
of maxilla

Zygomatic
arch

External
oblique
ridge
of mandible

Hyoid bone

Mandible
canal

FIG. **11-7** Anatomic landmarks identified in the oblique lateral projection of the mandibular ramus.

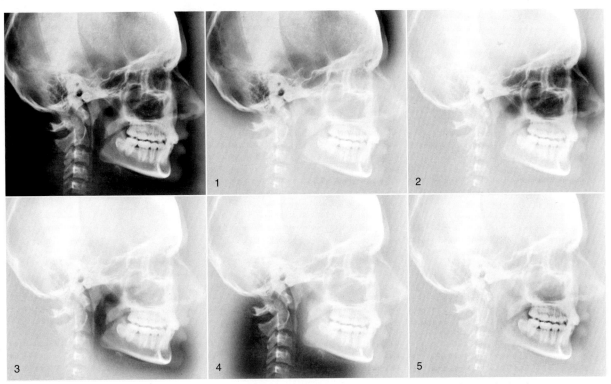

FIG. **11-8** Interrogating the lateral cephalometric projection. The radiograph in the upper left demonstrates the whole image. Subsequent radiographs correspond to the steps of interrogation.

In the calvarium, assess vessel grooves, sutures, and diploic space. Look for intracranial calcifications.

Step 2. Evaluate the upper and middle face. Identify the orbits, sinuses (frontal, ethmoid, and maxillary), pterygomaxillary fissures, pterygoid plates, zygomatic processes of the maxilla, anterior nasal spine, and hard palate (floor of the nose). Evaluate the soft tissues of the upper and middle face, nasal cavity (turbinates), soft palate, and dorsum of tongue.

Step 3. Evaluate the lower face. Follow the outline of the mandible, starting from the condylar and coronoid processes, to the rami, angles, and bodies, and finally to the anterior mandible. Evaluate the soft tissue of the lower face.

Step 4. Evaluate the cervical spine, airway, and area of the neck. Identify each individual vertebra, confirm that the skull–C1 and C1-C2 articulations are normal, and assess the general alignment of the vertebrae. Assess soft tissues of the neck, hyoid bone, and airway.

Step 5. Evaluate the alveolar bone and teeth.

- SMV PROJECTION (Fig. 11-9)

Step 1. Evaluate the calvarium and posterior cranial fossa. Assess the foramen magnum, atlas, dens, and occipital condyles. Identify the petrous ridge of the right and left temporal bones, the external auditory canals, and the mastoid air cells. In this and all subsequent steps, compare the right and left sides and look for symmetry.

Step 2. Evaluate the middle cranial fossa. Identify the foramina ovale and spinosum. Assess the clivus and sphenoid sinuses.

Step 3. Evaluate the upper and middle face. Assess the nasal cavity, nasal septum, maxillary and ethmoid sinuses, and orbits. Assess both the bony borders and antra or contents of these structures.

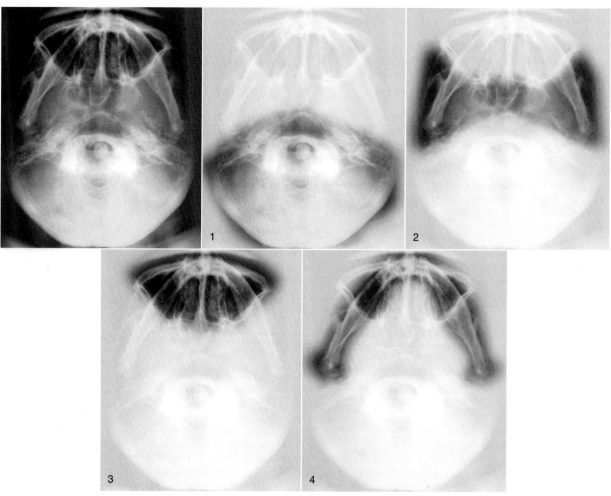

FIG. **11-9** Interrogating the submentovertex projection. The radiograph in the upper left demonstrates the whole image. Subsequent radiographs correspond to the steps of interrogation.

Step 4. Evaluate the mandible. Follow the outline from the right condylar head, coronoid process, ramus, angle, and body through the anterior mandible to the left body, angle, ramus, coronoid process, and condyle.

- **WATERS PROJECTION** (Fig. 11-10)

Step 1. Evaluate the calvarium and sutures starting in the left temporal area over the supraorbital ridges to the right temporal area. Look for intracranial calcifications. In this and all subsequent steps, compare the right and left sides and look for symmetry.

Step 2. Evaluate the orbits and the frontal sinuses. Identify the supraorbital and infraorbital rim, the inferior orbital foramen, the floor of the orbit, the zygomaticofrontal sutures, and the innominate line of the infratemporal fossa crossing on the lateral aspect of each orbit.

Step 3. Evaluate the maxillary sinuses and nasal cavity. Identify the superior, medial, and lateral walls and the floor of the maxillary sinuses; the nasal septum; and the floor and lateral walls of the nasal cavity. Try to identify the foramen rotundum projected towards the mesial wall of the sinus.

Step 4. Evaluate the zygomatic arches. Identify the frontal, maxillary, and temporal processes of the zygoma and the zygomaticofrontal suture. Confirm continuity of outlines and symmetry with the contralateral side.

Step 5. Evaluate the condylar and coronoid processes of the mandible. This is one of the best PA views of the coronoid process.

- **POSTEROANTERIOR PROJECTION** (Fig. 11-11)

Step 1. Evaluate the calvarium, sutures, and diploic space starting in the area of the left external auditory meatus (EAM), over the top of the calvarium, to the right EAM. Look for intracranial calcifications. Identify the mastoid air cells and petrous ridge of the right and left temporal bones. In this and all subsequent steps, compare the right and left sides and look for symmetry.

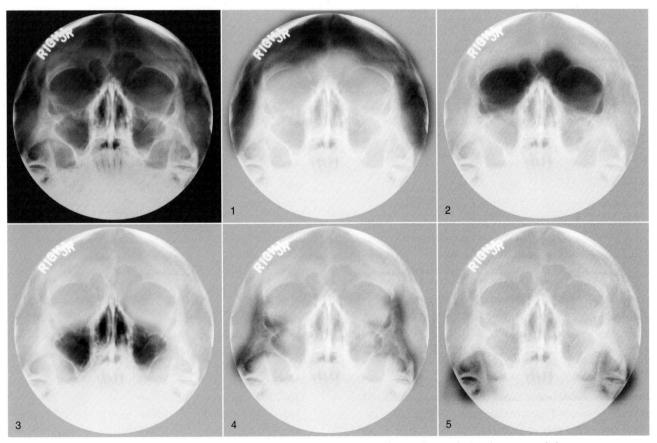

FIG. **11-10** Interrogating the Waters projection. The radiograph in the upper left demonstrates the whole image. Subsequent radiographs correspond to the steps of interrogation.

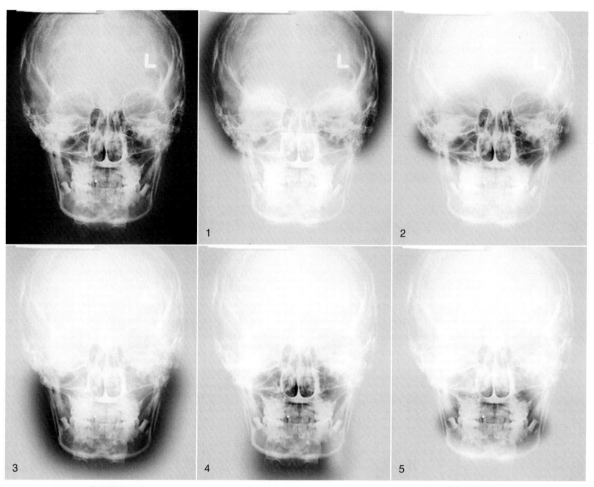

FIG. **11-11**　Interrogating the posteroanterior cephalometric projection. The radiograph in the upper left demonstrates the whole image. Subsequent radiographs correspond to the steps of interrogation.

Step 2. Evaluate the upper and middle face. Identify the orbits, sinuses (frontal, ethmoid, and maxillary), and zygomatic processes of the maxilla. Assess the nasal cavity, middle and inferior turbinates, nasal septum, and hard palate.

Step 3. Evaluate the lower face. Follow the outline of the mandible starting from the right condylar and coronoid processes, ramus, angle, and body through the anterior mandible to the left body, angle, ramus, coronoid process, and condyle.

Step 4. Evaluate the cervical spine. Identify the dens, the superior border of C2, and the inferior border of C1.

Step 5. Evaluate the alveolar bone and teeth.

- REVERSE-TOWNE PROJECTION (Fig. 11-12)

Step 1. Evaluate the calvarium and look for intracranial calcifications. Identify the foramen magnum and the posterior arch of the atlas. In this and all subsequent steps, compare the right and left sides and look for symmetry.

Step 2. Evaluate the middle cranial fossa, petrous ridges, and mastoid air cells. The anatomy in this area is difficult to discern. Look for displacement, interruption of outlines, radiolucencies, and loss of symmetry. Identify the odontoid process (dens) of the axis (C2) in the midline.

Step 3. Evaluate the nasal cavity. Identify the outline of the nasal cavity, the nasal septum, inferior and middle turbinates.

Step 4. Evaluate the condylar and coronoid process. In the open-mouth projection, the condylar head, including its superior surface and condylar neck, should be identified.

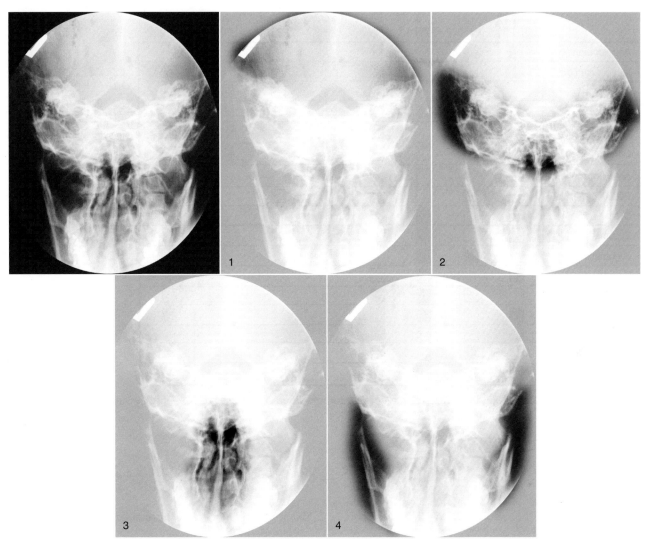

FIG. **11-12** Interrogating the reverse-Towne projection. The radiograph in the upper left demonstrates the whole image. Subsequent radiographs correspond to the steps of interrogation.

Selection Criteria

Keep in mind that although this section appears at the end of this chapter, in practice, selecting the appropriate extraoral radiographic examination is the *first* step in obtaining and interpreting a radiograph.

Extraoral radiographs are used to examine areas not fully covered by intraoral films or to evaluate the cranium, face (including the maxilla and mandible), or cervical spine for diseases, trauma, or abnormalities. Additionally, standardized extraoral radiographs taken with a cephalostat (and referred to as *cephalometric*

radiographs) are used for the evaluation of skeletal growth. Before obtaining an extraoral radiograph, it is essential to evaluate the patient's complaints and clinical signs in detail. The clinician must first decide which anatomic structures need to be evaluated and then select the appropriate projection(s). Usually, at least two radiographs taken at right angles to each another are obtained for spatial localization of pathology. Fig. 11-13 summarizes the use of extraoral radiographs for the evaluation of various anatomic structures. Although panoramic radiography is the subject of another chapter, it is included in Fig. 11-13 for comparison.

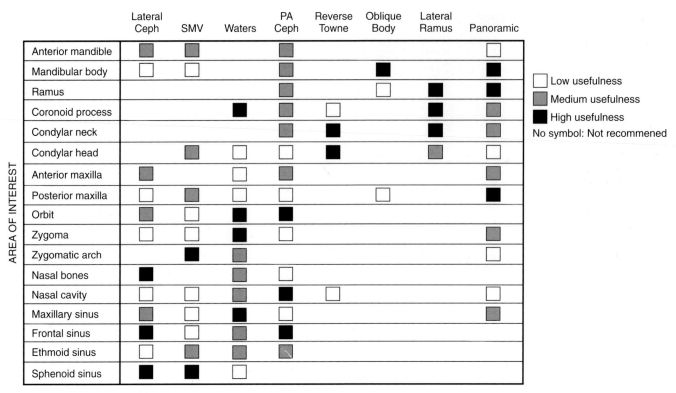

FIG. **11-13**   Relative usefulness of extraoral radiographic projections to display various anatomic structures.

BIBLIOGRAPHY

Ballinger PW, Frank ED: Merrill's atlas of radiographic positions and radiologic procedures, vol 2, ed 10, St. Louis, 2003, Mosby, pp. 353-399.

Kantor ML, Norton LA: Normal radiographic anatomy and common anomalies seen in cephalometric films, Am J Orthod Dentofac Orthop 91:414-26, 1987.

Keats TE, Anderson MW: Atlas of normal roentgen variants that may simulate disease, ed 7, St. Louis, 2001, Mosby, pp. 3-275.

Shapiro R: Radiology of the normal skull, Chicago, 1981, Year Book Medical.

Swischuk LE: Imaging of the cervical spine in children, New York, 2002, Springer-Verlag.

CHAPTER 12

Digital Imaging

JOHN B. LUDLOW ■ ANDRÉ MOL

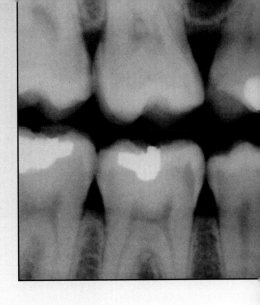

The advent of digital imaging has revolutionized radiology. This revolution is the result of both technologic innovation in image acquisition processes and the development of networked computing systems for image retrieval and transmission. Although adoption of computer and digital imaging technologies in dentistry has lagged somewhat behind medicine, we are seeing a steady increase in the use of these technologies, improvement of software interfaces, and introduction of new products. A number of forces are driving the shift from film to digital systems. The detrimental effects of inadequate film processing on diagnostic quality and the difficulty of maintaining high-quality chemical processing are well documented problems in dental radiography. Digital imaging eliminates chemical processing. Hazardous wastes in the form of processing chemicals and lead foil are eliminated with digital systems. Images can be electronically transferred to other health care providers without any alteration of the original image quality. In addition, digital intraoral receptors require less radiation than film, thus lowering the patient absorbed dose. However, current digital systems also have a number of disadvantages in comparison with film. The initial expense of setting up a digital imaging system is relatively high. Certain components such as the electronic x-ray receptor used in some intraoral systems are susceptible to rough handling and are costly to replace. Because digital systems utilize new or immature technologies, there is a risk—perhaps even a likelihood—of systems becoming obsolete or manufacturers going out of business. The excellent image quality and comparatively low cost of a properly exposed and processed film keeps film-based radiography competitive with digital alter-

natives. The trends, however, are certain: computers play a role in the majority of dental practices, and that role is expanding as a variety of functions from appointment scheduling, procedure billing, and patient charting are integrated into seamless practice management software solutions. It is no longer a matter of *if* but rather *when* the majority of dental practices will use digital imaging. Already during this time of transition, film-based practices will be confronted with digital images from practices that have implemented digital radiography. This chapter describes the characteristics of digital images, image receptors, display options, and storage devices. Additional attention is given to a discussion of processing digital images.

Analog Versus Digital

The term *digital* in digital imaging refers to the numeric format of the image content as well as its discreteness. Conventional film images can be considered an analog medium in which differences in the size and distribution of black metallic silver result in a continuous density spectrum. Digital images are numeric and discrete in two ways: (1) in terms of the spatial distribution of the picture elements (pixels) and (2) in terms of the different shades of gray of each of the pixels. A digital image consists of a large collection of individual pixels organized in a matrix of rows and columns (Fig. 12-1). Each pixel has a row and column coordinate that uniquely identifies its location in the matrix. The formation of a digital image requires several steps, beginning with analog processes. At each pixel of an electronic detector, the absorption of x rays generates

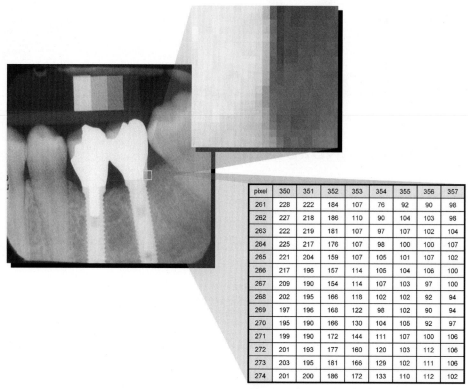

pixel	350	351	352	353	354	355	356	357
261	228	222	184	107	76	92	90	98
262	227	218	186	110	90	104	103	98
263	222	219	181	107	97	107	102	104
264	225	217	176	107	98	100	100	107
265	221	204	159	107	105	101	107	102
266	217	196	157	114	105	104	106	100
267	209	190	154	114	107	103	97	100
268	202	195	166	118	102	102	92	94
269	197	196	168	122	98	102	90	94
270	195	190	166	130	104	105	92	97
271	199	190	172	144	111	107	100	106
272	201	193	177	160	120	103	112	106
273	203	195	181	166	129	102	111	106
274	201	200	186	172	133	110	112	102

FIG. **12-1**   The digital image is made up of a large number of discrete picture elements (pixels). Their size is so small that the image appears smooth at normal magnification. The location of each pixel is uniquely identified by a row and column coordinate within the image matrix. The value assigned to a pixel represents the intensity (gray level) of the image at that location.

a small voltage. More x rays generate a higher voltage and vice versa. At each pixel, the voltage can fluctuate between a minimum and maximum value and is therefore an analog signal (Fig. 12-2, *A*). Production of a digital image requires a process called *analog-to-digital conversion (ADC)*. ADC consists of two steps: sampling and quantization. *Sampling* means that a small range of voltage values are grouped together as a single value (Fig. 12-2, *B*). Narrow sampling better mimics the original signal but leads to larger memory requirements for the resulting digital image (Fig. 12-2, *C*). Once sampled, the signal is *quantized,* which means that every sampled signal is assigned a value. These values are stored in the computer and represent the image. In order for the clinician to see the image, the computer organizes the pixels in their proper locations and gives them a shade of gray that corresponds to the number that was assigned during the quantization step.

To understand the strengths and weaknesses of digital radiography, we must establish which elements of the radiographic imaging chain stay the same and which ones change (Fig. 12-3). The use of digital detec-tors implies significant changes in how we acquire, store, retrieve, and display images. Although digital detectors also require adjustment of exposure factors, the essence of this part of the imaging chain (i.e., transmission and selective attenuation of x rays) is the same for digital detectors as it is for film. The physics of the interaction of x rays with matter and the effects of the projection geometry remain critically important for understanding the content of the radiographic image and for optimizing image quality, whether conventional or digital. Nevertheless, much of the focus of digital radiography has been on the performance of digital detectors since their development has been the driving force behind the digital transformation in dentistry.

Digital Detectors

CHARGE-COUPLED DEVICE (CCD)

The charge-coupled device (CCD) was the first direct digital image receptor to be adapted for intraoral imaging and was introduced to dentistry in 1987. The

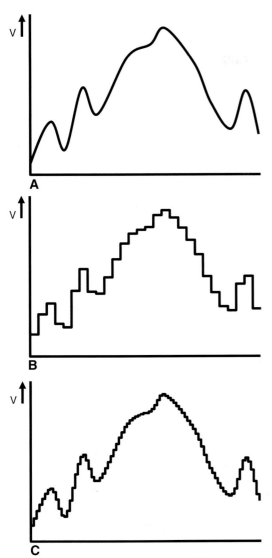

FIG. **12-2**   **A,** Illustration of an analog voltage signal coming from a detector. **B,** Sampling of the analog signal discards part of the signal. **C,** Sampling at a higher frequency preserves more of the original signal.

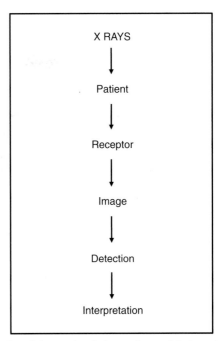

FIG. **12-3**   Schematic of the radiographic imaging chain.

CCD uses a thin wafer of silicon as the basis for image recording. The silicon crystals are formed in a picture element (pixel) matrix (Fig. 12-4). When exposed to radiation, the covalent bonds between silicon atoms are broken, producing electron-hole pairs (Fig. 12-5). The number of electron-hole pairs that are formed is proportional to the amount of exposure that an area receives. The electrons are then attracted toward the most positive potential in the device, where they create "charge packets." Each packet corresponds to one pixel. The charge pattern formed from the individual pixels in the matrix represents the latent image (Fig.

12-6). The image is read by transferring each row of pixel charges from one pixel to the next in a "bucket brigade" fashion. As a charge reaches the end of its row, it is transferred to a readout amplifier and transmitted as a voltage to the analog-to-digital converter located within or connected to the computer. Voltages from each pixel are sampled and assigned a numerical value representing a gray level. The silicon matrix and its associated readout and amplifying electronics are enclosed within a plastic housing to protect them from the oral environment. These elements of the detector consume part of the real estate of the sensor so that the active area of the sensor is smaller than its total surface area. Sensor bulk, while reduced by continued miniaturization of electronic components is a potential drawback of CCD detectors. In addition, most detectors incorporate an electronic cable to transfer data to the ADC. One manufacturer has produced a system that replaces the cable connection with a microwave transmitter. This frees the detector from a direct tether to the computer, but it necessitates some additional electronic components, thus increasing the overall bulk of the sensor. A number of manufacturers produce detectors with varying active sensor areas roughly corresponding to the different sizes of intraoral film. Detectors without flaws are relatively expensive to produce, and expense of the detector increases with increasing matrix size (total number of pixels). Pixel size varies from 20 microns to 70 microns. Smaller pixel

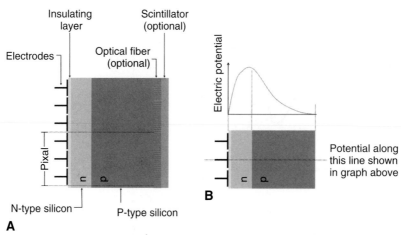

FIG. **12-4** **A,** Basic structure of the CCD: electrodes insulated from an n-p silicon sandwich. The surface of the silicon may incorporate a scintillating material to improve x-ray capture efficiency and fiberoptics to improve resolution. One pixel utilizes three electrodes. **B,** Excess electrons from the n-type layer diffuse into the p-type layer while excess holes in the p-type layer diffuse into the n-type layer. The resulting charge imbalance creates an electric field in the silicon with a maximum just inside the n-type layer.

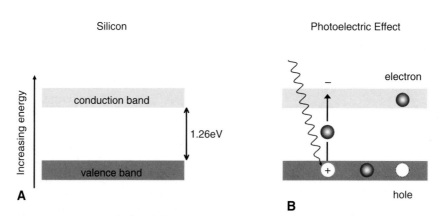

FIG. **12-5** **A,** Outer shells of the silicon atom showing an energy difference between the valence band and the conduction band. **B,** X-ray or light photons impart energy to valence electrons, releasing them into the conduction band. This generates an "electron-hole" charge pair.

size increases the cost of the receptor. Because CCDs are more sensitive to light than x rays, most manufacturers use a layer of scintillating material coated directly on the CCD surface or coupled to the surface by fiber optics. This increases the x-ray absorption efficiency of the detector. Gadolinium oxybromide compounds similar to those used in rare earth radiographic screens or cesium iodide are examples of scintillators that have been used for this purpose.

CCDs have also been made in linear arrays of a few pixels wide and many pixels long for panoramic and cephalometric imaging. In the case of panoramic units, the CCD is fixed in position opposite to the x-ray source with the long axis of the array oriented parallel to the fan-shaped x-ray beam. Some manufacturers provide CCD sensors that may be retrofitted to older panoramic units. Unlike film imaging, the mechanics for cephalometric imaging are different. Construction of a single CCD of a size that could simultaneously capture the area of a full skull would be prohibitively expensive. Combining a linear CCD array and a slit-shaped x-ray beam with a scanning motion permits scanning of the skull over several seconds. One disadvantage of this approach is the increased possibility of patient movement artifacts during the several seconds required to complete a scan.

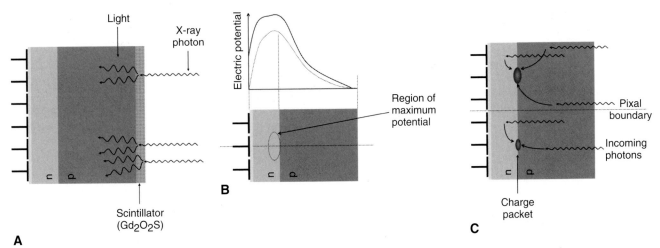

FIG. **12-6** **A,** X-ray photons are absorbed in the scintillating material and are converted to light photons. **B,** Light photons are absorbed in the silicon through photoelectric absorption; electrons released from the valence band collect selectively near the n-p layer interface, where the electric charge is at a maximum. A positive charge on the center electrode concentrates the collected electrons in the center of the pixel creating a charge packet. **C,** During CCD readout, the electrical potential of the pixel electrodes are sequentially modulated to shift the charge packet from pixel to pixel.

COMPLEMENTARY METAL OXIDE SEMICONDUCTORS (CMOS)

Complementary metal oxide semiconductor technology is the basis for typical consumer-grade video cameras. These detectors are silicon-based semiconductors but are fundamentally different from CCDs in the way that pixel charges are read. Each pixel is isolated from its neighboring pixels and is directly connected to a transistor. Like the CCD, electron-hole pairs are generated within the pixel in proportion to the amount of x-ray energy that is absorbed. This charge is transferred to the transistor as a small voltage. The voltage in each transistor can be addressed separately, read by the frame grabber, and then stored and displayed as a digital gray value. CMOS technology is widely used in the construction of computer central processing unit chips as well as video camera detectors, and the technology is less expensive than that used in the manufacture of CCDs. Only one manufacturer is currently utilizing the technology for intraoral applications (Fig. 12-7).

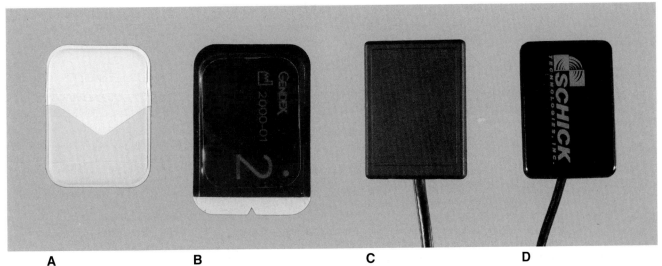

FIG. **12-7** **A,** Kodak #2 film. **B,** Gendex #2 PSP plate. **C,** Gendex #2 CCD sensor. **D,** Schick #2 CMOS sensor.

PHOTOSTIMULABLE PHOSPHOR PLATES (PSP)

Photostimulable phosphor plates (PSP) absorb and store energy from x rays and then release this energy as light (phosphorescence) when stimulated by other light of an appropriate wavelength. To the extent that the stimulating light and phosphorescent light wavelengths differ, the two may be distinguished and the phosphorescence can be quantified as a measure of the amount of x-ray energy that the material has absorbed. The photostimulable phosphor material used for radiographic imaging is "Europium-doped" barium fluorohalide. Barium in combination with iodine, chlorine, or bromine forms a crystal lattice. The addition of Europium (Eu^{+2}) creates imperfections in this lattice. When exposed to a sufficiently energetic source of radiation, valence electrons in Europium can absorb energy and move into the conduction band. These electrons migrate to nearby halogen vacancies (F-centers) in the fluorohalide lattice and may become trapped there in a metastable state. While in this state, the number of trapped electrons is proportional to x-ray exposure and represents a latent image. When stimulated by red light of around 600 nm, the barium fluorohalide releases trapped electrons to the conduction band. When an electron returns to the Eu^{+3} ion, energy is released in the green spectrum between 300 and 500 nm (Fig. 12-8). Fiberoptics conduct light from the PSP plate to a photomultiplier tube. The photomultiplier tube converts light into electrical energy. A red filter at the photomultiplier tube selectively removes the stimulating light, and the remaining green light is detected and converted to a varying voltage. The variations in voltage output from the photomultiplier tube correspond to variations in stimulated light intensity from the latent image. The voltage signal is quantified by an analog-to-digital converter and stored and displayed as a digital image. In

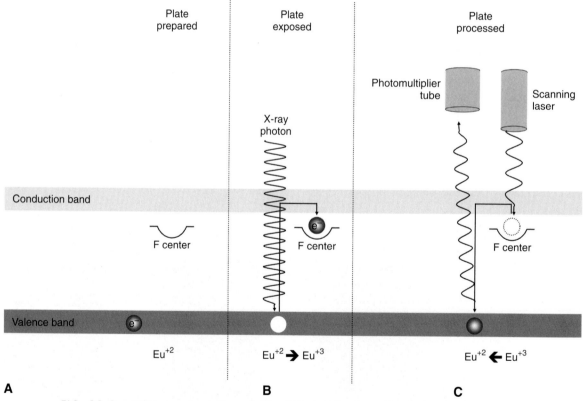

FIG. **12-8** *PSP image formation.* **A,** The PSP plate has been flooded with white light to return all electrons to the valence band. **B,** Exposure to x rays imparts energy to Europium valence electrons moving them into the conduction band. Some electrons become trapped at "F centers." **C,** A red scanning laser imparts energy to electrons at the F-centers promoting them to the conduction band from which many return to the valence band. With the electron's return to the valence band, energy is released in the form of light photons in the green spectrum. This light is detected by a photomultiplier tube or diode using a red filter to screen out the scanning laser light.

practice, the barium fluorohalide material is combined with a polymer and spread in a thin layer on a base material to create a photostimulable phosphor plate. For intraoral radiography a polyester base similar to radiographic film is used. When manufactured in standard intraoral sizes, these plates provide handling characteristics similar to intraoral film. PSP plates are also made in sizes commonly used for panoramic and cephalometric imaging. Some PSP processors accommodate a full range of intraoral and extraoral plate sizes. Other processors are limited to intraoral or extraoral formats.

Before exposure, PSP plates must be erased to eliminate "ghost images" from prior exposures (note that this is a different type of ghost image than that associated with panoramic radiography). This is accomplished by flooding the plate with a bright light source. Placing plates on a dental viewbox with the phosphor side of the plates facing the light for 1 or 2 minutes can accomplish this. More intense light sources can be used for shorter periods of time. Some PSP systems integrate automatic plate-erasing lights. Erased plates are placed in light-tight containers prior to exposure. In the case of intraoral plates, sealable polyvinyl envelopes that are impervious to oral fluids and light are used for packaging. For large format plates, conventional cassettes (without intensifying screens) are used. Following exposure, plates should be processed as soon as possible. Trapped electrons are spontaneously released over time. The rate of loss of electrons is greatest shortly after exposure. The rate varies depending on the composition of the storage phosphor and environmental temperature. Some phosphors lose 23% of their trapped electrons after 30 minutes and 30% after an hour. Because loss of trapped electrons is fairly uniform across the plate surface, early loss of charge does not typically result in clinically meaningful image deterioration. However, underexposed images may suffer noticeable image degradation. Adequately exposed images may be stored for 12 to 24 hours and retain acceptable image quality. A potentially more important source of latent image fading is exposure to ambient light during plate preparation for processing. A semi-dark environment is recommended for plate handling. The more intense the background light and the longer the exposure of the plate to this light, the greater is the loss of trapped electrons. Red safelights found in most darkrooms are not safe for exposed PSP plates, which are most sensitive to the red light spectrum.

Stationary Plate Scans

A number of approaches have been adopted for "reading" the latent images on PSP plates. An approach used by Soredex in its Digora system and Air Techniques in its ScanX system employs a rapidly rotating multifaceted mirror that reflects a beam of red laser light. As the mirror revolves, the laser light sweeps across the plate. The plate is advanced and the adjacent line of phosphor is scanned. The direction of the laser scanning the plate is termed the *fast scan direction*. The direction of plate advancement is termed the *slow scan direction*.

Rotating Plate Scans

An alternate approach to plate reading used by Gendex in the Denoptix system and by Orex in the Paxorama Xi system involves a rapidly rotating drum that holds the plate. The rotation of the drum past a fixed laser provides a rapid scan. Incremental movement of the laser in the slow scan direction allows image data to be acquired line by line.

Resolution in PSP systems is determined by a number of factors. The thickness of the phosphor material influences the diffusion of laser light. Thicker phosphor layers cause more diffusion and yield a lower resolution. On the other hand, a thicker layer enhances x-ray absorption efficiency, resulting in a faster image receptor. Resolution is inversely proportional to the diameter of the laser beam. Effective beam diameter is increased by vibration in the rotating mirror and drum scanner designs. Slow scan motion influences resolution by the increment of plate advancement. This increment may be adjusted to increase or reduce resolution in some systems.

FLAT PANEL DETECTORS

Flat panel detectors are being used for medical imaging but have also been used in prototypes of extraoral imaging devices. The detectors can provide relatively large matrix areas with pixel sizes less than 100 microns. This allows direct digital imaging of larger areas of the body, including the head. Two approaches have been taken in selecting x-ray sensitive materials for flat panel detectors. Indirect detectors are sensitive to visible light, and an intensifying screen (Gd_2O_2S or CsI) is used to convert x-ray energy into light. These devices are limited by the thickness of the intensifying screen. Thicker screens are more efficient but allow greater diffusion of light photons leading to image unsharpness. Direct detectors use a photoconductor material (selenium) with properties similar to silicon and a higher atomic number that permits more efficient absorption of x rays. Under the influence of an applied electrical field, the electrons that are freed during x-ray exposure of the selenium are conducted in a direct line to an underlying thin film transistor (TFT) detector element. Direct detectors using selenium (Z = 34) provide higher resolution but lower efficiency in comparison with indirect detectors using intensifying screens with gadolinium (Z = 64) or cesium (Z = 55). The electrical energy generated is proportional to the x-ray exposure and is stored at each pixel in a capacitor. The energy is released and read out by applying appropriate row and column voltages to a particular pixel's transistor. Currently, flat panel detectors are expensive and likely to be limited to specialized imaging tasks such as cone beam computed tomography.

Digital Detector Characteristics

CONTRAST RESOLUTION

Contrast resolution is the ability to distinguish different densities in the radiographic image. This is a function of the interaction of the attenuation characteristics of the tissues that are being imaged, the capacity of the image receptor to distinguish differences in numbers of x-ray photons coming from different areas of the subject, the ability of the computer display or other output to portray differences in density, and the ability of the observer to recognize those differences. Current digital detectors capture data at 8-, 10-, 12-, or 16-bit depths. The bit depth is a power of 2 (Fig. 12-9). This means that the detector can theoretically capture 256 (2^8) to 65,536 (2^{16}) different densities. In practice the actual number of meaningful densities that can be captured is limited by inaccuracies in image acquisition; these inaccuracies are given the generic term of *noise*. Regardless of the number of density differences that a detector can capture, conventional computer monitors are capable of displaying a gray scale of only 8 bits. Because operating systems such as Windows reserve a

number of gray levels for the display of system information, the actual number of gray levels that can be displayed on a monitor is 242. A more important limiting factor is the human visual system, which is capable of distinguishing only about 60 gray levels at any time under ideal viewing conditions. Considering the typical viewing environment in the dental operatory, the actual number of gray levels that can be distinguished falls to less than 30. Human visual limitations are also present for film viewing; however, the luminance (brightness) of a typical radiograph view box is much greater than that of a typical computer display. Therefore the ambient lighting of the room in which the image is viewed will theoretically have a lower impact on film than on digital displays.

SPATIAL RESOLUTION

Spatial resolution is the capacity for distinguishing fine detail. The theoretical limit of resolution is a function of picture element (pixel) size for digital imaging systems. Currently the highest resolution charge-coupled device detectors for dentistry have pixel sizes of approximately 20 microns. This compares with a silver grain size of 8 microns for intraoral film. Resolution is often measured and reported in units of line-pairs per millimeter. Test objects consisting of sets of very fine radiopaque lines separated from each other by spaces equal to the width of a line are constructed with a variety of line widths. A line and its associated space are called a *line pair (lp)*. At least two pixels are required to resolve a line pair, one for the line and one for the space. At 20 microns per pixel, a theoretical resolution of 25 lp/mm can be obtained. As was the case with contrast, actual resolutions are much lower in practice (Fig. 12-10). Typical observers are able to distinguish about 6 lp/mm without benefit of magnification. Intraoral film is capable of providing more than 20 lp/mm of resolution. Unless a film image is magnified, the observer is unable to appreciate the extent of the detail in the image. Current digital systems are capable of providing more than 7 lp/mm of resolution. Software displays of digital images permit magnification of images. A periapical image filling the display of a computer monitor may be magnified by a factor of 10× or more. At this level of magnification, the image takes on a building block pattern or pixilated appearance and the limits of resolution of the imaging system are evident.

DETECTOR LATITUDE

The ability of an imaging receptor to capture a range of x-ray exposures is termed *latitude*. A desirable quality

FIG. 12-9 *Contrast resolution.* Examples of gray scale ramps representing distinct gray levels from black to white. Bit depth controls the number of possible gray levels in the image. The actual number of distinct gray levels that are displayed is dependent on the output device and image processing. The perceived number of gray levels is influenced by viewing conditions and the visual acuity of the observer. **A,** 6 bits/pixel–64 gray levels. **B,** 5 bits/pixel–32 gray levels. **C,** 4 bits/pixel–16 gray levels. **D,** 3 bits/pixel–8 gray levels.

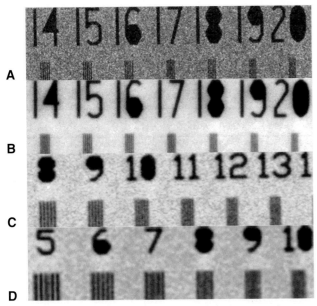

FIG. **12-10** *Images of a line-pair resolution test phantom made with various receptors.* **A,** Kodak Insight Film. **B,** Trophy RVGui–high resolution CCD. **C,** Gendex Denoptix PSP at 600 dpi. **D,** Gendex Denoptix PSP at 300 dpi.

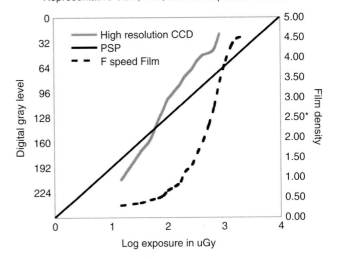

Representative CCD, PSP, and film exposure latitudes

*An optical density of 2.5 is generally considered the upper limit of useful clinical density in the absence of special illumination or "hot lighting" of films.

FIG. **12-11** Representative exposure latitudes of CCD, PSP, and intraoral film sensors. Note that the clinically useful optical density of film has an upper limit of 2.5. Use of a more intense view box or "hot lighting" can extend the upper end of the usable density range and expand useful film latitude.

in intraoral image receptors is the ability to record the full range of tissue densities, from gingiva to enamel. At the same time, subtle differences in density within these tissues should be visually apparent. The useful range of densities in film radiography is two orders of magnitude, from 0.5 to 2.5. The dynamic range of film actually extends for more than four orders of magnitude, but densities of 3 and 4, which transmit only 1/1,000th to 1/10,000th of the incident light, require intensified illumination or hot lighting to be distinguished from a density of 2.5. Such devices are not commonly used in general practice. The latitude of CCD and CMOS detectors is similar to film and can be extended with digital enhancement of contrast and brightness. Photostimulable phosphor receptors enjoy larger latitudes and have a linear response to five orders of magnitude of x-ray exposure (Fig. 12-11).

DETECTOR SENSITIVITY

Sensitivity of a detector is its ability to respond to small amounts of radiation. Intraoral film sensitivity is classified according to speed group using criteria developed by the International Organization for Standardization (ISO). Extraoral screen-film combinations use a classification system developed by Eastman Kodak. Currently there are no classification standards for dental digital x-ray receptors. As a result, reported sensitivity of systems by equipment manufacturers may exaggerate the per-

formance that can actually be achieved in routine practice. Useful sensitivity of digital receptors is affected by a number of factors including detector efficiency, pixel size, and system noise. Current PSP systems for intraoral imaging allow dose reductions of about 50% in comparison with F-speed film. High resolution CCD and CMOS systems achieve less dose reduction than lower resolution PSP systems. CCD and PSP systems for extraoral imaging require exposures similar to those needed for 200-speed screen-film systems.

Digital Image Display

CATHODE RAY TUBE (CRT)

Conventional computer monitors use cathode ray tube (CRT) designs. A beam of electrons emanating from an electron "gun" rapidly scans a phosphor-coated screen. The electron scan is horizontal and builds an image line by line. The image is repeated or refreshed at a rate of 60 times a second (Hz) or more to avoid the appearance of flicker. Color monitors utilize 3 electron guns, one each for red, blue, and green phosphors. The variable intensity of the electron beam is responsible for different shades of gray or color hue and intensity. High-quality monitors are able to display 256 different gray values or a combination of gray and color values. CRT displays involve conversion of digital information into analog voltages, which are supplied to the electron guns. Some loss of the original image information is inherent in the digital-to-analog conversion process. A number of factors affect the subjective quality of a monitor. The dot pitch is a measure of the distance between groups of subpixels (red, green, and blue phosphors) in the CRT. Smaller dot pitches on the order of 0.28 mm or less provide more pixels per area and sharper-looking images. The brightness of the monitor affects perceived contrast in the image. Brighter monitors are essential in working environments with greater amounts of ambient light. Over time, the color phosphors in a CRT fade, reducing the brightness of the monitor and the contrast within the image.

THIN FILM TRANSISTOR (TFT)

Thin film transistor (TFT) technology, which is used in flat panel detectors, is also used in laptop and flat panel computer displays. The process is somewhat reversed in that a signal is sent to the pixel's transistor, which in turn causes the associated liquid crystal display (LCD) to transmit light with an intensity proportional to the transistor voltage. Subpixels composed of red, green, and blue phosphors are subjected to varied voltages and in combination create a pixel output of a particular hue and intensity. The output of laptop displays is limited in intensity and does not have the dynamic range or contrast found in conventional desktop displays. The viewing angle of laptop displays is also limited, and the observer needs to be positioned squarely in front of the display for optimum viewing quality. Technologic innovation and improvement over early models have resulted in current laptop displays that are of sufficient quality to be used for typical dental diagnostic tasks. Desktop versions of TFT LCD displays have overcome brightness and viewing angle problems but consume more power and thus are not suited for laptop configurations. Some desktop flat panel displays are actually brighter than conventional CRT displays and have viewing angles as wide as 160 degrees. Some flat panel displays incorporate a digital video interface (DVI), which allows direct display of digital information without digital-to-analog conversion. These displays virtually eliminate signal loss and distortion from digital-to-analog conversion.

ELECTRONIC DISPLAY CONSIDERATIONS

The display of digital images on electronic devices is a fairly straightforward engineering issue. Positioning an image in the context of other diagnostic and demographic information and in useful relationships with other images is a more complex challenge that may vary according to diagnostic task, practice pattern, and practitioner preference. These challenges are answered with varying degrees of success by image display software. The quality, capabilities, and ease of use of display software vary from vendor to vendor, and these are numerous. Even with the same software the display of images can vary dramatically, depending on how the software handles resizing of windows or the size and resolutions of different displays. For instance, on some displays, it may be impossible to view a full mouth series of images on a single screen at normal magnification (100%). Software may permit reduction in image size or scrolling around the window to compensate for smaller display areas. These approaches are not as fast or flexible as shifting a film mount around on a view box. The visibility of electronic displays is degraded by many of the same elements which degrade viewing of film images. Bright background illumination from windows or other sources of ambient light reduce visual contrast sensitivity. Light reflecting off of a monitor surface may further reduce visibility of image contrast. Images are best viewed in an environment in which lighting is subdued and indirect.

HARD COPIES

Until all dental health care providers and third parties are able to send, receive, store, and display digital images from a variety of acquisition sources, there will be a need for a universal medium to exchange radiographic image information. With the development of digital photography as a mainstream technology, digital image printing has become an economical solution for making digital radiographs transferable. The question is whether the printed image provides adequate image quality to prevent loss of diagnostic information. Any time a digital image is modified, including the process of printing it in hard copy, there needs to be sufficient assurance that the image retains relevant diagnostic information. The requirements for quality vary with the diagnostic task at hand. For instance, assessment of the impaction status of a third molar puts a lower demand on the image quality than caries detection. Unfortunately, there is limited scientific evidence to support the diagnostic efficacy of printed images. The large number of variables that influence the quality of the printed image—for instance, the printing technology, printer quality, printer settings, and type of media—makes the printing process a much more complicated process than it initially appears to be. It is therefore imperative to use a printing system that is designed for its intended use and to follow the manufacturer's recommendations. The main types of printing technologies available for image printing include laser, inkjet, and dye-sublimation with the use of either film or paper.

Film Printers

Radiologists have traditionally relied on film images for common interpretive tasks. Most radiologists prefer film even for inherently digital technologies such as MR and CT imaging. There is something eminently satisfying about the feel of a 7-mil polyester sheet held between the thumb and forefinger. The crisp snap of a film being slipped under the hanging clips of a viewbox is an auditory stimulation akin to the crunch of autumn leaves underfoot. Unfortunately, high-quality film printers using laser or dye-sublimation technology are expensive, and low-cost alternatives suffer from reduced diagnostic quality. Current film transparencies produced with ink-jet technology appear to be suboptimal for tasks such as caries diagnosis.

Paper Printers

While printing on film allows radiographs to be evaluated in a traditional manner using the transmitted light of a view box, paper-printed digital radiographs require reflective light from a normally lit room. This offers a substantial advantage since most dental operatories are not well-equipped to control the ambient light level for viewing film images on a view box. Moreover, printing digital radiographs on paper allows the dentist to use technologies developed for the digital photography domain. Photographic printers vary widely in price and quality. Although more costly models usually provide higher print resolution, printer resolution is only one of many factors determining the final quality of the printed image. Inkjet printers are by far the most dominant in the market and offer the most economical alternative. Dye-sublimation printers provide excellent image quality but are generally more expensive. For any printing technology, the printing resolution is usually defined as the number of dots per inch (DPI) the printer can print. A printer with a higher DPI number is capable of laying the ink down more tightly than a printer with a lower DPI number. As a result, printers with a higher DPI number can print smaller objects and thus are said to have "higher resolution." The resolution of the digital radiograph can never be increased by a printer that prints at a higher resolution than that of the image itself. On the other hand, printing digital radiographs at a lower resolution will reduce the final resolution of the image.

IMAGE PROCESSING

Any operation that acts to improve, restore, analyze, or in some way change a digital image is a form of image processing. The use of digital imaging in dental radiography involves a variety of image processing operations. Some of these operations are integrated in the image acquisition and image management software and are hidden from the user. Others are controlled by the user with the intention to improve the quality of the image or to analyze its contents.

IMAGE RESTORATION

When the raw image data enter the computer, they are usually not yet ready for storage or display. A number of preprocessing steps need to be performed to correct the image for known defects and to adjust the image intensities so that they are suitable for viewing. For example, some of the pixels in a CCD sensor are always defective. The image is restored by substituting the gray values of the defective pixels with some weighted average of the gray values from the surrounding pixels. Depending on the quality of the sensor and the choices made by the manufacturer, a variety of other operations may be applied to the image before it becomes visible on the display. They are executed very rapidly and are unnoticed by the user. Most of the preprocessing operations are set by the manufacturer and cannot be changed.

IMAGE ENHANCEMENT

The term *image enhancement* implies that the adjusted image is an improved version of the original one. Most image enhancement operations are applied to make the image visually more appealing (subjective enhancement). This can be accomplished by increasing contrast, optimizing brightness, and reducing unsharpness and noise. Subjective image enhancement does not necessarily improve the accuracy of image interpretation. Image enhancement operations are often task-specific: what benefits one diagnostic task may reduce the image quality for another task. For example, increasing contrast between enamel and dentin for caries detection may make it more difficult to identify the contour of the alveolar crest. Image enhancement operations are also dependent on viewer preference.

Brightness and Contrast

Digital radiographs do not always effectively utilize the full range of available gray values. They can be relatively dark or light, and they can show too much contrast in certain areas or not enough. Although this can be judged visually, the image histogram is a convenient tool to examine which of the available gray values the image is using (Fig. 12-12). The minimum and maximum values and the shape of the histogram indi-

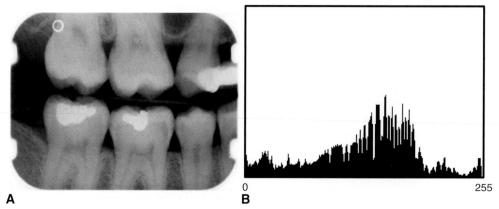

FIG. **12-12**   Digital image **(A)** with image histogram **(B)**. Horizontal axis represents image gray levels (8 bits–256 levels); vertical axis represents number of pixels. Each bar indicates the number of pixels in the image with that particular gray level.

cate the potential benefit of brightness and contrast enhancement operations. Digital imaging software commonly includes a histogram tool, as well as tools for the adjustment of brightness and contrast. Some also allow adjustment of the gamma value. Changing the gamma value of an image selectively enhances image contrast in either the brighter or darker areas of the image. Adjustment of brightness, contrast, and gamma value changes the original intensity values of the image (input) to new values (output). The operator can choose to make these changes permanent or to restore the image to its original settings. Fig. 12-13 is a graphic representation of the relationship between input values (horizontal axis) and output values (vertical axis) with the corresponding images and their histograms. Digital imaging software usually also includes tools for histogram equalization and contrast inversion. Histogram equalization is an enhancement operation that increases contrast between those image intensities abundantly present within the image while reducing contrast between image intensities that are used only sparsely. The actual effect of histogram equalization depends on the image content and may sometimes lead to unexpected degradation of image quality. Contrast inversion changes the radiographic positive image into a radiographic negative image. Although this may affect the subjective perception of the image content, the altered appearance is foreign to interpretive practice and has not shown to be useful.

The effect of contrast enhancement on the diagnostic value of digital radiographs is controversial. Some studies show substantial benefits of contrast enhancement operations, whereas others have found only limited value or no improvement at all. The effect of contrast enhancement cannot easily be predicted. The key to successful image enhancement is to selectively enhance relevant radiographic signs without simultaneously enhancing distracting signs. The development of such image processing operations requires careful consideration of the image content and the human visual perception system. Only under those conditions can one expect contrast enhancement to benefit the diagnostic value of the image.

Sharpening and Smoothing

The purpose of sharpening and smoothing filters is to improve image quality by removing blur or noise. Noise is often categorized as high-frequency noise (speckling) or low-frequency noise (gradual intensity changes). Filters that smooth an image are sometimes called *despeckling filters* because they remove high-frequency noise. Filters that sharpen an image either remove low-frequency noise or enhance boundaries between regions with different intensities (edge enhancement). For the purposeful application of filters, it is important to know what type of noise they reduce and how that affects radiographic features of interest. Without this knowledge, important radiographic features may degrade or disappear as noise is removed. Similarly, edge enhancement of radiographic features of interest may enhance noise. Sharpening and smoothing filters may make the dental radiographic images subjectively more appealing; however, there is no scientific evidence suggesting an increase in diagnostic value. The indiscriminate use of filters made available in most imaging software packages should be avoided if there is no scientific support for their clinical usefulness.

Color

Most digital systems currently on the market provide opportunities for color conversion of gray scale images, also called *pseudo-color*. Humans can distinguish many

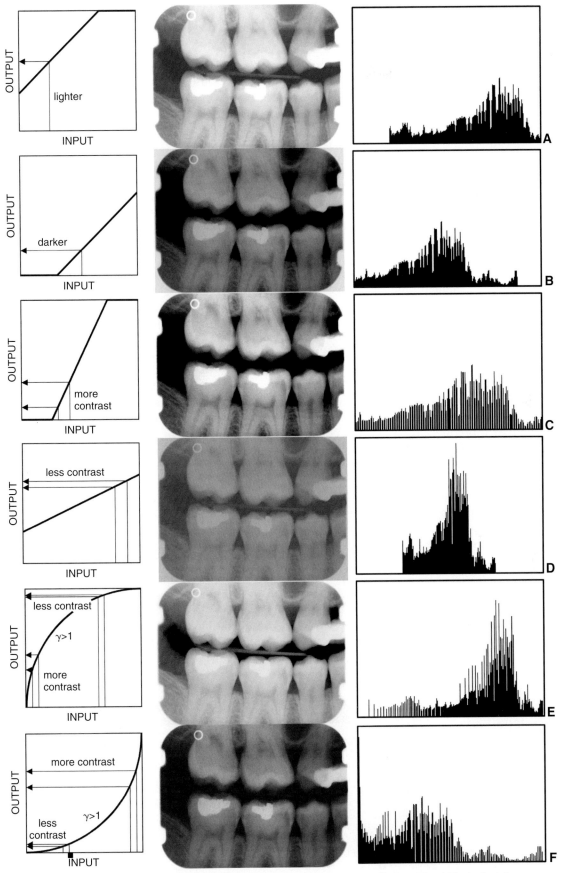

FIG. **12-13** Effect of brightness, contrast, and gamma adjustment as illustrated by image transformation graphs *(left),* digital images *(middle),* and image histograms *(right).* The image adjustments are relative to those of Fig. 12-12. **A,** Increase in brightness. **B,** Decrease in brightness. **C,** Increase in contrast. **D,** Decrease in contrast. **E,** Increase in gamma. **F,** Decrease in gamma.

more colors than shades of gray. Transforming the gray values of a digital image into various colors could theoretically enhance the detection of objects within the image. However, this works only if all the gray values representing an object are unique for that object. Since this is rarely the case, boundaries between objects may change and new boundaries may be created. In most cases this will distract the observer from seeing the real content of the image. Therefore, color conversion of radiographs is neither diagnostically nor educationally useful. Some useful applications of color exist. When objects can be uniquely identified based on a set of image features, color can be used to label or highlight these objects. The development of such criteria is a complex task, and only a limited number of successful studies have been reported in the literature.

Digital Subtraction Radiography

When two images of the same object are registered and the image intensities of corresponding pixels are subtracted, a uniform difference image is produced. If there is a change in the radiographic attenuation between the baseline and follow-up examination, this change shows up as a brighter area when the change represents gain and as a darker area when the change represents loss (Fig. 12-14). The strength of digital subtraction radiography (DSR) is that it cancels out the complex anatomic background against which this change occurs. As a result, the conspicuousness of the change is greatly increased. In order for DSR to be diagnostically useful, it is imperative that the baseline projection geometry and image intensities be reproduced.

The projection geometry is defined by the position and orientation of the x-ray source, the patient, and the detector, relative to one another. If the projection geometry used for the follow-up image is different from the projection geometry used for the baseline image, the subtraction image will show these differences. They can be difficult to distinguish from actual changes within the patient, or they may hide actual change. Perfect reproduction of the projection geometry would be ideal but is virtually impossible to achieve. Various types of changes in projection geometry are equally detrimental. Although most changes can be reversed through image processing, horizontal and vertical beam angulation changes cannot be reversed and should be reproduced as accurately as possible. Several image processing techniques have been developed to adjust for reversible projection errors and to minimize the effect of irreversible projection errors. The actual tolerance of changes in the projection geometry depends on how much actual change needs to be detected. Although exact reproduction of the projection geometry is not strictly necessary, some form of mechanical standardization will reduce the reliance on image processing and will generally produce better results.

Differences in image contrast and intensity between the baseline image and the follow-up image can hamper the detection task and make quantitative measurements unreliable. Fluctuations in the exposure factors and changes in projection geometry account for most of the discrepancies. When film is used as the image receptor, film processing variations are a main concern. Various methods have been used to match the intensities of baseline and follow-up images. All methods rely on either external or internal calibration.

Subtraction images are well-suited for acquiring quantitative information, such as linear, area, and density measurements. Methods used to make such measurements range from visual interpretation and manual measurement to computer-aided image analysis. Regardless of the analytic technique used, the detection and quantification of actual changes within the

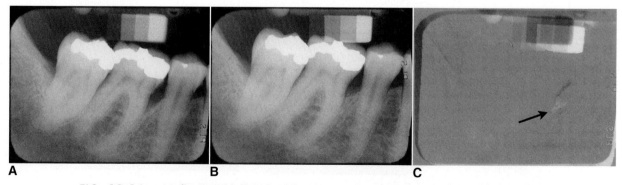

FIG. **12-14** *Application of digital subtraction radiography for detection and quantification of periodontal bone healing.* **A,** Baseline image. **B,** Standardized 1-year follow-up image. **C,** Subtraction image showing increase in bone *(arrow).*

patient requires that other factors affecting such measures are controlled.

IMAGE ANALYSIS

Image analysis operations are designed to extract diagnostically relevant information from the image. This information can range from simple linear measurements to fully automated diagnosis. The use of image analysis tools brings with it the responsibility to understand their limitations. The accuracy and precision of a measurement are limited by the extent to which the image is a truthful and reproducible representation of the patient and by the operator's ability to make an exact measurement.

Measurement

Digital imaging software provides a number of tools for image analysis. Digital rulers, densitometers, and a variety of other tools are readily available. These tools are usually digital equivalents of existing tools used in endodontics, orthodontics, periodontology, implantology, and other areas of dentistry (Fig. 12-15). Digital imaging has also added new tools that were not available with film-based radiography. The size and image intensity of any area within a digital radiograph can be measured. Tools are also being developed for measuring the complexity of the trabecular bone pattern. Such measurements can be useful as screening tools for

osteoporosis assessment and for the detection of other types of pathologies.

Diagnosis

One of the most challenging areas of research is the development of tools and procedures that automate the detection, classification, and quantification of radiographic signs of disease. The rationale for using such methods is to achieve early and accurate disease detection using reproducible and objective criteria. The development of automated image analysis operations is very complex and requires a thorough understanding of anatomy, pathology, and radiographic image formation. The three basic steps of image analysis are segmentation, feature extraction and object classification. Of these, segmentation is the most critical step. The goal of segmentation is to simplify the image and reduce it to its basic components. This involves subdividing the image, thus separating objects from the background. Objects of interest are defined by the diagnostic task, for example, a tooth, a carious lesion, a bone level, or an implant. When image segmentation results in the detection of an object, a variety of features can be measured that assist in determining what the object represents. Such features may include measures of size and shape, relative location, average density, homogeneity, and texture. A unique set of values for a certain combination of features can lead to classification of the object. Automated cephalometric landmark identification is an example of this technology. Other dental examples include caries detection, classification of periodontal disease, and detection and quantification of periapical bone lesions. The success of many of these applications is highly dependent on specific imaging parameters. Very few provide reliable results when used clinically. This underscores the complexity of the radiographic image interpretation process.

Image Storage

The use of digital imaging in dentistry requires an image archiving and management system that is very different from conventional radiography. Storage of diagnostic images on magnetic or optical media raises a number of new issues that must be considered. The file size of dental digital radiographs varies considerably, ranging from approximately 200 kB for intraoral images to as much as 6 MB for extraoral images. Storage and retrieval of these images in an average-size dental practice is not a trivial issue. Fortunately, the development of new storage media and the continuing decrease in the price of a unit of storage has alleviated the capacity issue in dental radiography. Hard drive

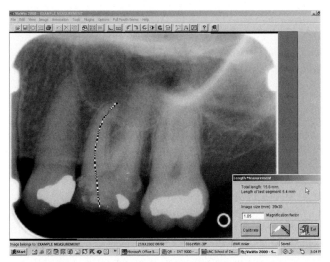

FIG. **12-15** Example of a measurement tool to determine the length of the crown and mesiobuccal root of the first molar. The measurement has been calibrated for a magnification factor of 1.05×. The digital measurement tool is more versatile than the analog ruler; however, for both types of measurement tools, the apparent length remains dependent on the projection geometry.

BOX 12-1
Digital Image Backup Considerations

- Type of backup media
- Time and method of backup
- Backup interval
- Storage location of backup media
- Recovery time
- Recovery reliability
- Future compatibility of backup technology

---

capacities of modern computers already exceed the storage needs of most dental practices.

The simplicity with which digital images can be modified through image processing poses a potential risk with respect to ensuring the integrity of the diagnostic information. Once in a digital format, critical image data can be deleted or modified. It is important that the software prevents the user from permanently deleting or modifying original image data, whether intentional or unintentional. Not all software programs provide such a safeguard. As the use of digital imaging in dentistry continues to expand, the implementation of standards for preserving original image data becomes urgent. It is also imperative that images and other important patient-related information are regularly stored on secondary external media. The use of computers for storing critical patient information mandates the design and use of a backup protocol. Box 12-1 shows some issues that need to be considered when designing a backup protocol. Backup media suitable for external storage of digital radiographs include external hard drives, digital tapes, CDs, and DVDs. All of these technologies are low in cost and have demonstrated reasonable reliability.

IMAGE COMPRESSION

The purpose of image compression is to reduce the size of digital image files for archiving or transmission. Particularly, the storage of extraoral images in a busy clinic may pose a challenge to storage capacity and speed of image access. The purpose of file compression is to significantly reduce the file size while preserving critical image information.

Compression methods are generally classified as lossless or lossy. *Lossless* methods do not discard any image data, and an exact copy of the image is reproduced after decompression. Most compression techniques take advantage of redundancies in the image, which can be expressed in simpler terms. The maximum com-

pression rate for lossless compression is usually less than 3:1. *Lossy* compression methods achieve higher levels of compression by discarding image data. Empirical evidence suggests that this does not necessarily affect the diagnostic quality of an image. Compression rates of 12:1 and 14:1 were shown to have no appreciable effect on caries diagnosis. For determining endodontic file length, a rate of 25:1 was diagnostically equivalent to the uncompressed image. A compression rate of 28:1 was acceptable for the subjective evaluation of image quality and the detection of artificial lesions in panoramic radiographs.

Version 3.0 of the DICOM (Digital Imaging and Communications in Medicine) standard adopted JPEG (Joint Photographic Experts Group) as the compression method, which provides a range of compression levels. Other types of image compression methods, such as wavelet compression, are being investigated for their use in medical imaging. Although the use of low and medium levels of lossy compression appear to have little effect on the diagnostic value of dental images, the application of lossy compression should be used with caution and only after evaluating its effect for specific diagnostic tasks. With the continuing increase in the capacity of storage media and the widespread use of high speed data communication lines, lossy compression of dental radiographs is rapidly becoming obsolete. At the same time, new digital image receptors are generating images with more and more pixels and more bits per pixel, thus increasing storage needs. Image compression negates to some extent the gain from such high-end detectors. Whether or not we need high resolution detectors and whether or not we can use image compression should be dictated by diagnostic criteria. Current evidence suggests that detector quality and moderate image compression have a limited impact on diagnostic outcomes.

Systems Compatibility

The development of digital imaging systems for dental radiography has largely been driven by industry. Manufacturers have adopted and developed technologies according to individual needs and philosophies. As a result, image formats among systems from different vendors are not standardized, and image archival, retrieval, and display systems are not compatible. Despite the proprietary nature of imaging software, it is not impossible to transfer images form one vendor's system to the other. Most systems provide image export and import tools using a variety of generic image formats, such as JPEG and TIFF (Tagged Image File Format). However, the process of transferring images through export-import procedures is somewhat cumbersome. It requires a number of steps, and the operator needs to ensure that the right images are imported into the proper patient folder. It can also not be assumed that the display and calibration of imported and native images will be the same. Clearly, exporting and importing is not the method of choice when digital imaging is going to be used on a large scale. It has long been recognized that the adoption of a standard for transferring images and associated information between digital imaging devices in medicine and dentistry is necessary. The American College of Radiology (ACR) and the National Electrical Manufacturers Association (NEMA) formed a joint committee to develop a standard for digital imaging systems. A large number of professional organizations have contributed to this complex development process, which has resulted in the current standard, known as the *Digital Imaging and Communications in Medicine (DICOM) standard*. Various dental organizations, including the American Dental Association, are playing an active role in defining aspects of the standard related to dentistry. The DICOM standard is not a static set of rules dictating to manufactures how to build imaging devices. Rather it is an evolving document addressing the interoperability of medical and dental imaging and information systems. Manufactures of digital imaging systems for dental radiography are responding to the call to adopt the DICOM standard. Not all systems are currently conforming to the DICOM standard, and those that do, do not necessarily conform to every aspect of the standard. The successful adoption of digital imaging in dentistry requires interoperability of all devices. It is likely that manufactures do not want to be left behind and that the market will weed out those that are *noncompliant*. Dentists using different vendors with DICOM–compliant imaging devices will be able to exchange images seamlessly.

Clinical Considerations

Some fundamental differences from film in the clinical handling of digital receptors should to be noted (Table 12-1). Because digital receptors are intended to be reusable, they must be handled with greater care than their film counterparts. Indeed, in certain situations film may be intentionally damaged through bending to accommodate patient anatomy. This is never the case with digital receptors. PSP plates are susceptible to bending and scratching during handling that induce permanent artifacts in the receptor. These artifacts obscure information of potential diagnostic importance and may necessitate disposal of the receptor and repeat imaging of the patient. Because of the inability of digital detectors to be bent to accommodate patient anatomy, new imaging strategies must be employed for some patients. It may not be possible to consistently capture the distal surface of the canine on premolar views. An additional projection may be required to adequately visualize this surface. A significant potential problem with current PSP systems is the inability to distinguish images that have been exposed backwards. Unlike film packets, which incorporate a lead foil with a characteristic embossed pattern that results in an underexposed image of the anatomy with the pattern artifact when exposed backwards, PSP images suffer little x-ray attenuation from the polyester base. It is much too easy for inattentive radiographers to mount these digital images on the contralateral position from their true side. One can image the liability that could occur from diagnosing and treating disease on the opposite side of the actual lesion. Infection control is also an issue with digital receptors. Digital receptors cannot be sterilized by conventional means. They may be disinfected by wiping with mild agents such as isopropyl alcohol but should not be immersed in disinfecting solutions. The adage that "you can autoclave a digital receptor...once" stems from the fact that heat will ruin electronic components in CCD and CMOS sensors and will distort the polyester base of PSP plates. Another potential drawback to drum-based PSP systems is the 2- to 5-minute cycle time required for plate scanning. During this time, no additional plates may be processed. With film and nondrum-based PSP scanners there is less delay between the time when additional films or plates may be "fed" into the processor. Although each of the preceding concerns are of potential importance, we should not overlook the advantage of eliminating chemical processing in digital systems. The time required to properly monitor and maintain a film processor is significant. Too often, insufficient attention is paid to this critical aspect of film radiography. Digital systems may not save the time gained by eliminating film processing, but they will eliminate the loss in diagnostic quality that occurs when insufficient time and effort is spent on film processing quality assurance.

Conclusion

Dental practitioners commonly ask, "Which is better, film or digital imaging?" There is no simple answer to this question (Tables 12-1 and 12–2). Reported technical properties of resolution, contrast, and latitude are confounded by a lack of standardization in the assessment of these characteristics. From a diagnostic stand-

TABLE 12-1
Clinical Comparison of Intraoral Imaging Alternatives

IMAGING STEP	FILM	CCD/CMOS	PSP
Receptor preparation	None	1) Place protective plastic sleeve over receptor 2) Receptor must be connected to computer and patient identifying information entered for acquisition/archiving software	1) "Erase" plates 2) Package plates in protective plastic envelope
Receptor placement	1) Numerous generic film holding devices are available 2) Film may be bent to accommodate anatomy	1) Specialized receptor holder specific for manufacturer's receptor may limit options 2) Receptor inflexibility and bulk limit placement options 3) Receptor cable must be carefully routed out of patient mouth 4) Patient discomfort more likely than with film or PSP	1) Many receptor holders used for film may be adapted for PSP plates 2) Bending of receptor may irreversibly damage it
Exposure	Simple exposure	Computer must be activated prior to exposure	Simple exposure
Processing	1) Dark, light-safe environment in form of darkroom or daylight loader required 2) Processor chemistry must be prepared or replenished 3) Chemical temperature must be warmed, or processing time must be adjusted to accommodate temperature 4) Films must be removed from wrapper; lead foil must be separated for recycling	Image acquisition and display is almost immediate	1) Dimly light environment desirable to prevent loss of image information 2) Processor must be programmed with patient and detector information so that images are identified, preprocessed, and stored properly 3) Protective wrapper must be removed from plates 4) Plates must be loaded on drum systems
Display preparation	1) Films may be placed in a variety of film mounts 2) Mounts must be labeled with patient identifying information	1) Software may be configured to place image in appropriate position in digital mount when exposures are made in a predetermined sequence; otherwise, images must be individually placed in mount 2) Images may need to be digitally rotated to achieve proper orientation	1) Images must be individually placed in mount 2) Images may need to be digitally rotated to achieve proper orientation
Display	1) A room with subdued lighting and a masked viewbox are optimal 2) Any light source (including the operatory window or ceiling light) will permit a quick evaluation of the image	Same considerations apply to all digital receptor types 1) A room with subdued lighting is optimal for interpretation activities 2) A computer and display with appropriate software are necessary; viewing is restricted to the location of the computer 3) Laptop computers increase flexibility of computer placement but may reduce display quality 4) Size of the display will restrict the numbers of images that may be viewed simultaneously; more time is required to open/close or expand contract images when interpreting a series of images	
Image duplication	Quality of duplication is always inferior to original and is sometimes nondiagnostic	1) Electronic copies may be stored on a variety of media without loss of image quality 2) Output on film or paper is inferior and is often nondiagnostic unless appropriate combinations of expensive printers and papers or film are used	

TABLE 12-2
Comparison of Physical Properties of Film, CCD, CMOS, and PSP Receptors

FEATURE	TECHNICAL COMMENT	CLINICAL COMMENT
Spatial resolution	Intraoral systems: Film > CCD = CMOS > PSP Panoramic systems: Film = CCD = PSP Cephalometric systems Film > CCD = PSP	The limits of resolution for digital systems are readily appreciated when magnifying these images. With magnification a "blocky" or "pixilated" appearance is evident. Resolution of panoramic systems is limited by mechanical motion to about 5 lp/mm.
Exposure latitude	PSP >> CCD = CMOS ≥ film	Because of the wide latitude of PSP and the automatic brightness and contrast "optimization" by image acquisition software, use of more x-ray exposure than is necessary is possible.
Receptor dimensions	For equivalent imaged area, Film = PSP < CCD = CMOS	The "active area" of CCD and CMOS receptors is smaller than the surface area because of other electronic components within in the plastic housing.
Time for image acquisition	CCD = CMOS << PSP = film	Rapid image acquisition may be important for endodontic procedures or during implant placement.
Image quality	Subjective quality is best with film when carefully exposed and well processed.	Digital and film imaging are not significantly different when used for common diagnostic tasks.
Image adjustment/ processing	Improves appearance of digital images.	Takes time; may not improve diagnostic performance.
Cost	Initial costs of digital systems are greater than film. Subsequent costs vary greatly depending on receptor wear and tear or abuse.	Manufacturer's estimates of life expectancy of reusable receptors are perhaps overly optimistic.
Reliability	Mechanical problems affect digital PSP and film systems. Software reliability varies greatly among manufacturers. Changes in unrelated computer components and software can cause digital systems to malfunction.	Digital systems fail when problems occur with receptors during image acquisition, or with computers during image processing, archiving, and display.
Image storage and retrieval	Data backup is critical for digital systems.	Films can be misfiled and lost or be damaged by poor storage conditions. Digital data can be lost as a result of failures in power supplies and/or storage media, as well as operator error.
Transmitting images to others	Rapidly done with digital images.	Facilitates communication between colleagues or with insurance companies.

point most studies suggest that digital performance is not statistically different from film for typical diagnostic tasks such as caries diagnosis. The "look and feel" of digital displays is distinctly different from film viewing, and some practitioners may find this difference disconcerting. A basic understanding of computers and mastery of common computing skills is essential for viewing digital images. Beyond this, learning the peculiarities and vagaries of a particular acquisition and display software will take time and may not be intuitive.

Multiple mouse clicks through multiple menus may be required to view a full mouth series of images. This may modestly increase the time required to complete the diagnostic process.

In selecting an imaging system, other issues should be considered. Digital images avoid environmental pollutants encountered with film processing, but what about the environmental impact associated with the disposal of broken or obsolete electronic equipment? The initial financial outlay for digital imaging hardware makes these systems more expensive than film. Manufacturers are quick to point out that the costs of film or digital systems should be amortized over the life of the equipment and consumables; however, the life expectancy of newer digital systems is highly speculative. Mishandling of digital system components can catastrophically shorten any projected life expectancy. And what price should we place on the ability to instantly transmit images and to integrate them into a fully electronic record? There are no universal answers to these questions. They must be asked and answered according to the needs and objectives of individual dental practices. As practice patterns and technology change with time, the answers will also change. Although the details of the image in our crystal ball have yet to resolve, the trends of increasing adoption of digital imaging and continuing technologic innovation makes the future of digital imaging in dentistry certain.

BIBLIOGRAPY

DIGITAL DETECTORS AND DISPLAYS

Abreu M Jr, Tyndall DA, Ludlow JB: Detection of caries with conventional digital imaging and tuned aperture computed tomography using CRT monitor and laptop displays, Oral Surg Oral Med Oral Pathol Oral Radiol Endod 88(2):234–8, 1999.

Abreu M Jr, Mol A, Ludlow JB: Performance of RVGui sensor and Kodak Ektaspeed Plus film for proximal caries detection, Oral Surg Oral Med Oral Pathol Oral Radiol Endod 91(3):381–5, 2001.

Borg E, Grondahl HG: On the dynamic range of different X-ray photon detectors in intra-oral radiography: a comparison of image quality in film, charge-coupled device and storage phosphor systems, Dentomaxillofac Radiol 25(2):82–8, 1996.

Couture RA, Hildebolt C: Quantitative dental radiography with a new photostimulable phosphor system, Oral Surg Oral Med Oral Pathol Oral Radiol Endod 89(4):498–508, 2000.

Hildebolt CF, Fletcher G, Yokoyama-Crothers N, Conover GL, Vannier MW: A comparison of the response of storage phosphor and film radiography to small variations in X-ray exposure, Dentomaxillofac Radiol 26(3):147–51, 1997.

Hildebolt CF, Couture RA, Whiting BR: Dental photostimulable phosphor radiography, Dent Clin North Am 44(2):273–97, 2000.

Kashima I, Sakurai T, Matsuki T, Nakamura K, Aoki H, Ishii M, Kanagawa Y: Intraoral computed radiography using the Fuji computed radiography imaging plate: correlation between image quality and reading condition, Oral Surg Oral Med Oral Pathol 78(2):239–46, 1994.

Sanderink GC, Miles DA: Intraoral detectors: CCD, CMOS, TFT, and other devices, Dent Clin North Am 44(2):249–55, v, 2000.

Van der Stelt PF: Principles of digital imaging, Dent Clin North Am 44(2):237–48, v, 2000.

Welander U, McDavid WD, Sanderink GC, Tronje G, Morner AC, Dove SB: Resolution as defined by line spread and modulation transfer functions for four digital intraoral radiographic systems, Oral Surg Oral Med Oral Pathol 78(1):109–15, 1994.

IMAGE PROCESSING

Analoui M: Radiographic image enhancement. Part I: spatial domain techniques, Dentomaxillofac Radiol 30:1–9, 2001.

Analoui M: Radiographic digital image enhancement. Part II: transform domain techniques. Dentomaxillofac Radiol 30:65–77, 2001.

Baxes GA: Digital Image Processing: Principles and Applications, New York, 1994, John Wiley & Sons.

Gonzalez R, Wintz P: Digital image processing, ed 2, 1987, Addison Wesley Publishing Co.

Gröndahl H-G, Gröndahl K, Webber R: A digital subtraction technique for dental radiography, Oral Surg Oral Med Oral Pathol 55:96–102, 1983.

Lehmann T, Gröndahl H-G, Benn D: Computer-based registration for digital subtraction in dental radiology, Dentomaxillofac Radiol 29:323–346, 2000.

Mol A: Image Processing tools for dental applications, Dent Clin North Amer 44:299–318, 2000.

Russ JC: The image process handbook, ed 4, Boca Raton, Fla, 2002, CRC Press.

Ruttimann U, Webber R, Schmidt E: A robust digital method for film contrast correction in subtraction radiography, J Periodont Res 21:486–495, 1986.

CHAPTER 13

Specialized Radiographic Techniques

NEIL L. FREDERIKSEN

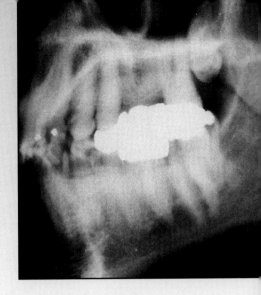

The techniques described in this chapter are used to address specific diagnostic tasks. Some have been available to clinicians for years; others are more recent innovations made possible through computer technology. Although general dental practitioners do not use most of these techniques routinely, all are used occasionally to aid in diagnosis of conditions in the oral cavity. For this reason, anyone involved in providing oral health care must have a basic understanding of these techniques, their operating principles, and their clinical applications.

Film Radiography

TOMOGRAPHY

Conventional film-based tomography, also called *body section radiography*, is a radiographic technique designed to image more clearly objects lying within a plane of interest. This is accomplished by blurring the images of structures lying outside the plane of interest through the process of motion "unsharpness." Since the introduction of computed tomography and magnetic resonance imaging, which have superior low-contrast resolution (ability to discriminate low density objects; e.g., soft tissue), film-based tomography has been used less frequently. Conventional tomography now is applied primarily to high-contrast anatomy, such as that encountered in temporomandibular joint (TMJ) and dental implant diagnostics.

Essential equipment for tomography includes an x-ray tube and radiographic film rigidly connected and capable of moving about a fixed axis or fulcrum (Fig. 13-1). The examination begins with the x-ray tube and film positioned on opposite sides of the fulcrum, which is located within the body's plane of interest (focal plane). As the exposure begins, the tube and film move in opposite directions simultaneously through a mechanical linkage. With this synchronous movement of tube and film, the images of objects located within the focal plane (at the fulcrum) remain in fixed positions on the radiographic film throughout the length of tube and film travel and are clearly imaged. On the other hand, the images of objects located outside the focal plane have continuously changing positions on the film; as a result, the images of these objects are blurred beyond recognition by motion unsharpness.

The objective of tomography, then, is to blur the images of structures not located in the focal plane both as much and as uniformly as possible. Blurring is greater under the following conditions:

- The farther the structure lies from the focal plane and the greater the distance between the structure and the film (determined by the physical location of the fulcrum within the object to be imaged and hence the diagnostic task to be accomplished)
- The more closely the long axis of the structure to be blurred is oriented perpendicular to the direction of tube travel (accomplished by the tomographic movement)
- The greater the amplitude of tube travel (determined by the tomographic angle or arc)

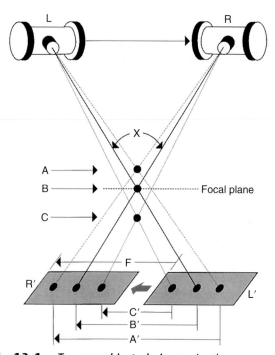

FIG. **13-1** *Tomographic techniques.* As the x-ray tube moves from left to right, the film moves in the opposite direction. In the figure, points *A* and *C* lie outside the focal plane (the plane that contains the fulcrum), whereas object *B* lies at the center of tube/film movement. Only objects that lie in the focal plane (i.e., *B*) remain in sharp focus because the image of *B* moves exactly the same distance (*B'*) as the film travels (*F*), and thus its image remains stationary on the film. The image of point *A* moves more than the film (distance *A'*) and the image of point *C* less than the film (distance *C'*); therefore the images of both are blurred. The figure illustrates a parallel movement of tube and film. *X* is the tomographic angle. The greater the tomographic angle, the thinner the plane of focus.

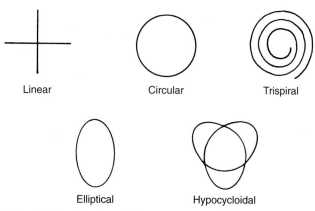

Linear

Circular

Trispiral

Elliptical

Hypocycloidal

FIG. **13-2** *Tomographic movements.* The more complex the motion, the smaller the likelihood the x-ray beam will strike an object of importance at the same tangent through the entire exposure. (Therefore blurring depends less on the orientation of the object under study.)

There are at least five types of tomographic movement: linear, circular, elliptical, hypocycloidal, and spiral (Fig. 13-2). Mechanically, the simplest tomographic motion is linear. Linear tomography can be accomplished in two ways: (1) the x-ray tube and film move in opposite directions about a fixed fulcrum in paths of travel parallel with one another or (2) both the x-ray tube and the film move along concentric arcs rather than in straight lines. Currently available x-ray units (Fig. 13-3) use both methods, which give similar results.

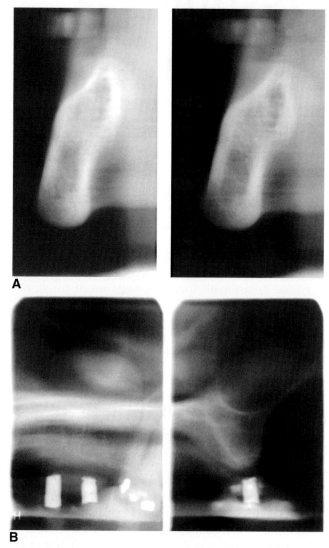

FIG. **13-3** *Linear tomographic images made by panoramic units.* **A,** Mandibular tomograms acquired using a Planmeca PM 2002 CC Proline panoramic unit. **B,** Maxillary tomograms in the premolar region acquired using an Instrumentarium Orthopantomograph 100 panoramic unit. Note the dome-shaped opacity in the floor of the maxillary sinus consistent with a mucous retention cyst. (**A,** Courtesy Planmeca, Inc., Roselle, IL; **B,** Courtesy Brad Potter, DDS, Augusta, Ga.)

The image quality of linear tomograms has several deficiencies compared with tomograms produced by other types of movement. With either type of linear motion the blurring pattern is irregular and incomplete leading to the recording of an image of an irregular plane of varying depth, the shape of which is dependent on the orientation of anatomic structures outside the presumed plane of focus to the central ray of the x-ray beam. These tomograms often appear streaked (Fig. 13-4). These streaks, called *false images* or *parasite lines,* represent the image of objects outside the focal plane whose long axis is oriented parallel with the movement of the tube. As a result, linear motion fails to satisfy a requirement for optimal blurring. In addition, with the parallel type of linear motion, the distance from the tube to the patient and the patient to the film is constantly changing, as is the angulation of the x-ray beam through the focal plane. This results in inconsistent magnification, dimensional instability, and nonuniform densities that may be seen across the linear tomographic image. Some equipment that uses the arc type of linear motion utilizes a slit beam of radiation like that employed in panoramic radiography. Images produced by this type of equipment may be distorted because magnification in the vertical plane is independent of that in the horizontal plane, just as in panoramic images. For some applications these deficiencies may be acceptable; if sharper tomographic images of more uniform density, consistent magnification, and dimensional stability are required, a multidirectional tomographic motion is necessary (Fig. 13-5).

The thickness of tissue in the focal plane is called the *tomographic layer.* The location of the tomographic layer within the object is determined by the position of the fulcrum and its width (described numerically as the *thickness of cut*) by the tomographic angle or arc (see Fig. 13-1). The relationship between the tomographic angle and the thickness of cut is inverse: the greater the tomographic angle, the thinner the thickness of cut. Selection of the tomographic angle, and hence the thickness of cut, depends on the objective of the diagnostic task and the type of tissue being examined.

Wide-angle tomography, which by definition uses tomographic angles greater than 10 degrees, allows visualization of fine structures that normally would be obscured by superimposition in conventional radiography. Using this technique, layers as thin as 1 mm can be imaged. A disadvantage of this technique, however, is that it produces images of decreased contrast. Subject contrast results partly from the different thickness of adjacent structures. Because wide-angle tomography reduces these differences by the thinness of its cut, subject contrast is decreased. Wide-angle tomography is most useful when tissues of greater physical density (another contributor to subject contrast), such as bone, are studied. Thus wide-angle tomography is an excellent technique for evaluating the maxilla and mandible before placing dental implants (Fig. 13-6).

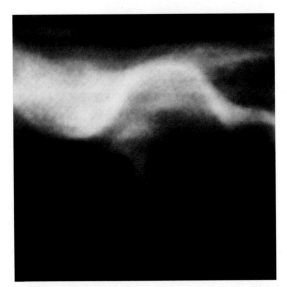

FIG. **13-4** *Linear tomogram of the TMJ.* Note the horizontal radiopaque streaks in this image. These streaks, called *parasite lines,* represent the blurred image of objects lying outside the focal plane. They are evident in the image when the long axes of objects located superficial or deep to the focal plane lie parallel with the path of the x-ray tube and film movement. Compare with Fig. 13-5.

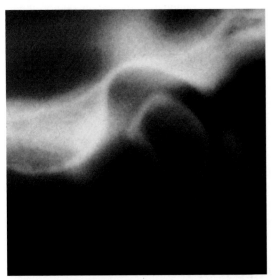

FIG. **13-5** *Spiral tomogram of the TMJ.* Complex tomographic movements result in maximal blurring of the images of objects lying superficial and deep to the plane of focus; the streaking parasite lines, therefore, are absent.

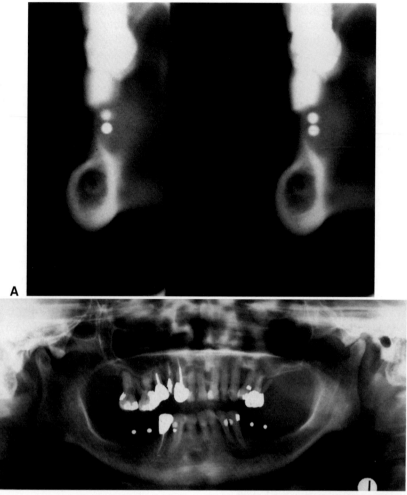

FIG. **13-6**   *Wide-angle tomograms made to evaluate the mandible before placement of a dental implant.* The mandibular right premolar-molar area in cross-section at the radiopaque markers is demonstrated on both the panoramic radiograph and the tomograms. Note the clarity with which the inferior alveolar canal is imaged in the tomograms acquired with a spiral movement. **A,** Each slice is 4 mm thick. **B,** The metallic markers are for orientation of the cross-sectional images.

Narrow-angle tomography uses an angle of less than 10 degrees. Called *zonography* because a relatively thick zone of tissue (up to 25 mm) is sharply imaged, it is particularly useful when subject contrast is low because of little difference in physical density between adjacent structures (Fig. 13-7). Because subject contrast is low in soft tissue, zonography is the preferred tomographic technique when this tissue is imaged.

STEREOSCOPY

Stereoscopy is not a new technique. J. MacKenzie Davidson introduced it in 1898, only 3 years after Röntgen's discovery of x rays. Over the next 30 to 40 years the technique grew in popularity among radiologists because of its educational value; understanding normal anatomy is simplified with stereoscopic images. Stereoscopy has also been used to determine the location of small intracranial calcifications and multiple foreign bodies in dense or thick body sections, cases in which the interpretation of images produced at right angles might be difficult, and to evaluate the relationships of margins of bony fractures. Despite these advantages, stereoscopy fell from favor for several reasons, among which were the introduction of more sophisticated and less time-consuming imaging techniques and, by the 1930s, a greater awareness of the possible adverse biologic effects of x rays.

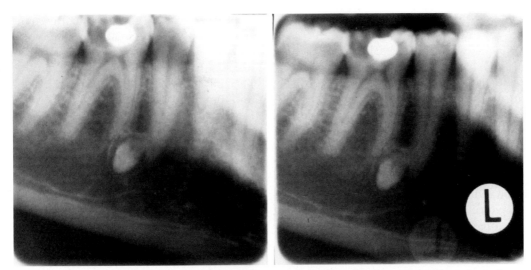

FIG. **13-7** *Narrow-angle tomograms (zonograms).* This pair of images, with a plane of focus tangent to the mandible, was made with narrow-angle tomographic techniques. The thick plane of focus (25 mm) allowed the supernumerary tooth and adjacent permanent teeth to be imaged clearly in one depth of the field. The diagnostic value of these images is increased by their having been made stereoscopically, allowing for localization of the supernumerary tooth relative to clinically erupted teeth. See also Fig. 13-8.

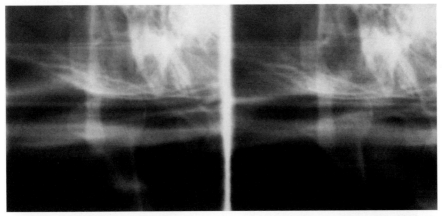

FIG. **13-8** *Posteroanterior rotational stereoscopic scanogram of the right TMJ.* Compared with a standard posteroanterior view of the condyle, this view demonstrates higher contrast and greater detail. The diagnostic value of such images is increased by their having been made stereoscopically, which allows for the perception of depth.

Stereoscopic imaging requires the exposure of two films, one for each eye, and thus delivers twice the amount of radiation to the patient. Between exposures the patient is maintained in position, the film is changed, and the tube is shifted from the right eye to the left eye position. Although the magnitude of the tube shift is empiric, it must be sufficient to form slightly different or discrepant images. A tube shift equal to 10% of the focal-film distance has been found to produce satisfactory results. After processing, the films commonly are viewed with a stereoscope that uses either mirrors or prisms to coordinate the accommodation and convergence of the viewer's eyes so that the brain can fuse the two images (Fig. 13-8; see also Fig. 13-7).

Stereoscopy currently enjoys a renewed interest for evaluation of bony pockets in patients with periodontal disease and the morphology of the temporomandibular joint area, determination of root configuration of teeth that require endodontic therapy, assessment of the relationship of the mandibular canal to the roots of unerupted mandibular third molars, and assessment of bone shape when placement of dental implants is considered.

SCANOGRAPHY

Scanography is a technique that uses a narrowly collimated, fan-shaped beam of radiation to scan an area of interest, sequentially projecting image data relative to this area onto a moving film, much the same as in panoramic radiography. Compared with images produced by standard radiography using round or rectangular collimation, scanograms demonstrate higher contrast with the perception of greater detail. Image contrast is greater in scanography because collimation of the x-ray beam reduces the amount of radiation scattered to the film during exposure. Therefore the major advantage of scanography over standard transmission radiography is image quality.

The Soredex Scanora (Soredex Inc., Milwaukee, WI) (see Fig. 10-11) is a commercially available x-ray unit capable of performing both rotational and linear scanography. In rotational scanography the beam of radiation rotates about a fixed axis that is predetermined based on the area to be imaged. The imaging sequence used by this unit results in the production of two or four scanograms, each made with the x-ray tube in a different position; thus multiple images are made,

any two of which can be viewed as stereoscopic pairs (see Fig. 13-8). Rotational scanography has been found to be as effective as intraoral periapical films in the assessment of periodontal disease and the detection of periapical lesions. In linear scanography the x-ray beam and film move in a linear fashion, scanning the area of interest. Linear scanography can be thought of as panoramic radiography that has been "straightened out." The Scanora system is capable of both posteroanterior and lateral linear scanning of the maxillofacial complex. Although these views are not produced stereoscopically, they have the advantage of optimal image contrast (Fig. 13-9).

Computed Tomography

In 1972 Godfrey Hounsfield announced the invention of a revolutionary imaging technique, which he referred to as *computerized axial transverse scanning*. With this technique he was able to produce an axial cross-sectional image of the head using a narrowly collimated, moving beam of x rays. A scintillation crystal detected the remnant radiation of this beam, and the

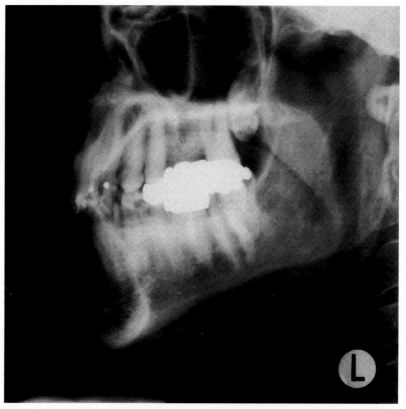

FIG. **13-9** *Lateral linear scanogram of the maxillofacial area.* Maximal image contrast is obtained by using linear scanning techniques rather than standard radiography.

resulting analog signal was fed into a computer, digitized, and analyzed by a mathematical algorithm and the data reconstructed as an axial tomographic image. The image produced by this technique was like no other x-ray image. Claimed to be 100 times more sensitive than conventional x-ray systems, it demonstrated differences between various soft tissues never before seen with x-ray imaging techniques. Since 1972 computed tomography has had many names, each of which referred to at least one aspect of the technique: "computerized axial tomography," "computerized reconstruction tomography," "computed tomographic scanning," "axial tomography," and "computerized transaxial tomography." Currently the preferred name is *computed tomography*, abbreviated as *CT.*

In its simplest form a CT scanner consists of a radiographic tube that emits a finely collimated, fan-shaped x-ray beam directed to a series of scintillation detectors or ionization chambers. Depending on the scanner's mechanical geometry, both the radiographic tube and detectors may rotate synchronously about the patient, or the detectors may form a continuous ring about the patient and the x-ray tube may move in a circle within the detector ring (Fig. 13-10). CT scanners that employ this type of movement for image acquisition are called *incremental scanners* because the final image set consists of a series of contiguous or overlapping axial images. More recently CT scanners have been developed that acquire image data in a spiral or helical fashion (Fig. 13-11). With these scanners, while the gantry containing the x-ray tube and detectors revolves around the patient, the table on which the patient is lying continuously advances through the gantry. This results in the acquisition of a continuous spiral of data as the x-ray beam moves down the patient. It is reported that, compared with incremental CT scanners, spiral scanners provide improved multiplanar image reconstructions, reduced examination time (12 seconds versus 5 minutes), and a reduced radiation dose (up to 75%). Regardless of the mechanical geometry, the transmission signal recorded by the detectors represents a composite of the absorption characteristics of all elements of the patient in the path of the x-ray beam.

The CT image is a digital image, reconstructed by computer, which mathematically manipulates the transmission data obtained from multiple projections (Fig. 13-12). For example, if one projection is made every one third of a degree, 1080 projections result during the course of a single 360-degree rotation of the scanner about the patient. Data derived from these 1080 projections (1080 projections constitute one scan) contain all the information necessary to construct a single image. The CT image is recorded and displayed as a matrix of individual blocks called *voxels* (volume

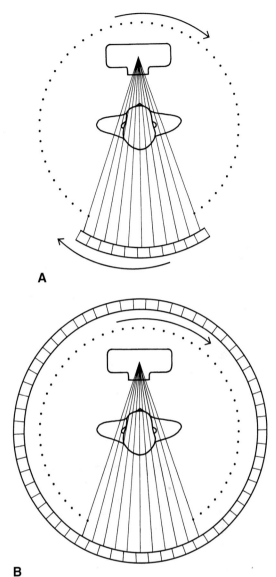

A

B

FIG. **13-10** *Mechanical geometry of CT scanners.* **A,** Both the x-ray tube and the detector array revolve around the patient. **B,** Only the x-ray tube rotates; radiation detection is accomplished by the use of a fixed circular array of as many as 1000 detectors.

elements). Each square of the image matrix is a pixel. Whereas the size of the pixel (about 0.1 mm) is determined partly by the computer program used to construct the image, the length of the voxel (about 1 to 20 mm) is determined by the width of the x-ray beam, which in turn is controlled by the prepatient and postpatient collimators. Voxel length is analogous to the tomographic layer in film tomography. For image display, each pixel is assigned a CT number representing density. This number is proportional to the degree to which the material within the voxel has attenuated the x-ray beam. It represents the absorption character-

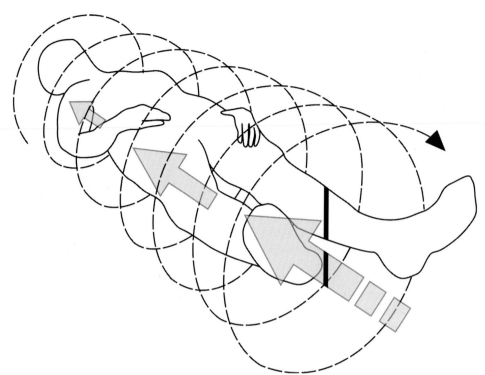

FIG. **13-11**   *Principles of helical CT.* As the patient is moved through the gantry, the continuously rotating x-ray tube and detector describe a helical or spiral path about the patient, acquiring image data as they rotate.

istics, or linear attenuation coefficient, of that particular volume of tissue in the patient. CT numbers, also known as *Hounsfield units* (named in honor of the inventor Godfrey Hounsfield), may range from −1000 to +1000, each constituting a different level of optical density. This scale of relative densities is based on air (−1000), water (0), and dense bone (+1000).

CT has several advantages over conventional film radiography and film tomography. First, CT completely eliminates the superimposition of images of structures outside the area of interest. Second, because of the inherent high-contrast resolution of CT, differences between tissues that differ in physical density by less than 1% can be distinguished; conventional radiography requires a 10% difference in physical density to distinguish between tissues. Third, data from a single CT imaging procedure consisting of either multiple contiguous or one helical scan can be viewed as images in the axial, coronal, or sagittal planes, depending on the diagnostic task. This is referred to as *multiplanar reformatted imaging*.

Primarily because of its high-contrast resolution and ability to demonstrate small differences in soft tissue density, CT has become useful for the diagnosis of disease in the maxillofacial complex (Fig. 13-13), including the salivary glands and TMJ. However,

with the advent of magnetic resonance imaging, which has proved superior to CT for depicting soft tissue, the use of CT scanning for assessment of internal derangements of the TMJ has decreased significantly. Additionally, CT has been shown to be useful for evaluation of patients before placement of endosseous oral implants. Despite the fact that similar information about maxillary and mandibular anatomy can be obtained with film tomography, CT allows reconstruction of cross-sectional images of the entire maxilla or mandible or both from a single imaging procedure.

Multiplanar CT imaging has made a significant contribution to diagnosis. However, these images are two-dimensional and require a certain degree of mental integration by the viewer for interpretation; this limitation has led to the development of computer programs that reformat data acquired from axial CT scans into three-dimensional images (3D CT).

Three-dimensional reformatting requires that each original voxel, shaped as a rectangular parallel piped or rectangular solid, be dimensionally altered into multiple cuboidal voxels. This process, called *interpolation*, creates sets of evenly spaced cuboidal voxels (cuberilles) that occupy the same volume as the original voxel (see Fig. 13-12). The CT numbers of the cuberilles rep-

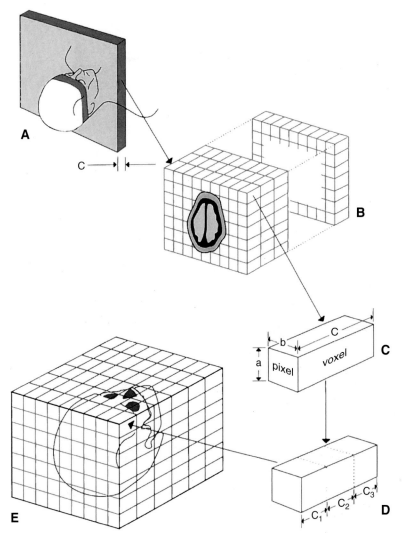

FIG. **13-12** *CT image formation.* **A,** Data for a single-plane image are acquired from multiple projections made during the course of a 360-degree rotation around the patient. Dimension c is controlled by prepatient and postpatient collimators. **B,** A single-plane image is constructed from absorption characteristics of the subject and displayed as differences in optical density, ranging from −1000 to +1000 Hounsfield units. Several planes may be imaged from multiple contiguous scans. **C,** The image consists of a matrix of individual pixels representing the face of a volume called a *voxel.* Although dimensions a and b are determined partly by the computer program used to construct the image, dimension c is controlled by the collimators as in **A. D,** Cuboid voxels can be created from the original rectangular voxel by computer interpolation. This allows the formation of multiplanar and three-dimensional images (**E**).

resent the average of the original voxel CT numbers surrounding each of the new voxels. Creation of these new cuboidal voxels allows the image to be reconstructed in any plane without loss of resolution by locating their position in space relative to one another. In construction of the 3D CT image, only cuberilles representing the surface of the object scanned are projected onto the viewing monitor. The surface formed by these cuberilles may then appear as if illuminated by a light source located behind the viewer. In this manner the visible surface of each pixel is assigned a gray-level value, depending on its distance from and orientation to the light source. Thus pixels that face the light source and/or are closer to it appear brighter than those that are turned away from the source and/or are farther away. The effects of this shading and the resulting

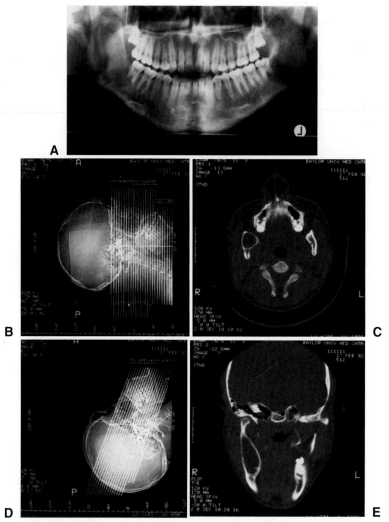

FIG. 13-13   **A,** Panoramic radiograph showing a unilocular radiolucent lesion involving the right mandibular ramus. **B,** Lateral scout radiograph for planning the location of contiguous CT scans. **C,** Reconstructed axial image at the level of scan 13 in **B**. Note the facilolingual extent of the radiolucent lesion on the right side. **D,** The patient is repositioned for oblique scans through the area of the lesion. **E,** Reconstructed oblique image at the level of scan 7 in **D**. Note the superior extent of the lesion into the condylar neck. (**B-E,** Courtesy Radiology Department, Baylor University Medical Center, Dallas, Texas.)

image perceived by the viewer have been described as similar to an artist's three-dimensional rendering of an object within a two-dimensional medium. Once constructed, 3D CT images may be further manipulated by rotation about any axis to display the structure imaged from many angles (Fig. 13-14). Also, external surfaces of the image can be removed electronically to reveal concealed deeper anatomy.

One of the first applications of 3D CT was the study of patients with suspected intervertebral disk hernia-

tion and spinal stenosis. Since that time 3D CT has been applied to craniofacial reconstructive surgery and has been used both for treatment of congenital and acquired deformities and for evaluation of intracranial tumors, benign and malignant lesions of the maxillofacial complex, cervical spine injuries, pelvic fractures, and deformities of the hands and feet. The availability of data in a three-dimensional format also has allowed the construction of life-sized models that can be used for trial surgeries and the construction of surgical stents

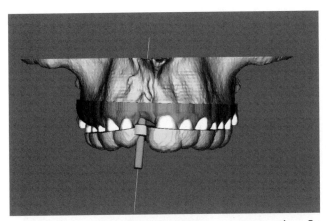

FIG. 13-14 *Three-dimensional image reconstruction.* By computer manipulation of the data acquired by a CT scanner, three-dimensional images can be reconstructed. This image has been reconstructed to show bone, soft tissue, and teeth. In addition, the image of a surgical guide showing its relation to supporting oral tissues has been reconstructed. The surgical guide will be used to direct the preparation of bone for the insertion of a dental implant. (Courtesy Materialise NV, Belgium.)

for guiding dental implant placement, as well as the creation of accurate implanted prostheses.

CT technology is being continually advanced. Imatron (San Francisco) has developed a CT scanner capable of acquiring data up to 10 times faster than conventional CT. Its Ultrafast CT, which has scan times on the order of 50 msec, is able to freeze cardiac and pulmonary motion, enhancing the quality without motion artifacts.

Cone Beam Radiography

Conventional film-based tomography and CT have been the techniques of choice for imaging bone and hard dental tissues of the jaws for the evaluation of pathosis, trauma, and treatment planning for dental implants. Within the last few years a new method called *cone-beam computed tomography (CBCT)* has been introduced that may prove to be more efficient and economical than either conventional tomography or CT for oral diagnostics.

CBCT uses a round or rectangular cone-shaped x-ray beam centered on a two-dimensional x-ray sensor to scan a 360-degree rotation about the patient's head. During the scan a series of 360 exposures or projections, one for each degree of rotation, is acquired, which provides the raw digital data for reconstruction of the exposed volume by computer algorithm. Depending on the equipment, scan times range from 17 seconds to a little more than 1 minute. Multiplanar

reformatting of the primary reconstruction allows for both three-dimensional images and two-dimensional images of any selected plane to be made. The visual resolving power of these systems varies up to about 2 lp/mm, four times that of CT. Final images may be printed on a 1:1 scale with geometric accuracy reported to be 2% or less.

CBCT equipment is less expensive than CT and has been reported to be free of the labor-intensive and costly service required by CT. Additionally, the radiation dose delivered to the patient as a result of one CBCT scan may be as little as 3% to 20% that of a conventional CT scan, depending on the equipment used and the area scanned.

Two systems, the 3D Accuitomo (J. Morita, Kyoto, Japan) and the NewTom Plus (Quantitative Radiology s.r.l, Verona, Italy), are commercially available. The 3D Accuitomo acquires 8 bit images at high resolution (having a cubic voxel 0.119 mm on a side) but its reconstruction volume is limited to a cylinder 3.0 cm high and 4.0 cm in diameter. The NewTom Plus captures 12 bit images of a larger volume (24 cm high, 26 cm in diameter) but at lower spatial resolution (cubic voxel 0.22 mm on a side). As a result, the 3D Accuitomo may display images including the area of 2 to 3 teeth in high detail while the NewTom Plus may display the entire maxilla and mandible (Fig. 13-15).

Magnetic Resonance Imaging

In contrast to the techniques described above, which use x rays for acquisition of information pertaining to an object studied, magnetic resonance imaging (MRI) uses nonionizing radiation from the radiofrequency (RF) band of the electromagnetic spectrum. To produce an MR image, the patient is placed inside a large magnet, which induces a relatively strong external magnetic field. This causes the nuclei of many atoms in the body, including hydrogen, to align themselves with the magnetic field. After application of an RF signal, energy is released from the body, detected, and used to construct the MR image by computer. The high contrast sensitivity of MRI to tissue differences and the absence of radiation exposure are the reasons MRI for the most part have replaced CT for imaging soft tissue. CT remains an important technique for imaging bony tissues.

The theory of MRI is based on the magnetic properties of an atom. Atomic nuclei spin about their axes much as the earth spins about its axis. In addition, individual protons and neutrons (nucleons), which make up the nuclei of atoms, each possess a spin, or angular momentum. In nuclei in which the protons and neutrons are evenly paired, the spin of each nucleon cancels

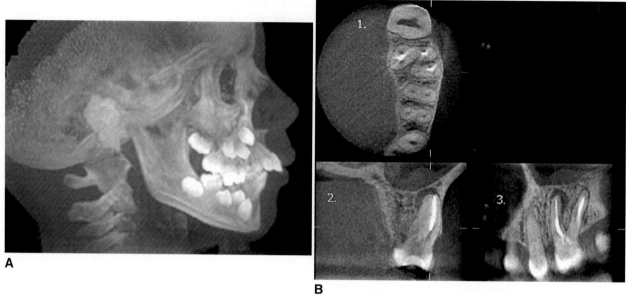

A

B

FIG. **13-15** *Cone-beam computed tomography.* Multiplanar reformatting of the primary image reconstruction allows for images of any body plane to be made. **A,** NewTom image showing lateral cephalometric view (8 bit image) with post-processing to reveal soft tissue of face, facial bones and developing dentition. **B,** 3D Accuitomo image of maxillary first molar with periapical disease at apex of mesiobuccal root, thickening of PDL at mid potion of distobuccal root and thickening of the mucoperiosteal lining of the maxillary sinus. Views 1-3 are in the axial, coronal and sagittal planes respectively. (**A** courtesy Aperio Services LLC, Sarasota, FL; **B** courtesy J. Morita USA, Inc., Irvine, CA and Dr. Edgar Hirsch.)

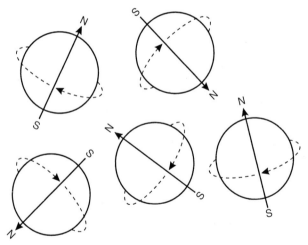

FIG. **13-16** A sample of hydrogen nuclei with net spins showing these dipoles to be randomly oriented.

that of another, producing a net spin of zero. In nuclei that contain an unpaired proton or neutron, a net spin is created. Because spin is associated with an electrical charge, a magnetic field is generated in nuclei with unpaired nucleons, causing these nuclei to act as magnets with north and south poles (magnetic dipoles).

The nucleus of the element hydrogen contains a single, unpaired proton and therefore acts as a magnetic dipole. A sample containing many hydrogen atoms would find these magnetic dipoles to be randomly oriented. This results in a total magnetization for the sample of zero (Fig. 13-16). In this natural state, if an external magnetic field is applied to the sample, all the hydrogen nuclear axes line up in the direction of the magnetic field, producing a quantity of net magnetization. However, not all north poles point in the same direction. Rather, two states are possible: *spin-up,* which parallels the external magnetic field, and *spin-down,* which is antiparallel with the field. Because more energy is required to align antiparallel with the magnetic field, those hydrogen nuclei are considered to be at a higher energy state than those aligned parallel with the field. Nuclei prefer to be in a lower energy state, and usually more are aligned parallel with the magnetic field (Fig. 13-17). Nuclei can be made to undergo transition from one energy state to another by absorbing or releasing a certain quantity of energy. Energy required for transition from the lower to the higher or from the higher to the lower energy level can be supplied or recovered in the form of electromagnetic energy in the RF portion of the electromagnetic spectrum. The tran-

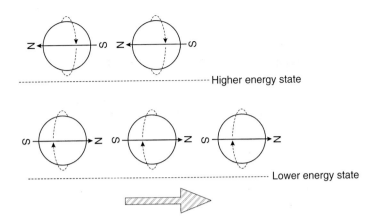

Externally applied magnetic field

FIG. **13-17** *Hydrogen nuclei in an external magnetic field.* Most nuclei are in the lower energy state and are aligned parallel with the magnetic field.

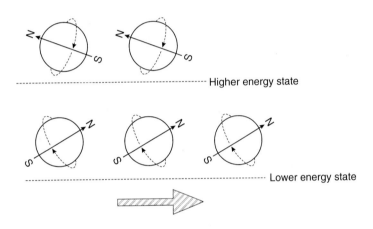

Externally applied magnetic field

FIG. **13-18** *Hydrogen nuclei in an external magnetic field.* The magnetic dipoles are not aligned exactly with the external magnetic field. Instead, the axes of spinning protons actually oscillate or wobble with a slight tilt from being absolutely parallel with the flux of the external magnet.

sition from one energy level to another is called *resonance.*

When an external magnetic field is applied to a sample of nuclei, their north and south poles do not align exactly with the direction of the magnetic field (Fig. 13-18). The axes of spinning protons actually oscillate or wobble with a slight tilt from a position absolutely parallel with the flux of the external magnet (Fig. 13-19). This tilting or wobbling, called *precession,* is similar to that of a spinning toy top, which does not spin in a perfectly upright position as it slows down, because of the effect of the earth's gravitational field. The axis of the spinning top wobbles about the direction of the local gravitational field, and the axis of the spinning

proton wobbles (or precesses) about the applied magnetic field. Because of the spin-up and spin-down states, the spinning protons precess together in the direction of their spin states, which can be visualized as two cones placed end to end (Fig. 13-20). The rate or frequency of precession is called the *resonant* or *Larmor frequency;* it depends on the species of nucleus and is proportional to the strength of the external magnetic field. The Larmor frequency of hydrogen is 42.58 MHz in a magnetic field of 1 Tesla (T). One Tesla is 10,000 times the earth's magnetic field. The magnetic field strengths used for MR imaging range from 0.1 to 4.0 T.

In summary, when nuclei are subjected to the flux of an external magnetic field, two energy states result:

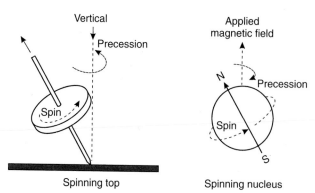

FIG. **13-19** *Precession.* The tilting or wobbling of the spinning hydrogen nuclei around the direction of the external magnetic field is called precession. The rate or frequency of precession is called the resonant or Larmor frequency. The Larmor frequency is specific for the nuclear species and depends on the strength of the external magnetic field.

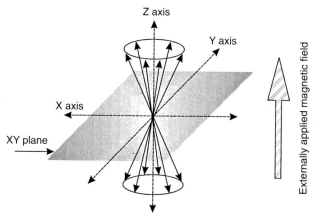

FIG. **13-20** *Spin-up and spin-down.* Because of the spin-up and spin-down states, the spinning hydrogen nuclei precess together in the direction of their spin states, which can be visualized as two cones placed end to end.

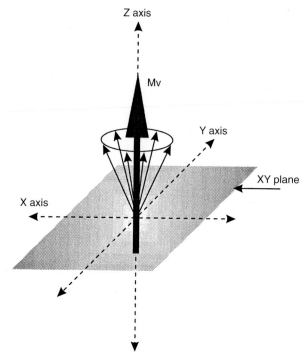

FIG. **13-21**   When hydrogen nuclei are subjected to the flux of an external magnetic field, two energy states result: spin-up, which is in the direction of the field, and spin-down, which is in the opposite direction of the field. The combined effect of these two energy states is a weak net magnetic moment, or magnetization vector (Mv), parallel with the applied magnetic field.

spin-up, which is in the direction of the field, and spin-down, which is in the opposite direction of the field. The combined effect of these two energy states is a weak net magnetic moment, or magnetization vector (Mv), parallel with the applied magnetic field (Fig. 13-21).

When energy in the form of an electromagnetic wave in the radiofrequency range from an RF antenna coil is directed to tissue with protons (hydrogen nuclei) that are aligned in the Z axis by an external static magnetic field (by the imaging magnet), the protons in the tissue that have a Larmor frequency matching that of the electromagnetic wave absorb energy and shift or rotate away from the direction induced by the imaging magnet (Fig. 13-22). The longer the RF pulse is applied, the greater the angle of rotation. If the pulse is of sufficient

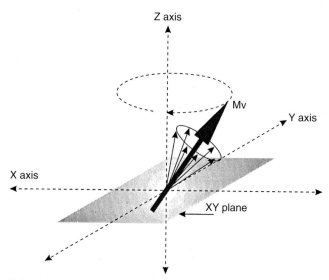

FIG. **13-22**   When energy in the form of an electromagnetic wave in the radiofrequency (RF) range from an RF antenna coil is directed to tissue with hydrogen nuclei that are aligned in the Z axis by an external static magnetic field, the protons in the tissue that have a Larmor frequency matching that of the electromagnetic wave absorb energy and shift or rotate away from the direction induced by the imaging magnet.

intensity (duration), it will rotate the net tissue magnetization vector into the transverse plane (XY plane), which is perpendicular to longitudinal alignment (Z axis), and cause all the protons to precess in phase. This is referred to as a *90-degree RF pulse* or a *flip angle of 90 degrees*. During an MR imaging sequence, many RF pulses with different intensities can be used, along with different times between repetitions of the pulse.

The net magnetization of the tissue in the transverse plane and the amount of transverse magnetization that exists at the termination of the RF pulse are equal to the amount of longitudinal magnetization that existed just before the pulse. Both are directly proportional to the strength of the static magnetic field and the number of hydrogen nuclei (protons) present in the tissue. At this precise moment, a maximal RF signal is induced in a receiver coil. The magnitude of this signal represents information about the overall concentration of hydrogen nuclei (proton density) in a sample of tissue, or about the number of hydrogen nuclei in a sample of different types of tissue. This signal depends not only on the presence or absence of hydrogen but also on the degree to which hydrogen is bound within a molecule. Tightly bound hydrogen atoms, such as those present in bone, do not align themselves with the external magnetic field and do not produce a usable signal. Loosely bound or mobile hydrogen atoms such as those present in soft tissues and liquids tilt and align to produce a detectable signal. The measure of the concentration of loosely bound hydrogen nuclei available to create the signal is referred to as the proton density or spin density of the tissue in question. The higher the concentration of these nuclei of loosely bound hydrogen atoms, the stronger the net magnetization at equilibrium and at all degrees of excitement, the more intense the recovered signal, and the lighter the MR image.

As soon as the radio waves (the resonant RF pulse) are turned off, two events occur simultaneously—the radiation of energy and the return of the nuclei to their original spin state at a lower energy. This process is called *relaxation,* and the energy loss is detected as a signal, which is called *free induction decay (FID):*

- First, the nuclei in transverse alignment begin to realign themselves with the main magnetic field (i.e., to relax), and net magnetization regrows to the original longitudinal orientation. Relaxation is accomplished by a transfer of energy from individual hydrogen nuclei (spin) to the surrounding molecules (lattice). The time constant that describes the rate at which net magnetization returns to equilibrium by this transfer of energy is called the *T1 relaxation time* or *spin-lattice relaxation time*. T1 varies with different tissues and the ability of nuclei to transfer their excess energy to their environment. A T1–weighted image

is produced by a short repetition time between RF pulses and a short signal recovery time. Because T1 is an exponential growth time constant, a tissue with a short T1 produces an intense MR signal, displayed as bright white in a T1–weighted image. A tissue with a long T1 produces a low-intensity signal and appears dark in the MR image.

- Second, the magnetic moments of adjacent hydrogen nuclei begin to interfere with one another; this causes the nuclei to dephase, with a resultant loss of transverse magnetization. The time constant that describes the rate of loss of transverse magnetization is called the *T2 relaxation time or transverse (spin-spin) relaxation time*. The transverse magnetization rapidly decays (exponentially) to zero, as do the amplitude and duration of the detected radio signal. A T2–weighted image is acquired using a long repetition time between RF pulses and a long signal recovery time. A tissue with a long T2 produces a high-intensity signal and is bright in the image. One with a short T2 produces a low-intensity signal and is dark in the image.

The FID relates signal intensity to time. A mathematical technique called the *Fourier transform* converts the relationship of signal intensity versus time to signal intensity versus resonant frequency, transforming the oscillating FID signal to a pulse of energy (current), the MR signal. When FIDs are received from a mixture of tissues, as is the case when a section of the body is examined, each volume of tissue generates a different radio signal at different frequencies. The antenna does not separate the individual signals; rather, they are summed to form a complex FID signal. The Fourier transform also separates the complex FID signal from the different tissues into its various frequency components. This procedure is coupled with reconstruction techniques similar to those used in CT to produce diagnostic images.

Image contrast among the various tissues in the body is manipulated in MRI by varying the rate at which the RF pulses are transmitted. A short repetition time (TR) of 500 msec between pulses and a short echo or signal recovery time (TE) of 20 msec produce a T1–weighted image; a long TR (2000 msec) and a long TE (80 msec) produce a T2–weighted image. For every diagnostic task, the operator must decide which imaging sequence will bring out optimal image contrast. T1–weighted images are called *fat images* because fat has the shortest T1 relaxation time and the highest signal relative to other tissues and thus appears bright in the image. High anatomic detail is possible in this type of image because of good image contrast. T1–weighted images are thus useful for depicting small anatomic regions (e.g., the TMJ), where high spatial resolution is required. T2–weighted images are called *water images* because water has the longest T2 relaxation time and thus appears bright in the image. In general, the T2 time of abnormal tissues is longer than that of normal tissues. Images with T2 weighting are most commonly used when the practitioner is looking for inflammatory or other pathologic changes. T1–weighted images are more commonly used to demonstrate anatomy. In practice, images often must be acquired with both T1 and T2 weighting to separate the several tissues by contrast resolution.

Localization of the MR image to a specific part of the body (selecting a slice) and the ability to create a three-dimensional image depend on the fact that the Larmor frequency of a nucleus is governed in part by the strength of the external magnetic field. When this strength is changed in a gradient across a body of tissue (selectively exciting the image slice), the Larmor frequency of individual nuclei or groups of nuclei (voxels) in the gradient also changes.

Three electromagnetic coils within the bore of the imaging magnet produce this magnetic gradient. The coils surround the patient and produce magnetic fields that oppose and redirect the magnetic flux in three orthogonal or right angle directions to delineate individual volumes of tissue (voxels), which are subjected to magnetic fields of unique strength. Partitioning the local magnetic fields tunes all the hydrogen protons in a particular voxel to the same resonant frequency. This is called *selective excitation*. When an RF pulse with a range of frequencies is applied, a voxel of tissue tuned to one of the frequencies is excited; when the RF radiation is terminated, the excited voxel radiates that distinctive frequency, identifying and localizing it. The bandwidth or spectrum of frequencies of the RF pulse and the magnitude of the slice-selecting gradient determine the slice thickness. Slice thickness can be reduced by increasing gradient strength or decreasing the RF bandwidth (frequency range).

MRI has several advantages over other diagnostic imaging procedures. First, it offers the best resolution of tissues of low inherent contrast. Although the x-ray attenuation coefficient may vary by no more than 1% between soft tissues, the spin density and T1 and T2 relaxation times may vary by up to 40%. Second, no ionizing radiation is involved with MRI. Third, because the region of the body imaged in MRI is controlled electronically, direct multiplanar imaging is possible without reorienting the patient. Disadvantages of MRI include relatively long imaging times and the potential hazard imposed by the presence of ferromagnetic metals in the vicinity of the imaging magnet. This latter disadvantage excludes from MRI any patient with implanted metallic foreign objects or medical devices that consist of or contain ferromagnetic metals (e.g., cardiac pacemakers, some cerebral aneurysm clips). Finally, some patients suffer from claustrophobia when positioned in a MRI machine.

Because of its excellent soft tissue contrast resolution, MRI has proved useful in a variety of circumstances (Fig. 13-23): diagnosing a suspected internal derangement of the TMJ and evaluating the treatment of that derangement after surgery; identifying and localizing orofacial soft tissue lesions; and providing images of salivary gland parenchyma.

Nuclear Medicine

Film radiography, CT, MRI, and diagnostic ultrasonography are considered morphologic imaging techniques; that is, each requires some specific structural difference or anatomic change for information to be recorded by an image receptor. In film radiography, for example, perception of an image depends on contrast, which in turn partly depends on the differential absorption of x rays. The dependence of x-ray imaging on differential absorption essentially limits this technique to a single variable (tissue electron density), which in turn is presented as a structural or anatomic difference. However, human disease can exist with no specific anatomic changes. Changes that are seen may simply be later effects of some biochemical process that remains undetected until physical symptoms develop. Radionuclide imaging (or functional imaging) provides the only means of assessing physiologic change that is a direct result of biochemical alteration (Fig. 13-24).

Radionuclide imaging is based on the radiotracer method, which assumes that radioactive atoms or molecules in an organism behave in a manner identical to that of their stable counterparts because they are chemically indistinguishable. Radiotracers allow measurement of tissue function in vivo and provide an early marker of disease through measurement of biochemical change. Radionuclide-labeled tracers are used in quantities well below amounts that are lethal to cells. However, in spite of the fact that radionuclide imaging is considered noninvasive, the radiation dose the patient receives as a result of intravenous injection of radionuclide-labeled tracers should be considered. It has been reported that injection of $3.7 \text{ X} \times 10^8 \text{Bq}$ of ^{99m}Tc-pertechnetate delivers a whole-body radiation dose of 1 mGy. This quantity is about one third the average annual effective dose resulting from natural radiation (see Chapter 3). Although many gamma-emitting isotopes have been used in radionuclide imaging, including iodine (^{131}I), gallium (^{67}Ga), and selenium (^{74}Se), the one most commonly used is technetium 99m (^{99m}Tc). As technetium pertechnetate, ^{99m}Tc mimics

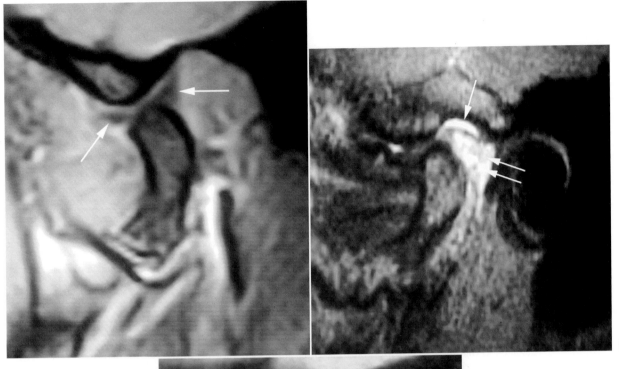

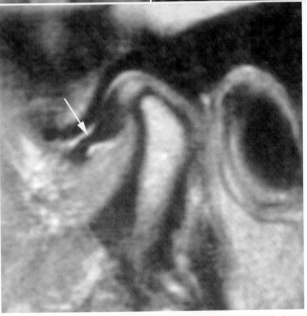

FIG. **13-23**　**A**, T1–weighted MR image of the TMJ. The MR signal depends not only on the presence or absence of hydrogen nuclei (protons) but also on the degree to which hydrogen is bound within a molecule. Tightly bound hydrogen atoms such as those in bone do not align themselves with the external magnetic field and do not produce a usable signal (the cortical outlines of the condyles appear black). In this image the jaw is partly open, as indicated by the location of the condyle relative to the articular eminence. The articular disk, which has a "bow tie" appearance *(arrows)*, is in a normal position relative to the translating condyle. **B**, T2–weighted MR image of the TMJ. Loosely bound or mobile hydrogen atoms such as those in soft tissues and liquids tilt and align, producing a detectable signal *(varying shades of gray)*. This image illustrates both inflammatory effluent in the superior joint space *(arrow)* and hyperemia caused by increased vasculature in the retrodiskal tissues *(double arrows)*. **C**, Proton or spin density MR image of the TMJ. The normal position of the posterior band of the articular disk is at the 11 to 12 o'clock position relative to the superior aspect of the condyle. In this image the disk is anteriorly displaced *(arrow)*, with the posterior band in the 9 o'clock position relative to the condylar head. **(B** and **C**, Courtesy Richard Harper, DDS, Dallas, Texas.)

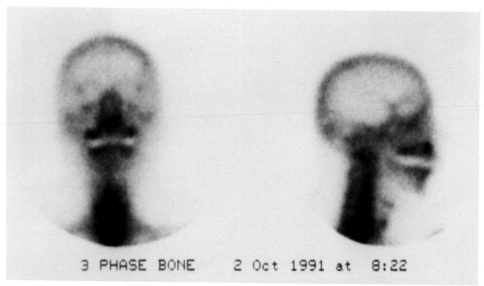

FIG. **13-24** *Radionuclide image.* The increased uptake of isotope in the region of the maxilla and mandible was attributed to an inflammatory response caused by poorly fitting complete dentures. (Courtesy Radiology Department, Baylor University Medical Center, Dallas, Tex.)

iodine distribution when injected intravenously. Additionally, when it is manipulated chemically and attached to other compounds, it can be used to perform scans of virtually every organ of the body.

The use of tracers for diagnostic imaging became possible with the development of, first, the rectilinear scanner and, later, the Anger or gamma scintillation camera. Both these instruments record the gamma emissions from patients injected with appropriate tracers. The cameras use a scintillation crystal that has the ability to fluoresce on interaction with gamma rays. This flash of light (or fluorescence) is detected by a photomultiplier tube that magnifies and amplifies the signal. The amplified signal is digitized and ultimately used to produce an image by computer algorithm. Use of a scintillation crystal for acquisition of data for image formation has led to the labeling of this technique as *scintigraphy.*

A stationary Anger camera or a rectilinear scanner is capable of producing a flat-plane image of an area or organ in question. Use of an Anger camera with the capacity to rotate 360 degrees about the patient or specialized ring detectors makes single photon emission computed tomography (SPECT) possible. In this technique, either multiple detectors or a single moving detector allows acquisition of data from a number of contiguous transaxial slices, similar to CT by x ray. These data can then be used to construct multiplanar images of the area of study.

An even more recent development than SPECT in the field of nuclear medicine is positron emission computed tomography (PET). PET, which is reported to have sensitivity nearly 100 times that of a gamma camera, relies on positron-emitting radionuclides generated in a cyclotron. After injection of the radionuclide into the patient, the isotope within the body's tissue emits a positron. This positron then interacts with a free electron and mutual annihilation occurs, resulting in the production of two 551 keV photons emitted at 180 degrees to each other. When electronically coupled opposing detectors simultaneously identify this pair of gamma photons, the annihilation event is known to have occurred along the line joining the two detectors. Raw PET scan data consist of a number of these coincidence lines, which are reorganized into projections that identify where activity is concentrated within the patient. The utility of PET is based not only on its sensitivity but also on the fact that the most commonly used radionuclides (^{11}C, ^{13}N, ^{15}O, ^{18}F) are isotopes of elements that occur naturally in organic molecules. Although fluorine does not technically fit into this category, it is a chemical substitute for hydrogen.

Ultrasonography

The phenomenon perceived as sound is the result of periodic changes in the pressure of air against the eardrum. The periodicity of these changes lies anywhere between 1500 and 20,000 cycles per second (hertz [Hz]). By definition, ultrasound has a periodicity greater than 20 kHz. Thus it is distinguished from other mechanical waveforms simply by having a vibratory frequency greater than the audible range. Diagnostic ultrasonography (sonography), the clinical application of ultrasound, uses vibratory frequencies in the range of 1 to 20 MHz.

Scanners used for sonography generate electrical impulses that are converted into ultra–high-frequency sound waves by a transducer, a device that can convert one form of energy into another—in this case, electrical energy into sonic energy. The most important component of the transducer is a thin piezoelectric crystal or material made up of a great number of dipoles arranged in a geometric pattern. A dipole may be thought of as a distorted molecule that appears to have a positive charge on one end and a negative charge on the other. Currently, the most widely used piezoelectric material is lead zirconate titanate (PZT). The electrical impulse generated by the scanner causes the dipoles in the crystal to realign themselves with the electrical field and thus suddenly change the crystal's thickness. This abrupt change begins a series of vibrations that produce the sound waves that are transmitted into the tissues being examined.

As the ultrasonic beam passes through or interacts with tissues of different acoustic impedance, it is attenuated by a combination of absorption, reflection, refraction, and diffusion. Sonic waves that are reflected back (echoed) toward the transducer cause a change in the thickness of the piezoelectric crystal, which in turn produces an electrical signal that is amplified, processed, and ultimately displayed as an image on a monitor. In this system the transducer serves as both a transmitter and a receiver. Current techniques permit echoes to be processed at a sufficiently rapid rate to allow perception of motion; this is referred to as *real-time imaging.*

In contrast to x-ray imaging, in which the image is produced by transmitted radiation, the reflected portion of the beam produces the image in sonography. The fraction of the beam that is reflected back to the transducer depends on the acoustic impedance of the tissue, which is a product of its density (and thus the velocity of sound through it) and the beam's angle of incidence. Because of its acoustic impedance, a tissue has a characteristic internal echo pattern. Consequently, not only can changes in echo patterns delineate different tissues, but they also can be correlated with pathologic changes in a tissue. Interpretation of sonograms, therefore, relies on knowledge of both the physical properties of ultrasound and the anatomy of the tissues being scanned (Figs. 13-25 and 13-26).

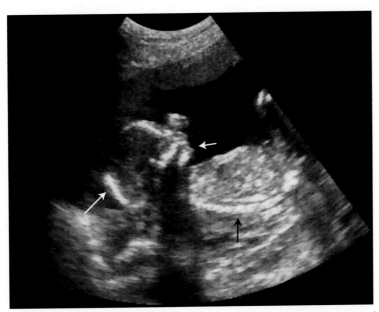

FIG. 13-25 Ultrasound image of 18-week male fetus. Fetal ultrasound is used to assess age of fetus, fetal heart beat, to screen for serious birth defects, and to assess the amount of amniotic fluid and size and position of fetus. Note normal calvarium on the left *(long arrow),* bright developing maxilla and mandible *(short arrow),* and the spinal cord below the abdomen *(black arrow)* and dark amniotic fluid above. A hand (of a future dentist?) is placed in front of the face. (Courtesy Dr. Alan Curtis, Tempe, AZ.)

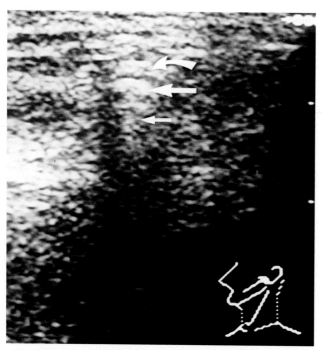

FIG. **13-26**   *Ultrasound image of the TMJ area.* Parasagittal image of the TMJ area showing the articular disk in its normal location superior to the condyle in the closed-mouth position. Glenoid fossa *(curved arrow),* articular disk *(long arrow),* and condyle *(short arrow).* (Courtesy Rüdiger Emshoff, MD, DMD, Innsbruck, Austria.)

BIBLIOGRAPHY

Bushberg JT et al: The essential physics of medical imaging, ed 2, Baltimore, 2002, Williams & Wilkins.

Curry TS et al: Christensen's physics of diagnostic radiology, ed 4, Philadelphia, 1990, Lea & Febiger.

Emshoff R et al: Ultrasonographic cross-sectional characteristics of muscles of the head and neck, Oral Surg Oral Med Oral Pathol Oral Radiol Endod 87:93-106, 1999.

Fahey FH: State of the art in emission tomography equipment, Radiographics 16:409, 1996.

Goldman LW, Fowlkes JB, editors: Categorical course in diagnostic radiology physics: CT and US cross-sectional imaging, Oak Brook, Ill, 2000, RSNA Publications.

Patton JA: MR imaging instrumentation and image artifacts, Radiographics 14:1083, 1994.

Reiderer SJ, Wood ML, editors: Categorical course in physics: the basic physics of MR imaging, Oak Brook, Ill, 1997, RSNA Publications.

CHAPTER 14

Guidelines for Prescribing Dental Radiographs

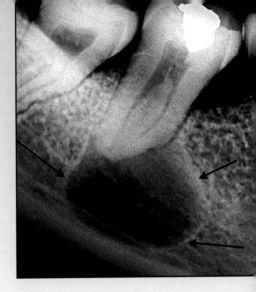

SHARON L. BROOKS ■ KATHRYN A. ATCHISON

The decision to conduct a radiographic examination should be based on the individual needs of the patient. These needs are determined by findings from the dental history and clinical examination and modified by patient age and general health. A radiographic examination is necessary when the history and clinical examination have not provided enough information for complete evaluation of a patient's condition and formulation of an appropriate treatment plan. Radiographic exposures are necessary only when, in the dentist's judgment, it is reasonably likely that the patient will benefit by the discovery of clinically useful information on the radiograph.

Role of Radiographs in Disease Detection and Monitoring

The goal of dental care is to preserve and improve patients' oral health while minimizing other health-related risks. Although the diagnostic information provided by radiographs may be of definite benefit to the patient, the radiographic examination does carry the potential for harm from exposure to ionizing radiation. One of the most effective means of reducing possible harm is to avoid making radiographs that will not contribute information pertinent to patient care. The judgment that underlies the decision to make a radiographic examination centers on several factors, including the following:

- Prevalence of the diseases that may be detected radiographically in the oral cavity
- Ability of the clinician to detect these diseases clinically and radiographically
- Consequences of undetected and untreated disease
- Impact of asymptomatic anatomic and pathologic variations detected radiographically on patient treatment.

As a general principle, radiographs are indicated when a reasonable probability exists that they will provide valuable information about a disease that is not evident clinically. Conversely, radiographs are not indicated when they are unlikely to yield information contributing to patient care. Radiographic information considered clinically useful includes data that are valuable in detecting disease and in monitoring the progression of known diseases.

For many clinical situations it is not readily apparent to the practitioner whether radiographs have a reasonable probability of providing valuable information. In these situations it is up to the practitioner's clinical judgment after weighing the patient factors to decide whether radiographs are indicated.

The philosophy of taking radiographs only when there is a high probability of obtaining clinically useful information has been advocated by all the organizations responsible for developing or endorsing guidelines for ordering radiographs. However, many dentists use radiographs as a screening tool, simply to see "what's there," without having a specific suspicion of disease arising from the dental history or clinical examination. There are probably a number of reasons for doing this. Some dentists feel that they have not provided an adequate service to their patients if they cannot assure them that they have searched diligently for disease with all reasonable diagnostic methods, including radiographs. They may state that having complete information, whether it affects the treatment plan or not, is of such benefit that it outweighs the risk of the radiation exposure. Other dentists raise medicolegal issues, stating fear of lawsuits if they fail to detect disease. Others express concern about the effect on the efficiency of the dental office of the extended examinations required for prescribing radiographs based on signs and symptoms.

The next few paragraphs will address these concerns.

Unlike their use in dentistry, screening radiographs are rarely used in medicine, with the exception of mammography for women above a certain age or with increased risk factors for breast cancer, and there is controversy over whether even this type of examination should be used as frequently as it is today. Breast cancer is a relatively common, yet serious disease that should be detected early, before the cancer becomes large enough to be found clinically. On the other hand, diseases of the jaws (with the exceptions of caries, periapical and periodontal disease) are rare and concentrated in certain ages, genders, and ethnicities. These diseases are unlikely to be discovered on routine screening radiographs before they have produced signs or symptoms that could be found on a thorough clinical examination and history. Periodontal disease can be diagnosed clinically, although radiographs are used to determine the extent of bone loss and presence of other factors that may affect prognosis. Periapical disease is usually associated with extensive restorations or caries that can be detected clinically. Dental caries on proximal surfaces, however, may not be detectable on clinical examination until it has reached an advanced stage; thus this is one occult disease for which screening radiographs are considered appropriate. Regarding the threat of lawsuits for failure to diagnose, dentists who follow guidelines on radiographs developed and/or endorsed by authoritative bodies that help establish the standard of care should have no concerns. While lawsuits can be filed for many reasons, it is unlikely that they will be successful if it can be shown that the practitioner did a *thorough* clinical examination and history and carefully considered the guidelines when determining whether to order radiographs.

Some dentists set up their practices such that new patients are automatically seen first by the dental hygienist, who takes a predetermined set of radiographs at the first appointment, before the dentist sees the patient. Although this may make efficient use of the dentist's time, it is contrary to the recommendations of the American Dental Association (ADA) that the selection of radiographs should be based on the findings of the clinical examination. Performing a thorough examination before radiographs are ordered should not be an insurmountable obstacle for an efficient dental practice.

Regarding the issue of cost versus benefit of radiographs, for any individual patient there is little risk of harm from a set of radiographs, even if no important diagnostic information is revealed. However, there is a large societal cost, both in terms of health-care dollars and radiation risk, if millions of dental patients receive unproductive radiographic examinations, as would happen if routine screening were widespread.

The philosophy of the authors of this chapter is that radiographs should be based on the need for diagnostic information for patients on a case-by-case basis. For that reason, the next section will discuss some of the clinical situations that may call for a radiographic examination.

CARIES

Dental caries is the most common dental disease, affecting people of all ages. Although the caries prevalence rates of developed countries have been decreasing since the 1970s, probably partially as a result of the widespread use of fluoride, increasing numbers of older adults are maintaining their teeth throughout their lifetime, leaving them at risk for developing both coronal and root caries. Although occlusal, buccal, and lingual carious lesions are reasonably easy to detect clinically, interproximal caries and caries associated with existing restorations are much more difficult to detect with only a clinical examination (see Chapter 16). Studies have repeatedly demonstrated that clinicians using radiographs detect caries not evident clinically, both in enamel and in dentin. Although a radiographic examination is very important for diagnosis of dental caries, the optimal frequency for such an examination should be based on such mitigating features such as the patient's age, medical condition, diet, oral hygiene practices, oral health status, and the nature of the caries process itself.

Carious lesions demonstrate one of three behaviors: progression, arrest, or regression. Only about 50% of lesions progress beyond the initial, just-detectable defect, and in most instances the lesions demonstrate a slow rate of progression through enamel (months to years). Mechanisms are also in use to enhance remineralization of early enamel lesions. However, the rate of caries progression is significantly faster in deciduous than in permanent enamel, and patients vary widely in their rates of formation of caries and in their rates of caries progression.

Because the presence of caries cannot be determined with confidence by clinical examination alone, it is necessary to expose patients periodically through bitewing radiography to monitor dental caries. The length of the exposure intervals varies considerably because of different patient circumstances. For most patients in good physical health with adequate oral hygiene, an infrequent radiographic examination is needed to monitor dental caries. However, if the patient history and clinical examination suggest that the individual has a relatively high caries experience, shorter intervals allow careful monitoring of disease.

PERIODONTAL DISEASES

Some form of periodontal disease affects most people at some point during their life, gingivitis more often in younger individuals and periodontitis more commonly in older adults. Periodontal diseases are responsible for a substantial portion of all teeth lost. A consensus exists among practitioners that radiographic examinations play an important role in the evaluation of patients with periodontal disease after the disease is initially detected on clinical examination (see Chapter 17). In addition to providing a picture of the extent of alveolar bone support for the dentition, radiographic examinations help demonstrate local factors that complicate the disease, including the presence of gingival irritants such as calculus and faulty restorations. Occasionally the length and morphology of roots, visible on periapical radiographs, are crucial factors in the prognosis of the disease. These observations suggest that when clinical evidence exists of periodontal disease, other than nonspecific gingivitis, it is appropriate to make radiographs, generally a combination of periapicals and bitewings, to help establish the severity of the disease. Follow-up radiographs after therapy is complete will help the clinician monitor the progression of disease and determine whether the destruction of alveolar bone has been halted.

DENTAL ANOMALIES

Abnormal formation of teeth may be manifested as deviations in number, size, and composition. These abnormalities in dental development occur more frequently, and are more likely to have a serious impact, in the permanent dentition than in the primary. The most frequently encountered anomalies are the presence of supernumerary teeth, usually mesiodens, or developmentally absent teeth, usually second premolars (see Chapter 18).

Few anomalies exist for which orthodontic treatment or surgical correction or modification must start at an early age. When the dentist suspects an abnormality requiring treatment, radiographs to confirm and localize it are not required until the time when the treatment is most appropriate. For example, a panoramic examination of a 5-year-old child to determine the presence or absence of permanent teeth may be ill-timed. Even though the examination provides evidence that one or more second premolars or lateral incisors are developmentally missing, this information usually does not influence the current treatment plan. When examination for dental anomalies is appropriate, consider both the radiation dose and anticipated diagnostic benefit. Select the projections that best demonstrate the required diagnostic information. A panoramic radiograph of the lower face is usually best for observing the presence or absence of teeth in all quadrants, although a periapical film or an occlusal film is sufficient for an examination limited to one area.

GROWTH AND DEVELOPMENT AND DENTAL MALOCCLUSION

Children and adolescents are often examined to assess the growth and development of the teeth and jaws. This assessment considers the relationship of one jaw to the other and to the soft tissues. An examination of occlusion, growth, and development requires an individualized radiographic examination that may include periapicals or a panoramic examination to supplement any radiographs ordered to assess dental disease. In addition, a patient of any age group who is being considered for orthodontic treatment may need other radiographs, such as a lateral or frontal cephalograph, occlusal view, carpal index, or temporomandibular joint (TMJ) radiograph, depending on the clinical findings (Fig. 14-1).

The dentist who is the primary provider of orthodontic treatment should select the number and type of radiographs needed. The needs of each patient should be considered individually. Selected radiographs should allow a maximal diagnostic yield with a minimal radiographic exposure after consideration of the clinical examination, the study of plaster models and photographs, and the optimal time to initiate treatment.

OCCULT DISEASE

Occult disease refers to disease that presents no clinical signs or symptoms. Occult diseases in the jaws include

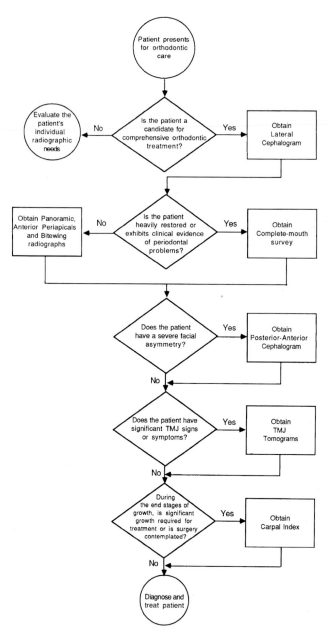

FIG. **14-1**   An example of a clinical algorithm to order radiographs for orthodontic patients. Selected radiographs are ordered after the dentist's consideration of the patient's history and clinical characteristics.

a combination of dental and intraosseous findings. Dental findings may include incipient carious lesions, resorbed or dilacerated roots, and hypercementosis. Intraosseous findings include osteosclerosis, unerupted teeth, periapical disease, and a wide variety of cysts and benign and malignant tumors (see Chapters 19-24). Small carious lesions, resorption of root structure, and bony lesions may go unnoticed until signs and symptoms develop.

Although the consequences of some occult diseases may be quite serious, most serious diseases are rare.

Often a historic or clinical sign or symptom of intraosseous disease suggests its presence. For instance, an unusual contour of bone or an absent third molar, not explained by a history of extraction, suggests the possibility of an impaction with the potential for an associated dentigerous cyst. Although patient history and clinical signs and symptoms do not always accurately predict the finding of dental and intraosseous findings, the majority of these true occult diseases are not clinically relevant or they are so rare that, except for caries as described previously, one need not obtain a radiographic examination of the jaws solely to screen for them in dentate individuals in the absence of unusual clinical signs or symptoms. Caries is an exception because of its much higher prevalence than other occult diseases.

There is considerable difference of opinion on whether asymptomatic edentulous patients presenting for routine denture construction should have screening radiographs taken to look for occult disease. Several studies have demonstrated a relatively large number of lesions on radiographs of edentulous patients, including retained root tips and areas of sclerotic bone, but almost all of these findings required no treatment and did not affect outcome of care. For that reason, some recommend no radiographs of edentulous patients if the clinical examination is negative for signs and symptoms of disease. Others still believe that screening radiographs of these patients are of value.

There has been increasing interest in the last few years in using panoramic radiographs to screen patients for the presence of calcified atheromas in the bifurcation of the carotid artery, a finding which indicates an increased risk for the development of a cerebrovascular accident (stroke). The general consensus at this time is that panoramic radiographs made for dental purposes should be evaluated for this calcification, particularly in patients over age 55, but that these radiographs should not be made simply to screen for atheromas without other dental indications. (See Chapter 27 for more details.)

JAW PATHOLOGY

Imaging of known jaw lesions, such as fibroosseous diseases or neoplastic diseases, before biopsy and definitive treatment is also important for appropriate management of the patient. For small lesions of the jaws, periapical and/or panoramic radiographs may be enough as long as the lesion can be seen in its entirety. If clinical evidence of swelling exists, some type of radiograph at 90 degrees to the original plane should be made to determine whether there is expansion of the jaw or perforation of the buccal or lingual cortical bone. If lesions are too large to fit on standard dental films, extend into the maxillary sinus or other portions of the head outside the jaws, or are suspected of malignancy, additional imaging such as computed tomography (CT) is appropriate before biopsy (see Chapter 13). This type of imaging can define the extent of the lesion, suggest an operative approach, and provide information about the nature of the lesion. The person performing the biopsy or managing the patient should order the advanced images to decrease confusion and increase coordination of care.

TEMPOROMANDIBULAR JOINT

Many types of diseases affect the TMJ, including congenital and developmental malformations of the mandible and cranial bones; acquired disorders such as disk displacement, neoplasms, fractures, and dislocations; inflammatory diseases that produce capsulitis or synovitis; and arthritides of various types, including rheumatoid and osteoarthritis. The goal of TMJ imaging, similar to that for imaging other body parts, should be to obtain new information that will influence patient care. Radiologic examination may not be needed for all patients with signs and symptoms referable to the TMJ region, particularly if no treatment is contemplated (see Chapter 25). The decision of whether and how to image the joints should depend on the results of the history and clinical findings, the clinical diagnosis, and results of prior examinations, as well as the tentative treatment plan and expected outcome.

The cost of the examination and the radiation dose should also influence the decision if more than one type of examination can provide the desired information. For example, information about the status of the osseous tissues can be obtained from panoramic radiographs, plain films, conventional tomography, CT, and magnetic resonance imaging (MRI). The subtlety of the expected findings and the amount of detail required should be considered when selecting the examination to perform. If soft tissue information such as disk position is necessary for patient care, MRI or arthrography is appropriate.

IMPLANTS

An increasingly common method of replacing missing teeth is with osseointegrated implants, metal screws that are inserted into the mandible or maxilla. Prosthetic appliances are then affixed to the screws after a period of healing. Preoperative planning is crucial to ensure success of the implants. The dentist must evaluate the adequacy of the height and thickness of bone for the desired implant; the quality of the bone, including the relative proportion of medullary and cortical bone; the location of anatomic structures such as the mandibular canal or maxillary sinus; and the presence of structural abnormalities such as undercuts that may affect placement or angulation of the implant (see Chapter 31).

Standard periapical and panoramic radiographs can supply information regarding the vertical dimensions of the bone in the proposed implant site. However, some type of cross-sectional imaging, either conventional tomography or CT, is recommended before implant placement for visualization of important anatomic landmarks, determination of size and path of insertion of implant, and evaluation of the adequacy of the bone for anchorage of the implant. Postoperative evaluation of implants may be needed at later times to judge healing, assess complete seating of fixtures, and ensure continued health of the surrounding bone.

PARANASAL SINUSES

Because dentists are not usually the primary providers of treatment for acute or chronic sinus disease, the necessity to perform sinus imaging may be limited in general dental practice. However, because sinus disease can present as pain in the maxillary teeth and because periapical inflammation of maxillary molars and premolars can also lead to changes in the mucosa of the maxillary sinus, circumstances occur in which the dentist needs to obtain an image of the maxillary sinus. Periapical and panoramic radiographs demonstrate the floor of the maxillary sinus well, but visualization of other walls requires additional imaging techniques such as occipitomental (Waters) view or CT. These radiographs are best ordered by the person treating the patient so that diagnostic and therapeutic measures may be coordinated (see Chapter 26).

TRAUMA

Patients who experience trauma to the oral region may visit a dentist for evaluation and management of the injuries. For proper management it is important to determine the full extent of the injuries. Periapical and/or panoramic radiographs are helpful for evaluation of fractures of the teeth. If a suspected root fracture is not visible on a periapical radiograph, a second radiograph made with a different angulation may be helpful. A fracture that is not perpendicular to the beam may not be detectable unless root resorption is present. Thus a tooth with a history of trauma should be monitored and evaluated radiographically on a periodic basis, even if the original radiograph is negative.

Fractures of the mandible can frequently be detected with panoramic radiographs, supplemented by images at 90 degrees such as a posteroanterior or reverse-Towne view (see Chapter 28). Trauma to the maxilla and midface may require CT for a thorough evaluation. Affected patients are more likely to report to a hospital emergency department than to a general dental office. The hospital may have a standard protocol for trauma cases. Ideally the clinician responsible for managing care determines the appropriate radiographs for the specific case.

Radiographic Examinations

After concluding that a patient requires a radiograph, the dentist should consider which radiographic examination is most appropriate to meet all the patient's diagnostic and treatment planning needs. A variety of radiographic projections is available. In choosing one, the dentist should consider the anatomic relationships, the size of the field, and the radiation dose from each view. Table 14-1 summarizes the more common types of radiographic examinations for general dental patients and factors to consider in choosing the most appropriate one. For example, a panoramic radiograph provides broad area coverage with moderate resolution. Intraoral films give more detailed information but a signifi-

cantly higher radiation dose per unit area exposed. The clinician must use clinical judgment to weigh these factors. Examples of all these radiographs can be found in previous chapters.

INTRAORAL RADIOGRAPHS

Intraoral radiographs are examinations made by placing the x-ray film within the patient's mouth during the exposure. These exposures offer the dentist a high-detail view of the teeth and bone in the area exposed. Such views are most appropriate for revealing caries and periodontal and periapical disease in a localized region. A complete-mouth or full-mouth examination (FMX) consists of periapical views of all the tooth-bearing regions as well as interproximal views (see Chapter 8).

Periapical Radiographs
Periapical views show all of a tooth and the surrounding bone and are very useful for revealing caries and periodontal and periapical disease. These views may be made of a specific tooth or region or as part of a FMX.

TABLE 14-1
Common Dental Radiographic Examinations and Their Properties

TYPE OF EXAMINATION	COVERAGE	RESOLUTION	RELATIVE EXPOSURE*	DETECTABLE DISEASE
Intraoral Radiographs				
Periapical	Limited	High	1	Caries, periodontal disease, occult disease
Bitewings	Limited	High	10	Caries, periodontal bone level
Full-mouth periapical	Limited	High	14-17	Caries, periodontal disease, dental anomalies, occult disease
Occlusal	Moderate	High	2.5	Dental anomalies, occult disease, salivary stones, expansion of jaw
Extraoral Radiographs				
Panoramic	Broad	Moderate	1-2	Dental anomalies, occult disease, extensive caries, periodontal disease, periapical disease, TMJ
Conventional tomography/slice	Moderate	Moderate	0.2-0.6	TMJ, implant site assessment
CT/head	Broad	High	25-800	Extent of craniofacial pathology, fracture, implants
MRI	Broad	Moderate	—	Soft tissue disease, TMJ
Skull	Broad	Moderate	30	Fracture, anatomic relation, jaw pathology

*The parameters assume use of F-speed film and rectangular collimation for periapical films, round collimation for bitewings and occlusal views, and rare-earth screens for panoramic examinations. With D-speed film the intraoral values are more than doubled compared with F-speed film, and with round collimation the periapical values increase by 2.5 times compared with rectangular collimation. Frederiksen N, Benson B, Sokolowski T: Effective dose and risk assessment from computed tomography of the maxillofacial complex, Dentomaxillofac Radiol 24:55, 1995; Scaf G et al: Dosimetry and cost of imaging osseointegrated implants with film-based and computed tomography, Oral Surg Oral Med Oral Pathol Oral Radiol and Endod 83:41, 1997; White SC: 1992 assessment of radiation risks from dental radiology, Dentomaxillofac Radiol 21:118, 1992.

Interproximal Radiographs

Interproximal views (bitewings) show the coronal aspects of both the maxillary and mandibular dentition in a region, as well as the surrounding crestal bone. These views are most useful for revealing proximal caries and evaluating the height of the alveolar bony crest. They can be made in either the anterior or posterior region of the mouth.

Occlusal Radiographs

Occlusal views are intraoral radiographs in which the film is positioned in the occlusal plane. They are often used in lieu of periapical views in children because the small size of the patient's mouth limits film placement. In adults, occlusal radiographs may supplement periapical views, providing visualization of a greater area of teeth and bone. They are useful for demonstrating impacted or abnormally placed maxillary anterior teeth or visualizing the region of a palatal cleft. Occlusal views may also demonstrate buccal or lingual expansion of bone or presence of a sialolith in the submandibular duct.

EXTRAORAL RADIOGRAPHS

Extraoral radiographs are examinations made of the orofacial region using films located outside the mouth. The relationships among patient position, film location, and beam direction vary, depending on the specific radiographic information desired. The standard technique for making several extraoral radiographs is discussed in Chapter 11. Only the panoramic radiograph is described here, because it has common use as a radiographic examination for general dental patients.

Panoramic Radiographs

Panoramic radiographs provide a broad view of the jaws, teeth, maxillary sinuses, nasal fossa, and TMJs (see Chapter 10). They show which teeth are present, their relative state of development, presence or absence of dental abnormalities, and many traumatic and pathologic lesions in bone. Panoramic radiographs are the technique of choice for initial examinations of edentulous patients. Because this system is an extraoral technique and uses intensifying screens, the resolution of the images is less than with the intraoral nonscreen films (see Chapter 4). Panoramic radiographs are also susceptible to artifacts from improper patient positioning that negatively affect the image. Consequently this system is generally considered inadequate for independent diagnosis of caries, root abnormalities, and periapical changes.

In the great majority of dental patients, oral disease involving the teeth or jawbones lies within the area imaged by periapical radiographs. Therefore, when a full-mouth set of radiographs is available, a panoramic examination is usually redundant because it does not add information that alters the treatment plan. However, situations may exist in which a panoramic radiograph may be preferred over a periapical examination, such as for a patient with unerupted third molars that are to be surgically removed. Panoramic views are most useful when the required field of view is large but the need for high resolution is of less importance. Although the selection of a radiographic examination should be based on the extent of the expected information it is likely to provide, the relatively low dose of radiation from the panoramic examination should also be a qualifying factor.

Advanced Imaging Procedures

A variety of advanced imaging procedures such as CT, MRI, ultrasonography, and nuclear medicine scans may be required in specific diagnostic situations. These techniques are discussed in Chapter 13, although in general the dentist refers the patient to a hospital or other imaging center for these procedures, rather than performing them in the dental office.

Guidelines for Ordering Radiographs

The dental profession has issued guidelines recommending which radiographs to make and how often to repeat them:
- Make radiographs only after a clinical examination.
- Order only those radiographs that directly benefit the patient in terms of diagnosis or treatment plan.
- Use the least amount of radiation exposure necessary to generate an acceptable view of the imaged area.

PREVIOUS RADIOGRAPHS

Most patients have been seen previously by a dentist and have already had radiographs made. These radiographs are helpful regardless of when they were exposed. If they are relatively recent, they may be adequate to the diagnostic problem at hand. Even if they were made so long ago that they are not likely to reflect the current status of the patient, they may still prove useful. These previous radiographs may demonstrate whether a condition has worsened, has remained unchanged, or has shown healing, such as in the progression of caries or periodontal disease.

ADMINISTRATIVE RADIOGRAPHS

Administrative radiographs are those made for reasons other than diagnosis, including those made for an insurance company or for an examining board. The authors believe that it is appropriate to expose patients only when it benefits their health care. Most administrative radiographs do not serve such an objective. Unfortunately, this recommendation is often not adhered to in practice, and dentists are left to sort out the most appropriate criteria to use in their practices.

Use of Guidelines to Order Dental Radiographs

At any time patients generally have a combination of diseases that the clinician must consider. Therefore guidelines specify not only which examinations to order but also which specific patient factors influence the number and type of x-ray films to order.

A panel of individuals was convened in the mid-1980s at the request of a branch of the Food and Drug Administration (FDA) to develop a set of guidelines (Table 14-2) for the making of dental radiographs. The panel addressed the topic of appropriate radiographs for an adequate evaluation of a new or recall asymptomatic patient seeking general dental care. The guidelines describe circumstances (patient age, medical and dental history, and physical signs) that suggest the need for radiographs. These circumstances are called *selection criteria*. The guidelines also suggest the types of radiographic examinations most likely to benefit the patient in terms of yielding diagnostic information. They recommend that radiographs not be made unless some expectation exists that they will provide evidence of diseases that will affect the treatment plan. The American Dental Association recommends use of the guidelines.

The guidelines that were developed by the FDA panel in the 1980s form the basis of the recommendations in this chapter. However, over the years some criticisms have arisen of certain portions of the guidelines, and recently interest has been expressed in revisiting, and perhaps revising, the document. Although some changes may be made in specific recommendations, it is unlikely that the basic principles underlying the guidelines will be altered. Therefore, the concepts should still be considered valid.

Central to the guidelines is the idea that dentists should expose patients to radiation only when they reasonably expect that the resulting radiograph will benefit patient care. Accordingly, two situations mandate a radiograph: some clinical evidence of an abnormality that requires further evaluation for a complete assessment or a high probability of disease that warrants a screening examination.

Selection criteria for radiographs are those signs or symptoms found in the patient history or clinical examination that suggest that a radiographic examination will yield clinically useful information. A key concept in the use of selection criteria is recognition of the need to consider each patient individually. Prescription of radiographs should be decided on an individual basis according to the patient's demonstrated need.

The guidelines include a description of clinical situations in which radiographs are likely to contribute to the diagnosis, treatment, or prognosis. Two examples highlight the differences between ordering radiographs for dental diseases with clinical signs and symptoms and dental diseases with no clinical indicators but high prevalences. In the first case, consider a patient with a hard swelling in the premolar region of the mandible with expansion of the buccal and lingual cortical plates. The clinical sign of swelling alerts the dentist to the need for a radiograph to determine the nature of the abnormality causing the swelling.

An example of the second situation is the patient who comes seeking general dental care after having not seen a dentist for many years. Even without clinical evidence of caries, bitewings are indicated because of the prevalence of dental caries in the population. Because this patient has not had interproximal radiographs for many years, it is reasonable to assume that the patient may benefit from the radiograph by the detection of interproximal caries. Although no clinical signs exist that predict the presence of caries, the dentist relies on clinical knowledge of the prevalence of caries to decide that this radiograph has a reasonable probability of finding disease.

Without some specific indication, it is inappropriate to expose the patient "just to see if there is something there." The major exception to this rule is the use of interproximal films for caries, in which no clinical signs exist of early lesions. The probability of finding occult disease in a patient with all permanent teeth erupted and no clinical or historic evidence of abnormality or risk factors is so low that making a periapical radiographic survey just to look for such disease is not indicated.

PATIENT EXAMINATION

The ordering of radiographs requires a reasonable expectation that they will provide information that will contribute to solving the diagnostic problem at hand. Accordingly, the first step is a careful examination of the patient, including transillumination of the anterior teeth to evaluate for interproximal decay. The clinical examination provides indications as to the nature and extent of the radiographic examination appropriate to the situation.

A team of dentists tested the ability of the ADA guidelines to reduce the number of intraoral radiographs while still offering adequate diagnostic information. This testing of the use of selection criteria demonstrated that a small but significant number of radiographic findings was not 100% covered in the anterior region if only posterior interproximal and selected periapical radiographs were used. The testing suggested that anterior interproximal radiographs or anterior periapicals are also indicated to detect interproximal caries and periodontal disease in the anterior region, specifically for patients with high levels of dental disease. A panoramic radiograph could be made in place of the periapical radiographs to supplement the posterior bitewings if the totality of the disease expected indicates a broad area of coverage and fine detail is not required.

In the guidelines patients are classified by stage of dental development, by whether they are being evaluated for the first time (without previous documentation) or being reevaluated during a recall visit, and by an estimate of their risk for having dental caries or periodontal disease. A footnote to Table 14-2 also outlines some other clinical findings that indicate when radiographs are likely to contribute to a complete description of the asymptomatic patient.

Applying these guidelines to the specific circumstances with each patient requires clinical judgment and an amalgamation of knowledge, experience, and concern. Clinical judgment is also required to recognize situations that are *not* described by the guidelines but in which patients will need radiographs nonetheless.

Initial Visit

The guidelines recommend that a child with primary dentition who is cooperative and has closed posterior contacts have only interproximal radiographs to examine for caries. Additional periapical views are recommended only in the case of clinically evident diseases and/or specific historic or clinical indications such as those listed at the footnote of Table 14-2. If the molar contacts are not closed, interproximal radiographs are not necessary because the proximal surfaces may be examined directly.

The guidelines recommend radiographic coverage of all tooth-bearing areas for a child with transitional dentition (after eruption of the first permanent tooth, 6 to 8 years of age). This usually consists of bitewings supplemented with either periapical or occlusal views (8 to 12 exposures) or a panoramic view. At this stage of development a panoramic projection is usually the view of choice because it offers the most general information with the lowest dose of ionizing radiation. Some clinicians express concern that complete coverage of all tooth-bearing areas is not warranted without a specific indication.

The guidelines group adolescents and dentate adults together to identify the kind and extent of appropriate radiographic examination. The guidelines recommend that these patients receive an individualized examination consisting of interproximal views and periapical views selected on the basis of specific historical or clinical indications. The presence of generalized dental disease often indicates the need for a full-mouth examination. Alternatively, the presence of only a few localized abnormalities or diseases suggests that a more limited examination consisting of interproximal and selected periapical views may suffice. In circumstances with no evidence of current or past dental disease, only interproximal views may be necessary for caries examination.

For the edentulous patient it may be appropriate to obtain a radiographic examination of all the tooth-bearing areas, either by periapical or panoramic radiographs. However, as discussed above, there is no consensus on this recommendation. If available, the panoramic projection usually provides the required information at a reduced radiation dose.

Recall Visit

Patients who are returning after initial care require careful examination before determining the need for radiographs. As at the initial examination, obtain selected periapical views if any of the historical or clinical signs or symptoms listed in the footnote to Table 14-2 are present and need further evaluation.

The guidelines recommend interproximal radiographs for recall patients to detect interproximal caries and monitor the status of alveolar bone loss. The optimal frequency for these views depends on the age of the patient and the probability of finding either of these two diseases. If the patient has clinically demonstrable caries or the presence of high-risk factors for caries (poor diet, poor oral hygiene, and those listed in the footnote to Table 14-2), then bitewings are exposed at fairly frequent intervals. Obtain bitewings for children at 6-month intervals until no carious lesions are clinically evident. For the adolescent at high risk for caries, the guidelines recommend bitewings at 6- to 12-month intervals; for the high-risk adult, at 12- to 18-month intervals. The recommended intervals are longer for individuals not at high risk for caries: 12 to

TABLE 14-2
Guidelines for Prescribing Dental Radiographs*

The recommendations in this table are subject to clinical judgment and may not apply to every patient. They are to be used by dentists only after reviewing the patient's health history and completing a clinical examination. They do not need to be altered because of pregnancy.

	CHILD	
	PRIMARY DENTITION (BEFORE ERUPTION OF FIRST PERMANENT MOLAR)	TRANSITIONAL DENTITION (AFTER ERUPTION OF FIRST PERMANENT MOLAR)
New Patient		
All new patients to assess dental diseases and growth and development	Posterior bitewing examination if proximal surfaces of primary teeth cannot be visualized or probed	Individualized radiographic examination consisting of periapical and/or occlusal views and posterior bitewings or panoramic examination and posterior bitewings
Recall Patient		
Clinical caries or high-risk factors for caries†	Posterior bitewing examination at 6-month intervals or until no carious lesions are evident	
No clinical caries and no high-risk factors for caries	Posterior bitewing examination at 12- to 24-month intervals if proximal surfaces of primary teeth cannot be visualized or probed	Posterior bitewing examination at 12- to 24-month intervals
Periodontal disease or history of periodontal treatment	Individualized radiographic examination consisting of selected periapical and/or bitewing radiographs for areas where periodontal disease (other than nonspecific gingivitis) can be demonstrated clinically	
Growth and development assessment	Usually not indicated	Individualized radiographic examination consisting of a periapical and/or occlusal or panoramic examination

*Clinical situations for which radiographs may be indicated include the following:

Positive historical findings:
1. Previous periodontal or endodontic therapy
2. History of pain or trauma
3. Familial history of dental anomalies
4. Postoperative evaluation of healing
5. Presence of implants

Positive clinical signs or symptoms:
1. Clinical evidence of periodontal disease
2. Large or deep restorations
3. Deep carious lesions
4. Malposed or clinically impacted teeth
5. Swelling
6. Evidence of facial trauma
7. Mobility of teeth
8. Fistula or sinus tract infection

9. Clinically suspected sinus pathology
10. Growth abnormalities
11. Oral involvement in known or suspected systemic disease
12. Positive neurologic findings in the head and neck
13. Evidence of foreign objects
14. Pain and/or dysfunction of the TMJ
15. Facial asymmetry

---

24 months for the child, 18 to 36 months for the adolescent, and 24 to 36 months for the adult. Note that individuals can change their risk category, going from high to low risk or the reverse. Similarly, patients with a history or clinical evidence of periodontal disease more serious than nonspecific gingivitis should have a combination of periapical and interproximal radiographs to allow appropriate monitoring at intervals dependent on the clinical findings.

A radiographic examination may be required in a number of other situations, such as for patients contemplating orthodontic treatment or patients with intraosseous lesions. The goal should be to obtain the necessary diagnostic information with the minimal radiation dose and financial cost, which can be substantial for advanced imaging procedures such as MRI. The dentist should determine specifically what type of information is needed and the most appropriate technique

for obtaining it. An example of a clinical algorithm for ordering radiographs before orthodontic treatment is shown in Fig. 14-1, using guidelines endorsed by the American Academy of Orthodontics. Because guidelines for ordering radiographs for other situations are not as well developed, the dentist must rely on clinical judgment.

SPECIAL CONSIDERATIONS

Pregnancy
Occasionally it is desirable to obtain radiographs of a woman who is pregnant. The x-ray beam is largely confined to the head and neck region in dental x-ray examinations; thus the fetal exposure is only about 1 μGy for a full-mouth examination. This exposure is quite small compared with that received normally from natural background sources. Accordingly, apply the guidelines

ADOLESCENT	ADULT	
PERMANENT DENTITION (BEFORE ERUPTION OF THIRD MOLARS)	**DENTULOUS**	**EDENTULOUS**
Individualized radiographic examination consisting of posterior bitewings and selected periapicals; a full-mouth intraoral radiographic examination is appropriate when patient presents with clinical evidence of generalized dental disease or a history of extensive dental treatment*	Full-mouth intraoral radiographic examination or panoramic examination	
Posterior bitewing examination at 6- to 12-month intervals or until no carious lesions are evident	Posterior bitewing examination at 12- to 18-month intervals	Not applicable
Posterior bitewing examination at 18- to 36-month intervals	Posterior bitewing examination at 24- to 36-month intervals	Not applicable
Individualized radiographic examination consisting of selected periapical and/or bitewing radiographs for areas where periodontal disease (other than nonspecific gingivitis) can be demonstrated clinically		Not applicable
Periapical or panoramic examination to assess developing third molars	Usually not indicated	Usually not indicated

16. Abutment for fixed or removable partial prosthesis
17. Unexplained bleeding
18. Unexplained sensitivity of teeth
19. Unusual eruption, spacing, or migration of teeth
20. Unusual tooth morphology, calcification, or color
21. Missing teeth with unknown reason

†Patients at high risk for caries may demonstrate any of the following

1. High level of caries experience
2. History of recurrent caries
3. Existing restorations of poor quality
4. Poor oral hygiene
5. Inadequate fluoride exposure
6. Prolonged nursing (bottle or breast)
7. Diet with high sucrose frequency
8. Poor family dental health
9. Developmental enamel defects
10. Developmental disability
11. Xerostomia
12. Genetic abnormality of teeth
13. Many multisurface restorations
14. Chemotherapy or radiation therapy

to pregnant patients just as with other patients, using an appropriate leaded apron to shield the abdominal area.

Radiation Therapy

Patients with a malignancy in the oral cavity or perioral region often receive radiation therapy for their disease. Some oral tissues receive 50 Gy or more. Although such patients are often apprehensive about receiving additional exposure, dental exposure is insignificant compared with what they have already received. The average skin dose from a dental radiograph is approximately 3 mGy, less if faster film or digital imaging is used. Furthermore, patients who have received radiation therapy may suffer from radiation-induced xerostomia and thus are at a high risk for developing radiation caries, which may produce serious consequences if extractions are needed in the future. Accord-

ingly, carefully follow patients who have had radiation therapy to the oral cavity because they are at special risk for dental disease.

EXAMPLES OF USE OF THE GUIDELINES

Consider the ways in which the guidelines can be applied to different clinical situations:
• The first visit of a 5-year-old boy to a dental office— A careful clinical examination reveals that the patient is cooperative and that the posterior teeth are in contact. Posterior bitewings are recommended to detect caries. If all of this patient's teeth are present, no evidence exists of decay, a reasonably good diet is being observed, and the parent(s) seem(s) well motivated to promote good oral hygiene, no further radiographic examination is required at this time. Radiographs for the detection of development abnor-

malities are not in order at this age because a complete appraisal cannot be made at 5 years. Even if it could be made, it is too early to initiate treatment for such abnormalities.

- A 25-year-old woman receiving a 6-month checkup after her last treatment for a fractured incisor—No caries is evident on interproximal radiographs made 6 months ago; currently no clinical signs suggest caries, nor does the patient have high-risk factors for caries. No evidence exists of periodontal disease or other remarkable signs or symptoms in general or associated with the recently fractured tooth. As long as the fractured incisor shows normal vitality testing, no radiographs are recommended for this patient. If the incisor is nonvital, expose a periapical view of this tooth.

- A 45-year-old man returning to the dentist's office after 1 year—At his last visit you placed two mesial, occlusal, distal (MOD) amalgam restorations on premolars and performed root canal therapy on number 30. The patient has a 5-mm pocket in the buccal furcation of number 3 but no other evidence of periodontal disease. The guidelines recommend that this patient receive interproximal radiographs to see whether he still has active caries and periapical views of numbers 3 and 30 to evaluate the extent of the periodontal disease and periapical disease, respectively.

- A 65-year-old woman coming to your office for the first time—No previous radiographs are available. A history exists of root canal therapy in two teeth, although the patient is not aware which teeth were treated. Clinical examination reveals multiple carious teeth, multiple missing teeth, and pockets of more than 3 mm involving most of the remaining teeth. The guidelines recommend a full-mouth examination, including interproximal radiographs, for this patient because of the high probability of finding caries, periodontal disease, and periapical disease.

BIBLIOGRAPHY

GUIDELINES FOR ORDERING RADIOGRAPHS

Åkerblom A, Rohlin M, Hasselgren G: Individualised restricted intraoral radiography versus full-mouth radiography in the detection of periradicular lesions, Swed Dent J 12:151, 1988.

Atchison KA, Luke LS, White SC: An algorithm for ordering pretreatment orthodontic radiographs, Am J Orthod Dentofac Orthop 102:29, 1992.

ADA Council on Scientific Affairs: An update on radiographic practices: information and recommendations, JADA 132:234, 2001.

Atchison KA et al: Assessing the FDA guidelines for ordering dental radiographs, JADA 126:1372, 1995.

Bohay RN, Stephens RG, Kogon SL: A study of the impact of screening or selective radiography on the treatment and post delivery outcome for edentulous patients, Oral Surg Oral Med Oral Pathol Oral Radiol Endod 86:353, 1998.

Brooks SL: A study of selection criteria for intraoral dental radiography, Oral Surg Oral Med Oral Pathol 62:234, 1986.

Brooks SL et al: Imaging of the temporomandibular joint: a position paper of the American Academy of Oral and Maxillofacial Radiology, Oral Surg Oral Med Oral Pathol Oral Radiol and Endod 83:609, 1997.

Bruks A et al: Radiographic examinations as an aid to orthodontic diagnosis and treatment planning, Swed Dent J 23:77, 1999.

Hollender L: Decision making in radiographic imaging, J Dent Educ 56:834, 1992.

Keur JJ: Radiographic screening of edentulous patients: sense or nonsense? A risk-benefit analysis, Oral Surg Oral Med Oral Pathol 62:463, 1986.

Luke LS et al: Orthodontic residents' indications for use of the lateral TMJ tomogram and the posteroanterior cephalogram, J Dent Educ 61:29, 1997.

Molander B: Panoramic radiography in dental diagnostics, Swed Dent J Suppl 119:1, 1996.

Pitts NB, Kidd EA: Some of the factors to be considered in the prescription and timing of bitewing radiography in the diagnosis and management of dental caries, J Dent 20:74, 1992.

Rushton VE, Horner K, Worthington HV: Routine panoramic radiography of new adult patients in general dental practice: relevance of diagnostic yield to treatment and identification of radiographic selection criteria, Oral Surg Oral Med Oral Pathol Oral Radiol Endod 93:488, 2002.

Stephens RG, Kogon SL: New U.S. guidelines for prescribing dental radiographs: a critical review, J Can Dent Assoc 56:1019, 1990.

Tyndall DA, Brooks SL: Selection criteria for dental implant site imaging: a position paper of the American Academy of Oral and Maxillofacial Radiology, Oral Surg Oral Med Oral Pathol Oral Radiol 89:630, 2000.

U.S. Department of Health and Human Services: The selection of patients for x-ray examinations: dental radiographic examinations, DHHS Publication FDA 88-8273, Rockville, MD, 1987.

White SC et al: Parameters of radiologic care: an official report of the American Academy of Oral and Maxillofacial Radiology, Oral Surg Oral Med Oral Pathol Oral Radiol Endod 91:498, 2001.

DISEASE DETECTION

Atchison K et al: Efficacy of the FDA selection criteria for radiographic assessment of the periodontium, J Dent Res 74:1424, 1995.

Backer Dirks O: Posteruptive changes in dental enamel, J Dent Res 45(suppl):503, 1966.

Carter LC et al: Use of panoramic radiography among an ambulatory dental population to detect patients at risk of stroke, JADA 128:977, 1997.

Friedlander AH: Identification of stroke-prone patients by panoramic and cervical spine radiography, Dentomaxillofac Radiol 24:160, 1995.

Hall WB: Decision making in periodontology, ed 3, St. Louis, 1998, Mosby.

Moles DR, Downer MC: Optimum bitewing examination recall intervals assessed by computer simulation, Commun Dent Health 17:14, 2000.

Reddy MS et al: Periodontal disease progression, J Periodontol 71:1583, 2000.

Shwartz M et al: A longitudinal analysis from bitewing radiographs of the rate of progression of approximal carious lesions through human dental enamel, Archs Oral Biol 29:529, 1984.

White SC et al: Clinical and historical predictors of dental caries on radiographs, Dentomaxillofac Radiol 24:121, 1995.

White SC et al: Efficacy of FDA guidelines for ordering radiographs for caries detection, Oral Surg Oral Med Oral Pathol 77:531, 1994.

RADIATION DOSAGE AND EFFECTS

Frederiksen N, Benson B, Sokolowski T: Effective dose and risk assessment from computed tomography of the maxillofacial complex, Dentomaxillofac Radiol 24:55, 1995.

Gonad doses and genetically significant dose from diagnostic radiology: U.S., 1964 and 1970, DHEW Publication (FDA) 76-8034, Washington, D.C., 1976.

Scaf G et al: Dosimetry and cost of imaging osseointegrated implants with film-based and computed tomography, Oral Surg Oral Med Oral Pathol Oral Radiol Endod 83:41, 1997.

White SC: 1992 assessment of radiation risks from dental radiology, Dentomaxillofac Radiol 21:118, 1992.

PART FIVE

Radiographic Interpretation of Pathology

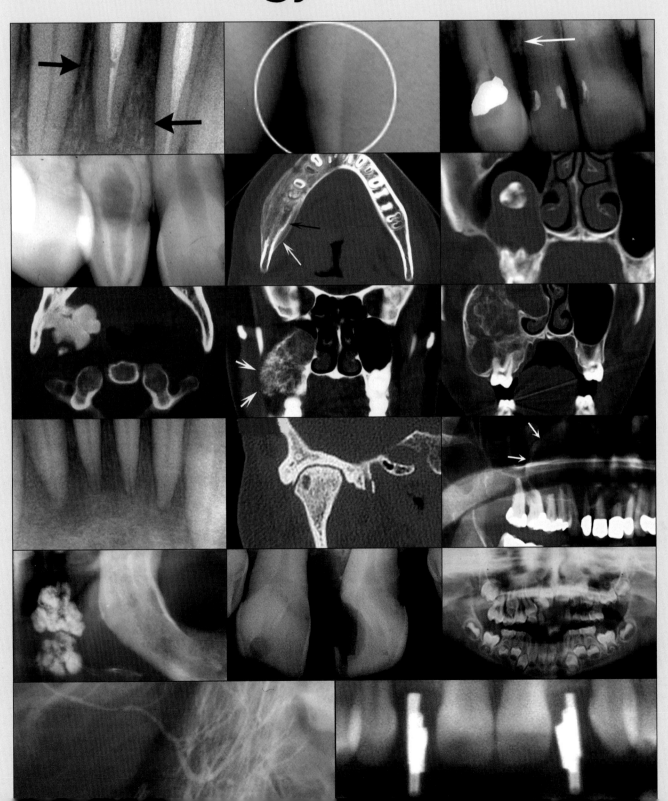

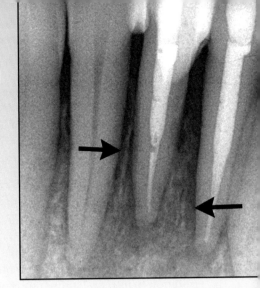

CHAPTER 15

Principles of Radiographic Interpretation

The objective of this chapter is to provide a step-by-step, analytic process that can be applied to the interpretation of diagnostic images. However, reading this chapter will not immediately bestow the ability to interpret radiographic films correctly; rather, it will equip the reader with a systematic method of image analysis. Proficiency comes only with practice.

Clinical Examination

Radiographs are prescribed when the dentist thinks that they are likely to offer useful diagnostic information that will influence the treatment plan. Often some clinical sign or symptom or finding from the patient's history indicates the need for a radiologic examination. This clinical information should be used first to select the type of radiographs and later to aid in their interpretation.

ACQUIRING APPROPRIATE DIAGNOSTIC IMAGES

An insufficient number or inadequate quality of radiographs limits the information available from diagnostic imaging. Because the general practitioner often is responsible both for prescribing and interpreting radiographs, inadequate films should be recognized and supplemental images obtained before proceeding with the analysis.

Quality of the Diagnostic Image

Before the analysis is started, the quality of the images is examined. Is the image distorted? For instance, if the image is elongated, greater error occurs in measuring the length of a root canal. Because of the inherent frequency of image distortion in panoramic films, this factor must always be taken into consideration. For example, a region of image magnification involving the mandibular condyle may be diagnosed erroneously as condylar hyperplasia. For this reason, a thorough knowledge of all possible image distortions is a prerequisite for analysis of panoramic images.

The practitioner also should check to see whether the density or contrast of the image has been degraded by exposure or developing errors. It may be impossible, for example, to diagnose osteoporosis in an overexposed image, or detail may be obscured in an underexposed film. If the images are of poor quality, it might be prudent to obtain better quality images before proceeding to the analysis.

Number and Type of Available Images

Initially the clinical examination indicates the number and types of films required (see Chapter 14). The interpretation of these films in turn may suggest the need for additional imaging. Caution should be exercised in attempting to make an interpretation based on a single film, especially if the only film is a panoramic view. Also, a bitewing or periapical projection often can be supplemented by another view produced by altering the horizontal or vertical angulation of the x-ray beam. For example, detection of recurrent caries around a heavily restored dentition may benefit from an additional view taken by altering the angle of the x-ray beam. One of the benefits of a full-mouth series of intraoral films is that it provides a second view of most areas at a slightly different angle.

Conventional dental radiography produces images in only two dimensions, usually in the mesiodistal direction. In some cases a view at right angles to the plane of the original film is beneficial. For instance, if a condylar neck fracture is suspected, a lateral view of the condylar region (e.g., a panoramic view) should be supplemented with an anteroposterior (AP) view. In a similar fashion, occlusal projections of the jaws can provide a supplementary right-angle view for the periapical film. Use of a vertex occlusal view follows this principle in establishing the location of impacted maxillary cuspids. In some cases an investigation requires other images in addition to intraoral radiography or panoramic images. Techniques such as tomography, sialography, arthrography, nuclear imaging, computed tomography, and magnetic resonance imaging may be required (see Chapter 13). These techniques are available through consultation with an oral and maxillofacial radiologist.

Diagnostic imaging should be completed before a biopsy procedure or treatment is provided. Diagnostic imaging can aid in the selection of the most appropriate anatomic site for a biopsy procedure. Also, the biopsy procedure may alter the tissue by inducing inflammatory changes, which in turn alter the imaging characteristics of the tissue. This compromises the diagnostic information that can be obtained, such as determining the extent of a disease.

Viewing Conditions

Ideally, viewing conditions should include the following characteristics:

- Ambient light in the viewing room should be reduced.
- Intraoral radiographs should be mounted in a film holder.
- Light from the viewbox should be of equal intensity across the viewing surface.
- The size of the viewbox should accommodate the size of the film. If the viewing area is larger than the film, an opaque mask should be used to eliminate all light from around the periphery of the film. This mask can be fabricated from a sheet of opaque material cut to fit the entire viewbox, leaving an opening for one film.
- An intense light source is essential for evaluating dark regions of the film.
- A magnifying glass allows detailed examination of small regions of the film.

Image Analysis

When the quality and number of films are satisfactory, analysis of the image begins.

SYSTEMATIC RADIOGRAPHIC EXAMINATION

The first step in image analysis is to use a systematic approach to identify all the normal anatomy present in an image or set of images. A profound knowledge of the variation of normal appearance is required to be able to recognize an abnormal appearance. Because no textbook can display all possible variations, the best learning method is to identify normal anatomy in every film analyzed. In this way the observer can build up a large mental database of the spectrum of normal anatomic appearances. An additional benefit of this procedure is that it forces the observer to examine the entire film. Practitioners should avoid limiting their attention to one particular region of the film; rather, all aspects of each image should be examined systematically. More than one abnormality may be present. For instance, a bitewing radiograph made to detect caries and alveolar bone loss also may reveal just the edge of an unsuspected intraosseous lesion that will be seen only if the dentist examines the radiograph thoroughly.

INTRAORAL IMAGES

For almost all dental patients, treatment planning includes some combination of periapical and bitewing images. We present here a systematic method for analyzing these images. This method may be used to analyze a single image or a full-mouth set. It is most important for the practitioner to develop a particular method and to use it regularly. A thorough examination is best accomplished when a specific sequence of analysis is used to enhance the scrutiny of all parts of images.

To follow the method presented here, examine the periapical images before the bitewing images, starting in the right maxilla and working across to the left, then dropping down and continuing in the left mandible to the right. Concentrate on one anatomic structure at a time. First, examine the bone. Identify all anatomic landmarks appropriate for the region. In the posterior maxilla, for example, examine the maxillary sinus, tuberosity, and zygomatic process of the maxilla. In what way does their appearance change as the angle of each projection is altered? Also examine the character of the trabecular bone. Are the density and size of the trabeculae normal for the region? Compare the same areas on adjacent images and with the corresponding area on images of the other side.

Next, make a second visual circuit through all the images, examining the bone of the alveolar process. Examine in particular the height of the alveolar crest relative to the teeth and its cortication. Loss of height of the alveolar bone (more than 1.5 mm from the adjacent cementoenamel junctions) may indicate active or past periodontal disease. Examine all regions of the alveolar process to gain an overall appreciation for the extent and severity of alveolar bone loss. Note any areas of erosion of the alveolar crest and the thickness of the overlying mucosa. Carcinomas arising from the epithelial covering may cause erosive lesions with ill-defined borders in the alveolar bone. Examine the trabecular pattern of the alveolar process. The lamina dura may be examined later together with the periodontal membrane space and tooth roots.

Finally, make a third visual circuit, examining the dentition and associated structures. Study each tooth in sequence, using all images available. Note the way the tooth's appearance and root structure change with different orientations of the x-ray beam. Count the teeth, looking for missing or supernumerary teeth. Examine the crowns for normal development of the enamel and for caries. Pay particular attention to the interproximal regions at or below the contact points. Check restorations carefully for signs of recurrent caries. Often lesions found on one view cannot be detected on another because of superimposition of the restoration. Examine the pulp chamber for size and contents. Examine the roots for shape and form to detect developmental or acquired abnormalities such as external resorption. Inspect the width of the periodontal ligament space around the roots of the tooth. The width should be fairly uniform, with very subtle widening toward the cervical region of the tooth. Examine particularly the lamina dura around each tooth. Is it intact? The most common abnormalities found in the bone are radiolucent or radiopaque lesions at the apices of teeth.

EXTRAORAL RADIOGRAPHY

The extraoral radiographs most commonly used in dentistry are panoramic images, cephalometric views, and examinations of the temporomandibular joint (TMJ). Specific methods for examining these images are covered in the chapters pertaining to these types of images. The same general principles of thorough, systematic coverage described earlier should be used. For viewing each of these types of images, it is important to develop a definite sequence that considers all the hard and soft tissues in the field. Always focus on one component at a time and examine it thoroughly. Only with such a pattern can the practitioner maximize the likelihood of detecting all abnormalities.

When an intraosseous lesion is identified, the following five steps should be used to analyze the lesion as fully as possible.

Analysis of Intraosseous Lesions

Two basic approaches can be used to analyze images of a lesion. One is the picture matching, or "Aunt Minnie," method. This involves trying to match the radiographic image with a mental picture or with an image in a favorite textbook, which would be similar to identifying your aunt Minnie in a picture because you are familiar with the appearance of your aunt Minnie. Although all radiologists probably use this technique to a certain extent, it has significant limitations. For instance, the observer's experience and memory limit the mental image of a particular disorder. Similarly, the appearance of different abnormalities in a textbook is limited by the author's knowledge and experience and, of course, by the number of images printed. Also, figures in a textbook usually represent the most ideal examples of the abnormality. For example, the term *periapical cemental dysplasia* often evokes a mental image of a radiolucent or mixed radiolucent-radiopaque lesion at the apex of a mandibular incisor because this appearance is the one used most often in textbooks (Figs. 15-1 and 15-2). Although this is a common location, this concept limits recognition and acceptance of this lesion in other areas of the jaws or where teeth have been extracted (Fig. 15-3). Therefore using this technique limits the scope of possible entities to be considered in the interpretation.

The preferred method of radiographic interpretation is presented here. It is a step-by-step analysis of all the radiographic characteristics of the abnormality and production of a radiographic interpretation based on these findings. This procedure helps ensure recognition and collection of all the information contained in the image and in turn improves the accuracy of interpretation.

STEP 1: LOCALIZE THE ABNORMALITY

Localized or generalized—Attempt to describe the anatomic location and limits of the abnormality. This information aids in starting to select various disease categories. Many abnormalities are localized to a specific region. If an abnormal appearance affects all the osseous structures of the maxillofacial region, generalized conditions such as metabolic or endocrine abnormalities of bone are considered. If the abnormality is localized, it may be unilateral or bilateral (Fig. 15-4). Often variations of normal anatomy are more commonly bilateral, whereas abnormal conditions are more commonly unilateral. For instance, a bilateral mandibular radiolucency may indicate normal anatomy, such as extensive submandibular gland fossa, whereas fibrous

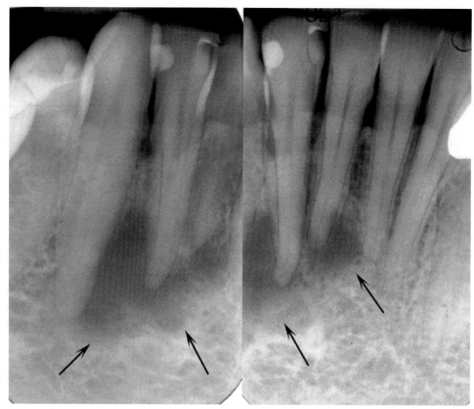

FIG. **15-1**   The typical location of lesions of periapical cemental dysplasia. Early lesions are radiolucent *(arrows)*.

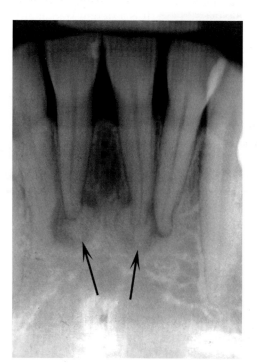

FIG. **15-2**   Late lesions of periapical cemental dysplasia have a more radiopaque interior surrounded by a more radiolucent margin.

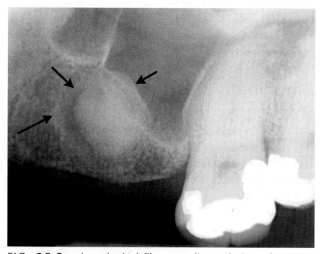

FIG. **15-3**   A periapical film revealing a lesion of cemental dysplasia left behind after extraction of the associated tooth.

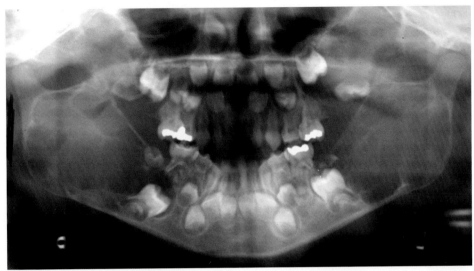

FIG. **15-4**   This lesion, cherubism, is bilateral, manifesting in both the left and right mandibular rami. Note that the mandibular molars have been displaced anteriorly on both sides.

dysplasia commonly is unilateral. However, a few abnormalities such as Paget's disease are always seen bilaterally in the mandible.

Position in the jaws—Is the abnormality in soft tissue, or is it contained within the jaws? When the lesion is in bone, the point of origin, or epicenter, can be estimated based on the assumption that the abnormality grew equally in every direction (this becomes less accurate with very large lesions). The point of origin may indicate the tissue types that compose the abnormality. However, determining the exact location may be difficult in some circumstances if the nature of the abnormality is not well defined. The following are a few examples:

- If the epicenter is coronal to a tooth, the lesion probably is composed of odontogenic epithelium (Fig. 15-5, *A*).
- If it is above the inferior alveolar nerve canal (IAC), the likelihood is greater that it is composed of odontogenic tissue (Fig. 15-6).
- If the epicenter is below the IAC, it is unlikely to be odontogenic in origin (Fig. 15-7).
- If it originates within the IAC, the tissue of origin probably is neural or vascular in nature (Fig. 15-8).
- The probability of cartilaginous lesions and osteochondromas occurring is greater in the condylar region.
- If the epicenter is within the maxillary antrum, the lesion is not of odontogenic tissue, as opposed to a lesion that has grown into the antrum from the alveolar process of the maxilla (Fig. 15-9).

Particular lesions tend to be found in specific locations:

- The epicenters of central giant cell granulomas commonly are located anterior to the first molars in the mandible and anterior to the cuspid in the maxilla.
- Osteomyelitis occurs in the mandible and rarely in the maxilla.
- Periapical cemental dysplasia occurs in the periapical region of teeth (see Figs. 15-1 and 15-2).

Single or multifocal—Establishing whether an abnormality is multifocal aids in interpretation because the list of possible multifocal abnormalities is short. Some examples are periapical cemental dysplasia, odontogenic keratocysts, metastatic lesions, multiple myeloma (Fig. 15-10), and leukemic infiltrates.

Occasionally exceptions to all these points occur. However, in the majority of cases these criteria will serve as a guide to an accurate interpretation.

Size—Finally, consider the size of the lesion. There are very few size restrictions for a particular lesion, but the size may aid in the differential diagnosis. For instance, a dentigerous cyst is often larger than a hyperplastic follicle.

STEP 2: ASSESS THE PERIPHERY AND SHAPE

Study the periphery of the lesion. Is the periphery well defined or ill defined? If an imaginary pencil can be used to draw confidently the limits of the lesion, the

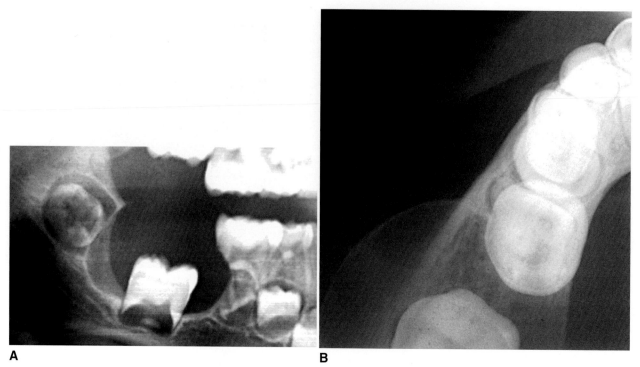

A   **B**

FIG. **15-5**   **A,** A cropped panoramic image of a lesion in which the epicenter is coronal to the unerupted mandibular first molar. **B,** An occlusal projection providing a right-angled view of the same lesion.

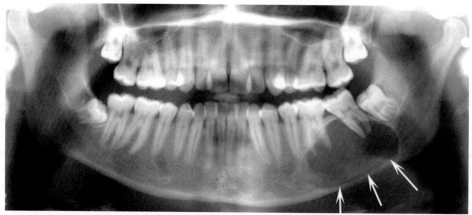

FIG. **15-6**   A panoramic image revealing a cystic ameloblastoma within the body of the left mandible. Note that the inferior alveolar nerve canal has been displaced inferiorly to the inferior cortex *(arrows),* indicating that the lesion started superior to the canal.

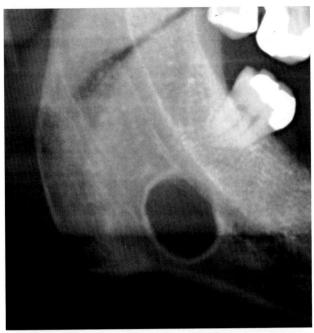

FIG. **15-7** A cropped panoramic image displaying a lesion (developmental salivary gland defect) below the inferior alveolar canal and thus unlikely to be of odontogenic origin.

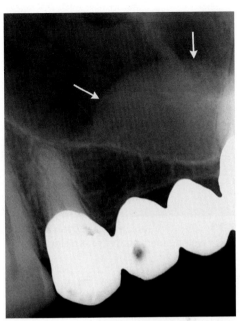

FIG. **15-9** The lack of a peripheral cortex on this benign cyst indicates that it originated in the sinus and not in the alveolar process. It therefore is unlikely to be of odontogenic origin.

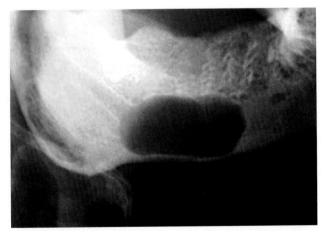

FIG. **15-8** A lateral oblique view of the mandible revealing a lesion within the inferior alveolar canal. The smooth fusiform expansion of the canal indicates a neural lesion.

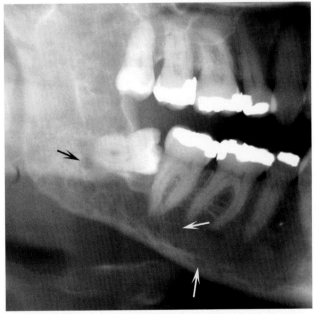

FIG. **15-10** A cropped panoramic film revealing several small punched-out lesions of multiple myeloma (*a few indicated by arrows*) involving the body and ramus of the mandible.

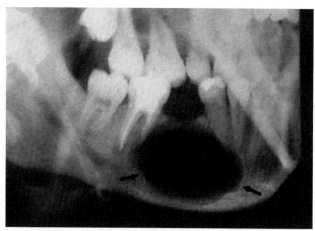

FIG. **15-11**   A lateral oblique projection of the mandible showing the well-defined border of a residual cyst.

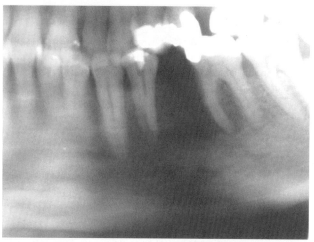

FIG. **15-12**   A cropped panoramic radiograph showing the poorly defined border of a malignant neoplasm which has destroyed bone between the first molar and first bicuspid.

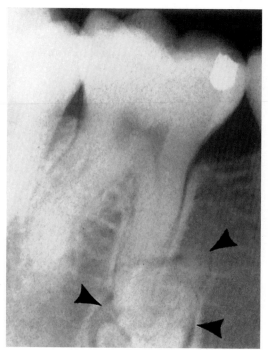

FIG. **15-13**   Note the thin, radiolucent periphery positioned between the internal radiopaque structure of this odontoma and the radiopaque outer cortical boundary.

margin is well defined (Fig. 15-11). Do not become concerned if some small regions are ill defined; these may be due to the shape or direction of the x-ray beam at that particular location. A well-defined lesion is one in which most of the periphery is well defined. In contrast, it is difficult to draw an exact delineation around most of an ill-defined periphery (Fig. 15-12). These two types of peripheries or borders can be further broken down under two subcategories: well-defined borders and ill-defined borders.

Well-Defined Borders

A punched-out border is one that has a sharp boundary in which no bone reaction is apparent immediately adjacent to the abnormality. This is analogous to punching a hole in a radiograph with a paper punch. The

border of the resulting hole is well defined, and the surrounding bone has a normal appearance up to the edge of the hole. This type of border sometimes is seen in multiple myeloma (see Fig. 15-10).

A corticated margin is a thin, fairly uniform radiopaque line of reactive bone at the periphery of a lesion. This is commonly seen with cysts (see Fig. 15-5).

A sclerotic margin is a wide, radiopaque border of reactive bone that usually is not uniform in width. This may be seen with periapical cemental dysplasia and may indicate a very slow rate of growth or the potential for the lesion to stimulate the production of surrounding bone (see Figs. 15-2 and 15-3).

A radiopaque lesion may have a soft tissue capsule, which is indicated by the presence of a radiolucent line at the periphery. This may be seen in conjunction with a corticated periphery, as is observed with odontomas and cementoblastomas (Figs. 15-13 and 15-14).

Ill-Defined Borders

A blending border is ill defined because of the gradual transition between normal-appearing bone trabeculae and the abnormal-appearing trabeculae of the lesion. The focus of this observation is on the trabeculae and not on the radiolucent marrow spaces. Some conditions with this type of margin are sclerosing osteitis (Fig. 15-15) and fibrous dysplasia.

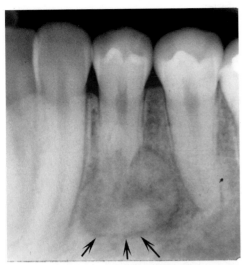

FIG. 15-14 A periapical film revealing a radiopaque mass associated with the root of the first bicuspid. Note the prominent radiolucent periphery *(arrows)* of this benign cementoblastoma.

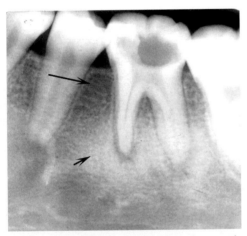

FIG. 15-15 In this periapical film there is a gradual transition from the dense trabeculae of sclerosing osteitis *(short arrow)* to the normal trabecular pattern near the crest of the alveolar process *(long arrow).* This is an example of an ill-defined, blending border.

An invasive border usually is associated with rapid growth and can be seen with malignant lesions. Usually an area of radiolucency representing bone destruction can be seen just behind the margin (Fig. 15-16). In contrast to the blending border, the focus of this observation is on the enlarging radiolucency at the expense of bone trabeculae. These borders have also been described as *permeative* because the lesion grows around existing trabeculae, producing radiolucent, fingerlike, or bay-type extensions at the periphery. This may result

in enlargement of the marrow spaces at the periphery (Fig. 15-17).

Shape

The lesion may have a particular shape, or it may be irregular. The following are some examples:

- A circular or fluid-filled shape, much like an inflated balloon, which sometimes is referred to as *hydraulic,* is characteristic of a cyst (see Fig. 15-5).
- A scalloped shape is a series of contiguous arcs or semicircles that may reflect the mechanism of growth (Fig. 15-18). This shape may be seen in cysts (e.g., odontogenic keratocysts), cystlike lesions (e.g., simple bone cysts), and some tumors. Occasionally a lesion with a scalloped periphery is referred to as *multilocular;* however, in this text the term *multilocular* is reserved for the description of the internal structure.

STEP 3: ANALYZE THE INTERNAL STRUCTURE

The internal appearance of a lesion can be classified into one of three basic categories: totally radiolucent, totally radiopaque, or mixed radiolucent and radiopaque (mixed density).

A radiolucent interior is common in cysts (see Fig. 15-5, *A*), and a totally radiopaque interior is observed in osteomas. The mixed density internal structure is seen as the presence of calcified structures against a radiolucent (black) backdrop. A challenging aspect of this analysis may be the decision concerning whether a calcified structure is in the internal aspect of the lesion or resides on either side. This is difficult to determine using images that are two-dimensional representations of three-dimensional structures. Examine the calcified structures and attempt to identify the structure by its shape, size, and pattern. For example, bone can be identified by the presence of trabeculae. Also, the degree of radiopacity may help, for instance enamel is more radiopaque than bone. The following is a list of the most radiolucent (top of the list) to the most radiopaque (bottom of the list) material seen in plain radiographs:

- Air, fat, and gas (most radiolucent)
- Fluid
- Soft tissue
- Bone marrow
- Trabecular bone
- Cortical bone and dentine
- Enamel
- Metal (most radiopaque)

This list is useful but its value may be compromised by the amount of material; for instance, a large amount cortical bone may be as radiopaque as enamel.

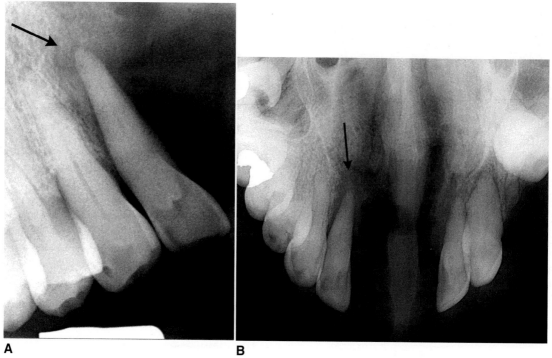

A   **B**

FIG. **15-16**   Periapical **(A)** and occlusal **(B)** films revealing a squamous cell carcinoma in the anterior maxilla. Note the invasive margin that extends beyond the lateral incisor *(arrow)* and the bone destruction immediately behind this margin.

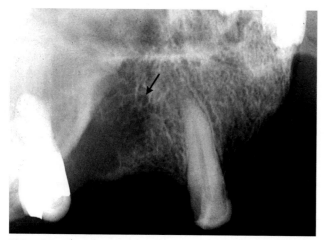

FIG. **15-17**   Occlusal view of a lesion revealing an ill-defined periphery with enlargement of the small marrow spaces at the margin *(arrow)*. This is characteristic of a malignant neoplasm, in this case a lymphoma.

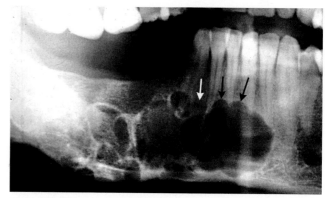

FIG. **15-18**   A cropped panoramic film of an odontogenic keratocyst displaying a scalloped border, especially around the apex of the associated teeth *(arrows)*.

The following list presents a few possible internal structures that may be seen in mixed density lesions:

- Abnormal bone may have a variety of trabecular patterns different from normal bone. These variations result from a difference in the number, length, width, and orientation of the trabeculae. For instance, in fibrous dysplasia the trabeculae usually are greater in number, shorter, and not aligned in response to applied stress to the bone but are randomly oriented, resulting in patterns described as have an orange-peel or a ground-glass appearance (Fig. 15-19). Another example is the stimulation of new bone formation on existing trabeculae in response to inflammation. This results in thick trabeculae, giving the area a more radiopaque appearance (see Fig. 15-15).

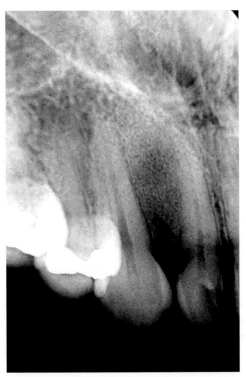

FIG. **15-19** A periapical film of a small lesion of fibrous dysplasia between the lateral incisor and cuspid demonstrating a change in bone pattern. Note the presence of a greater number of trabeculae per unit area and that the trabeculae are small and thin and randomly oriented in an orange-peel pattern.

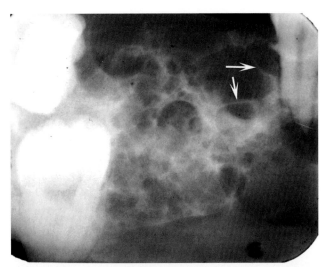

FIG. **15-20** A periapical film of an ameloblastoma. Notice the multilocular pattern created by septa *(arrows)* dividing the internal structure into small soap-bubble–like compartments.

- Septa represent residual bone that has been organized into long strands or walls. If these septa divide the internal structure into at least two compartments, the term *multilocular* is used. The length, width, and orientation of the septa can be assessed. For instance, curved, coarse septa may be seen in ameloblastoma and sometimes in odontogenic keratocysts (Fig. 15-20), giving the internal pattern a multilocular, "soap bubble" appearance. The septa seen in giant cell granulomas are described as wispy or granular; odontogenic myxomas may display a small number of straight, thin septa.
- Dystrophic calcification is a calcification that occurs in damaged soft tissue. This is most commonly seen in calcified lymph nodes that appear as dense, cauliflower-like masses in the soft tissue. In chronically inflamed cysts the calcification may have a very delicate, particulate appearance without a recognizable pattern.
- Cementum usually has a homogeneous, dense, amorphous structure and sometimes is organized into round or oval shapes (see Figs. 15-2 and 15-3).

- Tooth structure usually can be identified by the organization into enamel, dentin, and pulp chambers. Also, the internal density is equivalent to tooth structure and greater than the surrounding bone (see Fig. 15-13).

STEP 4: ANALYZE THE EFFECTS OF THE LESION ON SURROUNDING STRUCTURES

Evaluating the effects of the lesion on surrounding structures allows the observer to infer its behavior. The behavior may aid in identification of the disease, but this requires knowledge of the mechanisms of various diseases. For instance, inflammatory disease, as is seen in periapical osteitis, can stimulate bone resorption or formation. Bone formation may occur on the surface of existing trabeculae, resulting in thick trabeculae, which is reflected in the trabecular pattern and in an overall increase in the radiopacity of the bone (see Fig. 15-15). The term *space-occupying* is used to describe a lesion that slowly creates its own space by displacing teeth and other surrounding structures. The following sections give examples of effects on surrounding structures and the conclusions that may be inferred from the behavior of the lesions.

Teeth, Lamina Dura, and Periodontal Membrane Space

Displacement of teeth is seen more commonly with slower-growing, space-occupying lesions. The direction of tooth displacement is significant. Lesions with an epi-

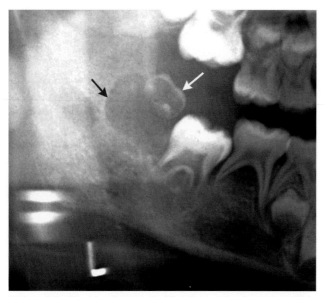

FIG. **15-21** Leukemic infiltration of the mandible showing coronal displacement of the developing second molar *(white arrow)* from the remnants of its crypt *(black arrow)*. Note the lack of a lamina dura around the apex of the first molar and widening of the periodontal ligament space around the second deciduous molar.

center above the crown of a tooth (i.e., follicular cysts and occasionally odontomas) displace the tooth apically (see Fig. 15-5, *A*). Lesions that start in the ramus, such as cherubism (see Fig. 15-4), may push teeth in an anterior direction. Some lesions grow in the papilla of developing teeth (i.e., lymphoma, leukemia, Langerhans' cell histiocytosis) and may push the developing tooth in a coronal direction (Fig. 15-21).

Widening of the periodontal membrane space may be seen with many different kinds of abnormalities. It is important to observe whether the widening is uniform or irregular and whether the lamina dura is still present. For instance, orthodontic movement of teeth results in widening of the periodontal membrane space, but the lamina dura remains intact. Malignant lesions can quickly grow down the ligament space, resulting in an irregular widening and destruction of the lamina dura (Fig. 15-22).

Resorption of teeth usually occurs with a more chronic or slowly growing process (see Fig. 15-5) and may result from chronic inflammation. Although tooth resorption is more commonly related to benign processes, malignant tumors occasionally resorb teeth.

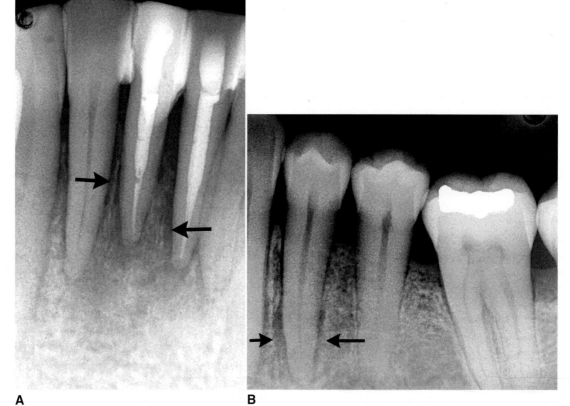

A   **B**

FIG. **15-22**   A and B, Periapical films revealing a malignant lymphoma that has invaded the mandible. Note the irregular widening of the periodontal ligament spaces *(arrows)*.

Surrounding Bone Density and Trabecular Pattern

The presence of reactive bone at the periphery of a lesion, whether corticated or sclerotic, usually signifies slow, benign growth and possibly the ability to stimulate osteoblastic activity in the surrounding bone (see Fig. 15-3).

Inferior Alveolar Nerve Canal and Mental Foramen

Some changes tend to be characteristic. For example, superior displacement of the inferior alveolar canal is strongly associated with fibrous dysplasia. Widening of the inferior alveolar canal with the maintenance of a cortical boundary may indicate the presence of a benign lesion of vascular or neural origin (see Fig. 15-8). Irregular widening with cortical destruction may indicate the presence of a malignant neoplasm growing down the length of the canal.

Outer Cortical Bone and Periosteal Reactions

The cortex of bone may remodel in response to a lesion. A slowly growing lesion may allow time for the outer periosteum to manufacture new bone so that the resulting expanded bone appears to have maintained an outer cortical plate (see Fig. 15-5). On the other hand, a rapidly growing lesion outstrips the ability of the periosteum to respond, and the cortical plate may be missing (see Fig. 15-12). Exudate from an inflammatory lesion can lift the periosteum off the surface of the cortical bone and then stimulate the periosteum to lay down new bone (Fig. 15-23). When this process occurs more than once, an onion-skin type of pattern can be seen. This is most commonly seen in inflammatory lesions and more rarely in some malignant lesions (e.g., leukemia) and in Langerhans' cell histiocytosis.

Some periosteal reactions are very specific, such as spiculated new bone formed at right angles to the outer cortical plate, which is seen with metastatic lesions of the prostate gland or in a radiating pattern in osteogenic sarcoma (Fig. 15-24).

STEP 5: FORMULATE A RADIOGRAPHIC INTERPRETATION

The preceding steps enable the observer to collect all the radiographic findings in an organized fashion. (Box 15-1 presents the process in abbreviated form.) Now the significance of each observation must be determined. The algorithm shown in Fig. 15-25 should be used as a dynamic guide to accommodate new observations and change incorrect concepts. The ability to give more significance to some observations over others comes with experience. For instance, in the analysis of a hypothetical lesion, the observations of tooth movement, tooth resorption, and an invasive destructive border are made. The effects on the teeth in this example may indicate a benign process; however, the invasive border and bone destruction are more important characteristics and indicate a malignant process. Avoid making an interpretation from a single observation. In the analysis, all the accumulated characteristics point the way to the diagnosis. Also, occasionally any algorithm may fail because lesions sometimes do not behave as expected.

Decision 1: Normal Versus Abnormal

Determine whether the structure of interest is a variation of normal or represents an abnormality. This is a crucial decision because variations of normal do not

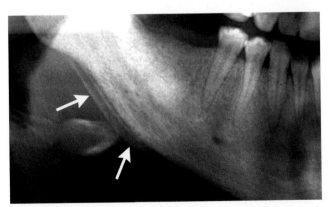

FIG. **15-23**   A panoramic image of osteomyelitis revealing at least two layers of new bone (*arrows*) produced by the periosteum at the inferior aspect of the mandible.

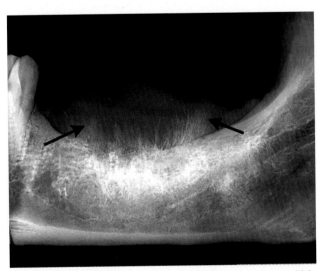

FIG. **15-24**   Specimen radiograph of a resected mandible with an osteosarcoma. Note the fine linear spicules of bone at the superior margin of the alveolar process.

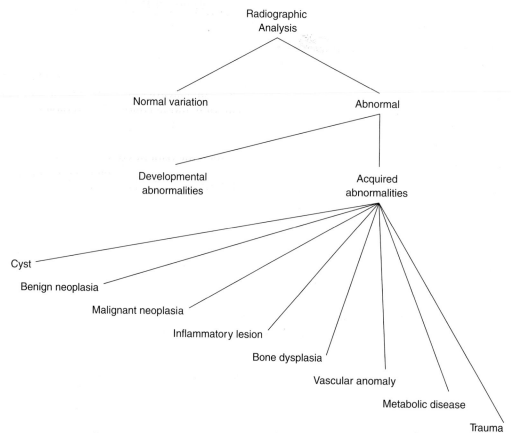

FIG. **15-25** An algorithm representing the diagnostic process that follows evaluation of the radiographic features of an abnormality.

require treatment or further investigation. However, as previously stated, to be proficient in the interpretation of diagnostic images, the practitioner needs an in-depth knowledge of the various appearances of normal anatomy.

Decision 2: Developmental Versus Acquired

If the area of interest is abnormal, the next step is to decide whether the radiographic characteristics (location, periphery, shape, internal structure, and effects on surrounding structures) indicate that the region of interest represents a developmental abnormality or an acquired change. For instance, the observation that a tooth has an abnormally short root leads to the pertinent question, "Did the tooth develop a short root, or was the root at one time of normal length?" If the answer is the latter, then the process must be external root resorption and hence an acquired abnormality. If the tooth merely developed a short root, the pulp canal should not be visible to the very end of the root because of normal apexification. In contrast, external root resorption may shorten the root, but the canal remains visible to the end of the root (Fig. 15-26).

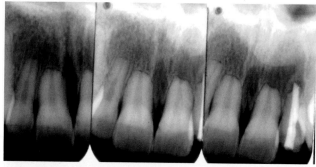

FIG. **15-26** Periapical films revealing external resorption of the maxillary incisors, which is acquired because of the wide pulp chambers at the apex of the roots of the teeth.

Decision 3: Classification

If the abnormality is acquired, the next step is to select the most likely category of acquired abnormality: cysts, benign tumors, malignant tumors, inflammatory lesions, bone dysplasias (fibroosseous lesions), vascular abnormalities, metabolic diseases, or physical changes such as fractures. Other chapters describe

> ### BOX 15-1
> ### *Analysis of Intraosseous Lesions*
>
> #### Step 1: Localize the Abnormality
> - Anatomic position (epicenter)
> - Localized or generalized
> - Unilateral or bilateral
> - Single or multifocal
>
> #### Step 2: Assess the Periphery and Shape
> **PERIPHERY**
> Well defined
> - Punched out
> - Corticated
> - Sclerotic
> - Soft tissue capsule
> Ill defined
> - Blending
> - Invasive
>
> **SHAPE**
> - Circular
> - Scalloped
> - Irregular
>
> #### Step 3: Analyze the Internal Structure
> - Totally radiolucent
> - Totally radiopaque
> - Mixed (describe pattern)
>
> #### Step 4: Analyze the Effects of the Lesion on Surrounding Structures
> - Teeth, lamina dura, periodontal membrane space
> - Inferior alveolar nerve canal and mental foramen
> - Maxillary antrum
> - Surrounding bone density and trabecular pattern
> - Outer cortical bone and periosteal reactions
>
> #### Step 5: Formulate a Radiographic Interpretation

the characteristic radiographic findings of these abnormalities. The analysis should strive at least to narrow the interpretation to one of these groups because this directs the next course of action for continued investigation and treatment. This is a good time to bring the clinical information such as patient history and clinical signs and symptoms into the decision-making process. Introducing this information at the end helps avoid the problem of trying to make the radiographic characteristics fit a preconceived diagnosis.

Decision 4: Ways to Proceed

After analyzing the images, the clinician must decide in what way to proceed. This may require further imaging, treatment, biopsy, or observation of the abnormality (watchful waiting). For example, if the lesion fits in the malignant category, the patient first should be referred to an oral and maxillofacial radiologist to complete the diagnostic imaging, thus permitting the radiologist to determine the extent of the lesion, and to select the biopsy site; then the patient should be referred to a surgeon for biopsy and treatment. Cemental dysplasia may not require any further investigation or treatment. In other cases a period of watchful waiting, followed by reexamination in a few months, may be indicated if the abnormality appears benign and no clear need for treatment exists.

With advanced training or experience in diagnostic imaging, the practitioner may be able to name one specific abnormality or at least make a short list of entities from one of the divisions of acquired abnormalities. It may be necessary to create a radiographic report for the purposes of documentation and communication with other clinicians.

The Radiographic Report

The radiographic report can be subdivided into the following subsections:

Patient and general information. This section appears at the beginning of the report and contains the following information: address of the radiology clinic; the date of the dictation; the referring clinician's name; clinic or address; the patient's name, age, and gender; and any numerical identification such as a clinic or medical registration number.

Imaging procedure. This section provides a list of the imaging procedures provided, along with the date of the examination. For example: Panoramic and intraoral maxillary standard occlusal films plus axial and coronal CT images of the mandible with administration of contrast made on February 20, 2002.

Clinical information. This optional section includes pertinent clinical information regarding the patient and is provided by the referring clinician or the clinician dictating the report if a clinical examination was made before proceeding to the radiological examination. The clinical information should be concise and to the point and summarize the relevant information. For example: Mass in floor of mouth, possible ranula, and patient has a history of lymphoma.

Findings (observations). This section is composed of an objective, detailed list of observations, without interpretation, made from the diagnostic images. Using the step-by-step analysis of the extent of the lesion, periphery and shape, internal structure, and effects on surrounding structures will ensure completeness.

Radiographic interpretation (or impression). This section should be shorter and provides an interpretation for the preceding observations. One should endeavor to provide a definitive interpretation, but when this is not possible, a short list of conditions (in order of likelihood) is acceptable. In some situations advice regarding additional studies, when required, and treatment may be included.

Finally, the name and signature of the clinician composing the report is included.

SELF-TEST

Using the following illustrated case, practice the analytic technique. Look at Fig. 15-5, *A* and *B*, and write down all your observations and the results of your diagnostic algorithm before reading the following section.

Description
Location. The abnormality is singular and unilateral, and the epicenter lies coronal to the mandibular first molar.

Periphery and shape. The lesion has a well-defined cortical boundary and a spherical or round shape. The periphery also attaches to the cementoenamel junction.

Internal structure. The internal structure is totally radiolucent.

Effects. This lesion has displaced the first molar in an apical direction, which reinforces the decision that the origin was coronal to this tooth. Also, the lesion has displaced the second molar distally and the second pre-

molar in an anterior direction. Apical resorption of the distal root of the second deciduous molar has occurred. The occlusal radiograph reveals that the buccal cortical plate has expanded in a smooth, curved shape, and a thin cortical boundary still exists.

Analysis. Making all the observations is an important first step; the following is an analysis built on these observations. To accomplish this next step, further knowledge of pathologic conditions and a certain amount of practice are required. The first objective is to select the correct category of diseases (e.g., inflammatory, benign tumor, cyst); at this point, try not to let all the names of specific diseases overwhelm you.

These images reveal an abnormal appearance. The coronal location of the lesion suggests that the tissue making up this abnormality probably is derived from a component of the dental follicle. The effects on the surrounding structures indicate that this abnormality is acquired. The displacement and resorption of teeth, intact peripheral cortex, curved shape, and radiolucent internal structure all indicate a slow-growing, benign, space-occupying lesion, most likely in the cyst category. Odontogenic tumors such as an ameloblastic fibroma may be considered but are less likely because of the shape. The most common type of cyst in a follicular location is a follicular or dentigerous cyst. Odontogenic keratocysts occasionally are seen in this location, but the tooth resorption and degree of expansion are not characteristic of that pathologic condition. Therefore the final interpretation is a follicular cyst, with odontogenic keratocyst and ameloblastic fibroma as possibilities in the differential diagnosis but less likely. Treatment usually is indicated for follicular cysts; therefore the patient is referred for surgical consultation.

BIBLIOGRAPHY

Worth HM: Principles and practice of oral radiologic interpretation, Chicago, 1972, Mosby.

CHAPTER 16

Dental Caries

ANN WENZEL

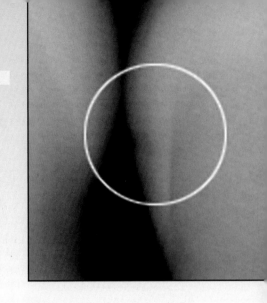

Dental caries is a multifactorial disease with interaction among three factors, the tooth, the microflora, and the diet. If not disturbed, bacteria accumulate at specific tooth sites to form what is known as *bacterial plaque (biofilm)*. The development of caries requires both the presence of bacteria and a diet containing fermentable carbohydrates. Caries is an infectious disease since it is the lactic acid produced by bacteria from the fermentation of carbohydrates that causes the dissolution, or demineralization, of the dental hard tissues. The mutans group of streptococci plays a central role in the demineralization. In the initial stages of the disease bacteria are located on the tooth surface. It is only after severe demineralization or cavity formation has occurred that bacteria penetrate into the hard tissues. The demineralized tooth surface, called the *carious lesion,* is thus not the disease but is a reflection of ongoing or past microbial activity in the plaque.

The initial carious lesion is a subsurface loss of mineral in the outer tooth surface. It appears clinically as a chalky white (indicating present activity) or an opaque or dark, brownish spot (indicating past activity). A lesion beneath active bacterial plaque will progress, slow or fast, but if this biofilm is removed or disturbed, the lesion will arrest. An arrested lesion may become re-active, however, and progress any time there is activity in the biofilm. Alternatively, remineralization in the outer parts of an arrested lesion can occur, for example, after the use of fluorides. Caries is therefore an ever-dynamic process.

The rate and extent of mineral loss depends on many factors. Mineral loss occurs faster in an active lesion when intercrystalline voids form. Demineraliza-tion may extend well into dentin before a breakdown of the outer surface (cavitation) occurs, resulting in a clinically visible cavity. With lesion progression and no intervention, demineralization may progress through the enamel, the dentin, and eventually into the pulp and may destroy the tooth (Fig. 16-1).

Use of Intraoral Radiographs

Radiography is useful for detecting dental caries because the caries process causes demineralization of enamel and dentin. The lesion is seen in the radiograph as a radiolucent (darker) zone since the demineralized area of the tooth does not absorb as many x-ray photons as the unaffected portion. It is important to keep in mind, though, that the lesion detected in the radiograph is merely a result of the bacterial activity on the tooth surface and radiography cannot reveal whether the lesion is active or arrested. An old inactive lesion will still appear as a demineralized "scar" in the hard tissues (Fig. 16-2). This is because remineralization takes place only in its outermost surface, as mineral-containing solutions from saliva cannot diffuse into the body of the lesion. Since the radiograph only mirrors the current extent of demineralization, one radiograph alone cannot distinguish between an active and an arrested lesion. Only a second radiograph taken at a later time can reveal whether the disease is active. When a decision is made to monitor a lesion, factors such as oral hygiene, fluoride exposure, diet, caries history, extent of restorative care, and age should be considered in determining the time interval between the radiographic examinations (see Chapter 14).

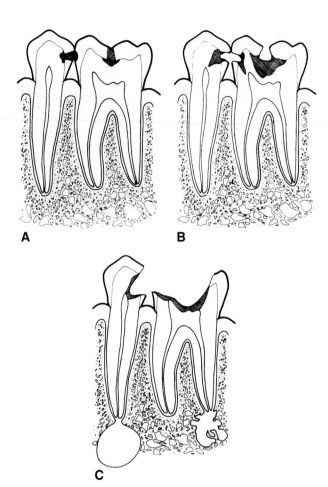

FIG. **16-1** **A,** Proximal and occlusal demineralization penetrating through tooth enamel and into the dentin. **B,** Proximal and occlusal tissue demineralization and cavitation nearing the pulp chamber of two vital teeth. **C,** Severe demineralization and cavitation reaching the pulp chamber, resulting in two nonvital pulps and periapical inflammatory disease.

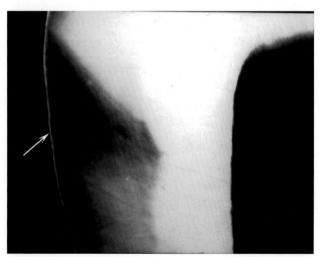

FIG. **16-2** Microradiograph of an inactive carious lesion *(dark region)* in enamel with an intact, well-mineralized surface *(arrow).*

Radiography is a valuable supplement to a thorough clinical examination of the teeth for detecting caries. A careful clinical examination assessing the carious activity on the tooth surface may be possible for smooth surfaces and to some extent for occlusal surfaces. However, when the surface is clinically intact—that is, no breakdown leading to cavitation has occurred—even the most meticulous examination may fail to reveal demineralization beneath the surface, including occlusal surfaces. Clinical access to proximal tooth surfaces in contact is quite limited. Indeed, numerous clinical studies have shown that a radiographic examination can reveal carious lesions both in occlusal and proximal surfaces that would otherwise remain undetected.

Radiographic Examination to Detect Caries

The bitewing projection is the most useful radiographic examination for detecting caries (see Chapter 8). The use of a film holder with a beam-aiming device (see Fig. 8-6) reduces the number of overlapping contact points and improves image quality, thus minimizing interpretation errors. Periapical radiographs are useful primarily for detecting changes in the periapical bone. Use of a paralleling technique for obtaining periapical radiographs increases the value of this projection in detecting caries of both anterior and posterior teeth, especially with heavily restored teeth.

Traditionally, size-2 "adult" films are used for a bitewing examination from the age of approximately 7 to 8 years onward. When it is necessary to examine all the contact surfaces from the cuspid to the most distal molar, usually two bitewing films per side are required (Fig. 16-3). The use of a single size-3 film often results in overlapping contact points and "cone-cut" images and is not recommended. In small children the size-0 or "child" film may be used (Fig. 16-4).

In recent decades there has been a dramatic decline in the prevalence of caries in all Western countries, leaving a smaller fraction of the population with rapidly progressing carious lesions. Accordingly, the interval between examinations should be customized for each individual patient and based on the perceived caries activity and susceptibility. For caries-free individuals the interval may be lengthened, whereas for caries-active individuals the interval should be shorter.

Radiographs used to detect carious lesions should be mounted in frames with dark borders and interpreted using a magnifying glass, particularly when evaluating the extent of small superficial lesions. Fig. 16-5 is a series of radiographs showing early lesions with and without magnification.

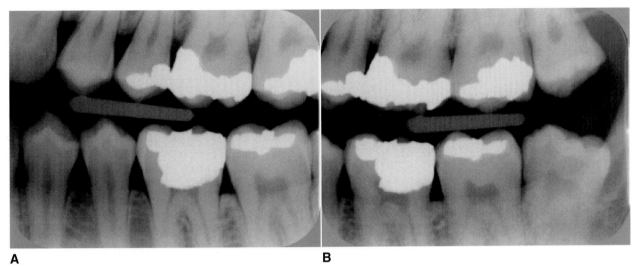

A   B

FIG. **16-3** Two bitewings from the patient's left side covering the surfaces from the distal surface of the canine to the distal surface of the most posterior molar.

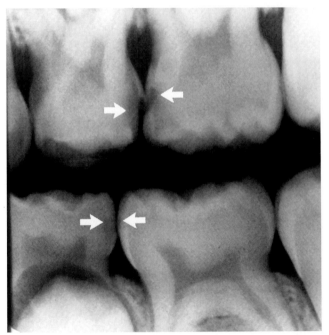

FIG. **16-4** Posterior bitewing using a size-0 film, demonstrating both permanent and deciduous teeth. Note the proximal carious lesions *(arrows)*.

Digital Image Receptors for a Bitewing Examination

Digital image receptors have recently become available for intraoral radiography. There are two different methods available: solid-state sensors (CCD and CMOS technology), in which a cord connects the receptor to the computer, and storage phosphors that use a film-like plate that is processed (scanned) after exposure. These receptors are described in Chapter 12. The holders available for bitewing examinations with phosphor plates appear similar to those for film, and recently universal sensor holders have also become available. However, there may be some problems when solid-state sensors are used for bitewing examination. First, the surface area of the sensor is smaller than the surface area of a size-2 film, resulting in the display of an average of three fewer interproximal tooth surfaces per bitewing image than with film. Furthermore, the stiffness and increased thickness of these sensors may result in more projection errors and retakes. When digital bitewing images are used, they should be displayed on a monitor in their full resolution (Fig. 16-6) for interpretation and viewed in a room with subdued light.

Radiographic Detection of Lesions

PROXIMAL SURFACES

The shape of the early radiolucent lesion in the enamel is classically a triangle with its broad base at the tooth surface (see Fig. 16-5), spreading along the enamel rods, but other appearances are common, such as a "notch," a dot, a band, or a thin line (Fig. 16-7). When the demineralizing front reaches the dentinoenamel junction (DEJ), it spreads along the junction, frequently forming the base of a second triangle with apex directed towards the pulp chamber. This triangle typically has a wider base than in the enamel and progresses

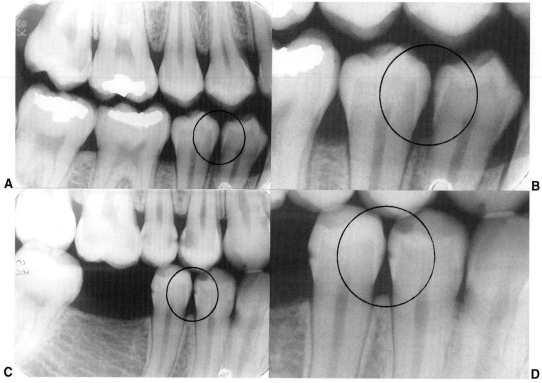

FIG. **16-5**   A magnifying glass is important for examining the extent of carious lesions. **A** and **C** are not magnified. **B** and **D** are magnified.

towards the pulp along the direction of the dentinal tubules. Again, more irregular shapes of decalcification may be seen (Fig. 16-8).

A lesion in proximal surfaces most commonly is found in the area between the contact point and the free gingival margin (Fig. 16-9). The fact that the lesion does not start below the gingival margin helps distinguish a carious lesion from cervical burnout (see Fig. 9-2). Close attention should be paid to intact proximal surfaces adjacent to a tooth surface with a restoration since occasionally this surface is inadvertently damaged during the restorative procedure and is thus at greater risk for caries (Fig. 16-10).

Because the proximal surfaces of posterior teeth are often broad, the loss of small amounts of mineral from incipient lesions and the advancing front of active lesions are often difficult to detect in the radiograph. Lesions confined to enamel may not be evident radiographically until approximately 30% to 40% demineralization has occurred. For this reason, the actual depth of penetration of a carious lesion is often deeper than seen radiographically.

Even experienced dentists often do not agree on the presence or absence of caries when examining the same set of radiographs, especially when the lesions are limited to the enamel. On occasion a lesion may be detected when the tooth surface is actually unaffected (a false-positive outcome). Various dental anomalies such as hypoplastic pits and concavities produced by wear can mimic the appearance of caries. In cases in which the demineralization is not yet radiographically visible, failure to detect the lesions is a false-negative outcome (Fig. 16-11). Approximately half of all proximal lesions in enamel cannot be detected by radiography. The possibility of false-positive diagnoses of small lesions, combined with the knowledge that caries progresses slowly in most individuals, argues for a conservative approach to caries diagnosis and treatment. A lesion extending into the dentin in the radiograph may be easier to detect with greater agreement among experienced observers. Occasionally demineralization in the enamel is not obvious, and a dentinal lesion is overlooked (see Fig. 16-8).

Potentially, a progressing proximal lesion may be arrested if cavitation has not developed. If cavitation has occurred, the lesion will always be active since the bacteria that colonize within the cavity cannot be removed. Unfortunately, the presence of cavitation cannot be accurately determined radiographically, although the greater the radiographic depth of the

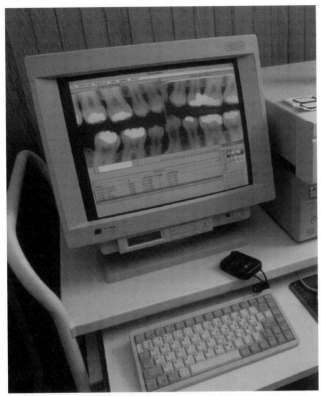

FIG. **16-6** Two bitewings captured on storage phosphor plates and displayed on a 17-inch monitor.

lesion, the greater the likelihood of cavitation. Since extensive demineralization must occur before the surface breaks down, the percentage of enamel lesions with surface cavitation is very small. Approximately half of lesions that are just into dentin have surface cavitation. The deeper the lesion has penetrated into dentin, the more likely it is cavitated, and dentinal lesions extending more than half way to the pulp are always cavitated. Temporarily separating proximal surfaces with orthodontic elastics or springs may allow direct inspection to determine whether there is cavitation. This method is easier in children than in adults.

The above considerations mean that operative treatment is usually not needed for lesions detected in enamel, and the dentist and the patient may arrest lesion progression with conservative intervention. Cavitated lesions, on the other hand, need operative treatment. For dentinal lesions, the decision whether to provide operative treatment is individualized for each patient. In cases in which it is decided to monitor the lesion, a follow-up radiograph should be taken to evaluate whether the lesion has arrested or is progressing. The interval between the radiographic examinations should also be determined individually, taking into account previous caries history, age, and not least, site

of the lesion, because the progression rate differs highly among the various tooth surfaces. Care should be taken to reproduce the same image geometry in the follow-up radiographs to provide a means of accurate comparison of depth of the lesion. When digital images are made with reproducible geometry, they can be superimposed and the information in the one image can be subtracted from the other (subtraction image), which displays the changes that have occurred between the two examinations (Fig. 16-12).

Progression of a lesion indicates the need for operative therapy. With highly motivated patients who clean the surface and with topical fluoride treatment, more than half of shallow dentinal lesions can be arrested, thus avoiding restorative therapy.

OCCLUSAL SURFACES

Carious lesions in children and adolescents most often occur on occlusal surfaces of posterior teeth. The demineralization process originates in enamel pits and fissures, where bacterial plaque can gather. The lesion spreads along the enamel rods and, if undisturbed, penetrates to the DEJ, where it may be seen as a thin radiolucent line between enamel and dentin.

Occlusal lesions commonly start in the sides of a fissure wall rather than at the base and then tend to penetrate nearly perpendicularly toward the DEJ. Early lesions appear clinically as chalky white, yellow, brown, or black discolorations of the occlusal fissures. Findings such as discolored fissures in a clinically intact occlusal surface suggest that a radiographic examination is indicated to determine whether a carious lesion exists. A clinical cavity is an indication that the lesion has already penetrated well into dentin. Therefore, a careful clinical examination must always precede the radiographic examination.

When an occlusal lesion is confined to enamel, the surrounding enamel often obscures the lesion. As the carious process progresses, a radiolucent line extends along the DEJ. As the lesion extends into the dentin, the margin between the carious and noncarious dentin is diffuse, and may obscure the fine radiolucent line at the DEJ. Therefore, false-positive detection rates may be as high as false-negative ones (Fig. 16-13). A false-negative outcome may not represent a severe mistake since in most cases the process progresses slowly and the lesion is detected at a later time. A false-positive outcome may result in a sound surface being irreversibly damaged. Also, when there is a sharply defined density difference, such as between enamel and dentin, there may appear to be a more radiolucent region immediately adjacent to the enamel. This is an optical illusion referred to as the *mach band*. This illusion can

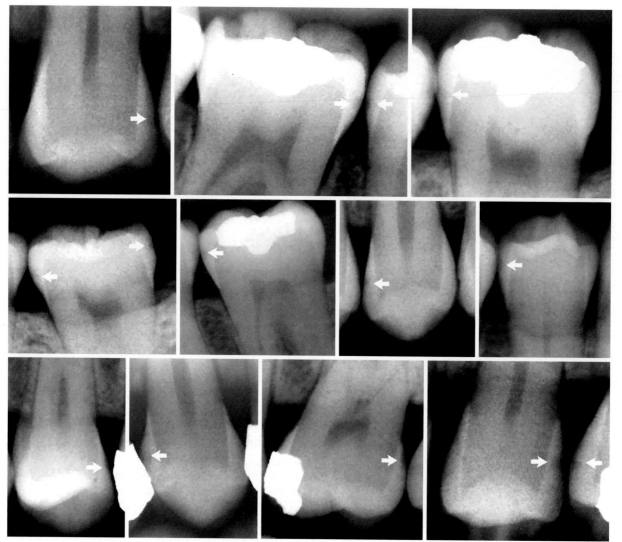

FIG. **16-7** *Incipient proximal enamel lesions.* Arrows indicate the areas showing demineralization. Note the shape, size, and location of these 14 early lesions.

contribute to the number of false-positive interpretations; therefore, when there are no clinical signs of a lesion, it is reasonable to observe these cases and withhold operative treatment.

The classic radiographic appearance of occlusal caries extending into the dentin is a broad-based, radiolucent zone, often beneath a fissure, with little or no apparent changes in the enamel. The deeper the occlusal lesion, the easier it is to detect on the radiograph (Fig. 16-14). This figure shows examples of occlusal caries with radiolucent changes indicating the need for operative treatment. A pitfall in the interpretation of dentinal occlusal lesions is superimposition of the image of the buccal pit, with or without a carious lesion, which may simulate an occlusal lesion (Fig. 16-15). Direct clinical inspection of the tooth most often

eliminates any such confusion. Occasionally demineralization in dentin may be quite extensive with a clinically intact surface and may only be detected radiographically.

As occlusal caries spreads through the dentin, it undermines the enamel, and eventually masticatory forces cause cavitation. Breakdown of the surface is clinically obvious if a thorough cleaning of the surface precedes the clinical examination.

Severe, rapidly progressing carious destruction of teeth is usually termed *rampant caries* and is usually seen in children with poor dietary and oral hygiene habits. This condition, however, is becoming increasingly rare because of widespread availability of water fluoridation and enlightened practices of good nutrition and hygiene. Rampant caries may also be seen in people suf-

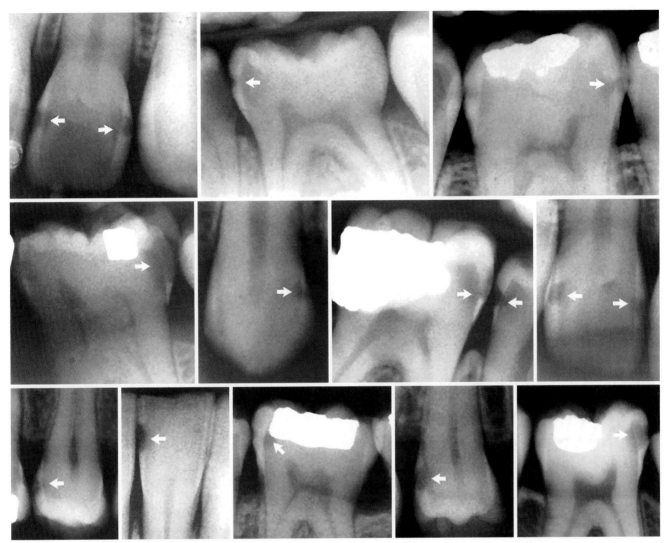

FIG. **16-8** *Dentinal proximal caries.* Note the size, shape, and location of these 15 lesions and the radiographic changes (increased radiolucency) of both enamel and dentin.

fering xerostomia. Radiographs (Fig. 16-16) of individuals with rampant caries demonstrate severe (advanced) carious destructions, especially of the mandibular anterior teeth.

BUCCAL AND LINGUAL SURFACES

Buccal and lingual carious lesions often occur in enamel pits and fissures of teeth. When small, these lesions are usually round; as they enlarge, they become elliptic or semilunar. They demonstrate sharp, well-defined borders.

It may be difficult to differentiate between buccal and lingual caries on a radiograph. When viewing buccal or lingual lesions, the clinician should look for a uniform noncarious region of enamel surrounding

the apparent radiolucency (see Fig. 16-15). This well-defined circular area represents parallel noncarious enamel rods surrounding the buccal or palatal lesion. It may at times be necessary to examine more than one view of the area, because the buccal or lingual lesion may be superimposed on the DEJ and suggest occlusal caries. Occlusal lesions, however, ordinarily are more extensive than lingual or buccal caries, and their outline is not as well defined. Clinical evaluation with visual and tactile methods is usually the definitive method of detecting buccal or lingual lesions.

ROOT SURFACES

Root surface lesions involve both cementum and dentin and are associated with gingival recession. The exposed cementum is relatively soft and usually only 20 to 50 μm thick near the cementoenamel junction, so it rapidly degrades by attrition, abrasion, and erosion. Root surface caries should be detected clinically, and often radiographs are not needed for diagnosis. In proximal root surfaces radiographic examination may reveal lesions that have gone undetected (Fig. 16-17). A pitfall in the detection of root lesions is that a surface may appear to be carious as a result of the cervical burnout phenomenon (see Fig. 9-2). The true caries lesion may be distinguished from the intact surface primarily by the absence of an image of the root edge and by the

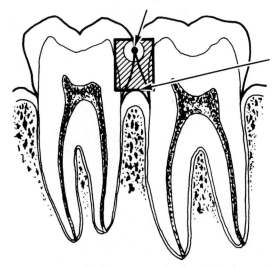

FIG. **16-9** *Proximal caries–susceptible zone.* This region extends from the contact point down to the height of the free gingival margin. It increases with recession of the alveolar bone and gingival tissues.

appearance of a diffuse rounded inner border where the tooth substance has been lost.

ASSOCIATED WITH DENTAL RESTORATIONS

A carious lesion developing at the margin of an existing restoration may be termed *secondary* or *recurrent caries.* It should be noted, though, that a lesion developing in a restored surface is most frequently a new primary demineralization, either because of faulty shaping or inadequate extension of the restoration leading to plaque accumulation (Fig. 16-18). These lesions (secondary caries) should be treated like any new caries lesion. It is important not to confuse secondary (primary) caries with residual caries, which is caries that remain if the original lesion is not completely removed.

A lesion next to a restoration may be obscured by the radiopaque image of the restoration. Thus the detection of secondary caries also depends on a careful clinical examination. Recurrent lesions at the mesiogingival and distogingival margins are most frequently detected radiographically. Examples of caries lesions next to dental restorations are seen in Fig. 16-18 on the mesial, distal, and occlusal borders of amalgam, gold, and composite dental restorations.

Restorative materials vary in their radiographic appearance depending on thickness, density, atomic number, and the x-ray beam energy used to make the radiograph. Some materials can be confused with caries. Older calcium hydroxide liners without barium, lead, or zinc (added to lend radiopacity) appear radiolucent and may resemble recurrent or residual caries.

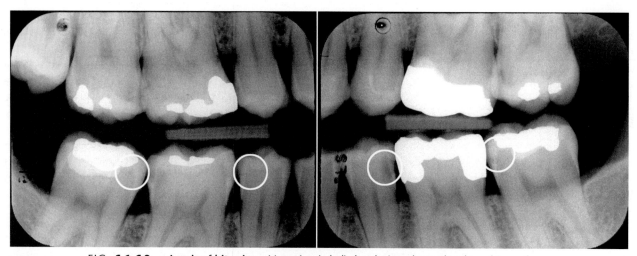

FIG. **16-10** *A pair of bitewings.* Note *(encircled)* that lesions have developed in surfaces adjacent to a restored surface but not in the same surfaces in the opposite side.

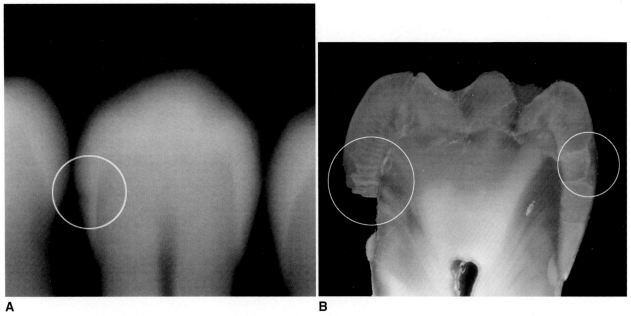

FIG. **16-11** **A,** Radiograph of an extracted tooth with a lesion just into dentin in the left side *(circle)* but no visible lesion in the right side. **B,** The same tooth after sectioning assessed under a microscope reveals lesions in both sides; the lesion in the right side is only in enamel.

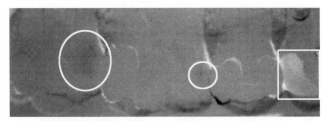

FIG. **16-12** Subtraction image made from two radiographs taken with 2 years' interval. The contours of four maxillary teeth can be seen. Between the two examinations a filling was placed *(rectangle)*, a new deep lesion has developed *(large circle)*, and a lesion has progressed from enamel into dentin *(small circle)*.

Despite the calcium present, the relatively large proportion of low atomic number material in calcium hydroxide causes its radiodensity to be similar to a carious lesion. Composite, plastic, or silicate restorations also may simulate lesions. It is often possible, however, to identify and differentiate these radiolucent materials from caries by their well-defined and smooth outline reflecting the preparation (Fig. 16-19).

AFTER RADIATION THERAPY

Patients who have received therapeutic radiation to the head and neck may suffer a loss of salivary gland function, leading to xerostomia (dry mouth). Untreated, this induces rampant destruction of the teeth, termed *radiation caries* (see Chapter 2). Typically, the destruction begins at the cervical region and may aggressively encircle the tooth, causing the entire crown to be lost, with only root fragments remaining in the jaws. The radiographic appearance of radiation caries is characteristic: radiolucent shadows appearing at the necks of teeth, most obvious on the mesial and distal aspects. Variations in the depth of destruction may be present, but generally there is uniformity within a given region of the mouth. Fig. 16-20 shows examples of radiation caries in patients with xerostomia following therapeutic radiation for cancer of the head and neck. Use of topical fluorides as remineralizing solutions and meticulous oral hygiene can markedly reduce the radiation damage to teeth resulting from xerostomia.

Alternative Diagnostic Tools to Detect Dental Caries

Other methods have been developed, in addition to clinical inspection and radiography, to detect carious lesions. These include light fluorescence (QLF), "Diagnodent" laser-light, fibre-optic transillumination

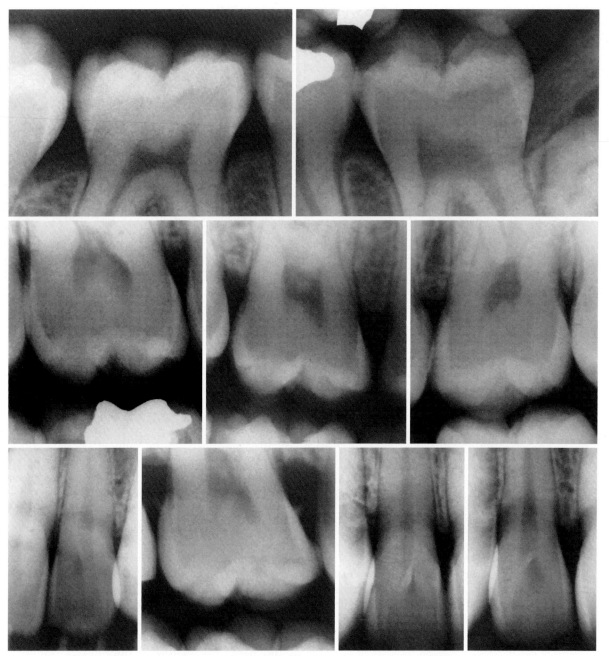

FIG. **16-13**   Little or no radiographic change, although clinically there were small occlusal lesions. Clinical observation is the definitive method for making treatment decision in these cases. Operative treatment is indicated only if the surface has a clinical cavity.

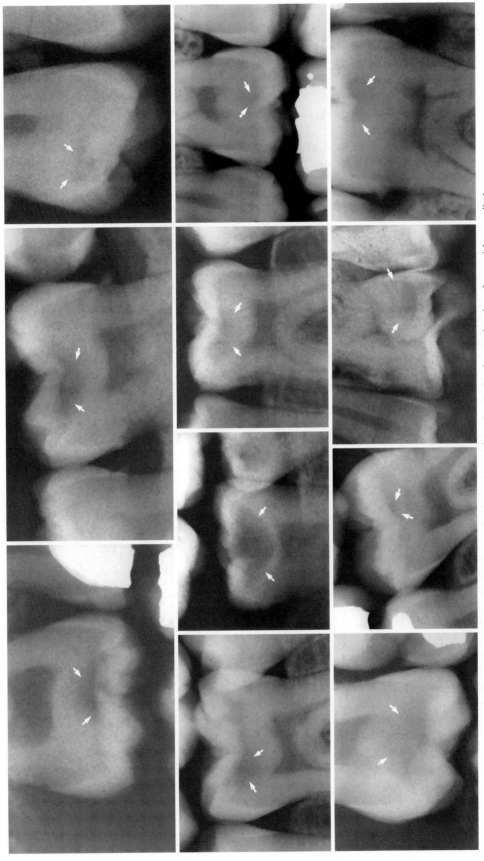

FIG. **16-14** Distinct radiolucencies within dentin in the occlusal surface with very little risk for a false-positive registration. Treatment is indicated whether or not a clinical cavity exists.

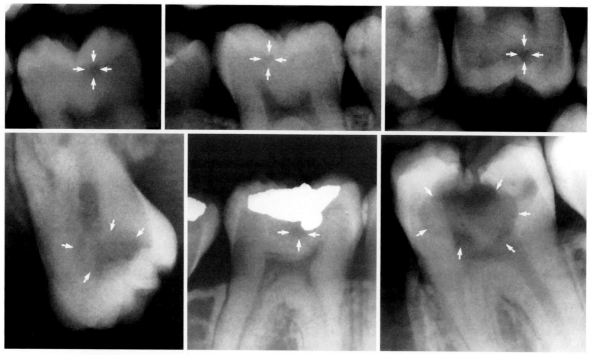

FIG. **16-15**   Note the uniform enamel surrounding the radiolucency. Clinical observation is the definitive method for making treatment decisions.

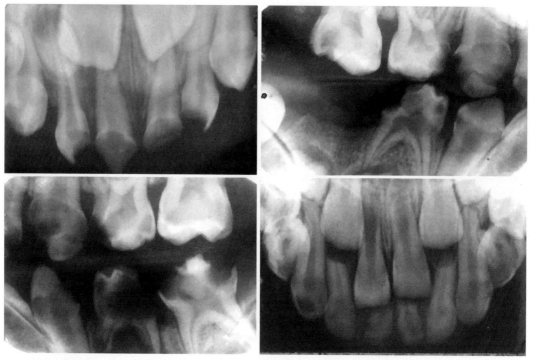

FIG. **16-16**   Rampant *(advanced)* caries in young children. (Courtesy Raphael Yeung, DDS, Alhambra, Calif.)

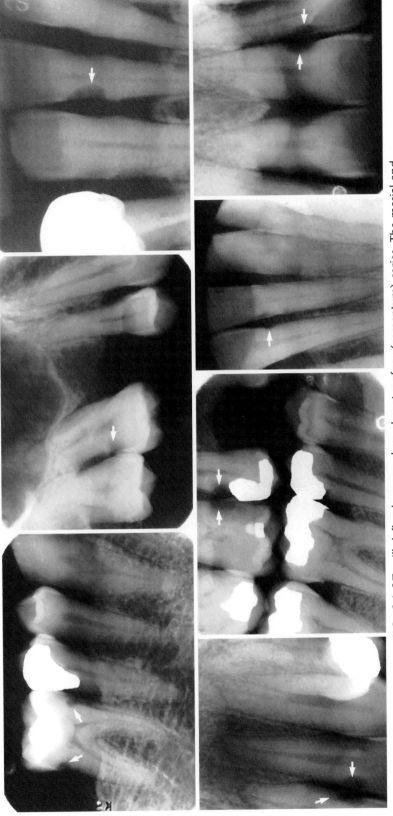

FIG. **16-17** Ill-defined, saucer-shaped root surface (cementum) caries. The mesial and distal portions of the root are exposed as a result of gingival recession.

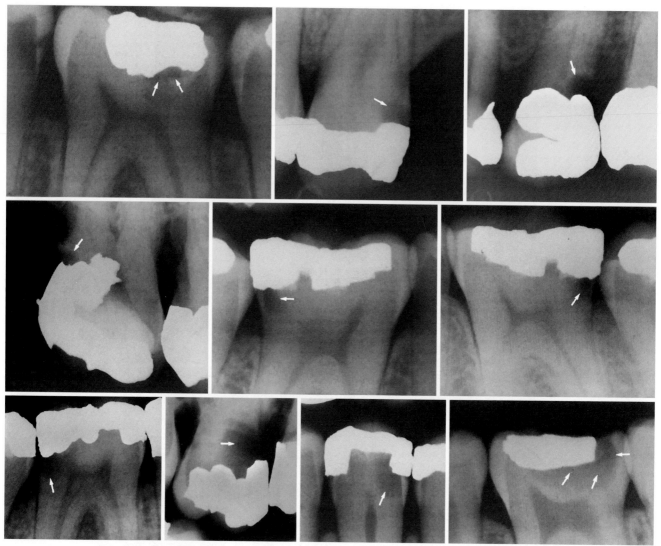

FIG. **16-18** *Recurrent carious lesions.* Note the increased radiolucency at the margins of existing restorations.

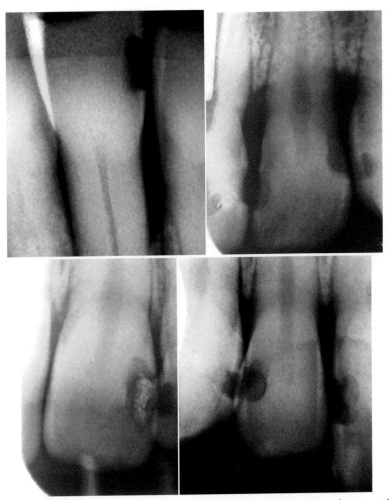

FIG. **16-19** *Restorative materials that resemble carious lesions.* Note the smooth classic outlines of these radiolucent areas, which are actually cavity preparations.

(FOTI), electrical conductance measurements (ECM), and ultrasound. QLF may be used to quantify mineral loss on smooth surfaces, whereas Diagnodent and ECM have been applied on occlusal surfaces. These two methods operate by displaying a value that provides quantitative information on the depth of the lesion. None of the methods can unequivocally distinguish between enamel and dentin lesions or between shallow and deep dentin lesions. Fiber optic trans-illumination (FOTI) has been used primarily for proximal surfaces but may also be applied to occlusal surfaces. FOTI is less sensitive than radiography for distinguishing shallow and deep lesions. ECM is better than FOTI in identifying occlusal caries in young children. There is little evidence yet that these methods can substitute traditional diagnostic methods in the clinic.

Treatment Considerations

Carious lesions in enamel require interceptive treatment but rarely operative treatment. The radiographic detection of small areas of demineralization require a decision of whether these represent active or inactive, arrested lesions. When the radiograph shows a lesion limited to enamel, the probability of cavitation is low and the prospect of arresting or reversing the caries process is good. Also, if the radiograph shows a lesion just into the dentin, treatment should include a means to stop the microbiologic activity and possibly reverse the demineralization process. Treatment of such lesions may include reductions in sugar intake, proper oral hygiene to reduce bacteria, and use of topical fluorides to inhibit microbiologic activity, retard demineralization, and promote remineralization of the outermost

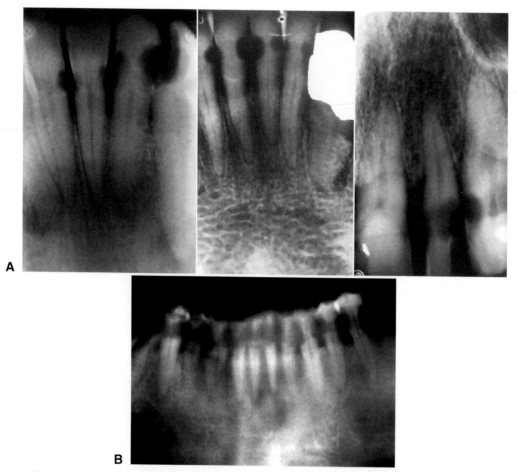

FIG. **16-20** *Examples of radiation caries.* Note the numerous large cervical carious lesions.

parts of the lesion. This may be successful if the surface of the tooth is intact and a follow-up radiograph shows no progression of the lesion. However, when the surface of a lesion is cavitated or follow-up radiographs reveal progression of the lesion, a restoration is required. Cavitated carious lesions require removal of the infected tissues and restoration of the tooth to form and function.

BIBLIOGRAPHY

American Dental Education Association: NIH Consensus Development Conference on Diagnosis and Management of Dental Caries Throughout Life, J Dent Educ 65, 2001.

Mandel ID: Caries prevention: current strategies, new directions, J Am Dent Assoc 127:1477, 1996.

Newbrun E: Cariology, ed 3, Baltimore, 1989, Williams & Wilkins.

Tanzer JM: Understanding dental caries: an infectious disease, not a lesion, Int J Oral Biol 22:205, 1997.

Thylstrup A, Fejerskov O: Textbook of Clinical Cariology, ed 2, Copenhagen, 1994, Munksgaard.

RADIOGRAPHIC CARIES DETECTION

De Araujo F et al: Diagnosis of approximal caries: radiographic versus clinical examination using tooth separation, Am J Dent 5:245, 1992.

Hintze H, Wenzel A: A two-film versus a four-film bite-wing examination for caries diagnosis in adults, Caries Res 33:380, 1999.

Hintze H, Wenzel A, Danielsen B: Behaviour of approximal carious lesions assessed by clinical examination after tooth separation and radiography: a 2.5-year longitudinal study in young adults, Caries Res 33:415, 1999.

Mejáre I, Källestål C, Stenlund H: Incidence and progression of approximal caries from 11 to 22 years of age in Sweden: a prospective radiographic study, Caries Res 33:93, 1999.

Mjör IA, Toffenetti F: Secondary caries: a literature review with case reports, Quintessence Int 31:165, 2000.

Nielsen LL, Hoernoe M, Wenzel A: Radiographic detection of cavitation in approximal surfaces of primary teeth using a digital storage phosphor system and conventional film, and the relationship between cavitation and radiographic lesion depth: an in vitro study, Int J Paediatr Dent 6:167, 1996.

Nyvad B, Fejerskov O: Assessing the stage of caries lesion activity on the basis of clinical and microbiological examination, Comm Dent Oral Epidemiol 25:69, 1997.

Petersson GH, Bratthall D: The caries decline: a review of reviews, Eur J Oral Sci 104:436, 1996.

Qvist V, Johannesen L, Bruun M: Progression of approximal caries in relation to iatrogenic preparation damage, J Dent Res 71:1370, 1992.

Ratledge DK, Kidd EAM, Beighton D: A clinical and microbiological study of approximal carious lesions. Part 1: the relationship between cavitation, radiographic lesion depth, the site specific gingival index and the level of infection of the dentine, Caries Res 35:3, 2001.

Wenzel A, Pitts N, Verdonschot EM, Kalsbeek H: Developments in radiographic caries diagnosis, J Dent 21:131, 1993.

Wenzel A: Current trends in radiographic caries imaging, Oral Surg Oral Med Oral Pathol Oral Radiol Endod 80:527, 1995.

Wenzel A: Digital radiography and caries diagnosis, Dentomaxillofac Radiol 27:3, 1998.

Wenzel A, Anthonisen PN, Juul MB: Reproducibility in the assessment of caries lesion behaviour: a comparison between conventional film and subtraction radiography, Caries Res 34:214, 2000.

White SC, Yoon DC: Comparative performance of digital and conventional images for detecting proximal surface caries, Dentomaxillofac Radiol 26:32, 1997.

TREATMENT DECISIONS

Bader JD, Shugars DA: What do we know about how dentists make caries-related treatment decisions? Comm Dent Oral Epidemiol 25:97, 1997.

de Vries H et al: Radiographic versus clinical diagnosis of approximal carious lesions, Caries Res 24:364, 1990.

Kidd EAM, Pitts NB: A reappraisal of the value of the bitewing radiograph in the diagnosis of posterior proximal caries, Br Dent J 1689:195, 1990.

Pitts NB: The use of bitewing radiographs in the management of dental caries: scientific and practical considerations, Dentomaxillofac Radiol 25:5, 1996.

Pitts NB: Diagnostic tools and measurements—impact on appropriate care, Comm Dent Oral Epidemiol 25:24, 1997.

Verdonschot EH et al: Developments in caries diagnosis and their relationship to treatment decisions and quality of care, Caries Res 33:32, 1999.

Woodward GL, Leake JL: The use of dental radiographs to estimate the probability of cavitation of carious interproximal lesions. Part I: evidence from the literature, J Can Dent Assoc 62:731, 1996.

CHAPTER 17

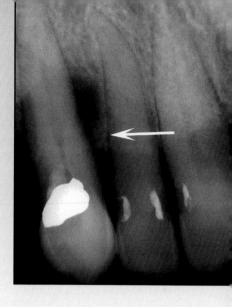

Periodontal Diseases

Several distinct, yet related disorders of the periodontium are collectively known as *periodontal disease*. The most common of these are gingivitis and periodontitis, which represent chronic infectious diseases. Essential components of these diseases are the presence of certain bacteria in plaque and the inflammatory host response. Gingivitis is a soft tissue inflammation involving the gingiva surrounding teeth. The transition to periodontitis entails the loss of soft tissue attachment and supporting bone of the involved teeth.

There are several other factors that may be involved with the etiology and the severity of periodontitis; these include systemic diseases such as diabetes, habits such as smoking, and in some instances, a genetic predisposition. Periodontitis has been subclassified into several types based primarily on the clinical manifestations. Some examples of these types are chronic, aggressive, necrotizing, those related to systemic disease, those related to abscess formation, and those in conjunction with endodontic lesions.

The causes of periodontal disease arise from an interplay of various host, bacterial, and environmental factors. The composition and type of plaque-forming bacteria, predominantly gram-negative bacteria, play an intimate role in the initiation of periodontal disease. These bacteria must have the ability to colonize the tooth and root surfaces, spread into the region between the root and the gingival margin, and in some cases invade the surrounding tissue. Also, the bacteria must be capable of causing damage to the host tissue either directly or more significantly indirectly by stimulating a host inflammatory reaction. The resulting inflammatory response causes loss of and apical migration of the epithelial attachment, resulting in pocket formation,

thus enhancing bacterial colonization. As part of the host response, the release of inflammatory mediators especially from neutrophils, is responsible for much of the injury to the surrounding soft tissue and stimulation of osteoclastic bone resorption.

The clinical manifestations of this interplay between bacterial plaque and the host tissue are clinical signs of inflammation. Gingivitis, seen as gingival swelling, edema, and erythema, is the most common first clinical sign, although some forms of periodontitis may be seen without gingivitis. Progression of these diseases leads to pocket formation, the universal manifestation of periodontal disease. Other clinical signs include bleeding, purulent exudate, edema, resorption of the alveolar crest, and tooth mobility. Rather than progressing smoothly from mild to moderate to severe, periodontitis often progresses in bursts. There are active periods of inflammation and tissue destruction followed by healing and quiescent periods (often years) of no appreciable change. The extent of disease activity is best measured by longitudinal probing of periodontal attachment level. This cycle of disease activity may repeat. The relative duration of the destructive and quiescent phases depends on the form of periodontitis, the nature of the bacterial pathogens, and the host response. Host factors such as systemic disease, age, immune system status, occlusal trauma, and stress influence the course of the disease. Spontaneous remission of the destructive process may even occur. The disease usually is painless, and most patients are unaware of its presence. Various forms of therapy are effective, including oral hygiene, scaling, and surgical treatment.

Those more prone to periodontal disease include smokers; older individuals; and people with poor education, neglected dental care, previous periodontal destruction, and system diseases such as diabetes. The prevalence of periodontal disease in the American population relies on the method of assessment and the threshold used. If loss of attachment by the formation of pockets measuring greater than 4 mm is used, the prevalence is about 23%. The incidence of adult periodontitis increases with age. The prevalence of aggressive periodontitis is less than 1%. It also appears that the prevalence of periodontal disease in the United States has declined in the last 30 years, but this may change with an increasing elderly population and an increase in retention of teeth.

Assessment of Periodontal Disease

CONTRIBUTIONS OF RADIOGRAPHS

Radiographs play an integral role in the assessment of periodontal disease. They provide unique information about the status of the periodontium and a permanent record of the condition of the bone throughout the course of the disease. Radiographs aid the clinician in identifying the extent of destruction of alveolar bone, local contributing factors, and features of the periodontium that influence the prognosis. Radiographs often are valuable in assessing specific points, which are presented in Box 17-1.

It is important to emphasize that the clinical and radiographic examinations are complementary. The clinical examination should include periodontal probing, a gingival index, mobility charting, and an evaluation of the amount of attached gingiva. Features that are not well delineated by the radiograph are most apparent clinically, and those that the radiograph best demonstrates are difficult to identify and evaluate clinically. Radiographs are an adjunct to the diagnostic process. Although a radiograph demonstrates advanced periodontal lesions well, other equally important changes in the periodontium may not be seen radiographically. Therefore a complete diagnosis of periodontal disease requires insight from a clinical examination of the patient combined with radiographic evidence.

LIMITATIONS OF RADIOGRAPHS

Radiographs may provide an incomplete presentation of the status of the periodontium. They have the following limitations:

1. Radiographs provide a two-dimensional view of a three-dimensional situation. Because the radiographic image fails to reveal the three-dimensional

BoX 17-1
Radiographic Assessment of Periodontal Conditions

Radiographs are especially helpful in the evaluation of the following points:
- Amount of bone present
- Condition of the alveolar crests
- Bone loss in the furcation areas
- Width of the periodontal ligament space
- Local initiating factors that cause or intensify periodontal disease
  - Calculus
  - Poorly contoured or overextended restorations
- Root length and morphology and the crown-to-root ratio
- Anatomic considerations
  - Position of the maxillary sinus in relation to a periodontal deformity
  - Missing, supernumerary, or impacted teeth
- Pathologic considerations
  - Caries
  - Periapical lesions
  - Root resorption

structure, bony defects overlapped by higher bony walls may be hidden. Also, because of overlapping tooth structure, only the interproximal bone is seen clearly. However, subtle changes in the density of the root structure (which is more radiolucent) may indicate bone loss on the buccal or lingual aspect of the tooth. Furthermore, use of multiple images made at different angulations, as in a full-mouth set, allows the viewer to use the buccal object rule to obtain three-dimensional information such as whether cortical plate loss has occurred on the buccal or lingual aspects.

2. Radiographs typically show less severe bone destruction than is actually present. The earliest (incipient) mildly destructive lesions in bone do not cause a sufficient change in density to be detectable.

3. Radiographs do not demonstrate the soft-tissue-to-hard-tissue relationships and thus provide no information about the depth of soft tissue pockets.

4. Bone level is often measured from the cementoenamel junction; however, this reference point is not valid in situations in which either overeruption or severe attrition with passive eruption exists.

For these reasons, although radiographs play an invaluable role in treatment planning, their use must be supplemented by careful clinical examination.

Technical Procedures

The usefulness of radiographs in the evaluation of periodontal disease can be improved by making radiographs with high technical quality. Interproximal (bitewing), in some cases vertical bitewings, and periapical radiographs are useful for evaluating the periodontium. This material is covered in greater detail in the chapters on projection geometry and intraoral radiographic technique (Chapters 5 and 8, respectively), but the features that are particularly important for imaging the alveolar bone are emphasized here.

FILM PLACEMENT AND BEAM ALIGNMENT

Place the film parallel with the long axis of the teeth or as near to this ideal position as the size and structure of the mouth permit. Direct the x-ray beam perpendicular to the long axis of the tooth and the plane of the film. These measures result in the best, undistorted images of the teeth and periodontal tissues. Interproximal (bitewing) images more accurately record the distance between the cementoenamel junction (CEJ) and the crest of the interradicular alveolar bone, because with interproximal views the beam is oriented at right angles to the long axis of the teeth, thus providing an accurate view of the relation of the height of the alveolar bone to the roots. Periapical views, especially in the posterior maxilla, may present a distorted view of the relationship between the teeth and the height of the alveolar bone, because the presence of the hard palate often requires the x-ray tube to be oriented slightly downward toward the posterior teeth to see the apices of these teeth. In this circumstance the level of the buccal alveolar bone may be projected near or even above the level of the lingual CEJ, thus making the bone height appear greater than it actually is.

The teeth will be depicted in their correct positions relative to the alveolar process when there is (1) no overlapping of the proximal contacts between crowns, (2) no overlapping of roots of adjacent teeth, and (3) overlapping of the buccal and lingual cusps of molars.

In recent years some periodontists have recommended the use of vertical interproximal radiographs for patients with periodontal disease. This method uses seven no. 2 films as vertical interproximal radiographs to cover the molar, premolar, canine, and midline regions. These views have the advantageous orientation of the interproximal views, yet show the reduced alveolar bone level even when bone loss has been considerable. Panoramic radiographs are not recommended for evaluation of periodontal disease because panoramic views tend to lead the clinician to underestimate minor marginal bone destruction and overestimate major destruction.

For radiography of the alveolar bone, a beam energy of 80 kVp should be used. Films that are slightly light are more useful for examining cortical margins of bone. A properly collimated beam reduces scattered radiation and improves image definition.

SPECIAL CONSIDERATIONS AND TECHNIQUES

The dentist must determine the optimal frequency of radiographic examination for patients with periodontal disease. Certainly, radiographs of all diseased areas must be available at the beginning of periodontal therapy to allow treatment planning and provide a baseline for later comparisons. The extent of continued disease activity, which can be determined clinically, should dictate the frequency of subsequent radiographic examinations.

Some clinicians have found it useful to superimpose fine wire grids when exposing radiographs to aid the measurement of relative bone height. Typically the grids form 1-mm squares (which show as fine, radiopaque lines on the resultant radiograph) that allow quantitative measurement of the position of the alveolar bone with respect to the dentition. This procedure can be useful in evaluating osseous changes over time but may be difficult because errors involved with the exact positioning of the film between examinations may lead to variations in image geometry.

In recent years computers and image-processing techniques have been used to enhance radiographs to achieve improved detection of alveolar bone loss associated with periodontal disease. The most widely used of these techniques is subtraction radiography (see Chapters 12 and 13). The advantage of this method is that it allows better detection of small amounts of bone loss between radiographs made at different times than may be achieved by visual inspection. However, radiographic subtraction is difficult to use because the images must be made with the same orientation of the primary x-ray beam, bone, and film at each examination, which is quite impractical and difficult to accomplish in general practice.

Normal Anatomy

The normal alveolar bone that supports the dentition has a characteristic radiographic appearance. A thin layer of opaque cortical bone often covers the alveolar crest. The height of the crest lies at a level approximately 1 to 1.5 mm below the level of the cementoenamel junctions (CEJs) of adjacent teeth. Between posterior teeth the alveolar crest also is parallel to a line connecting adjacent CEJs (Fig. 17-1). Between anterior teeth the alveolar crest usually is pointed and has a dense cortex. As between the posterior teeth, the alveolar crest between anterior teeth lies within 1 to 1.5 mm of a line connecting the adjacent CEJs (Fig. 17-2). A well-mineralized cortical outline of the alveolar crest indicates the absence of periodontitis activity. However, lack of a well-mineralized alveolar crest may be found in patients with or without periodontitis.

The alveolar crest is continuous with the lamina dura of adjacent teeth. In the absence of disease, this bony junction between the alveolar crest and lamina dura of posterior teeth forms a sharp angle next to the tooth root. The periodontal ligament space is often slightly wider around the cervical portion of the tooth root, especially in adolescents with erupting teeth. In this situation, if the lamina dura still forms a sharp, well-defined angle with the alveolar crest, the condition is a variant of normal and is not an indication of disease. The density of alveolar crests varies widely, and may be very thin at the crest. Therefore variation in density alone is not an indication of disease and may be a variation of normal.

Since gingivitis is an inflammatory condition confined to the gingiva, there are no significant changes to the underlying bone and therefore the radiographic appearance of the bone is normal.

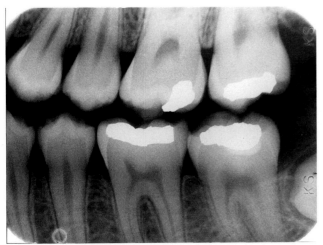

FIG. **17-1** The normal alveolar crest lies 1 to 1.5 mm below the adjacent CEJs and forms a sharp angle with the lamina dura of the adjacent tooth.

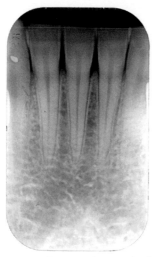

FIG. **17-2** Between the anterior teeth the alveolar crest normally is pointed and well corticated, coming to within 1 to 1.5 mm of the adjacent CEJs.

General Radiographic Features of Periodontal Disease

No matter the type of periodontal disease, the changes seen radiographically reflect changes seen with inflammatory lesions of bone. These changes can be divided into two aspects: changes in the morphology of the supporting alveolar bone and changes to the internal density and trabecular pattern. Changes in morphology become apparent because of loss of the interproximal crestal bone and bone overlapping the buccal or lingual aspects of the tooth roots. Changes to the internal aspect of the alveolar bone reflect a reduction or an increase in bone structure. A reduction is seen as an increase in radiolucency because of a decrease in number and density of existing trabeculae. An increase in bone is seen as an increase in radiopacity (sclerosis) as a result of an increase primarily in the thickness, density, and number of trabeculae. Similar to all inflammatory lesions of bone, periodontal disease usually involves a combination of bone loss and bone formation or sclerosis. However, acute early lesions display predominantly bone loss, whereas chronic lesions have a greater component of bone sclerosis. The following classifications are based in part on the radiographic appearance of periodontal disease.

Mild Periodontitis

The early lesions of adult periodontitis appear as areas of localized erosion of the interproximal alveolar bone crest (Fig. 17-3). The anterior regions show blunting of the alveolar crests and slight loss of alveolar bone height. The posterior regions may also show a loss of

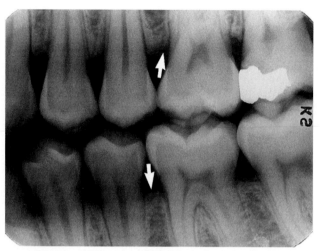

FIG. **17-3**   Initial periodontal disease is seen as a loss of cortical density *(arrows)* and a rounding of the junction between the alveolar crest and the lamina dura.

the normally sharp angle between the lamina dura and alveolar crest. In early periodontal disease, this angle may lose its normal cortical surface (margin) and appear rounded off, having an irregular and diffuse border. If only slight radiographic changes are apparent, the disease process may not be of recent onset because significant loss of attachment must be present for 6 to 8 months before radiographic evidence of bone loss appears. Also, variations in the x-ray beam's angle of projection can cause a slight change in the apparent

height of the alveolar bone. The presence of a mild lesion does not necessarily develop into a more severe lesion later. Small regions of bone loss on the buccal or lingual aspects of the teeth are much more difficult to detect.

Moderate Periodontitis

If the lesion of mild periodontitis progresses, the destruction of alveolar bone extends beyond early changes in the alveolar crest and may induce a variety of defects in the morphology of the alveolar crest. These patterns of bone loss have been divided into localized buccal or lingual cortical plate loss, generalized horizontal bone loss in a region, or localized vertical (angular) defects involving just one or two teeth. A radiograph is valuable in showing the extent and morphology of residual bone, but complete assessment of bone loss requires a clinical examination.

BUCCAL OR LINGUAL CORTICAL PLATE LOSS

The buccal or lingual cortical plate adjacent to the teeth may resorb. This type of loss is indicated by an increase in the radiolucency of the root of the tooth near the alveolar crest. The shape seen usually is a semicircular shadow with the apex of the radiolucency directed apically in relation to the tooth (Fig. 17-4).

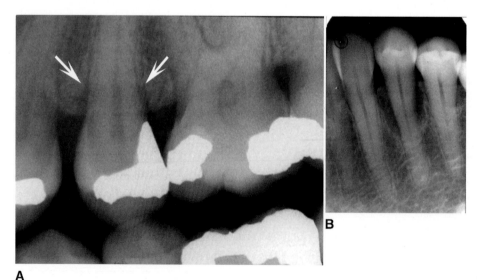

A

B

FIG. **17-4**   **A,** Example of a small bone loss of the alveolar crest lingual to the root of this maxillary second bicuspid *(arrows).* Note the roughly semicircular shape of the bone loss, resulting in the adjacent area of the tooth root being more radiolucent. **B,** Example of more profound loss of the lingual alveolar crest adjacent to this mandibular first bicuspid.

HORIZONTAL BONE LOSS

Horizontal bone loss is a term used to describe the radiographic appearance of loss in height of the alveolar bone around multiple teeth; the crest is still horizontal (i.e., parallel with the occlusal plane) but is positioned apically more than a few millimeters from the line of the cemental enamel junctions (CEJs). Horizontal bone loss may be mild, moderate, or severe, depending on its extent. Mild bone loss may be defined as approximately 1 mm of attachment loss, and moderate loss is anything greater than 1 mm up to the midpoint of the length of the roots or to the furcation level of the molars. Severe loss is anything beyond this point and often has evidence of furcation involvement of multirooted teeth. Care must be taken in using the CEJ as a reference point in cases of overeruption and severe attrition (Fig. 17-5). With overeruption the alveolar bone will not necessarily remodel to keep a normal relationship to the CEJ and similarly in passive eruption, which may accompany severe attrition.

In horizontal bone loss, the crest of the buccal and lingual cortical plates and the intervening interdental bone have been resorbed (Fig. 17-6). The extent of bone loss evident at a single examination does not indicate the current activity of the disease. For example, a patient who previously had generalized periodontal disease and subsequent successful therapy will likely always show bone loss but the bone level may remain stable.

VERTICAL OSSEOUS DEFECTS

The term *vertical* (or *angular*) *osseous defect* describes the types of bony lesions that are most commonly localized to one or two teeth. (An individual may have multiple osseous defects.) With these defects the crest of the remaining alveolar bone typically displays an oblique angulation to the line of the CEJs in the area of involved teeth.

Vertical osseous defects can be divided into two primary types. The interproximal crater is a two-walled, troughlike depression that forms in the crest of the interdental bone between adjacent teeth (Fig. 17-7). The infrabony defect is a vertical deformity within bone that extends apically along the root from the alveolar crest. This usually develops from bone loss extending down the root of the tooth and in its early form appears as abnormal widening of the periodontal ligament space at the CEJ (Fig. 17-8, *A*). The infrabony defect is described as *three-walled* (surrounded by three bony walls) when both buccal and lingual cortical plates remain; it is described as *two-walled* when one of these plates has been resorbed (Fig. 17-8, *B*) and as *one-walled* when both plates have been lost. The distinctions among these groups are important in designing the treatment plan.

Often infrabony defects are difficult or impossible to recognize on a radiograph because one or both of the cortical bony plates remain superimposed with the defect. Clinical and surgical inspections are the best means of determining the number of remaining bony

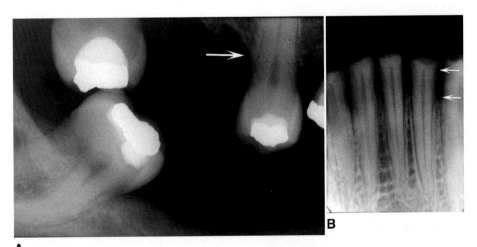

A

B

FIG. **17-5** **A,** This maxillary second bicuspid is overerupted; the etiology of the low bone level relative to the CEJ *(arrow)* is not necessarily due to periodontal disease. Similarly, **B** is an example of passive eruption secondary to severe attrition, and the apparent increase in the distance from the CEJ to the bone height *(arrows)* cannot be attributed to periodontal disease.

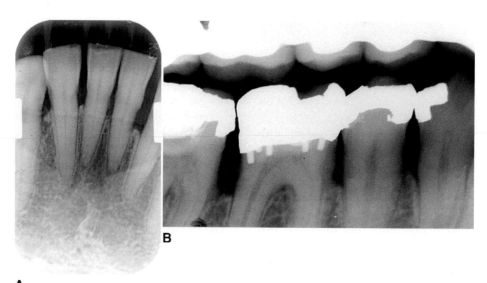

FIG. **17-6**   Horizontal bone loss is seen in the anterior region (**A**) and the posterior region (**B**) as a loss of the buccal and lingual cortical plates and interdental alveolar bone.

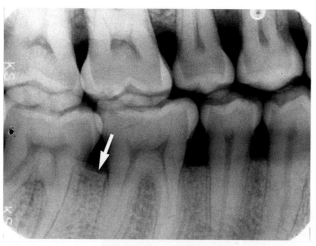

FIG. **17-7**   An interproximal crater, seen through a defect between the buccal and lingual cortical plates, shows as a radiolucency below the level of the crestal edges *(arrow)*.

walls. Visualization of the depth of pockets may be aided by inserting a gutta-percha point. The point follows the defect and appears on the radiograph because gutta-percha is relatively inflexible and radiopaque (Fig. 17-9).

SURROUNDING INTERNAL BONE CHANGES

As with all other inflammatory lesions, the inflammation may stimulate a reaction in the bone surrounding the periodontal lesion. The peripheral bone may appear more radiolucent or more sclerotic

(radiopaque), or more commonly, it may be a mixture of the two. Very rarely, no apparent change will be seen (see Fig. 17-8, *B*). A radiolucent change reflects loss of density and number of trabeculae, so that the trabeculae appear very faint; this is more commonly seen in early or acute lesions (Fig. 17-10, *A*). If the trabeculae are sufficiently decalcified, they may not appear in the radiographic image, although they are still present. This accounts for the apparent reformation of bone in some cases in which the acute inflammation resolves with successful treatment and the trabeculae remineralize. The sclerotic bone reaction appears radiopaque as a result of deposition of bone on existing trabeculae at the expense of the marrow, resulting in thicker trabeculae that may eventually be so dense as to appear as an amorphous radiopaque mass (Fig. 17-10, *B*). This sclerotic reaction may extend some distance from the periodontal lesion, sometimes to the inferior aspect of the mandible. Usually the surrounding bone reaction is a mixture of both bone loss and sclerosis.

Inflammatory products from a periodontal lesion can even extend through the cortex of the floor of the maxillary sinus to cause a regional mucositis (Fig. 17-11). In rare cases a periosteal reaction might be seen on the buccal or lingual aspect of the alveolar process.

Severe Periodontitis

In severe adult periodontitis the bone loss is so extensive that the remaining teeth show excessive mobility and drifting and are in jeopardy of being lost because

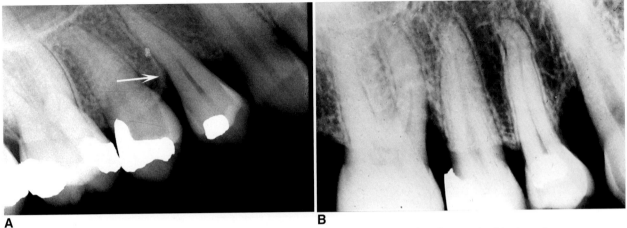

FIG. **17-8** **A,** Example of a developing vertical defect; note the abnormal widening of the periodontal ligament space *(arrow).* **B,** Maxillary periapical film reveals two examples of more severe vertical defects.

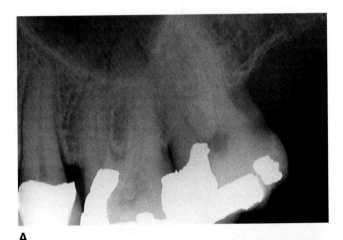

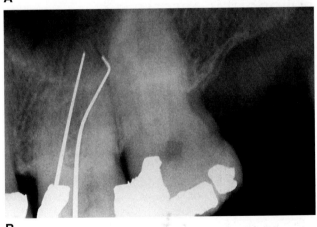

FIG. **17-9** Gutta-percha may be used to visualize the depth of infrabony defects. **A,** Radiograph fails to show the osseous defect without the use of the gutta-percha points. **B,** Radiograph reveals an osseous defect extending to the region of the apex. (Courtesy Dr. H. Takei, Los Angeles, CA.)

of inadequate support. Extensive horizontal bone loss or extensive vertical osseous defects may be present. As with moderate bone loss, the lesions seen during surgery usually are more extensive than is suggested by the radiographs alone.

OSSEOUS DEFORMITIES IN THE FURCATIONS OF MULTIROOTED TEETH

Progressive periodontal disease and its associated bone loss may extend into the furcations of multirooted teeth. As bone resorption extends down the side of a multirooted tooth, eliminating the bone covering the root, it can reach the level of the furcation and beyond. Widening of the periodontal ligament space at the apex of the interradicular bony crest of the furcation is strong evidence that the periodontal disease process involves the furcation (Fig. 17-12, *A*). If sufficient bone loss has occurred on the lingual and buccal aspects of a mandibular molar furcation, the radiolucent image of the lesion becomes prominent (Fig. 17-12, *B*). The bony defect may involve either the buccal or lingual cortical plate and extend under the roof of the furcation. In such a case, if the defect does not extend through to the other cortical plate, it appears more irregular and radiolucent than the adjacent normal bone. Using the buccal object rule with films of different angulations may make it possible to determine whether the buccal or the lingual cortical plate has been resorbed.

If the crestal bone is below the furcation but the disease process has not extended into the interradicular bone, the width of the periodontal membrane space appears normal. Also, the septal bone may appear more radiolucent but otherwise be normal. In the mandible

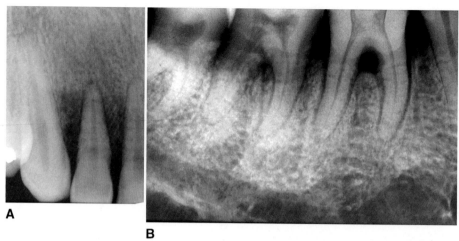

A   **B**

FIG. **17-10**   **A,** Example of a primarily radiolucent reaction around this maxillary lateral incisor. Note that the trabeculae toward the alveolar crest on the mesial and distal aspect of the tooth are barely perceptible. **B,** A periapical film revealing a predominantly sclerotic bone reaction to the periodontal disease. Note the individual thick trabeculae, especially mesial to the root of the first molar and the variation in density in other parts of the film due to the number and thickness of the trabeculae. The sclerotic reaction extends to the inferior alveolar canal.

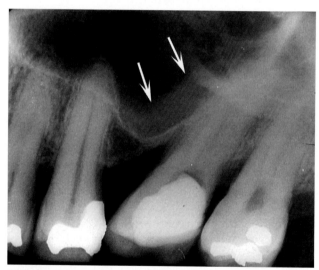

FIG. **17-11**   A periapical film revealing a localized mucositis within the maxillary sinus *(arrows)* immediately adjacent to a periodontal vertical defect.

the external oblique ridge may mask furcation involvement of the third molars. Convergent roots may also obscure furcation defects in maxillary and mandibular second and third molars.

Furcation defects involve maxillary molars about three times as often as mandibular molars. The loss of interradicular bone in the furcation of a maxillary molar may originate from the buccal, mesial, or distal surface of the tooth. The most common route for furcation involvement of the maxillary permanent first molar is from the mesial side. The image of furcation involvement is not as sharply defined around maxillary first molars as around mandibular molars because the palatal root is superimposed on the defect (Fig. 17-12, *C*). However, occasionally this pattern of bone destruction is prominent and appears as an inverted "J" shadow with the hook of the J extending into the trifurcation (Fig. 17-12, *D*).

PERIODONTAL ABSCESS

A periodontal abscess is a rapidly progressing, destructive lesion that usually originates in a deep soft tissue pocket. It occurs when the coronal portion of the pocket becomes occluded or when foreign material becomes lodged between a tooth and the gingiva. Clinically, pain and swelling are present in the region. If the lesion persists, a radiolucent region appears, often superimposed over the root of a tooth. A bridge of bone may be present over the coronal aspect of the lesion, separating it from the crest of the alveolar ridge (Fig. 17-13). After treatment, some of the lost bone may regenerate.

Aggressive Periodontitis

Aggressive periodontitis refers to periodontal disease with an aggressive and rapid nature that occurs in patients

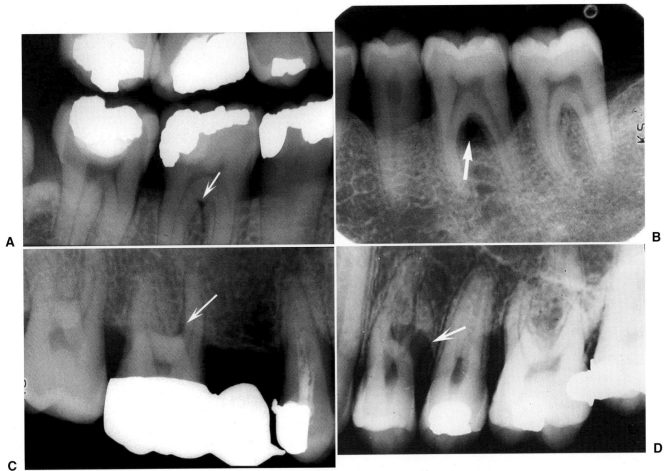

FIG. **17-12** **A,** A periapical film revealing very early furcation involvement of a mandibular molar characterized by slight widening of the periodontal ligament space in the furcation region. **B,** A periapical film revealing a profound radiolucent lesion within the furcation region *(arrow)* due to loss of bone in the furcation region as well as the buccal and lingual cortical plates. **C,** The angulation of this periapical view of a maxillary first molar projected the palatal root away from the trifurcation region revealing early widening of the furcation periodontal ligament space *(arrow).* **D,** Example of an inverted "J" shadow *(arrow)* resulting from bone destruction extending into the trifurcation region of a three-rooted maxillary first bicuspid.

under 30 years of age. The severity of the disease appears to be an exuberant reaction to a minimum amount of plaque accumulation and may result in early tooth loss. The term *aggressive periodontitis* replaces the formerly used term *early-onset periodontitis,* which included three classifications: localized juvenile periodontitis (LJP), generalized juvenile periodontitis (GJP), and rapidly progressing periodontitis (RPP). Aggressive periodontitis is subclassified into localized aggressive periodontitis (formerly LJP) and generalized aggressive periodontitis.

CLINICAL PRESENTATION

Localized aggressive periodontitis is associated with attachment loss involving the incisors and first molars. In this form the amount of bone loss correlates with the time of tooth eruption, in that the teeth that erupt first (incisors and first molars) have the most bone loss. This disease usually commences around puberty and the bone loss is rapid, up to 3 to 4 times that seen in chronic periodontitis. Of interest is the fact that there are usually very few signs of soft tissue inflammation or

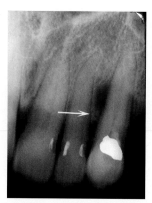

FIG. **17-13**   Example of a periodontal abscess related to the maxillary cuspid; note the well-defined area of bone loss over the midroot region of the tooth and extending in a mesial direction towards the lateral incisor. There appears to be a layer of bone (arrow) separating the area of bone destruction from the crest of the alveolar process.

plaque accumulation despite the presence of deep bony pockets. Often the patient will present with drifting and mobile incisors and early loss of first molars.

Generalized aggressive periodontitis can involve a variable number of teeth, from a least three to all of the dentition, and by definition is not confined to the first molars and incisors. This rapidly progressing disease usually affects individuals under 30 years of age. The gingiva

may appear normal as in the localized form or may present with exuberant inflammatory response. If there is a history of premature loss of deciduous teeth and the permanent teeth are rapidly lost soon after erupting, a possible diagnosis of Papillon-Lefèvre syndrome might be considered. This syndrome usually has an associated hyperkeratosis of palmer and planter surfaces.

Estimates of prevalence of localized aggressive periodontitis in the United States is 0.53%; for the generalized form, 0.13%. In a recent survey aggressive periodontitis was found in 10% of African-American, 5% of Hispanic, and 1.3% of white U.S. adolescents.

RADIOGRAPHIC APPEARANCE

The radiographic appearance of the bone loss in the localized aggressive periodontitis typically is vertical (Fig. 17-14). Maxillary teeth are involved slightly more often than mandibular teeth, and strong left-right symmetry is common. The generalized form of aggressive periodontitis can involve several teeth or all the dentition, and the rapid bone loss may be of the vertical or angular or horizontal pattern.

TREATMENT

Early identification and treatment of aggressive periodontitis is important because of the rapid progression

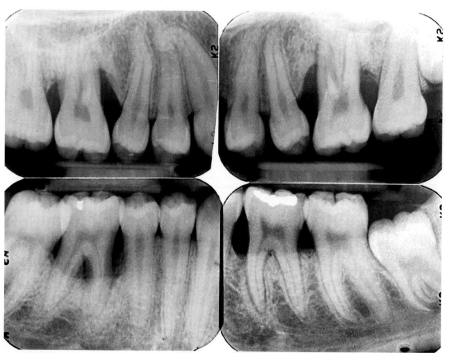

FIG. **17-14**   Typical vertical bone loss in juvenile periodontitis. Note the localization to the region of the first molars. (Courtesy Dr. T.D. Charbeneau, Dallas, Texas.)

of this condition and the associated tooth loss. The disease responds to total plaque control, just as adult periodontitis does. Treatment often consists of scaling, curettage, and administration of antibiotics.

Dental Conditions Associated With Periodontal Diseases

Various changes in the dentition and its supporting structures that frequently are associated with periodontal disease and may contribute to the exacerbation of the disease, include overhanging and faulty restorations, occlusal trauma, tooth mobility, open contacts, and local irritation. These conditions usually are apparent on radiographs.

OCCLUSAL TRAUMA

Traumatic occlusion causes degenerative changes in response to occlusal pressures that are greater than the physiologic tolerances of the tooth's supporting tissues. These lesions occur as a result of malfunction caused by excessive occlusal force on teeth or by normal forces on a periodontium compromised by bone loss. In addition to clinical symptoms such as increased mobility, wear facets, unusual response to percussion, and a history of contributing habits, there are associated radiographic findings that include widening of the periodontal ligament (PDL) space, widening of the lamina dura, bone loss, and an increase in the number and size of trabeculae. Other sequelae of traumatic occlusion include hypercementosis and root fractures. However, traumatic occlusion can be diagnosed only by clinical evaluation and not simply by the radiographic findings alone. Traumatic occlusion does not cause gingivitis or periodontitis, affect the epithelial attachment, or lead to pocket formation.

TOOTH MOBILITY

Widening of the PDL space suggests tooth mobility, which may result from occlusal trauma or a lack of bone support arising from advanced bone loss. If the affected tooth has a single root, the socket may develop an hourglass shape. If the tooth is multirooted, it may show widening of the PDL space at the apices and in the region of the furcation. These changes result when the tooth moves about an axis of rotation at some midpoint on the roots. In addition, the radiographic image of the lamina dura may appear broad and hazy and show increased density (osteosclerosis).

OPEN CONTACTS

When the mesial and distal surfaces of adjacent teeth do not touch, the patient has an open contact. This condition is potentially dangerous to the periodontium because of the potential for food debris to become trapped in the region. Trapped food particles may damage the soft tissue and induce an inflammatory response and contribute to the development of localized periodontal disease. Open contacts are associated with periodontal disease more than closed contacts. Similar potential situations in which periodontal disease may develop include discrepancies in the height of two adjacent marginal ridges or tipped teeth (Fig. 17-15). Abnormal tooth alignment does not cause periodontal disease but provides an environment in which the disease may develop because of difficulty in maintaining adequate oral hygiene.

LOCAL IRRITATING FACTORS

Other local factors that are radiographically apparent may provide an environment in which periodontal disease may develop or may aggravate existing periodontal disease. For instance, calculus deposits can prevent effective cleansing of a sulcus and lead to the progression of periodontal disease and enhance plaque formation. Similarly, defective restorations with overhanging or poorly contoured margins can lead to the accumulation of plaque, thus providing an environment

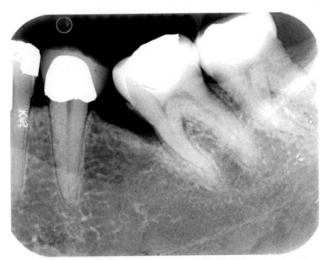

FIG. **17-15** The second molar has tipped mesially after loss of the first molar, creating an abnormal tooth alignment that was difficult for the patient to maintain and in this case developed localized periodontal disease. Note the calculus on the mesial surface of the second molar. The crown on the second premolar was constructed with an enlarged distal contour to stop further tipping of the molar.

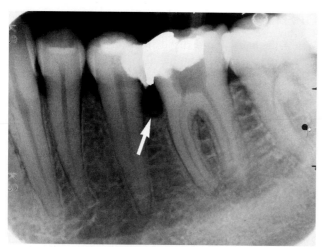

FIG. **17-16**   These overhanging restorations provided an environment suitable for the development of localized periodontal disease and subsequent bone loss *(arrow)*.

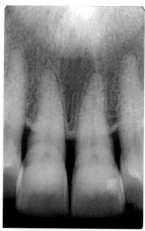

FIG. **17-17**   This periapical film is an example of a case in which the interproximal cortex has reformed after successful periodontal therapy.

in which periodontal disease may develop (Fig. 17-16). Radiographs often reveal these conditions.

Evaluation of Periodontal Therapy

Radiographs may show signs of successful treatment of periodontal disease. In some cases there may be reformation of the interproximal cortex (Fig. 17-17) and the normal sharp line angle between the cortex and lamina dura. The relatively radiolucent margins of bone that were undergoing active resorption before treatment may become more sclerotic (radiopaque) after successful therapy. In cases in which there has been considerable mineral loss of the cancellous bone (radiolucent) so that the bone is not radiographically apparent and successful treatment has resulted in remineralization so that the bone becomes visible in the radiographic image, the false impression may be given that bone has actually grown into periodontal defects. In many cases there will be no apparent radiographic changes after successful treatment. Also, radiographs do not disclose the therapeutic elimination of (radiolucent) soft tissue periodontal pockets; healing, therefore, is best assessed by clinical evaluation.

Sequential radiographs made with different beam angulations may give the false impression that bone has grown into the periodontal defects. Therefore in a longitudinal study, effort should be made to duplicate the image geometry as well as to ensure ideal exposure and processing variables. For instance, too high an x-ray exposure or too long a developing time increases the density of the image (more radiolucent) and thin bone such as the alveolar crest may not be apparent, giving the false impression that the bone has been resorbed. Alternatively, underexposed or underdeveloped films may give the false impression of bone growth.

The clinical crown-to-tooth ratio is a useful criterion not only for determining the nature of the restorative treatment to be performed on a tooth but also for deciding on the prognosis of an individual tooth. It is a measure of the tooth's bony support, relating the proportion of tooth length beyond the level of bone (clinical crown) to that supported by the lowest level of bone (bony investment). Teeth have an unfavorable crown-to-root ratio when the length of the tooth out of bone exceeds the length of root supported by bone.

Differential Diagnosis

The vast majority of cases of bone loss around teeth are caused by periodontal diseases. This fact can make the clinician less attentive to the possibility of other diseases with similar manifestations, which should always be considered in the differential diagnosis. Occasionally, more serious diseases are missed or recognized late. The most likely clinical sign of disease other than periodontal disease is the presence of one or a few adjacent loose teeth when the rest of the mouth shows no signs of periodontal disease. Radiographically, suspicion should be heightened if the bone destruction does not have the pattern or morphology normally associated with periodontal disease. Squamous cell carcinoma of the alveolar process occasionally is treated as periodontal disease, resulting in an unfortunate delay in diagnosis and treatment. This malignancy may display characteristics that suggest its true nature, such as extensive bone destruction of a localized region or invasive characteristics (see Chapter 22), or it may mimic periodontal disease. In some cases only the clinical characteristics of the lesion and the failure to respond to treatment indicate the presence of malignancy.

Any lesion of bone destruction that has ill-defined borders and a lack of peripheral bone response (sclerosis) should be viewed with suspicion. Another disease to be considered is Langerhans' cell histiocytosis (eosinophilic granuloma). Often this disease may manifest as single or multiple regions of bone destruction around the roots of teeth, similar to periodontal disease. The condition may appear similar to juvenile periodontitis except that the bone destruction does not correlate with the time of tooth eruption, as is seen in periodontitis. Also, in histiocytosis the midroot region is the epicenter of bone destruction, which gives early lesions an "ice cream scoop" appearance (see Chapter 23). The alveolar crest may remain intact.

Effect of Systemic Diseases on Periodontal Disease

Although systemic diseases do not cause periodontal disease, they do influence its course by interfering with the natural defenses against irritants or limiting the body's capacity to repair. Although any systemic disease may have some influence on other body systems, only a few appear to influence the periodontium and periodontal treatment. These include diabetes mellitus, hematologic disorders (e.g., monocytic conditions and, less often, myelogenous leukemia, neutropenia, hemophilia, abnormal bleeding, and nonhemophilic polycythemia vera), genetic and hereditary disturbances (e.g., Papillon-Lefèvre syndrome, Down syndrome, hypophosphatemia, Chédiak-Higashi syndrome), hormonal changes (e.g., puberty, pregnancy, menopause), and stress.

ACQUIRED IMMUNODEFICIENCY SYNDROME

The incidence and severity of periodontal disease is high in patients with acquired immunodeficiency syndrome (AIDS). In these individuals the disease process is characterized by a rapid progression that leads to bone sequestration and loss of several teeth. These patients may not respond to standard periodontal therapy.

DIABETES MELLITUS

Diabetes mellitus is the most common and important systemic disease to influence the onset and course of periodontal disease. Uncontrolled, it may result in protein breakdown, degenerative vascular changes, lowered resistance to infection, and increased severity of infections. Consequently, patients with diabetes are more disposed to develop periodontal disease than are those with normal glucose metabolism. Patients with uncontrolled diabetes and periodontal disease also show more severe and rapid alveolar bone resorption and are more prone to develop periodontal abscesses. In patients whose diabetes is under control, periodontal disease responds normally to traditional treatment.

BIBLIOGRAPHY

CLINICAL CHARACTERISTICS OF PERIODONTAL DISEASES

Armitage GC: Clinical evaluation of periodontal diseases, Periodontol 2000 7:39, 1995.

Armitage GC: Periodontal diseases: diagnosis, Ann Periodontol 1:1, 1996.

Herrera C et al: The periodontal abscess (I). Clinical and microbiological findings, J Clin Periodontol 27:387, 2000.

Newman MG, Takei HH, Carranza FA: Carranza's Clinical Periodontology, ed 9, Philadelphia, 2002, WB Saunders.

Page RC: Periodontal research: implications for the future of academic dentistry, J Dent Educ 47:226, 1983.

Page RC, Schroeder HE: Periodontitis in man and other animals, Basel, 1982, S Karger.

Walsh TF et al: The relationship of bone loss observed on panoramic radiographs with clinical periodontal screening, J Clin Periodontol 24:153, 1997.

EPIDEMIOLOGY

American Academy of Periodontology, Research, Science, and Therapy Committee: Epidemiology of periodontal diseases, J Periodontol 67:935, 1996.

Beck JD et al: Prevalence and risk indicators for periodontal attachment loss in a population of older community-dwelling blacks and whites, J Periodontol 61:521, 1990.

Brown LJ et al: Evaluating the periodontal status of US employed adults, J Am Dent Assoc 121:226, 1990.

Melvin WL et al: The prevalence and sex ratio of juvenile periodontitis in a young racially mixed population, J Periodontol 62:330, 1991.

Papapanou PH: Periodontal diseases: epidemiology, Ann Periodontol 1:1, 1996.

ETIOLOGY

Bergström J et al: Cigarette smoking and periodontal bone loss, J Periodontol 62:242, 1991.

Bimstein E, Garcia-Godoy F: The significance of age, proximal caries, gingival inflammation, probing depths, and the loss of lamina dura in the diagnosis of alveolar bone loss in the primary molars, ASDC J Dent Child 61:125, 1994.

Fox CH: New considerations in the prevalence of periodontal disease, Curr Opin Dent 2:5, 1992.

Page RC et al: Advances in the pathogenesis of periodontitis: summary of developments, clinical implications and future directions, Periodontol 2000 14:216, 1997.

Salvi GE et al: Influence of risk factors on the pathogenesis of periodontitis, Periodontol 2000 14:173, 1997.

Schwartz Z et al: Mechanisms of alveolar bone destruction in periodontitis, Periodontol 2000 14:158, 1997.

Van Dyke TE, Serhan: Resolution of inflammation: a new paradigm for the pathogenesis of periodontal diseases, J Dent Res 82:82, 2003.

RADIOGRAPHIC MANIFESTATIONS

Goodson JM et al: The relationship between attachment level loss and alveolar bone loss, J Clin Periodontol 11:348, 1984.

Gutteridge DL: The use of radiographic techniques in the diagnosis and management of periodontal diseases, Dentomaxillofac Radiol 24:107, 1995.

Jeffcoat MK et al: Radiographic diagnosis in periodontics, Periodontol 2000 7:54, 1995.

Khocht A et al: Screening for periodontal disease: radiographs vs PSR, J Am Dent Assoc 127:749, 1996.

Koral SM et al: Alveolar bone loss due to open interproximal contacts in periodontal disease, J Periodontol 52:477, 1981.

Kugelberg CF et al: Periodontal healing after impacted lower third molar surgery: a retrospective study, Int J Oral Surg 14:29, 1985.

Mann J et al: Investigation of the relationship between clinically detected loss of attachment and radiographic changes in early periodontal disease, J Clin Periodontol 12:247, 1985.

Nielsen IM et al: Interproximal periodontal intrabony defects: prevalence, localization, and etiological factors, J Clin Periodontol 7(3):187, 1980.

Rams TE et al: Utility of radiographic crestal lamina dura for predicting periodontitis disease activity, J Clin Periodontol 21:571, 1994.

Rushton VE, Horner K: The use of panoramic radiology in dental practice, J Dent 24:185, 1996.

Tammisalo T et al: Detailed tomography of periapical and periodontal lesions: diagnostic accuracy compared with periapical radiography, Dentomaxillofac Radiol 25:89, 1996.

Waite IM et al: Relationship between clinical periodontal condition and the radiological appearance at first molar sites in adolescents: a 3-year study, J Clin Periodontol 21:155, 1994.

AGGRESSIVE PERIODONTITIS

Albandar JM et al: Dental caries and tooth loss in adolescents with early onset periodontitis, J Periodontol 67:960, 1996.

Albandar JM et al: Clinical features of early onset periodontitis, J Am Dent Assoc 128:1393, 1997.

Brown LJ et al: Early onset periodontitis: progression of attachment loss during 6 years, J Periodontol 67:968, 1996.

Liljenberg B, Lindhe J: Juvenile periodontitis: some microbiological, histopathological, and clinical characteristics, J Clin Periodontol 7:48, 1980.

Loe H, Brown LJ: Early onset periodontitis in the United States of America, J Periodontol 62:608, 1991.

Page RC et al: Rapidly progressive periodontitis: a distinct clinical condition, J Periodontol 54:197, 1983.

Page RC et al: Clinical and laboratory studies of a family with a high prevalence of juvenile periodontitis, J Periodontol 56:602, 1985.

RADIOGRAPHIC TECHNIQUE

Bragger I: Radiographic diagnosis of periodontal disease progression, Curr Opin Periodontol 3:59, 1996.

Duckworth J et al: A method for the geometric and densitometric standardization of intraoral radiographs, J Periodontol 54:435, 1983.

Gröndahl K et al: Influence of variations in projection geometry on the detectability of periodontal bone lesions: a comparison between subtraction radiography and conventional radiographic technique, J Clin Periodontol 11:411, 1984.

Pepelassi EA, Diamanti-Kipioti A: Selection of the most accurate method of conventional radiography for the assessment of periodontal osseous destruction, J Clin Periodontol 24:557, 1997.

Reed B, Polson A: Relationships between bitewing and periapical radiographs in assessing crestal alveolar bone levels, J Periodontol 55:22, 1984.

SUBTRACTION RADIOGRAPHY

Eickholz P, Hausmann E: Evidence for healing of periodontal defects 5 years after conventional and regenerative therapy: digital subtraction and bone level measurements, J Clin Periodontol 29:922, 2002.

Griffiths GS et al: Use of an internal standard in subtraction radiography to assess initial periodontal bone changes, Dentomaxillofac Radiol 25:76, 1996.

Gröndahl HG, Gröndahl K: Subtraction radiography for the diagnosis of periodontal bone lesions, Oral Surg 55:208, 1983.

Jeffcoat MK: Diagnosing periodontal disease: new tools to solve an old problem, J Am Dent Assoc 122:55, 1991.

Stassinakis A et al: Accuracy in detecting bone lesions in vitro with conventional and subtracted direct digital imaging, Dentomaxillofac Radiol 24:232, 1995.

Nummikoski PV et al: Clinical validation of a new subtraction radiography technique for periodontal bone loss detection, J Periodontol 71:598, 2000.

OCCLUSAL TRAUMA

Burgett FG: Trauma from occlusion: periodontal concerns, Dent Clin North Am 39:301, 1995.

Wank GS, Kroll YJ: Occlusal trauma: an evaluation of its relationship to periodontal prostheses, Dent Clin North Am 25:511, 1981.

SYSTEMIC DISEASE

Emrich LJ et al: Periodontal disease in non-insulin-dependent diabetes mellitus, J Periodontol 62:123, 1991.

Farzim I, Edalat M: Periodontosis with hyperkeratosis palmaris and plantaris (the Papillon-Lefèvre syndrome): a case report, J Periodontol 45:316, 1974.

Nelson RG et al: Periodontal diseases and NIDDM in Pima Indians, Diabetes Care 13:836, 1990.

Rateitschak-Pluss EM, Schroeder HE: History of periodontitis in a child with Papillon-Lefèvre syndrome, J Periodontol 55:35, 1984.

Winkler JR et al: Clinical description and etiology of HIV–associated periodontal disease. In Robinson PB, Greenspan JS, editors: Prospectus on oral manifestations of AIDS, Littleton, MA, 1988, PSG Publishing.

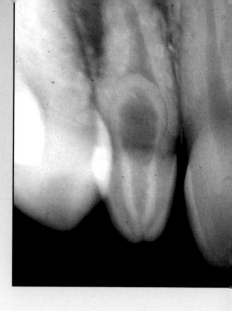

CHAPTER 18

Dental Anomalies

Dental anomalies include variations in normal number, size, eruption, or morphology of the teeth. In this chapter these anomalies have been divided into developmental abnormalities and acquired abnormalities. The term *developmental* indicates that a particular anomaly occurred during the formation of the tooth or teeth. Given the complexities and interactions involved in tooth development, from initiation at about the sixth week in utero to eruption, the small number of various anomalies is surprising. Most of the defects considered are inherited. In contrast, acquired abnormalities result from changes to teeth after normal formation. For instance, teeth that form abnormally short roots represent a developmental anomaly, whereas the shortening of normal tooth roots by external resorption represents an acquired change.

Developmental Abnormalities

NUMBER OF TEETH

SUPERNUMERARY TEETH

Synonyms
Hyperdontia, distodens, mesiodens, parateeth, peridens, and supplemental teeth

Definition
Supernumerary teeth are those that develop in addition to the normal complement. The tooth form may be normal or abnormal. When the extra teeth have normal morphology, the term *supplemental* is sometimes used. Although the cause is unknown, the tendency is familial. Most cases are polygenetic and represent initial

spontaneous gene mutations. When the anomaly is restricted to supernumerary teeth, it is inherited as an autosomal recessive trait. The supernumerary teeth that occur between the maxillary central incisors are mesiodens (Fig. 18-1); those occurring in the molar area are *parateeth*. Those that erupt distal to the third molar are called *distodens* or *distomolar teeth* (Fig. 18-2). Also, supernumerary teeth that erupt ectopically either buccally or lingually to the normal arch are *peridens*.

Clinical Features
Supernumerary teeth occur in 1% to 4% of the population. Although they may develop in both dentitions, they are more common in the permanent. Supernumerary teeth may occur anywhere in either jaw. Single teeth are most common in the anterior maxilla (mesiodens) and in the maxillary molar region. Multiple supernumerary teeth occur most frequently in the premolar regions, usually in the mandible (Fig. 18-3). The mandibular counterpart of the mesiodens is rare. Supernumerary teeth occur twice as often in males and have a greater incidence in Asians and Native Americans. They usually do not erupt but are discovered radiographically. Occasionally a patient may appear clinically to be missing one or more teeth; however, an appropriate radiographic examination may reveal a supernumerary tooth interfering with normal tooth eruption (Fig. 18-4). When a supernumerary tooth is erupted and clinically evident, it is commonly positioned outside the normal arch because of space restriction.

Radiographic Features
The radiographic features of the supernumerary tooth may vary from normal-appearing tooth structure to a

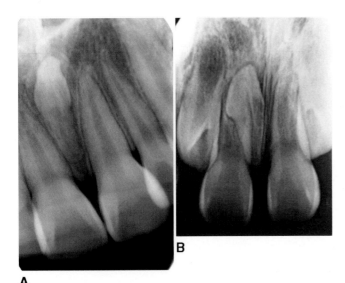

A

FIG. **18-1**   A and B, Examples of inverted mesiodens.

conical tooth form and, in extreme cases, to grossly deformed tooth structure. The size varies but the tooth usually is smaller than the surrounding normal dentition. The supernumerary tooth is easily identified by counting and identifying all the teeth. The supernumerary tooth can interfere with normal eruption; therefore the radiograph often reveals an unerupted permanent tooth in close proximity to the supernumerary tooth. Radiographs may reveal supernumerary teeth in the deciduous dentition (Fig. 18-5) after 3 or

4 years of age, when the deciduous teeth have formed. They may be detected in the permanent dentition of children older than 9 to 12 years.

Care must be taken not to miss supernumerary teeth in the panoramic image, especially when the image of the tooth is distorted as a result of the position of the tooth outside the focal trough, for instance, in the palate. Besides the periapical intraoral examination, occlusal radiographs aid in determining the location and number of unerupted supernumerary teeth.

Differential Diagnosis

Multiple supernumerary teeth have been associated with a number of syndromes. For instance, multiple teeth, especially bicuspids, have been associated with cleidocranial dysplasia (see Chapter 29). Supernumerary teeth have also been reported in Gardner's syndrome (see Chapter 21).

Management

The management of supernumerary teeth depends on many factors, including their potential effect on the developing normal dentition, their position and number, and the complications that may result from surgical intervention. If they erupt, they can cause malalignment of the normal dentition. Those that remain in the jaws may cause root resorption or interfere with the normal eruption sequence. Follicles of unerupted supernumerary teeth occasionally develop into dentigerous cysts. All of the preceding factors

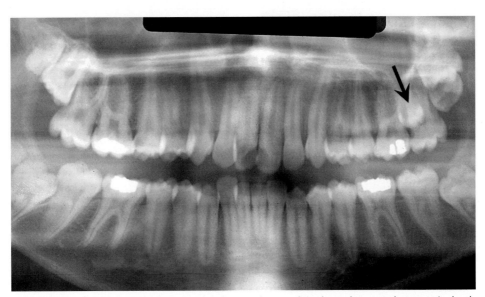

FIG. **18-2**   In this panoramic image distomolars or fourth molars can be seen in both maxillary quadrants as well as a supplemental molar in the left maxilla, bringing the total to five molars in this quadrant.

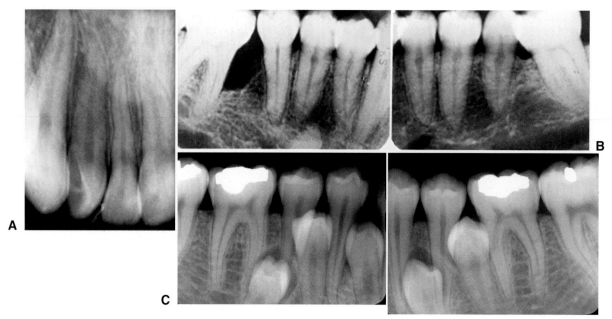

FIG. **18-3**   Supernumerary or supplemental lateral incisors, **A**, and premolars, **B** and **C**.

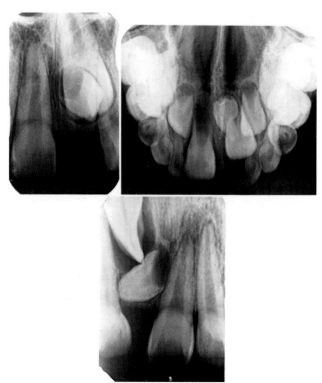

FIG. **18-4**   Examples of mesiodens that interfered with the eruption and caused impaction of permanent teeth.

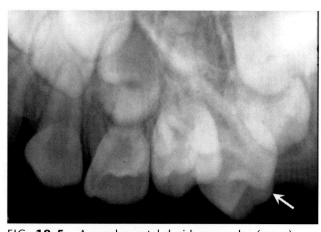

FIG. **18-5**   A supplemental deciduous molar *(arrow).*

influence the decision to either remove a supernumerary tooth or keep it under observation.

MISSING TEETH

Synonyms

Hypodontia, oligodontia, and anodontia

Definition

The expression of developmentally missing teeth may range from the absence of one or a few teeth *(hypodontia),* to the absence of numerous teeth *(oligodontia),* to the failure of all teeth to develop *(anodontia).*

Developmentally missing teeth may also be the result of numerous independent pathologic mechanisms that can affect the orderly formation of the dental lamina (e.g., orofaciodigital syndrome), failure of a tooth germ to develop at the optimal time, lack of necessary space imposed by a malformed jaw, and a genetically determined disproportion between tooth mass and jaw size.

Clinical Features

Hypodontia in the permanent dentition, excluding third molars, is found in 3% to 10% of the population. Hypodontia is more frequently found in Asians and Native Americans. Although missing primary teeth are relatively uncommon, when one tooth is missing, it is usually a maxillary incisor. The most commonly missing teeth are third molars, second premolars (Fig. 18-6), and maxillary lateral and mandibular central incisors. The absence may be either unilateral or bilateral. Children who have developmentally missing teeth tend to have more than one tooth absent and more than one morphologic group (incisors, premolars, and molars) involved.

Radiographic Features

Missing teeth are recognized by identifying and counting the existing teeth. However, it must be kept in mind that the development of teeth may vary markedly among patients. Eruption of some teeth may be developmentally delayed by a number of years after the established time (especially mandibular second bicuspids)

and others may show evidence of development as late as a year after the contralateral tooth.

Differential Diagnosis

A tooth may be considered to be developmentally missing when it cannot be discerned clinically or radiographically and no history exists of its extraction. Anodontia or oligodontia frequently occurs in patients with ectodermal dysplasia (Fig. 18-7). This inherited disorder results in the absence of at least two ectodermally derived structures, such as sweat glands, hair, skin, nails, and teeth. The severity of the condition is variable and may result in multiple missing teeth and malformed teeth, often having a conical shape or a notable decrease in size. Many other syndromes and conditions may interfere with the development of teeth.

Management

Missing teeth, abnormal occlusion, or altered facial appearance may cause some patients psychologic distress. If the extent of hypodontia is mild, the associated changes may likewise be slight and manageable by orthodontics. In more severe cases restorative, implant, and prosthetic procedures can be undertaken.

SIZE OF TEETH

A positive correlation exists between tooth size (mesiodistal diameter × buccolingual diameter) and body height. Males also have larger primary and

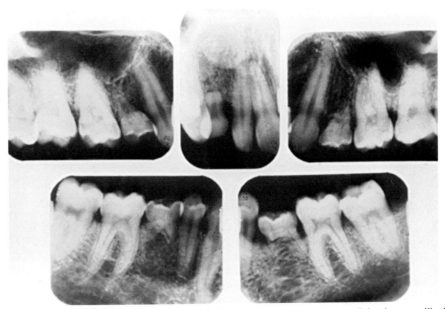

FIG. **18-6** Developmental absence of all maxillary premolars and both mandibular second premolars. Note the retention of the maxillary primary canine as a result of the posterior position of the maxillary permanent canine.

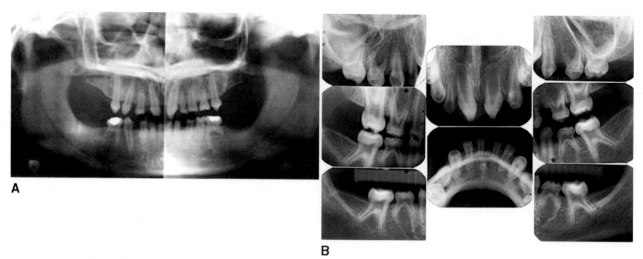

FIG. **18-7**   **A** and **B**, Examples of ectodermal dysplasia displaying various degrees of missing and malformed teeth.

permanent teeth than females. Beyond these normal variations, however, individuals may occasionally develop unusually large or small teeth.

MACRODONTIA

Definition

In macrodontia the teeth are larger than normal. When the teeth are of normal size but occur in smaller-than-normal jaws, the condition is relative macrodontia. Macrodontia may rarely affect the entire dentition, but more commonly it involves a group of teeth, individual contralateral teeth, or a single tooth (Fig. 18-8). The presence of a hemangioma (either intraosseous or in the soft tissues) can result in an increase in the size and advanced development of adjacent teeth. Also localized true macrodontia can occur in hemihypertrophy of the face. True generalized macrodontia may also occur with pituitary gigantism. The cause of macrodontia is unknown.

The large size of the teeth is apparent on clinical examination. Associated crowding, malocclusion, or impaction may occur.

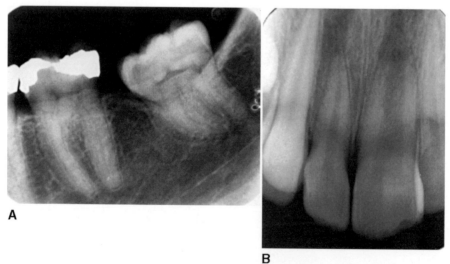

FIG. **18-8**   *Macrodontia is a condition that results in enlarged teeth.* **A**, The macrodont molar shows an increased mesiodistal dimension. **B**, The macrodont central incisor shows enlargement of both its mesiodistal and longitudinal dimension. (**A**, Courtesy Dr. B. Gratt, Los Angeles, CA.)

Radiographic Features

Radiographs reveal the increased size of both erupted and unerupted macrodont teeth. The crowding may cause impaction of other teeth. The shape of the tooth is usually normal, but some cases may exhibit a mildly distorted morphology.

Differential Diagnosis

The macrodont may resemble gemination or fusion. When fusion occurs, there is a missing tooth. In gemination all the teeth may be present and often evidence exists of a division or cleft of the coronal or root segment of the tooth. However, the differentiation of these three conditions may not influence the treatment provided.

Management

In most cases macrodontia does not require treatment. Orthodontic treatment may be necessary, however, in the case of malocclusion.

MICRODONTIA

Definition

In microdontia the involved teeth are smaller than normal. As with macrodontia, microdontia may involve all the teeth or be limited to a single tooth or group of teeth. Relative microdontia can also occur. In this condition normal-sized teeth develop in an individual with large jaws. Generalized microdontia is extremely rare, although it does occur in some patients with pituitary dwarfism. Supernumerary teeth are frequently microdont. Also, the lateral incisors and third molars, which often are developmentally missing, may be small.

Clinical Features

The involved teeth are noticeably small and may have altered morphology. Microdont molars may have altered shape—from five to four cusps in mandibular molars and from four to three in upper molars (Fig. 18-9). Microdont lateral incisors are also smaller and peg-shaped (Fig. 18-10).

Radiographic Features

The shape of these small teeth may be normal, but more frequently they are malformed.

Differential Diagnosis

The recognition of small teeth indicates the diagnosis. The number and distribution of microdonts may also suggest consideration of syndromes (e.g., congenital heart disease, progeria).

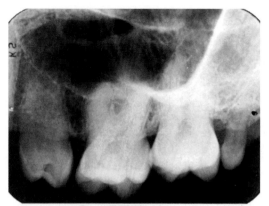
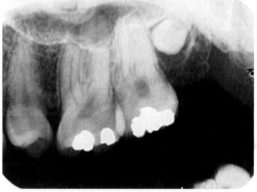

FIG. **18-9** Microdontia of the maxillary third molars, showing reduction in both the size and number of cusps.

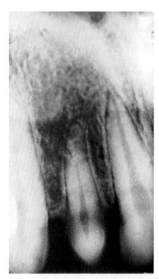

FIG. **18-10** Microdontia of the maxillary lateral incisor results in a characteristic peg-shaped deformity.

Management

Restorative or prosthetic treatment may be considered to create a more normal-appearing tooth, especially when considering esthetic concerns in the anterior dentition.

ERUPTION OF TEETH

TRANSPOSITION

Definition
Transposition is the condition in which two teeth have exchanged positions.

Clinical Features
The most frequently transposed teeth are the permanent canine and first premolar (more often than the lateral incisor). Second premolars infrequently lie between first and second molars. The transposition of central and lateral incisors is rare. Transposition in the primary dentition has not been reported. It can occur with hypodontia, supernumerary teeth, or the persistence of a deciduous predecessor.

Radiographic Features
Radiographs reveal transposition when the teeth are not in their usual sequence in the dental arch (Fig. 18-11).

Differential Diagnosis
Transposed teeth are usually easily recognized.

Management
Transposed teeth are frequently altered prosthetically to improve function and esthetics.

ALTERED MORPHOLOGY OF TEETH

FUSION

Synonym
Synodontia

Definition
Fusion of teeth results from the combining of adjacent tooth germs, resulting in union of the developing teeth. Some authors believe that fusion results when two tooth germs develop so close together that as they grow, they contact and fuse before calcification. Others contend that a physical force or pressure generated during development causes contact of adjacent tooth buds. The genetic basis for the anomaly is probably autosomal dominant with reduced penetrance. Males and females experience fusion in equal numbers, and the incidence is higher in Asians and Native Americans.

Clinical Features
Fusion usually causes a reduced number of teeth in the arch. It occurs in deciduous and permanent dentitions, although it is more common between deciduous teeth. When a deciduous canine and lateral incisor fuses, the corresponding permanent lateral incisor may be absent. Fusion is more common in anterior teeth of both the permanent and deciduous dentition (Fig. 18-12). Fusion may be total or partial depending on the stage of odontogenesis and the proximity of the developing teeth. The result can vary from a single tooth of about normal size to a tooth of nearly twice the normal size. A bifid crown may exist, or two recognizable teeth may be joined by dentin or enamel. The crowns of fused teeth usually appear to be large and single, or an incisocervical groove of varying depth or a bifid crown occurs.

Radiographic Features
Radiographs disclose the unusual shape or size of the entire tooth. The true nature and extent of the union are frequently more evident on the radiograph than can be determined by clinical examination. Fused teeth may show an unusual configuration of the pulp chamber, root canal, or crown.

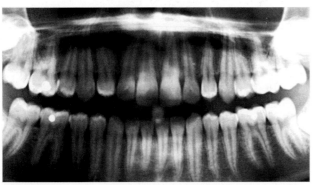

FIG. **18-11**   A cropped panoramic image demonstrating bilateral transposition of the maxillary canines and first bicuspids.

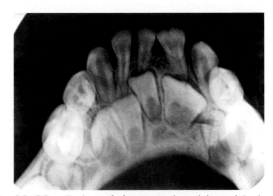

FIG. **18-12**   Fusion of the central and lateral incisors in both the primary and the permanent dentition. Note the reduction in number of teeth and the increased width of the fused tooth mass.

Differential Diagnosis

The differential diagnosis for fused teeth includes gemination and macrodontia. Fusion may be differentiated from gemination by the reduced number of teeth, except in an unusual case, in which the fusion is between a supernumerary tooth and a normal tooth. The differentiation is usually academic because little difference exists in the treatment provided.

Management

The management of a case of fusion depends on which teeth are involved, the degree of fusion, and the morphologic result. If the affected teeth are deciduous, they may be retained as they are. If the clinician contemplates extraction, it is important first to determine whether the succedaneous teeth are present. In the case of fused secondary teeth, the fused crowns may be reshaped with a restoration that mimics two independent crowns. The morphology of fused teeth requires radiographic evaluation before they are reshaped. Endodontic therapy may be necessary and perhaps may be difficult or impossible if the root canals are of unusual shape. In some cases it is most prudent to leave the teeth as they are.

CONCRESCENCE

Definition

Concrescence occurs when the roots of two or more teeth are united by cementum. It may involve either primary or secondary teeth. Although its cause is unknown, many authorities suspect that space restriction during development, local trauma, excessive occlusal force, or local infection after development may play an important role. If the condition occurs during development, it is called *true concrescence;* if later, it is *acquired concrescence.*

Clinical Features

Maxillary molars are the teeth most frequently involved, especially a third molar and a supernumerary tooth. Involved teeth may fail to erupt or may erupt incompletely. The sexes are equally affected.

Radiographic Features

A radiographic examination may not always distinguish between concrescence and teeth that are in close contact or are simply superimposed (Fig. 18-13). When the condition is suspected on a radiograph and extraction of one of the teeth is being considered, additional

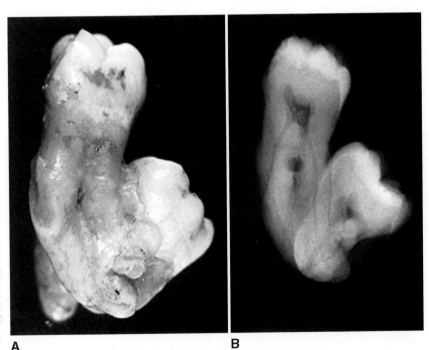

A　　　　　　　　　　**B**

FIG. **18-13**　**A,** Concrescence occurs when two teeth are joined by a mass of cementum. **B,** Extraction of one tooth may result in the unintended removal of the second because cementum is often not well visualized radiographically. (Courtesy Dr. R. Kienholz, Dallas, Texas.)

projections at different angles may be obtained to better delineate the condition.

Differential Diagnosis

It is usually impossible to determine radiographically with certainty whether the teeth whose root images are superimposed are actually joined. Is the periodontal membrane space continuous around each root? If the roots are joined, it may not be possible to tell whether the union is by cementum or by dentin (fusion).

Management

Concrescence affects treatment only when the decision is made to remove one or both of the involved teeth. This condition complicates the extraction. The clinician should warn the patient that an effort to remove one might result in the unintended and simultaneous removal of the other.

GEMINATION

Synonym

Twinning

Definition

Gemination is a rare anomaly that arises when the tooth bud of a single tooth attempts to divide. The result may be an invagination of the crown, with partial division, or in rare cases complete division throughout the crown and root, producing identical structures. Complete twinning results in a normal tooth plus a supernumerary tooth in the arch. Its cause is unknown, but some evidence exists that it is familial.

Clinical Features

Gemination more frequently affects the primary teeth, but it may occur in both dentitions, usually in the incisor region. It can be detected clinically after the anomalous tooth erupts. The occurrence in males and females is about equal. The enamel or dentin of geminated teeth may be hypoplastic or hypocalcified.

Radiographic Features

Radiographs reveal the altered shape of the hard tissue and pulp chamber of the germinated tooth. Radiopaque enamel outlines the clefts in the crowns and invaginations and thus accentuates them. The pulp chamber is usually single and enlarged and may be partially divided (Fig. 18-14). In the rare case of premolar gemination, the tooth image suggests a molar with an enlarged crown and two roots.

Differential Diagnosis

The differential diagnosis of gemination includes fusion. If the malformed tooth is counted as one, individuals with gemination have a normal tooth count, whereas those with fusion are seen to be missing a tooth.

Management

A geminated tooth in the anterior region may compromise arch esthetics. Areas of hypoplasia and invagination lines or areas of coronal separation represent caries-susceptible sites that may in time result in pulpal infection. Affected teeth can cause malocclusion and lead to periodontal disease. Consequently the affected tooth may be removed (especially if it is deciduous), the crown(s) may be restored or reshaped, or the tooth may

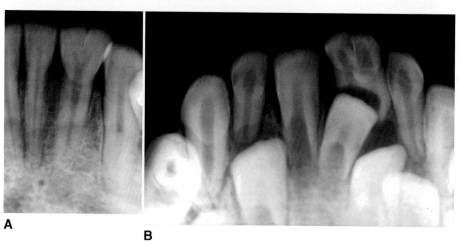

FIG. 18-14   **A,** Gemination of a mandibular lateral incisor showing bifurcation of the crown and the pulp chamber. **B,** Almost complete gemination of a deciduous lateral incisor.

be left untreated and periodically examined to preclude the development of complications. Before treatment is initiated on primary teeth, the status of the succedaneous teeth and configuration of their root canals should be determined radiographically.

TAURODONTISM

Definition

Taurodont teeth have longitudinally enlarged pulp chambers. The crown is of normal shape and size, but the body is elongated and the roots are short. The pulp chamber extends from a normal position in the crown throughout the length of the extended body, leading to an increased distance between the cementoenamel junction and the furcation. Taurodontism may occur in either the permanent or primary dentition (or both). Although some evidence of the trait can be seen in any

tooth, it is usually fully expressed in the molars and less often in the premolars. Single or multiple teeth may show taurodont features, unilaterally or bilaterally and in any combination of teeth or quadrants.

Clinical Features

Because the body and roots of taurodont teeth lie below the alveolar margin, the distinguishing features of these teeth are not recognizable clinically.

Radiographic Features

The distinctive morphology of taurodont teeth is quite apparent on radiographs. The peculiar feature is an extension of the rectangular pulp chamber into the elongated body of the tooth (Fig. 18-15). The shortened roots and root canals are a function of the long body and normal length of the tooth. The size of the crown is normal.

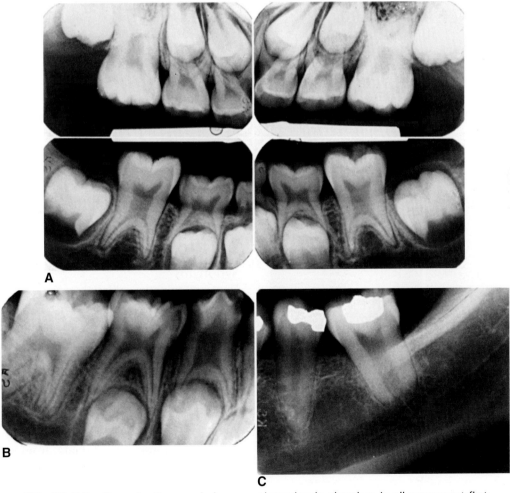

FIG. **18-15** Taurodontia, revealed as an enlarged pulp chamber, in all permanent first molars (**A**), in a primary first molar (**B**), and in a permanent molar (**C**).

Differential Diagnosis

The image of the taurodont tooth is characteristic and easily recognized radiographically. The developing molar may appear similar; however, the identification of the wide apical foramina and incompletely formed roots helps in the differential diagnosis. Taurodontism has been reported with greater frequency in trisomy 21 syndrome.

Management

Taurodont teeth do not require treatment.

DILACERATION

Definition

Dilaceration is a disturbance in tooth formation that produces a sharp bend or curve in the tooth. One of the oldest concepts is that it is probably the result of mechanical trauma to the calcified portion of a partially formed tooth. Although this may occur, especially to the maxillary incisors, most cases are likely to be true developmental anomalies. The angular distortion may occur anywhere in the crown or root.

Clinical Features

Most cases of radicular dilaceration are not recognized clinically. If the dilaceration is so pronounced that the tooth does not erupt, the only clinical indication of the defect is a missing tooth. If the defect is in the crown of an erupted tooth, it may be readily recognized as an angular distortion (Fig. 18-16).

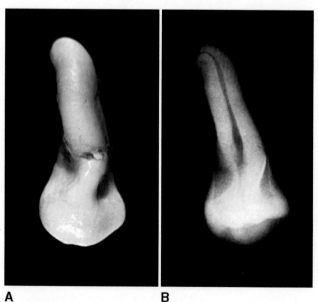

A   B

FIG. **18-16   A,** Dilaceration of the crown may be readily recognized clinically. **B,** Radiograph of the specimen in **A.** (Courtesy Dr. R. Kienholz, Dallas, Texas.)

Radiographic Features

Radiographs provide the best means of detecting a radicular dilaceration. The condition occurs most often in permanent maxillary premolars. One or more teeth may be affected. If the roots bend mesially or distally, the condition is clearly apparent on a periapical radiograph (Fig. 18-17). When the roots are bent buccally (labially) or lingually, the central ray passes approximately parallel with the deflected portion of the root. The dilacerated portion then appears at the apical end of the unaltered root as a rounded opaque area with a dark shadow in its central region cast by the apical foramen and root canal (an appearance like a bull's-eye). The periodontal ligament (PDL) space around this dilacerated portion may be seen as a radiolucent halo (Fig. 18-18), and the radiopacity of this segment of root is greater than the rest of the root. In some cases, especially in the maxilla, the geometry of the projections may preclude the recognition of a dilaceration.

Differential Diagnosis

Occasionally dilacerated roots are difficult to differentiate from fused roots, condensing osteitis, or a dense bone island. They can usually be identified, however, by obtaining radiographs exposed from different angles.

Management

The dilacerated root generally does not require treatment because it provides adequate support. If it must be extracted for some other reason, its removal can be complicated, especially if the surgeon is not prepared with a preoperative radiograph. In contrast, dilacerated crowns are frequently restored with a prosthetic crown to improve esthetics and function.

DENS IN DENTE

Synonyms

Dens invaginatus, dilated odontome, and gestant odontome

Definition

Dens in dente results from an infolding of the outer surface into the interior of a tooth. This can occur in either the crown or the root during tooth development and may involve the pulp chamber or root canal, resulting in deformity of either the crown or the root. These anomalies are seen most often in tooth crowns. Coronal invaginations usually originate from an anomalous infolding of the enamel organ into the dental papilla. In a mature tooth the result is a fold of hard tissue within the tooth characterized by enamel lining the fold (Fig. 18-19). The most extreme form of this anomaly is referred to as the *dilated odontome*.

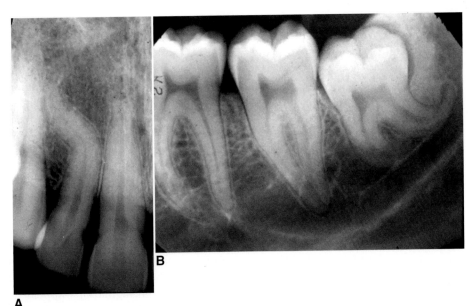

FIG. **18-17**   **A,** Dilaceration of the root of a maxillary lateral incisor. **B,** Dilaceration of the root of a mandibular third molar.

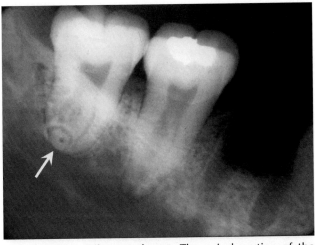

FIG. **18-18**   *Dilacerated root.* The apical portion of the root of this third molar is bent buccally or lingually into the plane of the central ray. Note the halo in the apical region, produced by the PDL space giving a "bull's-eye" appearance *(arrow).*

When dens in dente involves a root (radicular dens invaginatus), it appears to be the result of an invagination of Hertwig's epithelial root sheath. This results in an accentuation of the normal longitudinal root groove. In contrast to the coronal type (lined with enamel), the radicular-type defect is lined with cementum. If the invagination retracts and is cut off, it leaves a longitudinal structure of cementum, bone, and remnants of PDL within the pulp canal. The structure often extends for most of the root length. In other cases the

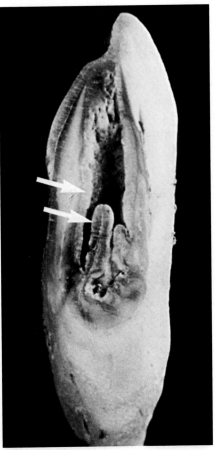

FIG. **18-19**   Dens in dente is characterized by an infolding of enamel into the tooth. This sectioned canine with a dens in dente shows enamel *(arrows)* folded into the tooth's interior.

root sheath may bud off a saclike invagination that produces a circumscribed cementum defect in the root. Mandibular first premolars and second molars are especially prone to develop the radicular variety of this invagination anomaly.

Little difference in the frequency of occurrence exists among white and Asian people. If all grades of expression of invagination, mild to severe, are included, the condition is found in approximately 5% of these two racial groups. The condition appears to be rare in blacks. No sexual predilection exists. Although no specific mode of inheritance seems to fit all the data, a high degree of inheritability seems to exist.

Clinical Features

Coronal dens in dente may be identified clinically as a pit at the incisal edge or the cingulum. The pit in the cingulum may be particularly broad and deep, especially when these features occur in the lateral incisor. Often the lingual marginal ridges or cingula are prominent. In most cases, however, the dens in dente is not large, and crown morphology appears normal. Dens in dente occurs most frequently in the permanent maxillary lateral incisors, followed by (in decreasing frequency) the maxillary central incisors, premolars, and canines and less often in the posterior teeth. Invagination is rare in the crowns of mandibular teeth and in deciduous teeth. It occurs symmetrically in about half the cases. Concomitant involvement of the central and lateral incisors may occur.

The clinical importance of dens invaginatus results from the risk of pulpal disease. Although enamel lines the coronal defect, it is frequently thin, often of poor quality, and even missing in some areas. Furthermore, the cavity is usually separated from the pulp chamber by a relatively thin wall and opens into the oral environment through a narrow constriction. The pit is often difficult to keep clean, and consequently, it offers conditions favorable for the development of caries. Such carious lesions are difficult to detect clinically and will rapidly involve the pulp. In addition, sometimes fine canals extend between the invagination and the pulp chamber, resulting in pulpal disease even in the absence of caries.

Radiographic Features

Most cases of dens in dente are discovered radiographically. The infolding of the enamel lining is more radiopaque than the surrounding tooth structure and can easily be identified (Fig. 18-20). Less frequently the radicular invaginations appear as poorly defined, slightly radiolucent structures running longitudinally within the root. The defects, especially the coronal variety, may vary in size and shape from small and superficial to large and deep. If a coronal invagination is extensive, the crown is almost invariably malformed; when the crown is malformed, the apical foramen is usually wide (Fig. 18-21). A frequent cause of an open apical foramen is the cessation of root development that occurs as a result of death of the pulpal tissue. In the most severe form (dilated odontome) the tooth is severely deformed, having a circular or oval shape with a radiolucent interior (Fig. 18-22). Dens in dente can be identified in the radiographic image even before the tooth erupts.

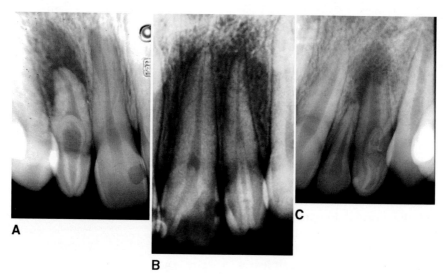

FIG. 18-20   Dens in dente is seen radiographically as a radiopaque infolding of enamel into the tooth's pulp chamber. **A-C,** Various degrees of involvement of the maxillary lateral incisors.

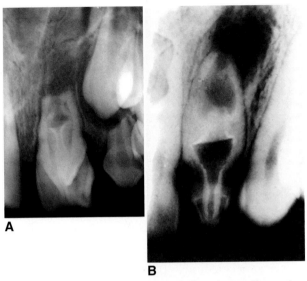

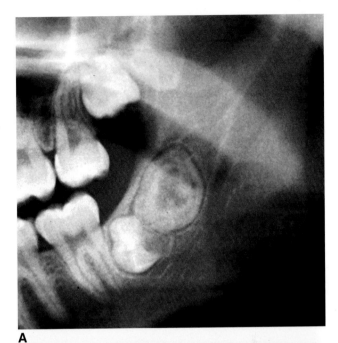

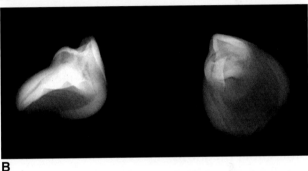

FIG. **18-21** **A** and **B**, Examples of severe malformations of dens in dente. These usually result in necrosis of the pulp, open apices, and periapical inflammatory lesions.

FIG. **18-22** **A**, A dilated odontome is positioned just posterior to the developing mandibular third molar in this panoramic film. **B**, The specimen radiographs represent two views of a dilated odontome.

Differential Diagnosis

The appearance and usual occurrence in incisors are so characteristic that, once recognized, little probability exists that the anomaly will be confused with another condition.

Management

Although it is important to evaluate every case individually, the placement of a prophylactic restoration in the defect is typically the treatment of choice and should ensure a normal life span for the tooth. Failure of early identification and hence treatment may result in premature tooth loss or the requirement for root canal therapy.

DENS EVAGINATUS

Synonym

Leong's premolar

Definition

In contrast to the dens in dente, dens evaginatus is the result of an outfolding of the enamel organ. The result is an enamel-covered tubercle, usually in or near the middle of the occlusal surface of a premolar or occasionally a molar (Fig. 18-23). Canines are rarely affected. The frequency of occurrence of dens evaginatus is highest in Asians and Native Americans.

Clinical Features

Clinically, dens evaginatus appears as a tubercle of enamel on the occlusal surface of the affected tooth. A polyplike protuberance exists in the central groove or lingual ridge of a buccal cusp. Dens evaginatus may occur bilaterally and usually in the mandible. The tubercle often has a dentin core, and a very slender pulp horn frequently extends into the evagination. After the tubercle is worn down by the opposing teeth, it appears as a small circular facet with a small black pit in the center (Fig. 18-24, *B*). Wear, fracture, or indiscriminate surgical removal of this tubercle may precipitate a pulpal infection. In rare cases a microscopic direct communication may occur between the pulp and the oral cavity through this tubercle. In these instances the pulp may become infected shortly after eruption.

Radiographic Features

The radiographic image shows an extension of a dentin tubercle on the occlusal surface unless the tubercle is

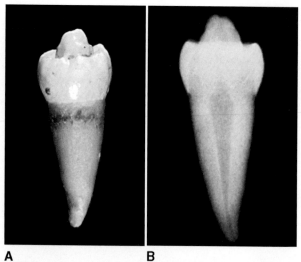

FIG. 18-23   **A,** Dens evaginatus, seen as a tubercle in the mandibular premolar. **B,** Radiograph of the specimen. (Courtesy Dr. R. Kienholz, Dallas, Texas.)

already worn down. The dentin core is usually covered with opaque enamel. A fine pulp horn may extend into the tubercle, but this may not be visible radiographically. If the tubercle has been worn to the point of pulpal exposure or has fractured, pulpal necrosis may result (see Fig. 18-24). This is indicated by an open apical foramen and periapical radiolucency.

Differential Diagnosis

The clinical and radiographic appearance may be characteristic or may be difficult to visualize if the tubercle has been worn down to the occlusal surface.

Management

If the tubercle causes any occlusal interference or shows evidence of marked abrasion, it should probably be removed under aseptic conditions and the pulp capped, if necessary. Such a precaution may preclude pulpal exposure and infection as the result of accidental fracture or advanced abrasion.

AMELOGENESIS IMPERFECTA

Definition

Amelogenesis imperfecta is a developmental disturbance that interferes with normal enamel formation. It leads to marked changes in the enamel of all or nearly all the teeth in both dentitions. Most forms are autosomal dominant or recessive, but two types are X-linked. Amelogenesis imperfecta is not related to any time or period of enamel development or any clinically demonstrable alteration (disease or dietary abnormality) in

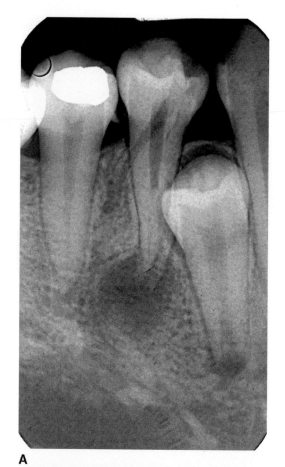

A

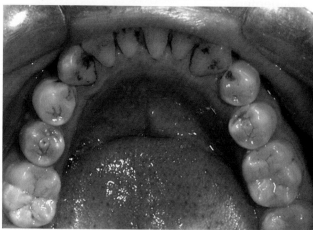

B

FIG. 18-24   **A,** Periapical film of mandibular first bicuspid with a dens evaginatus and apical rarefying osteitis. **B,** Clinical photograph of another case with dens evaginatus involving both mandibular second bicuspids, since the tubercles have been worn down there is now a black pit representing communication with the pulp chamber.

other tissues. The enamel may lack the normal prismatic structure, being laminated throughout its thickness or at the periphery. As a result these teeth are more resistant to decay. The dentin and root form are usually normal. Eruption of the affected teeth is often delayed, and a tendency for impaction exists. Although at least 14 variants of the condition have been described, four general types have characteristic clinical or radiographic appearances: a hypoplastic type, a hypomaturation type, a hypocalcified type, and a hypomaturation-hypocalcified type associated with taurodontism.

Clinical Features

Hypoplasia. As a result of some defect in ameloblasts, the enamel of the affected teeth fails to develop to its normal thickness. It is so thin that the dentin shows through and imparts a yellowish-brown color to the tooth. In the various hypoplastic forms the enamel may be pitted, rough, or smooth and glossy. The crowns of the teeth may not have the usual contour of enamel but rather have a roughly square shape. The reduced enamel thickness also causes the teeth to be undersized, with lack of contact between adjacent teeth (Fig. 18-25). The occlusal surfaces of the posterior teeth are relatively flat with low cusps. This is a result of the attrition of cusp tips that were initially low and not fully formed. An anterior open bite may be noted.

Hypomaturation. In the hypomaturation form of amelogenesis imperfecta, the enamel has a normal thickness but a mottled appearance. It is softer than normal (density comparable to dentin) and may crack away from the crown. Its color may range from clear to cloudy white, yellow, or brown. In one form of hypomaturation the teeth appear to be snow-capped (with white opaque enamel).

Hypocalcification. Hypocalcification of teeth is more common than the hypoplastic variety of amelogenesis imperfecta. The crowns of the teeth are normal in size and shape when they erupt because the enamel is of regular thickness (Fig. 18-26). However, because the enamel is poorly mineralized (less dense than dentin), it starts to fracture away shortly after it comes into function. This creates clinically recognizable defects. The soft enamel abrades rapidly and the softer dentin also wears down rapidly, resulting in a grossly worn tooth, sometimes to the level of the gingiva. An explorer point under pressure can penetrate the soft enamel; yet caries in these worn teeth is unusual. The hypocalcified enamel has increased permeability and becomes stained and darkened. The teeth of a young person with

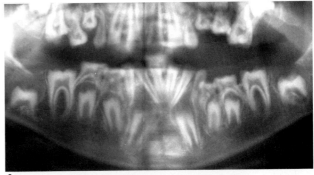

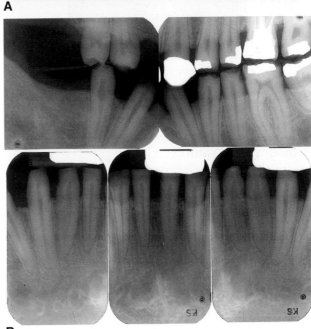

B

FIG. **18-25** **A,** A cropped panoramic film of amelogenesis imperfecta (generalized hypoplastic form) with absence of enamel; note that without the normal tooth crowns the follicular spaces appear large. **B,** Intraoral films of another case of amelogenesis imperfecta; note the very thin enamel layer.

generalized hypomineralization of the enamel are frequently dark brown from food stains.

Hypomaturation/hypocalcification. This classification indicates a combination of hypomaturation and hypocalcification that involves both the permanent and deciduous dentition. If the dominant defect is hypomaturation, then the term *hypomaturation-hypocalcification* is used. The enamel is usually mottled and discolored (yellow and brown). The enamel has the same radiopacity as the dentin. When the dominant defect is hypocalcification, the term *hypocalcification-hypomaturation* is used. The appearance of the teeth is similar, but the enamel is thin.

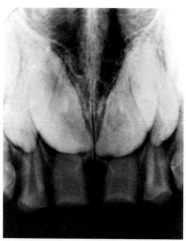

FIG. **18-26**   Amelogenesis imperfecta (generalized hypo-mineralized form). Note the reduced enamel density and the rapid abrasion of the crowns of primary teeth.

Radiographic Features

Identification of amelogenesis imperfecta is made primarily by clinical examination. Although this condition manifests radiographically, the radiographic features substantiate the clinical impression. The radiographic signs of hypoplastic amelogenesis imperfecta include a square shape of the crown, a relatively thin opaque layer of enamel, and low or absent cusps. The density of the enamel is normal. Pitted enamel appears as sharply localized areas of mottled density, quite different from the image cast by a tooth that is normal in shape and density. The hypomaturation form demonstrates a normal thickness of the enamel, but its density is the same as that of dentin. In the hypocalcified forms the enamel thickness is normal, but its density is even less (more radiolucent) than that of dentin. With advanced abrasion, obliteration of the pulp chambers may complicate recognition of the radiographic picture.

Differential Diagnosis

If advanced abrasion is present and secondary dentin obliterates the pulp chambers, the radiographic picture of the amelogenesis imperfecta appears similar to that of dentinogenesis imperfecta. However, the presence of bulbous crowns and narrow roots, the relatively normal density of any remaining enamel, and the obliteration of pulp chambers and root canals, in the absence of marked attrition, are characteristic of dentinogenesis imperfecta (see the following section) and should distinguish it from amelogenesis imperfecta.

Management

Appropriate treatment for amelogenesis imperfecta is restoration of the esthetics and function of the affected teeth.

DENTINOGENESIS IMPERFECTA

Synonym

Hereditary opalescent dentin*

Definition

Dentinogenesis imperfecta is a developmental disturbance primarily of the dentin. Enamel may be thinner than normal in this condition. Dentinogenesis imperfecta is an autosomal dominant disturbance of high penetrance and occurs with equal frequency in both sexes. Both the deciduous and permanent dentition may show this defect.

Two types of dentinogenesis imperfecta exist. Type I is associated with osteogenesis imperfecta (see following description). The tooth roots and pulp chambers are generally small and underdeveloped. The lesion affects the primary dentition more severely than the permanent teeth. Type II lesions are similar to type I lesions but affect only the dentin without any skeletal defects. The expression of type II lesions is variable, and occasionally individuals show enlarged pulp chambers in the primary teeth.

Clinical Features

The appearance of the teeth with dentinogenesis imperfecta is characteristic. They show a high degree of amberlike translucency and a variety of colors from yellow to blue-gray. The colors change according to whether the teeth are observed by transmitted light or reflected light. The enamel easily fractures from the teeth and the crowns wear readily. In adults the teeth may frequently wear down to the gingiva. The exposed dentin becomes stained. The color of the abraded teeth may change to dark brown or even black. Some patients demonstrate an anterior open bite.

Radiographic Features

The images of the crowns in patients with dentinogenesis imperfecta are usually of normal size, but a constriction of the cervical portion of the tooth gives the crown a bulbous appearance. Radiographs may reveal slight to marked attrition of the occlusal surface. The roots are usually short and slender. Types I and II show partial or complete obliteration of the pulp chambers. Early in development, the teeth may appear to have large pulp

---

*Although the terms *dentinogenesis imperfecta* and *hereditary opalescent dentin* have been used interchangeably for more than 40 years, evidence suggests they are two distinct entities. Dentinogenesis imperfecta is the dental defect that accompanies osteogenesis imperfecta, whereas hereditary opalescent dentin is an isolated defect. These conditions share common clinical, radiographic, and dental features. For convenience, the author refers to the defect as *dentinogenesis imperfecta*, which is the term that most dentists associate with this condition.

chambers, but these are quickly obliterated by the formation of dentin. Ultimately the root canals may be absent or threadlike (Fig. 18-27). Occasional periapical radiolucencies are seen in association with sound teeth without evidence of pulpal involvement, which may occur from microscopic communication between residual pulp and the oral cavity. These lesions do not occur as frequently as in dentin dysplasia. The architecture of the bone in the maxilla and mandible is normal.

Differential Diagnosis
See the following section on the differential diagnosis of dentin dysplasia.

Management
The placement of prosthetic crowns on the affected teeth is usually unsuccessful unless they have good root support. The teeth should not be extracted from patients 5 to 15 years of age. It is generally preferable to place full overdentures on the teeth to prevent alveolar resorption. In adults extraction of the teeth and their replacement can be recommended.

OSTEOGENESIS IMPERFECTA

Osteogenesis imperfecta is a hereditary disorder characterized by osseous fractures. The pathogenesis is believed to be an inborn error in the synthesis of type I collagen, which results in brittle bones. It is usually transmitted as an autosomal dominant trait. Patients may have blue sclera, wormian bones (bones in skull sutures), skeletal deformities, and progressive osteopenia. Dentinogenesis imperfecta is found in approximately 25% of cases. In addition, oral findings may include class III malocclusions and an increased incidence of impacted first and second molars.

DENTIN DYSPLASIA

Definition
Dentin dysplasia is an autosomal dominant trait that resembles dentinogenesis imperfecta. It is rarer than dentinogenesis imperfecta (1:100,000 compared with 1:8000). Two types have been described, type I (radicular) and type II (coronal) dentin dysplasia. In type I

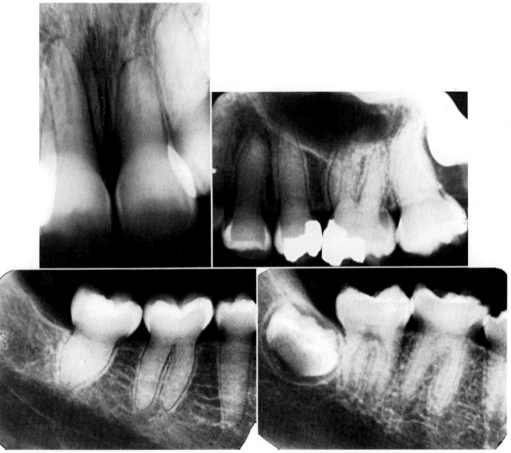

FIG. **18-27** Dentinogenesis imperfecta characteristically shows a constriction in the cervical portion of the root, a bulbous crown, short roots, and a reduced size of the pulp chamber and root canals.

disease, the most marked alterations are found in the appearance of the roots. In type II disease, changes in the crown are most clearly seen in the altered shape of the pulp chambers.

Clinical Features

Clinically, teeth with dentin dysplasia have characteristic features. In the radicular pattern (type I) the teeth have mostly normal color and shape in both dentitions. Occasionally a slight bluish-brown translucency is apparent. Teeth in patients with the type I defect are often misaligned in the arch, and patients may describe drifting and state that the teeth exfoliate with little or no trauma. In the coronal pattern (type II) the crowns of primary teeth appear to be of the same color, size, and contour as those in dentinogenesis imperfecta. The permanent teeth are normal in these respects. Apparently no other distinctive clinical features exist. Although not universally accepted, reports exist that primary teeth rapidly abrade.

Radiographic Features

In type I (radicular dentin dysplasia) the roots of all teeth, primary and permanent, are either short or abnormally shaped (Fig. 18-28). The roots of primary

teeth may be only thin spicules. The pulp chambers and root canals completely fill in before eruption. The extent of obliteration of the pulp chambers and canals is variable. In addition, about 20% of teeth with type I disease have periapical radiolucencies, which are described as either cysts or granulomas. This is likely the result of microscopic communication between the residual pulp and the oral cavity. Association of these periapical radiolucencies with noncarious teeth is an important feature for recognition of this particular entity.

In type II (coronal dentin dysplasia), obliteration of the pulp chamber (Fig. 18-29) and reduction in the caliber of the root canals occurs after eruption (at least by 5 or 6 years). These changes are not seen before

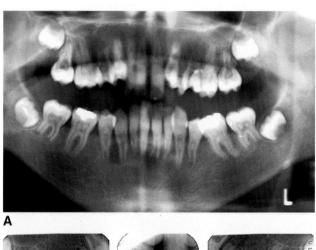

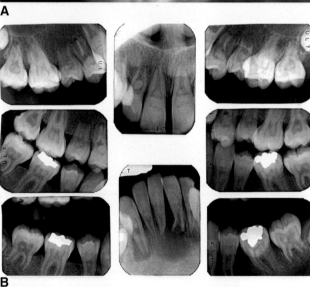

FIG. 18-29   Dentin dysplasia, type II. A panoramic film **(A)** and periapical films **(B)** of the same case show obliteration of the pulp chamber, reduction in the caliber of root canals, and pulp stones obscuring the flame-shaped pulp chambers associated with dentin dysplasia, type II (coronal dentin dysplasia). Periapical inflammatory lesions are associated with some of the mandibular anterior teeth.

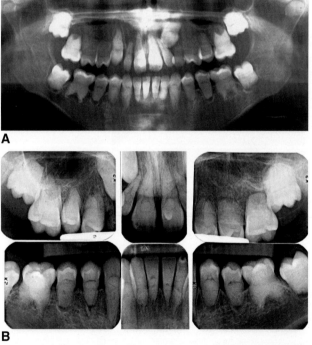

FIG. 18-28   Dentin dysplasia, type I. A panoramic film **(A)** and periapical films **(B)** of the same case show the short and poorly developed roots, obliterated pulp chambers and root canals, and periapical inflammatory lesions associated with dentin dysplasia, type I (radicular).

eruption. As the chambers of the molars are being filled with hypertrophic dentin, the pulp chambers may become flame-shaped and may have multiple pulp stones. Occasionally the anterior teeth and premolars develop a pulp chamber that is thistle-tube in shape because of its extension into the root. The roots of the coronal variety are normal in shape and proportions.

Differential Diagnosis

The differential diagnosis for dentin dysplasia may include only one other entity, dentinogenesis imperfecta. Because these two conditions seem to form a continuum, their differentiation may be difficult at first. Both entities can produce altered color and occluded pulp chambers. In type II dentin dysplasia, however, the pulp chambers do not fill in before eruption. Also, finding a thistle-tube–shaped pulp chamber in a single-rooted tooth strengthens the probability of dentin dysplasia. In addition, crown size can help distinguish between the two: the teeth in dentinogenesis imperfecta have typical bulbous shaped crowns with a constriction in the cervical region, whereas the crowns in dentin dysplasia are usually of normal shape, size, and proportions. If the roots are short and narrow, the condition is likely to be dentinogenesis imperfecta. On the other hand, normal-appearing roots or practically no roots at all should suggest dentin dysplasia. Periapical rarefying osteitis in association with noncarious teeth are more commonly seen in dentin dysplasia.

Management

Teeth with type I dentin dysplasia have such poor root support that prosthetic replacement is about the only practical treatment. On the other hand, teeth that are of normal shape, size, and support (type II) can be crowned if they seem to be rapidly abrading. At the same time the esthetics of discolored anterior teeth can be improved by prosthetic treatment.

REGIONAL ODONTODYSPLASIA

Synonym
Odontogenesis imperfecta

Definition

Regional odontodysplasia is a relatively rare condition in which both enamel and dentin are hypoplastic and hypocalcified. The result is localized arrest in tooth development. Typically, regional odontodysplasia affects only a few adjacent teeth in a quadrant. They may be either primary or permanent teeth. If the primary teeth are affected, their successors are usually involved. Although many theories exist regarding the etiology of this condition, its cause is unknown.

Clinical Features

Teeth affected with regional odontodysplasia are small and mottled brown as a result of staining of the hypocalcified hypoplastic enamel. They are especially susceptible to caries, are brittle, and are subject to fracture and pulpal infection. Central incisors are most often affected, with lateral incisors and canines also occasionally showing the defect (most often in the maxilla). Eruption of the defective teeth is often delayed and in severe cases they may not erupt.

Radiographic Features

The radiographic images of teeth with regional odontodysplasia have a ghostlike appearance. The pulp chambers are large and the root canals wide because the hypoplastic dentin is thin, just serving to outline the image of the root (Fig. 18-30). The poorly outlined roots are short. The enamel is, likewise, thin and less dense than usual, sometimes so thin and poorly mineralized that it may not be evident on the radiograph. The tooth is little more than a thin shell of hypoplastic enamel and dentin. Teeth that do not erupt are so hypomineralized and hypoplastic that they appear to be resorbing.

Differential Diagnosis

The malformed teeth occasionally seen in one of the expressions of dentinogenesis imperfecta may occasionally be confused with those in regional odontodysplasia. However, the fact that the dentinogenesis imperfecta trait usually carries a history of familial involvement, in contrast to odontodysplasia (which is not hereditary), is an important distinguishing feature. Also the enamel in regional odontodysplasia is obviously hypoplastic, which is not the case in dentinogenesis imperfecta. Finally, only a few teeth of either dentition in an isolated segment of the arch are affected in regional odontodysplasia, whereas the type of dentinogenesis imperfecta that resembles regional odontodysplasia involves all primary teeth.

Management

With the advent of newer restorative materials, it is recommended to retain and restore the affected teeth as much as possible. Unerupted teeth should be retained during the period of skeletal growth. Severely damaged permanent teeth that become pulpally involved may require removal and replacement.

ENAMEL PEARL

Synonyms
Enamel drop, enamel nodule, and enameloma

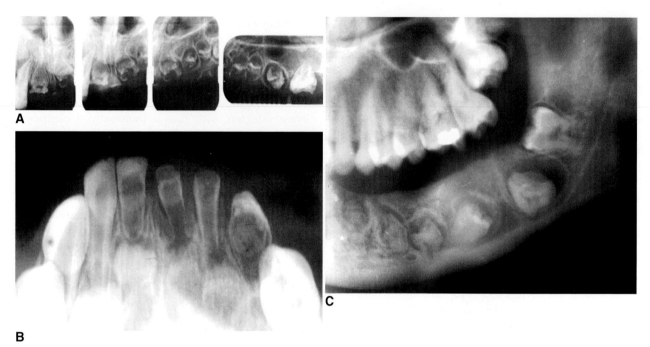

FIG. **18-30**   Regional odontodysplasia revealing poor mineralization of both enamel and dentin. **A,** Involvement of the left maxillary dentition. **B,** Involvement of the primary incisors and cuspids. **C,** Involvement of the left mandibular cuspids and first and second molars; note the lack of eruption and hypoplasia of enamel and dentin expressed mainly as short roots.

Definition

The enamel pearl is a small globule of enamel 1 to 3 mm in diameter that occurs on the roots of molars (Fig. 18-31). It is found in about 3% of the population, probably formed by Hertwig's epithelial root sheath before the epithelium loses its enamel-forming potential. Usually only one pearl develops, but occasionally more develop. Enamel pearls may have a core of dentin and rarely a pulp horn extending from the chamber of the host tooth.

Clinical Features

Most enamel pearls form below the crest of the gingiva and are not detected during a clinical examination. However, they develop at the trifurcation of a maxillary molar (usually third molar) or the bifurcation of a mandibular molar. Some lie at or just apical to the cementoenamel junction. Those that form on the maxillary molars are usually at the mesial or distal aspect, in contrast to those on the mandibular molars, which are most often buccal or lingual. Usually no clinical symptoms are associated with their presence, although they may predispose to periodontal pocket formation and subsequent periodontal disease.

Radiographic Features

The enamel pearl appears smooth, round, and comparable in degree of radiopacity to the enamel covering the crown (Fig. 18-32). Occasionally the dentin casts a small, round, radiolucent shadow in the center of the radiopaque sphere of enamel. If projected over the crown, it may be obscured.

Differential Diagnosis

It is possible to mistake an enamel pearl for an isolated piece of calculus or a pulp stone. The differentiation between a pulp stone and an enamel pearl can be made by increasing the vertical angle of projection to move the image of the enamel pearl away from the pulp chamber. If the opacity is calculus, it is usually clinically detectable. Occasionally oblique views of maxillary or mandibular molars may cause superimposition of a portion of the roots in the region of the furcation, producing a density that appears similar to an enamel pearl. In this case, producing another image at a slightly different horizontal angle eliminates this radiopaque region.

Management

As a rule, the recognition that a radiopaque mass superimposed on the tooth is an enamel pearl precludes the necessity for treatment. The clinician can remove the mass if its location at the cementoenamel junction predisposes to periodontal disease. The possibility must always be considered that it may contain a pulp horn.

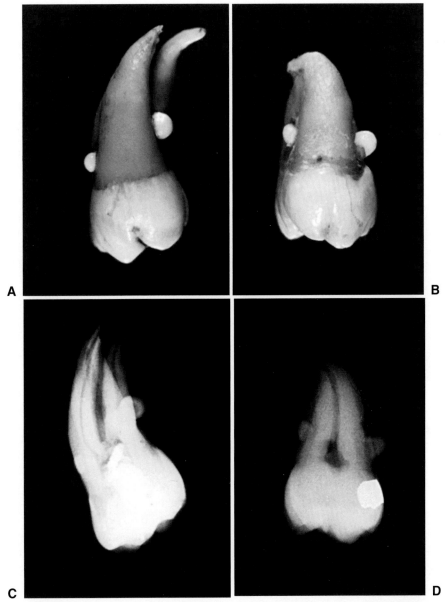

FIG. **18-31** A and **B,** Enamel pearls are small outgrowths of enamel and dentin seen in the furcation area of a tooth. **C** and **D,** Radiographs of these teeth. (Courtesy Dr. R. Kienholz, Dallas, TX.)

TALON CUSP

Definition

The talon cusp is an anomalous hyperplasia of the cingulum of a maxillary or mandibular incisor. It results in the formation of a supernumerary cusp. Normal enamel covers the cusp and fuses with the lingual aspect of the tooth. Any developmental grooves that are present may become caries-susceptible areas. The cusp

may or may not contain an extension (horn) of the pulp. No apparent racial association exists.

Clinical Features

The talon cusp is infrequently encountered. It may be found in either sex and on both primary and permanent incisors. It varies in size from that of a prominent cingulum to that of a cusplike structure extending to the level of the incisal edge. When viewed from its incisal edge, an incisor bearing the cusp is T-shaped, with the top of the T representing the incisal edge. Although it usually occurs as an isolated entity, its incidence has been reported to be increased in teeth related to cleft palate syndromes and in association with other anomalies.

Radiographic Features

The radiopaque image of a talon cusp is superimposed on that of the crown of the involved incisor (Fig. 18-33). Its outline is smooth, and a layer of normal-

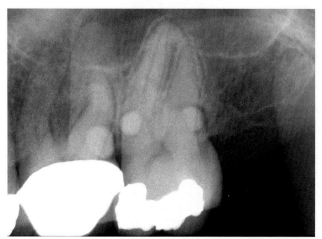

FIG. 18-32   Three enamel pearls (one attached to the first molar and two on the second molar) are apparent in this periapical film.

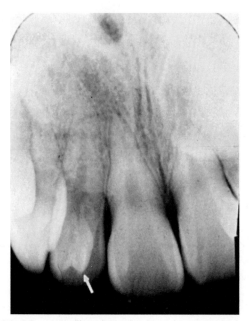

FIG. 18-33   Maxillary lateral incisor bearing a talon cusp *(arrow)*. Note that the tooth also has two enamel invaginations. (Courtesy Dr. R.A. Cederberg, Dallas, TX.)

appearing enamel is generally distinguishable. The radiograph may not reveal a pulp horn. The cusp is often apparent radiographically before eruption and may simulate the presence of a supernumerary tooth.

Differential Diagnosis

The appearance of a talon cusp is quite distinctive. Although it may not be distinguishable from a supernumerary tooth with a single film, using a second image with either the parallax or the buccal object technique can demonstrate a connection to the tooth.

Management

If developmental grooves are present where the cusp fuses with the lingual surface of the incisor, treatment may be required to prevent the development of decay. If the cusp is large, it may pose an esthetic or occlusal problem. Slowly removing the cusp over a long period may stimulate the formation of secondary dentin and prevent exposure of a pulp horn.

TURNER'S HYPOPLASIA

Synonym

Turner's tooth

Definition

Turner's hypoplasia is a term used to describe a permanent tooth with a local hypoplastic defect in its crown. This defect may have been caused by the extension of a periapical infection from its deciduous predecessor or by mechanical trauma transmitted through the deciduous tooth. If the trauma (whether infectious or mechanical) takes place while the crown is forming, it may adversely affect the ameloblasts of the developing tooth and result in some degree of enamel hypoplasia or hypomineralization.

Clinical Features

Turner's hypoplasia most often affects the mandibular premolars, generally because of the relative susceptibility of the deciduous molars to caries, their proximity to the developing premolars, and their relative time of mineralization. The severity of the defect depends on the severity of the infection or mechanical trauma and on the stage of development of the permanent tooth. It may disturb matrix formation or calcification, in which case the result varies from a hypoplastic defect to a hypomineralization spot in the enamel. The hypomineralized area may become stained, and the tooth usually shows a brownish spot on the crown. If the insult is severe enough to cause hypoplasia, the morphology of the crown may show pitting or a more pronounced defect.

Radiographic Features

The enamel irregularities associated with Turner's hypoplasia alter the normal contours of the affected tooth and are often apparent on a radiograph (Fig. 18-34). The involved region of the crown may appear as an ill-defined radiolucent region. A stained hypomineralized spot may not be apparent because there is an insufficient difference in the degree of radiopacity between the spot and the crown of the tooth. Also, the hypomineralized areas may become remineralized by continued contact with saliva.

Differential Diagnosis

Other conditions that result in deformation of the tooth crown, such as the delivery of high doses of therapeutic radiation, should be considered, although usually several adjacent teeth are involved. Small defects may simulate the appearance of carious lesions but can be easily differentiated with clinical inspection.

Management

If a radiograph of a tooth affected by Turner's hypoplasia shows that the tooth has good root support, the esthetics and function of the deformed crown can be restored.

CONGENITAL SYPHILIS

Definition

About 30% of people with congenital syphilis develop dental hypoplasia that involves the permanent incisors and first molars. Development of primary teeth is seldom disturbed. The affected incisors are called *Hutchinson's teeth* and the molars, *mulberry molars*. The changes characteristic of the condition seem to result from a direct infection of the developing tooth because the spirochete of syphilis has been identified in the tooth germ.

Clinical Features

The affected incisor has a characteristic screwdriver-shaped crown, with the mesial and distal surfaces tapering from the middle of the crown to the incisal edge (Fig. 18-35). The effect is that the edge may be no wider than the cervical area of the tooth. The incisal edge is also frequently notched. Although maxillary central incisors usually demonstrate these syphilitic changes, the maxillary lateral and mandibular central incisors may also be involved.

As with incisor crowns, the crowns of affected first molars are quite characteristic, being usually smaller than normal and sometimes even smaller than second molar crowns. The most distinctive feature is the constricted occlusal third of the crown, with the occlusal surface no wider than the cervical portion of the tooth. The cusps of these molars are also reduced in size and poorly formed. The enamel over the occlusal surface is hypoplastic, unevenly formed in irregular globules, like the surface of a mulberry.

Radiographic Features

The characteristic shapes of the affected incisor and molar crowns can be identified in the radiographic image. Because the crowns of these teeth form at about 1 year of age, radiographs may reveal the dental features of congenital syphilis 4 to 5 years before the teeth erupt.

Management

Hutchinson's teeth and mulberry molars often do not require dental treatment. Esthetic restorations may be

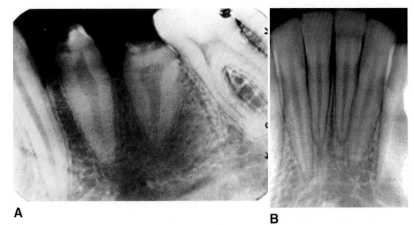

A **B**

FIG. **18-34** **A,** Turner's hypoplasia, demonstrated as an extensive malformation and hypomineralization of the crowns of both premolars. **B,** A band of hypoplasia extending around the crown of the mandibular left central incisor.

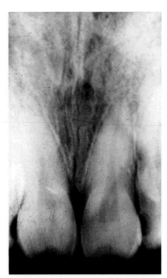

FIG. **18-35**   Congenital syphilis may induce a developmental malformation of the maxillary central incisors characterized by tapering of the mesial and distal surfaces toward the incisal edge with notching of the incisal edge.

used to correct the hypoplastic defects as indicated clinically.

Acquired Abnormalities

Acquired changes of the dentition, those that are initiated after development of the tooth, range in severity from changes that have no clinical significance to those that cause tooth loss. In the latter case, early detection and treatment is required to preserve the tooth.

ACQUIRED PATHOLOGIC CONDITIONS

ATTRITION

Definition
Attrition is the physiologic wearing away of the dentition resulting from occlusal contacts between the maxillary and mandibular teeth. It occurs on the incisal, occlusal, and interproximal surfaces. Interproximal wear causes the contact points to become flattened into interproximal surfaces. Attrition occurs in more than 90% of young adults and is generally more severe in men than women. Its extent depends on the abrasiveness of the diet, salivary factors, mineralization of the teeth, and emotional tension. Physiologic attrition is a component of the aging process. When the loss of dental tissue becomes excessive, however, as from bruxism, the attrition becomes pathologic.

Clinical Features
The tooth wear patterns from attrition are characteristic. Wear facets first appear on cusps and marginal oblique and transverse ridges. The incisal edges of the maxillary and mandibular incisors show evidence of broadening. The wear facets on the occlusal surfaces of molars become more pronounced, with the lingual cusps of maxillary teeth and the buccal cusps of mandibular posteriors showing the most wear. When the dentin is exposed, it usually becomes stained and the color contrast between stained dentin and enamel highlights the areas of attrition. The incisal edges of mandibular incisors tend to become pitted because the dentin wears more rapidly than its surrounding enamel. In the case of pathologic attrition the patterns of wear are generally not as uniformly progressive as those described for physiologic attrition. The wear facets develop at a faster rate. It is important to emphasize, however, that *physiologic attrition* is a relative term and its clinical manifestations vary with the customs (dietary and otherwise) of the population in question.

Radiographic Features
The radiographic appearance of attrition results in a change in the normal outline of the tooth structure, altering the normal curved surfaces into flat planes. The crown is shortened and is bereft of the incisal or occlusal surface enamel (Fig. 18-36). Often a number of adjacent teeth in each arch show this wear pattern. Reduction in the size of the pulp chambers and canals may occur because attrition stimulates the deposition of secondary dentin. This may result in complete obliteration of the pulp chamber and canals. A simultaneous widening of the PDL space frequently occurs if the

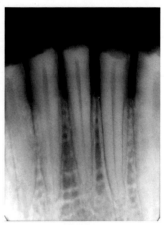

FIG. **18-36**   Attrition is the physiologic wearing away of tooth structure. Note the severe wearing of almost the total coronal aspect of these mandibular incisors.

tooth is mobile. Occasionally evidence of hypercementosis is present.

Differential Diagnosis

Recognition of physiologic attrition is usually not difficult given the characteristic history, location, and extent of wear. The general pattern is predictable and familiar.

Management

Physiologic attrition does not require treatment.

ABRASION

Abrasion is the nonphysiologic wearing away of teeth by contact with foreign substances. It results from friction induced by factitious habits or occupational hazards. A clinical examination usually readily reveals it. Although many causes exist, two occur with moderate frequency and can usually be eliminated: improper tooth brushing and improper or excessive use of dental floss. Other causes include pipe smoking, opening hairpins with the teeth, improper use of toothpicks, denture clasps, and cutting thread with the teeth.

TOOTHBRUSH INJURY

Clinical Features

Toothbrush abrasion is probably the most frequently observed type of injury and is usually the result of improper technique, most frequently a back-and-forth movement of the brush with heavy pressure. This causes the bristles to assume a wedge-shaped arrangement between the crowns and the gingiva. The brushing wears a V-shaped groove into the cervical area of the tooth, usually involving enamel and the softer root surface.

Abraded teeth may become sensitive as the dentin is exposed. The abraded areas are usually most severe at the cementoenamel junction on the labial and buccal surfaces of maxillary premolars, canines, and incisors, in approximately that order. The enamel generally limits the coronal extension of abrasion. The lesions are more common and more pronounced on the left side for a right-handed person, and vice versa. The deposition of secondary dentin opposite the abraded areas usually keeps pace with the destruction at the surface, so pulpal exposure is rarely a complication.

Radiographic Features

The radiographic appearance of toothbrush abrasion is radiolucent defects at the cervical level of teeth. These defects have well-defined semilunar shapes with borders of increasing radiopacity. The pulp chambers

of the more seriously involved teeth are frequently partially or completely obliterated. The most common location of this injury is the premolar areas, usually in the upper arch.

DENTAL FLOSS INJURY

Clinical Features

Excessive and improper use of dental floss, particularly in conjunction with toothpaste, may result in abrasion of the dentition (Fig. 18-37). The most frequent site is the cervical portion of the proximal surfaces just above the gingiva.

Radiographic Features

The radiographic appearance of dental floss abrasion is narrow semilunar radiolucency in the interproximal surfaces cervical area. Most often the radiolucent grooves on the distal surfaces of the teeth are deeper than those on the mesial surfaces, probably because it is easier to exert more pressure in a forward direction by pulling than by pushing the floss backward into the mouth.

Differential Diagnosis

Dental floss abrasion is readily identified by its clinical and radiographic appearance. Its location provides some evidence regarding the nature of the cause. This can be verified by the patient history. On occasion the

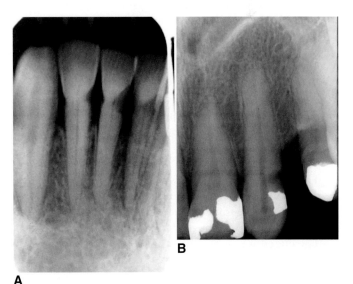

FIG. 18-37 **A,** Abrasion of the cervical portion of these teeth is evident from excessive (and improper) use of dental floss. Note the obliteration of the pulp chambers and reduction in size of the root canals. **B,** Abrasion on the distal aspect of the maxillary cuspid due to a denture clasp.

radiolucencies simulate carious lesions located at the cervical region of the tooth. The differential diagnosis is accomplished with clinical inspection.

Management

The primary treatment recommended for abrasion is elimination of the causative agents or habits. Extensively abraded areas can be restored.

EROSION

Definition

Erosion of teeth results from a chemical action not involving bacteria. Although in many cases the cause is not apparent, in others it is obviously the contact of acid with teeth. The source of the acid may be (1) chronic vomiting or acid reflux from gastrointestinal disorders or (2) a diet in which the individual consumes large amounts of acidic foods, citrus fruits, or carbonated beverages. Some occupations involve contact with acids that can induce dental erosion. The location of the erosion, the pattern of eroded areas, and the appearance of the lesion usually provide clues as to the origin of the decalcifying agent. Regurgitated acids attack lingual surfaces; dietary acids primarily demineralize labial surfaces.

Clinical Features

Dental erosion is usually found on incisors, often involving multiple teeth. The lesions are generally smooth, glistening depressions in the enamel surface, frequently near the gingiva. Erosion may result in so much loss of enamel that a pink spot shows through the remaining enamel.

Radiographic Features

Areas of erosion appear as radiolucent defects on the crown. Their margins may be either well defined or diffuse. A clinical examination usually resolves any questionable lesions.

Differential Diagnosis

The diagnosis of erosion is based on the recognition of dished-out or V-shaped defects in the buccal and labial enamel and dentinal surfaces. The margins of a restoration may project above the remaining tooth surface. The edges of lesions caused by erosion are usually more rounded off than those caused by abrasion.

Management

With abrasion, erosion is managed with identification and removal of the causative agent. If the cause is chronic vomiting from a psychologic disorder, a daily fluoride rinse should be prescribed during counseling

therapy. If the cause is unknown, management depends solely on restoration of the defect. This prevents additional damage, possible pulp exposure, and objectionable esthetic appearance.

RESORPTION

Resorption is the removal of tooth structure by osteoclasts, referred to as *odontoclasts* when they are resorbing tooth structure. Resorption is classified as internal or external on the basis of the surface of the tooth being resorbed. External resorption affects the outer tooth surface, and internal resorption affects the inner surface of the pulp chamber and canal. These two types differ in their radiographic appearance and treatment. The resorption discussed here is not that associated with the normal loss of deciduous teeth. Although the etiology of most resorptive lesions remains unknown, at least presumptive evidence exists that some lesions are the sequelae of chronic infection (inflammation), excessive pressure and function, or factors associated with local tumors and cysts.

INTERNAL RESORPTION

Definition

Internal resorption occurs within the pulp chamber or canal and involves resorption of the surrounding dentin. This results in enlargement of the size of the pulp space at the expense of tooth structure. This condition may be transient and self-limiting or progressive. The etiology of the recruitment and activation of odontoclasts is unknown but may be related to inflammation of the pulpal tissues. Internal resorption has been reported to be initiated by acute trauma to the tooth, direct and indirect pulp capping, pulpotomy, and enamel invagination.

Clinical Features

Internal resorption may affect any tooth in either the primary or secondary dentition. It occurs most frequently in permanent teeth, usually in central incisors and first and second molars. The resorption most commonly begins during the fourth and fifth decades and is more common in males. When the lesion is in the pulp chamber of the crown, it may enlarge until the crown has a dark shadow. If the enlarging pulp perforates the dentin and involves the enamel, it may appear as a pink spot. If the condition is not intercepted, it may perforate the crown, with hemorrhagic tissue projecting from the perforation, and lead to infectious pulpitis. When the lesion occurs in the root of a tooth, it is for the most part clinically silent. If the resorption is extensive, it may weaken the tooth and result in a fracture. It is also possible that the pulp may expand into the periodontal ligament and communicate with a deep periodontal pocket or the gingival sulcus, also leading to pulpal infection.

Radiographic Features

Radiographs can reveal symptomless early lesions of internal resorption. The lesions are radiolucent and round, oval, or elongated within the root or crown and continuous with the image of the pulp chamber or canal. The outline is usually sharply defined and smooth or slightly scalloped. The result is an irregular widening of the pulp chamber or canal (Fig. 18-38). It is characteristically homogeneously radiolucent, without bony trabeculation or pulp stones. However, the internal structure may seem to be apparent, if the

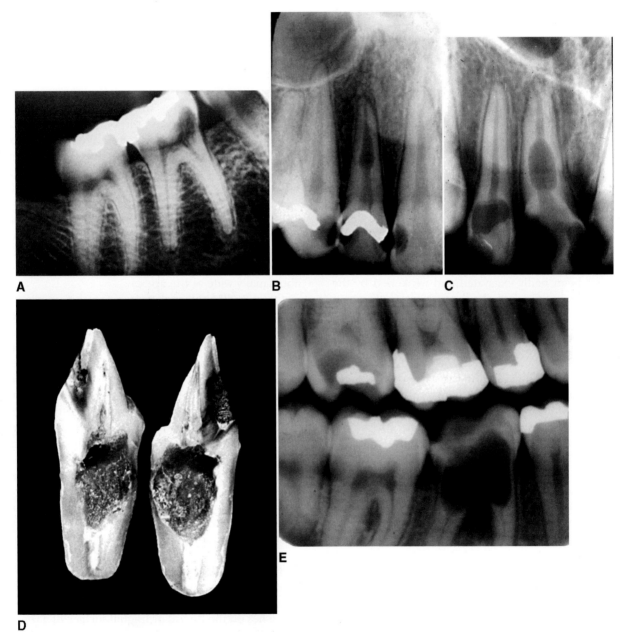

FIG. **18-38** Internal root resorption may be seen in the crown. **A,** In this example the connection to the pulp chamber is not obvious. **B** and **C,** Examples where the margins of the internal resorption are continuous with the pulp canal. **D,** A sectioned incisor (after crown reduction); note the large area of internal root resorption. **E,** Example of extensive resorption involving a mandibular first molar.

surface of the resorbed tooth structure is very irregular and has a scalloped texture. In some cases virtually the whole pulp may enlarge within a tooth, although more commonly the lesion remains localized.

Differential Diagnosis

The most common lesions to be confused with internal root resorption are dental caries on the buccal or lingual surface of a tooth and external root resorption. Carious lesions have more diffuse margins than lesions caused by internal root resorption. Clinical inspection quickly reveals caries on the buccal or lingual surface of a tooth. Also, the mesial and distal surfaces of the pulp chamber and canal can usually be separated from the borders of the carious lesion. With internal root resorption, however, the image of the resorption cannot be separated from the pulp chamber or canal by altering the horizontal angulation of the x-ray beam.

Management

The treatment for internal resorption depends on the condition of the tooth. If the process has not led to a serious weakening defect in the structure, filling the root canal halts the resorption. If the expanding pulp has not structurally compromised the tooth but a perforation of the root has occurred, the perforated surface can be surgically exposed and retrofilled. If the tooth has been badly excavated and weakened by the resorption, extraction may be the only alternative.

EXTERNAL RESORPTION

Definition

In external resorption odontoclasts resorb the outer surface of the tooth. This most commonly involves the root surface but may also involve the crown of an unerupted tooth. The resorption may involve cementum and dentin and in some cases gradually extends to the pulp. Because the recruitment of odontoclasts requires an intact blood supply, only sections of the tooth with soft tissue coverage are susceptible to this resorption. This resorption may occur to a single tooth, multiple teeth, or, in rare cases, all of the dentition. In many cases the etiology is unknown but in others causes can be attributed to localized inflammatory lesions, reimplanted teeth, tumors and cysts, excessive mechanical (orthodontic) and occlusal forces, and impacted teeth.

Clinical Features

External resorption is usually not recognized because often no characteristic signs or symptoms exist. Even when considerable loss of tooth structure occurs, the tooth in question is frequently firm and immobile in the dental arch. In advanced resorption, some nonspecific pain or fracture of the resorbed root occurs.

External resorption may appear at the apex of the tooth or on the lateral root surface, although it most commonly occurs in the apical and cervical regions. It is slightly more prevalent in mandibular teeth than in maxillary teeth and involves primarily the central incisors, canines, and premolars. External root resorption is common. One study of 18- to 25-year-old men and women found that all patients exhibited some degree of external root resorption in four or more teeth.

Radiographic Features

Common sites for external root resorption are the apical and cervical regions. When the lesion begins at the apex, it generally causes a smooth resorption of the tooth structure resulting in blunting of the root apex (Fig. 18-39). Almost always the bone and lamina dura follow the resorbing root and present a normal appearance around this shortened structure. When external root resorption occurs as the result of a periapical inflammatory lesion, the lamina dura is lost around the apex. After normal apexification (constriction of the walls of the pulp canal at the apex) of the pulp canal, it is very difficult or impossible to see the canal exit the apex of the tooth. However, if resorption of the apical region has occurred, the pulp canal is visible and is abnormally wide at the apex.

Occasionally external root resorption involves the lateral aspects of roots (Fig. 18-40). Such lesions tend to be irregular, may involve one side more than the other, and occur in any tooth. A common cause of external resorption on the side of a root is the presence of an unerupted adjacent tooth. Examples of such include resorption of the distal aspect of the roots of an upper second molar by the crown of the adjacent third molar and resorption of the root of a permanent central or lateral incisor, or both, by an unerupted maxillary canine. External resorption of an entire tooth can occur when the tooth is unerupted and completely embedded in bone (Fig. 18-41), usually involving the maxillary canine or third molar. In such instances the entire tooth, including the root and crown, may undergo resorption.

Differential Diagnosis

External root resorption on the apex or lateral surface of a root is radiographically self-evident. When the lesion lies on the buccal or lingual surface of a root and above the level of the adjacent bone, the differential diagnosis includes caries and internal resorption. Internal resorption characteristically appears as an expansion of the pulp chamber or canal. In the case of external resorption the image of the normal intact pulp

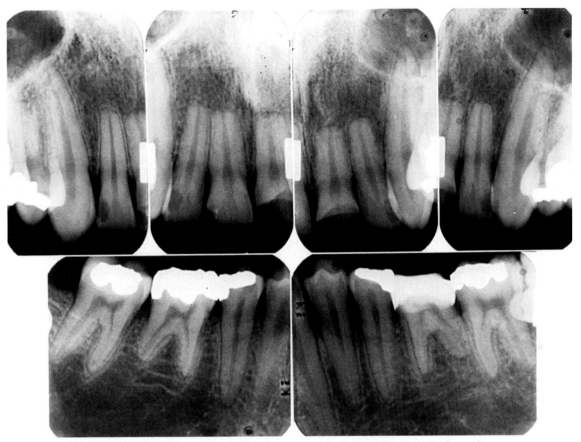

FIG. **18-39** External root resorption results in a loss of tooth structure from the apex. Note the wide openings of the pulp canals and the intact lamina dura.

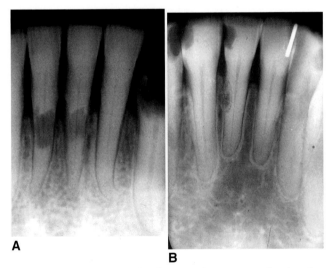

A

B

FIG. **18-40** **A,** Example of external root resorption involving the buccal or lateral surface of the root of the mandibular central incisors which appears as a sharply defined radiolucency confined to the root surfaces. **B,** Example of external root resorption of a mandibular central incisor; note that bone has replaced the resorbed root, sometimes referred to as *inostosis.*

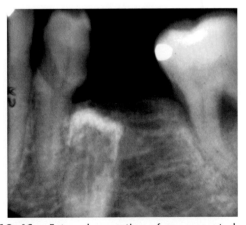

FIG. **18-41** External resorption of an unerupted second bicuspid, both enamel and dentin have been resorbed; note residual enamel of the crown and a hint of a pulp chamber.

chamber or canal may be traced through the radiolucent area of external resorption. Also, projections made at different angles can be compared. The location of the radiolucency caused by external root resorption moves with respect to the pulp canal, whereas the image of internal resorption remains fixed to the canal.

Management

When the cause of external root resorption is known, the treatment is usually to remove the etiologic factors. This may mean cessation of excessive mechanical forces, removal of an adjacent impacted tooth, or eradication of a cyst, tumor, or source of inflammation. If the area of resorption is broad and on an accessible surface of the root (such as at the cervical location), curettage of the defect and the placement of a restoration usually stops the process.

SECONDARY DENTIN

Definition

Secondary dentin is that deposited in the pulp chamber after the formation of primary dentin has been completed. This is a normal aging process and results from such stimuli as chewing or slight trauma. Secondary dentin also develops after chronic trauma from such pathologic conditions as moderately progressive caries, trauma, erosion, attrition, abrasion, or a dental restorative procedure. This specific stimulus promotes a more rapid and localized coronal response than that seen as a result of normal aging. The term *tertiary dentin* has

been suggested to identify dentin specifically initiated by stimuli other than the normal aging response and normal biologic function.

Clinical Features

The response of odontoblasts in producing secondary dentin reduces the sensitivity of teeth to stimuli from the external environment. In elderly individuals with extensive secondary dentin formation, this reduced sensitivity may be especially pronounced. Similarly, the formation of an additional layer of dentin between the pulp and a region of insult reduces the sensitivity often experienced by individuals with recent dental restorations or coronal fractures.

Radiographic Features

Radiographically, secondary dentin is indistinguishable from primary dentin. It is visible as a reduction in size of the normal pulp chamber and canals (Fig. 18-42). When secondary dentin formation results from the normal aging process, the result is a generalized reduction in pulp chamber and canal size, maintaining a relatively normal shape. Often there remains only a thin, narrow pulp chamber and canal. The pulp horns usually disappear relatively early, followed by a reduction in size of the pulp chamber and narrowing of the canals. When more specific stimuli initiate secondary dentin formation, it begins in the region adjacent to the source of stimuli and alters the normal shape of the pulp chamber. Although formation of secondary dentin may continue until the pulp appears to be

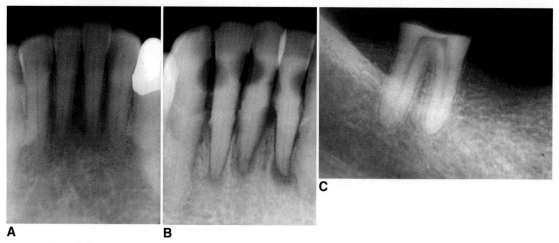

FIG. **18-42**   **A**, Normal formation of secondary dentin causes recession of the pulp chamber and narrowing of the canal. **B**, Secondary dentin has obliterated the pulp chamber and narrowed the pulp canal likely secondary to the carious lesions. **C**, Secondary dentin formation has obliterated the pulp chamber stimulated by the severe attrition of the coronal aspect of this molar.

completely obliterated, histologic studies show that even in these extreme cases, a small thread of viable pulp tissue remains.

Differential Diagnosis

Secondary dentin is recognized indirectly by the reduction in size of the pulp chamber. This appearance differs from the pulp stone. The pulp stone (see the following description) simply occupies some pulp chamber or canal space, but it has a round to oval shape (conforming to the chamber).

Management

Secondary dentin per se does not require treatment. The precipitating cause is removed if possible and the tooth restored when appropriate.

PULP STONES

Definition

Pulp stones are foci of calcification in the dental pulp. They are probably apparent microscopically in more than half the teeth of young people and in almost all the teeth of people older than 50 years of age. Although most are microscopic, they vary in size, with some as large as 2 or 3 mm in diameter, almost filling the pulp chamber. Only these larger concretions are radiographically apparent. Although the larger masses represent only 15% to 25% of pulpal calcification, they are a common radiographic finding and may appear in a single tooth or several teeth. Their cause is unknown, and no firm evidence exists that they are associated with any systemic or pulpal disturbance.

Clinical Features

Pulp stones are not clinically discernible.

Radiographic Features

The radiographic appearance of pulp stones is quite variable; they may be seen as radiopaque structures within pulp chambers or root canals or extending from the pulp chamber into the root canals (Fig. 18-43). No uniform shape or number exists. They may be round or oval; and some, occupying most of the pulp chamber, will conform to its shape. In rare instances the canal remodels and increases its girth to accommodate a large stone. Also, pulp stones may occur as a single dense mass or as several small radiopacities. Their outline, likewise, varies from sharply defined to a more diffuse margin. They occur in all tooth types but most commonly in molars.

Differential Diagnosis

Although pulp stones are variable in size and form, their recognition is usually not difficult. However, in some cases differentiation from pulpal sclerosis is difficult.

Management

Pulp stones do not require treatment.

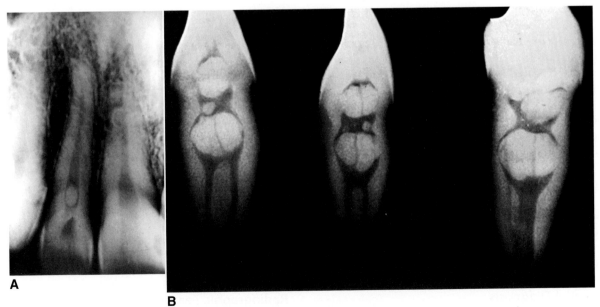

A

B

FIG. **18-43** Pulp stones may be found as isolated calcifications in the pulp (**A**) or may cause deformation of pulp chamber and canals (**B**).

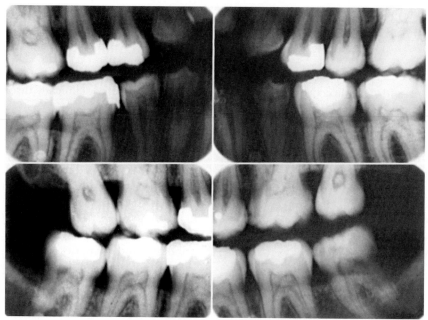

FIG. **18-44**   Pulpal sclerosis is seen as diffuse calcification of the pulp chamber and canals.

PULPAL SCLEROSIS

Definition

Pulpal sclerosis is another form of calcification in the pulp chamber and canals of teeth. In contrast to pulp stones, pulpal sclerosis is a diffuse process. Its specific cause is unknown, although its appearance correlates strongly with age. About 66% of all teeth in individuals between the ages of 10 and 20 years, as well as 90% of all teeth in individuals between the ages of 50 and 70 years, show histologic evidence of pulpal sclerosis. Histologically the pattern of calcification is amorphous and unorganized, being evident as linear strands or columns of calcified material paralleling blood vessels and nerves in the pulp.

Clinical Features

Pulpal sclerosis is a clinically silent process without clinical manifestation.

Radiographic Features

Early pulpal sclerosis, a degenerative process, is not radiographically demonstrable. Diffuse pulpal sclerosis produces a generalized, ill-defined collection of fine radiopacities throughout large areas of the pulp chamber and pulp canals (Fig. 18-44).

Differential Diagnosis

The differential diagnosis includes small pulp stones, but this differentiation is academic because neither condition requires treatment.

Management

Pulpal sclerosis does not require treatment. As with pulp stones, its only importance may be that it can cause difficulty in the performance of endodontic therapy when such a procedure is indicated for other reasons.

HYPERCEMENTOSIS

Definition

Hypercementosis is excessive deposition of cementum on the tooth roots. In most cases its cause is unknown. Occasionally it appears on a supraerupted tooth after the loss of an opposing tooth. Another cause of hypercementosis is inflammation, usually resulting from periapical inflammatory lesions. In this condition, cementum is deposited on the root surface adjacent to the apex. Occasionally hypercementosis has been associated with teeth that are in hyperocclusion or that have been fractured. Finally, hypercementosis occurs in patients with Paget's disease of bone (see Chapter 23) and with hyperpituitarism (gigantism and acromegaly).

Clinical Features

Hypercementosis does not cause any clinical signs or symptoms.

Radiographic Features

Hypercementosis is evident radiographically as an excessive buildup of cementum around all or part of a root (Fig. 18-45). The outline is usually smooth but on

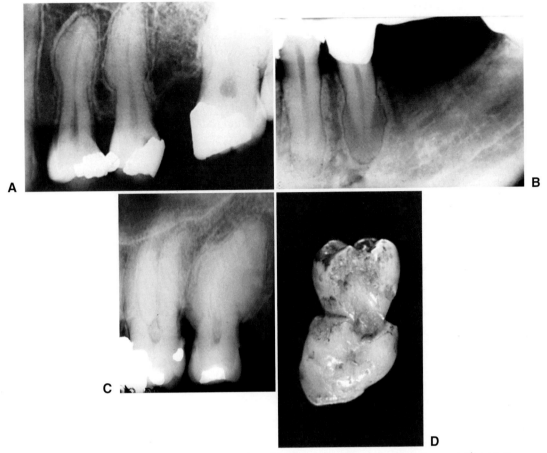

FIG. **18-45** A-C, Hypercementosis is evident as a buildup of cementum on the root surface of teeth. Note the continuity of the lamina dura and the PDL space that encompasses the extra cementum. **D,** Extracted molar, showing extensive hypercementosis. (**D,** Courtesy Dr. R. Kienholz, Dallas, TX.)

occasion may be seen as an irregular enlargement of the root. It is most evident at the apical end and is usually seen as a mildly irregular accumulation of cementum. This cementum is slightly more radiolucent than dentin. Of importance is the fact that the lamina dura and PDL space encompass the extra dentin. In the case of Paget's disease the hypercementosis is usually very exuberant and irregular in outline.

Differential Diagnosis

The differential diagnosis may include any radiopaque structure that is seen within the vicinity of the root, such as enostosis or mature cemental dysplasia. The differentiating characteristic is the presence of the periodontal membrane space around the hypercementosis. There may be a resemblance to a small benign cementoblastoma. Occasionally a severely dilacerated root may have the appearance of hypercementosis.

Management

Hypercementosis itself requires no treatment. If a related condition such as a periapical inflammatory lesion exists, treatment may be necessary. Perhaps the primary significance of hypercementosis relates to the difficulty that the root configuration can pose if extraction is indicated.

BIBLIOGRAPHY

DEVELOPMENTAL ABNORMALITIES

Bergsma D, editor: Birth defects compendium, ed 2, New York, 1979, Alan R Liss.

Dixon GH, Stewart RE: Genetic aspects of anomalous tooth development. In Steward RE, Prescott GH, editors: Oral facial genetics, St. Louis, 1976, Mosby.

Pindborg JJ: Pathology of the dental hard tissues, N Engl J Med 301:13, 1979.

Schulze C: Developmental abnormalities of the teeth and jaws. In Gorlin RJ, Goldman HM, editors: Thoma's oral pathology, ed 6, vol 1, St. Louis, 1970, Mosby.

Witkop CJ Jr, Rao S: Inherited defects in tooth structure. In Bergsma D, editor: Birth defects. XI. Orofacial structures, vol 7, no 7, Baltimore, 1971, Williams & Wilkins.

Worth HM: Principles and practice of oral radiologic interpretation, Chicago, 1963, Year Book Medical Publishers.

SUPERNUMERARY TEETH

Grahnen H, Lindahl B: Supernumerary teeth in the permanent dentition: a frequency study, Odontol Rev 12:290, 1961.

Grimanis GA, Kyriakides AT, Spyropoulos ND: A survey on supernumerary molars, Quintess Int 22:989, 1991.

Niswander JD: Effects of heredity and environment on development of the dentition, J Dent Res 42:1288, 1963.

Rao SR: Supernumerary teeth. In Bergsma D, editor: Birth defects compendium, ed 2, New York, 1979, Alan R Liss.

Yusof WZ: Non-syndrome multiple supernumerary teeth: literature review, J Can Dent Assoc 56:147, 1990.

DEVELOPMENTALLY MISSING TEETH

al-Emran S: Prevalence of hypodontia and developmental malformation of permanent teeth in Saudi Arabian school children, Br J Orthod 17:115, 1990.

Garn SM, Lewis AB: The relationship between third molar agenesis and reduction in tooth number, Angle Orthod 32:14, 1962.

Keene HJ: The relationship between third molar agenesis and the morphologic variability of the molar teeth, Angle Orthod 35:289, 1965.

Levin LS: Dental and oral abnormalities in selected ectodermal dysplasia syndromes, Birth Defects 24:205, 1988.

O'Dowling IB, McNamara TG: Congenital absence of permanent teeth among Irish school-children, J Ir Dent Assoc 36:136, 1990.

MACRODONTIA

Garn SM, Lewis AB, Kerewsky BS: The magnitude and implications of the relationship between tooth size and body size, Arch Oral Biol 13:129, 1968.

TRANSPOSITION

Schacter H: A treated case of transposed upper canine, Dent Res 71:105, 1951.

FUSION

Hagman FT: Anomalies of form and number, fused primary teeth, a correlation of the dentitions, J Dent Child 55:359, 1988.

Sperber GH: Genetic mechanisms and anomalies in odontogenesis, J Can Dent Assoc 33:433, 1967.

GEMINATION

Tannenbaum KA, Alling EE: Anomalous tooth development: case report of gemination and twinning, Oral Surg 16:883, 1963.

TAURODONTISM

Bixler D: Heritable disorders affecting dentin. In Steward RE, Prescott GA, editors: Oral facial genetics, St. Louis, 1976, Mosby.

DENS IN DENTE

Oehlers FAC: The radicular variety of dens invaginatus, Oral Surg 11:1251, 1958.

Rushton MA: A collection of dilated composite odontomes, Br Dent J 63:65, 1937.

Soames JV, Kuyebi TA: A radicular dens invaginatus, Br Dent J 152:308, 1982.

DENS EVAGINATUS

Oehlers FA, Lee KW, Lee EC: Dens invaginatus (invaginated odontome), Dent Pract 17:239, 1967.

Sykaras SN: Occlusal anomalous tubercle on premolars of a Greek girl, Oral Surg 38:88, 1974.

Yip WW: The prevalence of dens invaginatus, Oral Surg 38:80, 1974.

AMELOGENESIS IMPERFECTA

Crawford PJ, Aldred MJ: X-linked amelogenesis imperfecta: presentation of two kindreds and a review of the literature, Oral Surg 73:449, 1992.

Toller PA: A clinical report of six cases of amelogenesis imperfecta, Oral Surg 12:325, 1959.

Witkop CJ Jr: Amelogenesis imperfecta, dentinogenesis imperfecta and dentin dysplasia revisited: problems in classification, J Oral Pathol 17:547, 1988.

Witkop CJ Jr, Saulk JJ: Heritable defects of enamel. In Stewart RE, Prescott GA, editors: Oral facial genetics, St. Louis, 1976, Mosby.

DENTINOGENESIS IMPERFECTA

Schwartz S, Tsipouras P: Oral findings in osteogenesis imperfecta, Oral Surg 57:161, 1984.

Winter GB: Hereditary and idiopathic anomalies of tooth number, structure, and form, Dent Clin North Am 13:355, 1969.

Witkop CJ Jr: Hereditary defects in enamel and dentin. Proceedings of the First International Congress on Human Genetics, Acta Genet Stat Med 7:236, 1957.

DENTIN DYSPLASIA

O'Carroll MK, Duncan WK, Perkins TM: Dentin dysplasia: review of the literature and a proposed subclassification based on radiographic findings, Oral Surg 72:119, 1991.

Richardson AS, Fantin TD: Occlusal anomalous dysplasia of dentin: report of a case, J Can Dent Assoc 36:189, 1970.

Shields EP, Bixler D, El-Kafraevy AM: A proposed classification for heritable human dentin defects with a description of a new entity, Arch Oral Biol 18:543, 1973.

Witkop CJ Jr: Hereditary defects of dentin, Dent Clin North Am 19:25, 1975.

REGIONAL ODONTODYSPLASIA

Crawford PJ, Aldred MJ: Regional odontodysplasia: a bibliography, J Oral Pathol Med 18:251, 1989.

ENAMEL PEARL

Moskow BS, Canut PM: Studies on root enamel. II. Enamel pearls: a review of their morphology, localization, nomenclature, occurrence, classification, histogenesis, and incidence, J Clin Periodontol 17:275, 1990.

TALON CUSP

Meskin LH, Gorlin RJ: Agenesis and peg-shaped permanent lateral incisors, J Dent Res 42:1476, 1963.

Natkin E, Pitts DL, Worthington P: A case of talon cusp associated with other odontogenic abnormalities, J Endod 9:491, 1983.

TURNER'S HYPOPLASIA

Via WF Jr: Enamel defects induced by trauma during tooth formation, Oral Surg 25:49, 1968.

CONGENITAL SYPHILIS

Bradlaw RV: Dental stigmata of prenatal syphilis, Oral Surg 6:147, 1953.

Putkonen P: Dental changes in congenital syphilis, Acta Derm Venereol 42:44, 1962.

Sarnat BG, Shaw NG: Dental development in congenital syphilis, Am J Orthod 29:270, 1943.

ACQUIRED ABNORMALITIES

Baden E: Environmental pathology of the teeth. In Gorlin RJ, Goodman HM, editors: Thoma's oral pathology, ed 6, vol 1, St. Louis, 1970, Mosby.

Mitchell DF, Standish SM, Fast TB: Oral diagnosis/oral medicine, Philadelphia, 1978, Lea & Febiger.

Pindborg JJ: Pathology of the dental hard tissues, Philadelphia, 1970, WB Saunders.

Shafer WG, Hine MK, Levy BM: Oral pathology, ed 4, Philadelphia, 1983, WB Saunders.

ATTRITION

Johnson GK, Sivers JE: Attrition, abrasion, and erosion: diagnosis and therapy, Clin Prev Dent 9:12, 1987.

Murphy TR: Reduction of the dental arch by approximal attrition: quantitative assessment, Br Dent J 116:483, 1964.

Russell MD: The distinction between physiological and pathological attrition: a review, J Ir Dent Assoc 33:23, 1987.

Seligman DA, Pullinger AG, Solberg WK: The prevalence of dental attrition and its association with factors of age, gender, occlusion, and TMJ symptomatology, J Dent Res 67:1323, 1988.

ABRASION

Bull WH et al: The abrasion and cleaning properties of dentifrices, Br Dent J 125:331, 1968.

Erwin JC, Buchner CM: Prevalence of tooth root exposure and abrasion among dental patients, Dent Items Interest 66:760, 1944.

EROSION

Bruggen ten Cate JH: Dental erosion in industry, Br J Industr Med 25:249, 1968.

Stafne EC, Lovestedt SA: Dissolution of tooth substance by lemon juice, acid beverages, and acid from some other sources, J Am Dent Assoc 34:586, 1949.

RESORPTION

Bakland LK: Root resorption, Dent Clin North Am 36:491, 1992.

Bennett TG, Paleway SA: Internal resorption, post-pulpotomy type, Oral Surg 17:228, 1964.

Goldman HM: Spontaneous intermittent resorption of teeth, J Am Dent Assoc 49:522, 1954.

Massler M, Perreault JG: Root resorption in the permanent teeth of young adults, J Dent Child 21:158, 1954.

Phillips JR: Apical root resorption under orthodontic therapy, Angle Orthod 20:1, 1955.

Simpson HE: Internal resorption, J Can Dent Assoc 30:355, 1964.

Solomon CS, Notaro PJ, Kellert M: External root resorption: fact or fancy, J Endod 15:219, 1989.

Stafne EC, Austin LT: Resorption of embedded teeth, J Am Dent Assoc 32:1003, 1945.

Tronstad L: Root resorption: etiology, terminology, and clinical manifestations, Endod Dent Traumatol 4:241, 1988.

SECONDARY DENTIN

Kuttler Y: Classification of dentin into primary, secondary and tertiary, Oral Surg 12:966, 1959.

PULP STONES

Moss-Salentijn L, Hendricks-Klyvert M: Calcified structures in human dental pulps, J Endod 14:184, 1988.

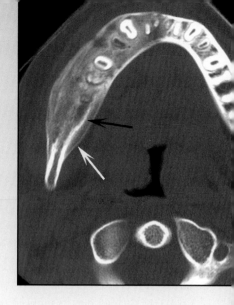

CHAPTER 19

Inflammatory Lesions of the Jaws

LINDA LEE

Inflammatory lesions are by far the most common pathologic condition of the jaws. The jaws are unique from other bones of the body in that the presence of teeth creates a direct pathway for infectious and inflammatory agents to invade bone by means of caries and periodontal disease. The body responds to chemical, physical, or microbiologic injury with inflammation. The inflammatory response destroys or walls off the injurious stimulus and sets up an environment for repair of the damaged tissue.

Under normal conditions, bone metabolism represents a balance of osteoclastic bone resorption and osteoblastic bone production. This is a complex, interdependent relationship in which osteoblasts mediate the resorptive activity of the osteoclasts. Mediators of inflammation (cytokines, prostaglandins, and many growth factors) tip this balance to favor either bone resorption or bone formation. For the purposes of this chapter, all inflammatory conditions of bone, regardless of the specific etiology, are considered to represent a spectrum or continuum of conditions with different clinical features (e.g., site, severity, duration).

When the initial source of inflammation is a necrotic pulp and the bony lesion is restricted to the region of the tooth, the condition is called a *periapical inflammatory lesion*. When the infection spreads in the bone marrow and is no longer contained to the vicinity of the tooth root apex, it is called *osteomyelitis*. Another source of inflammatory lesion in bone is extension of inflammation into bone from the overlying soft tissues; this type of lesion includes periodontal lesions (see Chapter 17) and pericoronitis, an inflammation that arises in the tissues surrounding the crown of a partially erupted tooth. It must be emphasized that the names of the various inflammatory lesions tend to describe their clinical and radiologic presentations and behavior; however, all have the same underlying disease mechanism.

General Clinical Features

The four cardinal signs of inflammation—redness, swelling, heat, and pain—may be observed in varying degrees with inflammation of the jaws. Acute lesions are those of recent onset. The onset typically is rapid, and these lesions cause pronounced pain, often accompanied by fever and swelling. Chronic lesions are characterized by a prolonged course with a longer insidious onset and pain that is less intense. Fever may be intermittent and low-grade, and swelling may occur gradually. In fact, some chronic, low-grade infections may not produce any significant clinical symptoms.

General Radiographic Features

LOCATION

With periapical inflammatory lesions, which are pathologic conditions of the pulp, the epicenter typically is located at the apex of a tooth. However, lesions of pulpal origin also may be located anywhere along the root surface because of accessory canals or perforations caused by root canal therapy or root fractures. Periodontal lesions have an epicenter that is located at the alveolar crest. If periodontal bone loss is severe, the bone inflammatory changes may extend to the root furcation level or even to the root apex. Osteomyelitis, a diffuse, uncontained inflammation of the bone, most commonly is found in the posterior mandible. The maxilla rarely is involved.

PERIPHERY

Most often the periphery is ill defined, with a gradual blending of normal trabecular pattern into a sclerotic pattern, or the normal trabecular pattern may gradually fade into a radiolucent region of bone loss.

INTERNAL STRUCTURE

The internal structure of inflammatory lesions presents a spectrum of appearances. Cancellous bone may respond to an insult by tipping the bone metabolic balance either in favor of resorption (giving the area a radiolucent appearance) or toward bone formation (resulting in a radiopaque or sclerotic appearance). Usually there is a combination of these two reactions. The radiolucent regions may show no evidence of previous trabeculation or a very faint pattern of trabeculation. The increased radiopacity is caused by an increase in bone formation on existing trabeculae. Radiographically these trabeculae appear thicker and more numerous, replacing marrow spaces. In acute disease, resorption typically predominates; with a chronic disease, excessive bone formation leads to an overall radiopaque, sclerotic appearance. In cases of osteomyelitis, careful examination of the x-ray films may reveal sequestra, which appear as ill-defined areas of radiolucency containing a radiopaque island of nonvital bone.

EFFECTS ON SURROUNDING STRUCTURES

The effects of inflammation on surrounding cancellous bone include stimulation of bone formation, resulting in a sclerotic pattern, or bone resorption, resulting in radiolucency. The periodontal ligament space involved in the lesion will be widened; this widening is greatest at the source of the inflammation. For example, with periapical lesions the widening is greatest around the apical region of the root; in periodontal disease the widening is greatest at the alveolar crest. With chronic infections, root resorption may occur and cortical boundaries may be resorbed. The periosteal component of bone, whether on the surface of the jaws or lining the floor of the maxillary sinus, also responds to inflammation. The periosteum contains a layer of pluripotential lining cells that, under the right conditions, differentiate into osteoblasts and lay down new bone. Inflammatory exudate from infection within the bone can penetrate the cortex, lift up the periosteum from the surface of the bone, and stimulate the periosteum to produce new bone. Because inflammatory exudate is a fluid, the periosteum is lifted from the surface of bone in a manner that positions the periosteum almost parallel to the surface of the bone; thus the layer of new bone is almost parallel to the bone surface.

Periapical Inflammatory Lesions

Synonyms

Periapical inflammatory lesions have been called *acute apical periodontitis, chronic apical periodontitis, periapical abscess,* and *periapical granuloma.* Radiolucent presentations have been called *rarefying osteitis,* whereas radiopaque presentations have been called *sclerosing osteitis, condensing osteitis,* and *focal sclerosing osteitis.* Chapter 20 presents a discussion of periapical cysts of inflammatory origin (radicular cysts).

Definition

A *periapical inflammatory lesion* is defined as a local response of the bone around the apex of a tooth that occurs secondary to necrosis of the pulp or through destruction of the periapical tissues by extensive periodontal disease (Fig. 19-1). The pulpal necrosis may occur secondary to pulpal invasion of bacteria through caries or trauma. In Fig. 19-1, the periapical inflammatory lesion is characterized by apical periodontitis, an inflammatory process that may histologically represent either a periapical abscess or a periapical granuloma. Toxic metabolites from the necrotic pulp exit the root apex to incite an inflammatory reaction in the periapical periodontal ligament and surrounding bone

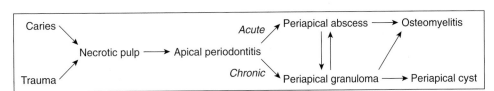

FIG. **19-1** Interrelationship of possible results of periapical inflammation.

(apical periodontitis). This reaction is characterized histologically by an inflammatory infiltrate composed predominantly of lymphocytes mixed with polymorphonuclear neutrophils. Depending on the severity of the response, the neutrophils may collect to form pus, resulting in an apical abscess. This result is categorized as acute inflammation. Alternatively, in an attempt to heal from apical periodontitis, the body stimulates the formation of granulation tissue mixed with a chronic inflammatory infiltrate composed predominantly of lymphocytes, plasma cells, and histiocytes, giving rise to *periapical granuloma.* Entrapped epithelium (the rests of Malassez) may proliferate to form a radicular or apical cyst. Acute exacerbations of the chronic lesions may occur intermittently.

If the surrounding bone marrow becomes involved with the inflammatory reaction through the spread of pyogenic organisms, the localized periapical abscess may transform into osteomyelitis. The exact point at which a periapical inflammatory lesion becomes osteomyelitis is not easily determined or defined. The size of the area of inflammation is not as important as the severity of the reaction. However, considering the size of the lesion as one factor, periapical inflammatory lesions usually involve only the local bone adjacent to the apex of the tooth, and osteomyelitis involves a larger area of bone. Periapical lesions occasionally may be large, but the epicenter of the lesion remains in the vicinity of the tooth apex. If the periapical lesion extends farther, so that the lesion no longer is centered on the tooth apex, osteomyelitis may be considered as a possible diagnosis. The distinction between periapical inflammation and osteomyelitis can be made if sequestra are detected radiographically. Progression from periapical inflammation to osteomyelitis is relatively rare, and other factors play a role in its development, such as a decrease in the host defenses and an increase in the virulence of pathogenic microorganisms.

Clinical Features

The symptoms of periapical inflammatory lesions can range across a broad spectrum, from being asymptomatic, to an occasional toothache, to severe pain with or without facial swelling, fever, and lymphadenopathy. A periapical abscess usually manifests with severe pain; mobility and sometimes elevation of the involved tooth; swelling; and tenderness to percussion. Palpation of the apical region elicits pain. Spontaneous drainage into the oral cavity through a fistula (parulis) may relieve the acute pain. In rare cases a dental abscess may manifest with systemic symptoms (e.g., fever, facial swelling, lymphadenopathy) along with the pain. The acute lesion may evolve into a chronic one (periapical granuloma or cyst), which may be asymptomatic except for

intermittent flare-ups of "toothache" pain, which mark the acute exacerbation of the chronic lesion. Patients often have a history of intermittent pain. The associated tooth may be asymptomatic, or it may be sensitive to percussion and mobile. More often, however, the periapical lesion arises in the chronic form *de novo;* in this case it may be asymptomatic. It is important to understand that the clinical presentation does not necessarily correlate with the histologic or radiographic findings.

Radiographic Features

The radiographic features of periapical inflammatory lesions vary depending on the time course of the lesion. Because very early lesions may not show any radiographic changes, diagnosis of these lesions relies solely on the clinical symptoms (Fig. 19-2). More chronic lesions may show lytic (radiolucent) or sclerotic (radiopaque) changes, or both.

Location. In most cases the epicenter of periapical inflammatory lesions is found at the apex of the involved tooth (Fig. 19-3). The lesion usually starts within the apical portion of the periodontal ligament space. Less often, such lesions are centered around another region of the tooth root. This may occur because of accessory pulpal canals, perforation of the root structure from instrumentation of the pulp canal, and root fracture.

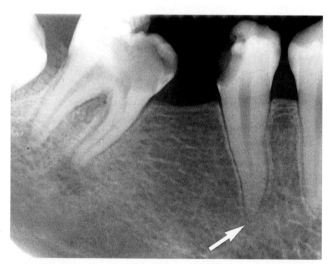

FIG. **19-2**   A very early lesion involving the pulp of the second bicuspid without significant change in the periapical bone *(arrow).* In contrast, note the loss of the lamina dura and periapical bone at the apex of the mesial root of the second molar. Also note the subtle halo of sclerotic bone reaction around this apical radiolucency.

Periphery. In most instances the periphery of periapical inflammatory lesions is ill defined, showing a gradual transition from the surrounding normal trabecular pattern into the abnormal bone pattern of the lesion (Figs. 19-1 and 19-4). Rarely the periphery may be well defined, with a sharp transition zone and an appearance suggesting a cortical boundary.

Internal Structure. Early periapical inflammatory lesions may show no radiographic change in the normal bone pattern. The earliest detectable change is loss of bone density, which usually results in widening of the periodontal ligament space at the apex of the tooth and later involves a larger diameter of surrounding bone. At this early stage no evidence may be seen of a sclerotic bone reaction (see Fig. 19-1). Later in the evolution of the disease, a mixture of sclerosis and rarefaction (loss of bone giving a radiolucent appearance) of normal bone occurs (see Fig. 19-4). The percentage of these two bone reactions varies. When most of the lesion consists of increased bone formation, the term *periapical sclerosing osteitis* is used (Fig. 19-5); when most of the lesion is undergoing bone resorp-tion, the term *periapical rarefying osteitis* is used (see Fig. 19-3). The area of greatest bone destruction usually is centered on the apex of the tooth, with the sclerotic pattern located at the periphery. The radiolucent regions may be bereft of any bone structure or may have a faint outline of trabeculae. Close inspection of sclerotic regions reveals

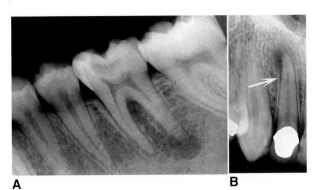

A   **B**

FIG. **19-3** Periapical inflammatory lesions associated with a mandibular first molar **(A)** and a maxillary lateral incisor **(B).** Note that in both cases the epicenter of bone destruction is located at the apex of the root. Also, note gradual widening of the periodontal membrane space *(arrow)* characteristic of an inflammatory lesion.

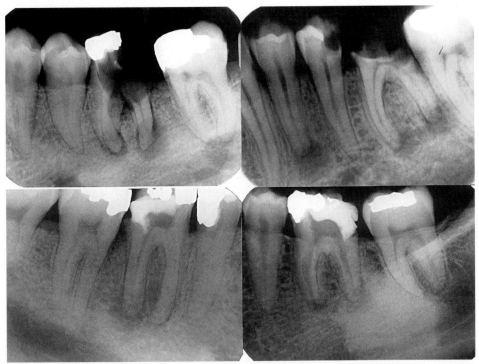

FIG. **19-4** *Several examples of a mixture of rarefying and sclerosing osteitis.* Note the similarity of the pattern, composed of a radiolucent region at the apex of the tooth surrounded by a radiopaque reaction of sclerotic dense bone. Also note that most often a gradual transition occurs from the sclerotic bone reaction to the more normal surrounding bone pattern.

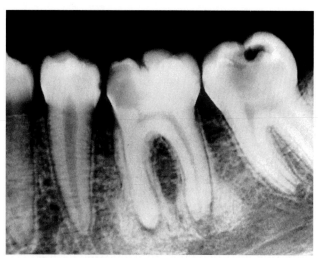

FIG. **19-5**   *Periapical sclerosing osteitis associated with the first molar.* This is called a *sclerosing lesion* because most of the lesion is bone formation, resulting in a very radiopaque density. Note, however, the small region of bone loss next to the root apex and the widening of the periodontal membrane space.

thicker than normal trabeculae and sometimes an increase in the number of trabeculae per unit area. In chronic cases the new bone formation may result in a very dense sclerotic region of bone, obscuring individual trabeculae. Occasionally the lesion may appear to be composed entirely of sclerotic bone (sclerosing osteitis), but usually some evidence exists of widening of the apical portion of the periodontal membrane space (see Fig. 19-5).

Effects on Surrounding Structures. As mentioned previously, periapical inflammatory lesions may stimulate either the resorption of bone or the manufacture of new bone. The lamina dura around the apex of the tooth usually is lost. The sclerotic reaction of the cancellous bone may be limited to a small region around the tooth apex or in some cases may be extensive. In rare instances in the mandible the sclerotic reaction may extend to the inferior cortex. In chronic cases external resorption of the apical region of the root may occur. If the lesion is long-standing, the pulp canal may appear wider than adjacent teeth. This is a result of the death of odontoblasts and subsequent cessation of the formation of secondary dentin, which occurs naturally with time to diminish the caliber of the pulp canal slowly.

Nearby cortical boundaries may be destroyed, such as a segment of the floor of the maxillary antrum, the floor of the nasal fossa, or the buccal or lingual plates

of the alveolar process immediately adjacent to the root apex. These lesions are capable of producing an inflammatory periosteal reaction, most notably in the adjacent floor of the maxillary antrum. This usually results in a thin layer of new bone within the maxillary antrum, sometimes referred to as a *halo shadow* (Fig. 19-6). A regional mucositis may be present within the adjacent segment of the maxillary antrum. Periosteal reaction may also occur on the buccal or lingual surfaces of the alveolar process and in rare cases on the inferior aspect of the mandible.

Differential Diagnosis

The two types of lesions that most often must be differentiated from periapical inflammatory lesions are periapical cemental dysplasia (PCD) and an enostosis (dense bone island, osteosclerosis) at the apex of a tooth. In the early radiolucent phase of PCD, the radiographic characteristics may not reliably differentiate this lesion from a periapical inflammatory lesion (Fig. 19-7). The differential diagnosis may rely solely on the clinical examination, including a test of tooth vitality. With long-standing periapical inflammatory lesions, the pulp chamber of the involved tooth may be wider than the adjacent teeth. More mature PCD lesions may show evidence of a dense, radiopaque structure within the radiolucency, which helps in the differential diagnosis. Also, a common site for PCD is the mandibular anterior teeth. External root resorption is more common with inflammatory lesions than with PCD. When enostosis is centered on the root apex, it may mimic an inflammatory lesion. However, the periodontal ligament space around the apex of the tooth has a normal uniform width (Fig. 19-8). Also, the periphery of an enostosis usually is well defined and does not blend gradually with surrounding trabeculae.

Small, radiolucent periapical lesions with a well-defined periphery simulating a cortex may be either periapical granulomas or cysts (radicular cysts). Differentiation may not be possible unless other characteristics of a cyst are present such as displacement of adjacent structures and expansion of the outer cortical boundaries of the jaw. Lesions larger than 1 cm in diameter usually are radicular cysts. If the patient has had endodontic treatment or apical surgery, a periapical radiolucency may remain that may resemble periapical rarefying osteitis (Fig. 19-9). In either case the destroyed bone may not be replaced with normal bone but with scar tissue. The differential diagnosis cannot be made on radiologic grounds alone; thus the clinical signs and symptoms must take precedence.

In rare cases metastatic lesions and malignancies such as leukemia may grow in the periapical segment of the periodontal membrane space. Close inspection

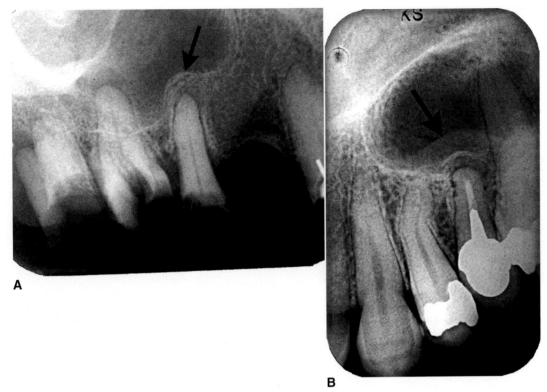

A

B

FIG. **19-6** *Periostitis emanating from the floor of the maxillary antrum that arises secondary to apical inflammatory lesions.* **A,** Laminated type of periostitis *(arrow).* **B,** Periostitis and mucositis. The mucositis is characterized by a slight radiopaque band *(arrow).*

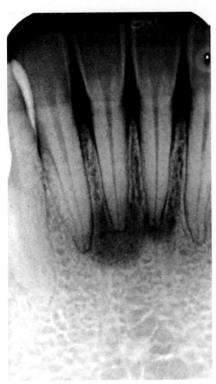

FIG. **19-7** Two early lesions of PCD related to the apical region of the mandibular central incisors. Note the similarity to apical rarefying osteitis.

of the surrounding bone may reveal other small regions of malignant bone destruction.

Management

Standard dental treatment of periapical lesions includes root canal therapy or extraction with the intention of eliminating the necrotic material in the root canal and hence the source of inflammation. If left untreated, the tooth may become asymptomatic because of drainage established through the carious lesion or a parulis. However, the possibility always exists that the lesion will spread to involve a larger area of bone, resulting in osteomyelitis, or into the surrounding soft tissue, which may result in a space infection or cellulitis.

Pericoronitis

Synonym
Operculitis

Definition
The term *pericoronitis* refers to inflammation of the tissues surrounding the crown of a partially erupted tooth.

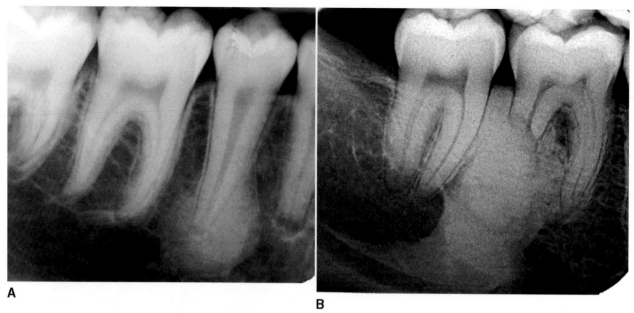

FIG. **19-8**   *Enostosis (dense bone island) in periapical positions.* **A,** Enostosis around the apex of a second bicuspid. Note that the periodontal membrane space is uniform in width. **B,** Enostosis associated with apical root resorption of a vital tooth. The most common site of enostosis and root resorption is the mesial or distal root of mandibular first molars.

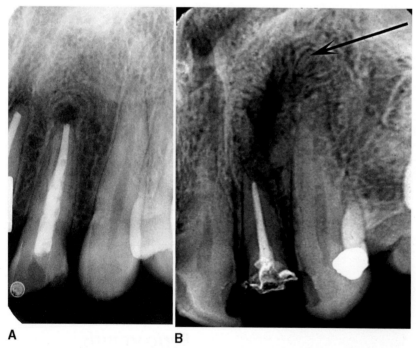

FIG. **19-9**   **A,** Radiolucent apical scar left after successful endodontic treatment. **B,** Healing periapical inflammatory lesion associated with the apical region of a maxillary lateral incisor. Note the radiating, spokelike pattern of new bone forming from the periphery of the lesion.

It is most often seen in association with the mandibular third molars in young adults. The gingiva surrounding the erupted portion of the crown becomes inflamed when food or microbial debris becomes trapped under the soft tissue. The gingiva subsequently becomes swollen and may become secondarily traumatized by the opposing occlusion. This inflammation may extend into the bone surrounding the crown of the tooth.

Clinical Features

Patients with pericoronitis typically complain of pain and swelling. Trismus is a common presentation when the partially erupted tooth is a lower third molar, and usually pain is felt on occlusion. An ulcerated operculum is usually the source of the pain. Pericoronitis can affect patients of any age or gender but is most commonly seen during the time of eruption of the third molars in young adults.

Radiographic Features

The radiologic signs of pericoronitis can range from no changes when the inflammatory lesion is confined to the soft tissues, to localized rarefaction and sclerosis, to osteomyelitis in the most severe cases.

Location. When bone changes are associated with pericoronitis, they are centered on the follicular space or the portion of the crown still embedded in bone or in close proximity to bone. The mandibular third molar region is the most common location.

Periphery. The periphery of pericoronitis is ill defined, with a gradual transition of the normal trabecular pattern into a sclerotic region.

Internal structure. The internal structure of bone adjacent to the pericoronitis most often is sclerotic with thick trabeculae. An area of bone loss or radiolucency immediately adjacent to the crown may be seen that enlarges the follicular space (Fig. 19-10). If this lesion spreads considerably, the internal pattern becomes consistent with osteomyelitis (see the next section).

Effects on surrounding structures. As with the periapical inflammatory lesions, pericoronitis may cause the typical changes of sclerosis and rarefaction of surrounding bone. In extensive cases evidence of periosteal new bone formation may be seen at the inferior cortex, the posterior border of the ramus, and along the coronoid notch of the mandible.

Differential Diagnosis

The differential diagnosis of pericoronitis includes other mixed density or sclerotic lesions that can exist

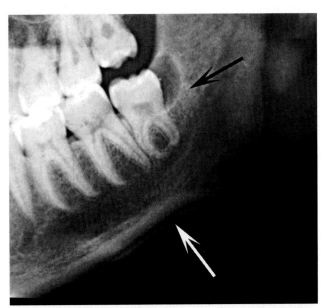

FIG. **19-10** *Panoramic view of a case of pericoronitis related to a partially erupted third molar.* Note the sclerotic bone reaction adjacent to the follicular cortex *(black arrow)* and the periosteal reaction *(white arrow)*.

adjacent to the crown of a partially erupted third molar. These include enostosis and fibrous dysplasia. The clinical symptoms indicative of an inflammatory lesion usually exclude these conditions. Neoplasms to be considered include the sclerotic form of osteosarcoma and, in older patients, squamous cell carcinoma. The occurrence of squamous cell carcinoma in the midst of a preexisting inflammatory lesion may be difficult to identify. Features characteristic of malignant neoplasia, such as profound cortical bone destruction and invasion, aid with the diagnosis.

Management

The aim of treatment of pericoronitis is removal of the partially erupted tooth. However, in the acute phase, when trismus may prevent adequate access, antibiotic therapy and reduction in occlusion of the opposing tooth should relieve the symptoms until definitive treatment is provided.

Osteomyelitis

Definition

Osteomyelitis is inflammation of bone. The inflammatory process may spread through the bone to involve the marrow, cortex, cancellous portion, and periosteum. In the jaws pyogenic organisms that reach the bone marrow from abscessed teeth or postsurgical infection usually cause osteomyelitis. However, in some instances no source of infection can be identified, and hematogenous spread is presumed to be the origin. In some patients no infectious organisms can be identified, possibly because of previous antibiotic therapy or inadequate methods of bacterial isolation. Bacterial colonies also may be present in small, isolated pockets of bone that may be missed during sampling.

In patients with osteomyelitis, the bacteria and their products stimulate an inflammatory reaction in bone, causing destruction of the endosteal surface of the cortical bone. This destruction may progress through the cortical bone to the outer periosteum. In young patients, in whom the periosteum is more loosely attached to the outer cortex of bone than it is in adults, the periosteum is lifted up by the inflammatory exudate and new bone is laid down. This periosteal reaction is a characteristic but not pathognomonic feature of osteomyelitis. The hallmark of osteomyelitis is the development of sequestra. A sequestrum is a segment of bone that has become necrotic because of ischemic injury caused by the inflammatory process.

Numerous forms of osteomyelitis have been described. For the sake of simplicity, we group them into two major phases—acute and chronic—recognizing that these represent two ends of a continuum without a definite separating boundary in the process of bone inflammation. Other forms of osteomyelitis have been described as separate and distinct clinico-pathologic entities with unique radiographic features. These are Garré's osteomyelitis and diffuse sclerosing osteomyelitis. We consider these two forms as part of the same continuum. Garré's osteomyelitis is an exuberant periosteal response to inflammation. Diffuse sclerosing osteomyelitis is a chronic form of osteomyelitis with a pronounced sclerotic response. It is important to understand that all these variations of osteomyelitis have the same underlying process of bone's response to inflammation. The features expressed by each subtype represent only variations in the type and degree of bone reaction.

Osteomyelitis may resolve spontaneously or with appropriate antibiotic intervention. However, if the condition is not treated or is treated inadequately, the infection may persist, continue to spread and become chronic in about 20% of patients. Some chronic systemic diseases, immunosuppressive states, and disorders of decreased vascularity may predispose an individual to the development of osteomyelitis. For example, osteopetrosis, sickle cell anemia, and acquired immunodeficiency syndrome (AIDS) have been documented as underlying factors in the development of osteomyelitis.

Acute Phase

Synonyms
Acute suppurative osteomyelitis, pyogenic osteomyelitis, subacute suppurative osteomyelitis, Garré's osteomyelitis, proliferative periostitis, periostitis ossificans

Definition
The acute phase of osteomyelitis is caused by infection that has spread to the bone marrow. With this condition, the medullary spaces of the bone contain an inflammatory infiltrate consisting predominantly of neutrophils and, to a lesser extent, mononuclear cells. In the jaws the most common source of infection is a periapical lesion from a nonvital tooth. Infection also can occur as a result of trauma or hematogenous spread.

The changes described by Garré may accompany acute osteomyelitis. It is believed that the inflammatory exudate spreads subperiosteally, elevating the periosteum and stimulating formation of new bone. This condition is more common in younger people because in these individuals the periosteum is loosely attached to the bone surface and has greater osteogenic potential.

Clinical Features
The acute phase of osteomyelitis can affect people of all ages, and it has a strong male predilection. It is much more common in the mandible than in the maxilla, possibly because of the poorer vascular supply to the mandible. The typical signs and symptoms of acute osteomyelitis are rapid onset, pain, swelling of the adjacent soft tissues, fever, lymphadenopathy, and leukocytosis. The associated teeth may be mobile and sensitive to percussion. Purulent drainage also may be present. Paresthesia of the lower lip in the third division of the fifth cranial nerve distribution is not uncommon.

Radiologic Examination
In addition to a complete examination using plain films (panoramic, intraoral periapical, and occlusal films), the following additional modalities may be employed. A two-phase nuclear medicine study composed of a technetium bone scan followed by a gallium citrate scan may help to confirm the diagnosis. With inflammatory lesions, a positive result on the technetium scan indicates increased bone metabolic activity, and a positive result on the gallium scan in the same location indicates an inflammatory cell infiltrate. Computed tomography (CT) is the imaging method of choice. CT reveals more bone surface for detecting periosteal new bone and is the best imaging method for detecting sequestra (Fig. 19-11). MRI imaging has been employed using T2 weighted images to display abnormal bone marrow edema.

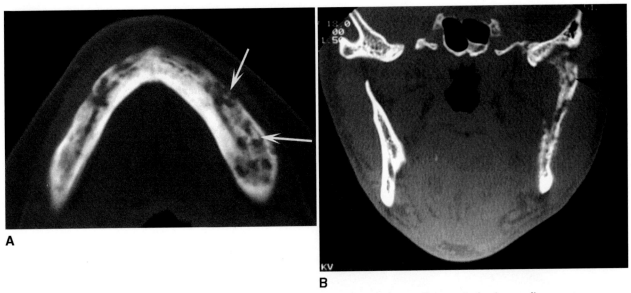

FIG. **19-11** *CT image of multiple sequestra.* **A**, An axial scan (bone window) revealing multiple sequestra *(arrows)*, and **B**, a coronal scan (bone window) demonstrating a sequestrum *(arrow)* in two different cases of chronic osteomyelitis.

Radiographic Features

Very early in the disease, no radiographic changes may be identifiable. The bone may be filled with inflammatory exudate and inflammatory cells and may show no radiographic change.

Location. The most common location is the posterior body of the mandible. The maxilla is a rare site.

Periphery. Acute osteomyelitis most often presents an ill-defined periphery with a gradual transition to normal trabeculae.

Internal structure. The first radiographic evidence of the acute form of osteomyelitis is a slight decrease in the density of the involved bone, with a loss of sharpness of the existing trabeculae. In time the bone destruction becomes more profound, resulting in an area of radiolucency in one focal area or in scattered regions throughout the involved bone (Fig. 19-12). Later, the appearance of sclerotic regions becomes apparent. Sequestra may be present but usually are more apparent and numerous in chronic forms (Fig. 19-13). Sequestra can be identified by closely inspecting a region of bone destruction (radiolucency) for an island of bone. This island of nonvital bone may vary in size from a small dot (smaller sequestra usually are seen in young patients) to larger segments of radiopaque bone.

Effects on surrounding structures. Acute osteomyelitis can stimulate either bone resorption or bone formation. Portions of cortical bone may be resorbed. An inflammatory exudate can lift the periosteum and stimulate bone formation. Radiographically, this appears as a thin, faint, radiopaque line adjacent to and almost parallel or slightly convex to the surface of the bone. A radiolucent band separates this periosteal new bone from the bone surface (Fig. 19-14). As the lesion develops into a more chronic phase, cyclic and periodic acute exacerbations may produce more inflammatory exudate, which again lifts the periosteum from the bone surface and stimulates the periosteum to form a second layer of bone. This is detected radiographically as a second radiopaque line almost parallel to the first and separated from it by a radiolucent band. This process may continue and may result in several lines (an onion-skin appearance), and eventually a massive amount of new bone may be formed. This is referred to as *proliferative periostitis* and is seen more often in children (Fig. 19-15). The effects on the teeth and lamina dura may be the same as those described for periapical inflammatory lesions.

Differential Diagnosis

The differential diagnosis of the acute phase of osteomyelitis may include fibrous dysplasia, especially in children. Aside from the clinical signs of acute infection, the most useful radiographic characteristic to distinguish osteomyelitis from fibrous dysplasia is the way the enlargement of the bone occurs. The new bone that enlarges the jaws in osteomyelitis is laid down by the periosteum and therefore is on the outside of the outer

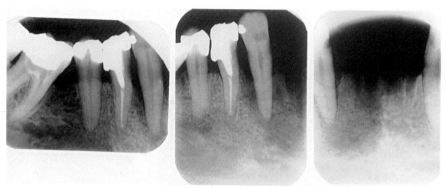

FIG. **19-12** Acute osteomyelitis involving the body of the right mandible, with initial blurring of bony trabeculae. (Courtesy Lars Hollender, DDS, PhD, Seattle, Wash.)

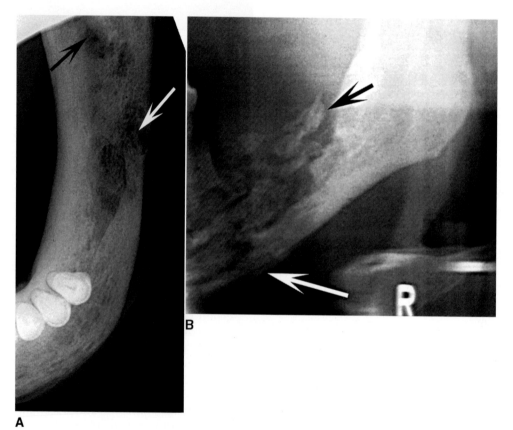

FIG. **19-13** Examples of sequestra. **A,** Occlusal film demonstrates small sequestra as radiopaque islands of bone in radiolucent regions in the chronic phase of osteomyelitis *(arrows)*. **B,** Panoramic film reveals large sequestra *(black arrow)* and a periosteal reaction at the inferior border of the mandible in a case of chronic osteomyelitis *(white arrow)*.

cortical plate. In fibrous dysplasia the new bone is manufactured on the inside of the mandible; thus the outer cortex, which may be thinned, is on the outside and contains the lesion. This point of differentiation is important because the histologic appearance of a biopsy of new periosteal bone in osteomyelitis may be similar to that of fibrous dysplasia, and the condition may be reported as such.

Malignant neoplasia (e.g., osteosarcoma, squamous cell carcinoma) that invades the mandible at times may be difficult to differentiate from the acute phase of osteomyelitis, especially if the malignancy has been secondarily infected via an oral ulcer; this may result in a mixture of inflammatory and malignant radiographic characteristics. If part of the inflammatory periosteal bone has been destroyed, the possibility of a malignant neoplasm should be considered. The differential diagnosis may include other lesions that can cause bone destruction and may stimulate a periosteal reaction that is similar to that seen in inflammatory lesions. Langerhans' cell histiocytosis causes lytic ill-defined

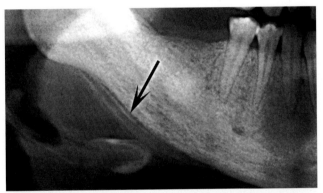

FIG. **19-14** Osteomyelitis of the mandible with a periosteal reaction located at the inferior cortex. Note the radiolucent line *(arrow)* between the inferior cortex of the mandible and the first layer of periosteal new bone. A second radiolucent line separates the second layer of new bone from the first layer.

bone destruction and often results in the formation of periosteal reactive new bone. This lesion rarely stimulates a sclerotic bone reaction such as that seen in osteomyelitis. Leukemia and lymphoma may stimulate a similar periosteal reaction.

Management

As with all inflammatory lesions of the jaws, removal of the source of inflammation is the primary goal of therapy. Antimicrobial treatment is the mainstay of treatment of acute osteomyelitis, along with establishing drainage. This may entail removal of a tooth, root canal therapy, or surgical incision and drainage.

CHRONIC PHASE

Synonyms

Chronic diffuse sclerosing osteomyelitis, chronic non-suppurative osteomyelitis, chronic osteomyelitis with proliferative periostitis, Garré's chronic nonsuppurative sclerosing osteitis

Definition

The chronic phase of osteomyelitis may be a sequela of inadequately treated acute osteomyelitis, or it may arise *de novo. Diffuse sclerosing osteomyelitis* refers to chronic osteomyelitis in which the balance in bone metabolism is tipped toward increased bone formation, producing a subsequent sclerotic radiographic appearance. The

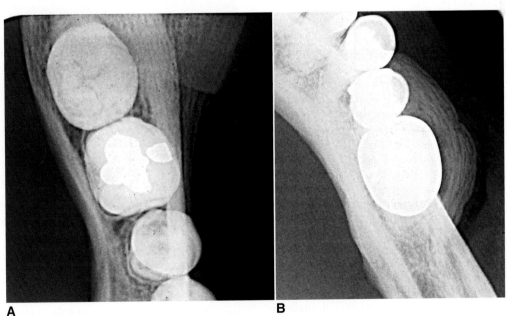

A   **B**

FIG. **19-15** **A** and **B**, Proliferative periostitis resulting from inflammatory lesions. Note the multiple layers of new bone on the buccal aspect of the mandible, resulting in an onion-skin appearance.

symptoms of the chronic form generally are less severe and have a longer history than those of the acute form. They include intermittent, recurrent episodes of swelling, pain, fever, and lymphadenopathy. As with the acute form, paresthesia and drainage with sinus formation also may occur. In some cases pain may be limited to the advancing front of the osteomyelitis, or the patient may have little or no pain. Histologically, a chronic inflammatory infiltrate may be seen within the medullary spaces of bone; however, this may be quite sparse, with only fibrosis of the marrow seen with scattered regions of inflammation. At this stage of the disease, the offending etiologic agent rarely is found because culture results usually are negative. If left untreated, osteomyelitis can spread and involve both sides of the mandible. Further spread into the temporomandibular joint may cause a septic arthritis, and ear infections and infection of the mastoid air cells also may develop.

Radiologic Examination

If chronic osteomyelitis is suspected from the clinical examination, in addition to a complete series of plain films, CT is the imaging method of choice. CT, with the ability to demonstrate sequestra (see Fig. 19-11) and periosteal new bone, is important for a correct diagnosis and allows accurate staging of the disease, which is important for future assessment of healing. MR imaging is not as useful because of the lack of bone marrow edema; however, it may be of use during acute exacerbation of the disease. Scintigraphy using bone scans, gallium, or labeled white blood cells is not particularly useful for differential diagnosis. Bone scans indicate increased bone formation, which is nonspecific, and often gallium scans (which highlight inflammatory cells) are not positive because of a very low population of inflammatory cells. The amount of bone activity assessed with bone scans using SPECT (single-photon emission computed tomography) has been used to monitor healing. There are also reports of the use of positron emission tomography (PET) to detect a high cellular metabolic rate in tissues, but this type of imaging is nonspecific.

Radiographic Features

Location. As in the acute phase of osteomyelitis, the most common site is the posterior mandible.

Periphery. The periphery may be better defined than in the acute phase, but it is still difficult to determine the exact extent of chronic osteomyelitis. Usually a gradual transition is seen between the normal surrounding trabecular pattern and the dense granular pattern characteristic of this disease. When the disease

is active and is spreading through bone, the periphery may be more radiolucent and have poorly defined borders.

Internal structure. The internal structure comprises regions of greater and lesser radiopacity compared with surrounding normal bone. Most of the lesion usually is composed of the more radiopaque or sclerotic bone pattern (Fig. 19-16). In older, more chronic lesions the internal bone density can be exceedingly radiopaque and equivalent to cortical bone. In these cases no

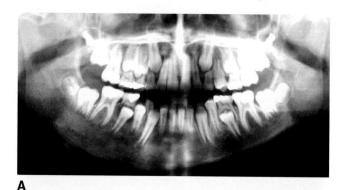

A

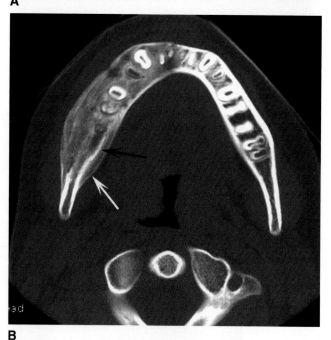

B

FIG. **19-16** *Chronic osteomyelitis.* **A,** This panoramic film demonstrates chronic osteomyelitis of the patient's right mandible. Note the increase in density and size of the right mandible compared with the left side. **B,** An axial CT image using bone window of the mandible of the same case. Note the increase in bone density, width of the mandible and the new periosteal bone formation *(white arrow)* and evidence of the original cortex *(black arrow).*

obvious regions of radiolucency may be seen. In other cases, small regions of radiolucency may be scattered throughout the radiopaque bone. A close inspection of the radiolucent regions may reveal an island of bone or sequestrum within the center (Fig. 19-17). Often the sequestrum appears more radiopaque than the surrounding bone. Detection may require illumination of the radiolucent regions of the film with an intense light source. CT is superior for revealing the internal structure and sequestra, especially in cases with very dense sclerotic bone. The bone pattern usually is very granular, obscuring individual bone trabeculae.

Effects on surrounding structures. Chronic osteomyelitis often stimulates the formation of periosteal new bone, which is seen radiographically as a single radiopaque line or a series of radiopaque lines (similar to onion skin) parallel to the surface of the cortical bone. Over time the radiolucent strip that separates this new bone from the outer cortical bone surface may be filled in with granular sclerotic bone. When this occurs, it may not be possible to identify the original cortex, which makes it difficult to determine whether the new bone is derived from the periosteum. After a considerable amount of time the outer contour of the mandible also may be altered, assuming an abnormal shape, and the girth of the mandible may be much larger than on the unaffected side. The roots of teeth may undergo

external resorption, and the lamina dura may become less apparent as it blends with the surrounding granular sclerotic bone. If a tooth is nonvital, the periodontal ligament space usually is enlarged in the apical region. In patients with extensive chronic osteomyelitis, the disease may slowly spread to the mandibular condyle and into the joint, resulting in a septic arthritis. Further spread may involve the inner ear and mastoid air cells. Chronic lesions may develop a draining fistula, which may appear as a well-defined break in the outer cortex or in the periosteal new bone (Fig. 19-18).

Differential Diagnosis

Very sclerotic, radiopaque chronic lesions of osteomyelitis may be difficult to differentiate from fibrous dysplasia, Paget's disease, and osteosarcoma. In children, osteomyelitis with a proliferative periosteal response may be misinterpreted as fibrous dysplasia (see the Differential Diagnosis section under Acute Phase). Differentiation of the chronic form of osteomyelitis may be even more difficult if considerable remodeling and loss of a distinct original cortex have occurred. In these cases, inspection of the bone surface at the most peripheral part of the lesion may reveal subtle evidence of periosteal new bone formation. The presence of sequestra indicates osteomyelitis. Paget's disease affects the entire mandible, which is rare in osteomyelitis. Periosteal new bone formation and sequestra are not seen in Paget's disease. Dense, granular bone may be seen in some forms of osteosarcoma, but usually evidence of bone destruction is found.

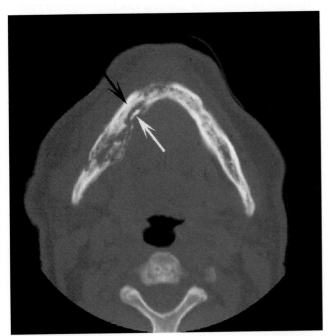

FIG. 19-17 An axial CT image using bone window of chronic osteomyelitis with a mixture of increased bone density *(black arrow)*, areas of radiolucency, and presence of sequestra *(white arrow)*.

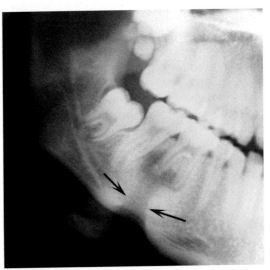

FIG. 19-18 A fistulous tract extending inferiorly from the apex of the first molar through the inferior cortex of the mandible *(arrows)*.

A characteristic spiculated (sunray-like) periosteal response also may be seen. As mentioned in the section on acute osteomyelitis, other entities such as Langerhans' cell histiocytosis, leukemia, and lymphoma may stimulate a similar periosteal response, but these usually produce evidence of bone destruction characteristic of malignant tumors.

The imaging method of choice for aiding in the differential diagnosis is CT because of its ability to reveal sequestra and periosteal new bone.

Management

Chronic osteomyelitis tends to be more difficult to eradicate than the acute form. In cases involving an extreme osteoblastic response (very sclerotic mandible), the subsequent lack of a good blood supply may work against healing. Hyperbaric oxygen therapy and creative modes of long-term antibiotic delivery have been used with limited success. Surgical intervention, which may include sequestrectomy, decortication, or resection, often is necessary. The probability of successful treatment, especially when using long-term antibiotic therapy with decortication, is greater in the first 2 decades of life.

Diagnostic Imaging of Soft Tissue Infections

Diagnostic imaging may be used to confirm the presence and extent of soft tissue infections. Magnetic resonance imaging (MRI) and CT may be used to differentiate soft tissue neoplasia from inflammatory lesions. MRI can be used in the T2 or T1 with gadolinium and fat suppression modes to detect the presence of soft tissue edema. CT usually is used with intravenous contrast. The CT image characteristics that suggest the presence of a soft tissue inflammation include abnormal fascial planes, thickening of the overlying skin and adjacent muscles, streaking of the fat planes, and abnormal collections of gas in the soft tissue (Fig. 19-19). Over time the contrast between soft tissue planes may disappear, and the presence of an abscess may become evident as a well-defined region of low density surrounded by a wide border of contrast-enhanced (more radiopaque) tissue.

Osteoradionecrosis

Definition

Osteoradionecrosis refers to an inflammatory condition of bone (osteomyelitis) that occurs after the bone has been exposed to therapeutic doses of radiation usually given for a malignancy of the head and neck region. It is characterized by the presence of exposed bone for a period of at least 3 months occurring at any time after the delivery of the radiation therapy. Doses above 50 Gy usually are required to cause this irreversible damage. Bone that has been irradiated is hypocellular and hypovascular. The lack of sufficient vascularity results in a hypoxic environment in which adequate healing of bone is not possible. Although infection may be a contributing factor, it is not necessarily the primary insult after the radiation damage has occurred. In many cases dental extraction and denture trauma after radiation therapy have been implicated as etiologic factors. Secondary infection is common, further fomenting the inflammatory reaction. Because of the difficulty of management, this serious complication of radiation therapy carries a high morbidity.

Clinical Features

The mandible is much more commonly affected than the maxilla. This is likely due to the microanatomy and reduced vasculature of this bone. The posterior mandible is affected more often than the anterior portion. The posterior body of the mandible is more frequently in the direct field of the radiation treatment because primary tumors and metastatic lesions in lymph nodes being treated are commonly adjacent to this part of the mandible. Loss of mucosal covering and exposure of bone is the hallmark of osteoradionecrosis. Pathologic fracture also may occur. The exposed bone becomes necrotic as a result of loss of vascularity from the periosteum and subsequently sequestrates, often leading to exposure of more bone. Pain may or may not be present. Intense pain may occur, with intermittent swelling and drainage extraorally. However, many patients experience no pain with bone exposure.

Radiologic Examination

The prescription of diagnostic imaging is the same as used for chronic-phase osteomyelitis, with CT being the imaging modality of choice.

Radiographic Features

The radiographic features of osteoradionecrosis have many similarities to those of chronic osteomyelitis, and the reader is referred to that section for a detailed description. The following is a description of the radiographic changes seen in bone that has received a considerable amount of therapeutic radiation. The presence of osteoradionecrosis cannot always be diagnosed radiographically, and often clinically obvious signs of exposed necrotic bone may not be accompanied by significant radiologic changes.

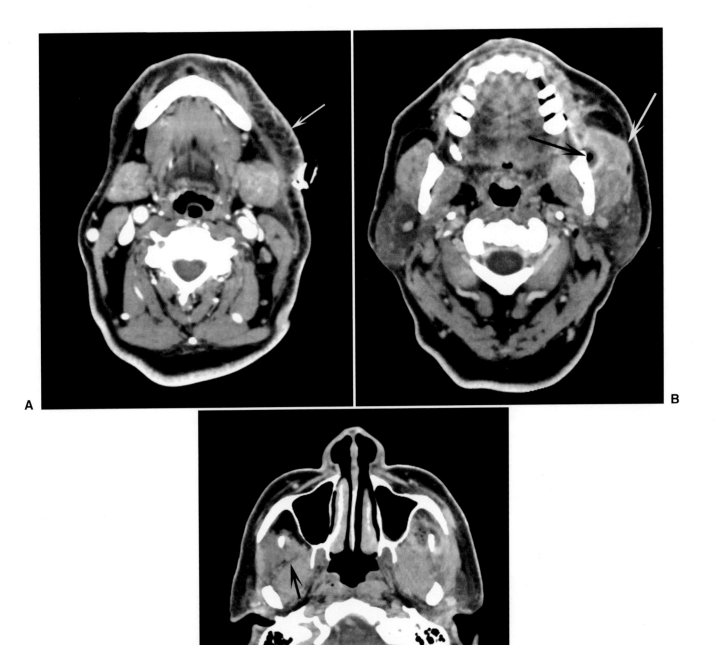

FIG. **19-19** Three axial CT images, using a contrast medium, of a soft tissue infection demonstrating streaking (reticulation pattern) of the fat planes and thickening of the skin *(arrow)* **(A)**; thickening of the masseter muscle *(white arrow)* and a radiolucent pocket of gas *(black arrow)* **(B)**; and loss of distinctive soft tissue planes, for example, individual muscles defined by fat planes [the lateral border of the normal lateral pterygoid muscle *(arrow)* is not apparent on the opposite effected side] **(C)**. (Courtesy Stuart White, DDS, Los Angeles, Calif.)

Location. The mandible, especially the posterior mandible, is the most common location for osteoradionecrosis. The maxilla may be involved in some cases.

Periphery. The periphery is ill defined and similar to that in osteomyelitis. If the lesion reaches the inferior border of the mandible, irregular resorption of this bony cortex often occurs.

Internal structure. A range of bone formation to bone destruction occurs, with the balance heavily toward more bone formation, giving the affected bone an overall sclerotic or radiopaque appearance. This is very similar to chronic osteomyelitis. The bone pattern is granular. Scattered regions of radiolucency may be seen, with and without central sequestra. The affected maxillary bone may also be very sclerotic and have areas of bone resorption (Fig. 19-20).

Effects on surrounding structures. Inflammatory periosteal new bone formation is uncommon, possibly because of the deleterious effects of radiation on potential osteoblasts in the periosteum. In very rare cases the periosteum appears to have been stimulated to produce bone, resulting in new bone formation on the outer cortex in an unusual shape. Radiation exposure may also stimulate the resorption of bone, especially in the maxilla, which may be similar in appearance to bone destruction caused by a malignant neoplasm. The most common effect on the surrounding bone is the stimulation of sclerosis.

Differential Diagnosis

Bone resorption, stimulated by high levels of irradiation, may simulate bone destruction from a malignant neoplasm, especially in the maxilla. For this reason, the detection of a recurrence of the malignant neoplasm (usually squamous cell carcinoma) in the presence of osteoradionecrosis may be very difficult. If recurrence is suspected, CT and MR imaging may be used to detect an associated soft tissue mass. Differentiation from other sclerotic lesions, as in chronic osteomyelitis, is less difficult because of the history of radiation therapy.

Management

The treatment of osteoradionecrosis currently is unsatisfactory. Decortication with sequestrectomy and hyperbaric oxygen with antibiotics have shown limited success because of poor healing after surgery. Conservative approaches with the aim of therapy to maintain the integrity of the lower border of the mandible and to keep the site free of infection and the patient free of pain may in the long term prove more successful. Fortunately, the incidence of osteoradionecrosis has declined because preventive therapy has proved quite effective. Removal of teeth that have significant periodontal disease or have a poor prognosis before radiation treatment and excellent oral and denture hygiene are the mainstays of preventive treatment.

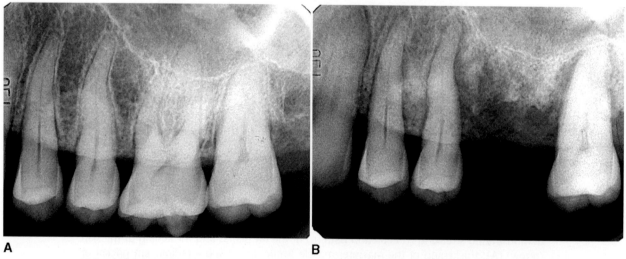

A   **B**

FIG. **19-20** *Osteoradionecrosis of the maxilla.* This periapical film was taken before radiotherapy **(A)**, and within 6 months of receiving the radiation **(B)**. Note the combination of bone sclerosis and profound bone destruction around the teeth and alveolar crest.

BIBLIOGRAPHY

PERIAPICAL INFLAMMATORY LESIONS

Heersche JNM: Bone cells and bone turnover: the basis for pathogenesis. In Tam CS et al, editors: Metabolic bone disease: cellular and tissue mechanisms, Boca Raton, Fla, 1989, CRC Press.

Shafer WG et al: A textbook of oral pathology, Philadelphia, 1983, WB Saunders.

Stern MH et al: Quantitative analysis of cellular composition of human periapical granuloma, J Endocrinol 7:117, 1981.

PERICORONITIS

Blakey GH et al: Clinical/biological outcomes of treatment for pericoronitis, J Oral Maxillofac Surg 54:1150, 1996.

OSTEOMYELITIS

Becker W: Imaging osteomyelitis and the diabetic foot. Q J Nucl Med 43(1):9-20, 1999.

Cotran RS et al: Pathologic basis of disease, ed 4, Philadelphia, 1989, WB Saunders.

Guhlmann A, et al: Chronic osteomyelitis: detection with FDG PET and correlation with histopathologic findings, Radiology 206(3):749-54, 1998.

Ledermann HP, et al: Pitfalls and limitations of magnetic resonance imaging in chronic posttraumatic osteomyelitis, Eur Radiol 10(11):1815-23, 2000.

Morrison WB, et al: Osteomyelitis of the foot: relative importance of primary and secondary MR imaging signs, Radiology 207(3):625-32, 1998.

Nordin U et al: Antibody response in patients with osteomyelitis of the mandible, Oral Surg Oral Med Oral Pathol 79:429, 1995.

Orpe E, et al: Radiographic features of osteomyelitis of the jaws, Dentomaxillofac Radiol 25:125, 1996.

Petrikowski CG, et al: Radiographic differentiation of osteogenic sarcoma, osteomyelitis, and fibrous dysplasia of the jaws, Oral Surg Oral Med Oral Pathol 80:747, 1995.

Van Merkesteyn JP, et al: Diffuse sclerosing osteomyelitis of the mandible: clinical radiographic and histologic findings in twenty-seven patients, J Oral Maxillofac Surg 46:825, 1988.

Wannfors K: Chronic osteomyelitis of the jaws, Stockholm, 1990, Gotab (thesis).

Wannfors K, Hammarstrom L: Infectious foci in chronic osteomyelitis of the jaws, Int J Oral Surg 14:493, 1985.

Wood RE, et al: Periostitis ossificans versus Garré's osteomyelitis. I. What did Garré really say? Oral Surg Oral Med Oral Pathol 65:773, 1988.

OSTERADIONECROSIS

Curi MM, Dib LL: Osteoradionecrosis of the jaws: a retrospective study of the background factors and treatment in 104 cases, J Oral Maxillofac Surg 55:540, 1997.

Hermans R, et al: CT findings in osteoradionecrosis of the mandible, Skeletal Radiol 25:31, 1996.

Hutchison IL, et al: The investigation of osteoradionecrosis of the mandible by ^{99m}Tc-methylene diphosphonate radionuclide bone scans, Br J Oral Maxillofac Surg 28(3):143-9, 1990.

Marx RE: Osteoradionecrosis: a new concept of its pathophysiology, J Oral Maxillofac Surg 41:283, 1983.

Wong JK et al: Conservative management of osteoradionecrosis, Oral Surg Oral Med Oral Pathol 84:16, 1997.

CHAPTER 20

Cysts of the Jaws

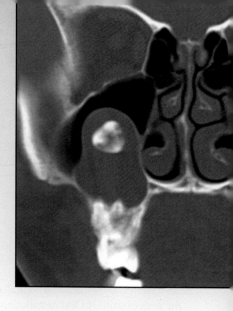

A *cyst is a pathologic cavity filled with fluid,* lined by epithelium, and surrounded by a definite connective tissue wall. The cystic fluid either is secreted by the cells lining the cavity or derives from the surrounding tissue fluid.

Clinical Features

Cysts occur more often in the jaws than in any other bone because most cysts originate from the numerous rests of odontogenic epithelium that remain after tooth formation. Cysts are radiolucent lesions, and the prevalent clinical features are swelling, lack of pain (unless the cyst becomes secondarily infected or is related to a nonvital tooth), and missing teeth, especially third molars.

Radiographic Features

LOCATION

Cysts may occur centrally (within bone) in any location in the maxilla or mandible but are rare in the condyle and coronoid process. Odontogenic cysts are found most often in the tooth-bearing region. In the mandible, they originate above the inferior alveolar nerve canal. Odontogenic cysts may grow into the maxillary antrum. Some nonodontogenic cysts also originate within the antrum (see Chapter 26). A few cysts arise in the soft tissues of the orofacial region.

PERIPHERY

Cysts that originate in bone usually have a periphery that is well defined and corticated (characterized by a fairly uniform, thin, radiopaque line). However, a secondary infection or a chronic state can change this appearance into a thicker, more sclerotic boundary.

SHAPE

Cysts usually are round or oval, resembling a fluid-filled balloon. Some cysts may have a scalloped boundary.

INTERNAL STRUCTURE

Cysts often are totally radiolucent. However, long-standing cysts may have dystrophic calcification, which can give the internal aspect a sparse, particulate appearance. Some cysts have septa, which produce multiple loculations separated by these bony walls or septa. Cysts that have a scalloped periphery may appear to have internal septa. Occasionally the image of structures that are positioned on either side of the cyst may overlap the internal aspect of the cyst, giving the false impression of internal structure.

EFFECTS ON SURROUNDING STRUCTURES

Cysts grow slowly, sometimes causing displacement and resorption of teeth. The area of tooth resorption often has a sharp, curved shape. Cysts can expand the mandible, usually in a smooth, curved manner, and change the buccal or lingual cortical plate into a thin cortical boundary. Cysts may displace the inferior alveolar nerve canal in an inferior direction or invaginate the maxillary antrum, maintaining a thin layer of bone that separates the internal aspect of the cyst from the antrum.

Odontogenic Cysts

RADICULAR CYST

Synonyms
Periapical cyst, apical periodontal cyst, or dental cyst

Definition
A radicular cyst is a cyst that most likely results when rests of epithelial cells (Malassez) in the periodontal ligament are stimulated to proliferate and undergo cystic degeneration by inflammatory products from a nonvital tooth.

Clinical Features
Radicular cysts are the most common type of cyst in the jaws. They arise from nonvital teeth (i.e., teeth that have lost vitality because of extensive caries, large restorations, or previous trauma). Often radicular cysts produce no symptoms unless secondary infection occurs. A cyst that becomes large may cause swelling. On palpation the swelling may feel bony and hard if the cortex is intact, crepitant as the bone thins, and rubbery and fluctuant if the outer cortex is lost. The incidence of radicular cysts is greater in the third to sixth decades and shows a slight male predominance.

Radiographic Features
Location. In most cases the epicenter of a radicular cyst is located approximately at the apex of a nonvital tooth (Fig. 20-1). Occasionally it appears on the mesial or distal surface of a tooth root, at the opening of an accessory canal, or infrequently in a deep periodontal pocket. Most radicular cysts (60%) are found in the maxilla, especially around incisors and canines. Because of the distal inclination of the root, cysts that arise from the maxillary lateral incisor may invaginate the antrum. Radicular cysts may also form in relation to a nonvital deciduous molar and be positioned buccal to the developing bicuspid.

Periphery and shape. The periphery usually has a well-defined cortical border (Fig. 20-2). If the cyst becomes secondarily infected, the inflammatory reaction of the surrounding bone may result in loss of this cortex (see Fig. 20-1, *B*) or alteration of the cortex into a more sclerotic border. The outline of a radicular cyst usually is curved or circular unless it is influenced by surrounding structures such as cortical boundaries.

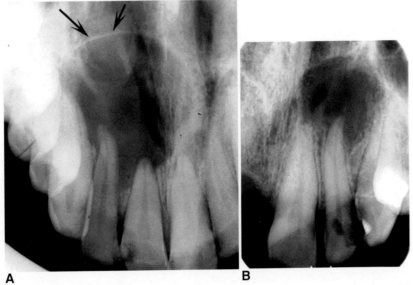

A   **B**

FIG. **20-1** *Radicular cysts.* In **A**, note that the epicenter is apical to the lateral incisor and the presence of a peripheral cortex *(arrows).* In **B**, note the lack of a well-defined peripheral cortex as this cyst was secondarily infected and that the root canal of the lateral incisor is abnormally wide as it is visible at the root apex.

Internal structure. In most cases the internal structure of radicular cysts is radiolucent. Occasionally, dystrophic calcification may develop in long-standing cysts, appearing as sparsely distributed, small particulate radiopacities.

Effects on surrounding structures. If a radicular cyst is large, displacement and resorption of the roots of adjacent teeth may occur. The resorption pattern may have a curved outline. In rare cases the cyst may resorb the roots of the related nonvital tooth. The cyst may invaginate the antrum, but there should be evidence of a cortical boundary between the contents of the cyst and the internal structure of the antrum. The outer cortical plates of the maxilla or mandible may expand in a curved or circular shape (Fig. 20-3). Cysts may displace the mandibular alveolar nerve canal in an inferior direction.

Differential Diagnosis

Differentiation of a small radicular cyst from an apical granuloma may be difficult and in some cases impossible. A round shape, a well-defined cortical border, and a size greater than 2 cm in diameter are more characteristic of a cyst. An early radiolucent stage of periapical cemental dysplasia, a radiolucent apical scar, and a periapical surgical defect should also be considered in the differential diagnosis. The patient's history helps with the differentiation. Radicular cysts that originate from the maxillary lateral incisor and are positioned between the roots of the lateral incisor and the cuspid may be difficult to differentiate from an odontogenic keratocyst or a lateral periodontal cyst. The vitality of the involved tooth should be tested. A nonvital tooth may have a larger pulp chamber than neighboring teeth because of the lack of secondary dentin, which normally forms with time in the pulp chamber and canal of a vital tooth (see Fig. 20-1).

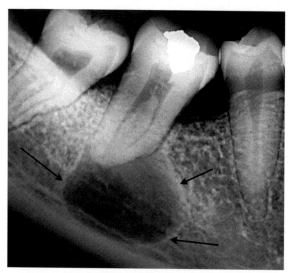

FIG. **20-2** A periapical film of a radicular cyst reveals a lesion with a well-defined cortical boundary *(arrows)*. Note that the presence of the inferior cortex of the mandible has influenced the circular shape of the cyst.

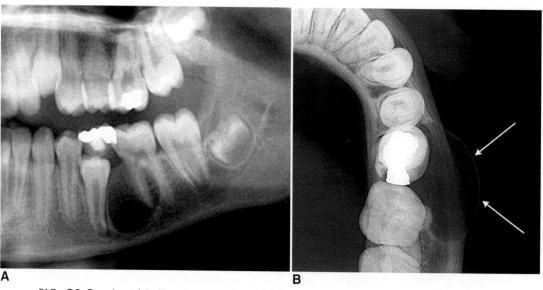

A   B

FIG. **20-3** A and B, Two images of a radicular cyst originating from a nonvital deciduous second molar show expansion of the buccal cortical plate to a circular or hydraulic shape *(arrows)* and displacement of the adjacent permanent teeth.

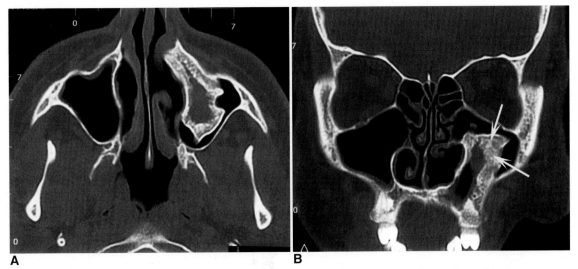

FIG. **20-4** Axial **(A)** and coronal **(B)** CT images using bone algorithm of a collapsing radicular cyst within the sinus. Note the unusual shape and the fact that new bone *(arrows)* is being formed from the periphery *(arrows)* toward the center. (Courtesy of Drs. S. Ahing and T. Blight, University of Manitoba.)

A large radicular cyst that has invaginated the maxillary antrum may collapse and start filling in with new bone (Fig. 20-4). With biopsy, the histologic analysis may result in an erroneous diagnosis of ossifying fibroma or a benign fibroosseous lesion. Radiographically, the important feature is that the new bone always forms first at the periphery of the cyst wall as the cyst shrinks and not in the center of the cyst; this is a different pattern of bone formation than is seen with benign fibroosseous lesions.

Management

Treatment of a tooth with a radicular cyst may include extraction, endodontic therapy, and apical surgery. Treatment of a large radicular cyst usually involves surgical removal or marsupialization. The radiographic appearance of the periapical area of an endodontically treated tooth should be checked periodically to make sure that normal healing is occurring (Fig. 20-5). Characteristically, new bone grows into the defect from the periphery, sometimes resulting in a radiating pattern resembling the spokes of a wheel. However, in a few cases normal bone may not fill the defect, especially if a secondary infection or a considerable amount of bone destruction occurred. Recurrence of a radicular cyst is unlikely if it has been removed completely.

RESIDUAL CYST

Definition

A residual cyst is a cyst that remains after incomplete removal of the original cyst. The term *residual* is used

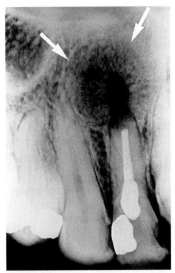

FIG. **20-5** A radicular cyst that is healing after endodontic treatment. Arrows show the original outline of the cyst; note that the new bone grows toward the center from the periphery.

most often for a radicular cyst that may be left behind most commonly after extraction of a tooth.

Clinical Features

A residual cyst usually is asymptomatic and often is discovered on radiographic examination of an edentulous area. However, there may be some expansion of the jaw or pain in the case of secondary infection.

Radiographic Features

Location. Residual cysts occur in both jaws, although they are found slightly more often in the mandible. The epicenter is positioned in a periapical location. In the mandible the epicenter is always above the inferior alveolar nerve canal (Fig. 20-6).

Periphery and shape. A residual cyst has a cortical margin unless it becomes secondarily infected. Its shape is oval or circular.

Internal structure. The internal aspect of a residual cyst typically is radiolucent. Dystrophic calcifications may be present in long-standing cysts.

Effects on surrounding structures. Residual cysts can cause tooth displacement or resorption. The outer cortical plates of the jaws may expand. The cyst may invaginate the maxillary antrum or depress the inferior alveolar nerve canal.

Differential Diagnosis

Without the patient's history and previous radiographs, the clinician may have difficulty determining whether a solitary cyst in the jaws is a residual cyst. Other examples of common solitary cysts include odontogenic keratocysts. A residual cyst has greater potential for expansion compared with an odontogenic keratocyst. The epicenter of a Stafne developmental salivary gland defect is located below the mandibular canal (and thus is unlikely to be odontogenic in nature).

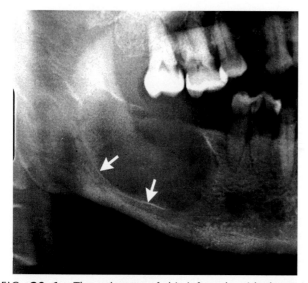

FIG. **20-6**   The epicenter of this infected residual cyst is above the inferior alveolar nerve canal and has displaced the canal in an inferior direction *(arrows)*. Note that the cortical boundary is not continuous around the whole cyst.

Management

The treatment for residual cysts is surgical removal or marsupialization, or both, if the cyst is large.

DENTIGEROUS CYST

Synonym

Follicular cyst

Definition

A dentigerous cyst is a cyst that forms around the crown of an unerupted tooth. It begins when fluid accumulates in the layers of reduced enamel epithelium or between the epithelium and the crown of the unerupted tooth. An eruption cyst is the soft tissue counterpart of a dentigerous cyst.

Clinical Features

Dentigerous cysts are the second most common type of cyst in the jaws. They develop around the crown of an unerupted or supernumerary tooth. The clinical examination reveals a missing tooth or teeth and possibly a hard swelling, occasionally resulting in facial asymmetry. The patient typically has no pain or discomfort. About 4% of individuals with at least one unerupted tooth have a dentigerous cyst. Dentigerous cysts around supernumerary teeth account for about 5% of all dentigerous cysts, most developing around a mesiodens in the anterior maxilla.

Radiographic Features

Location. The epicenter of a dentigerous cyst is found just above the crown of the involved tooth, which usually is the mandibular or maxillary third molar or the maxillary canine, the teeth most commonly affected (Fig. 20-7). An important diagnostic point is that this cyst attaches at the cementoenamel junction. Some dentigerous cysts are eccentric, developing from the lateral aspect of the follicle so that they occupy an area beside the crown instead of above the crown (see Fig. 20-7, *D*). Cysts related to maxillary third molars often grow into the maxillary antrum and may become quite large before they are discovered. Cysts attached to the crown of mandibular molars may extend a considerable distance into the ramus.

Periphery and shape. Dentigerous cysts typically have a well-defined cortex with a curved or circular outline. If infection is present, the cortex may be missing.

Internal structure. The internal aspect is completely radiolucent except for the crown of the involved tooth.

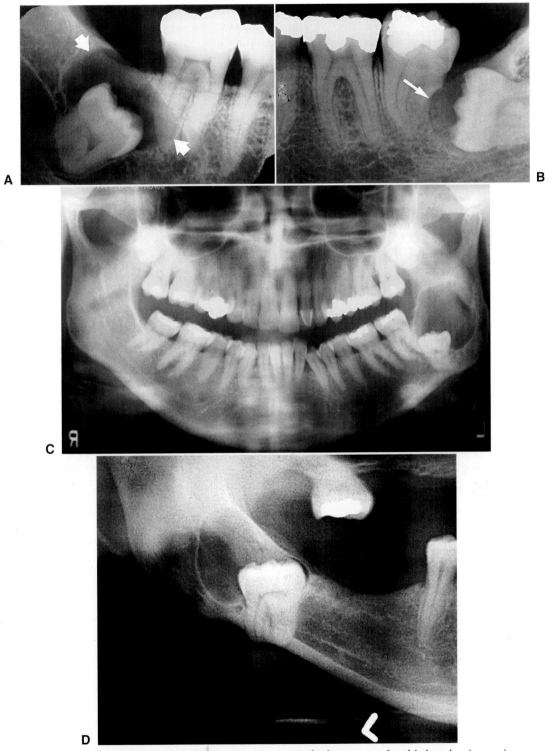

FIG. **20-7**   *Dentigerous cysts.* **A,** A cyst surrounds the crown of a third molar *(arrows)*; note the resorption of the distal root of the second molar *(arrow)* **(B). C,** A cyst that involves the ramus of the mandible. **D,** A dentigerous cyst that is expanding distally from the involved third molar.

Effects on surrounding structures. A dentigerous cyst has a propensity to displace and resorb adjacent teeth (Fig. 20-8). It commonly displaces the associated tooth in an apical direction (Fig. 20-9). The degree of displacement may be considerable. For instance, maxillary third molars or cuspids may be pushed to the floor of the orbit (see Fig. 20-8), and mandibular third molars may be moved to the condylar or coronoid regions or to the inferior cortex of the mandible (Fig. 20-10). The floor of the maxillary antrum may be displaced as the cyst invaginates the antrum, and the cyst may displace the inferior alveolar nerve canal in an inferior direction. This slow-growing cyst often expands the outer cortical boundary of the involved jaw.

Differential Diagnosis

Because the histopathologic appearance of the lining epithelium is not specific, the diagnosis relies on the radiographic and surgical observation of the attachment of the cyst to the cementoenamel junction. A histopathologic examination must always be done to eliminate other possible lesions in this location.

One of the most difficult differential diagnoses to make is between a small dentigerous cyst and a hyperplastic follicle. A cyst should be considered with any evidence of tooth displacement or considerable expansion of the involved bone. The size of the normal follicular space is 2 to 3 mm. If the follicular space exceeds 5 mm, a dentigerous cyst is more likely. If uncertainty remains,

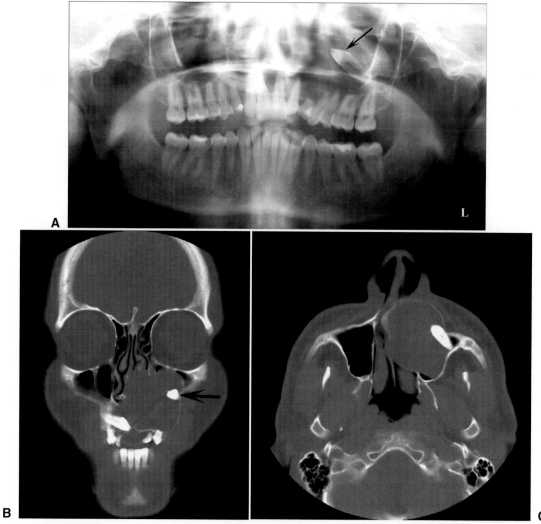

FIG. **20-8**   **A,** This panoramic image reveals the presence of a large dentigerous cyst associated with the left maxillary cuspid *(arrow),* which has been displaced. Notice the displacement and resorption of other teeth in the left maxilla. **B** and **C,** Coronal and axial CT images of the same case showing superior-lateral displacement of the cuspid, expansion of the anterior wall of the maxilla and expansion of the cyst into the nasal fossa.

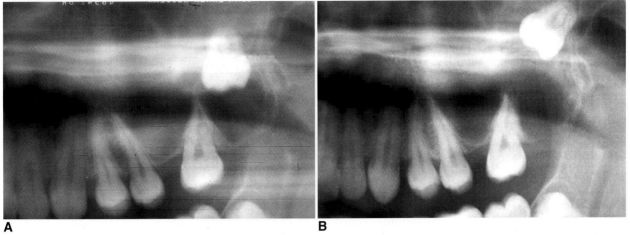

FIG. **20-9** **A** and **B,** These panoramic films of the same case taken several years apart demonstrate superior-posterior displacement of a maxillary third molar by a dentigerous cyst.

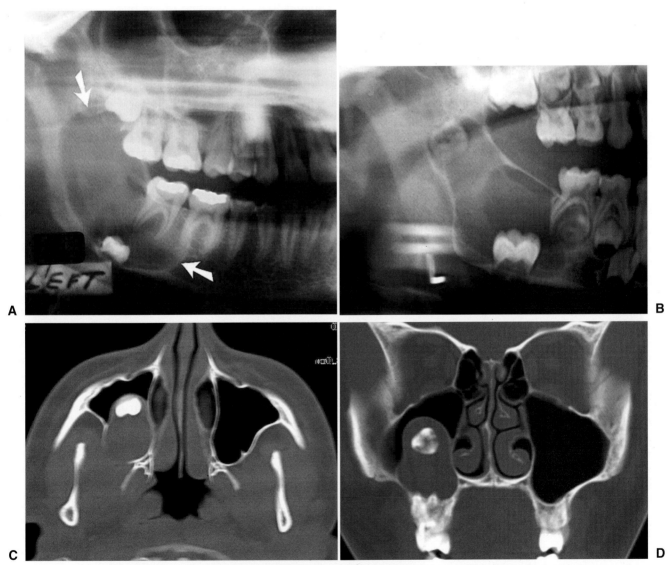

FIG. **20-10** *Dentigerous cysts displacing teeth.* **A,** The third molar has been displaced to the inferior cortex. **B,** The second molar has been displaced into the ramus by a cyst associated with the first molar. Axial **(C)** and coronal **(D)** CT images using bone algorithm reveal a maxillary third molar displaced into the space occupied by the maxillary antrum.

the region should be reexamined in 4 to 6 months to detect any increase in size or any influence on surrounding structures characteristic of cysts.

The differential diagnosis also may include an odontogenic keratocyst, an ameloblastic fibroma, and a cystic ameloblastoma. An odontogenic keratocyst does not expand the bone to the same degree as a dentigerous cyst, is less likely to resorb teeth, and may attach farther apically on the root instead of at the cementoenamel junction. It may not be possible to differentiate a small ameloblastic fibroma or cystic ameloblastoma from a dentigerous cyst if there is no internal structure. Other rare lesions that may have a similar pericoronal appearance are adenomatoid odontogenic tumors and calcified odontogenic cysts, both of which can surround the crown and root of the involved tooth. Evidence of a radiopaque internal structure should be sought in these two lesions. Occasionally a radicular cyst at the apex of a primary tooth surrounds the crown of the developing permanent tooth positioned apical to it, giving the false impression of a dentigerous cyst associated with the permanent tooth. This occurs most often with the mandibular deciduous molars and the developing bicuspids. In these cases the clinician should look for deep caries or extensive restorations in a primary tooth that would indicate a radicular cyst.

Management

Dentigerous cysts are treated by surgical removal, which may include the tooth as well. Large cysts may be treated by marsupialization before removal. The cyst lining should be submitted for histologic examination because ameloblastomas have been reported to occur in the cyst lining. In addition, squamous cell carcinoma has been reported to arise from the cyst lining of chronically infected cysts. Mucoepidermoid carcinoma also has been reported.

BUCCAL BIFURCATION CYST

Synonyms

Mandibular infected buccal cyst, paradental cyst, or inflammatory collateral dental cyst

Definition

The source of epithelium probably is the epithelial cell rests in the periodontal membrane of the buccal bifurcation of mandibular molars. The histopathologic characteristics of the lining are not distinctive. The etiology of proliferation is unknown; one theory holds that inflammation is the stimulus, but inflammation is not always present. The World Health Organization includes these cysts under inflammatory cysts.

It is unclear whether the paradental cyst of the third molar and the buccal bifurcation cyst (associated with first and second molars) are the same entity. The buccal bifurcation cyst (BBC) is certainly a distinct clinical entity. An associated enamel extension into the furcation region of third molars with paradental cysts has not been documented with molars involved in a BBC. Also, the inflammatory component associated with paradental cysts is not always present with BBCs.

Clinical Features

A common sign is the lack of or a delay in eruption of a mandibular first or second molar. On clinical examination the molar may be missing or the lingual cusp tips may be abnormally protruding through the mucosa, higher than the position of the buccal cusps. The first molar is involved more frequently than the second molar. The teeth are always vital. A hard swelling may be present buccal to the involved molar, and if it is secondarily infected, the patient has pain. The age of detection is younger, within the first 2 decades for a BBC and in the third decade for a paradental cyst of the third molar.

Radiographic Features

Location. The mandibular first molar is the most common location of a BBC, followed by the second molar. The cyst occasionally is bilateral. It is always located in the buccal furcation of the affected molar (Fig. 20-11). On periapical and panoramic films the lesion may appear to be centered a little distal to the furcation of the involved tooth.

Periphery and shape. In some cases the periphery is not readily apparent, and the lesion may be a very subtle radiolucent region superimposed over the image of the roots of the molar. In other cases the lesion has a circular shape with a well-defined cortical border. Some cysts can become quite large before they are detected.

Internal structure. The internal structure is radiolucent.

Effects on surrounding structures. The most striking diagnostic characteristic of a BBC is the tipping of the involved molar so that the root tips are pushed into the lingual cortical plate of the mandible (see Fig. 20-11, *B* and *C*) and the occlusal surface is tipped toward the buccal aspect of the mandible (see Fig. 20-11, *A*). This accounts for the lingual cusp tips being positioned higher than the buccal tips. This tipping may be detected in a panoramic or periapical film if the image of the occlusal surface of the affected tooth is apparent, whereas the unaffected teeth are not. The best diagnostic film is the cross-sectional (standard) mandibular

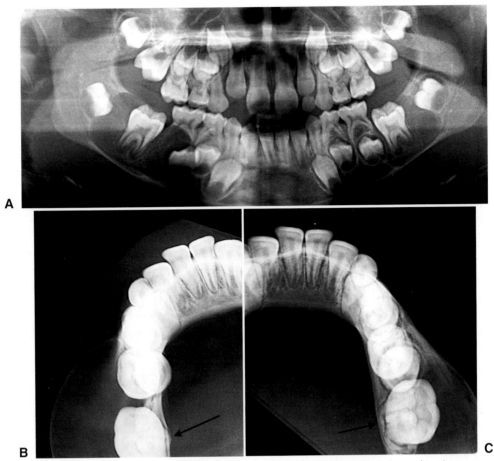

FIG. **20-11** *Bilateral buccal bifurcation cysts.* **A,** A panoramic image showing cysts related to the mandibular first molars. Note that the occlusal surface of each tooth has been tipped in relation to the other teeth and that adjacent teeth have been displaced. **B** and **C,** Occlusal films of the same case. Note the circular expansion of the buccal cortex and the displacement of the roots of the first molars into the lingual cortical plate *(arrows).*

occlusal projection, which demonstrates the abnormal position of the root apex. If the cyst is large enough, it may displace and resorb the adjacent teeth and cause a considerable amount of smooth expansion of the buccal cortical plate. If the cyst is secondarily infected, periosteal new bone formation is seen on the buccal cortex adjacent to the involved tooth.

Differential Diagnosis

Diagnosis of a BBC relies entirely on clinical and radiographic information. The major differential diagnosis includes lesions that could elicit an inflammatory periosteal response on the buccal aspect of mandibular molars such as a periodontal abscess or Langerhans' cell histiocytosis. The fact that only a BBC tilts the molar as described helps to differentiate it from other lesions. Also in the differential diagnosis is the dentigerous cyst.

However, the epicenter of a dentigerous cyst is different because a BBC starts near the bifurcation region of the tooth and does not surround the crown, as does a dentigerous cyst.

Management

A BBC usually is removed by conservative curettage, although some cases have resolved without intervention. The involved molar should not be removed. BBCs do not recur.

ODONTOGENIC KERATOCYST

Synonym

It is a commonly held view that primordial cysts are odontogenic keratocysts. However, this view is not universally accepted.

Definition

An odontogenic keratocyst (OKC) is a noninflammatory odontogenic cyst that arises from the dental lamina. Unlike other cysts, which are thought to grow solely by osmotic pressure, the epithelium in an OKC appears to have innate growth potential, much as in a benign tumor. This difference in the mechanism of growth gives OKCs a different radiographic appearance. The epithelial lining is distinctive because it is keratinized (hence the name) and thin (4 to 8 cells thick). Occasionally budlike proliferations of epithelium grow from the basal layer into the adjacent connective tissue wall. Also, islands of epithelium in the wall may give rise to satellite microcysts. The inside of the cyst often contains a viscous or cheesy material derived from the epithelial lining.

Clinical Features

OKCs account for about one tenth of all cysts in the jaws. They occur in a wide age range, but most develop during the second and third decades, with a slight male predominance. The cysts sometimes form around an unerupted tooth. OKCs usually have no symptoms, although mild swelling may occur. Pain may occur with secondary infection. Aspiration may reveal a thick, yellow, cheesy material (keratin). It is important to note that, unlike other cysts, OKCs have a high propensity for recurrence, possibly because of small satellite cysts or fragments of epithelium left behind after surgical removal of the cyst.

Radiographic Features

Location. The most common location of an OKC is the posterior body of the mandible (90% occur posterior to the canines) and ramus (more than 50%) (Fig. 20-12). The epicenter is located superior to the inferior alveolar nerve canal. This type of cyst occasionally has the same pericoronal position as, and is indistinguishable from, a dentigerous cyst (see Fig. 20-12).

Periphery and shape. As with other cysts, OKCs usually show evidence of a cortical border unless they have become secondarily infected. The cyst may have a smooth round or oval shape identical to that of other cysts, or it may have a scalloped outline (a series of contiguous arcs) (see Figs. 20-12 and 20-14, *C*).

Internal structure. The internal structure most commonly is radiolucent. The presence of internal keratin does not increase the radiopacity. In some cases curved internal septa may be present, giving the lesion a multilocular appearance (Fig. 20-13; see also Fig. 20-12).

Effects on surrounding structures. An important characteristic of the OKC is its propensity to grow along the internal aspect of the jaws, causing minimal expansion

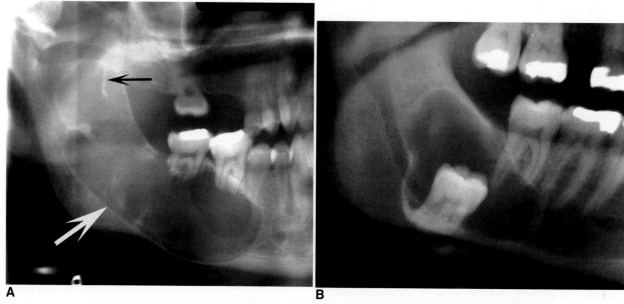

A   **B**

FIG. **20-12**   **A,** Panoramic image shows a large keratocyst occupying the ramus and body of the mandible; note the septa *(black arrow),* inferiorly displaced mandibular canal *(white arrow),* and the root resorption. The keratocyst in **B** has a pericoronal position relative to the impacted third molar and the distal margin has a scalloped shape.

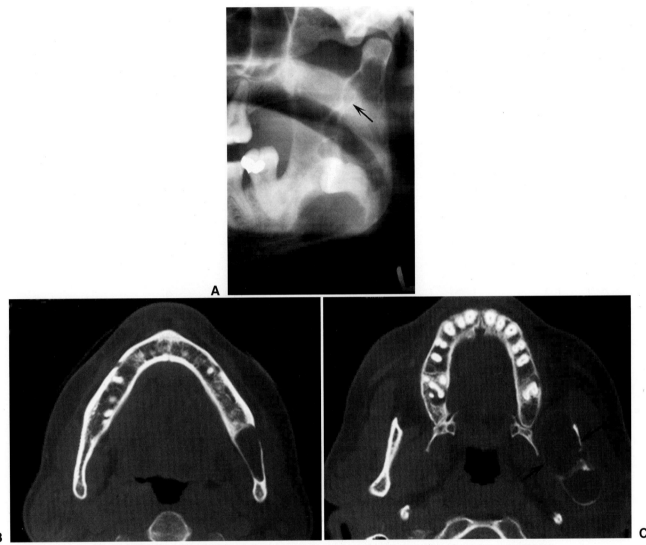

FIG. **20-13**   **A**, Cropped panoramic image of a keratocyst occupying the mandibular ramus; note the septa *(arrow)*. **B** and **C**, Axial CT images using bone algorithm of the same case demonstrating very little expansion in the body **(B)** but significant expansion in the upper ramus in **C** *(arrows)*.

(Fig. 20-14). This occurs throughout the mandible except for the upper ramus and coronoid process, where considerable expansion may occur (see Fig. 20-13, *C*). Occasionally the expansion of large cysts may exceed the ability of the periosteum to form new bone, thus allowing the cyst wall to contact soft tissue peripheral to the outer cortex of the mandible (Fig. 20-15). The relatively slight expansion common with these cysts probably contributes to their late detection, which occasionally allows them to reach a large size. OKCs can displace and resorb teeth but to a slightly lesser degree than dentigerous cysts. The inferior alveolar nerve canal may be displaced inferiorly. In the maxilla this cyst can invaginate and occupy the entire maxillary antrum.

Differential Diagnosis

When in a pericoronal position, an OKC may be indistinguishable from a dentigerous cyst. The cyst is likely to be an OKC if the cyst is connected to the tooth at a point apical to the cementoenamel junction or if no expansion of the cortical plates has occurred. The typical scalloped margin and multilocular appearance of the OKC may resemble an ameloblastoma, but the latter has a greater propensity to expand. An OKC may

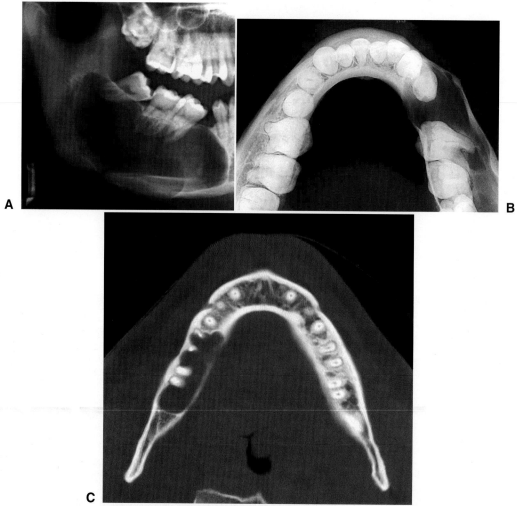

FIG. **20-14**   A large keratocyst occupying most of the right body and ramus of the mandible. **A,** Note that, despite the cyst's size, the buccal and lingual cortical plates of the mandible have expanded only slightly, as can be seen in the occlusal film **(B). C,** An axial image of a keratocyst within the body of the mandible; note the lack of expansion and the cyst scalloping between the roots of the teeth.

show some similarity to an odontogenic myxoma, especially in the characteristics of mild expansion and multilocular appearance. A simple bone cyst often has a scalloped margin and minimal bone expansion, as with an OKC; however, the margins of a simple bone cyst usually are more delicate and often difficult to detect. If several OKCs are found (which occurs in 4% to 5% of cases), these cysts may constitute part of a basal cell nevus syndrome.

Management

If an OKC is suspected, referral to a radiologist for a complete radiologic examination is advisable. Because this cyst has a propensity to recur, an accurate determination of the extent and location of any cortical perforations with soft tissue extension is best achieved with computed tomography. In the case of multiple cysts and the possibility of basal cell nevus syndrome, a thorough radiologic examination is required. This allows accurate determination of the number of cysts and other osseous characteristics that confirm the diagnosis.

Surgical treatment may vary and can include resection, curettage, or marsupialization to reduce the size of large cysts before surgical excision. More attention usually is devoted to complete removal of the walls of the cyst to reduce the chance of recurrence. After sur-

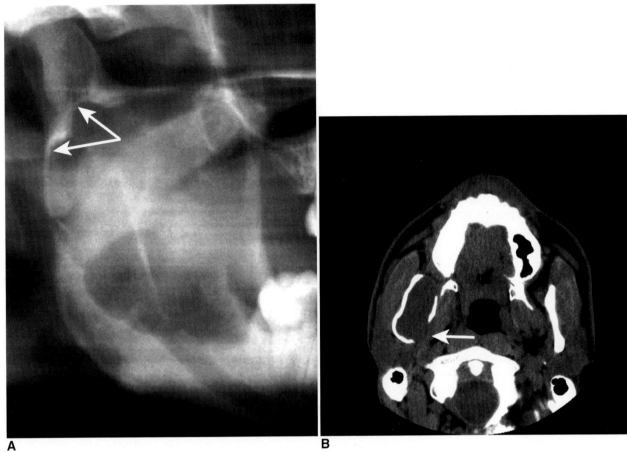

FIG. **20-15** **A,** Cropped panoramic image revealing a large keratocyst occupying most of the ramus; note the scalloping margin *(arrows)*. **B,** This axial CT using soft tissue window of the same case showing perforation of the medial cortex and contacting the medial pterygoid muscle *(arrow)*.

gical treatment, it is important to make periodic post treatment clinical and radiographic examinations to detect any recurrence. Recurrent lesions usually develop within the first 5 years but may be delayed as long as 10 years.

BASAL CELL NEVUS SYNDROME

Synonyms

Nevoid basal cell carcinoma syndrome or Gorlin-Goltz syndrome

Definition

The term *basal cell nevus syndrome* comprises a number of abnormalities such as multiple nevoid basal cell carcinomas of the skin, skeletal abnormalities, central nervous system abnormalities, eye abnormalities, and multiple OKCs. It is inherited as an autosomal dominant trait with variable expressivity.

Clinical Features

Basal cell nevus syndrome starts to appear early in life, usually after 5 years of age and before 30 years of age, with the development of jaw cysts and skin basal cell carcinomas. The lesions occur as multiple OKCs of the jaws, usually appearing in multiple quadrants and earlier in life than solitary OKCs. The recurrence rate of OKCs in this syndrome appears to be higher than with the solitary variety. The skin lesions are small, flattened, flesh-colored or brown papules that can occur anywhere on the body but are especially prominent on the face, neck, and trunk. Occasionally basal cell carcinomas form later in life than the jaw cysts or not at all. Skeletal anomalies include bifid rib (most common) and other costal abnormalities such as agenesis, deformity, and synostosis of the ribs, kyphoscoliosis, vertebral fusion, polydactyly, shortening of the metacarpals, temporal and temporoparietal bossing, minor hypertelorism, and mild prognathism. Calcification of the falx cerebri and other parts of the dura occur early in life.

Radiographic Features
Location. The location is the same as that of solitary OKCs, as described previously. The multiple keratocysts may develop bilaterally and can vary in size from 1 mm to several centimeters in diameter (Fig. 20-16).

Other radiographic features. See the preceding radiographic description of OKCs. In addition, a radiopaque line of the calcified falx cerebri may be prominent on the posteroanterior skull projection. Occasionally this calcification may appear laminated.

Differential Diagnosis
The presence of a cortical boundary and other cystic characteristics differentiate basal cell nevus syndrome from other abnormalities characterized by multiple radiolucencies (e.g., multiple myeloma). Cherubism appears as bilateral multilocular lesions but usually has significant jaw expansion, which is not characteristic of basal cell nevus syndrome. Also, cherubism pushes posterior teeth in an anterior direction, a distinctive characteristic. Occasionally patients with multiple dentigerous cysts may show some similarities, but dentigerous cysts are more expansile.

Management
The keratocysts are treated more aggressively than other solitary OKCs because there appears to be an even greater propensity for recurrence. It is reasonable to examine the patient yearly for new and recurrent cysts. A panoramic film serves as an adequate

screening film. Referral for genetic counseling may be appropriate.

LATERAL PERIODONTAL CYST
Definition
Lateral periodontal cysts are thought to arise from epithelial rests in periodontium lateral to the tooth root. This condition usually is unicystic, but it may appear as a cluster of small cysts, a condition referred to as botryoid odontogenic cysts. It has been postulated that the lateral periodontal cyst is the intrabony counterpart of the gingival cyst in the adult.

Clinical Features
The lesions usually are asymptomatic and less than 1 cm in diameter. The disorder has no apparent sexual predilection, and the age distribution extends from the second to the ninth decades (the mean age is about 50 years). If these cysts become secondarily infected, they will mimic a lateral periodontal abscess.

Radiographic Features
Location. Fifty percent to 75% of lateral periodontal cysts develop in the mandible, mostly in a region extending from the lateral incisor to the second premolar (Fig. 20-17).

Occasionally these cysts appear in the maxilla, especially between the lateral incisor and the cuspid.

Periphery and shape. A lateral periodontal cyst appears as a well-defined radiolucency with a prominent cortical boundary and a round or oval shape. Rare large cysts have a more irregular shape.

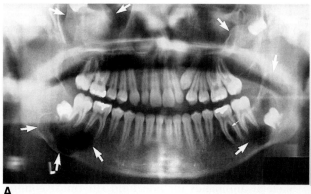 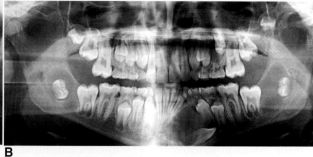

A   **B**

FIG. **20-16**   Multiple OKCs associated with nevoid basal cell carcinoma syndrome. **A,** Upper arrows point to opacified maxillary antra; smaller arrow indicates the extension of one of the mandibular cysts *(lower arrows)* into the bifurcation region of a mandibular molar. **B,** Five cysts are present, which are related to the mandibular third molars and left cuspid and to the maxillary left second premolar and third molar.

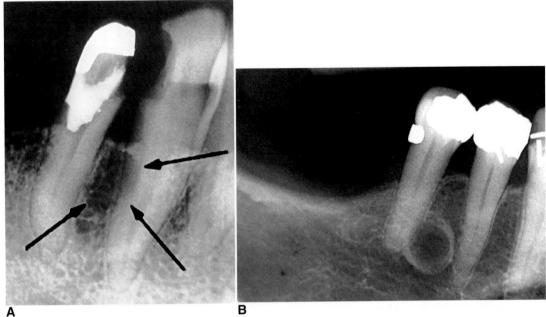

FIG. 20-17 Lateral periodontal cysts in the mandibular premolar region. **B** has the classic well-defined cortical border, whereas **A** does not.

Internal structure. The internal aspect usually is radiolucent. The botryoid variety may have a multilocular appearance.

Effects on surrounding structures. Small cysts may efface the lamina dura of the adjacent root. Large cysts can displace adjacent teeth and cause expansion.

Differential Diagnosis
Because the location and radiographic appearance of a lateral periodontal cyst are similar in other conditions, the following lesions should be included in the differential diagnosis: a small OKC, mental foramen, small neurofibroma or a radicular cyst at the foramen of a lateral (accessory) pulp canal. The multiple (botryoid) cysts with a multilocular appearance may resemble a small ameloblastoma.

Management
Lateral periodontal cysts usually do not require sophisticated imaging because of their small size. Excisional biopsy or simple enucleation is the treatment of choice, since these cysts do not tend to recur.

CALCIFYING ODONTOGENIC CYST
Synonyms
Calcifying epithelial odontogenic cyst or Gorlin cyst

Definition
Calcifying odontogenic cysts are uncommon, slow-growing, benign lesions. They occupy a spectrum ranging from a cyst to an odontogenic tumor, with characteristics of a cyst alone or sometimes those of a solid neoplasm (epithelial proliferation and a tendency to continue growing). The World Health Organization now categorizes calcifying odontogenic cysts as benign tumors. This lesion may manufacture calcified tissue identified as dysplastic dentin, and in some instances the lesion is associated with an odontoma. This lesion also sometimes contains a more solid component that gives it an appearance resembling an ameloblastoma, although it does not behave like one.

Clinical Features
Calcifying odontogenic cysts have a wide age distribution that peaks at 10 to 19 years of age, with a mean age of 36 years. A second incidence peak occurs during the seventh decade. Clinically, the lesion usually appears as a slow-growing, painless swelling of the jaw. Occasionally the patient complains of pain. In some cases the expanding lesion may destroy the cortical plate, and the cystic mass may become palpable as it extends into the soft tissue. The patient may report a discharge from such advanced lesions. Aspiration often yields a viscous, granular, yellow fluid.

Radiographic Features

Location. At least 75% of calcifying odontogenic cysts occur in bone, with a nearly equal distribution between the jaws. Most (75%) occur anterior to the first molar, especially associated with cuspids and incisors, where the cyst sometimes manifests as a pericoronal radiolucency.

Periphery and shape. The periphery can vary from well defined and corticated with a curved, cystlike shape to ill defined and irregular.

Internal structure. The internal aspect can vary in appearance. It may be completely radiolucent; it may show evidence of small foci of calcified material that appear as white flecks or small smooth pebbles; or it may show even larger, solid, amorphous masses (Fig. 20-18). In rare cases the lesion may appear multilocular.

Effects on surrounding structures. Occasionally (20% to 50% of cases) the cyst is associated with a tooth (most commonly a cuspid) and impedes its eruption. Displacement of teeth and resorption of roots may occur. Perforation of the cortical plate may be seen radiographically with enlarging lesions.

Differential Diagnosis

When no internal calcifications are evident and this lesion has a pericoronal position, it may be indistinguishable from a dentigerous cyst. Other lesions that have internal calcifications to be considered include an adenomatoid odontogenic tumor, ameloblastic fibroodontoma, and calcifying epithelial odontogenic tumor. The common position for the calcifying odontogenic cyst is not common for either the fibroodontoma or the calcifying epithelial odontogenic tumor. Finally, long-standing cysts may have dystrophic calcification, giving a similar appearance.

Management

Although this cyst does have some neoplastic characteristics, such as a tendency for continued growth, the treatment should be enucleation and curettage. Because clinicians generally have little experience with the more solid neoplastic variants, it is wise to follow treatment with periodic radiographic evaluation for recurrence.

Nonodontogenic Cysts

NASOPALATINE DUCT CYST

Synonyms

Nasopalatine canal cyst, incisive canal cyst, nasopalatine cyst, median palatine cyst, or median anterior maxillary cyst

Definition

The nasopalatine canal usually contains remnants of the nasopalatine duct, a primitive organ of smell, as well as the nasopalatine vessels and nerves. Occasionally a cyst forms in the nasopalatine canal when these embryonic epithelial remnants of the nasopalatine duct undergo proliferation and cystic degeneration.

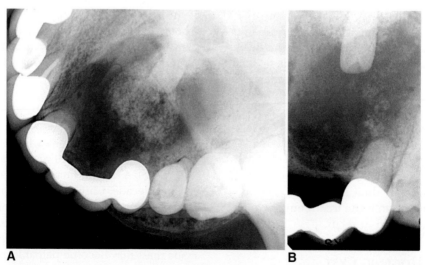

FIG. **20-18** A and B, Calcifying odontogenic cyst related to the lateral incisor. Note the well-defined, corticated border, internal calcifications, and resorption of part of the root of the central incisor.

Clinical Features

Nasopalatine duct cysts account for about 10% of jaw cysts. The age distribution is broad, with most cases being discovered in the fourth through sixth decades. The incidence is three times higher in males. Most of these cysts are asymptomatic or cause such minor symptoms that they are tolerated for long periods. The most frequent complaint is a small, well-defined swelling just posterior to the palatine papilla. This swelling usually is fluctuant and blue if the cyst is near the surface. The deeper nasopalatine duct cyst is covered by normal-appearing mucosa unless it is ulcerated from masticatory trauma. If the cyst expands, it may penetrate the labial plate and produce a swelling below the maxillary labial frenum or to one side. The lesion also may bulge into the nasal cavity and distort the nasal septum. Pressure from the cyst on the adjacent nasopalatine nerves that occupy the same canal may cause a burning sensation or numbness over the palatal mucosa. In some cases cystic fluid may drain into the oral cavity through a sinus tract or a remnant of the nasopalatine duct. The patient usually detects the fluid and reports a salty taste.

Radiographic Features

Location. Most nasopalatine duct cysts are found in the nasopalatine foramen or canal. However, if this cyst extends posteriorly to involve the hard palate (Fig. 20-19), it often is referred to as a median palatal cyst. If it expands anteriorly between the central incisors, destroying or expanding the labial plate of bone and causing the teeth to diverge, it sometimes is referred to as a median anterior maxillary cyst. This cyst may not always be positioned symmetrically.

Periphery and shape. The periphery usually is well defined and corticated and is circular or oval in shape. The shadow of the nasal spine sometimes is superimposed on the cyst, giving it a heart shape.

Internal structure. Most nasopalatine duct cysts are totally radiolucent. Some rare cysts may have internal dystrophic calcifications, which may appear as ill-defined, amorphous, scattered radiopacities.

Effects on surrounding structures. Most commonly this cyst causes the roots of the central incisors to diverge, and occasionally root resorption occurs (Fig. 20-20). Seen from a lateral perspective, the cyst may expand the labial cortex as well as the palatal cortex (Fig. 20-21). The floor of the nasal fossa may be displaced in a superior direction.

Differential Diagnosis

The most common differential diagnosis is a large incisive foramen. A foramen larger than 6 mm may simulate the appearance of a cyst. However, a clinical examination should reveal the expansion characteristic of a cyst and other changes that occur with a space-occupying lesion, such as displacement of teeth. A lateral view of the anterior maxilla, using an occlusal film held outside the mouth and against the cheek, also can help in making the differential diagnosis, as can a cross-sectional (standard) occlusal view. If doubt still exists, comparison with previous images may be useful, or aspiration may be attempted, or another image may be made in 6 months to 1 year to assess any change in size. A radicular cyst or granuloma associated with a central incisor is similar in appearance to an asymmetric nasopalatine cyst. The presence or absence of the lamina dura and enlargement of the periodontal ligament space around the apex of the central incisor indicate an inflammatory lesion. A vitality test of the central incisor may be useful. A second periapical view taken at a different horizontal angulation should show an altered position of the image of a nasopalatine duct cyst, whereas a radicular cyst should remain centered about the apex of the central incisor.

Management

The appropriate treatment for a nasopalatine cyst is enucleation, preferably from the palate to avoid the nasopalatine nerve. If the cyst is large and the danger exists of devitalizing the tooth or creating a naso-oral or antro-oral fistula, the surgeon may elect to marsupialize the cyst.

NASOLABIAL CYST

Synonym

Nasoalveolar cyst

Definition

The exact origin of nasolabial cysts is unknown. They may be fissural cysts arising from the epithelial rests in fusion lines of the globular, lateral nasal, and maxillary processes. Alternatively, the source of the epithelium may be from the embryonic nasolacrimal duct, which initially lies on the bone surface.

Clinical Features

When this rare lesion is small, it may produce a very subtle, unilateral swelling of the nasolabial fold and may elicit pain or discomfort. When large, it may bulge into the floor of the nasal cavity, causing some obstruction, flaring of the alae, distortion of the nostrils, and fullness of the upper lip. If infected, it may drain into the

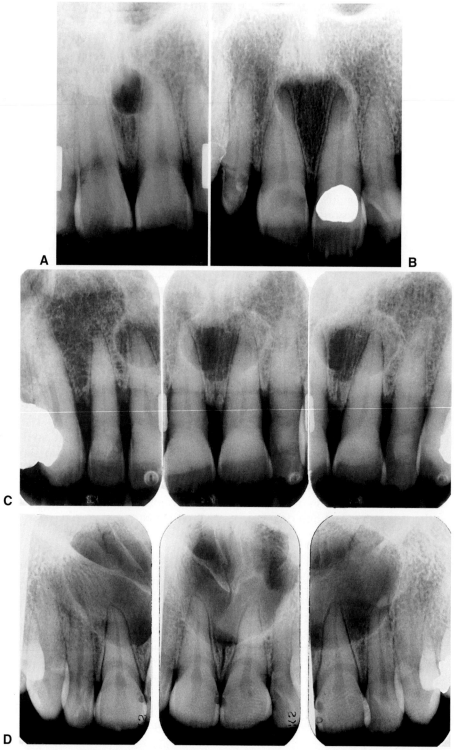

FIG. **20-19** *Nasopalatine duct cysts.* Note the uniform periodontal membrane space around all the apices. **A** through **D** show variations in size. The differential diagnosis of a smaller cyst with a normal nasopalatine foramen may be difficult.

nasal cavity. It usually is unilateral, but bilateral lesions have occurred. The age of detection ranges from 12 to 75 years, with a mean age of 44 years. About 75% of these lesions occur in females.

Radiographic Features

Location. Nasolabial cysts are primarily soft tissue lesions located adjacent to the alveolar process above the apices of the incisors. Because this is a soft tissue

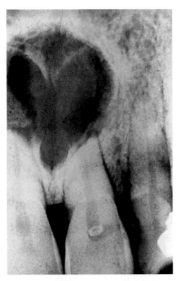

FIG. **20-20** A nasopalatine canal cyst causing external root resorption of a maxillary central incisor.

lesion, plain radiographs may not show any detectable changes. The investigation could include either computed tomography (CT) or magnetic resonance imaging (MRI), both of which can provide an image of soft tissues (Fig. 20-22).

Periphery and shape. Thin axial CT images using the soft tissue algorithm with contrast reveal a circular or oval lesion with slight soft tissue enhancement of the periphery.

Internal structure. In CT images using the soft tissue algorithm the internal aspect appears homogeneous and relatively radiolucent compared with the surrounding soft tissues.

Effects on surrounding structures. Occasionally a cyst causes erosion of the underlying bone (Fig. 20-23), producing an increased radiolucency of the alveolar process beneath the cyst and apical to the incisors. Also, the usual outline of the inferior border of the nasal fossa may become distorted, resulting in a posterior bowing of this margin.

Differential Diagnosis

The swelling caused by an infected nasolabial cyst may simulate an acute dentoalveolar abscess. It is important to establish the vitality of the adjacent teeth. This cyst may also resemble a nasal furuncle if it pushes upward into the floor of the nasal cavity. A large mucous extravasation cyst or a cystic salivary adenoma should

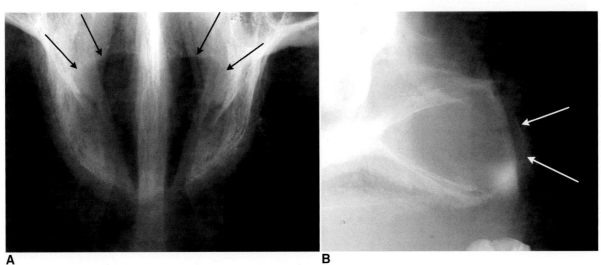

A **B**

FIG. **20-21** A nasopalatine canal cyst viewed from two perspectives: **(A)** a standard occlusal view and **(B)** from the lateral aspect, which is created by placing the film outside the mouth against the cheek and directing the x-ray beam at a tangent to the labial surface of the central incisors.

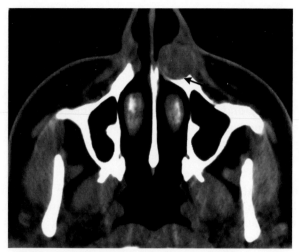

FIG. **20-22**　Nasolabial cyst shown in an axial CT image using a soft tissue algorithm. Note the well-defined periphery and the erosion of the labial aspect of the alveolar process *(arrow)*.

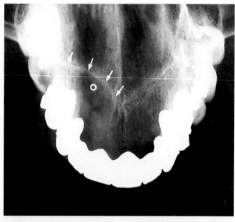

FIG. **20-23**　*Occlusal view of a nasolabial cyst.* The radiograph shows erosion of the alveolar bone *(o)* and elevation of the floor of the nasal fossa *(arrows)*. (From Montenegro Chineallato LE, Demante JH: Oral Surg 58:729, 1984.)

also be considered in the differential diagnosis of an uninfected nasolabial cyst.

Management

The nasolabial cyst should be excised through an intraoral approach. These cysts do not tend to recur.

DERMOID CYST

Definition

Dermoid cysts are a cystic form of a teratoma thought to be derived from trapped embryonic cells that are totipotential. The resulting cysts are lined with epidermis and cutaneous appendages and filled with keratin or sebaceous material (and in rare cases with bone, teeth, muscle, or hair, in which case they are properly called *teratomas*).

Clinical Features

Dermoid cysts may develop in the soft tissues at any time from birth, but they usually become clinically apparent between 12 and 25 years of age, about equally distributed between the sexes. The swelling, which is slow and painless, can grow to several centimeters in diameter, and when located in the neck or tongue, it may interfere with breathing, speaking, and eating. Depending on how deep the cyst is positioned in the neck, it can deform the submental area. On palpation these cysts may be fluctuant or doughy, according to their contents. Because they usually are in the midline, they do not affect the teeth.

Radiographic Features

Because dermoid cysts are soft tissue cysts, diagnostic imaging is best accomplished by CT or MRI.

Location. A dermoid cyst is a rare developmental anomaly that may occur anywhere in the body. About 10% or fewer arise in the head and neck, and only 1% to 2% develop in the oral cavity. Of these, about 25% occur in the floor of the mouth and on the tongue. They may be midline or lateral in location.

Periphery and shape. The periphery of the lesion usually is well defined by more radiopaque soft tissue of this cyst compared with surrounding soft tissue, as seen in CT scans.

Internal structure. Dermoid cysts seldom have any internal mineralized structures when they occur in the oral cavity; therefore they are radiolucent on conventional radiographs. However, a CT scan of the area may reveal a soft tissue multilocular appearance (Fig. 20-24). If teeth or bone form in the cyst, their radiopaque images, with characteristic shapes and densities, are apparent on the radiograph.

Differential Diagnosis

Lesions that are clinically similar to dermoid cysts are ranula (unilateral or bilateral blockage of Wharton's ducts), thyroglossal duct cysts, cystic hygromas, branchial cleft cysts, cellulitis, tumors (lipoma and liposarcoma), and normal fat masses in the submental area.

Management

Dermoid cysts do not recur after surgical removal.

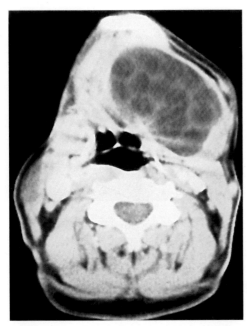

FIG. **20-24** CT scan of a dermoid cyst showing an encapsulated mass on the left and several soft tissue loculations. (From Hunter TB et al: Am J Roentgenol 141:1229, 1983.)

FORMER CYSTS

In recent years it has become clear that some names used to describe distinct entities are no longer valid. These names include *primordial cysts* (now recognized largely to be odontogenic keratocysts [OKCs]), *median palatal cysts* (now recognized as a variant of the nasopalatine duct cyst), and *median mandibular* and *globulomaxillary cysts* (because the entrapment of epithelium theory is no longer accepted). Globulomaxillary cysts are now recognized to be radicular or lateral periodontal cysts or OKCs.

Cystlike Lesions

Simple bone cysts are included in this chapter because of their historic classification and because the characteristics and behavior seen in diagnostic imaging are cystic in nature. However, it is important to remember that these lesions are not true cysts.

SIMPLE BONE CYST

Synonyms
Traumatic bone cyst, hemorrhagic bone cyst, extravasation cyst, progressive bone cavity, solitary bone cyst, or unicameral bone cyst

Definition
A simple bone cyst (SBC) is a cavity within bone that is lined with connective tissue. It may be empty, or it may contain fluid. However, because it has no epithelial lining, it is not a true cyst. The etiology of SBCs is unknown, although they may be a localized aberration in normal bone remodeling or metabolism. This theory is supported indirectly by the fact that these bony cavities often occur inside lesions of cemento-osseous dysplasia and fibrous dysplasia. No evidence exists to support a traumatic cause.

Clinical Features
SBCs are very common lesions. Most occur in the first 2 decades of life, with a mean age of 17 years. The lesion shows a male predominance of approximately 2:1. Multiple SBCs can develop, especially when the disorder occurs with cemento-osseous dysplasia. The occurrence of SBCs in cemento-osseous dysplasia is seen in an older population, with a mean age of 42 years, and with a female predominance of 4:1. SBCs are asymptomatic in most cases, but occasionally pain or tenderness may be present, especially if the cyst has become secondarily infected. Expansion of the mandible or tooth movement is possible but unusual. The teeth in the affected region usually are vital. Most SBCs are discovered only by chance, during radiographic examinations, and for this reason they can become quite large. There is no significant incidence of pathologic fractures. When aspiration is productive, usually only a few milliliters of straw-colored or serosanguineous fluid are obtained.

Radiographic Features
Location. Almost all SBCs are found in the mandible (Fig. 20-25); in rare cases they develop in the maxilla. The lesion can occur anywhere in the mandible but is seen most often in the ramus and posterior mandible in older patients. SBCs also frequently occur with cemento-osseous and fibrous dysplasia.

Periphery and shape. The margin may vary from a well-defined, delicate cortex to an ill-defined border that blends into the surrounding bone. The boundary usually is better defined in the alveolar process around the teeth than in the inferior aspect of the body of the mandible. The shape most often is smooth and curved, like a cyst, with an oval or scalloped border. The lesion often scallops between the roots of the teeth (see Fig. 20-25).

Internal structure. The internal structure is totally radiolucent, but occasionally it may appear multilocular, although the lesion does not contain true septa.

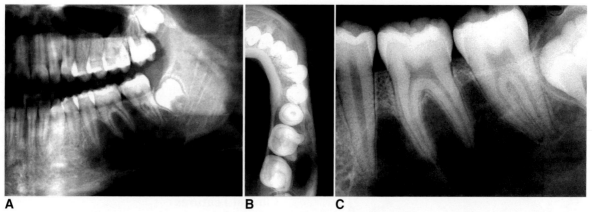

FIG. 20-25 Panoramic film demonstrating a simple bone cyst **(A)**, an occlusal film **(B)**, and a periapical film **(C)**. The occlusal film shows that no expansion has occurred in the buccal or lingual cortical plates. Note that, except for the superior border, the borders are ill-defined and that the lesion has scalloped around the teeth and thinned the inferior border of the mandible but the lamina dura is still present.

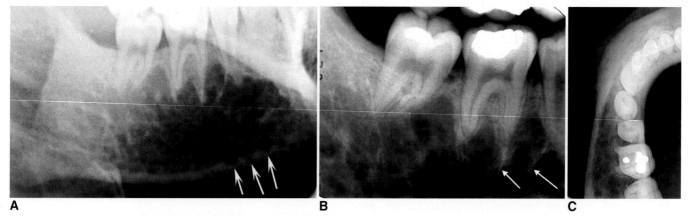

FIG. 20-26 An SBC has a multilocular appearance in this lateral oblique view of the mandible **(A)**. The periapical view **(B)** appears to show internal septa *(arrows)* because of the scalloping of the endosteal surface of the cortical plates, as is seen in the inferior cortex *(arrows)* in **A** and of the endosteal surface of the buccal cortex in the occlusal view **(C)**.

This appearance is the result of pronounced scalloping of the endosteal surface of either the buccal or lingual plates (Fig. 20-26). The ridges of bone produced by the scalloping give the appearance of septa on a lateral view of the mandible.

Effects on surrounding structures. In most cases these lesions have no effect on the surrounding teeth, although rare cases of tooth displacement and resorption have been documented. Often the lesion involves all the bone around the roots of the teeth but leaves the lamina dura intact or only partly disrupted (Fig. 20-27). Similarly, the sparing of the cortical boundary of the crypt around a developing tooth is characteristic. As previously mentioned, these lesions have a propensity to scallop the endosteal surface of the outer cortex of

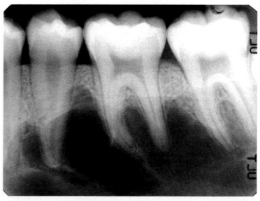

FIG. 20-27 An SBC in which the lamina dura is maintained on most root surfaces involved with the lesion, except for the mesial surface of the distal root tip of the first molar.

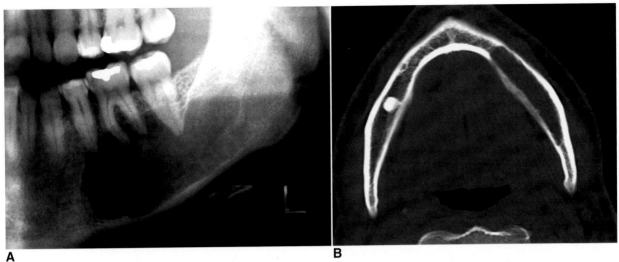

A **B**

FIG. **20-28** A and B, An SBC extending from the first bicuspid posteriorly to the base of the ramus and occupying most of the mandible. Considering the extent of the lesion, very little expansion of the buccal or lingual cortical plates has occurred, as can be seen in the axial CT image **(B)** using bone algorithm.

the mandible. SBCs also have a tendency to grow along the long axis of the bone, causing minimal expansion (Fig. 20-28). However, expansion of the involved bone can occur and is more common with larger lesions (Fig. 20-29).

Differential Diagnosis

An SBC may have an appearance similar to that of a true cyst, especially an odontogenic keratocyst (OKC). This is because OKCs tend to grow along bone with very little expansion and often have scalloped borders similar to those of an SBC. However, OKCs usually have a more definite cortical boundary, resorb and displace teeth, and occur in an older age group. Because the SBC may remove bone around teeth without affecting the teeth, there may be a tendency to include a malignant lesion in the differential. However, maintenance of some lamina dura and the lack of an invasive periphery and bone destruction should be enough to remove this category of diseases from consideration.

The diagnosis relies primarily on radiographic and surgical observations because the histopathologic aspects are not characteristic. These lesions occasionally heal spontaneously. A biopsy and analysis of a healing cyst may falsely indicate the presence of an ossifying fibroma or fibrous dysplasia because of the formation of new immature bone (Fig. 20-30).

Management

The customary treatment is a conservative opening into the lesion and careful curettage of the lining; this usually initiates bleeding and subsequent healing.

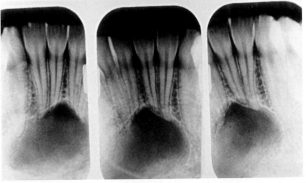

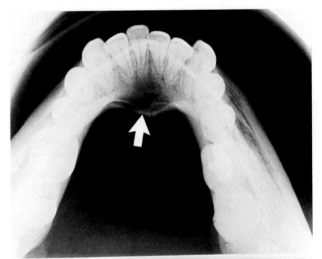

FIG. **20-29** An SBC (arrow) positioned in the anterior of the mandible. Note that the superior aspect of the peripheral cortex is better defined than the inferior border and that evidence exists of some expansion of the mandible's lingual cortex, which in part may due to muscle attachment at the genial tubercles.

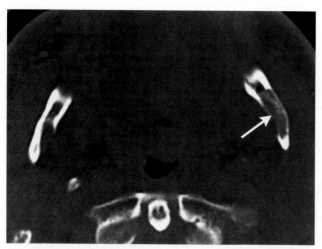

FIG. 20-30 An axial CT image using a bone algorithm displaying a small SBC in the process of healing *(arrow)*. Note the fine internal granular bone and very slight expansion of the ramus.

Spontaneous healing has been reported. Periodic follow-up radiographic examinations are advisable, especially if the patient declines treatment. These lesions can recur, but it is rare.

BIBLIOGRAPHY

Shear M: Cysts of the jaws: recent advances, J Oral Pathol 14:43, 1985.

Shear M: Developmental odontogenic cysts: an update, J Oral Pathol Med 23:1, 1994.

ODONTOGENIC CYSTS

Radicular cyst

Stockdale CR, Chandler NP: The nature of the periapical lesion: a review of 1108 cases, J Dent 16(3):123, 1988.

Syrjauanen S et al: Radiological interpretation of the periapical cysts and granulomas, Dentomaxillofac Radiol 11:89, 1982.

Toller PA: Origin and growth of cysts of the jaws, Ann R Coll Surg Engl 40:306, 1967.

Wood RE et al: Radicular cysts of primary teeth mimicking premolar dentigerous cysts: report of three cases, ASDC J Dent Child 55(4):288, 1988.

Residual cyst

High AS, Hirschmann PN: Age changes in residual cysts, J Oral Pathol 15:524, 1986.

Schwimmer AM et al: Squamous cell carcinoma arising in residual odontogenic cyst: report of a case and review of literature, Oral Surg 72(2):218, 1991.

Dentigerous cyst

Daley TD, Wysocki GP: The small dentigerous cyst, Oral Surg Oral Med Oral Pathol Oral Radiol Endod 79:77, 1995.

Lustmann J, Bodner L: Dentigerous cysts associated with supernumerary teeth, Int J Oral Maxillofac Surg 17(2):100, 1988.

Main DMG: Follicular cysts of mandibular third molar teeth: radiological evaluation of enlargement, Dentomaxillofac Radiol 18:156, 1989.

Maxymiw WG, Wood RE: Carcinoma arising in a dentigerous cyst: a case report and review of the literature, J Oral Maxillofac Surg 49(6):639, 1991.

Buccal bifurcation cyst

Bohay RN, Weinberg S: The paradental cyst of the mandibular permanent first molar: report of a bilateral case, J Dent Child Sept-Oct:361, 1992.

Fowler CB, Brannon RB: The paradental cyst: a clinicopathologic study of six new cases and review of the literature, J Oral Maxillofac Surg 47:243, 1989.

Packota GV et al: Paradental cysts on mandibular first molars in children: report of five cases, Dentomaxillofac Radiol 19:126, 1990.

Shear M: Cysts of the oral regions, Bristol, UK, 1976, John Wright & Sons.

Stoneman DW, Worth HM: The mandibular infected buccal cyst—molar area, Dent Radiogr Photogr 56:1, 1983.

Odontogenic keratocyst

Brannon RB: The odontogenic keratocyst: a clinicopathological study of 312 cases. I. Clinical features, Oral Surg 42:54, 1976.

Browne RM: The odontokeratocyst: clinical aspects, Br Dent J 128:225, 1970.

Frame JW, Wake MJC: Computerized axial tomography in the assessment of mandibular keratocysts, Br Dent J 153:93, 1982.

Kakarantza-Angelopoulou E, Nicolatou O: Odontogenic keratocysts: clinicopathologic study of 87 cases, J Oral Maxillofac Surg 48(6):593, 1990.

Kondell PA, Wiberg J: Odontogenic keratocysts: a follow-up study of 29 cases, Swed Dent J 12(1-2):57, 1988.

Partridge M, Towers JF: The primordial cyst (odontogenic keratocyst): its tumor-like characteristics and behavior, Br J Oral Maxillofac Surg 25:271, 1987.

Shear M: The aggressive nature of the odontogenic keratocyst: is it a benign cystic neoplasm?: Part 1, Oral Oncol 38:219, 2002.

Basal cell nevus syndrome

Angelopoulou E, Angelopoulos AP: Lateral periodontal cyst: review of the literature and report of a case, J Periodontol 61(2):126, 1990.

Donatsky O et al: Clinical, radiographic, and histologic features of the basal cell nevus syndrome, Int J Oral Surg 5:19, 1976.

Evans DC et al: The incidence of Gorlin syndrome in 173 consecutive cases of medulloblastoma, Br J Cancer 64(5):959, 1991.

Gorlin RJ: Nevoid basal cell carcinoma syndrome, Medicine 66(2):98, 1987.

Lateral periodontal cyst

Regezi JA et al: The pathology of head and neck tumors: cysts of the jaw. XII, Head Neck Surg 4:48, 1981.

Shear M, Pindborg JJ: Microscopic features of the lateral periodontal cyst, Scand J Dent Res 83:103, 1975.

Weathers DR, Waldron CA: Unusual multilocular cysts of the jaws (botryoid odontogenic cysts), J Periodontol 41:249, 1970.

Wysocki GP et al: Histogenesis of the lateral periodontal cyst and the gingival cyst of the adult, Oral Surg 50:327, 1980.

Calcifying odontogenic cyst

Altini M, Farman AG: The calcifying odontogenic cyst: eight new cases and a review of the literature, Oral Surg 20:751, 1975.

Fejerskov O, Krough J: The calcifying ghost cell odontogenic tumor or the calcifying odontogenic cyst, J Oral Pathol 1:272, 1972.

Freedman PD et al: Calcifying odontogenic cyst, Oral Surg 40:93, 1975.

Hirshberg A et al: Calcifying odontogenic cyst associated with odontoma, J Oral Maxillofac Surg 52:555, 1994.

Saito I et al: Calcifying odontogenic cyst: case reports, variations, and tumorous potential, J Nihon Univ Sch Dent 24:69, 1982.

NONODONTOGENIC CYSTS

Nasopalatine duct cyst

Abrams AM et al: Nasopalatine cysts, Oral Surg 16:306, 1963.

Allard RHB et al: Nasopalatine duct cyst, Int J Oral Surg 10:447, 1981.

Hartziotis J: Median palatine cyst: report of a case, J Oral Surg 24:343, 1966.

Nortjé CJ, Farman AG: Nasopalatine duct cyst: an aggressive condition in adolescent Negroes from South Africa? Int J Oral Surg 7:65, 1978.

Nasolabial cyst

Roed-Petersen B: Nasolabial cysts, Br J Oral Surg 7:85, 1970.

Seward GR: Nasolabial cysts and their radiology, Dent Pract 12:154, 1962.

Walsh-Waring GP: Nasoalveolar cysts: aetiology, presentation, and treatment, J Laryngol Otol 81:263, 1967.

Dermoid cyst

Seward GR: Dermoid cysts of the floor of the mouth, Br J Oral Surg 3:36, 1965.

CYSTLIKE LESIONS

Simple bone cyst

Feinberg S et al: Recurrent "traumatic" bone cysts of the mandible, Oral Surg 57:418, 1984.

Kaugars GE, Cale AE: Traumatic bone cyst, Oral Surg Oral Med Oral Pathol 63:318, 1987.

Saito Y et al: Simple bone cyst: a clinical and histopathologic study of fifteen cases, Oral Surg Oral Med Oral Pathol 74:487, 1992.

Sapp PJ, Stark ML: Self-healing traumatic bone cysts, Oral Surg Oral Med Oral Pathol 69:597, 1990.

JH Damante JH et al: Spontaneous resolution of simple bone cysts, Dentomaxillofac Radiol 31:182, 2002.

CHAPTER 21

Benign Tumors of the Jaws

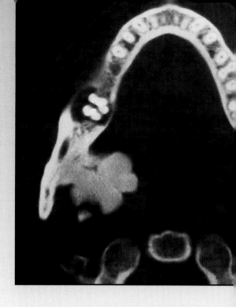

Benign tumors represent a new uncoordinated growth that generally has the following characteristics. Benign tumors are slow-growing and spread by direct extension and not by metastases. They tend to resemble the tissue of origin histologically. For example, an ameloblastoma, a tumor thought to be derived from odontogenic epithelium is often is composed of cells that resemble ameloblasts. It is thought that benign tumors have unlimited growth potential. Often hamartomas are included in the category of benign tumors. However, hamartomas are overgrowths of disorganized normal tissue that have a limited growth potential. For example, an odontoma is a hamartoma of dental tissue (disorganized enamel, dentin, and pulp tissues) derived from the dental follicle that stops growing at approximately the same time as other normal dental tissues. Included in this chapter are hyperplasias. *Hyperplasia* refers to a growth formed by an increase in the number of cells of a tissue; hyperplasias differ from hamartomas in that the tissue is in a normal arrangement. Hyperplasia is generally thought to be a reaction to a stimulus such as inflammation. Therefore, both of these entities have limited growth potential and tend to regress when the stimulus is removed.

Clinical Features

Benign tumors typically have an insidious onset and grow slowly. These tumors usually are painless, do not metastasize, and are not life threatening unless they interfere with a vital organ by direct extension.

Benign tumors are usually detected clinically by enlargement of the jaws or are found during a radi-ographic examination. Sometimes the radiologic examination is performed to try to discover the reason for the lack of development of a tooth.

Radiographic Examination

Once the clinician has made a preliminary diagnosis of the presence of a tumor, a full radiologic examination should be made to fully document the extent and characteristics of the lesion. This may entail further films, such as intraoral and occlusal radiographs or a panoramic film. For central bone lesions the addition of computed tomography is essential for assessing the effects on the surrounding osseous structures. If the lesion originates in soft tissue or has extended from bone into the surrounding soft tissue, the magnetic resonance imaging may be required.

A thorough radiologic examination will provide information regarding the extent of the lesion and sometimes the characteristics are so specific that a preliminary diagnosis of the type of benign tumor can be made. On the other hand, the imaging characteristics of the lesion may fail to indicate the type of tumor. A thorough workup will also indicate the most favorable biopsy site. The radiological examination should always be completed before the biopsy procedure.

Radiographic Features

The following general features suggest the presence of a benign neoplasm.

LOCATION

Because many tumors have a specific anatomic predilection, the location of a particular neoplasm is important in establishing the differential diagnosis. For example, odontogenic lesions occur in the alveolar processes above the inferior alveolar nerve canal, where tooth formation occurs. Vascular and neural lesions may originate inside the mandibular canal, arising from the neurovascular tissues. Cartilaginous tumors occur in jaw locations where residual cartilaginous cells lie, such as around the mandibular condyle.

PERIPHERY AND SHAPE

Benign tumors enlarge slowly by formation of additional internal tissue. Because of this, the radiographic borders of benign tumors appear relatively smooth, well defined, and sometimes corticated. If the tumor produces a calcified product—for example, abnormal tooth material or abnormal bone—the most mature part of the tumor will be in the central region with the most immature aspect at the periphery. This sometimes results in a radiolucent band of soft tissue or capsule at the periphery where the calcified product has not yet formed; this band separates the more mature internal radiopaque portion from the surrounding normal bone.

INTERNAL STRUCTURE

The internal structure may be completely radiolucent or radiopaque or may be a mixture of radiolucent and radiopaque tissues. If the lesion contains radiopaque elements, these structures usually represent either residual bone or a calcified material that is being produced by the tumor. For instance curved septa that are characteristic in ameloblastoma represent residual bone trapped inside the tumor that has remodeled into curved septa. The ameloblastoma does not produce bone. On the other hand the osteoblastoma often has an internal granular radiopaque pattern produced by the abnormal bone that is actually being manufactured by the tumor. Often the internal pattern is characteristic for specific types of tumors and may help with the diagnosis. A totally radiolucent internal structure is not as useful as an aid to the diagnosis.

EFFECTS ON SURROUNDING STRUCTURES

The manner in which a tumor affects adjacent tissues may suggest a benign behavior. For example, a benign tumor exerts pressure on neighboring structures, resulting in the displacement of teeth or bony cortices. If the growth is slow enough, there will be adequate time for the outer cortex to remodel in response to the pressure, resulting in an appearance that the cortex has been displaced by the tumor (Fig. 21-1). This is caused by simultaneous resorption of bone along the inner surface (endosteal) of the cortex and deposition of bone along the outer cortical surface by the periosteum (Fig. 21-2). Through this remodeling process, the cortex maintains its integrity and resists perforation. Benign tumors may also cause bodily displacement of nearby teeth (Fig. 21-3). The movement of teeth adjacent to benign tumors is slow because these lesions grow slowly.

The roots of teeth may be resorbed by either benign or malignant tumors, but root resorption more commonly is associated with benign processes. The benign tumors especially likely to resorb roots are ameloblas-

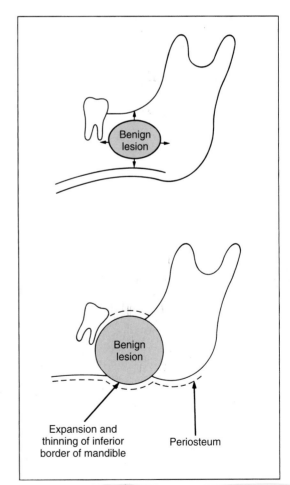

FIG. **21-1** Benign lesions growing in bone tend to be round or oval. They grow by displacing adjacent tissues. (From Matteson SR et al: Dent Radiogr Photogr 57:35, 1985.)

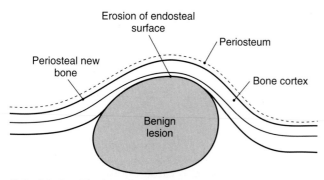

FIG. **21-2**   The host bone of a benign tumor may expand as a result of outward remodeling of its cortical borders. As the benign tumor extends toward the periphery of the bone, the periosteum lays down new bone along the outer cortex, thereby maintaining the integrity of the cortex.

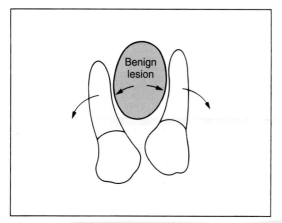

FIG. **21-3**   A benign lesion usually grows slowly, causing displacement of adjacent teeth. (From Matteson SR et al: Dent Radiogr Photogr 57:35, 1985.)

tomas, ossifying fibromas, and central giant cell granulomas. Benign tumors tend to resorb the adjacent root surfaces in a smooth fashion. Bone dysplasias such as fibrous dysplasia do not usually resorb teeth. When root resorption is associated with malignant tumors, the resorption is usually in smaller quantities causing thinning of the root into a "spiked" shape.

Hyperplasias

Bony hyperplasias are included in this chapter but are not considered tumors because of the normal arrangement of the tissue, limited growth potential, and in some cases, the fact that this growth is in response to a stimulus. Bony hyperplasias are growths of normal new bone that sometimes occur in characteristic locations. In dentistry the terms *exostosis* and *hyperostosis*

are both used to describe a bony growth that occurs on the surface of normal bone. It should be noted that in medicine the term *exostosis* often is used for a surface bony growth with a cartilage cap (osteochondroma). Therefore the term *hyperostosis* may be preferred to avoid confusion.

TORUS PALATINUS

Synonym
Palatine torus

Definition
Torus palatinus is a bony protuberance (hyperostosis) that occurs in the middle third of the midline of the hard palate.

Clinical Features
Torus palatinus, the most common of the exostoses, occurs in about 20% of the population, although various studies have shown marked differences in racial groups. It develops about twice as often in women as in men and more often in Native Americans, Eskimos, and Norwegians. Although it may be discovered at any age, it is rare in children. Torus palatinus usually begins developing in young adults before 30 years of age and is thought to arise through an interplay of genetic and environmental factors. The base of the bony nodule extends along the central portion of the hard palate, and the bulk reaches downward into the oral cavity. The size and shape of a torus palatinus can vary, and these lesions have been described as flat, lobulated, nodular, or mushroom-like (Fig. 21-4, *A*). Normal mucosa covers the bony mass and may appear pale and sometimes ulcerated when traumatized. Patients often are unaware of this hyperplasia, and those who do discover it may insist that it occurred suddenly and has been growing rapidly.

Radiographic Features
Location.   On maxillary periapical or panoramic radiographs, a torus palatinus appears as a dense radiopaque shadow below and attached to the hard palate. It may be superimposed over the apical areas of the maxillary teeth, especially if the torus has developed in the middle or anterior regions of the palate. The image of a palatal torus may project over the roots of the maxillary molars (Fig. 21-4, *B*) but the shadow will usually move in its position relative to the roots of the teeth if another film is taken with a different horizontal or vertical angulation of the central ray (Fig. 21-5).

Periphery and shape.   The border of the radiopaque shadow usually is well defined and may have a convex or a lobulated outline (Fig. 21-6).

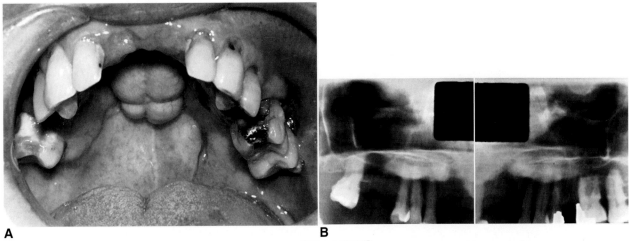

FIG. **21-4**   **A,** A clinical photograph of torus palatinus. **B,** A panoramic radiograph shows the radiopaque shadow of torus palatinus above the maxillary premolars and canine. (Courtesy Ronald Baker, DDS, Chapel Hill, N.C.)

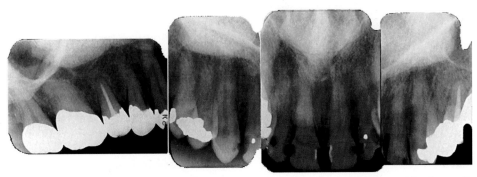

FIG. **21-5**   Maxillary periapical radiographs show a radiopaque area with the well-defined borders of torus palatinus.

Internal structure. The internal aspect is homogeneously radiopaque.

Treatment

A torus palatinus usually does not require treatment, although removal may be necessary if a maxillary denture is to be made.

TORUS MANDIBULARIS

Synonym
Mandibular torus

Definition
Torus mandibularis is a hyperostosis that protrudes from the lingual aspect of the mandibular alveolar process, usually near the premolar teeth.

Clinical Features
Tori occur less often on the lingual surface of the mandible than on the palate, with the former

occurring in about 8% of the population. These tori develop singly or multiply, unilaterally, or bilaterally (usually bilaterally), and most often in the premolar region. The size also varies, ranging from an outgrowth that is just palpable to one that contacts a torus on the opposite side. In contrast to torus palatinus, torus mandibularis develops later, being first discovered in middle-aged adults. However, it has the same gender predilection as torus palatinus. In women the occurrence of torus mandibularis correlates with that of torus palatinus, but this apparently is not the case in men. As with torus palatinus, torus mandibularis may occur more often in those of Mongoloid ancestry.

Genetic and environmental factors seem to be involved in the development of torus mandibularis, but masticatory stress is reported as an essential factor underlying its formation. The high prevalence among Eskimos and other subarctic peoples who make extraordinary chewing demands on their teeth seems to support this suggestion. Also, a patient with a torus

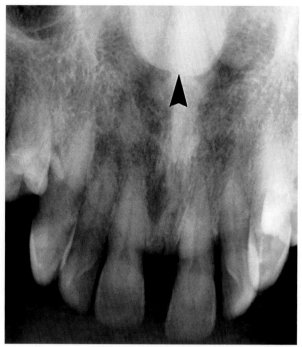

FIG. 21-6 An occlusal radiograph of torus palatinus (*arrowhead*).

mandibularis has, on average, more teeth present than a patient without a torus.

Radiographic Features

Location. Recognition of mandibular tori relies on their appearance and location. Their presence bilaterally reinforces this impression although they can occur unilaterally. On mandibular periapical radiographs, a torus mandibularis appears as a radiopaque shadow, usually superimposed on the roots of premolars and molars and occasionally over a canine or incisor. It usually is superimposed over about three teeth.

Periphery. Mandibular tori are sharply demarcated anteriorly on periapical films and are less dense and less well defined as they extend posteriorly (Fig. 21-7). There is no margin between the periphery of the torus and the surface of the mandible as the torus is continuous with the mandibular cortex.

Internal structure. On occlusal radiographs a mandibular torus appears as radiopaque and homogeneous (Fig. 21-8).

Treatment

A torus mandibularis usually does not require treatment, although removal may be necessary if a mandibular denture is planned.

OTHER EXOSTOSES

Synonym
Hyperostoses

Definition
In addition to the torus other exostoses may occur at other sites in the jaws. These are usually small regions of osseous hyperplasia of cortical bone and occasionally internal cancellous bone and usually occur on the surface of the alveolar process.

Clinical Features
Exostoses may develop most commonly on the buccal surface of the maxillary alveolar process, usually in the canine or molar area. They may also occur on the palatal surface or crest and less commonly on the mandibular alveolar process. Occasionally they will grow on the crest under a pontic of a fixed bridge. Exostoses are less common than mandibular or palatine tori, may attain a large size, and may be solitary or multiple. They are nodular, pedunculated, or flat prominences on the surface of the bone. They are covered with a normal mucosa and are bony hard on palpation. No published data indicate their actual incidence or whether they occur more often in one gender. As with the exostoses described previously, they appear to be more prevalent in Native Americans.

Radiographic Features
Location. The maxillary alveolar process is the most common location and usually the image overlaps the roots of the adjacent teeth.

Periphery. The periphery of an exostosis is usually well defined, smoothly contoured, with a curved border (Fig. 21-9). However, some may have poorly defined borders that blend radiographically into the surrounding normal bone.

Internal structure. The internal aspect of an exostosis usually is homogeneous and radiopaque. Although large exostoses can have an internal cancellous bone pattern, they most often consist only of cortical bone.

Treatment
Exostoses usually do not require treatment.

ENOSTOSES

Synonyms
Dense bone island and periapical idiopathic osteosclerosis

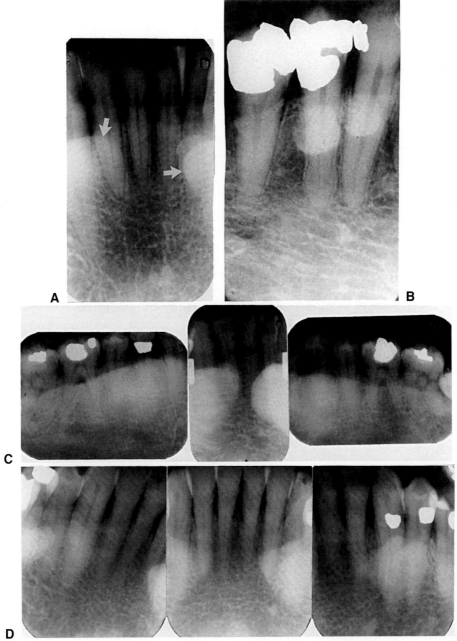

FIG. **21-7** Mandibular tori usually are seen as dense radiopacities *(arrows)* in the canine region (**A**) and the premolar region (**B**). **C**, Large mandibular tori are seen from the molar region to the midline. **D**, Note the common appearance of mandibular tori on these anterior periapical radiographs.

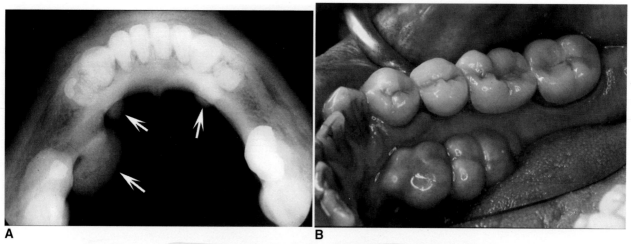

FIG. 21-8   **A,** An occlusal radiograph shows an unusual case of mandibular tori *(arrows)* in which the number and size are not symmetrical between the sides. **B,** A clinical picture of a different case. Note that the tori extend from the region of the cuspid to the first molar. **(B,** Courtesy of Dr. Bernard Friedland, Harvard University.)

Definition

Enostoses are the internal counterparts of exostoses. They are localized growths of compact bone that extend from the endosteal (inner) surface of cortical bone into the cancellous bone.

Clinical Features

Enostoses are asymptomatic.

Radiographic Features

Location. Enostoses are more common in the mandible than in the maxilla. They occur most often in the premolar-molar area (Fig. 21-10), although their existence does not correlate with the presence or absence of teeth.

Periphery. The periphery is usually well defined but occasionally blends with the trabeculae of the surrounding bone. There is no trace of a radiolucent margin or capsule as the radiopaque dense bone island abuts directly against normal bone.

Internal structure. The internal aspect of an enostosis usually is uniformly radiopaque without any characteristic pattern but sometimes, depending on its form and thickness, there may be patches of more radiolucent areas.

Effects on surrounding structures. In rare instances an area of enostosis is located periapical to a tooth root and is associated with external root resorption (see Fig. 21-10, *C*). The tooth most often involved

is the mandibular first molar. In all circumstances the tooth is vital and the root resorption appears to be self-limiting. In very rare cases enostosis can inhibit the eruption of a tooth and even displace a tooth.

Differential Diagnosis

Several radiopaque lesions must be considered in forming a differential diagnosis. Periapical cemental dysplasia can be differentiated by the presence of its radiolucent periphery. When an area of enostosis is located at the root apex, it may resemble periapical sclerosing osteitis. However, in periapical osteitis there is an associated widening of the periapical portion of the periodontal membrane space. Also, periapical osteitis should be centered on the root apex of the tooth and extend in a more symmetrical form in every direction. Finally, an inflammatory lesion may have an apparent etiology such as a large restoration or carious lesion. There may be some similarity to hypercementosis or a benign cementoblastoma, but in both cases there should be a soft tissue (radiolucent) capsule at the periphery. Enostosis are often static but may increase in size, especially when there is active growth of the jaws. If several areas of enostosis (five or more) are present, multiple polyposis syndromes (e.g., Gardner's syndrome) should be considered.

Treatment

Enostosis does not require treatment. If multiple, the patient's family history should be reviewed for incidences of cancer of the intestine.

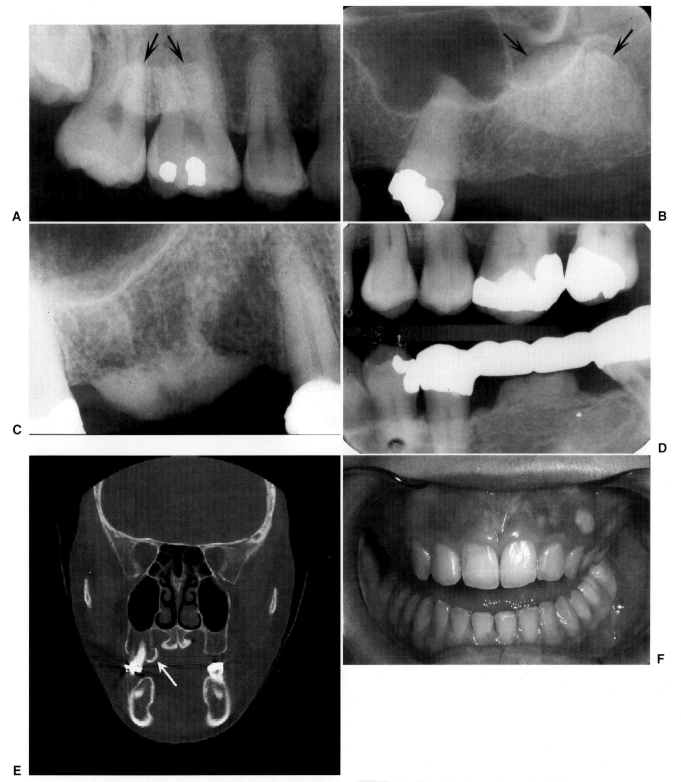

FIG. **21-9**   **A,** A periapical film of a region of hyperostosis on the buccal aspect of the maxillary alveolar process, seen as a region of slight increase in radiopacity overlapping the roots of the molars *(arrows).* **B,** Another example overlapping an edentulous ridge. **C,** An example occurring on the crest of the alveolar ridge. **D,** Example occurring under a bridge pontic. **E,** A coronal CT image of hyperostosis located on the palatal aspect of the right maxillary alveolar process. Note the presence of a maxillary torus. **F,** A clinical photograph of a small hyperostosis occurring on the labial surface of the maxillary alveolar ridge.

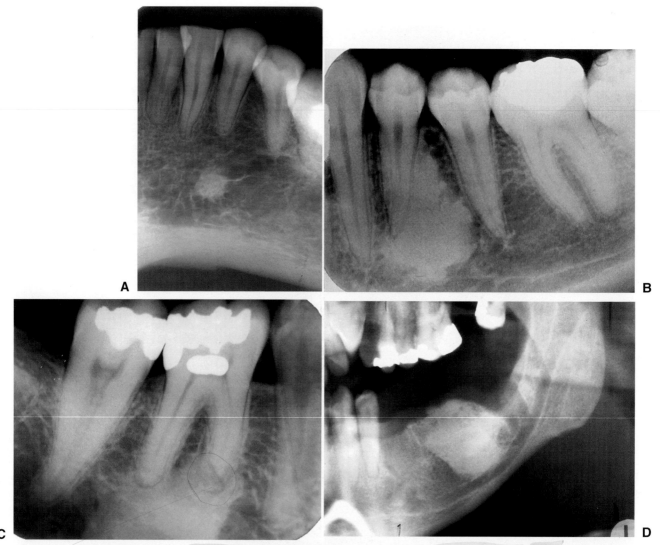

FIG. **21-10**   **A,** A small enostosis (dense bone island) apical to the first bicuspid. Note the lack of a soft tissue capsule and that some of the surrounding trabeculae appear to merge into the radiopaque mass. **B,** A larger dense bone island between the bicuspids. Note the normal appearing periodontal membrane space. **C,** Example apical to the first molar, causing external root resorption of the mesial root. **D,** A large dense bone island occupying the body of the left mandible.

Mesial Root resorption

Benign Tumors

The benign neoplasias are separated into two major groups: odontogenic tumors and nonodontogenic tumors.

ODONTOGENIC TUMORS

Odontogenic tumors arise from the tissues of the odontogenic apparatus. According to the World Health Organization (WHO), these tumors can be classified into three categories depending on the type of tissue that comprises each tumor: (1) tumors of odontogenic epithelium, (2) mixed tumors of both odontogenic epithelium and odontogenic ectomesenchyme (connective tissue), and (3) tumors composed of primarily ectomesenchyme. Odontogenic tumors comprise 1.3% to 15% of all oral tumors. The following text presents benign jaw tumors according to their tissues of origin. This format should assist the reader in learning to correlate the radiographic appearance of tumors with the underlying pathologic basis of the disease process.

ODONTOGENIC EPITHELIAL TUMORS

AMELOBLASTOMA

Synonyms

Adamantinoma, adamantoblastoma, adontomes embryolastiques, and epithelial odontoma

Definition

The ameloblastoma, a true neoplasm of odontogenic epithelium, is a persistent and locally invasive tumor; it has an aggressive but benign growth characteristics. The ameloblastoma represents about 1% of all oral odontogenic epithelial tumors and 11% of all odontogenic tumors. It is an aggressive neoplasm that arises from remnants of the dental lamina and dental organ (odontogenic epithelium). Malignant forms of this neoplasm do exist and are discussed in Chapter 22. Ameloblastomas may be divided into solid or multicystic types or unicystic types. The unicystic variant may develop as a single entity or may form from the epithelial lining of a dentigerous cyst; this is called a *mural* ("within the wall") *ameloblastoma* (Fig. 21-11). The existence of peripheral (soft tissue location) forms of this neoplasm is well documented.

Clinical Features

There is a slight predilection for this lesion to occur in men, and it develops more often in blacks. Although it may be found in the young (3 years) and in individuals older than 80 years, most patients are between 20 and 50 years, with the average age at discovery about 40 years.

Ameloblastomas grow slowly, and few, if any, symptoms occur in the early stages. The tumor is frequently discovered during a routine dental examination. Usually the patient eventually notices gradually increasing facial asymmetry. Swelling of the cheek, gingiva, or hard palate has been reported as the chief complaint in 95% of untreated maxillary ameloblastomas. The mucosa over the mass is normal, but teeth in the involved region may be displaced and become mobile. Generally patients with ameloblastomas do not have pain, paresthesia, fistula, ulcer formation, or tooth mobility, but these features have been described. As the tumor enlarges, palpation may elicit a bony hard sensation or crepitus as the bone thins. If the lesion destroys overlying bone, the swelling may feel firm or fluctuant. As it grows, this tumor can cause bony expansion and sometimes erosion through the adjacent cortical plate with subsequent invasion of the adjacent soft tissues.

An untreated tumor may grow to great size and is more of a concern in the maxilla, where it can extend into vital structures and reach into the cranial base. Tumors that develop in the maxilla may extend into the paranasal sinuses, orbit, nasopharynx, or vital structures at the base of the skull. Recurrence rates are higher in older patients and in those with multilocular lesions. As seen with other jaw tumors, local recurrence, whether detected radiographically or histologically, may have a more aggressive character than the original tumor.

Radiographic Features

Location. Most ameloblastomas (80%) develop in the molar-ramus region of the mandible, but they may extend to the symphyseal area. Most lesions that occur

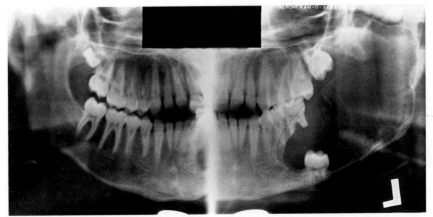

FIG. **21-11**   A unicystic ameloblastoma developing occlusal to the left second mandibular molar causing expansion of the mandibular body and ramus to the sigmoid notch and condylar neck, as well as inferior displacement of the mandibular second molar and root resorption of the alveolar left first molar. (Courtesy E.J. Burkes, DDS, Chapel Hill, N.C.)

in the maxilla are in the third molar area and extend into the maxillary sinus and nasal floor. In either jaw this tumor can originate in an occlusal position to a developing tooth (see Fig. 21-11).

Periphery. The ameloblastoma is usually well defined and frequently delineated by a cortical border. The border is often curved and in small lesions the border and shape may be indistinguishable from a cyst (Fig. 21-12). The periphery of lesions in the maxilla is usually more ill defined.

Internal structure. The internal structure varies from totally radiolucent (see Fig. 21-12) to mixed with the presence of bony septa creating internal compartments. These septa are usually coarse and curved and originate from normal bone that has been trapped within the tumor. Because this tumor frequently has internal cystic components, these septa are often remodeled into curved shapes providing a honeycomb (numerous small compartments or loculations) or soap bubble (larger compartments of variable size) patterns (Fig. 21-13). Generally the loculations are larger in the posterior mandible and smaller in the anterior mandible.

Effects on surrounding structures. There is pronounced tendency for ameloblastomas to cause exten-

sive root resorption (Fig. 21-14). Tooth displacement is common. Because a common point of origin is occlusal to a tooth, some teeth may be displaced apically. An occlusal radiograph may demonstrate cystlike expansion and thinning of an adjacent cortical plate, leaving a thin "eggshell" of bone (Fig. 21-15). Actual perforation of bone into the surrounding soft tissues or anatomic spaces is a late feature of ameloblastoma (Fig. 21-16). Unicystic types of ameloblastoma may cause extreme expansion of the mandibular ramus and often the anterior border of the ramus is no longer visible in the panoramic image (Fig. 21-17).

Recurrent Ameloblastoma

Ameloblastomas may recur when the initial surgical procedure inadequately removes the entire tumor. Recurrent tumor has a characteristic appearance of multiple small cystlike structures with very course sclerotic cortical margins (Fig. 21-18) and sometimes separated by normal bone.

Additional Imaging

If a preliminary diagnosis of ameloblastoma is made, CT imaging is highly recommended. CT imaging can not only confirm the diagnosis but also accurately demonstrate the anatomic extent of the tumor (see Fig. 21-16). Of importance is the ability of CT imaging to detect perforation of the outer cortex and invasion into the surrounding soft tissues. If soft tissue invasion is extensive, MRI will provide superior images of the nature and extent of the invasion. CT examination is essential in the postsurgical follow-up assessment of ameloblastoma.

Differential Diagnosis

Small unilocular ameloblastomas that are located around the crown of an unerupted tooth often cannot be differentiated from a dentigerous cyst. Since the appearance of the internal bony septa is important for the identification of ameloblastoma, other types of lesions that also have internal septa (such as the odontogenic keratocyst, giant cell granuloma, odontogenic myxoma, and ossifying fibroma) may have a similar appearance. The odontogenic keratocyst may contain curved septa but usually the keratocyst tends to grow along the bone without marked expansion, which is characteristic of ameloblastomas. Giant cell granulomas generally occur anterior to the molars, occur in a younger age group, and have more granular and ill-defined septa. Odontogenic myxomas may have similar-appearing septa; however, there are usually one or two thin, sharp, straight septa, characteristic of the myxoma. Even the presence of one such septum may indicate a myxoma. Also myxomas are not as expansile

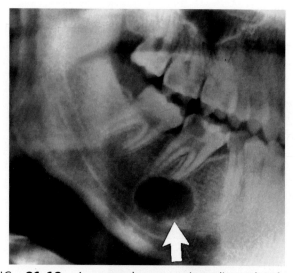

FIG. **21-12** A cropped panoramic radiograph of an ameloblastoma *(arrow)* that has a unicystic appearance in the body of the right mandible. The lesion, which has a well-defined, corticated border, has caused apical root resorption of the mesial root of tooth no. 31. This lesion easily could be misdiagnosed as a radicular cyst. (Courtesy E.J. Burkes, DDS, Chapel Hill, N.C.)

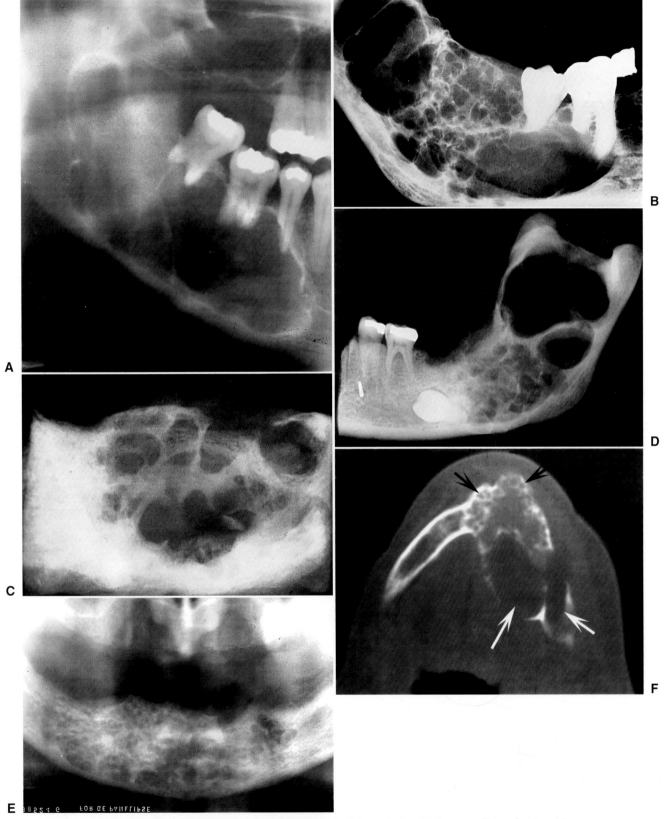

FIG. **21-13** Multilocular ameloblastoma. **A,** A large lesion in the mandibular body and ramus shows only a few rather straight septa. **B,** Lateral radiograph of a resected mandibular specimen containing a multilocular ameloblastoma. Note the course, curved septa. **C,** Another surgical specimen of an ameloblastoma. **D,** A large multilocular lesion in the right mandibular ramus. **E,** A cropped panoramic image showing small loculations that are more common in the anterior mandible. **F,** An axial CT image using bone algorithm showing a large ameloblastoma. Note the smaller loculations in the anterior mandible *(black arrows)* and the larger loculations in the posterior mandible *(white arrows)*.

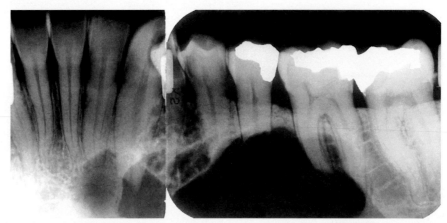

FIG. **21-14** Root resorption of the premolars and canine adjacent to a radiolucent ameloblastoma in the left mandible.

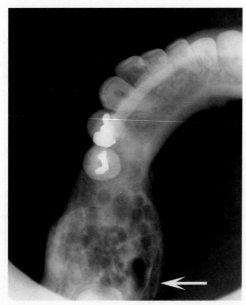

FIG. **21-15** An occlusal film demonstrating expansion of the lingual cortex with maintenance of a thin outer shell of bone *(arrow)*.

as ameloblastomas and tend to grow along the bone. The septa in ossifying fibroma are usually wide, granular, and ill defined. Also, look for the presence of small irregular trabeculae.

Treatment

The most common treatment is surgical resection. The surgical procedure should take into account the tendency of the neoplasm to invade adjacent bone beyond its apparent radiographic margins. CT and MRI are useful in determining the exact extent of the tumor. If the ameloblastoma is relatively small, it may be removed completely by an intraoral approach and larger lesions may require resection of the jaw. The maxilla is usually treated more aggressively because of the tendency of ameloblastoma to invade adjacent vital structures. Radiation therapy may be used for inoperable tumors, especially those in the posterior maxilla.

CALCIFYING EPITHELIAL ODONTOGENIC TUMOR

Synonyms

Pindborg tumor and ameloblastoma of unusual type with calcification

Definition. Calcifying epithelial odontogenic tumors are rare neoplasms. They account for about 1% of odontogenic tumors. These tumors usually are located within bone and produce a mineralized substance within amyloid-like material. Calcifying epithelial odontogenic tumors have a distinctive microscopic appearance with epithelium that resembles the stratum intermedium of the enamel organ.

Clinical Features

A calcifying epithelial odontogenic tumor (CEOT) is less aggressive than the ameloblastoma and is found in about the same age group. Rarely this tumor may have an extraosseous location. The neoplasm is somewhat more common in men, and patients range in age from 8 to 92 years, with an average age of about 42 years (considerably younger in men and somewhat older in women). Jaw expansion is a regular feature and usually only symptom. Palpation of the swelling reveals a hard tumor.

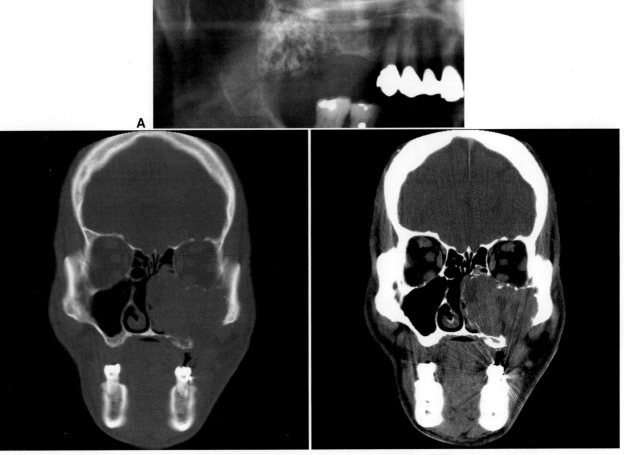

FIG. **21-16**   **A,** A cropped panoramic image of an ameloblastoma involving the left maxilla. Note the multilocular appearance in the tuberosity region. It is not possible to determine the extent of the lesion with the panoramic film. **B** and **C,** The same coronal CT image slices using both bone and soft tissue algorithms of the same case. Note the aggressive nature of the tumor as it has invaded the sinus and nasal fossa and destroyed the lateral aspect of the maxilla.

Radiographic Features

Location. As with ameloblastomas, calcifying epithelial odontogenic tumors have a definite predilection for the mandible, with a ratio of at least 2:1, and most develop in the premolar-molar area, with a 52% association with an unerupted or impacted tooth. In about half of cases, radiographs taken early in the development of these tumors reveal a radiolucent area around the crown of a mature, unerupted tooth.

Periphery. The border may have a well-defined cystlike cortex. In some tumors the boundary may be irregular and ill defined.

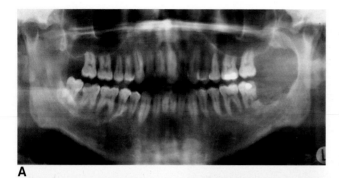

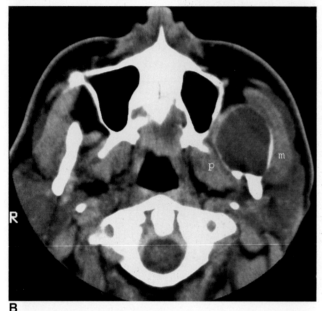

FIG. **21-17** **A,** A panoramic film of a unicystic ameloblastoma occupying the left mandibular ramus. Note the absence of the anterior border of the ramus. **B,** An axial CT image using soft tissue algorithm showing significant expansion towards the masseter *(m)* and lateral pterygoid *(p)* muscles.

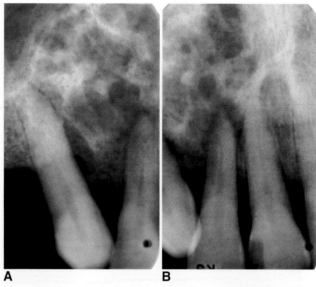

FIG. **21-18** Periapical films of a recurrent ameloblastoma of the right maxilla. Note the sclerotic margins of the small cystic lesions.

Differential Diagnosis

Lesions with completely radiolucent internal structure may mimic dentigerous cysts or even ameloblastomas. Other lesions with radiopaque foci, including adenomatoid odontogenic tumor, ameloblastic fibro-odontoma, and calcifying odontogenic cyst, may have similar appearances. However, the prominent location of the CEOT and the age of the patient will help in the differential diagnosis.

Treatment

The treatment of the CEOT is more conservative than the ameloblastoma, with local resection.

MIXED TUMORS (OF ODONTOGENIC EPITHELIUM AND ODONTOGENIC ECTOMESENCHYME)

ODONTOMA
Synonyms

Compound odontoma, compound composite odontoma, complex odontoma, complex composite odontoma, odontogenic hamartoma, calcified mixed odontoma, and cystic odontoma

Definition

The term *odontoma* is used to identify a tumor that is radiographically and histologically characterized by the production of mature enamel, dentin, cementum, and pulp tissue. These components are seen in various states

Internal structure. The internal aspect may appear unilocular or multilocular with numerous scattered, radiopaque foci of varying size and density. The most characteristic and diagnostic finding is the appearance of radiopacities close to the crown of the embedded tooth (Fig. 21-19). In addition, small, thin, opaque trabeculae may cross the radiolucency in many directions.

Effects on surrounding structures. Calcifying epithelial odontogenic tumors may displace a developing tooth or prevent its eruption. Associated expansion of the jaw with maintenance of a cortical boundary may also occur.

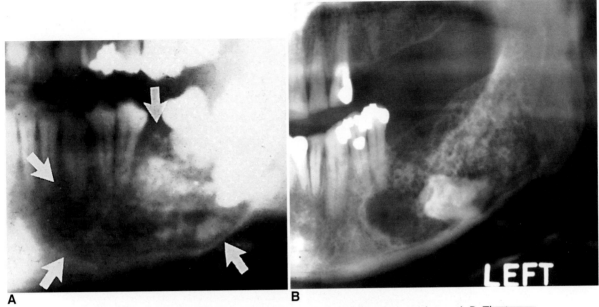

FIG. **21-19** **A,** Calcifying odontogenic tumor, or Pindborg tumor *(arrows).* **B,** The tumor appears as a mixed radiolucent-radiopaque lesion associated with an unerupted tooth. (**A,** Courtesy M. Gornitsky, DDS, Montreal, Canada; **B** courtesy Dr. D. Lanigan, University of Saskatchewan.)

of histodifferentiation and morphodifferentiation. Because of its limited and slow growth and well-differentiated tooth tissue, this lesion is considered to be a hamartoma and not a true tumor.

The structural relationship of the component tissues may vary from nondescript masses of dental tissue referred to as a complex odontoma to multiple well-formed teeth (denticles) of a compound odontoma. A dilated odontoma has been described as another type of odontoma; however, this is a single structure that actually may be the most severe expression of a dens in dente.

Clinical Features

Odontomas are the most common odontogenic tumor. They often interfere with the eruption of permanent teeth (Fig. 21-20). The lesion shows no gender predilection, and most begin forming while the normal dentition is developing. Odontomas develop and mature while the corresponding teeth are forming and cease development when the associated teeth complete development. Most odontomas occur in the second decade of life and many times are found during investigation of delayed eruption of adjacent teeth or retained primary teeth. In rare cases odontomas form with primary teeth. If left untreated, they persist although do not continue to increase in size and may be detected later in life. Compound odontomas are about twice as

common as the complex type. Although the compound variety forms equally between men and women, 60% of complex odontomas occur in women. In rare circumstances a compound odontoma may erupt into the oral cavity of a child.

Radiographic Features

Location. More of the compound variety of odontomas (62%) occur in the anterior maxilla in association with the crown of an unerupted canine. In contrast, 70% of complex odontomas are found in the mandibular first and second molar area.

Periphery. The borders of odontomas are well defined and may be smooth or irregular. These lesions have a cortical border and immediately inside and adjacent to the cortical border is a soft tissue capsule.

Internal structure. The contents of these lesions are largely radiopaque. Compound odontomas have a number of toothlike structures or denticles that look like deformed teeth (Fig. 21-21). Complex odontomas contain an irregular mass of calcified tissue (see Fig. 21-20). The degree of radiopacity is equivalent to or exceeds adjacent tooth structure and may vary in the degree of radiopacity from one region to another, reflecting variations in amount and type of hard tissue

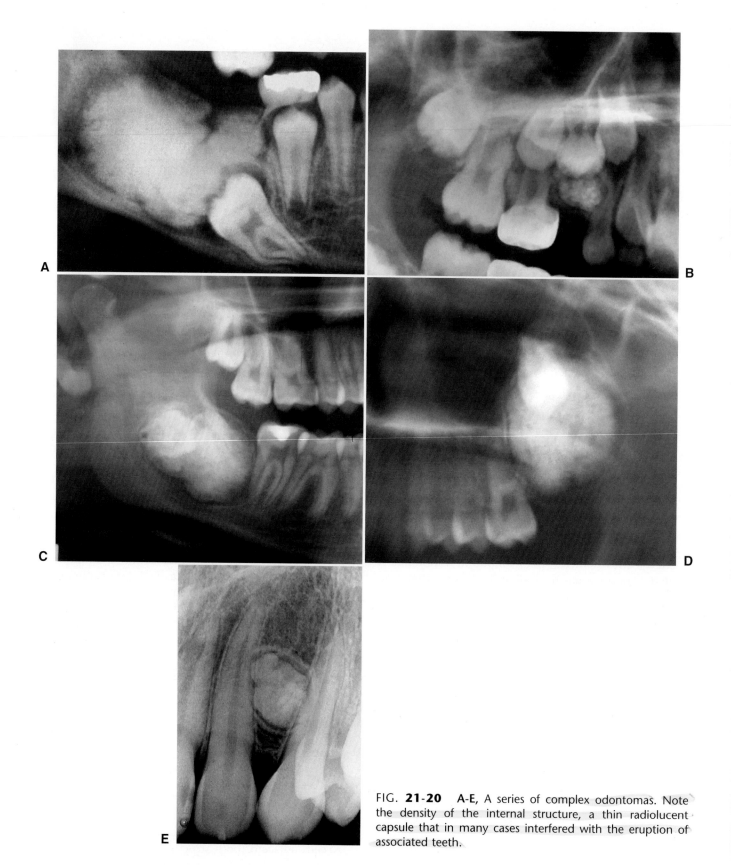

FIG. **21-20**   A-E, A series of complex odontomas. Note the density of the internal structure, a thin radiolucent capsule that in many cases interfered with the eruption of associated teeth.

that has been formed. A dilated odontoma has a single calcified structure with a more radiolucent central portion that has an overall form like a donut (Fig. 21-22).

Effects on surrounding structures. Odontomas can interfere with the normal eruption of teeth. Most odontomas (70%) are associated with abnormalities such as impaction, malpositioning, diastema, aplasia, malformation, and devitalization of adjacent teeth. Large complex odontomas may cause expansion of the jaw with maintenance of the cortical boundary.

Differential Diagnosis

A toothlike appearance of the radiopaque structures within a well-defined lesion leads to easy recognition of a compound odontoma. Complex odontomas differ from cemento-ossifying fibromas by their tendency to associate with unerupted molar teeth and because they usually are more radiopaque than cemento-ossifying fibromas. Odontomas may also develop in much younger patients than cemento-ossifying fibromas. Periapical cemental dysplasia may resemble complex odontomas but are usually multiple and centered on the periapical region of teeth. However, if the

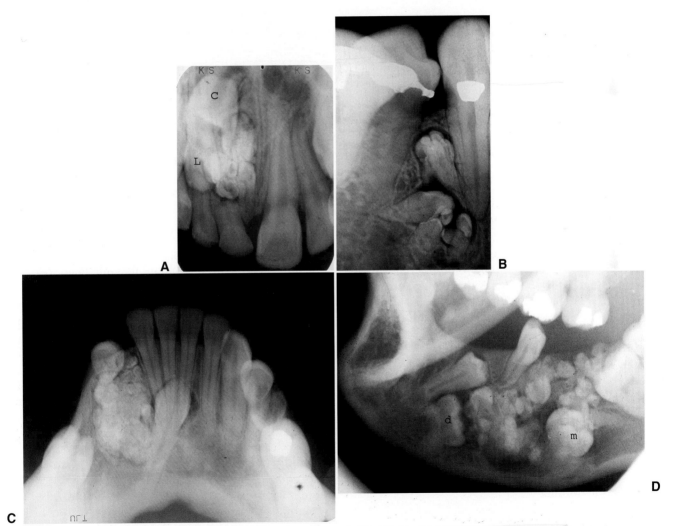

FIG. **21-21** Several examples of compound odontomas. Note the numerous internal components and the radiolucent capsule. **A,** An example in the anterior maxilla which has interfered with the eruption of the central incisor **(C)** and the lateral incisor *(L),* **B** within the mandible, **C** within the anterior mandible interfering with the eruption of the cuspid, and **D** within the mandible interfering with the eruption of the first premolar, deciduous molar *(d),* and the first molar *(m).*

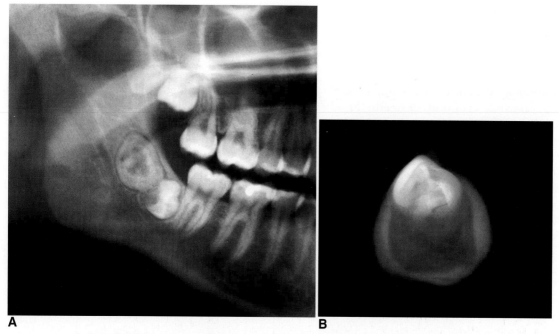

FIG. 21-22   **A,** A cropped panoramic image demonstrating a dilated odontoma positioned immediately distal to the unerupted third molar. **B,** A radiograph of a specimen. Note part of the odontoma resembles a tooth crown.

cemental dysplastic lesion is solitary and located in an edentulous region of the jaws, the differential diagnosis may be more difficult. The periphery of cemental dysplasia usually has a wider uneven sclerotic border, whereas odontomas have a well-defined cortical border and usually the soft tissue capsule is more uniform and better defined with odontomas than in cemental dysplasia. Areas of enostosis, although radiopaque, do not have a soft tissue capsule, as is seen with odontomes.

Treatment
Complex and compound odontomas are usually removed by simple excision. They do not recur and are not locally invasive.

AMELOBLASTIC FIBROMA
Synonyms
Soft odontoma, soft mixed odontoma, mixed odontogenic tumor, fibroadamantoblastoma, and granular cell ameloblastic fibroma

Definition
Ameloblastic fibromas are benign, mixed odontogenic tumors. They are characterized by neoplastic proliferation of maturing and early functional ameloblasts, as well as the primitive mesenchymal components of the dental papilla. Enamel, dentin, and cementum are not formed in this tumor.

Clinical Features
The behavior of ameloblastic fibromas is completely benign. Complete agreement has not been reached regarding sex predilection. Most of these tumors occur between 5 and 20 years of age, during the period of tooth formation, with an average age of about 15 years. They usually produce a painless, slow-growing expansion, and displacement of the involved teeth (Fig. 21-23).

Although the most common symptom is swelling or occlusal pain, the tumor may be discovered on a routine dental radiograph. It may be associated with a missing tooth.

Radiographic Features
Location. Ameloblastic fibromas usually develop in the premolar-molar area of the mandible. In some cases the tumor may involve the ramus and extend forward to the premolar-molar area. A common location is near the crest of the alveolar process (Fig. 21-24) or in a follicular relationship with an unerupted tooth (located occlusal to the tooth), or it may arise in an area where a tooth failed to develop.

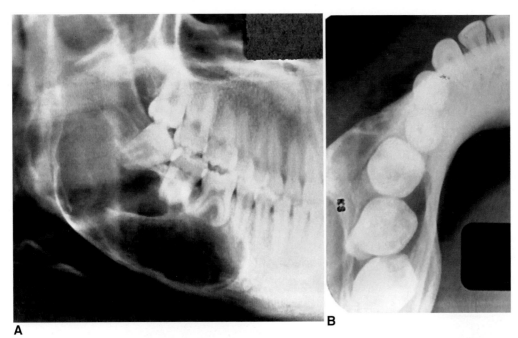

FIG. **21-23**   An ameloblastic fibroma in the body and ramus of the right mandible.
A, A panoramic radiograph. **B,** An occlusal radiograph showing mediolateral expansion of
the mandible adjacent to the lesion.

Periphery. The borders of an ameloblastic fibroma are well defined and often corticated in a manner similar to that of a cyst.

Internal structure. An ameloblastic fibroma is more commonly unilocular (totally radiolucent) (Fig. 21-25) but may be multilocular with indistinct curved septa (see Fig. 21-23).

Effects on surrounding structures. If the lesion is large, there may be expansion with an intact cortical plate. The associated tooth or teeth may be inhibited from normal eruption or may be displaced in an apical direction.

Differential Diagnosis

A common difficulty will occur in differentiating a small tumor with a follicular relationship to an unerupted tooth from a small dentigerous cyst or a hyperplastic follicle. In fact the radiological features may not allow the differentiation between these three entities. This tumor may have similar features to an ameloblastoma; however, the ameloblastic fibroma occurs at an earlier age and the septa in an ameloblastoma are more defined and coarse. In fact the septa in ameloblastic fibroma are infrequent and often very fine. Giant cell

granulomas may appear multilocular, but these tumors usually have an epicenter anterior to the first molar and the septa are characteristically granular and ill defined. Odontogenic myxomas can appear multilocular but usually a few sharp straight septa can be identified, which are not characteristic of ameloblastic fibromas and myxomas usually occur in an older age group.

Treatment. Ameloblastic fibromas are benign, and the rate of recurrence is low. A conservative surgical approach, including enucleation and mechanical curettage of the surrounding bone, is reported to be successful for these cases.

AMELOBLASTIC FIBRO-ODONTOMA

Definition

An ameloblastic fibro-odontoma is a mixed tumor with all the elements of an ameloblastic fibroma but with scattered collections of enamel and dentine. Some authorities consider the ameloblastic fibro-odontoma to be an early stage of a developing odontoma; however, there is compelling evidence that the ameloblastic fibro-odontoma is a separate entity and has a more neoplastic behavior than the odontoma. On the other hand, some lesions are probably incorrectly identified

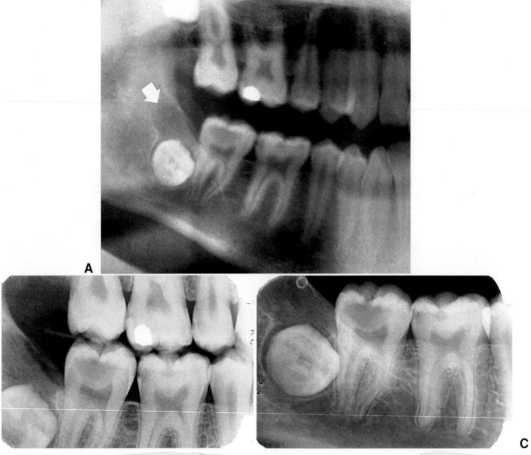

FIG. **21-24**   An ameloblastic fibroma. **A,** An ameloblastic fibroma seen as a radiolucency above the unerupted third molar *(arrow).* **B,** A bitewing radiograph of the same lesion. **C,** A periapical radiograph. (Courtesy G. Sanders, DDS, LaCrosse, Wisc.)

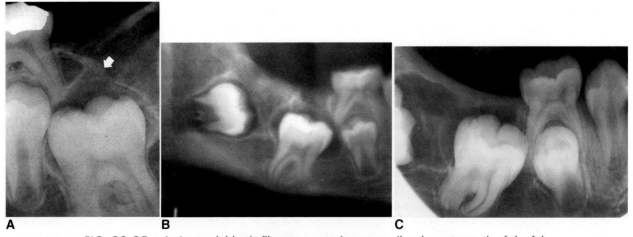

FIG. **21-25**   **A,** An ameloblastic fibroma appearing as a unilocular outgrowth of the follicle of the unerupted first permanent molar. A cropped panoramic image **(B)** and a periapical film **(C)** illustrating an ameloblastic fibroma associated with the crowns of the first and second molars.

as ameloblastic fibro-odontomas, when they are really developing odontomas.

Clinical Features. The clinical features are similar to odontomas, often associated with a missing tooth or tooth that has failed to erupt. Occasionally, this tumor takes the position of a missing tooth. This tumor appears during the same age as odontomas and ameloblastic fibromas with no particular sex predilection.

Radiographic Features
Location. Most cases occur in the posterior aspect of the mandible. The epicenter of the lesion is usually occlusal to a developing tooth or toward the alveolar crest.

Periphery. This tumor is usually well defined and sometimes corticated.

Internal structure. The internal structure is mixed, with the majority of the lesion being radiolucent. Small lesions may appear as enlarged follicles with only one or two small, discrete radiopacities. Larger lesions may have a more extensive calcified internal structure (Fig. 21-26). In some cases these small calcifications have a round shape with a radiopaque enamel-like margin, giving a shape similar to a small doughnut. Most often an associated impacted tooth is present.

Differential Diagnosis
If calcification is not detected, this tumor cannot be differentiated from an ameloblastic fibroma. Differentiation from a developing odontoma may be difficult, but generally these tumors have a greater soft tissue component (radiolucent) than an odontoma. It may be argued that given time, the amount of hard tissue will increase; however, the distribution of hard tissue is different. A complex odontoma, which shares a common location, usually has one mass of disorganized tissue in the center, whereas the ameloblastic fibro-odontoma will usually have multiple scattered mature small pieces of dental hard tissue. Although the compound odontoma has multiple denticles, the posterior mandible is a rare location and the organization of the tooth material in ameloblastic fibro-odontomes is never organized enough to resemble a tooth. Finally, the ameloblastic fibro-odontomas do not occur early enough compared with odontomas to be considered a precursor.

Treatment
Usually conservative enucleation is used, although recurrence has been reported.

ADENOMATOID ODONTOGENIC TUMOR
Synonyms
Adenoameloblastoma and ameloblastic adenomatoid tumor

Definition
Adenomatoid odontogenic tumors are uncommon, nonaggressive tumors of odontogenic epithelium. This lesion, first reported by Stafne, has distinctive clinical and microscopic features and behavior patterns that sharply differ from ameloblastomas. The origin of adenomatoid odontogenic tumors may be from enamel organ epithelium, and it is classified as a mixed tumor because dentinoid material and occasionally enamel matrix is manufactured. Adenomatoid odontogenic tumors comprise 3% of all oral tumors. Both central and peripheral tumors occur. The central tumors are divided into the follicular type (those associated with the crown of an embedded tooth) and the extra-follicular type (those with no embedded tooth). Approximately 73% of central lesions are the follicular type.

Clinical Features
Adenomatoid odontogenic tumors appear in the age range of 5 to 50 years; however, about 70% occur in the second decade, with an average age of 16 years. The tumor has a 2:1 female predilection. The follicular type is diagnosed somewhat earlier than the extra-follicular type, probably because the failure of the associated tooth to erupt is noted. The tumor is slow-growing, and presents as a gradually enlarging, painless swelling or asymmetry, often associated with a missing tooth.

Radiographic Features
Location. At least 75% of adenomatoid odontogenic tumors occur in the maxilla (Fig. 21-27). The incisor-canine-premolar region, especially the canine region, is the usual area involved in both jaws. It occurs more commonly in the maxilla. This tumor may have a follicular relationship with an impacted tooth; however, often it does not attach at the cementoenamel junction but surrounds a greater part of the tooth, most often a canine (Fig. 21-28).

Periphery. The usual radiographic appearance is a well-defined corticated or sclerotic border.

Internal structure. Radiographically, radiopacities develop in about two thirds of cases. One tumor may be completely radiolucent, another may contain faint radiopaque foci (see Fig. 21-28), and some may show dense clusters of ill-defined radiopacities. Occasionally

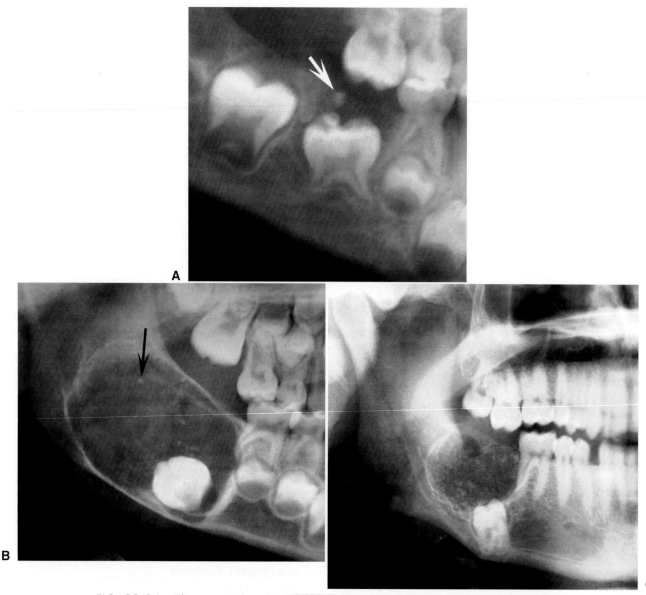

FIG. **21-26**   Three examples of ameloblastic fibro-odontoma. **A,** A cropped panoramic film with a lesion occlusal to a second deciduous molar. The lesion is ill defined and radiolucent except for two small radiopacities *(arrow).* **B,** A cropped panoramic image of a well-defined radiolucent lesion with only a few scattered radiopacities. **C,** A cropped panoramic image of a lesion with a larger number of radiopacities.

the calcifications are small and with well-defined borders, like a cluster of small pebbles (see Fig. 21-28, *B*). Intraoral radiographs may be required to demonstrate the calcifications within the lesion, which may not be seen on panoramic radiographs. Microscopic studies have verified that the size, number, and density of small radiopacities in the central radiolucency of the lesion vary from tumor to tumor and seem to increase with age.

Effects on surrounding structures. As the tumor enlarges, adjacent teeth are displaced. Root resorption is rare. This lesion also may inhibit eruption of an involved tooth. Although some expansion of the jaw may occur, the outer cortex is maintained.

Differential Diagnosis
When this tumor is completely radiolucent and has a follicular relationship with an impacted tooth, the

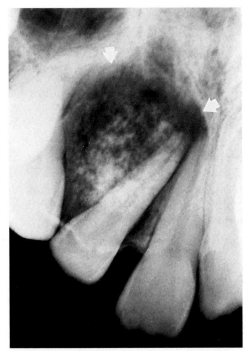

FIG. **21-27** An adenomatoid odontogenic tumor in the region of the right maxillary canine and lateral incisor. Calcification is present within the tumor mass, and the canine and lateral incisor have been displaced by the lesion. (Courtesy R. Howell, DDS, Morgantown, W.V.)

differentiation from a follicular cyst or a pericoronal odontogenic keratocyst may be difficult. If the attachment of the radiolucent lesion is more apical than the cementoenamel junction, a follicular cyst can be discounted. However, this would not exclude an odontogenic keratocyst. If there is a calcified product (radiopacities) in this tumor, other lesions with calcifications might be entertained in the differential diagnosis. The maxillary and mandibular anterior regions are also common sites for calcifying odontogenic cysts. It may not be possible to differentiate the extrafollicular type of adenomatoid odontogenic tumor from the calcifying odontogenic cyst. The ameloblastic fibro-odontoma and the calcifying epithelial odontogenic tumor occur more commonly in the posterior mandible.

Treatment

Conservative surgical excision is adequate because the tumor is not locally invasive, is well encapsulated, and is separated easily from the bone. The theory that adenomatoid odontogenic tumors are hamartomas is supported by the innocuous behavior of the lesion, because as with odontomas, adenomatoid odontogenic tumors stop developing about the time tooth structures complete their growth. The recurrence rate is 0.2%.

MESENCHYMAL TUMORS (ODONTOGENIC ECTOMESENCHYME)

ODONTOGENIC MYXOMA
Synonyms

Myxoma, myxofibroma, and fibromyxoma

Definition

Odontogenic myxomas are uncommon, accounting for only 3% to 6% of odontogenic tumors. They are

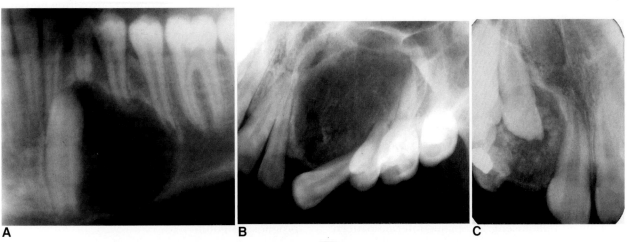

FIG. **21-28** Examples of adenomatoid odontogenic tumor with various amount of internal calcification. **A,** A cropped panoramic film with a totally radiolucent lesion associated with a mandibular cuspid. **B,** A lesion with sparse pebble-like calcifications associated with a maxillary cuspid. **C,** A lesion related to a maxillary lateral incisor with abundant calcification.

benign, intraosseous neoplasms that arise from odontogenic ectomesenchyme and resemble the mesenchymal portion of the dental papilla. These myxomas are not encapsulated and tend to infiltrate the surrounding cancellous bone but do not metastasize. They have a loose, gelatinous consistency and show microscopic characteristics similar to those of soft tissue myxomas of the extremities. Odontogenic myxomas develop only in the bones of the facial skeleton. The theory that this lesion develops from odontogenic rather than nonodontogenic ectomesenchyme is supported by the fact that it appears only in the jaws, it affects young people, it occasionally is related to a tooth that failed to erupt or is missing, and in some cases odontogenic epithelium can be detected microscopically.

Clinical Features

If odontogenic myxomas have a gender predilection, they slightly favor females. Although the lesions can occur at any age, more than half arise in individuals between 10 and 30 years; they rarely occur before age 10 or after age 50. The tumor grows slowly and may or may not cause pain. Eventually it causes swelling and may grow quite large if left untreated. It may also invade the maxillary sinus. Recurrence rates as high as 25% have been reported. This high rate may be explained by the lack of encapsulation of the tumor, its poorly defined boundaries, and the extension of nests or pockets of myxoid (jellylike) tumor into trabecular spaces, where they are difficult to detect and remove surgically.

Radiographic Features

Location. Myxomas more commonly affect the mandible by a margin of 3:1. In the mandible these tumors occur in the premolar and molar areas and only rarely in the ramus and condyle (non–tooth-bearing areas). Myxomas in the maxilla usually involve the alveolar process in the premolar and molar regions and the zygomatic process.

Periphery. The lesion usually is well defined, and it may have a corticated margin but most often is poorly defined, especially in the maxilla (Fig. 21-29).

Internal structure. When it occurs pericoronally with an impacted tooth, an odontogenic myxoma may have a cystlike, unilocular outline, although the majority have a mixed radiolucent-radiopaque internal pattern. Residual bone trapped within the tumor will remodel into curved and straight, course or fine septa. The presence of these septa gives the tumor a multilocular appearance. A characteristic septa identified with this

tumor is a straight, thin-etched septa (see Fig. 21-29, *C*). These have been described as making a tennis-racket–like or stepladder-like pattern, but this pattern is rarely seen. In reality, the majority of the septa are curved and course, but the finding of one or two of these straight septa will help in the identification of this tumor (Fig. 21-30; see also Fig. 21-29).

Effects on surrounding structures. When growing in a tooth-bearing area, it displaces and loosens teeth, but rarely causes resorption of teeth. The lesion also frequently scallops between the roots of adjacent teeth similar to a simple bone cyst. This tumor has a tendency to grow along the involved bone without the same amount of expansion seen with other benign tumors.

Additional Imaging

CT and, in particular, MRI can help in establishing the intraosseous extent of the tumor and thus guide the surgeon in planning the resection margins. The high tissue signal characteristic of this tumor in T2 weighted MR images is particularly useful in establishing tumor extent and the presence of a recurrent tumor (Fig. 21-31).

Differential Diagnosis

Because odontogenic myxomas most often have a multilocular internal pattern, the differential diagnosis should include other multilocular lesions such as ameloblastomas, central giant cell granulomas, and central hemangiomas. The finding of characteristic thin, straight septa with less-than-expected bone expansion is very useful in the differential. On occasion a small area of expansion with straight septa may be projected over an intact outer bony cortex and give a spiculated appearance seen in osteogenic sarcomas (see Fig. 21-29, *C*). Careful inspection of this area of expansion will reveal a thin but intact outer cortex that would not be seen in osteogenic sarcoma. On occasion the odontogenic fibroma will have the same radiographic characteristics and cannot be reliably differentiated from the myxoma.

Treatment

Odontogenic myxomas are treated by resection with a generous amount of surrounding bone to ensure removal of myxomatous tumor that infiltrates the adjacent marrow spaces. With appropriate treatment, the prognosis is good.

BENIGN CEMENTOBLASTOMA

Synonyms

Cementoblastoma and true cementoma

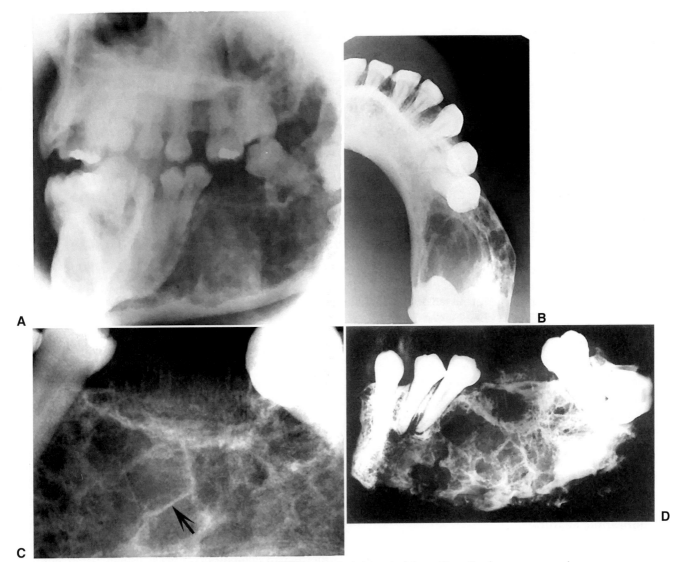

FIG. **21-29** An odontogenic myxoma. **A,** A lateral oblique film of a large myxoma in the body of the mandible. **B,** An occlusal view shows slight buccal expansion considering the size of the lesion. **C,** A periapical view shows a multilocular pattern. Note the one straight sharp septa *(arrow)*. Also note the fine straight septa emanating from the crest of the edentulous alveolar ridge; these may simulate the appearance of spiculation seen in malignant tumors. **D,** A lateral radiograph of a surgical specimen from the same patient.

Definition

Benign cementoblastomas are slow-growing, mesenchymal neoplasms composed principally of cementum. The tumor manifests as a bulbous growth around and attached to the apex of a tooth root. Its histologic characteristics are similar to osteoblastomas and some authors consider cementoblastomas to be osteoblastomas. Putative cementoblasts that compose this tumor produce cementum-like material and abnormal bone. The tumor most often develops with permanent teeth but in rare cases occurs with primary teeth.

Clinical Features

Although statistical data suggest that benign cementoblastomas are uncommon, many believe that they occur more often than published accounts indicate. The

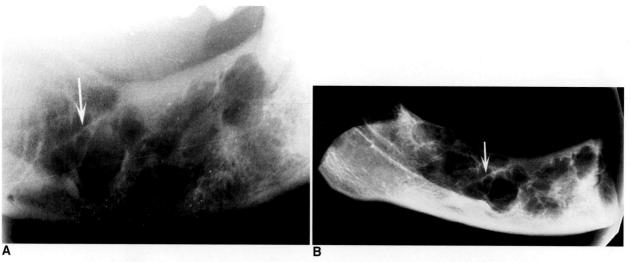

FIG. **21-30**   An odontogenic myxoma with ill-defined borders occupying the body of the mandible. Note the lack of expansion for the size of the lesion. **A,** A lateral oblique radiograph. **B,** A lateral radiograph of the surgical specimen of the same case. Note the sharp straight septa *(arrow).*

lesion is more common in males than females, and the ages of reported patients range from 12 to 65 years, although most patients are relatively young. There is no racial predilection. The tumor usually is a solitary lesion that is slow-growing but that may eventually displace teeth. The involved tooth is vital and often painful. The pain seems to vary from patient to patient and can be relieved by antiinflammatory drugs.

Radiographic Features

Location. Benign cementoblastomas occur more often in the mandible (78%) and form most commonly on a premolar or first molar (90%).

Periphery. The lesion is a well-defined radiopacity with a cortical border and then a well-defined radiolucent band just inside the cortical border.

Internal structure. Benign cementoblastomas are mixed radiolucent-radiopaque lesions in which the majority of the internal structure is radiopaque. The resulting pattern may be amorphous or may have a wheel spoke pattern (Fig. 21-32). The density of the cemental mass usually obscures the outline of the enveloped root. This central radiopaque mass as mentioned is surrounded by a radiolucent band indicating that the tumor is maturing from the central aspect to the periphery.

Effects on surrounding structures. If the root outline is apparent, in most cases various amounts of external resorption can be seen. If large enough, this tumor can cause expansion of the mandible but with an intact outer cortex.

Differential Diagnosis

The most common lesion to simulate this appearance is a solitary lesion of periapical cemental dysplasia. The differential may be difficult in some cases, and the presence or absence of symptoms or observation of the lesion over a period of time may be required. In general the radiolucent band around the benign cementoblastoma is usually better defined and more uniform than with cemental dysplasia. Also, in the first molar region the cementoblastoma has a more rounded shape than cemental dysplasia. Other lesions that may be included in the differential diagnosis are periapical sclerosing osteitis, enostosis, and hypercementosis. However, periapical sclerosing osteitis and enostosis do not have a soft tissue capsule, as does the benign cementoblastoma. Hypercementosis should be surrounded by a periodontal membrane space, which is usually thinner than the soft tissue capsule of the benign cementoblastoma, and there is no root resorption or jaw expansion with hypercementosis.

Treatment

Benign cementoblastomas are apparently self-limiting and rarely recur after enucleation. Simple excision and extraction of the associated tooth are sufficient treatment. In some cases the tumor may be ampu-

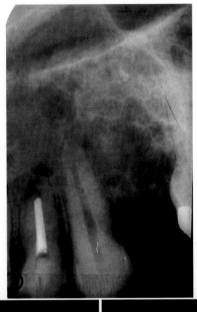

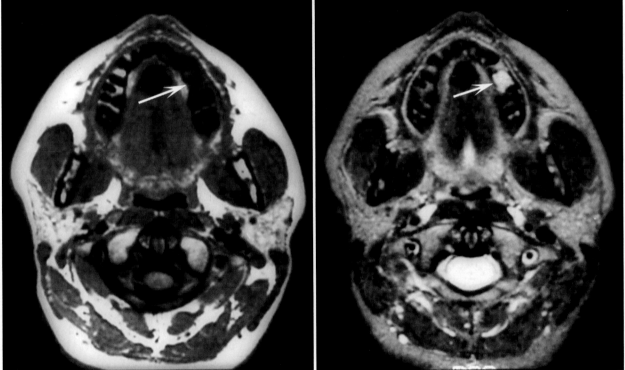

FIG. **21-31**   **A,** A periapical film taken to investigate a possible recurrence of an odontogenic myxoma in the alveolar process between the cuspid and the first molar after treatment by surgical curettage. **B,** MR axial image using T1 weighting, showing a low signal *(black)* from the segment of the alveolar process between the cuspid and molar. **C,** MR axial image of the same image slice as B but using T2 weighting resulting in a high signal *(white)* from the same alveolar segment, which is characteristic of an odontogenic myxoma and confirming the presence of a recurrence.

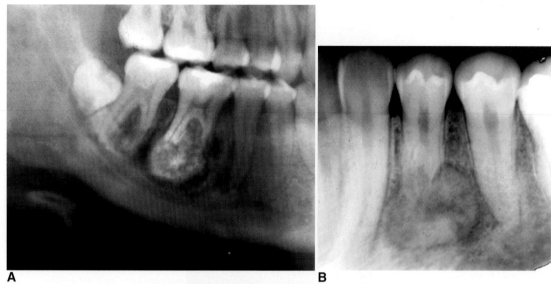

FIG. **21-32**   A cementoblastoma. **A,** A portion of a panoramic radiograph showing a large, bulbous, radiopaque mass associated with the apical portion of the mandibular right first molar. A radiolucent band can be seen surrounding the mass, and root resorption of the molar roots has occurred. **B,** A periapical radiograph of a lesion associated with a bicuspid. (Courtesy B. Pynn, Canada.)

tated from the tooth, which is then treated endodontically.

CENTRAL ODONTOGENIC FIBROMA

Synonyms
Simple odontogenic fibroma and odontogenic fibroma (World Health Organization [WHO] type)

Definition
Central odontogenic fibromas are rare neoplasms that sometimes are divided into two types according to histologic appearance: the simple type contains mature fibrous tissue with sparsely scattered odontogenic epithelial rests; the WHO type, which is more cellular, has more epithelial rests and may contain calcifications that resemble dysplastic dentin, cementum, or osteoid. One theory is that these types merely represent a spectrum and that odontogenic myxoma may be a part of this range.

Clinical Features
Most cases of central odontogenic fibromas occur between the ages of 11 and 39 years. The neoplasm shows a definite female preponderance, with a reported ratio of 2.2:1. Affected patients may be asymptomatic or may have swelling and mobility of the teeth.

Radiographic Features
Location. Central odontogenic fibromas occur slightly more often in the mandible, the most prevalent site being the molar-premolar region. They are also prevalent in the maxilla anterior to the first molar.

Periphery. The periphery usually is well defined.

Internal structure. Smaller lesions usually are unilocular, and larger lesions have a multilocular pattern. The internal septa may be fine and straight, as in odontogenic myxomas, or it may be granular, resembling those seen in giant cell granulomas. Some lesions are totally radiolucent, whereas unorganized internal calcification has been reported in others.

Effects on surrounding structures. A central odontogenic fibroma may cause expansion with maintenance of a thin cortical boundary or on occasion can grow along the bone with minimum expansion similar to an odontogenic myxoma. Tooth displacement is common, and root resorption has been reported.

Differential Diagnosis
The histologic features may resemble those of a central (originating in bone) desmoplastic fibroma if no epithelial rests are apparent. Desmoplastic fibromas are

more aggressive and tend to break through the peripheral cortex and invade surrounding soft tissue. The septa in desmoplastic fibroma will be very thick, straight, and angular. If thin, straight septa are present in the odontogenic fibroma, it may not be possible to differentiate this neoplasm from an odontogenic myxoma on radiographic criteria alone. If granular septa are present, the radiographic appearance may be identical to that of a giant cell granuloma.

Treatment
Central odontogenic fibromas are treated with simple excision. These lesions have a very low recurrence rate.

NONODONTOGENIC TUMORS

BENIGN TUMORS OF NEURAL ORIGIN

NEURILEMOMA
Synonym
Schwannoma

Definition
A central neurilemoma is a tumor of neuroectodermal origin, arising from the Schwann cells that make up the inner layer covering the peripheral nerves. Although rare, it is the most common intraosseous nerve tumor. This tumor has practically no potential for malignant transformation.

Clinical features. Neurilemomas grow slowly, can occur at any age (but most commonly arise in the second and third decades), and occur with equal frequency in both males and females. The mandible and

sacrum are the most common sites. These lesions cause few symptoms other than those related to the location and size of the tumor. The usual complaint is a swelling. Although pain is uncommon unless the tumor encroaches on adjacent nerves, paresthesia may arise, especially with lesions originating in the inferior alveolar canal. Pain, when present, usually develops at the site of the tumor; if paresthesia occurs, it is felt anterior to the tumor.

Radiographic Features
Location. Neurilemomas most often involve the mandible, with fewer than 1 in 10 cases occurring in the maxilla. The tumor most often is located within an expanded inferior alveolar nerve canal posterior to the mental foramen (Fig. 21-33).

Periphery. In keeping with its slow growth rate, the margins of this tumor are well defined and usually corticated as it expands the cortical walls of the inferior alveolar canal. Small lesions may appear cystlike but more commonly are fusiform in shape as the tumor expands the canal.

Internal structure. The internal structure is uniformly radiolucent. When lesions have a scalloping outline, this may give a false impression of a multilocular pattern.

Effects on surrounding structures. If the tumor reaches either the mandibular foramen or mental foramen, it can cause enlargement of the foramen. Expansion of the inferior alveolar canal is slow and thus the outer

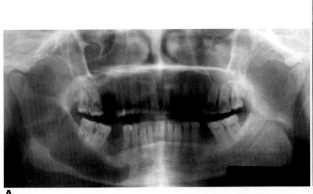
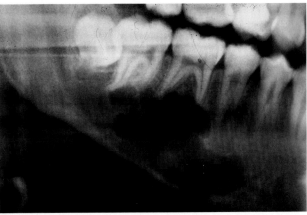

FIG **21-33**   **A,** A panoramic film of a large neurilemoma expanding all of the inferior alveolar nerve canal from the mandibular to the mental foramen. **B,** A cropped panoramic image of a smaller tumor.

cortex of the canal is maintained and the expansion of the canal is usually localized with a definite epicenter unless the lesion is large. The expanding tumor may cause root resorption of adjacent teeth (see Fig. 21-33).

Differential Diagnosis

Because neurilemomas most commonly originate within the inferior alveolar canal, vascular lesions such as a hemangioma or arteriovenous fistula should be considered. However, neurilemomas have an epicenter while vascular lesions will usually cause more of a uniform widening of the whole canal and do not have an obvious epicenter and usually change the course of the canal, most commonly to a serpiginous shape. Only neural tumors and vascular lesions originate within the inferior alveolar canal, but malignant lesions that grow down and enlarge the canal should be in the differential diagnosis. When this happens, the appearance is different with an irregular widening and destruction of the cortical boundaries of the canal.

Treatment

Excision is usually the treatment of choice. These lesions generally do not recur if completely removed. A capsule usually is present, facilitating surgical removal, although occasionally preservation of the nerve may not be possible. However, periodic examination is indicated to check for recurrence.

NEUROMA

Synonyms

Amputation neuroma and traumatic neuroma

Definition

Despite its name, a neuroma is not a neoplasm. Rather, it is an overgrowth of severed nerve fibers attempting to regenerate with abnormal proliferation of scar tissue after a fracture involving a peripheral nerve. As a result, the proliferating nerve forms a disorganized collection of nerve fibers composed of varying proportions of axons, perineural connective tissue, Schwann cells, and scar tissue. The original nerve damage may be the result of mechanical or chemical irritation of the nerve caused by fracture, orthognathic surgery, removal of a tumor or cyst, extrusion of endodontic cement, dental implants, or tooth extraction.

Clinical Features

Central neuromas are slow-growing, reactive hyperplasias that seldom become large, rarely exceeding 1 cm in diameter. They may cause a variety of symptoms, including severe pain resulting from pressure applied as the tangled mass enlarges in its bony cavity or as the result of external trauma. The patient may have reflex neuralgia, with pain referred to the eyes, face, and head.

Radiographic Features

The radiographic features of a neuroma relate to the extent and shape of the proliferating mass of neural tissue.

Location. The most common location is the mental foramen, followed by the anterior maxilla and the posterior mandible.

Periphery. Neuromas usually have well-defined, corticated borders. They may occur in various shapes, depending on the amount of resistance to expansion offered by the surrounding bone. In the mandible the tumor usually forms in the mandibular canal.

Internal structure. The internal structure is totally radiolucent.

Effects on surrounding structures. Some expansion of the inferior alveolar nerve canal may occur.

Differential Diagnosis

It is not possible to differentiate this lesion from other benign neural tumors.

Treatment

Treatment is recommended because neuromas tend to continue to enlarge. They also may cause pain. Regardless of the type of injury that precipitates development of the neuroma, recurrence is uncommon after simple excision.

NEUROFIBROMA

Synonym

Neurinoma

Definition

Neurofibromas are moderately firm, benign, well-circumscribed tumors caused by proliferation of Schwann cells in a disorderly pattern that includes portions of nerve fibers, such as peripheral nerves, axons, and connective tissue of the sheath of Schwann. As neurofibromas grow, they incorporate axons. In contrast, neurilemomas are composed entirely of Schwann cells and grow by displacing axons.

Clinical Features

The central lesion of a neurofibroma may be the same as the multiple lesions that develop in von Recklinghausen's disease. Central lesions also may occur in that syndrome but are rare. Neurofibromas can occur at any age but usually are found in young patients. Neurofibromas associated with the mandibular nerve may produce pain or paresthesia. Neurofibromas also may expand and perforate the cortex; causing swelling that is hard or firm to palpation.

Radiographic Features
Location. Central neurofibromas may occur in the mandibular canal, in the cancellous bone, and below the periosteum.

Periphery. As with neurilemomas, the margins of the radiolucency in neurofibromas usually are sharply defined and may be corticated. However, despite the benign nature and slow growth of the neurofibroma, some of these lesions have indistinct margins.

Internal structure. The tumors usually appear unilocular but on occasion may have a multilocular appearance.

Effects on surrounding structures. A neurofibroma of the inferior dental nerve shows a fusiform enlargement of the canal (Fig. 21-34).

Differential Diagnosis
Differentiation from other types of neural lesions may not be possible. This tumor can be differentiated from vascular lesions because the expansion of the canal is in a fusiform shape, whereas vascular lesions enlarge the whole canal and alter its path.

Treatment
Solitary central lesions that have been excised seldom recur. However, it is wise to re-examine the area periodically, because these tumors are not encapsulated and some undergo malignant change.

NEUROFIBROMATOSIS
Synonym
von Recklinghausen's disease

Definition
Neurofibromatosis is a syndrome consisting of café au lait spots on the skin, multiple peripheral nerve tumors, and a variety of other dysplastic abnormalities of the skin, nervous system, bones, endocrine organs, and blood vessels. The two major classifications are NF-1, a generalized form, and NF-2, a central form. Oral lesions may occur as part of NF-1 or may be solitary and are called *segmental* or *forme fruste manifestations* (Fig. 21-35). Recent observations of abnormal fat tissue in close association with changes in the osseous structure of the mandible support the theory that a mesodermal dysplasia is part of the spectrum of changes that may be observed in NF-1 lesions.

Clinical Features
Neurofibromatosis is one of the most common genetic diseases, occurring in 1 in every 3000 births and present in about 30 people per 10,000 population. The peripheral nerve tumors are of two types, schwannomas and neurofibromas. Some manifestations are congenital,

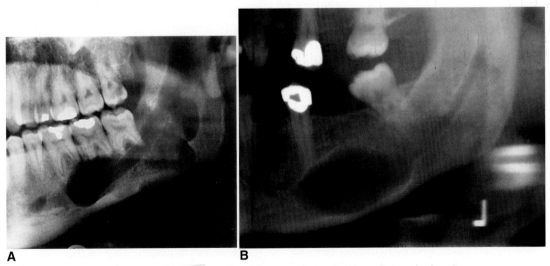

A   **B**

FIG. **21-34**   A neurofibroma. **A,** A portion of a panoramic radiograph showing a neurofibroma forming in the mandibular body along the path of the mandibular canal. **B,** A cropped panoramic image of a neurofibroma within the body of the left mandible. Note the fusiform shape as the tumor expands the canal.

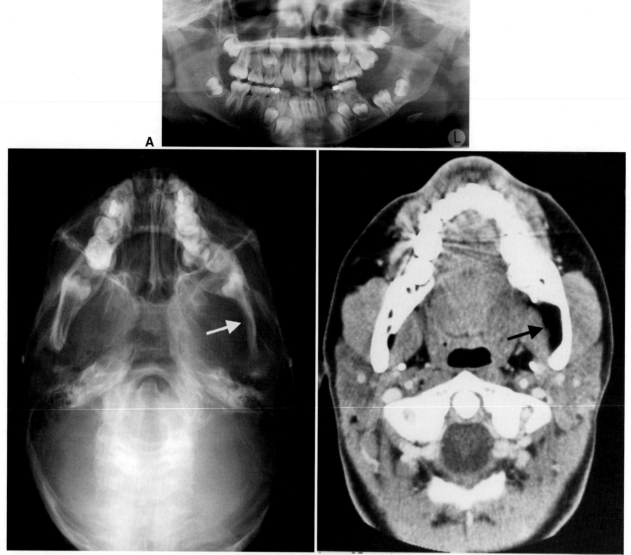

FIG **21-35**   An example of segmental neurofibromatosis involving the mandible. **A,** A panoramic film demonstrating enlargement of the left coronoid notch, enlargement of the mandibular foramen, and interference of the eruption of the first and second molars. **B,** A basal skull view of the same case revealing thinning and bowing of the ramus in a lateral direction *(arrow)*. **C,** CT axial image using soft tissue algorithm showing fatty tissue adjacent to the abnormal ramus *(arrow)*.

but most appear gradually during childhood and adult life. Café-au-lait spots become larger and more numerous with age; most patients eventually have more than six spots larger than 1.5 cm in diameter. Other skin lesions include freckles; soft, pedunculated, cutaneous neurofibromas; and firm, subcutaneous neurofibromas.

Radiographic Features

The radiographic changes in the jaws with neurofibromatosis can be characteristic. These changes include

the following alterations in the shape of the mandible: enlargement of the coronoid notch in either or both the horizontal and vertical dimensions; an obtuse angle between the body and the ramus; deformity of the condylar head; lengthening of the condylar neck; and lateral bowing and thinning of the ramus, as seen in basal skull views (see Fig. 21-35). Changes in mandibular morphology can continue to increase in severity through the second decade. Other radiographic changes include enlargement of the mandibular canal and mental and mandibular foramina and an increased incidence of branched mandibular canal. Erosive changes to the outer contour of the mandible and interference with normal eruption of the molars also may occur. Abnormal accumulations of fatty tissue within deformities of the mandible have been observed in images produced by computed tomography (CT) (see Fig 21-35, *C*).

Treatment

Most patients live a normal life with few or no symptoms. Small cutaneous and subcutaneous neurofibromas can be removed if they are painful, but large plexiform neurofibromas should be left alone. Malignant conversion of these lesions has occurred in rare cases.

Mesodermal Tumors

OSTEOMA

Definition

Osteomas can form from membranous bones of the skull and face. The cause of the slowly growing osteoma is obscure, but the tumor may arise from cartilage or embryonal periosteum. It is not clear whether osteomas are benign neoplasms or hamartomas. This lesion may be solitary or multiple occurring on a single bone or on numerous bones. Osteomas originate from the periosteum and may occur either externally or within the paranasal sinuses (Fig. 21-36). It is more common in the frontal and ethmoid sinuses than in the maxillary sinuses (see Chapter 26). Structurally, osteomas can be divided into three types: those composed of compact bone (ivory), those composed of cancellous bone, and those composed of a combination of compact and cancellous bone.

Clinical Features

Osteomas can occur at any age but most frequently are found in individuals older than 40 years. The only symptom of a developing osteoma is the asymmetry caused by a bony, hard swelling on the jaw. The swelling is painless until its size or position interferes with function. The osteomas are attached to the cortex of the jaw by a pedicle or along a wide base. The mucosa covering the tumor is normal in color and freely movable. Cortical type osteomas develop more often in men, whereas women have the highest incidence of the cancellous type. Although most osteomas are small, some may become large enough to cause severe damage, especially those that develop in the frontoethmoid region.

Radiographic Features

Location. The mandible is more commonly involved than the maxilla. Osteomas are found most frequently on the posterior aspect of the mandible commonly on the lingual side of the ramus or on the inferior mandibular border below the molars (Fig. 21-37). Other locations include the condylar and coronoid

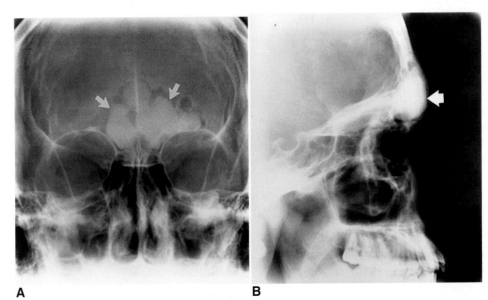

A   **B**

FIG. **21-36** An osteoma in the frontal sinus. **A,** A Caldwell view shows a large, amorphous mass in the frontal sinus *(arrows)*. **B,** A lateral view shows an osteoma occupying most of the space in the sinus *(arrow)*. (Courtesy G. Himadi, DDS, Chapel Hill, N.C.)

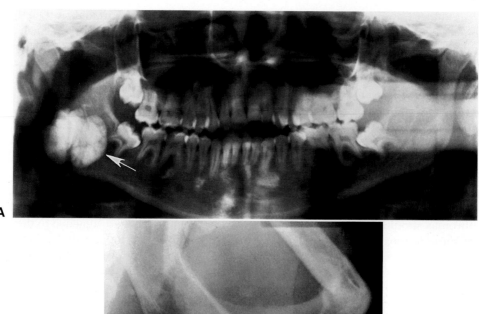

FIG. 21-37   An osteoma. **A,** A panoramic radiograph shows an osteoma in the right mandibular angle region *(arrow)*. **B,** An oblique lateral jaw radiograph shows a solid radiopaque osteoma attached to the inferior border of the mandible *(arrow)*. **(A,** From Matteson SR et al: Semin Adv Oral Radiol Dent Radiol Photogr 57(1-4):1, 1985.)

regions. The mandibular lesion may be exophytic, extending outward into adjacent soft tissues (Fig. 21-38). The lesions also occur in the paranasal sinuses, especially the frontal sinus.

Periphery.   Osteomas have well-defined borders.

Internal structure. Osteomas composed solely of compact bone are uniformly radiopaque; those containing cancellous bone show evidence of internal trabecular structure.

Effects on surrounding structures.   Large lesions can displace adjacent soft tissues, such as muscles, and cause dysfunction.

Differential Diagnosis

Usually the appearance is characteristic and does not present a problem with diagnosis. However, osteomas involving the condylar head can be difficult to differentiate from osteochondromas, osteophytes, or condy-

lar hyperplasia, and those involving the coronoid process may be similar to osteochondromas. A small osteoma may be similar in appearance to a torus or a large hyperostosis (exostosis).

Treatment

Unless the osteoma interferes with normal function or presents a cosmetic problem, this lesion may not require treatment. In such cases the osteoma should be kept under observation. Resection of osteomas is possible and may be difficult if the osteoma is of the cortical (ivory) type.

GARDNER'S SYNDROME

Synonym

Familial multiple polyposis

Definition

Gardner's syndrome is a type of familial multiple polyposis, in which there is an associated neoplasm. This syndrome is a hereditary condition characterized

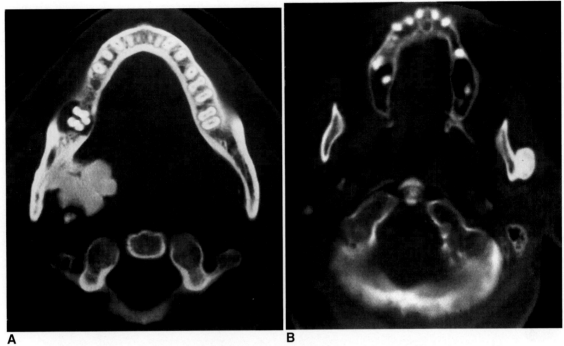

FIG. **21-38** CT scans of osteomas. **A,** An osteoma on the lingual side of the mandibular ramus. **B,** An osteoma on the lateral side of the mandibular ramus.

by multiple osteomas, multiple enostosis (dense bone islands), cutaneous sebaceous cysts, subcutaneous fibromas, and multiple polyps of the small and large intestine. The associated osteomas appear during the second decade. They are most common in the frontal bone, mandible, maxilla, and sphenoid bones (Fig. 21-39). A significant feature of familial multiple polyposis is the strong predilection of the intestinal polyps to undergo malignant conversion, making early detection of the syndrome important. Because the osteomas and enostosis often develop before the intestinal polyps, early recognition of the syndrome may be a lifesaving event. Occasionally osteomas may not be present but the presence of five or more areas of enostosis may indicate the presence of a familial multiple polyposis syndrome (Fig. 21-40). Multiple unerupted supernumerary and permanent teeth in both jaws also occur with Gardner's syndrome. Multiple osteomas may occur as isolated findings in the absence of the diseases associated with Gardner's syndrome.

Treatment

The removal of osteomas is not generally necessary unless the tumors interfere with normal function or present a cosmetic concern. It is most important to recognize the relationship of multiple osteomas and enostosis with familial multiple polyposis syndromes for early diagnosis. A family history of intestinal cancer may

also help. These patients should be referred to their family physician for examination for intestinal polyposis and treatment.

CENTRAL HEMANGIOMA

Definition

A hemangioma is a proliferation of blood vessels creating a mass that resembles a neoplasm, although in many cases it is actually a hamartoma. Hemangiomas can occur anywhere in the body but are most frequently noticed in the skin and subcutaneous tissues. The central (intraosseous) type most often is found in the vertebrae and skull. It rarely develops in the jaws, as fewer than 50 mandibular hemangiomas and an even smaller number of maxillary lesions have been reported. The lesions may be developmental or traumatic in origin.

Clinical Features

Hemangiomas are more prevalent in females than males, the ratio being 2:1. This tumor occurs most commonly in the first decade but may occur later in life. Enlargement is slow, producing a nontender expansion of the jaw that occurs over several months or years. The swelling may or may not be painful, is not tender, and usually is bony hard. Pain, if present, probably is the throbbing type. Some tumors may be compressible or pulsate, and a bruit may be detected on auscultation.

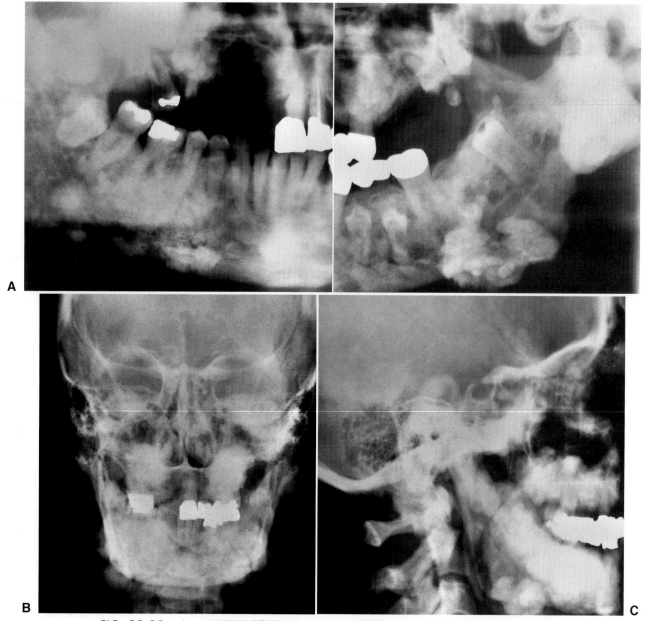

FIG. **21-39**   An osteoma with Gardner's syndrome. **A,** A panoramic radiograph shows several osteomas and enostoses throughout both jaws. Note the impacted mandibular left second premolars. **B,** A posteroanterior radiograph shows numerous osteomas. **C,** A lateral cephalometric radiograph of the same patient.

Anesthesia of the skin supplied by the mental nerve may occur. The lesion may cause loosening and migration of teeth in the affected area. Bleeding may occur from the gingiva around the neck of the affected teeth. These teeth may demonstrate rebound mobility; that is, when depressed into their sockets, they rebound to their original position within several minutes because of the pressure of the vascular network around the

tooth. Aspiration with a syringe produces arterial blood that may be under considerable pressure.

Radiographic Features

Location. Hemangiomas affect the mandible about twice as often as the maxilla. In the mandible the most common site is the posterior body and ramus and within the inferior alveolar canal.

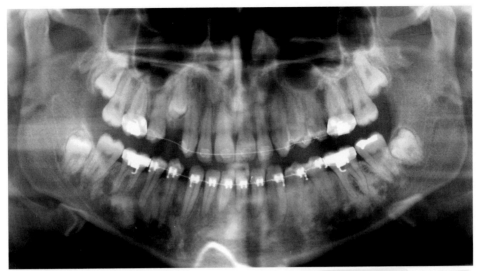

FIG. **21-40** A panoramic film of a patient with familial multiple polyposis syndrome. Note the multiple dense bone islands throughout the jaws; one has interfered with the eruption of the maxillary right first bicuspid.

Periphery. In some instances the periphery is well defined and corticated, and in other cases it may be ill defined and even simulate the appearance of a malignant tumor. This variation probably is related to the amount of residual bone present around the blood vessels. The formation of linear spicules of bone emanating from the surface of the bone in a sunray-like appearance can occur when the hemangioma breaks through the outer cortex and displaces the periosteum (Fig. 21-41).

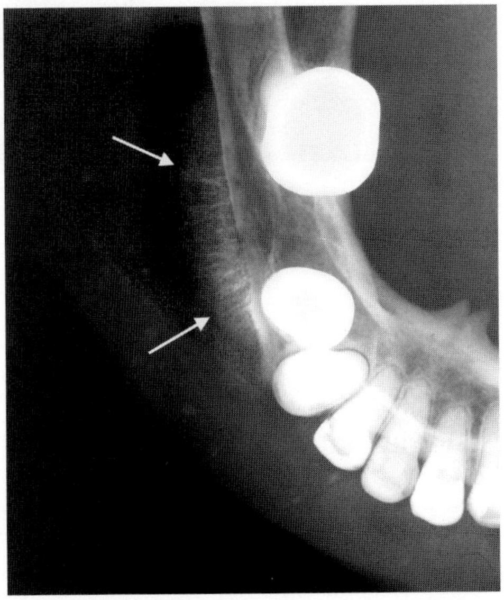

Internal structure. When there is residual bone trapped around the blood vessels, the result may be a multilocular appearance. Small radiolucent locules may resemble enlarged marrow spaces surrounded by coarse, dense, and well-defined trabeculae (Fig. 21-42). These internal trabeculae may produce a honeycomb

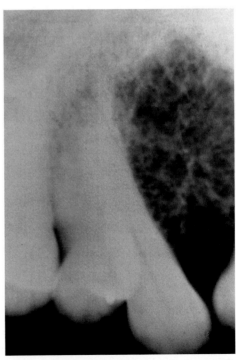

FIG. **21-41** An occlusal film of a case of a central hemangioma of the mandible with adjacent spiculation *(arrows),* which has a very similar appearance to the spiculation seen in osteogenic sarcoma.

FIG. **21-42** A hemangioma in the anterior maxilla shows a coarse trabecular pattern. (Courtesy E.J. Burkes, DDS, Chapel Hill, N.C.)

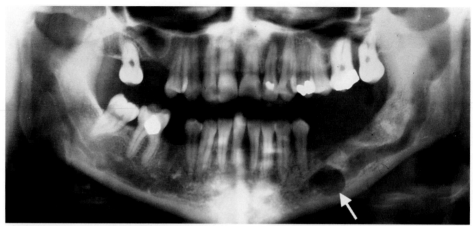

FIG. **21-43**   A panoramic film of a vascular lesion. Note that the whole width of the left inferior alveolar canal is enlarged, that it has an irregular abnormal path, and that the mental foramen has been enlarged *(arrow)*.

pattern composed of small circular radiolucent spaces that represent blood vessels oriented in the same direction of the x-ray beam. When the inferior alveolar canal is involved, the whole canal is increased in width and often the normal path of the canal is altered into a serpiginous shape sometimes creating a multilocular appearance (Fig. 21-43). Some lesions may be totally radiolucent. When the hemangioma involves soft tissue the formation of phleboliths (small areas of calcification or concretions found in a vein with slow blood flow) may occur within surrounding soft tissues (Fig. 21-44). They develop from thrombi that become organized and mineralized and consist of calcium phosphate and calcium carbonate.

Effects on surrounding structures.   The roots of teeth in the region of the vascular lesion often are resorbed or displaced. When the lesion involves the inferior alveolar nerve canal, the canal can be enlarged along its entire length and its shape may be changed to a serpiginous path. The mandibular and mental foramen may be enlarged. Hemangiomas can influence the growth of bone and teeth. The involved bone may be enlarged and have coarse, internal trabeculae. Also, developing teeth may be larger and erupt earlier when in an intimate relationship with a hemangioma (Fig. 21-45).

Differential Diagnosis

Hemangiomas should be considered in the differential diagnosis of multilocular lesions involving the body of the ramus and body of the mandible. Demonstration of involvement of the inferior alveolar canal is an important indicator of a vascular lesion. In most cases,

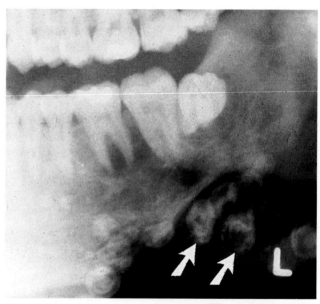

FIG. **21-44**   A soft tissue hemangioma with phleboliths *(arrows)*.

soft tissue changes suggest a vascular lesion. When a hemangioma produces a sunray spiculated bone pattern at its periphery, the appearance may be difficult to differentiate from an osteogenic sarcoma (see Fig. 21-41).

Treatment

Central hemangiomas should be treated without delay, because trauma that disrupts the integrity of the affected jaw may result in lethal exsanguination. Specifically, embolization (introduction of inert materials

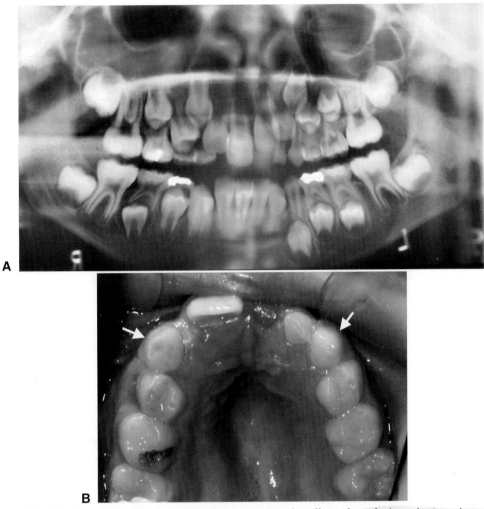

FIG. **21-45**   **A,** A panoramic film demonstrating the effect of a soft tissue hemangioma on the developing dentition. Note that the root development and eruption of the right cuspids and bicuspids are significantly advanced compared to the left side. **B,** An occlusal photograph from the same case. Note the difference in size of the maxillary deciduous cuspids.

into the lesion by a vascular route), surgery (en bloc resection with ligation of the external carotid artery), and sclerosing techniques have been used singly or together.

ARTERIOVENOUS FISTULA

Synonyms
A-V defect, A-V shunt, A-V aneurysm, and A-V malformation

Definition
An arteriovenous (A-V) fistula, an uncommon lesion, is a direct communication between an artery and a vein

that bypasses the intervening capillary bed. It usually results from trauma, but in rare instances may be a developmental anomaly. An arteriovenous fistula can occur anywhere in the body—in soft tissue, in the alveolar process, and centrally in the jaw. The head and neck are the most common sites.

Clinical Features
The clinical appearance of a central arteriovenous aneurysm can vary considerably, depending on the extent of bone or soft tissue involvement. The lesion may expand bone, and a mass may be present in the extraosseous soft tissue. The soft tissue swelling may

have a purple discoloration. Palpation or auscultation of the swelling may reveal a pulse. On the other hand, neither the bone nor the soft tissue may be expanded, and no pulse may be clinically apparent. Aspiration produces blood. Recognition of the hemorrhagic nature of these lesions is of utmost importance, because extraction of an associated tooth may be immediately followed by life-threatening bleeding.

Radiographic Features

Location. These lesions most commonly develop in the ramus and retromolar area of the mandible and involve the mandibular canal.

Periphery. The margins usually are well defined and corticated.

Internal structure. A tortuous path of an enlarged vessel in bone may give a multilocular appearance. Otherwise the lesion is radiolucent.

Effects on surrounding structures. Both central lesions and those in adjacent soft tissue can erode bone, resulting in well-defined (cystlike) lesions in the bone. Changes in the inferior alveolar canal may occur, as described in the preceding section on hemangiomas.

Additional Imaging

CT with contrast injection is a useful method for aiding the differential diagnosis of any vascular lesion and other neoplasms of the jaws (Fig. 21-46). An imaging modality called *MR angiography* is now being used routinely to document the size, extent, and vessels involved with the vascular lesion. Angiography, a radiographic procedure performed by injecting a radiopaque contrast agent into the blood vessels and making radiographs, provides the same information and is usually used when interventional therapy is planned in conjunction with the angiography (Fig. 21-47).

Differential Diagnosis

Occasionally the radiographic appearance is not specific for the A-V aneurysm. The differential diagnosis is similar to hemangiomas and includes multilocular lesions. However, association with the inferior alveolar canal is important in the differentiation.

Treatment

An A-V aneurysm is treated surgically.

OSTEOBLASTOMA

Synonym

Giant osteoid osteoma

Definition

An osteoblastoma is an uncommon, benign tumor of osteoblasts with areas of osteoid and calcific tissue. This tumor occurs most often in the spine of a young person. Agreement apparently is increasing that if osteoblastomas and osteoid osteomas are different lesions, they differ only in size and morphologic and histologic features. For example, the osteoid trabeculae in an osteoblastoma generally are larger (broader and longer), with wider trabecular spaces than those in an osteoid osteoma. An osteoblastoma is usually less painful, and it has more osteoclasts. In addition, benign osteoblastomas are considered more aggressive lesions. On the level of their ultrastructures, the two lesions essentially are similar or at least closely related.

Clinical Features

Both osteoblastomas and osteoid osteomas are rare in the jaws. The male-to-female ratio is 2:1, and the average age of occurrence is 17 years, with most lesions occurring in the second and third decades of life. Clinically, patients often report pain and swelling of the affected region; however, the pain is more severe in osteoid osteomas and is often relieved by salicylates.

Radiographic Features

Location. Osteoblastomas are found both in the tooth-bearing regions and commonly around the temporomandibular joint (within the condyle or the temporal bone).

Periphery. The borders may be diffuse or may show some sign of a cortex. Lesions often have a soft tissue capsule around the periphery indicating that this tumor is more mature in the central regions where there is evidence of abnormal bone (Fig. 21-48).

Internal structure. The internal structure may be entirely radiolucent in early developing tumors or may show varying degrees of calcific material. The internal calcification may take the form of a sunray pattern or fine granular bone trabeculae.

Effects on surrounding structures. Osteoblastomas can expand bone, but usually a thin outer cortex is maintained. This lesion may invaginate the maxillary sinus or the middle cranial fossa.

Differential Diagnosis

An important differential diagnosis may be a well-defined osteogenic sarcoma, because the histological appearance may be very similar. The differentiation may rely on the benign features of the osteoblastoma as revealed in the radiographic images. Osteoblastomas

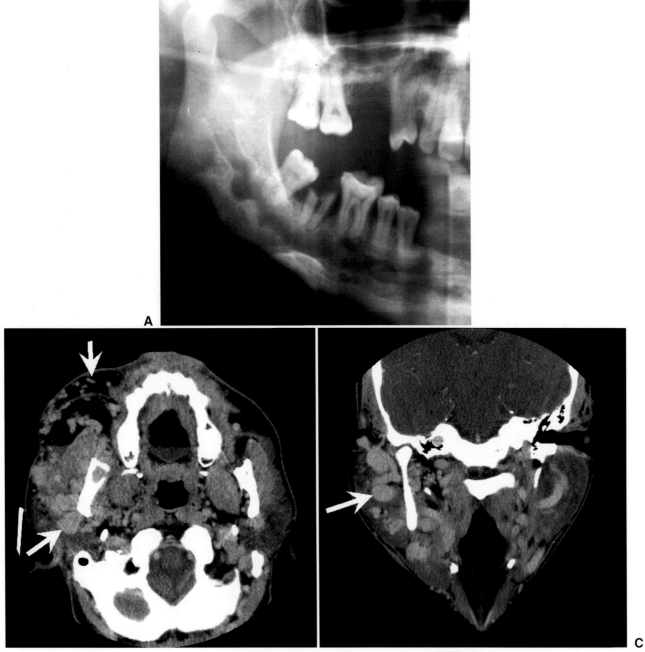

FIG. **21-46**   **A,** A panoramic film of a patient with an A-V malformation. Note the enlarged and irregular inferior alveolar canal. **B** and **C,** Axial and coronal CT images using soft tissue algorithm and after intravascular contrast was administered, which will cause the blood vessels to be more radiopaque *(arrows).*

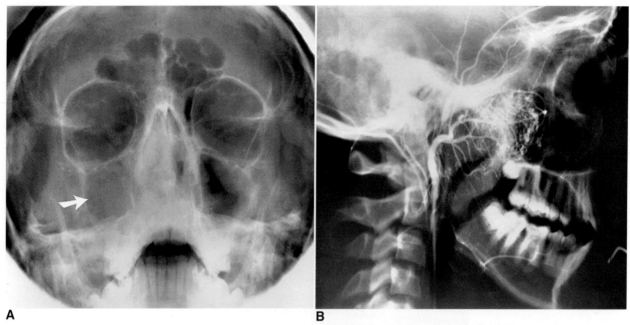

FIG. 21-47   A vascular lesion in the right maxillary sinus. **A,** A Waters radiograph shows the opacified maxillary antrum *(arrow).* **B,** Note the tumor vascularization in this angiogram. A radiopaque dye has been injected into the vasculature to enhance visualization. (Courtesy G. Himadi, DDS, Chapel Hill, N.C.)

do not normally break through cortical boundaries and invade surrounding soft tissue. Osteoid osteomas are usually smaller and have an associated sclerotic bone reaction at the periphery. Sometimes the appearance of an osteoblastoma may be similar to a large area of cemental dysplasia. Both have a soft tissue capsule but the osteoblastoma behaves more aggressively like a tumor.

Treatment
Osteoblastomas are treated with curettage or local excision. Recurrences have been described, and in a few cases the differentiation from a low-grade osteosarcoma may be difficult.

OSTEOID OSTEOMA
Definition
An osteoid osteoma is a benign tumor that is extremely rare in the jaws. Its true nature is not known, but some investigators think it is a variant of osteoblastoma. The tumor has an oval or round, tumor-like core usually only about 1 cm in diameter, although some may reach 5 or 6 cm. This core consists of osteoid and newly formed trabeculae within highly vascularized, osteogenic connective tissue. The tumor usually develops within the outer cortex but may form within the cancellous bone. There is a sclerotic bone reaction

around the periphery, often thinner in lesions within the cancellous bone.

Clinical Features
Osteoid osteomas occur most often in young people, usually males between the ages of 10 and 25 years. They seldom occur before 4 years or after 40 years. This condition affects at least twice as many males as females. Most of the lesions occur in the femur and tibia; the jaws are rarely involved. Severe pain in the bone that can be relieved by antiinflammatory drugs is characteristic. In addition, the soft tissue over the involved bony area may be swollen and tender.

Radiographic Features
Location.   The lesion is most common in the cortex of the limb bones. In those that do occur in the jaws, somewhat more develop in the body of the mandible.

Periphery.   The margins are well defined by a rim of sclerotic bone (Fig. 21-49).

Internal structure.   The internal aspect of young lesions is composed of a small ovoid or round radiolucent area (core). In more mature lesions the central radiolucency may have a radiopaque foci representing abnormal bone.

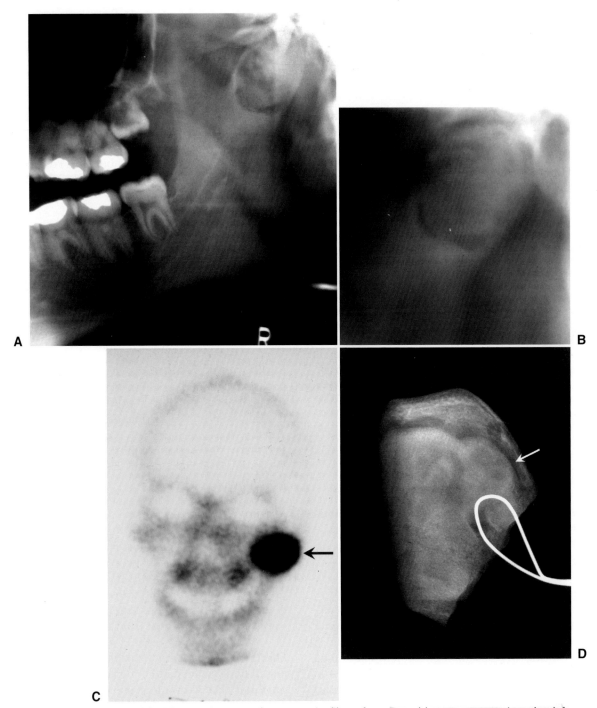

FIG. **21-48** **A,** A cropped panoramic film of an osteoblastoma occupying the left condyle. Note the enlargement of the condyle and presence of a soft tissue capsule surrounding an internal structure of granular bone. **B,** A tomograph of the left condyle. **C,** A technetium bone scan demonstrating increased bone activity in the left condyle *(arrow).* **D,** A radiograph of the surgical specimen. Note the internal granular bone surrounded by a soft tissue capsule *(arrow).*

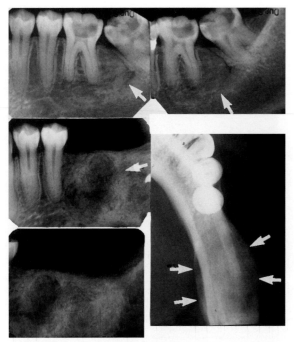

FIG. **21-49** An osteoid osteoma *(arrow)* appears as a mixed radiolucent-radiopaque lesion in the molar region; the lesion has caused expansion of the buccal and lingual cortex of the mandible *(arrows)*. (Courtesy A. Shawkat, DDS, Radcliff, Ky.)

Effects on surrounding structures. As previously mentioned, this tumor can stimulate a sclerotic bone reaction and cause thickening of the outer cortex by stimulating periosteal new bone formation.

Differential Diagnosis

Osteoid osteomas are extremely rare in the jaws. A clinician who suspects that a sclerotic lesion is an osteoid osteoma should also consider sclerosing osteitis, cemento-ossifying fibroma, benign cementoblastoma, and cemental dysplasia. The presence of a central radiolucency usually eliminates enostosis or osteosclerosis. Scintigraphy using a bone scan will help in the differential diagnosis by revealing considerable vascularity in the blood pool phase and a very high comparative bone metabolism.

Treatment

Complete excision currently is the recommended treatment, because this often relieves the pain and cures the disease. Although spontaneous remission can occur in some cases, the data are insufficient for identifying such cases in advance.

DESMOPLASTIC FIBROMA OF BONE

Synonym

Aggressive fibromatosis (usually reserved for tumors that originate in soft tissue)

Definition

A desmoplastic fibroma of bone is an aggressive, infiltrative neoplasm that produces abundant collagen fibers. It is composed of fibroblast-like cells that have ovoid or elongated nuclei in abundant collagen fibers. The lack of pleomorphism of the cells is important.

Clinical Features

Patients usually complain of facial swelling, pain (in rare cases), and sometimes dysfunction, especially when the neoplasm is close to the joint. The lesion occurs most often in the first two decades of life, with a mean reported age of 14 years. Although it originates in bone, the tumor may invade the surrounding soft tissue extensively. It also may occur as part of Gardner's syndrome.

Radiographic Features

Location. Desmoplastic fibromas of bone may occur in the mandible or maxilla, but the most common site is the ramus and posterior mandible.

Periphery. The periphery most often is ill defined and has an invasive characteristic commonly seen in malignant tumors.

Internal structure. The internal aspect may be totally radiolucent, especially when the lesion is small. Larger lesions appear to be multilocular with very coarse, thick septa. These wide septa may be straight or may have an irregular shape (Fig. 21-50). In T1 weighted MRI scans the internal structure has a low signal, which helps in determining intraosseous extent because of the contrast with the high signal from the bone marrow.

Effects on surrounding structures. Desmoplastic fibromas of bone can expand bone and often break through the outer cortex, invading the surrounding soft tissue. Usually CT or MRI is required to determine the exact soft tissue extent of the lesion.

Differential Diagnosis

Distinguishing this neoplasm from a fibrosarcoma may be difficult during the histologic examination. The radiographic appearance may not be helpful because a desmoplastic fibroma often has the appearance of a malignant neoplasm. However, the presence of coarse, irregular, and sometimes straight septa may help support the correct diagnosis. The appearance of these

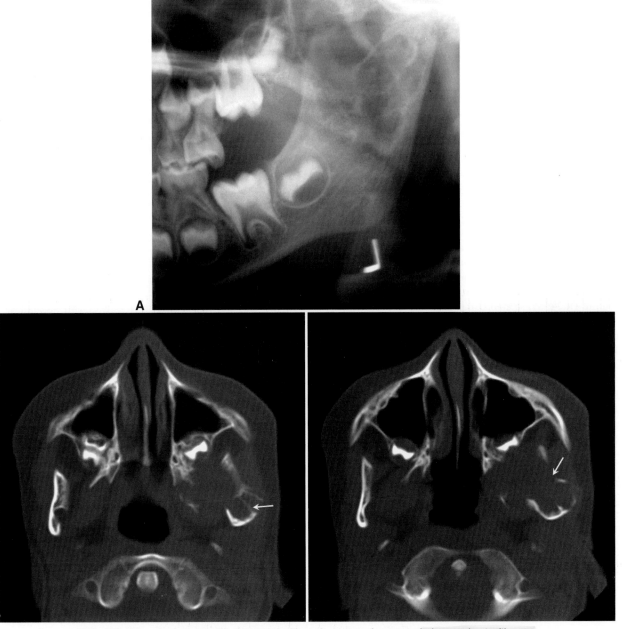

FIG. **21-50** **A,** A cropped panoramic film of a case of a central desmoplastic fibroma centered within the left condyle and ramus. **B,** An axial CT image using bone algorithm revealing thick straight septa *(arrow).* **C,** Another CT image at a higher level revealing that the tumor has broken through the anterior cortex of the condylar head.

septa also helps differentiate the lesion from other multilocular tumors. Very small lesions may resemble simple bone cysts.

Treatment

Resection of this neoplasm with adequate margins is recommended because of its high recurrence rate. Patients who have been treated for the condition should be followed closely with frequent radiologic examinations.

BIBLIOGRAPHY

Daley TD et al: Relative incidence of odontogenic tumors and oral and jaw cysts in a Canadian population, Oral Surg Oral Med Oral Pathol 77:276, 1994.

Gorlin RJ et al: Odontogenic tumors: clinical behavior in man and domesticated animals, Cancer 14:73, 1961.

Hoffman S et al: Intraosseous and parosteal tumors of the jaws, atlas of tumor pathology, series 2, fascicle 24, Washington, DC, 1987, Armed Forces Institute of Pathology.

Krishnan Unni K: Dahlin's bone tumors: general aspects and data on 11,087 cases, ed 5, Philadelphia, 1996, Lippincott-Raven.

Pindborg J, Kramer IRA: Histological typing of odontogenic tumours, jaw cysts, and allied lesions, International Histological Classification of Tumors, no 5, Geneva, 1971, World Health Organization.

Regezi JA et al: Odontogenic tumors: an analysis of 706 cases, J Oral Surg 36:771, 1978.

SUGGESTED READINGS

TORUS PALATINUS

Eggan S et al: Variation in torus palatinus prevalence in Norway, Scand J Dent Res 102:54, 1994.

Gorsky M et al: Prevalence of torus palatinus in a population of young and old Israelis, Arch Oral Biol 41:623, 1996.

Haugen LK: Palatine and mandibular tori; a morphologic study in the current Norwegian population, Acta Odontol Scand 50:65, 1992.

TORUS MANDIBULARIS

Eggen S, Natvig B: Concurrence of torus mandibularis and torus palatinus, Scand J Dent Res 102:60, 1994.

ENOSTOSIS

McDonnel D: Dense bone island: a review of 107 patients, Oral Surg Oral Med Oral Pathol 76:124, 1993.

Petrikowski GC, Peters E: Longitudinal radiographic assessment of dense bone islands of the jaws, Oral Surg Oral Med Oral Pathol Oral Radiol Endod 83:627, 1997.

AMELOBLASTOMA

Atkinson CH et al: Ameloblastoma of the jaw: a reappraisal of the role of megavoltage irradiation, Cancer 53:869, 1984.

Heffez L et al: The role of magnetic resonance imaging in the diagnosis and management of ameloblastoma, Oral Surg Oral Med Oral Pathol 65:212, 1988.

Ueta E et al: Intraosseous carcinoma arising from mandibular ameloblastoma with progressive invasion and pulmonary metastasis, Int J Oral Maxillofac Surg 25:370, 1996.

Weissman JL et al: Ameloblastoma of the maxilla: CT and MR appearance, Am J Neuroradiol 14:223, 1993.

ADENOMATOID ODONTOGENIC TUMOR

Dare A et al: Limitation of panoramic radiography in diagnosing adenomatoid odontogenic tumors, Oral Surg Oral Med Oral Pathol 77:662, 1994.

Giansanti JS et al: Odontogenic adenomatoid tumor (adenoameloblastoma), Oral Surg Oral Med Oral Pathol 30:69, 1969.

Hicks MJ et al: Pathology consultation: adenomatoid and calcifying epithelial odontogenic tumors, Ann Otol Rhinol Laryngol 102:159, 1993.

Philipsen HP et al: Adenomatoid odontogenic tumor: biologic profile based on 499 cases, J Oral Pathol Med 20:149, 1991.

Stafne EC: Epithelial tumors associated with developmental cysts of the maxilla, Oral Surg 1:887, 1948.

Vitkus R, Meltzer JA: Repair of defect following the removal of a maxillary adenomatoid odontogenic tumor using guided tissue regeneration: a case report, J Periodontol 67:46, 1996.

CALCIFYING EPITHELIAL ODONTOGENIC TUMOR

Franklin CD, Pindborg JJ: The calcifying epithelial odontogenic tumor: a review and analysis of 113 cases, Oral Surg Oral Med Oral Pathol 42:753, 1976.

Pindborg JJ: The calcifying epithelial odontogenic tumor: review of literature and report of extraosseous case, Acta Odontol Scand 24:419, 1966.

Vap OR et al: Pindborg tumor: the so-called calcifying epithelial odontogenic tumor, Cancer 25:629, 1970.

COMPOUND ODONTOMA

Haishima K et al: Compound odontomes associated with impacted maxillary primary central incisors: report of 2 cases, Int J Pediatr Dent 4:251, 1994.

Kaugars GE et al: Odontomas, Oral Surg Oral Med Oral Pathol 67:172, 1989.

Nik-Hussein NN, Majid ZA: Erupted compound odontoma, Ann Dent 52:8, 1993.

AMELOBLASTIC FIBROMA

Dallera P et al: Ameloblastic fibroma: a follow-up of six cases, Int J Oral Maxillofac Surg 25:199, 1996.

Trodahl JN: Ameloblastic fibroma: a survey of cases from the Armed Forces Institute of Pathology, Oral Surg Oral Med Oral Pathol 33:547, 1972.

ODONTOGENIC MYXOMA

Cohen MA, Mendelsohn DB: CT and MR imaging of myxofibroma of the jaws, J Comput Assist Tomogr 14:281, 1990.

Peltola J et al: Odontogenic myxoma: a radiographic study of 21 tumours, Br J Oral Maxillofac Surg 32:298, 1994.

Zachariades N, Papanicolaou S: Treatment of odontogenic myxoma, Ann Dent 6:34, 1987.

BENIGN CEMENTOBLASTOMA

Berwick JE et al: Benign cementoblastoma, J Oral Maxillofac Surg 48:208, 1990.

Jelic JS et al: Benign cementoblastoma: report of an unusual case and analysis of 14 additional cases, J Oral Maxillofac Surg 51:1037, 1993.

Ruprecht A, Ross AS: Benign cementoblastoma (true cementoblastoma), Dentomaxillofac Radiol 12:31, 1983.

Ulmansky M et al: Benign cementoblastoma: a review and five new cases, Oral Surg Oral Med Oral Pathol 77:48, 1994.

CENTRAL ODONTOGENIC FIBROMA

Gardner DG: Central odontogenic fibroma: current concepts, J Oral Pathol Med 25:556, 1996.

Handlers JP et al: Central odontogenic fibroma: clinicopathologic features of 19 cases and review of the literature, J Oral Maxillofac Surg 49:46, 1991.

Kaffe I, Buchner A: Radiologic features of central odontogenic fibroma, Oral Surg Oral Med Oral Pathol 78:811, 1994.

HEMANGIOMA

Lund BA, Dahlin DC: Hemangiomas of the mandible and maxilla, J Oral Surg 22:234, 1964.

OSTEOMA

Earwaker J: Paranasal osteomas: a review of 46 cases, Skeletal Radiol 22:417, 1993.

Matteson S et al: Advanced imaging methods, Crit Rev Oral Biol Med 7:346, 1996.

Thakker NS et al: Florid oral manifestations in an atypical familial adenomatous polyposis family with late presentation of colorectal polyps, J Oral Pathol Med 25:459, 1996.

Williams SC et al: Gardner's syndrome: case report and discussion of the manifestations of the disorder, Clin Nucl Med 19:668, 1994.

NEUROFIBROMATOSIS

D'Ambrosia JA et al: Jaw and skull changes in neurofibromatosis, Oral Surg Oral Med Oral Pathol 66:391, 1988.

Lee L et al: Radiographic features of the mandible in neurofibromatosis: a report of 10 cases and review of the literature, Oral Surg Oral Med Oral Pathol Oral Radiol Endod 81:361, 1996.

Shapiro SD et al: Neurofibromatosis: oral and radiographic manifestations, Oral Surg 58:493, 1984.

OSTEOBLASTOMA

Brady CL, Bronne RM: Benign osteoblastoma of the mandible, Cancer 30:329, 1977.

Lucas DR et al: Osteoblastoma: clinicopathologic study of 306 cases, Hum Pathol 25:117, 1994.

DESMOPLASTIC FIBROMA OF BONE

Gebhardt MC et al: Desmoplastic fibroma of bone: a report of eight cases and review of the literature, J Bone Joint Surg Am 67A:732, 1985.

Hopkins KM et al: Desmoplastic fibroma of the mandible: review and report of two cases, J Oral Maxillofac Surg 54:1249, 1996.

Zachariades N, Papanicolaou S: Juvenile fibromatosis, J Craniomaxillofac Surg 16:130, 1987.

CHAPTER 22

Malignant Diseases of the Jaws

ROBERT E. WOOD

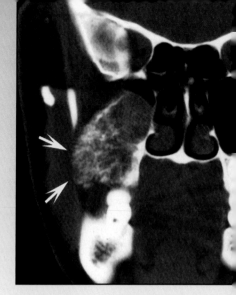

Definition

Malignant tumors represent an uncontrolled growth of tissue. Unlike benign neoplasms, they are more locally invasive, have a greater degree of anaplasia, and have the ability to metastasize regionally to lymph nodes or distantly to other sites. Malignant tumors that arise de novo are termed *primary tumors,* and those that originate from distant primary tumors are referred to as *secondary* or *metastatic malignancy.* Cancers may be caused by viruses, significant radiation exposure, genetic defects, and exposure to carcinogenic chemicals. For instance, using tobacco is strongly associated with oral carcinoma.

The most convenient method of classification of cancers is based on histopathology. In this chapter the malignancies that commonly affect the jaws have been divided into four categories: carcinomas (lesions of epithelial origin), metastatic lesions from distant sites, sarcomas (lesions of mesenchymal origin), and malignancies of the hematopoietic system. Unusual malignant tumors have been omitted to concentrate on more common lesions that a general practitioner may encounter.

Clinical Features

The following clinical signs and symptoms suggest that a lesion may be malignant: displaced teeth, loosened teeth over a short time, foul smell, ulceration, presence of an indurated or rolled border, exposure of underlying bone, sensory or motor neural deficits, lymphadenopathy, weight loss, dysgeusia, dysphagia, dysphonia, hemorrhage, lack of normal healing, and pain or rapid swelling with no demonstrable dental cause. Most oral cancers occur in men aged 50 years and older; however, malignant tumors may occur at any age in either gender.

Dentists must watch vigilantly for the possibility of malignancy in their patients. Because the prevalence of oral malignancy is low, many general practitioners practice years without encountering a patient who has a malignant tumor. This rarity may make a dentist less likely to recognize a malignant condition when it does exist. Lack of attention to this possibility may result in delayed diagnosis, delayed treatment, increased need for aggressive treatment with added morbidity, and in the worst case, premature death.

Radiographic Examination

Radiology plays a number of important roles in the management of the patient with cancer. First, diagnostic images may aid in the establishment of an initial diagnosis of a tumor. Diagnostic imaging also aids in the appropriate staging of disease from early small cancers to large cancers that have spread. Appropriate radiologic investigations assist the surgeon or radiation oncologist to determine the anatomic spread of the tumor so that it can be excised or irradiated adequately. Radiologic investigation has the potential to determine the presence of osseous involvement from soft tissue tumors and allow the practitioner to assess the involvement of lymph nodes and treatment outcome. Finally, a thorough radiographic dental examination plays a part in the management of the cancer survivor, who often is rendered xerostomic, neutropenic, and susceptible to dental caries, periodontal disease, and systemic infection.

RADIOGRAPHIC FEATURES

The following features may suggest the presence of a malignant tumor. The absence of visible radiologic signs as described does not preclude malignancy; it only implies that no visible radiographic signs exist.

Location

Primary and metastatic malignant tumors may occur anywhere in the oral and maxillofacial region. Primary carcinomas are more commonly seen in the tongue, floor of mouth, tonsillar area, lip, soft palate, or gingiva and may invade the jaws from any of these sites. Sarcomas are more common in the mandible and in posterior regions of both jaws. Metastatic tumors are most common in the posterior mandible and maxilla. Some metastatic lesions grow at the apices of teeth or in the follicles of developing teeth (Fig. 22-1, D).

Periphery and Shape

The typical appearance of the periphery (border) of a malignant lesion is an ill-defined border with lack of cortication and absence of encapsulation (a soft tissue or radiolucent periphery). This infiltrative border has uneven extensions of bone destruction. Fingerlike extension of the tumor occurs in many directions; this extension is followed by osseous destruction producing a region of radiolucency (Fig. 22-1, A). Evidence of osseous destruction with adjacent soft tissue mass is highly suggestive of malignancy (Fig. 22-1, B). Such a mass may exhibit a smooth or ulcerated peripheral border if cast against a radiolucent background. The shape of a malignant tumor of the jaw is irregular.

Internal Structure

Because most malignancies do not produce bone or stimulate the formation of reactive bone, their internal aspect is radiolucent in most instances. Occasionally, residual islands of bone are present, resulting in a pattern of patchy destruction with some scattered residual internal osseous structure. Some tumors, such as metastatic prostate or breast lesions, can induce bone formation, resulting in an abnormal-appearing internal osseous architecture, whereas others, such as osteogenic sarcomas, produce abnormal bone giving the involved bone a sclerotic (radiopaque) appearance.

Effects on Surrounding Structures

Malignancy is destructive, often rapidly so. The effect on surrounding structures mirrors this behavior. Slower-growing benign tumors or cysts may resorb tooth roots or displace teeth in a bodily fashion without causing loose teeth. In contrast, rapidly growing malignant lesions generally destroy supporting alveolar bone so that teeth may appear to be floating in space (Fig. 22-1, F).

Occasionally root resorption is present; this is more common in sarcomas. Internal trabecular bone is destroyed, as are cortical boundaries such as the sinus floor (Fig. 22-1, B), inferior border of the mandible, follicular cortices, and the cortex of the inferior alveolar neurovascular canal. Because malignant tumors tend to grow rapidly, they invade by means of the easiest routes, such as through the maxillary antrum or through the periodontal ligament space around teeth, resulting in irregular widening with destruction of the lamina dura (Fig. 22-1, C); they also may spread through the inferior alveolar neurovascular canal, causing similar widening. Where the tumor has destroyed the outer cortex of bone, usually no periosteal reaction occurs; however, some tumors stimulate unusual periosteal new bone formation (Fig. 22-1, E). Lesions such as osteosarcoma and metastatic prostate lesions, as well as other tumors, can stimulate the formation of thin straight spicules of bone, giving a "hair-on-end" or sunburst appearance. If there is a secondary inflammatory lesion coexisting with the malignancy, a periosteal reaction normally associated with an inflammatory lesion (e.g., "onion skin–like") may be seen.

Carcinomas

SQUAMOUS CELL CARCINOMA ARISING IN SOFT TISSUE

Synonym

Epidermoid carcinoma

Definition

Squamous cell carcinoma, the most common oral malignancy, may be defined as a malignant tumor originating from surface epithelium. It is characterized initially by invasion of malignant epithelial cells into the underlying connective tissue with subsequent spread into deeper soft tissues adjacent bone local-regional lymph nodes and ultimately to distant sites such as the lung, liver, and skeleton.

Clinical Features

Squamous cell carcinoma appears initially as white or red (sometimes mixed) irregular patchy lesions of the affected epithelium. With time, these lesions exhibit central ulceration; a rolled or indurated border, which represents peripheral invasion of malignant cells; and palpable infiltration into adjacent muscle or bone. Pain may be variable, and regional lymphadenopathy characterized by rubbery-hard lymph nodes that may be tethered to underlying structures may be present.

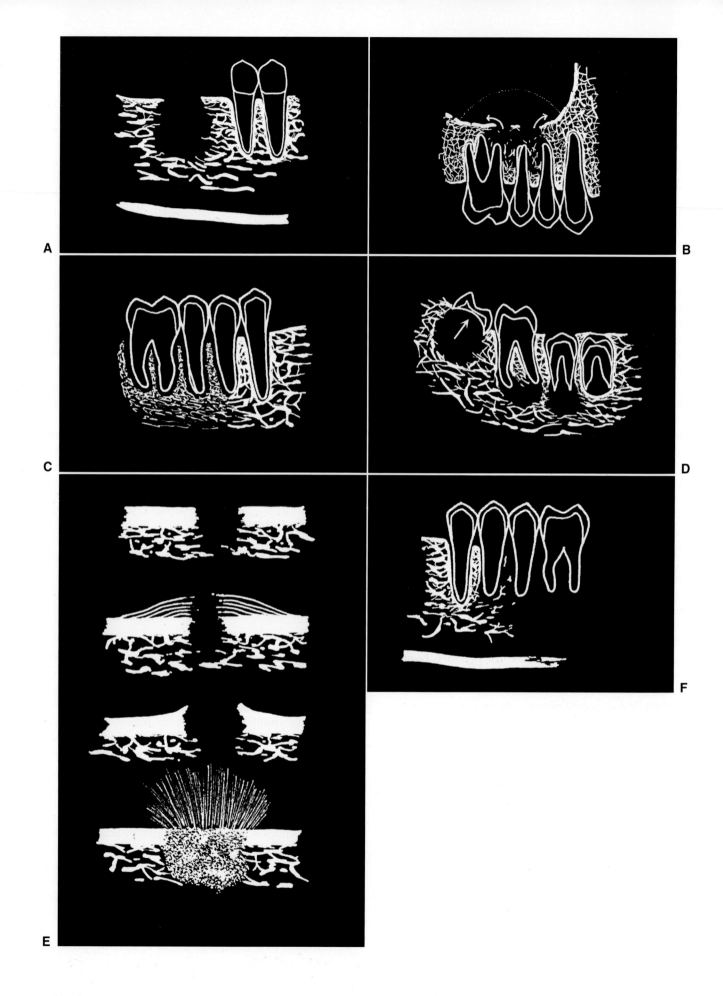

FIG. **22-1** Radiologic features of oral malignancy. **A,** Ill-defined invasive borders followed by bone destruction. **B,** Destruction of the cortical boundary (floor of maxillary antrum) with an adjacent soft tissue mass *(arrows)*. **C,** Tumor invasion along the periodontal membrane space, causing irregular thickening of this space. **D,** Multifocal lesions located at root apices and in the papilla of a developing tooth, destroying the crypt cortex and displacing the developing tooth in an occlusal direction *(arrow)*. **E,** Four types of effects on cortical bone and periosteal reaction, from top to the bottom: cortical bone destruction without periosteal reaction, laminated periosteal reaction with destruction of the cortical bone and the new periosteal bone, destruction of cortical bone with periosteal reaction at the periphery forming Codman's triangles, and a spiculated or sunray type of periosteal reaction. **F,** Bone destruction around existing teeth, producing an appearance of teeth floating in space.

Other clinical features include a soft tissue mass, paresthesia, anesthesia, dysesthesia, pain, foul smell, trismus, grossly loosened teeth, or hemorrhage. Large lesions can obstruct the airway, the opening of the eustachian tube (leading to diminished hearing), or the nasopharynx. Patients often report a significant weight loss and feel unwell. Males are more commonly affected than females. The condition is often fatal if untreated. Most squamous cell carcinomas occur in persons older than 50 years.

Radiographic Features

Location. Squamous cell carcinoma commonly involves the lateral border of the tongue. Therefore a common site to observe bone invasion is the posterior mandible. Lesions of the lip and floor of the mouth may invade the anterior mandible. Lesions involving attached gingiva and underlying alveolar bone may mimic inflammatory disease such as periodontal disease. This malignancy is also seen on the tonsils, soft palate, and buccal vestibule. It is uncommon on the hard palate.

Periphery and shape. Squamous cell carcinoma may erode into underlying bone from any direction, producing a radiolucency that is polymorphous and irregular in outline. Invasion occurs in one half of cases and is characterized most commonly by an ill-defined, non-corticated border (Fig. 22-2). Rarely the border may appear smooth without a cortex, indicating underlying erosion rather than invasion. If bone involvement is extensive, the periphery appears to have fingerlike extensions preceding a zone of impressive osseous destruction. If pathologic fracture occurs, the borders

show sharpened thinned bone ends with displacement of segments and an adjacent soft tissue mass. Sclerosis in underlying osseous structures (likely from secondary inflammatory disease) may be seen in association with erosions from surface carcinomas.

Internal structure. The internal structure of squamous cell carcinoma in jaw lesions is totally radiolucent; the original osseous structure can be completely lost. Occasionally small islands of residual normal trabecular bone are visible within this central radiolucency.

Effects on surrounding structures. Evidence of invasion of bone around teeth may first appear as widening of the periodontal ligament space with loss of adjacent lamina dura. Teeth may appear to float in a mass of radiolucent soft tissue bereft of any bony support. In extensive tumors this soft tissue mass may grow with the teeth in it as "passengers," so teeth are grossly displaced from their normal position. Tumors may grow along the inferior neurovascular canal and through the mental foramen, resulting in an increase in the width and loss of the cortical boundary of this canal. Destruction of adjacent normal cortical boundaries such as the floor of the nose, maxillary sinus, or buccal or lingual mandibular plate may occur. The posterior aspect of the maxilla may also be effaced. The inferior border of the mandible may be thinned or destroyed. If the tumor is extensive, pathologic fracture may occur.

Differential Diagnosis

Squamous cell carcinoma is discernible from other malignancies by its clinical and histologic features. Occasionally it is difficult to differentiate inflammatory lesions such as osteomyelitis from squamous cell carcinoma, especially when oral bacteria secondarily infect the tumor. Both osteomyelitis and squamous cell carcinoma are destructive, leaving islands of osseous structure that may appear to be consistent with sequestra. Evidence of profound bone destruction or invasive characteristics helps to identify the presence of a malignancy when a mixture of inflammatory changes and carcinoma exists. Osteomyelitis usually produces some periosteal reaction, whereas squamous cell carcinoma does not. In cases of osteoradionecrosis, where the patient has had prior malignancy, periosteal new bone is absent. If osseous destruction is present, the differentiation of this condition from squamous cell carcinoma requires advanced imaging and biopsy.

Management

Oral squamous cell carcinoma is usually managed using a combination of surgery and radiation therapy. The choice of which modality to use depends on the

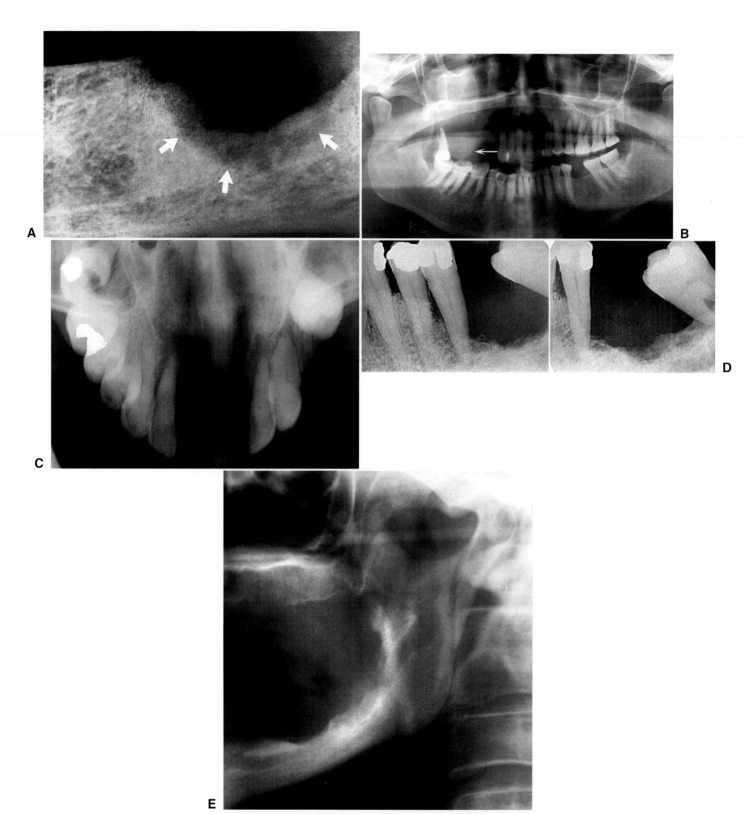

FIG. **22-2**   A through **E**, Squamous cell carcinoma *(arrows),* resulting in irregular destruction of bone. Note the destruction of the right alveolar process and floor of maxillary sinus and the soft tissue mass *(arrow)* in **B.** In the occlusal film image (**C**) the anterior floor of the nose has been destroyed (note lack of anterior nasal spine), as well as the anterior alveolar process. **D,** The supporting alveolar bone has been destroyed from around the teeth. **E,** Displays destruction of the anterior border of the mandibular ramus by a squamous cell carcinoma.

protocol of the treating center and the location and severity of the tumor. Generally, if an adequate margin of normal tissue can be obtained, surgery is the usual treatment, followed by radiation treatment. An alternative is to use radiation as the primary treatment followed by surgical salvage. Currently, there is a trend is to add concomitant chemotherapy as an adjunct to either radiation or surgical treatment, which requires the dental practitioner to be aware of changes in the patient's circulating blood count prior to any invasive dental treatment including scaling.

SQUAMOUS CELL CARCINOMA ORIGINATING IN BONE

Synonyms

Primary intraosseous carcinoma, intraalveolar carcinoma, primary intraalveolar epidermoid carcinoma, primary epithelial tumor of the jaw, central squamous cell carcinoma, primary odontogenic carcinoma, intramandibular carcinoma, odontogenic carcinoma, and central mandibular carcinoma

Definition

Primary intraosseous carcinoma is a squamous cell carcinoma arising within the jaw that has no original connection with the surface epithelium of the oral mucosa. Primary intraosseous carcinomas are presumed to arise from intraosseous remnants of odontogenic epithelium. Carcinoma from surface epithelium, odontogenic cysts, or distant sites (metastases) must be excluded.

Clinical Features

These neoplasms are rare and may remain silent until they have reached a fairly large size. Pain, pathologic fracture, and sensory nerve abnormalities such as lip paresthesia and lymphadenopathy may occur with this tumor. It is more common in men and in patients in their fourth to eighth decade of life. The surface epithelium is invariably normal in appearance.

Radiographic Features

Location. The mandible is far more commonly involved than the maxilla, with most cases being present in the molar region (Fig. 22-3) and less frequently in the anterior aspect of the jaws. Because the lesion is by definition associated with remnants of the dental lamina, it originates only in tooth-bearing parts of the jaw.

Periphery and shape. The periphery of the majority of lesions is ill-defined, although some have been described as well-defined. They are most often rounded or irregular in shape and have a border that demon-

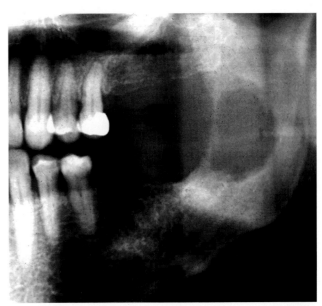

FIG. **22-3** This primary intraosseous carcinoma in the left mandible exhibits no internal structure, a poorly defined periphery, and thinning of the overlying mandibular bone.

strates osseous destruction and varying degrees of extension at the periphery. The degree of raggedness of the border may reflect the aggressiveness of the lesion. If sufficient in size, pathologic fracture occurs, with its associated step defects, thinned cortical borders, and subsequent soft tissue mass.

Internal structure. The internal structure is wholly radiolucent with no evidence of bone production and very little residual bone left within the center of the lesion. If the lesion is small, overlying buccal or lingual plates may cast a shadow that may mimic the appearance of internal trabecular bone.

Effects on surrounding structures. These lesions are capable of causing destruction of the antral or nasal floors, loss of the cortical outline of the mandibular neurovascular canal, and effacement of the lamina dura. Root resorption is unusual. Teeth that lose both lamina dura and supporting bone appear to be floating in space.

Differential Diagnosis

If the lesions are not aggressive and have a smooth border and radiolucent area, they may be mistaken for periapical cysts or granulomas. Alternately, if lesions are not centered about the apex of a tooth, occasionally it is difficult to differentiate this condition from odontogenic cysts or tumors. If the border is obviously infiltrative with extensive bone destruction, a metastatic lesion must be excluded, as well as multiple myeloma, fibrosarcoma, and carcinoma arising in a dental cyst. Examination of the oral cavity and especially the surface epithelium assists in differentiating this condition from surface squamous cell carcinoma.

Management

Generally these tumors are excised with their surrounding osseous structure in an en bloc resection. Radiation and chemotherapy may be used as adjunctive therapies.

SQUAMOUS CELL CARCINOMA ORIGINATING IN A CYST

Synonyms

Epidermoid cell carcinoma and carcinoma ex odontogenic cyst

Definition

Squamous cell carcinoma arising in a preexisting dental cyst is uncommon and excludes invasion from surface epithelial carcinomas, metastatic tumors, and primary intraosseous carcinoma. This condition may arise from inflammatory periapical, residual, dentigerous, and odontogenic keratocysts. Histologically the lining squamous epithelium of the cyst gives rise to the malignant neoplasm.

Clinical Features

The most common presenting sign or symptom associated with this condition is pain. The pain may be characterized as dull and of several months' duration. Swelling is occasionally reported. Pathologic fracture may occur, as may fistula formation and regional lymphadenopathy. If the upper jaw is involved, sinus pain or swelling may be present.

Radiographic Features

Location. This tumor may occur anywhere an odontogenic cyst is found, namely, the tooth-bearing portions of the jaws. Most cases occur in the mandible (Fig. 22-4), with a few cases reported in the anterior maxilla.

Periphery and shape. The radiologic picture of squamous cell carcinoma originating in a cyst mirrors the histologic findings. Because the lesion arises from a cyst, the shape is often round or ovoid. If it is a small lesion in a cyst wall, the periphery may be mostly well defined and even corticated. In this case the radiographic differentiation from a normal cyst is impossible. As the malignant tissue progressively replaces cyst lining, the smooth border is lost or becomes ill-defined.

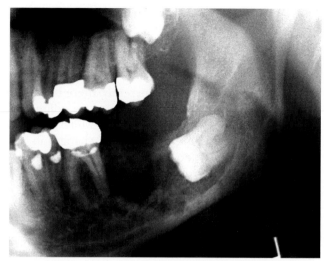

FIG. 22-4 Carcinoma arising in a preexisting dentigerous cyst related to the mandibular left third molar shows absence of a cyst cortex, invasion into adjacent bone, and ill-defined borders.

The advanced lesion has an ill-defined, infiltrative periphery that lacks any cortication. Its shape becomes less "hydraulic" in appearance and more diffuse.

Internal structure. This lesion lacks any ability to produce bone. It is wholly radiolucent, perhaps more so than invasive surface carcinoma, owing to prior osteolysis from the cyst.

Effects on surrounding structures. Carcinoma arising in dental cysts is capable of thinning and destroying the lamina dura of adjacent teeth or adjacent cortical boundaries such as the inferior border of the jaw or floor of the nose. It can produce complete destruction of the alveolar process.

Differential Diagnosis

If a dental cyst is infected, it may lose its normal cortical boundary and appear ragged and identical to a malignant lesion arising in a preexisting cyst. However, inflamed cysts usually show a reactive peripheral sclerosis because of inflammatory products present in the cyst lumen. This is not normally present in a cyst, which has undergone malignant transformation. Nevertheless, the two may be difficult to differentiate radiologically, and therefore cysts should always be submitted for histologic examination. Multiple myeloma may appear as a solitary lesion and may be difficult to distinguish, especially if the lesion has a cystic, well-defined shape. Metastatic disease may be similar, although it is commonly multifocal.

Management

The treatment of squamous cell carcinoma originating in a cyst is identical to that described with primary intraosseous carcinoma.

CENTRAL MUCOEPIDERMOID CARCINOMA

Synonym

Mucoepidermoid carcinoma

Definition

Central mucoepidermoid carcinoma is an epithelial tumor arising in bone, likely originating from pluripotential odontogenic epithelium or from a cyst lining. It is histologically indistinguishable from its soft tissue counterpart. The criteria for diagnosis of a central mucoepidermoid tumor are the presence of intact cortical plates, radiographic evidence of bone destruction, and typical histologic findings consistent with mucoepidermoid tumor. Additionally, the practitioner must exclude the possibility of an invasive overlying mucoepidermoid tumor or odontogenic tumor.

Clinical Features

Unlike other malignant tumors of the jaws, the central mucoepidermoid tumor is more likely to mimic a benign tumor or cyst. The most common complaint is of a painless swelling. The swelling may have been present for months or even years and has been reported to cause facial asymmetry. Occasionally it may feel as if teeth have been moved or a denture may no longer fit. Tenderness rather than severe pain may also be present. Paresthesia of the inferior alveolar nerve as well as spreading of the lesion to regional lymph nodes has been reported. Central mucoepidermoid tumor, unlike other oral malignancies, is more common in females than males.

Radiographic Features

Location. The lesion is twice as common in the mandible as the maxilla, usually occurring in the premolar and molar region with a few cases reported in the anterior mandible. The lesion most commonly occurs above the mandibular canal, similar to odontogenic tumors.

Periphery and shape. Mucoepidermoid tumor presents as a unilocular or multilocular expansile mass (Fig. 22-5). The border is most often well defined and well corticated and often crenated or undulating in nature, which is similar to benign odontogenic tumors. The peripheral cortication may be impressively thick, which belies its malignant nature. Rarely the periphery is not corticated and has a more malignant appearance.

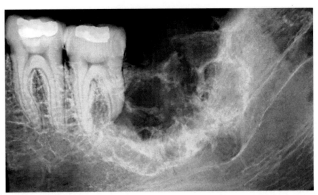

FIG. **22-5** The multilocular radiolucency in this radiograph has displaced the mandibular canal and destroyed the superior crest of the alveolar process and the distal supporting bone of the second molar.

Internal structure. The internal structure has features like those of a benign odontogenic tumor such as an ameloblastoma. Lesions are often described as being multilocular or having either a soap-bubble or honeycomb internal structure, implying the presence of compartments separated by thin or thick cortical septa. This bone is not produced by the tumor, but is merely remodeled residual bone taking the form of septa.

Effects on surrounding structures. Mucoepidermoid tumor is capable of causing expansion of adjacent normal bony walls. The buccal and lingual cortical plates, inferior border of the mandible, and alveolar crest are usually intact; however, they may be thinned and grossly displaced. The mandibular canal may be depressed or pushed laterally or medially. These characteristics are more similar to benign tumors than malignant tumors. Teeth remain largely unaffected by this disease, although adjacent lamina dura may be lost.

Differential Diagnosis

The differential diagnosis of this lesion reflects its lack of features commonly associated with oral malignancy. The chief differential is ameloblastoma, with which it shares similarities in its peripheral and internal features. It may not be possible to differentiate the two. Odontogenic myxoma and central giant cell granuloma also may be confused with mucoepidermoid tumor, as may other odontogenic cysts or tumors.

Management

Mucoepidermoid carcinoma is treated surgically with en bloc resection encompassing a margin of adjacent normal bone. Neck dissection and postoperative radiation therapy may be required to control spread to lymph nodes.

MALIGNANT AMELOBLASTOMA AND AMELOBLASTIC CARCINOMA

Definition

Malignant ameloblastoma is defined as an ameloblastoma exhibiting the histologic criteria of a malignant neoplasm, such as increased and abnormal mitosis and hyperchromatic, large, pleomorphic nuclei. The histologic features may not correlate with the clinical behavior. On the other hand, ameloblastic carcinoma is an ameloblastoma with typical benign histologic features that is deemed malignant because of its biologic behavior, namely, metastasis.

Clinical Features

Clinically these lesions may behave as benign ameloblastomas, exhibiting a hard expansile mass of the jaw with displaced and perhaps loosened teeth and normal overlying mucosa. Tenderness of the overlying soft tissue has been reported. Metastatic spread may be to the cervical lymph nodes, lung, or other viscera, as well as to the skeleton, especially the spine. Local extension may occur into adjacent bones, connective tissue, or salivary glands. These tumors occur most commonly between the first and sixth decades of life and are more common in males than females.

Radiographic Features

Location. These lesions are more common in the mandible than in the maxilla, with most occurring in the premolar and molar region, where ameloblastoma is typically found.

Periphery and shape. Similar to ameloblastoma, a well-defined border occurs with cortication, presence of crenations, or scalloping of the border. Malignant ameloblastoma may show some of the signs more commonly seen in malignant neoplasms, namely, loss of and subsequent breaching of the cortical boundary, invading into the surrounding soft tissue.

Internal structure. The lesions are either unilocular or, more commonly, multilocular, giving the appearance of a honeycomb or soap-bubble pattern as seen in benign ameloblastomas. Most of the septa are robust and thick.

Effects on surrounding structures. Teeth may be moved bodily by the tumor and may exhibit root resorption similar to a benign tumor. Bony borders may be effaced or breached, and as in benign ameloblastoma, the lesions may erode lamina dura and displace normal anatomic boundaries such as the floor of the nose and maxillary sinus. The mandibular neurovascular canal may be displaced or eroded.

Differential Diagnosis

The differential diagnosis of this lesion should include benign ameloblastoma, odontogenic keratocyst, odontogenic myxoma, and central mucoepidermoid tumor, from which malignant ameloblastoma may not be distinguishable radiologically. If the lesion is locally invasive and this is apparent radiologically, a diagnosis of carcinoma arising in a dental cyst should be entertained. If the patient is young and the location of the lesion is anterior to the second permanent molar, central giant cell granuloma may mimic some of its radiologic features. Often the final diagnosis is the result of histologic evaluation or the detection of metastatic lesions.

Management

These lesions are most often treated with en bloc surgical resection. However, many may not be discovered to be malignant until the time of the first surgery or even later. Because the histologic appearance of these lesions may mimic benign ameloblastoma, the initial treatment often is inadequate. In addition, the metastatic lesions may not appear for many months or years after treatment of the primary tumor, adding another reason for treatment failure.

Metastatic Tumors

Synonym
Secondary malignancy

Definition

Metastatic tumors represent the establishment of new foci of malignant disease from a distant malignant tumor usually by way of the blood vessels. An interesting feature of these lesions is that metastatic lesions in the jaws usually arise from sites that are anatomically inferior to the clavicle. Metastatic lesions of the jaws usually occur when the distant primary lesion is already known, although on occasion the presence of a metastatic tumor may herald the presence of a silent primary lesion. Jaw involvement accounts for less than 1% of metastatic malignancies found elsewhere, with most affecting the spine, pelvis, skull, ribs, and humerus. Most frequently the tumor is a type of carcinoma, the most common primary sites being the breast, kidney, lung, colon and rectum, prostate, thyroid, stomach, melanoma, testes, bladder, ovary, and cervix. In children the tumors include neuroblastoma, retinoblastoma, and Wilms' tumor. Metastatic carcinoma must be differentiated from the more common locally invading squamous carcinoma.

Clinical Features

Metastatic disease is more common in patients in their fifth to seventh decade of life. Patients may complain of dental pain, numbness or paresthesia of the third branch of the trigeminal nerve, pathologic fracture of the jaw, or hemorrhage from the tumor site.

Radiographic Features

Location. The posterior areas of the jaws are more commonly affected (Fig. 22-6, *A*), the mandible being favored over the maxilla. The maxillary sinus may be the next most common site, followed by the anterior hard palate and mandibular condyle. Frequently metastatic lesions of the mandible are bilateral (Fig. 22-6, *B* and *C*). Also, lesions may be located in the periodontal ligament space (sometimes at the root apex), mimicking periapical and periodontal inflammatory disease, or in the papilla of a developing tooth.

Periphery and shape. Metastatic lesions may be moderately well demarcated but have no cortication or encapsulation at their tumor margins; they may also have ill-defined invasive margins (see Fig. 22-6, *A*). The lesions are not usually round but polymorphous in shape. Both prostate and breast lesions may stimulate bone formation of the adjacent bone, which will be sclerotic. The tumor may begin as a few zones of osseous destruction separated by normal bone. After a time these small areas coalesce into a larger, ill-defined mass and the jaw may become enlarged.

Internal structure. Lesions are generally radiolucent, in which case the internal structure is a combination of residual normal trabecular bone in association with areas of bone lysis. If sclerotic metastases are present (i.e., prostate and breast), the normally ragged radiolucent area may appear as an area of patchy sclerosis, the result of new bone formation. The origin of this new bone is not the tumor but stimulation of surrounding normal bone. If the tumor is seeded in multiple regions of the jaw, the result is a multifocal appearance (multiple small radiolucent lesions) with normal bone between the foci. Significant dissemination of metastatic tumor may give the jaws a general radiolucent appearance occasionally mimicking osteopenia.

Effects on surrounding structures. Metastatic carcinomas may stimulate a periosteal reaction that usually takes the form of a spiculated pattern (prostate and neuroblastoma). Typical of malignancy, the lesion effaces the lamina dura and can cause an irregular increase in the width of the periodontal ligament space. If the tumor has seeded in the papilla of a developing tooth, the cortices of the crypt may be totally or partially destroyed. Teeth may seem to be floating in a soft tissue mass and may be in an altered position because of loss of bony support. Extraction sockets may fail to heal and may increase in size. Resorption of teeth is rare (sometimes associated with multiple myeloma and chondrosarcoma); this is more common in benign lesions. The cortical bone of adjacent structures such as the neurovascular canal, sinus, and nasal fossa is destroyed. On occasion the tumor breaches the outer cortical plate of the jaws and extends into surrounding soft tissues or presents as an intraoral mass (Fig. 22-6, *E*).

Differential Diagnosis

In most cases a known primary malignancy is present, and the diagnosis of metastasis is straightforward. Multiple myeloma may be confused with metastatic tumors; however, the border of multiple myeloma is usually better defined than in metastatic disease. When a lesion starts within the periodontal ligament space of a tooth, the appearance may be identical to that of a periapical inflammatory lesion. A point of differentiation is that the periodontal ligament space widening from inflammation is at its greatest width and centered about the apex of the root. In contrast, the malignant tumor usually causes irregular widening, which may extend up the side of the root. An odontogenic cyst, if secondarily infected, may have an ill-defined border, giving a similar appearance to a metastatic lesion. Invasion of the jaws by primary tumors of the overlying epithelium such as squamous cell carcinoma may be indistinguishable from metastatic disease but can be differentiated by clinical examination.

Management

The presence of a metastatic tumor in the jaw indicates a poor prognosis. If metastatic disease is present, in the majority of cases the patient will usually die within 1 to 2 years. If the radiographic appearance is suspicious, an opinion from a dental radiologist should be sought and tissue submitted for histologic analysis. Nuclear medicine may be employed to detect other metastatic lesions. Isolated malignant deposits, if symptomatic, may be treated with localized high-dose radiation treatment. In the rare occasion that the jaw is the first diagnosed site of malignant spread, it is imperative that the patient be referred quickly to an oncologist so that the primary lesion can be found and anticancer treatment can be delivered promptly. This treatment may take the form of chemotherapy, radiation therapy, surgery, immunotherapy, or hormone treatment.

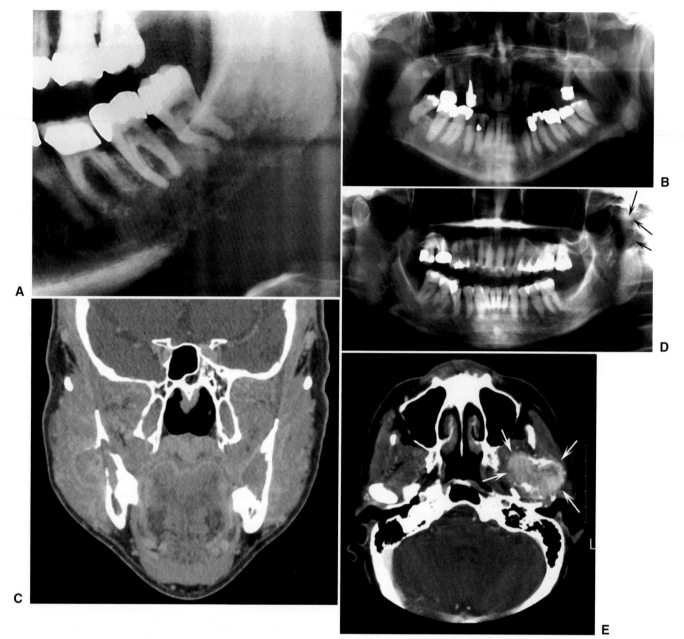

FIG. **22-6** Metastatic carcinomas. **A,** Metastatic breast carcinoma surrounding the apical half of the second and third molar roots and extending inferiorly. It has destroyed the inferior border of the mandible. **B,** Bilateral metastatic lesions from the lung destroying the mandibular rami. **C,** Coronal CT image using soft tissue algorithm of the same case. **D,** Destruction of the left mandibular condyle *(arrows)* from a thyroid metastatic lesion. **E,** Axial CT image using soft tissue algorithm of the same case showing invasion into surrounding soft tissue *(arrows).*

Sarcomas

OSTEOSARCOMA

Synonym
Osteogenic sarcoma

Definition
Osteosarcoma is a malignant neoplasm of bone in which osteoid is produced directly by malignant stroma as opposed to adjacent reactive bone formation. The three major histologic types are chondroblastic, osteoblastic, and fibroblastic osteosarcoma. The cause of osteosarcoma is unknown, but genetic mutation and viral causes have been suggested. It is also known to occur in association with Paget's disease and fibrous dysplasia after therapeutic irradiation.

Clinical Features
Osteosarcoma of the jaws is quite rare and accounts for approximately 7% of all osteosarcomas. Despite its rarity, the dentist may be the first health professional who observes a tumor involving the jaws. The lesion occurs in all racial groups worldwide and in males twice as frequently as females. Jaw lesions typically occur with a peak in the fourth decade, about 10 years later on average than long bone lesions. The most commonly reported symptom or sign is swelling, which may be present as long as 6 months before diagnosis; the swelling is usually rapid. Other indicators are pain, tenderness, erythema of overlying mucosa, ulceration, loose teeth, epistaxis, hemorrhage, nasal obstruction, exophthalmos, trismus, and blindness. Hypoesthesia has also been reported in cases involving neurovascular canals.

Radiographic Features
Location. The mandible is more commonly affected than the maxilla. Although the lesion can occur in any part of either jaw, the posterior mandible, including the tooth-bearing region, angle, and vertical ramus, is most commonly affected. The posterior areas are also more commonly affected in the maxilla, with the most frequent sites being the alveolar ridge, antrum, and palate. The lesion may cross the midline.

Periphery and shape. Osteosarcoma has an ill-defined border in most instances. When viewed against normal bone, the lesion is usually radiolucent with no peripheral sclerosis or encapsulation. If the lesion involves the periosteum directly or by extension, one may see the typical sunray spicules or "hair-on-end" trabeculae (Fig. 22-7). This occurs when the periosteum is displaced, partially destroyed, and disorganized. If the periosteum is elevated and maintains its osteogenic potential but is breached in the center, a Codman's triangle at the edges is formed (see Fig. 22-1, *E*). Even more rarely, laminar periosteal new bone may be present. In many cases, extension is even more prominent, and a soft tissue mass is visible radiographically.

Internal structure. Osteosarcoma may be entirely radiolucent, mixed radiolucent-radiopaque, or quite radiopaque. The internal osseous structure may take the appearance of granular- or sclerotic-appearing bone, cotton balls, wisps, or honeycombed internal structures in areas with adjacent destruction of the pre-existing osseous architecture. Whatever the resultant internal structure, the normal trabecular structure of the jaws is lost.

Effects on surrounding structures. Widening of the periodontal membrane is associated with osteosarcoma but is also seen in other malignancies (Fig. 22-8). The antral or nasal wall cortices may be lost in maxillary lesions. Mandibular lesions may destroy the cortex of the neurovascular canal and adjacent lamina dura. Alternatively, the neurovascular canal may be symmetrically widened and enlarged. Effects on the periosteum are discussed under the discussion on periphery.

Differential Diagnosis
If internal structure is minimal or absent, fibrosarcoma or metastatic carcinoma may appear similar to osteosarcoma. If osseous structure is visible, the practitioner should also consider chondrosarcoma. If spiculated periosteal new bone is present, prostate and breast metastases should be considered. Comprehensive physical examination and laboratory tests assist in determining whether the lesion is primary or metastatic. Benign tumors such as ossifying fibroma and benign conditions such as fibrous dysplasia may mimic osteosarcoma. The former conditions, however, are usually better demarcated and have a more uniform internal structure. The histopathology of osteosarcoma may be interpreted as a benign fibroosseous lesion, and in these cases, the correct diagnosis may rely on the radiographic characteristics alone. Ewing's sarcoma, solitary plasmacytoma, and even osteomyelitis share some of the radiographic characteristics of osteosarcoma. Osteosarcoma is generally not associated with signs of infection.

Management
The management of osteosarcoma is resection with a large border of adjacent normal bone. This may be possible in orthopedic cases but may be complicated by the presence of important adjacent anatomic structures in

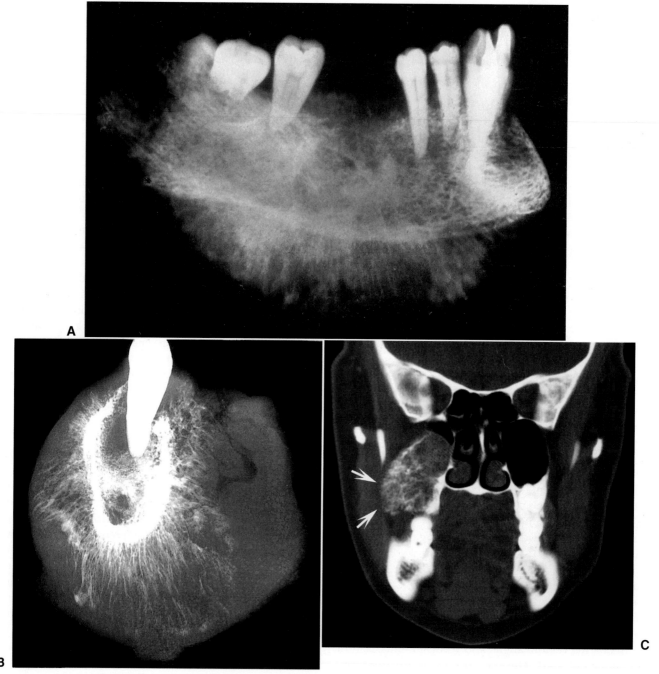

FIG. 22-7   A and B, Radiographs of a resected mandible of a 25-year-old man with osteosarcoma, showing sunray spicules. C, Coronal CT image of an osteosarcoma of the maxilla; note the spiculated bone formation extending laterally from the maxilla (arrows).

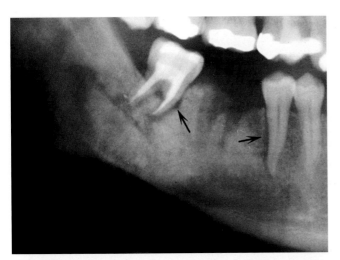

FIG. **22-8** Cropped panoramic image of an osteosarcoma occupying the body of the right mandible. Note the widened ligament spaces *(arrows)* and that the density of the mandible in the first molar region is greater than normal due to abnormal bone formation from the tumor.

the head and neck. Generally radiation therapy and chemotherapy are used only for controlling metastatic spread or for palliation.

CHONDROSARCOMA

Synonym
Chondrogenic sarcoma

Definition
Chondrosarcoma is a malignant tumor of cartilaginous origin. The four histologic subtypes, which develop most commonly in the craniofacial region, are the clear cell, dedifferentiated, myxoid, and mesenchymal forms. They may occur centrally within bone, on the periphery of bone, or less commonly, in soft tissue. They can arise directly from cartilage or may occur within benign cartilaginous tumors. In the case of the latter, they are termed *secondary chondrosarcomas.*

Clinical Features
Chondrosarcomas generally occur at any age, although they are more common in adults (mean age 47 years). They affect males and females equally. A patient with chondrosarcoma may have a firm or hard mass of relatively long duration. Enlargement of these lesions may cause pain, headache, and deformity. Less frequent signs and symptoms include hemorrhage from tumor or from the necks of the teeth, sensory nerve deficits, proptosis, and visual disturbances. Invariably the tumors are covered with normal overlying skin or

mucosa unless secondarily ulcerated. If chondrosarcoma occurs in or near the temporomandibular joint region, trismus or abnormal joint function may result.

Radiographic Features
Location. Chondrosarcomas in the facial bones are unusual, accounting for about 10% of all cases. They occur in the mandible and maxilla with equal frequency. Maxillary lesions typically occur in the anterior region in areas where cartilaginous tissues may be present in the maxilla. Mandibular lesions occur in the coronoid process, condylar head and neck (Fig. 22-9, *B* and *C*), and occasionally the symphyseal region.

Periphery and shape. Chondrosarcomas are slow-growing tumors, and their radiologic signs may be misleading and benign in nature. The lesions are generally round, ovoid, or lobulated. Generally their borders are well defined and at times corticated, whereas at other times they meld with adjacent normal bone. Occasionally peripheral periosteal new bone may be present perpendicular to the original cortex, giving the so-called *sunray* or *hair-on-end* appearance. Uncommonly these lesions are ill defined and invasive. Aggressive lesions such as these have infiltrative, ill-defined, and noncorticated borders.

Internal structure. Chondrosarcomas usually exhibit some form of calcification within their center, giving them a mixed radiolucent-radiopaque appearance. At times this mixture takes the form of moth-eaten bone alternating with islands of residual bone unaffected by tumor. Lesions are rarely completely radiolucent. The central radiopaque structure has been described as flocculent, implying snowlike features. This diffuse calcification may be superimposed on a bony background that resembles granular or ground-glass–appearing abnormal bone (see Fig. 22-9, *A*). Careful examination of these areas of flocculence may reveal a central radiolucent nidus, which is probably cartilage surrounded by calcification. The result is rounded or speckled areas of calcification.

Effects on surrounding structures. Chondrosarcoma, being relatively slow-growing, often expands normal cortical boundaries rather than rapidly destroying them. In mandibular cases the inferior border or alveolar process may be grossly expanded while still maintaining its cortical covering. Maxillary lesions may push the walls of the maxillary sinus or nasal fossa and impinge on the infratemporal fossa. Lesions of the condyle cause its expansion and perhaps remodeling of the corresponding articular fossa and eminence. If lesions occur in the articular disk region, a widened

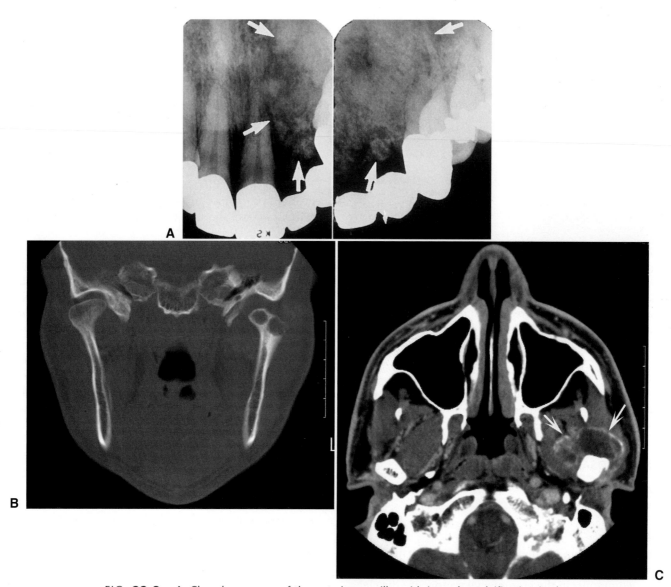

FIG. **22-9** **A,** Chondrosarcoma of the anterior maxilla, with irregular calcification in the internal structure of the tumor *(arrows).* **B,** Coronal CT image using bone algorithm of a chondrosarcoma involving the mandibular condyle; note the two areas of bone destruction. **C,** Axial CT scan using soft tissue algorithm, demonstrating the soft tissue extent of the lesion *(arrows)* and sparse calcifications. (**A,** Courtesy L. Hollender, DDS, Seattle, Wash.)

joint space may be present with corresponding remodeling of the condylar neck. Erosion of the articular fossa may also occur. If lesions occur near teeth, root resorption and tooth displacement may occur, as may widening of the periodontal membrane space.

Differential Diagnosis

Osteosarcoma is often radiographically indistinguishable from chondrosarcoma. Although the typical calcifications of chondrosarcoma may be absent from osteosarcoma, the two share many other radiologic features. Fibrous dysplasia may also be difficult to differentiate from chondrosarcoma because similarities in the internal pattern. (The radiopaque portion of fibrous dysplasia is abnormal bone and not calcification. The calcifications in chondrosarcoma represent calcified cartilage.) Generally, the periphery of fibrous dysplasia is better defined and its margin with adjacent teeth differs from that of chondrosarcoma. For instance, fibrous dysplasia alters the bone pattern up to and including the lamina dura, leaving a normal or thin periodontal ligament space. The greatest danger results from the misleading benign characteristics of chondrosarcoma, which may delay correct diagnosis.

Management

The management of chondrosarcoma is surgical. Radiation therapy and chemotherapy generally have no role to play. Patients with chondrosarcomas have a relatively good 5-year survival rate but poor 10-year survival rate.

EWING'S SARCOMA

Synonyms

Endothelial myeloma and round cell sarcoma

Definition

Ewing's sarcoma is of indeterminate histogenesis. It is a tumor of long bones and is relatively rare in the jaws. Lesions arise in the medullary portion of the bone and spread to the endosteal and later periosteal surfaces.

Clinical Features

Ewing's sarcoma is most common in the second decade of life with most patients being between the ages of 5 and 30 years. Males are twice as likely to manifest the disease as females. In addition, multicentric lesions have been reported. Other reported findings at the time of presentation include, in descending frequency, swelling, pain, loose teeth, paresthesia, exophthalmos, ptosis, epistaxis, ulceration, shifted teeth, trismus, and sinusitis. Cervical lymphadenopathy has also been reported.

Radiographic Features

Location. Mandibular cases outnumber maxillary cases by about 2 to 1, with the highest frequency found in posterior areas in both jaws. Generally the lesions develop within the marrow space first and then extend to involve overlying cortical plates. This neoplasm rarely occurs in the jaws.

Periphery and shape. Ewing's sarcoma is a radiolucency that is poorly demarcated and never corticated. Its advancing edge destroys bone in an uneven fashion, resulting in a ragged border. The lesions are usually solitary and may cause pathologic fracture with adjacent radiographically visible soft tissue masses (Fig. 22-10). They may be round or ovoid but generally have no typical shape.

Internal structure. Ewing's sarcoma is a destructive process with little induction of bone formation. Because it commences on the internal aspect of the bone and involves the endosteal and periosteal surfaces later in its course, it is usually entirely radiolucent.

Effects on surrounding structures. Ewing's sarcoma may stimulate the periosteum to produce new bone. This is usually the result of gross disturbances to the overlying periosteum and takes the form of Codman's triangle or the sunray or hair-on-end spiculation. Laminar

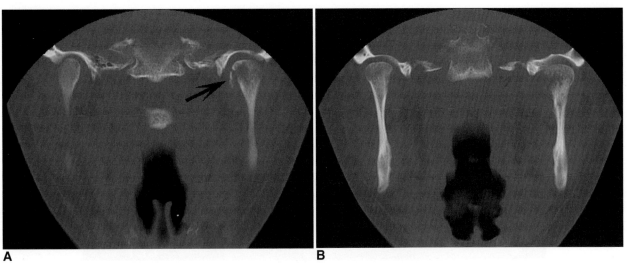

A   **B**

FIG. **22-10** A and B, Coronal CT images using bone algorithm, demonstrating Ewing's sarcoma involving the left mandibular condyle; note the irregular margins, destruction of the medial cortex of the condyle, and a small pathological fracture *(arrow).*

periosteal new bone formation has been reported to occur but is not a common feature of active Ewing's sarcoma lesions. Adjacent normal structures such as the mandibular neurovascular canal, inferior border of the mandible, and alveolar cortical plates may be effaced. If the lesion abuts teeth or tooth follicles, the cortices of these structures are destroyed. This tumor does not characteristically cause root resorption, although it does destroy the supporting bone of adjacent teeth.

Differential Diagnosis

Inflammatory or infectious lesions such as osteomyelitis of the jaw may share some of the radiographic features of Ewing's sarcoma. Although both lesions are radiolucent, osteomyelitis is likely to have demonstrable sequestra present within the confines of the lesion, whereas Ewing's sarcoma does not. Inflammatory lesions contain some sign of reactive bone formation, resulting in some sclerosis internally or at the periphery, and differ in the associated periosteal bone formation.

Another destructive process that occurs in the same part of the bone is eosinophilic granuloma of the jaw. This condition is associated with laminar periosteal bone reaction, whereas Ewing's sarcoma in the jaw is not. The other central primary malignancies of bone such as osteosarcoma, chondrosarcoma, and fibrosarcoma may be difficult to differentiate from this condition.

Management

Too few cases of maxillofacial Ewing's sarcoma have been managed at any single treatment center for any specific treatment policy to have been adopted. Surgery, radiation therapy, and chemotherapy may be used alone or in combination.

FIBROSARCOMA

Definition

Fibrosarcoma is a neoplasm composed of malignant fibroblasts that produce collagen and elastin. The etiology is unknown, although it may arise secondarily in tissues that have received therapeutic levels of radiation.

Clinical Features

These lesions occur equally in males and females with a mean age in the fourth decade. A slowly to rapidly enlarging mass is the usual presenting symptom. The mass may be within bone, in which case it usually is accompanied by pain. Peripheral lesions or those exiting from bone may invade local soft tissues, causing a bulky, clinically obvious lesion. If central or peripheral lesions reach a large size, pathologic fracture may occur. If fibrosarcomas involve the course of peripheral nerves, sensory-neural abnormalities may occur. Overlying mucosa, although initially normal, may become erythematous or ulcerated. Involvement of the temporomandibular joint or paramandibular musculature is often accompanied by trismus.

Radiographic Features

Location. Most cases of fibrosarcoma of the jaws occur in the mandible, with the greatest number of these occurring in the premolar-molar region.

Periphery and shape. Fibrosarcomas have ill-defined borders that are best described as ragged (Fig. 22-11). They are poorly demarcated and noncorticated and lack any semblance of a capsule. These tumors are

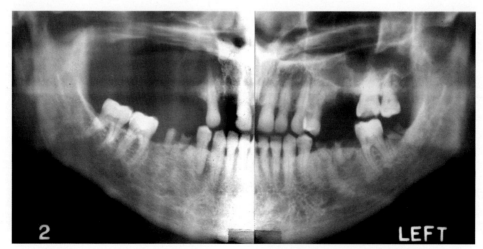

FIG. **22-11**   A fibrosarcoma involving the right maxillary sinus has destroyed the cortical boundaries of the sinus, zygomatic process, hard palate and posterior maxilla, and the alveolar process in this panoramic film.

generally shaped in a fashion that suggests that they have grown along a bone; therefore they tend to be elongated through the marrow space. The radiographic border may underestimate the extent of the tumor because these lesions typically are infiltrative. If soft tissue lesions occur adjacent to bone, they may cause a saucer-like depression in the underlying bone or invade it as would a squamous cell carcinoma. Finally, sclerosis may occur in the adjacent normal bone whether the fibrosarcoma is peripheral to bone or central.

Internal structure. Fibrosarcomas have little internal structure. In most cases the lesions are entirely radiolucent. If the lesions have been present for some time and are not overly aggressive, either residual jawbone or reactive osseous bone formation occurs.

Effects on surrounding structures. The most common effect on adjacent structures is destruction. In the mandible, the alveolar process, inferior border of the jaw, and cortices of the neurovascular canal are lost. In the maxilla, the inferior floor of the maxillary sinus, posterior wall of the maxilla, and nasal floor can be destroyed. In either jaw, lamina dura and follicular cortices are obliterated. Destruction of the outer cortical plate is usually accompanied by a protruding soft tissue mass. Root resorption is uncommon. Teeth are more likely to be grossly displaced and lose their support bone so that they appear to be floating in space. In addition, widening of the periodontal membrane space occurs with this tumor, as in other malignancies. Periosteal reaction is uncommon; however, if the lesion disrupts the periosteum, a Codman's triangle or sunray spiculation may be evident.

Differential Diagnosis
This solitary, ragged radiolucency with little internal structure is difficult to differentiate from other central malignancies. If the lesion does not cause enlargement of the jaw, the practitioner must rule out metastatic carcinoma, multiple myeloma, and primary or secondary intraosseous carcinoma. Another possibility is a grossly infected dental cyst, although this condition usually shows some degree of induced peripheral sclerosis in adjacent bone. If a fibrosarcoma exhibits enlargement of the affected jaw with an associated soft tissue mass, other sarcomas such as chondrosarcoma or osteosarcoma (both usually have internal structure) should be ruled out. Ewing's sarcoma and radiolucent osteosarcomas may not be distinguishable from this tumor. Finally, peripheral invasive squamous cell carcinoma shares some of these radiologic features, but its ulcerative surface features differentiate it from fibrosarcoma, which usually lacks these.

Management
The management of fibrosarcoma is chiefly surgical. A wide margin of adjacent normal bone is taken if anatomically possible. Radiation therapy and chemotherapy are usually reserved for palliation.

Malignancies of the Hematopoietic System

MULTIPLE MYELOMA
Synonyms
Myeloma, plasma cell myeloma, and plasmacytoma

Definition
Multiple myeloma is a malignant neoplasm of plasma cells. It is the most common malignancy of bone in adults. Single lesions are called *plasmacytoma*, and multiple lesions are termed *multiple myeloma*.

Clinical Features
Multiple myeloma is a fatal systemic malignancy. A patient with multiple myeloma is usually between the ages of 35 and 70 years (mean age 60 years). The patient may complain of fatigue, weight loss, fever, bone pain, and anemia, although the typical presenting feature is low back pain. Secondary signs include amyloidosis and hypercalcemia. In half of all patients, characteristic Bence Jones protein is present in the urine, which causes the urine to be foamy. The disease is more common in men. When this clonal cellular proliferation occurs, these cells occupy first cancellous and later cortical bone, replacing the normally radiopaque bone with areas of radiolucency.

Orally, patients may complain of dental pain, swelling, hemorrhage, paresthesia, and dysesthesia, or they may have no complaints. The number of patients with demonstrable radiologic findings in the jaws at the time of diagnosis is relatively small.

Radiographic Features
Location. Multiple myeloma (Fig. 22-12) is seen more frequently in the mandible than the maxilla but is uncommon in either. The incidence of jaw involvement has been reported to vary from 2% to 78%. In the mandible the posterior body and ramus is favored. Maxillary lesions usually appear in posterior sites.

Periphery and shape. The periphery of multiple myeloma lesions is well defined but not corticated and lack any sign of bone reaction (Fig. 22-13). The lesions have been described as appearing "punched out." However, many appear ragged and even infiltrative.

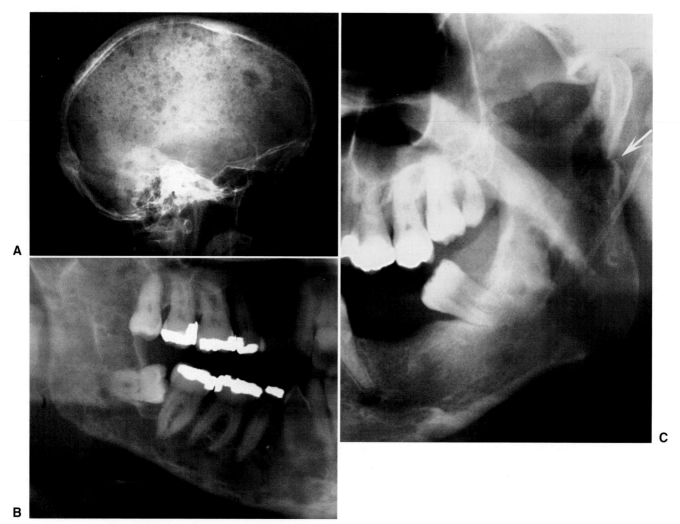

FIG. **22-12**   Multiple myeloma, seen as multiple circular radiolucent lesions in the skull **(A)**. In a different case **(B)** multiple small lesions of multiple myeloma are present through the body and ramus of the mandible in this cropped panoramic image. **C,** Cropped panoramic image shows a solitary lesion in the condylar neck region and a pathologic fracture *(arrow)*.

Some lesions have an oval or cystic shape. Untreated or aggressive areas of destruction may become confluent, giving the appearance of multilocularity. If the lesion is located in the periapical periodontal ligament space, it may have a border similar to that seen in inflammatory or infectious periapical disease. Soft tissue lesions have been reported in the jaws and nasopharynx. When visible on radiographs, they appear as smooth-bordered soft tissue masses, possibly with underlying bone destruction.

Internal structure.   No internal structure is radiographically visible. Occasionally islands of residual bone, yet unaffected by tumor, give the appearance of the presence of new trabecular bone within the mass. Very rarely the lesions appear radiopaque internally.

Effects on surrounding structures.   If a good deal of bone mineral is lost, teeth may appear to be "too opaque" and may stand out conspicuously from their osteopenic background. Lamina dura and follicles of impacted teeth may lose their typical corticated surrounding bone in a manner analogous to that seen in hyperparathyroidism. The same may be said of the mandibular neurovascular canal, which, although usually visible, loses its cortical boundary in whole or in

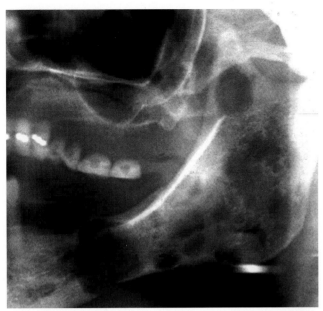

FIG. **22-13** Panoramic radiograph depicting multiple areas of well-defined bone destruction lacking any cortical boundary. The lesions are multiple and separate and appear to be "punched out," typical of changes seen in multiple myeloma. (Courtesy G. Petrikowski, DDS, Toronto, Ontario, Canada.)

part. These changes are profound when there is associated renal disease. Mandibular lesions may cause thinning of the lower border of the mandible or endosteal scalloping. Any cortical boundary may be effaced if lesions involve them. Periosteal reaction is uncommon, but if present, it takes the form of a single radiopaque line or more rarely a sunray appearance.

Differential Diagnosis

The most likely disease to be mistaken for multiple myeloma is the radiolucent form of metastatic carcinoma. Knowledge of a prior malignancy in a patient may help differentiate multiple myeloma from metastatic carcinoma. Osteomyelitis, if severe, may yield a radiologic picture similar to that of multiple myeloma; however, a visible cause for it usually exists. In addition, inflammatory lesions and infections in general cause sclerosis in adjacent bone, whereas multiple myeloma does not. Simple bone cysts may be bilateral in the mandible and therefore may be mistaken for multiple myeloma. They are usually corticated in part and characteristically interdigitate between the roots of the teeth in a much younger population. Generalized radiolucency of the jaws may be caused by hyperparathyroidism but is differentiated based on abnormal blood chemistry. However, brown tumors of hyperparathyroidism,

if present with generalized radiolucency of the jaws and similar symptomology, can readily be confused with multiple myeloma radiographically. Other metabolic diseases such as thalassemia, Gaucher's disease or oxalosis may cause many of the changes similar to multiple myeloma that are observed on dental radiographs but may be ruled out on the basis of the medical history.

Management

The management of multiple myeloma is usually chemotherapeutic, with or without autologous or allogeneic bone marrow transplantation. Radiation therapy may be used for treatment of symptomatic osseous lesions when palliation is required.

Non-Hodgkin's Lymphoma

Synonyms

Malignant lymphoma and lymphosarcoma

Definition

Non-Hodgkin's lymphoma is a malignant tumor of cells normally resident in the lymphatic system. In general, lymphomas occur within lymph nodes; however, extranodal sites such as bone, skin, gastrointestinal mucosa, tonsils, and Waldeyer's ring can be involved. The term *non-Hodgkin's lymphoma* describes a family of heterogeneous tumors of varying type and severity. The classification of these diseases is difficult, and numerous means exist of subdividing these tumors. Currently the working formulation for clinical usage classifies tumors based on their histologic appearance into low-grade, intermediate-grade, or high-grade tumors, with the last classification being the most aggressive.

Clinical Features

Non-Hodgkin's lymphoma occurs in all age groups but is rare in patients in the first decade. The maxillary sinus, palate, tonsillar area, and bone may be sites of primary or secondary lymphoma spread. Lesions occurring outside lymph nodes in the head and neck are present in as much as 1 out of 5 cases. Patients may feel unwell, experiencing night sweats, pruritus, and weight loss. Palpable painless swelling, lymphadenopathy, and sensorineural deficits may accompany isolated lesions of the jaws. Lesions present for some time may cause pain and ulceration. Teeth resident in a lymphoma may become mobile, as the supporting bone is lost.

Radiographic Features

Location. Most non-Hodgkin's lymphomas of the head and neck occur in the lymph nodes. Those that are extranodal are likely to affect the maxillary sinus, posterior mandible, and maxillary regions.

Periphery and shape. Most non-Hodgkin's lymphomas initially take the shape and form of the host bone. If untreated, however, they are capable of causing destruction of the overlying cortex (Fig. 22-14). They may appear rounded or multiloculated and lack a defining outer cortex. Generally the borders are ill defined and invasive. Occasionally, lymphoma appears as multiple areas of destruction, which likely appear as fingerlike extensions of malignant tumor cells in a buccal or lingual direction. Visible lesions occurring in the maxillary sinus or nasopharynx have a smooth periphery.

Internal structure. The internal structure of lymphoma is almost always entirely radiolucent. It is rare to see reactive bone formation. Occasionally patchy radiopacity may be present, but this is rare.

Effects on surrounding structures. In maxillary sinus lesions the antral walls may be effaced and a soft tissue mass may be visible radiographically, either internally within the sinus or external to the maxillary sinus. Lesions involving the mandible destroy the cortex of the neurovascular canal. This tumor has a propensity to grow in the periodontal ligament space of mature teeth (Fig. 22-15). The cortex of the crypts of developing teeth may be lost when the lymphoma is located in the developing papilla, and the involved teeth may be displaced in an occlusal direction and exfoliated. Periosteal reaction is not common but may take the form of laminated or spiculated bone formation. With the advent of soft tissue imaging with MRI, it has become apparent that this tumor has a habit of growing along soft tissue spaces (fat layers) and along the surface of bone.

Differential Diagnosis

Multiple myeloma and metastatic carcinoma are easily confused with non-Hodgkin's lymphoma of the jaws. However, Ewing's sarcoma and Langerhans' histiocytosis, although also capable of producing the same effects, occur in a slightly younger age group. Osteolytic osteosarcoma and any of the central squamous cell carcinomas may not be radiographically distinguishable from non-Hodgkin's lymphoma. Squamous cell carcinoma arising in the maxillary sinus may be difficult to differentiate from lymphoma of the maxillary sinus. Other lesions that can displace developing teeth in an occlusal direction include leukemia and Langerhans' histiocytosis. Differentiation from apical rarefying osteitis may be difficult; however, careful inspection of the radiographic film may reveal the presence of an infiltrative border and adjacent bone destruction.

Management

The management of extranodal or isolated nodal disease is radiation therapy with or without concomitant chemotherapy. Treatment depends on histologic variants and the location and extent of disease.

BURKITT'S LYMPHOMA

Synonym

African jaw lymphoma

Definition

Burkitt's lymphoma is a high-grade B cell lymphoma that differs from other B cell lymphomas with respect to its histologic appearance and clinical behavior. It was first described by Denis Burkitt in East Africa as *African jaw lymphoma.*

Two separate forms of the disease have been described: the endemic African Burkitt's lymphoma and the American form. The latter is not characterized by jaw involvement (although it occurs), but by involvement of abdominal viscera. African Burkitt's lymphoma affects young children, whereas American Burkitt's lymphoma affects adolescents and young adults. Cases of endemic and nonendemic Burkitt's tumor have been described throughout the world.

Clinical Features

The disease affects more males than females. Clinically the hallmark of this tumor is rapidity of growth, with a tumor doubling time of less than 24 hours. It may involve children as young as 2 years and adults in their seventh decade, although it is primarily a disease of youth. Jaw tumors are rapidly growing and cause facial deformity very early in their course. They are capable of blocking nasal passages, displacing orbital contents, causing gross facial swelling, and eroding through skin. These rapidly growing tumors are more characteristic of African Burkitt's lymphoma than the American form and cause pain and paresthesia. Teeth may become rapidly loosened and alveolar bone grossly distended. Paresthesia of the inferior alveolar nerve or other sensory facial nerves is common.

Radiographic Features

Location. Extranodal disease is the norm in Burkitt's tumor. African cases may involve one jaw or both the maxilla and mandible and affect the posterior parts of the jaws. By contrast, American cases may not involve the facial bones but are more likely to affect the abdominal viscera and testes.

Periphery and shape. The lesions may begin as multiple, ill-defined, noncorticated radiolucencies, which

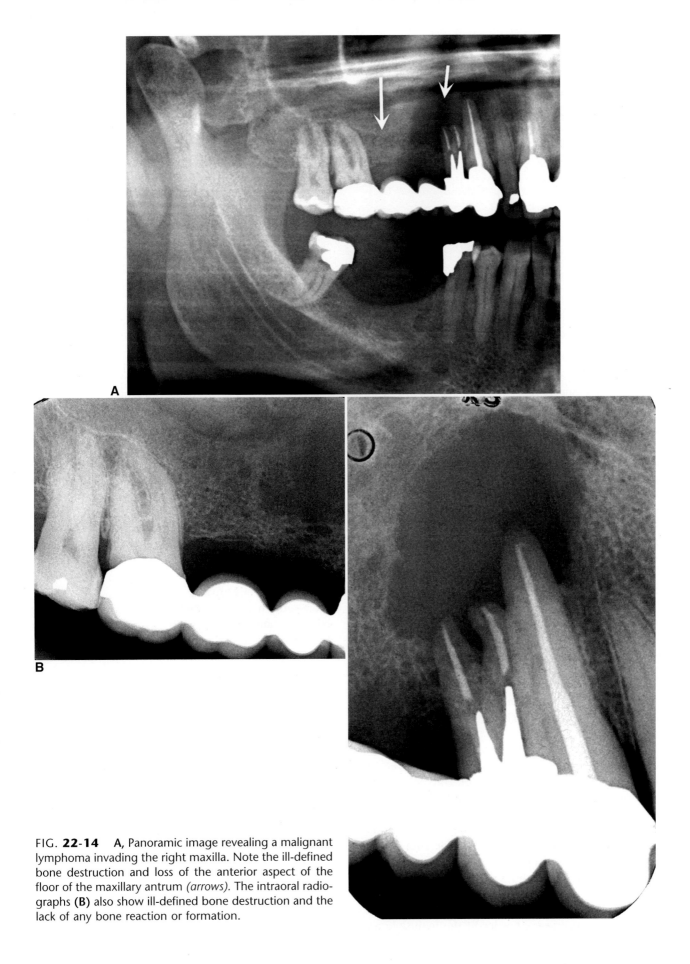

FIG. **22-14** **A,** Panoramic image revealing a malignant lymphoma invading the right maxilla. Note the ill-defined bone destruction and loss of the anterior aspect of the floor of the maxillary antrum *(arrows).* The intraoral radiographs **(B)** also show ill-defined bone destruction and the lack of any bone reaction or formation.

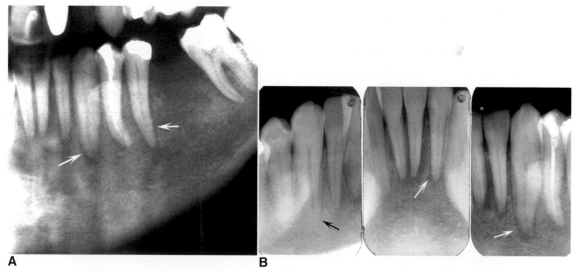

FIG. 22-15 Cropped panoramic image **(A)** revealing an ill-defined lymphoma invading the left body of the mandible; note the irregular widening of the periodontal ligament spaces *(arrows)* and intraoral films of the same case **(B)**. Note the widened periodontal ligament spaces *(white arrows)* compared with the normal periodontal ligament space of the right mandibular cuspid *(black arrow)*.

later coalesce into larger, ill-defined radiolucencies with an expansile periphery. They are of no specific shape, although they expand rapidly and have been likened to a balloon. This expansion breaches its outer cortical limits, causing gross balloon-like expansion with thinning of adjacent structures and production of a soft tissue tumor mass adjacent to the osseous lesion. Lesions that abut the orbital contents or the maxillary sinus may show a smooth surface soft tissue mass radiologically.

Internal structure. Burkitt's lymphoma does not produce bone and rarely induces production of reactive bone within its center. For this reason, the lesions are radiolucent in almost all cases. It is particularly radiolucent in the jaw of a child.

Effects on surrounding structures. Erupted teeth in the area of Burkitt's tumor are grossly displaced, as are developing tooth crypts. Tumor cells within the crypt may displace the developing tooth bud to one side of its crypt. A tumor that is located apical to a developing tooth may cause it to be displaced such that it appears to erupt with little if any root formation. After tumor involvement of the developing dental structures occurs, root development ceases. Lamina dura of teeth in the area is destroyed, and cortical boundaries such as the maxillary sinus, nasal floor, orbital walls, and inferior border of the mandible are thinned and later destroyed. The cortex of the inferior

alveolar canal is lost, although it is difficult to see in the normal pediatric patient in any case. If periosteum is involved, the border may show sunray spiculation, although this is rare. Cases that involve the orbit displace the orbital contents, seen both clinically and radiologically.

Differential Diagnosis

Metastatic neuroblastoma may give similar changes clinically and radiologically, as may Ewing's tumor. Osteolytic osteosarcoma can grow rapidly and may be indistinguishable from Burkitt's tumor on clinical and radiologic grounds. Cherubism has more internal structure, does not breach bony borders, is bilateral, and grows much more slowly. Finally, non-Hodgkin's lymphoma must be considered, although it occurs in a much older age group in most cases.

Management

The management of Burkitt's tumor is chemotherapeutic. Chemotherapy regimens vary from geographic locales, but the tumor is exquisitely sensitive to combinations of chemotherapeutic agents.

LEUKEMIA

Synonyms

Acute myelogenous leukemia, acute lymphoblastic leukemia, chronic myelogenous leukemia, and chronic lymphocytic leukemia

Definition

Leukemia is a malignant tumor of hematopoietic stem cells. These malignant cells displace normal bone marrow constituents and spill out into the peripheral blood. They are subdivided into acute leukemias and chronic leukemias and further subdivided by the cell of origin. The acute leukemias occur with a bimodal age distribution, with very young patients and very old patients being the most commonly affected. Most cases of leukemia are associated with nonrandom chromosomal abnormalities.

Clinical Features

The patient with chronic leukemia may have no presenting signs or complaints. Acute leukemia patients generally feel unwell with weakness and bone pain. They may exhibit pallor, spontaneous hemorrhage, hepatomegaly, splenomegaly, lymphadenopathy, and fever. Oral symptoms are generally absent but if present include loose teeth, petechiae, ulceration, and boggy, enlarged gingiva.

Radiographic Features

Radiologic signs associated with chronic leukemia are comparatively rare.

Location. Leukemia affects the entire body, because it is a malignancy of bone marrow, which discharges malignant cells into circulating blood. Its manifestations in the jaws may be seen more often in areas of developing teeth. Frequently, leukemia may be localized around the periapical region of a tooth, giving the appearance of a rarefying osteitis.

Periphery and shape. Leukemia must be considered a systemic malignancy, and as such its oral radiologic features may be present bilaterally as ill-defined, patchy radiolucent areas. With time and lack of treatment, these patchy areas may coalesce to form larger areas of ill-defined radiolucent regions of bone (Fig. 22-16). The teeth may appear to stand out conspicuously from their surrounding, osteopenic bone.

Internal structure. The internal structure of leukemia is characterized by patchy areas of radiolucency and generalized radiolucency of the bone. Rarely, granular bone may be seen within these lesions. Occasionally, foci of leukemic cells may be present as a mass that may behave like a localized malignant tumor. These lesions are called *chloromas* and are rare in the jaws.

Effects on surrounding structures. Leukemia does not cause expansion of bone, although occasionally a single layer of periosteal new bone may be seen in association with the disease, this being uncommon in chronic leukemia. Developing teeth in their crypts and teeth undergoing eruption may be displaced in an occlusal direction (Fig. 22-17) or into the oral cavity before root development. Less commonly, developing teeth may be displaced from their normal position. The result of this is premature loss of teeth. The lamina dura and cortical outlines of follicles may be effaced. If lesions

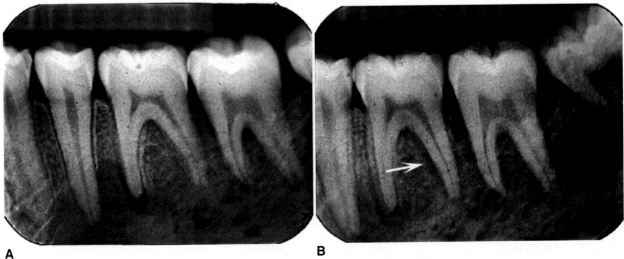

A   **B**

FIG. **22-16**   A and B, Periapical radiographs of the left mandible illustrating multifocal areas of bone destruction and widening of portions of the periodontal ligament space *(arrow)* characteristic of infiltration of the mandible with leukemia.

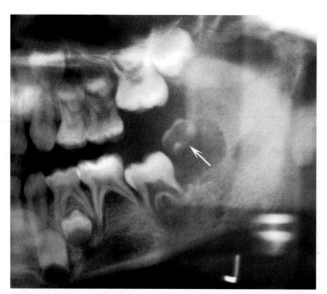

FIG. **22-17** Cropped panoramic film demonstrating occlusal displacement of the developing mandibular second molar out of its follicle *(arrow).*

affect the periodontal structures, the crestal bone may be lost.

Differential Diagnosis

Generally, by the time oral radiologic signs of leukemia are present, a medical diagnosis has been reached. However, the development of radiologic changes may be the first indication of the relapse of treatment. Occasionally lymphoma or neuroblastoma may mimic some of the features of destruction seen in leukemia. Metabolic disorders may be considered in those cases in which generalized rarefaction of bone is seen. These conditions are all excluded based on blood testing. With apical lesions, careful examination of the involved tooth clinically and radiologically typically shows no apparent cause for rarefying osteitis.

Management

The management of leukemia is primarily through a combination of chemotherapy with or without allogeneic or autologous bone marrow transplantation. Some chronic leukemias are managed with low-dose chemotherapy.

Dental Radiology for the Cancer Survivor

The cancer survivor requires dental treatment just as any other patient. For the cancer survivor, dental radi-

ologic examination may be more important than for a healthy patient receiving a routine examination. Some patients who have received a full course of radiation therapy are concerned about the additional exposure from a dental radiographic examination. Such patients should be assured that this exposure is not a danger, because the small dose associated with dental radiographic examinations is negligible compared with the radiation dose received from cancer therapy.

The patient treated for head and neck malignancy with radiation therapy is prone to develop postradiation dental caries and osteoradionecrosis. Careful clinical examination and a thorough dental radiologic examination may be required periodically to ensure that the remaining dentition and periodontal apparatus is in good shape. Radiation caries occur in many patients and appear clinically different from typical dental caries. If untreated, these carious teeth become nonvital and may cause infection in the underlying jaw. If they require extraction, healing can be expected to be slow and occasionally osteoradionecrosis may result.

The role of radiology in these patients, however, is not restricted to examination of the teeth and supporting structures. Equally important is the monitoring of the outcome of treatment and specifically the examination of dental radiographs for evidence of tumor recurrence, development of metastases, and osteoradionecrosis.

BIBLIOGRAPHY

SQUAMOUS CELL CARCINOMA

Casiglia J, Woo SB: A comprehensive review of oral cancer, Gen Dent 49:72, 2001.

Carter RL: Patterns and mechanisms of spread of squamous carcinomas of the oral cavity, Clin Otolaryngol 15:185, 1990.

Marchetta FC, Sako K, Murphy JB: The periosteum of the mandible and intraoral carcinoma, Am J Surg 122:711, 1971.

McGregor AD, MacDonald D: Routes of entry of squamous cell carcinoma to the mandible, Head Neck Surg 10:284, 1988.

Noyek AM et al: The radiologic diagnosis of malignant tumors of the paranasal sinuses and related structures, J Otolaryngol 6:399, 1977.

O'Brien CJ et al: Invasions of the mandible by squamous carcinomas of the oral cavity and oropharynx, Head Neck Surg 8:247, 1986.

SQUAMOUS CELL CARCINOMA ORIGINATING IN BONE

Ariji E et al: Central squamous cell carcinoma of the mandible: computed tomographic findings, Oral Surg Oral Med Oral Pathol 77:541, 1994.

Elzay RP: Primary intra-osseous carcinoma of the jaws, Oral Surg Oral Med Oral Pathol 54:299, 1982.

Yoshikazu S et al: Primary intra-osseous carcinoma: review of the literature and diagnostic criteria, J Oral Maxillofac Surg 52:580, 1994.

SQUAMOUS CELL CARCINOMA ORGINATING IN A CYST

Dabbs DJ et al: Squamous cell carcinoma arising in recurrent odontogenic keratocyst, Head and Neck 16:375, 1994.

Eversole LR, Sabre WR, Lovin S: Aggressive growth and neoplastic potential of odontogenic cysts, Cancer 35:270, 1975.

Kaffe I et al: Radiological features of primary intra-osseous carcinoma of the jaws: analysis of the literature and report of a new case, Dentomaxillofac Radiol 27:209, 1998.

van der Wal, KGH, de Visscher JGAM, Eggink HF: Squamous cell carcinoma arising in a residual cyst, Int J Oral Maxillofac Surg 23:350, 1993.

MUCOEPIDERMOID CARCINOMA

Bilge OM, Dayi E: Central mucoepidermoid carcinoma of the jaws: review of the literature and case report, Ann Dentistry 51:36, 1992.

Browand BC, Waldron CA: Central mucoepidermoid tumors of the jaws: report of nine cases and review of the literature, Oral Surg Oral Med Oral Pathol 40:631, 1975.

Freije JE et al: Central mucoepidermoid carcinoma of the mandible, Otolaryngol Head Neck Surg 112:453, 1995.

Lopez JI, Elizalde JM, Landa S: Central mucoepidermoid carcinoma: report of a case and review of the literature, Pathol Res Pract 189:365, 368, 1993.

Sidoni A et al: Central mucoepidermoid carcinoma of the mandible, J Oral Maxillofac Surg 54:1242, 1996.

MALIGNANT AMELOBLASTOMA AND AMELOBLASTIC CARCINOMA

Ameerally P, McGurk M, Shaheen O: Atypical ameloblastoma: report of three cases and review of the literature, Br J Oral Maxillofac Surg 34:235, 1996.

Buff SJ et al: Pulmonary metastasis from ameloblastoma of the mandible: report of a case and review of the literature, J Oral Surg 38:374, 1980.

Slootweg PJ, Muller H: Malignant ameloblastoma or ameloblastic carcinoma, Oral Surg Oral Med Oral Pathol 57:168, 1984.

METASTATIC TUMORS

Ciola B: Oral radiographic manifestations of a metastatic prostatic carcinoma, Oral Surg 52:105, 1981.

Mast HL, Nissenblatt MJ: Metastatic colon carcinoma to the jaw: a case report and review of the literature, J Surg Oncol 34:202, 1987.

Mucitelli DR, Zuna RE, Archard HO: Hepatocellular carcinoma presenting as an oral cavity lesion, Oral Surg Oral Med Oral Pathol 66:701, 1988.

Nevins A et al: Metastatic carcinoma of the mandible mimicking periapical lesion of endodontic origin, Endod Dent Traumatol 4:238, 1988.

Redman RS, Behrens AS, Calhoun NR: Carcinoma of the lung presenting as a mandibular metastasis, J Oral Maxillofac Surg 40:745, 1982.

Vigneul JC et al: Metastatic hepatocellular carcinoma of the mandible, J Oral Maxillofac Surg 40:745, 1982.

OSTEOGENIC SARCOMA

Batsakis JG: Osteogenic and chondrogenic sarcomas of the jaws, Ann Otol Rhinol Laryngol 96:474, 1987.

Chindia ML: Osteosarcoma of the jaw bones, Oral Oncol 37:545, 2001.

Clark JL et al: Osteosarcoma of the jaw, Cancer 51:2311, 1983.

Gardner DG, Mills DM: The widened periodontal ligament of osteosarcoma of the jaws, Oral Surg 41:652, 1976.

Seeger LL, Gold RH, Chandnani VP: Diagnostic imaging of osteosarcoma, Clin Orthop Rel Res 270:254, 1991.

Vener J, Rice DH, Newman AN: Osteosarcoma and chondrosarcoma of the head and neck, Laryngoscope 94:240, 1984.

CHONDROSARCOMA

Garrington GE, Collett WK: Chondrosarcoma. I. A selected literature review, J Oral Pathol 17:1, 1988.

Garrington GE, Collett WK: Chondrosarcoma. II. Chondrosarcoma of the jaws: analysis of 37 cases, J Oral Pathol 17:12, 1988.

Gorsky M, Epstein JB: Craniofacial osseous and chondromatous sarcomas in British Columbia: a review of 34 cases, Oral Oncol 36:27, 2000.

Hertzanu Y et al: Chondrosarcoma of the head and neck—the value of computed tomography, J Surg Oncol 28:97, 1985.

Vener J, Rice D, Newman AN: Osteosarcoma and chondrosarcoma of the head and neck, Laryngoscope 94:240, 1984.

EWING'S SARCOMA

Dahlin DC, Coventry MB, Scanlon PW: Ewing's sarcoma, J Bone Joint Surg 2:185, 1961.

Greer RO, Mierau GW, Favara BE: Tumors of the head and neck in children, New York, 1983, Praeger.

Wood RE et al: Ewing's sarcoma, Oral Surg Oral Med Oral Pathol 69:120, 1990.

FIBROSARCOMA

Dahlin DC: Bone tumors, Springfield, Ill, 1981, Charles C Thomas.

Huvos AG: Bone tumors, Philadelphia, 1979, WB Saunders.

O'Day RA, Soule EH, Goresg RJ: Soft tissue sarcomas of the oral cavity, Mayo Clin Proc 39:169, 1964.

Slootweg PJ, Miller H: Fibrosarcoma of the jaws, J Maxillofac Surg 12:157, 1984.

Taconis WK, van Rijssel TG: Fibrosarcoma of the jaws, Skeletal Radiol 15:10, 1986.

van Blarcom CW, Masson JMK, Dahlin DC: Fibrosarcoma of the mandible, Oral Surg 32:428, 1971.

RHABDOMYOSARCOMA

Bras J, Batsakis JG, Luna MA: Rhabdomyosarcoma of the oral soft tissues, Oral Surg 64:585, 1987.

Grieman RB, Katsikeris NK, Symington JM: Rhabdomyosarcoma of the maxillary sinus. Review of the literature and report of a case, J Oral Maxillofac Surg 46:1090, 1988.

Masson JK, Soule EH: Embryonal rhabdomyosarcoma of the head and neck. Report of 88 cases, Am J Surg 110:585, 1965.

Sekhar Ms, Desai S, Kumar GS: Alveolar Rhabdomyosarcoma Involving The Jaws: A Case Report. J Oral Maxillofac Surg. 58:1062, 2000.

Stobbe GD, Dargeon HW: Embryonal rhabdomyosarcoma of the head and neck in children and adolescents, Cancer 3:826, 1950.

MULTIPLE MYELOMA

Furutani M, Ohnishi M, Tanaka Y: Mandibular involvement in patients with multiple myeloma, J Oral Maxillofac Surg 52:23, 1994.

Huvos AG: Bone tumors, Philadelphia, 1979, WB Saunders.

Kaffe I, Ramon Y, Hertz M: Radiographic manifestations of multiple myeloma in the mandible, Dentomaxillofac Radiol 15:31, 1986.

Witt C: Radiographic manifestations of multiple myeloma in the mandible: a retrospective study of 77 patients, J Oral Maxillofac Surg. 55:450, 1997.

NON-HODGKIN'S LYMPHOMA

Dahlin DC: Bone tumors, ed 3, Springfield, Ill, 1981, Charles C Thomas.

Daramola JO, Ajagbe HA: Presentation and behavior of primary malignant lymphoma of the oral cavity in adult Africans, J Oral Med 1983; 38(4):177-9.

Maxymiw WG, Goldstein M, Wood RE: Extranodal non-Hodgkin's lymphoma of the maxillofacial region: analysis of 88 consecutive cases, SADJ. 56:524, 2001.

BURKITT'S LYMPHOMA

Adatia AK: Radiology of Burkitt's tumour in the jaws, East Afr Med J 43:290, 1966.

Adatia AK: Significance of jaw lesions in Burkitt's lymphoma, Br Dent J 145:263, 1978.

Burkitt DA: Sarcoma involving the jaws in African children, Br J Surg 46:218, 1958.

Levine PH et al: The American Burkitt's lymphoma registry: eight years' experience, Cancer 49:1016, 1982.

Sariban E, Donahue A, Magrath IT: Jaw involvement in American Burkitt's lymphoma, Cancer 53:1777, 1984.

LEUKEMIA

Curtis AB: Childhood leukemias: initial oral manifestations, JADA 83:159, 1971.

Ficarra G et al: Granulocytic sarcoma (chloroma) of the oral cavity: a case with a leukemic presentation, Oral Surg 53:709, 1987.

Greer RO, Mierau GW, Favara BE: Tumors of the head and neck in children, New York, 1983, Praeger Scientific.

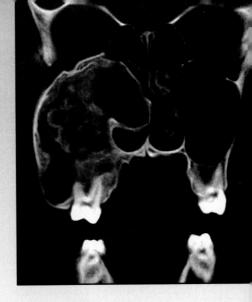

CHAPTER 23

Diseases of Bone Manifested in the Jaws

This chapter discusses disorders of bone that do not easily fit into well-defined categories of disease.

Bone Dysplasias

Bone dysplasias constitute a group of conditions in which normal bone is replaced with fibrous tissue containing abnormal bone or cementum. These lesions must be differentiated from tumors, because the treatment is very different. *Fibroosseous lesion* is a commonly used term that includes the following bone dysplasias, as well as neoplasms and other lesions of bone.

FIBROUS DYSPLASIA

Definition
Fibrous dysplasia results from a localized change in normal bone metabolism that leads to the replacement of all the components of cancellous bone by fibrous tissue containing varying amounts of abnormal-appearing bone. Histologically, this results in the appearance of numerous short, irregularly shaped trabeculae of woven bone. These trabeculae are not aligned in response to stress but rather have a random orientation. This histologic appearance is responsible for the internal pattern seen in radiographs. Fibrous dysplasias may be solitary or multiple (Jaffe type) or may occur in another multiple form associated with McCune-Albright syndrome, which usually comprises polyostotic fibrous dysplasia, cutaneous pigmentation (café au lait spots), and hyperfunction of one or more of the endocrine glands.

Clinical Features
The solitary (monostotic) form of fibrous dysplasia, which accounts for 70% of all cases, is the type that most often involves the jaws. The most common sites (in order) are the ribs, femur, tibia, maxilla, and mandible. The multiple (polyostotic) form usually is found in children less than 10 years, whereas monostotic disease typically is discovered in a slightly older age group. The lesions usually become static when skeletal growth stops, but proliferation may continue, particularly in the polyostotic form. The lesions may become active in pregnant females or with the use of oral contraceptives; this condition has been reported to occur after surgical intervention in young patients. Studies of the sex distribution of fibrous dysplasia show no sexual predilection except for McCune-Albright syndrome, which affects females almost exclusively. Symptoms of the disease may be mild or absent. Monostotic fibrous dysplasia often is discovered as an incidental radiographic finding. Patients with jaw involvement first may complain of unilateral facial swelling or an enlarging deformity of the alveolar process. Pain and pathologic fractures are rare. If extensive craniofacial lesions have impinged on nerve foramina, neurologic symptoms such as anosmia (loss of the sense of smell), deafness, or blindness may develop.

Radiographic Features
Location. Fibrous dysplasia involves the maxilla almost twice as often as the mandible and occurs more frequently in the posterior aspect. Lesions more commonly are unilateral (Fig. 23-1) except for very rare extensive lesions of the maxillofacial region that are bilateral.

485

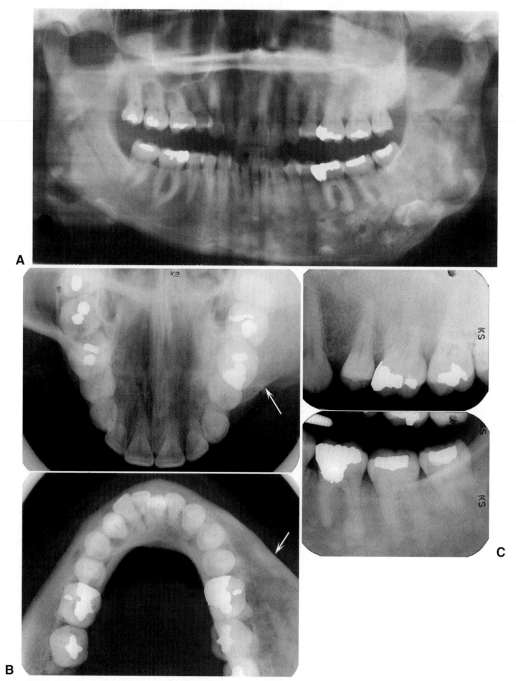

FIG. **23-1**   **A,** Unilateral fibrous dysplasia involving the left maxilla and mandible. **B,** Note the expansion of the lateral aspect of the maxilla and mandible *(arrow)* and the increased bone density caused by an increase in the number of internal trabeculae. **C,** Periapical films show a mixed radiolucent-radiopaque internal structure; however, the overall radiopacity is greater than on the right side of the jaws.

Periphery. The periphery of fibrous dysplasia lesions most commonly is ill defined, with a gradual blending of normal trabecular bone into an abnormal trabecular pattern. Occasionally the boundary between normal bone and the lesion can appear sharp and even corticated, especially in young lesions (Fig. 23-2).

Internal structure. The density and trabecular pattern of fibrous dysplasia lesions vary considerably. The variation is more pronounced in the mandible and more homogeneous in the maxilla. The internal aspect of bone may be more radiolucent, more radiopaque, or a mixture of these two variations compared with normal bone (see Fig. 23-1). The internal density is more

radiopaque in the maxilla and the base of the skull. Early lesions may be more radiolucent (Fig. 23-3) than mature lesions and in rare cases may appear to have granular internal septa, giving the internal aspect a multilocular appearance.

The abnormal trabeculae usually are shorter, thinner, irregularly shaped, and more numerous than normal trabeculae. This creates a radiopaque pattern that can vary; it may have a granular appearance ("ground-glass" appearance, resembling the small fragments of a shattered windshield), a pattern resembling the surface of an orange (peau d'orange), a wispy arrangement (cotton wool), or an amorphous, dense pattern (Fig. 23-4). A distinctive characteristic is the

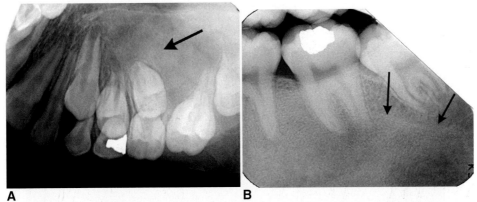

FIG. 23-2 **A,** Fibrous dysplasia in the posterior maxilla, with an ill-defined anterior margin that blends into the normal bone pattern in the region of the unerupted cuspid. The internal pattern is granular *(arrow)*. **B,** In contrast, the margin of this case of mandibular fibrous dysplasia has a well-defined, almost corticated margin *(arrows)*.

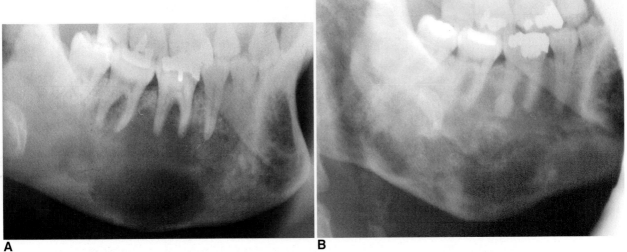

FIG. 23-3 Fibrous dysplasia in the mandible. **A,** Early radiolucent stage. **B,** Same case, 18 years later shows a more mature radiopaque appearance.

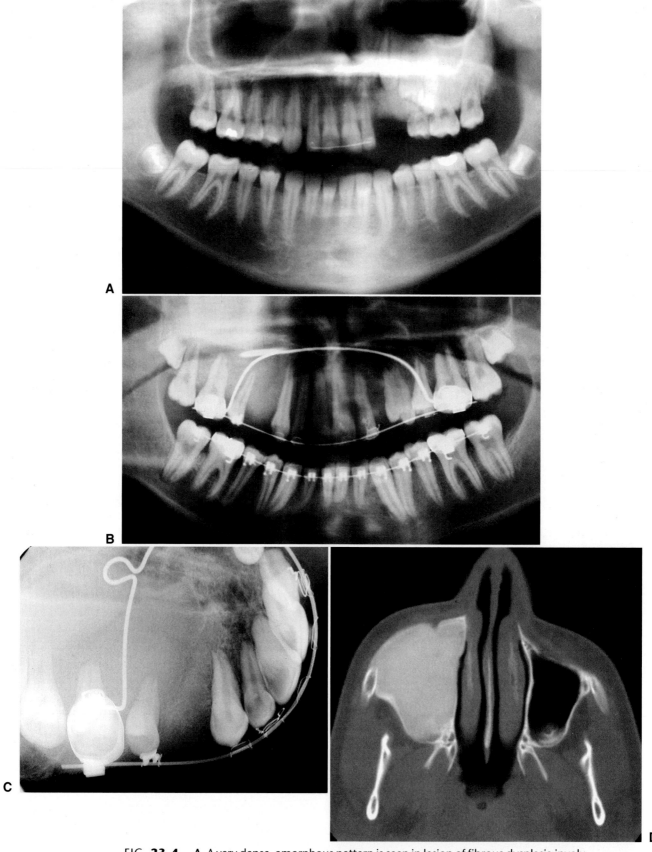

FIG. **23-4**   **A,** A very dense, amorphous pattern is seen in lesion of fibrous dysplasia involving the left maxilla and preventing the normal eruption of the cuspid and the bicuspids. Panoramic **(B)**, occlusal **(C)**, axial **(D)**, and coronal **(E)** CT images of an example of fibrous dysplasia with a homogeneous dense pattern that occupies most of the right maxillary sinus.

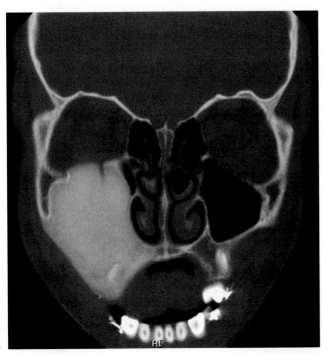

E

FIG. **23-4**—*cont'd*

organization of the abnormal trabeculae into a swirling pattern similar to a fingerprint (Fig. 23-5). Occasionally radiolucent regions resembling cysts may occur in mature lesions of fibrous dysplasia. These are bone cavities that are analogous to simple bone cysts (Fig. 23-6).

Effects on surrounding structures. If the fibrous dysplasia lesion is small, it may have no effect on surrounding structures (subclinical variety). The effects on the involved bone may include expansion with maintenance of a thinned outer cortex (Fig. 23-7). Fibrous dysplasia may expand into the antrum by displacing its cortical boundary and subsequently occupying part or most of the maxillary sinus. Extension into the maxillary antrum usually occurs from the lateral wall, and the last section of the sinus to be involved usually is the most posterosuperior portion. Cortical boundaries such as the floor of the antrum may be changed into the abnormal bone pattern. Often the bone surrounding the teeth is altered without affecting the dentition, and a distinct lamina dura disappears because this bone also is changed into the abnormal bone pattern (see Fig. 23-5). If the fibrous dysplasia increases the bone density, the periodontal ligament space may appear to be very narrow. Fibrous dysplasia can displace teeth or interfere with normal eruption, complicating orthodontic therapy. In rare cases, some root resorption may occur. Fibrous dysplasia appears to be unique in its ability to

displace the inferior alveolar nerve canal in a superior direction (Fig. 23-8).

Differential Diagnosis

Other diseases can alter the bone pattern in a similar fashion. Metabolic bone diseases such as hyperparathyroidism may produce a similar pattern. However, these diseases are polyostotic and bilateral and, unlike fibrous dysplasia, do not cause bone expansion. Paget's disease may produce a similar pattern and may cause expansion, but it occurs in an older age group, and when it involves the mandible, the whole mandible is involved, unlike the unilateral tendency of fibrous dysplasia. Occasionally periapical cemental dysplasia may show a similar bone pattern, but the distribution is different in that it often is bilateral, with an epicenter in the periapical region. Furthermore, periapical cemental dysplasia also occurs in an older age group. With spontaneous healing of a simple bone cyst, the radiographic and histologic appearance of the new bone may be very similar to that of fibrous dysplasia.

Of paramount importance is the differentiation of osteomyelitis and osteogenic sarcoma because of both radiologic and histologic similarities. Osteomyelitis may result in enlargement of the jaws, but the additional bone is generated by the periosteum; therefore the new bone is laid down on the surface of the outer cortex, and close examination may reveal evidence of the original cortex within the expanded portion of the jaw. Fibrous dysplasia, in contrast, expands the internal aspect of bone, displacing and thinning the outer cortex so that the remaining cortex maintains its position at the outer surface of the bone. The identification of sequestra aids in the identification of osteomyelitis. Osteogenic sarcoma may produce a similar pattern but should show malignant radiologic features (see Chapter 22).

Some difficulty may arise in differentiating cemento-ossifying fibroma of the maxilla, especially the juvenile ossifying fibroma type. If the bone pattern is altered around the teeth without displacement of the teeth from one specific epicenter, the lesion probably is fibrous dysplasia. The shape of the bone expansion of fibrous dysplasia into the antrum reflects the original outer contour of the antral wall, which is different from the more convex extension of a neoplasm.

Management

In most cases the radiographic characteristics of fibrous dysplasia and the clinical information are sufficient to allow the practitioner to make a diagnosis without a biopsy. There are reports of exaggerated growth from stimulation of a lesion during surgical intervention in young patients. A consultation with a dental radiologist

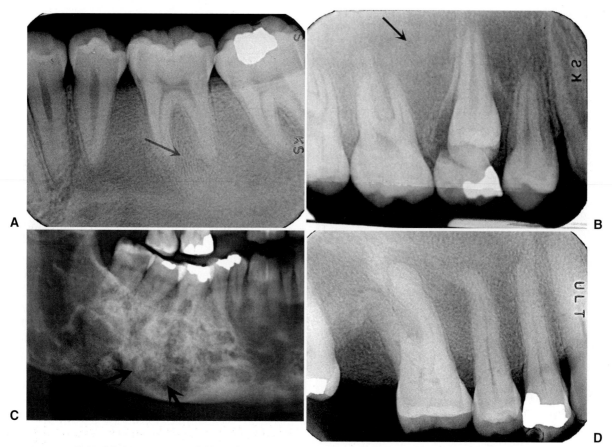

FIG. **23-5** A series of films showing a variety of internal patterns of fibrous dysplasia. **A**, A fingerprint pattern around the roots of the first molar *(arrow)*. Note the change in the lamina dura around the molars into the abnormal bone pattern. **B**, A granular or ground-glass pattern *(arrow)*. **C**, A cotton wool pattern. Note the almost circular radiopaque regions *(arrows)*. **D**, An orange-peel pattern.

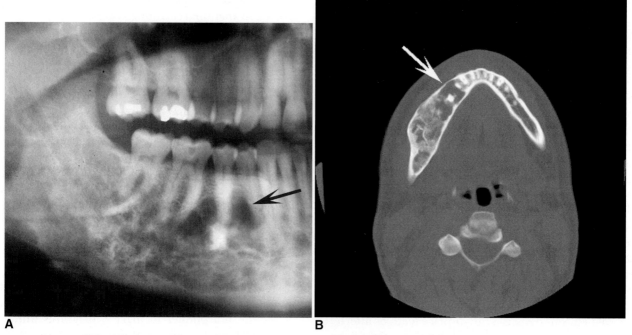

FIG. **23-6** **A**, A cropped panoramic image of fibrous dysplasia of the mandible. A cyst-like radiolucent lesion is in the region of the bicuspids *(arrow)*. **B**, An axial CT using bone algorithm of the same case also revealing the same simple bone-like cyst *(arrow)*.

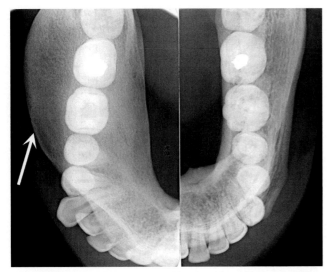

FIG. **23**-7 Occlusal views of both sides of the mandible of the same patient. Note the expansion of the right side of the mandible caused by fibrous dysplasia. The outer cortical plates have been displaced and thinned but are still intact *(arrow)*.

is advisable. The radiologist may supplement the examination with computed tomography (CT), which can give a more accurate, three-dimensional representation of the extent of the lesion and can serve as a precise baseline study for future comparisons. It is reasonable to continue occasional monitoring of the lesion or ask the patient to report any changes. With most lesions, growth is complete at skeletal maturation; therefore orthodontic treatment and cosmetic surgery may be delayed until this time. Sarcomatous changes are unusual but have been reported, especially if therapeutic radiation has been given. In the case of female patients, hormonal changes from pregnancy or the use of oral contraceptives may stimulate growth or result in the development of lesions within the area of fibrous dysplasia, such as aneurysmal bone cysts or giant cell granulomas.

CEMENTO-OSSEOUS DYSPLASIAS

Periapical cemental dysplasia and florid osseous dysplasia are essentially the same process but are separated on the basis of the extent of involvement of the jaws.

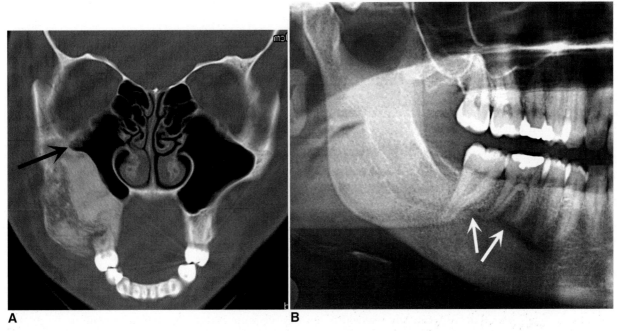

A   **B**

FIG. **23**-8   **A,** A coronal CT scan using bone algorithm of a maxillary lesion of fibrous dysplasia. The lesion has caused the lateral wall of the maxilla to expand into the maxillary antrum. The shape of the lateral wall of the sinus has maintained the zygomatic recess *(arrow).* **B,** Mandibular fibrous dysplasia that has displaced the inferior alveolar nerve canal in a superior direction *(arrows).*

PERIAPICAL CEMENTAL DYSPLASIA

Synonyms

Cementoma, fibrocementoma, sclerosing cementoma, periapical osteofibrosis, periapical fibrous dysplasia, and periapical fibroosteoma

Definition

Periapical cemental dysplasia (PCD) is a localized change in normal bone metabolism that results in the replacement of the components of normal cancellous bone with fibrous tissue and cementum-like material, abnormal bone (similar to that seen in fibrous dysplasia), or a mixture of the two. By definition the lesion is located near the apex of a tooth.

Clinical Features

PCD is a common bone dysplasia that typically occurs in middle age, the mean age being 39 years. It occurs nine times more often in females than in males and almost three times more often in blacks than in whites. It also is seen frequently in Asians. The involved teeth are vital, and the patient usually has no history of pain or sensitivity. The lesions usually come to light as an incidental finding during a periapical or panoramic radiographic examination made for other purposes. The lesions can become quite large, causing a notable expansion of the alveolar process, and may continue to enlarge slowly.

Radiographic Features

Location. The epicenter of a PCD lesion usually lies at the apex of a tooth (Fig. 23-9). In rare cases the epicenter is slightly higher and over the apical third of the root. The condition has a predilection for the periapical bone of the mandibular anterior teeth, although any tooth can be involved, and in rare cases the maxillary teeth may be involved (Fig. 23-10). In most cases the lesion is multiple and bilateral, but occasionally a solitary lesion arises. If the involved teeth have been extracted, this lesion can still develop but the periapical location is less evident (Fig. 23-11). In these cases the term *cemental dysplasia* may be more appropriate.

Periphery and shape. In most cases the periphery of a PCD lesion is well defined. Often a radiolucent border of varying width is present, surrounded by a band of sclerotic bone that also can vary in width (Fig. 23-12). The sclerotic bone represents a reaction of the immediate surrounding bone. The lesion may be irregularly shaped or may have an overall round or oval shape centered over the apex of the tooth.

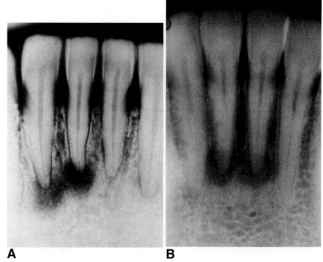

FIG. 23-9 PCD: radiolucent stage. The lamina dura around the central incisor has been lost in **A**, but the periodontal membrane space can still be seen in **B**.

Internal structure. The internal structure varies, depending on the maturity of the lesion. In the early stage, normal bone is resorbed and replaced with fibrous tissue that usually is continuous with the periodontal ligament (causing loss of the lamina dura). Radiographically, this appears as a radiolucency at the apex of the involved tooth (see Fig. 23-9).

In the mixed stage, radiopaque tissue appears in the radiolucent structure. This material usually is amorphous; has a round, oval, or irregular shape; and is composed of cementum or abnormal bone (see Fig. 23-12). These structures sometimes are called *cementicles*; however, this is a radiographic term that does not necessarily represent the histologic appearance. In rare cases the radiopaque material resembles the abnormal trabecular patterns seen in fibrous dysplasia (Fig. 23-13).

In the mature stage, the internal aspect may be totally radiopaque without any obvious pattern. Usually a thin, radiolucent margin can be seen at the periphery, because this lesion matures from the center outward (Fig. 23-14). Occasionally this radiolucent margin is not apparent, which makes the differential diagnosis more difficult. The internal structure may appear dramatically radiolucent if cavities resembling simple bone cysts form within the cemental lesions (Fig. 23-15). In some cases the simple bone cyst extends beyond the margin of the cemental lesion.

Effects on surrounding structures. The normal lamina dura of the teeth involved with the lesion is lost, making

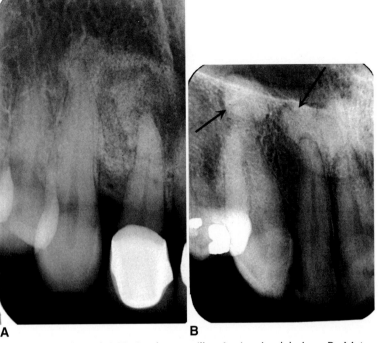

FIG. **23-10** Examples of PCD in the maxilla. **A**, A mixed lesion. **B**, Mature lesions *(arrows)*.

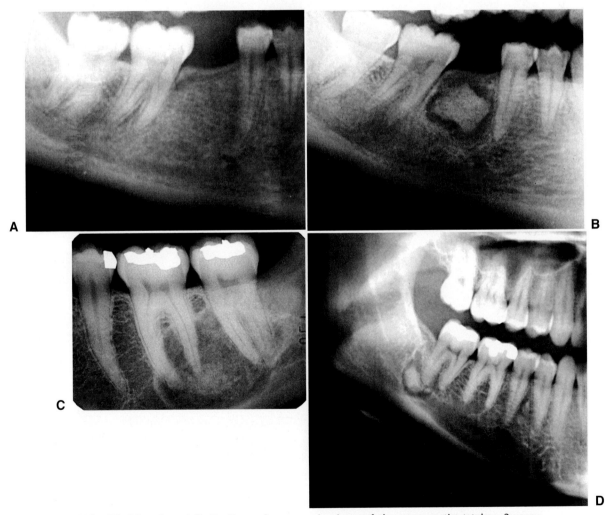

FIG. **23-11** **A** and **B**, Portions of panoramic views of the same patient taken 3 years apart. Note the development of a solitary lesion of PCD in the apical region of the first molar extraction site. **C** and **D**, Solitary lesions in the posterior mandible.

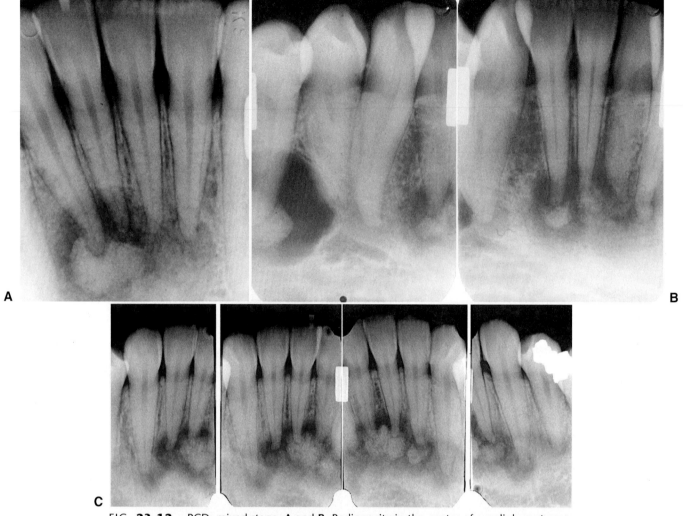

FIG. 23-12 PCD: mixed stage. **A** and **B,** Radiopacity in the center of a radiolucent area. **C,** Multiple lesions. Note the band of sclerotic bone reaction at the periphery of the lesion.

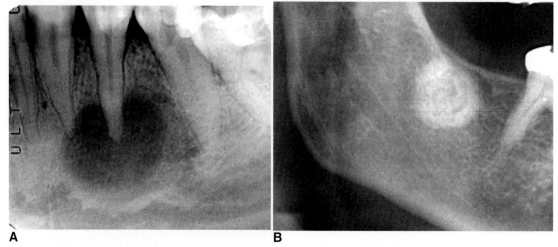

FIG. 23-13 **A,** PCD with a fibrous dysplasia type of internal bone pattern. **B,** A swirling internal pattern of cemental dysplasia.

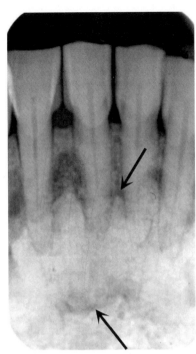

FIG. **23-14** The mature stage of PCD. Note the thin, radiolucent periphery *(arrows)*.

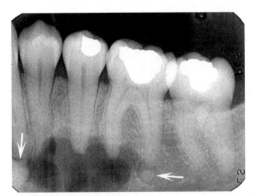

FIG. **23-15** A simple bone cyst within an area of PCD; only a few regions of cementum-like tissue remain *(arrows)*.

the periodontal ligament space either less apparent or giving it a wider appearance (see Fig. 23-9). The tooth structure usually is not affected, although in rare cases some root resorption may occur. Also, occasionally hypercementosis occurs on the root of a tooth positioned within the lesion. Some lesions stimulate a sclerotic bone reaction from the surrounding bone. Small lesions do not cause expansion of the involved jaw. However, larger lesions may cause expansion of the jaw, an area that is always bordered by a thin, intact outer cortex similar to that seen in fibrous dysplasia. This lesion may elevate the floor of the maxillary antrum.

Differential Diagnosis

In early (radiolucent) PCD lesions, the most important differential diagnosis is periapical rarefying osteitis. Occasionally PCD cannot be distinguished from this inflammatory lesion by radiographic characteristics alone. In these cases the final diagnosis must rely on clinical information such as testing of the vitality of the involved tooth.

In the mixed and late forms of PCD the differential diagnosis may include a benign cementoblastoma. This tumor is solitary and usually is attached to the surface of the root, which may be partly resorbed. The presence or absence of clinical symptoms may help distinguish PCD from benign cementoblastoma. Another lesion to consider is an odontoma. Odontomas often start occlusal to a tooth and prevent its eruption, but some odontomas may have a periapical position. The organization of the internal aspect into toothlike structures and the identification of enamel (very radiopaque) can help in the differential diagnosis. Also, the peripheral cortex and soft tissue capsule of an odontoma are more uniform in width and better defined than is the periphery of PCD. In mature PCD lesions, the appearance may resemble that of a dense bone island. The finding of a radiolucent periphery, even if very slight, indicates a diagnosis of PCD. Solitary lesions may be difficult to differentiate from a cemento-ossifying fibroma. Cases that have been quiescent and then suddenly start to grow aggressively suggest that there may be a continuum between the category of cemento-osseous dysplasia and cemento-osseous tumors.

Management

The diagnosis of PCD can be made on the basis of the appropriate radiologic and clinical characteristics. In fact, a possible complication of biopsy is secondary infection, which may occur in lesions that have abundant cementum formation and poor vascularity. Normally treatment is not required. However, if the teeth have been removed and if considerable atrophy of the alveolar ridge has occurred, these segments of cementum may reach the mucosal surface, much in the same way as stones become exposed in old, worn concrete. These pieces of cementum can perforate the mucosa when positioned under a denture, and the result is secondary infection. If this occurs, the pieces of cementum may have to be removed surgically because they can act as sequestra in osteomyelitis.

FLORID OSSEOUS DYSPLASIA

Synonyms

Florid cemento-osseous dysplasia, gigantiform cementoma, and familial multiple cementomas

Definition

Florid osseous dysplasia (FOD) appears be a widespread form of PCD. Normal cancellous bone is replaced with dense, acellular cemento-osseous tissue in a background of fibrous connective tissue. The lesion has a poor vascular supply, a condition that likely contributes to its susceptibility to infection. In some cases a familial trend can be seen. No clear definition indicates when multiple regions of PCD should be termed *FOD*. However, if PCD is identified in three or four quadrants or is extensive throughout one jaw, it usually is considered to be FOD.

Clinical Features

Several key similarities exist between FOD and PCD, including the age, sex, and racial profiles of patients and comparable radiographic and histologic appearances. Most patients with FOD are female and middle-aged (the mean age being 42 years), although the age range is broad. The condition shows a marked predilection for blacks and Asians. Often FOD produces no symptoms and is found incidentally during a radiographic examination. Occasionally patients complain of intermittent, poorly localized pain in the affected bone, especially when a simple bone cyst has developed within the lesion. Extensive lesions often have an associated bony swelling. If the lesions become secondarily infected, features of osteomyelitis may develop, including mucosal ulceration, fistulous tracts with suppuration, and pain. In fact, historically FOD that was secondarily infected was diagnosed as chronic sclerosing osteomyelitis without the identification of the underlying bone dysplasia. Teeth in the involved bone are vital unless other dental disease coincidentally affects them.

Radiographic Features

Location. FOD lesions usually are bilateral and present in both jaws (Fig. 23-16). However, when they are present in only one jaw, the mandible is the more common location. The epicenter is apical to the teeth, within the alveolar process and usually posterior to the cuspid. In the mandible, lesions occur above the inferior alveolar canal.

Periphery. The periphery usually is well defined and has a sclerotic border that can vary in width, very similar to PCD. The soft tissue capsule may not be apparent in mature lesions.

Internal structure. The density of the internal structure can vary from an equal mixture of radiolucent and radiopaque regions to almost complete radiopacity. Some prominent radiolucent regions may be present, which usually represent the development of a simple bone cyst (Fig. 23-17). These cysts may enlarge with time even beyond the boundary of the lesion into the surrounding normal bone or may fill in with abnormal dysplastic cemento-osseous tissue. The radiopaque regions can vary from small oval and circular regions (cotton-wool appearance) to large, irregular, amorphous areas of calcification. These calcified masses are similar in appearance to those seen in mature PCD lesions.

Effects on surrounding structures. Large FOD lesions can displace the inferior alveolar nerve canal in an inferior direction. FOD also can displace the floor of the antrum in a superior direction and can cause enlargement of the alveolar bone by displacement of the buccal and lingual cortical plates. The roots of associated teeth may have a considerable amount of hypercementosis, which may fuse with the abnormal surrounding cemental tissue of the lesion. Extraction of these teeth may be difficult.

Differential Diagnosis

The fact that FOD is bilateral and centered in the alveolar process helps in the differentiation from other lesions. Paget's disease of bone may also show cotton wool–type radiopaque regions with associated hypercementosis. However, Paget's disease affects the bone of the entire mandible, whereas FOD is centered above the inferior alveolar canal. Furthermore, Paget's disease often is polyostotic, involving other bones as well as the jaws. The well-defined nature of FOD, with its radiolucent periphery and surrounding sclerotic border, also is useful in making the differential diagnosis.

Another disease that may resemble FOD is chronic sclerosing osteomyelitis. Regions of cementum may appear that are similar to the sequestrum seen in osteomyelitis. CT imaging can aid in the differential diagnosis. Another confusing factor may be the development of a secondary osteomyelitis that may mask the underlying FOD.

Management

Under normal circumstances, FOD does not require treatment, although there is value in obtaining a panoramic film to establish the extent of the disease. Unlike with fibrous dysplasia, no age limit is apparent for the cessation of growth of FOD. Because of the propensity to develop secondary infections in FOD, the patient should be encouraged to maintain an effective oral hygiene program to avoid odontogenic infections. Also, if the teeth are extracted and severe atrophy of the alveolar process occurs, as in PCD, the cementum masses emerge and the pressure of the overlying denture may cause dehiscence in the mucosa, resulting

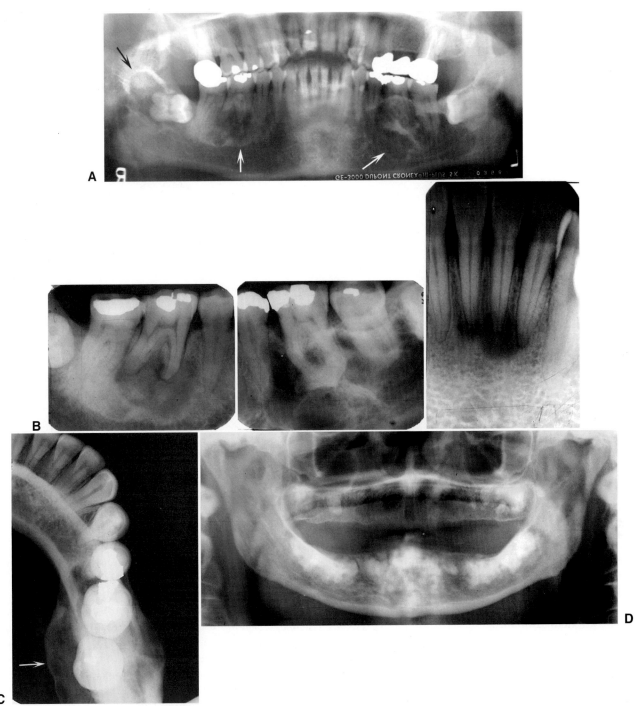

FIG. **23-16** FOD. **A,** Three mixed radiopaque-radiolucent lesions in the periapical regions throughout the jaws *(arrows)*; note that although the right third molar is horizontally impacted, the lesion still has a periapical relationship. **B,** A composite of periapical films of the same case. Note the appearance of the lesions involving the mandibular incisors (not apparent in the panoramic film), which appear identical to periapical cemental dysplasia. **C,** An occlusal film of the left mandibular lesion showing expansion of the medial cortical plate *(arrow).* **D,** A panoramic film of a different case showing multiple, very mature almost totally radiopaque lesions in edentulous jaws. Note that the epicenter of all lesions is above the inferior alveolar canal.

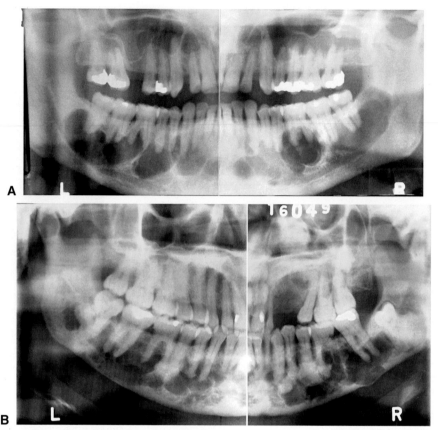

FIG. **23-17**   FOD associated with multiple simple bone cysts. **A,** Large cysts occupy most of the bone involved with the FOD lesions. **B,** Another example of multiple simple bone cysts in lesions of FOD.

in osteomyelitis. If this occurs, the avascular cemental masses become large sequestra. The osteomyelitis may spread slowly throughout the jaw from one region of FOD to another. It may be necessary to remove large areas of cemental tissue, leaving very little residual bone for prosthetic treatment.

Other Lesions of Bone

CEMENTO-OSSIFYING FIBROMA

Synonyms
Ossifying fibroma and cementifying fibroma

Definition
Cemento-ossifying fibroma (COF) is classified as and behaves like a benign bone neoplasm. However, it appears in this chapter because it often is considered to be a type of fibroosseous lesion. This bone tumor consists of highly cellular, fibrous tissue that contains varying amounts of abnormal bone or cementum-like

tissue. In the past this lesion was classified as two different entities depending on whether bone or cementum was the predominant calcified product. When the histologic appearance of most of the calcified tissue was of irregular trabeculae of woven bone, the term *ossifying fibroma* was used. The resulting internal pattern may be very similar to or indistinguishable from fibrous dysplasia. One distinguishing feature that may be present is a soft tissue capsule at the periphery not seen in fibrous dysplasia. When the predominant calcified component was cementum, the term *cementifying fibroma* was used. However, the microscopic appearance of an ossifying fibroma and a cementifying fibroma can be very similar, and the two are now thought to represent a spectrum of one disease and are combined under the name *cemento-ossifying fibroma*.

Juvenile ossifying fibroma is a very aggressive form of COF that occurs in the first 2 decades of life. Although the histopathologic definition of this entity is controversial, the radiologic appearance has similarities to that of COF.

Clinical Features

The clinical features of COF can vary from indolent to aggressive behavior. The characteristics are more like those of a tumor than a bone dysplasia. COF can occur at any age but usually is found in young adults. Females are affected more often than males. The disease usually is asymptomatic at the time of discovery. Occasionally facial asymmetry develops. Displacement of the teeth may be an early clinical feature, although most lesions are discovered during routine dental examinations. In cases of juvenile ossifying fibroma, rapid growth may occur in a young patient, resulting in deformity of the involved jaw.

Radiographic Features

Location. COF appears almost exclusively in the facial bones and most commonly in the mandible, typically inferior to the premolars and molars and superior to the inferior alveolar canal. In the maxilla it occurs most often in the canine fossa and zygomatic arch area.

Periphery. The borders of COF lesions usually are well defined. A thin, radiolucent line, representing a fibrous capsule, may separate it from surrounding bone (Fig. 23-18). Sometimes the bone next to the lesion develops a sclerotic border.

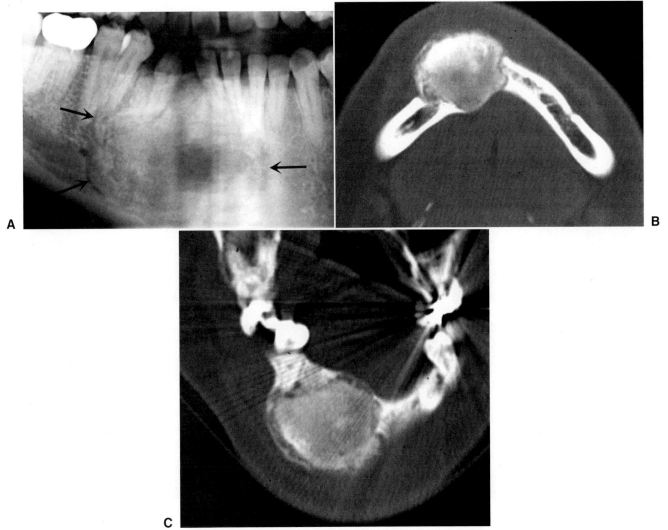

FIG. **23-18** A cementifying fibroma depicted in a panoramic film *(arrows)* **(A)**, an axial CT scan **(B)**, and a coronal CT scan **(C)**. Note the homogeneous, radiopaque internal structure and the radiolucent band at the periphery.

Internal structure. The internal structure of a COF lesion is a mixed radiolucent-radiopaque density with a pattern that depends on the amount and form of the manufactured calcified material. In some instances the internal structure may appear almost totally radiolucent with just a hint of calcified material. In the type that contains mainly abnormal bone, the pattern may be similar to that seen in fibrous dysplasia, or a wispy (similar to stretched tufts of cotton) or flocculent pattern (similar to large, heavy snowflakes) may be seen (Fig. 23-19). Lesions that produce more cementum-like material may contain solid, amorphous radiopacities (cementicles) similar to those seen in cemental dysplasia (see Fig. 23-18).

Effects on surrounding structures. COF can be distinguished from the previously mentioned bone dysplasias by its tumorlike behavior. This is reflected in the growth of the lesion, which tends to be concentric within the medullary part of the bone with outward expansion approximately equal in all directions. This can result in displacement of teeth or of the inferior alveolar canal and expansion of the outer cortical plates of bone. A significant point is that the outer cortical plate, although displaced and thinned, remains intact. The COF lesion can grow into and occupy the entire maxillary sinus (Fig. 23-20), expanding its walls outward; however, a bony partition always exists between the internal aspect of the remaining sinus and the tumor. The lamina dura of involved teeth usually is missing, and resorption of teeth may occur.

Differential Diagnosis

The differential diagnosis of COF includes lesions with a mixed radiolucent-radiopaque internal structure. The differentiation from fibrous dysplasia can be very difficult. The boundaries of a COF lesion usually are better defined, and these lesions occasionally have a soft tissue capsule and cortex, whereas fibrous dysplasia usually blends in with surrounding bone. The internal structure of fibrous dysplasia lesions may be more homogeneous and show less variation. Both types of lesions can displace teeth, but COF displaces from a specific point or epicenter. Fibrous dysplasia rarely resorbs teeth. The

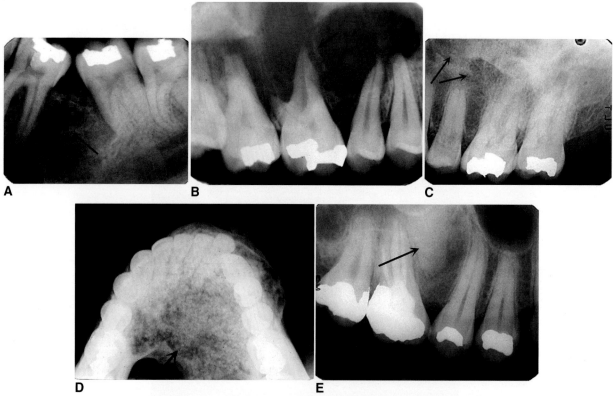

FIG. **23-19** Various bone patterns seen in COFs. **A,** A wispy trabecular pattern *(arrow)*. **B,** Most of this pattern is radiolucent with a few wispy trabeculae *(arrow)*. **C,** A fibrous dysplasia granular-like pattern *(arrows)*. **D,** A flocculent pattern with larger tufts of bone formation *(arrow)*. **E,** A solid, radiopaque, cementum-like pattern *(arrow)*.

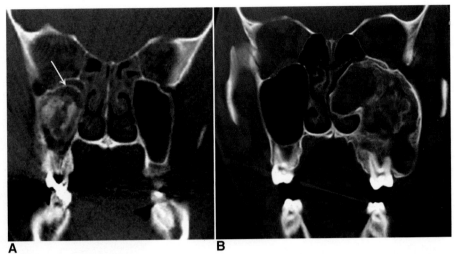

FIG. **23-20** Large COFs involving the maxilla. **A,** A coronal CT scan of a lesion invaginating the maxillary antrum. Note that unlike in fibrous dysplasia, the peripheral border of the lesion *(arrow)* does not parallel the original shape of the antrum. **B,** A coronal CT scan of a larger lesion expanding the maxilla, occupying all of the maxillary antrum, and extending into the nasal fossa.

expansion of the jaws associated with COF is more concentric about a definite epicenter, but fibrous dysplasia enlarges the bone while distorting the overall shape to a smaller degree; in other words, the expanded bone still resembles normal morphology.

Great difficulty may arise in differentiating juvenile ossifying fibroma from fibrous dysplasia when the lesion involves the maxillary antrum. Fibrous dysplasia usually displaces the lateral wall of the maxilla into the maxillary antrum, maintaining the outer shape of the wall, whereas an ossifying fibroma has a more convex shape as it extends into the maxillary antrum (see Figs. 23-8 and 23-20). Also, fibrous dysplasia may change the bone around the teeth without displacing them from an obvious epicenter of a concentrically growing benign tumor. The importance of this differentiation lies in the treatment, which is resection for an ossifying fibroma and observation for fibrous dysplasia.

The differential diagnosis of the type of COF that produces mainly cementum-like material from PCD may be difficult, especially with large single lesions of PCD. However, cemental dysplasia usually is multifocal, whereas COF is not. Also, the presence of a simple bone cyst is a characteristic of cemental dysplasia. COF behaves in a more tumorlike fashion, with the displacement of teeth. A wide sclerotic border is more characteristic of the slow-growing cemental dysplasia.

Other lesions to be considered include those that may have internal calcifications similar to the pattern seen in COF. These include calcifying odontogenic cysts, calcifying epithelial odontogenic (Pindborg) tumors, and adenomatoid odontogenic tumors.

Occasionally the diagnosis of osteogenic sarcoma is considered. However, characteristics suggesting a malignant lesion should be seen, such as cortical bone destruction and invasion into the surrounding soft tissues and along the periodontal ligament space.

Management

The prognosis of COF is favorable with surgical enucleation or resection. Large lesions require a detailed determination of the extent of the lesion, which can be obtained with CT imaging. Even if the lesion has reached appreciable size, it usually can be separated from the surrounding tissue and completely removed. Recurrence after removal is unlikely.

CENTRAL GIANT CELL GRANULOMA

Synonyms

Giant cell reparative granuloma, giant cell lesion, and giant cell tumor

Definition

Central giant cell granuloma (CGCG) is thought to be a reactive lesion to an as-yet-unknown stimulus and not a neoplastic lesion. However, radiographically the characteristics of the lesion are similar to those of a benign tumor, and occasionally maxillary lesions may have some malignant type characteristics. The histologic appearance consists primarily of fibroblasts, numerous vascular channels, multinucleated giant cells, and macrophages. The relationship of the benign giant cell tumor to the giant cell granuloma is controversial and unclear.

Clinical Features

CGCG is a common lesion in the jaws that affects mostly adolescents and young adults; at least 60% of cases occur in individuals under 20 years of age. The most common presenting sign of CGCG is painless swelling. Palpation of the suspect bone area may elicit tenderness, although in a minority of cases the patient may complain of pain. The overlying mucosa may have a purple color. Some of these lesions cause no symptoms and are found only on routine examination. The lesion usually grows slowly, although it may grow rapidly, creating the suspicion of a malignancy.

Radiographic Features

Location. Lesions develop in the mandible twice as often as in the maxilla. The epicenter of the lesion usually is anterior to the first molar, although large lesions can extend posterior to the first molar. Most maxillary lesions arise anterior to the cuspid. Lesions can cross the midline of the mandible.

Periphery. Because this neoplasm grows relatively slowly, it usually produces a well-defined radiographic margin in the mandible. In most cases the periphery shows no evidence of cortication. Lesions in the maxilla may have ill-defined, almost malignant-appearing, borders.

Internal structure. Some CGCG lesions show no evidence of internal structure (Fig. 23-21), especially small lesions. Other cases have a subtle granular pattern of calcification that may require a bright light source behind the film to enable visualization. Occasionally this granular bone is organized into ill-defined, wispy septa (Fig. 23-22). If present, these granular septa are characteristic of this lesion, especially if they emanate at right angles from the periphery of the lesion. This characteristic is even stronger if a small indentation of the expanded cortical margin is seen at the point where this right-angle septum originates (Fig. 23-23). In some instances the septa are better defined and divide the internal aspect into compartments, creating a multilocular appearance.

Effects on surrounding structures. Giant cell granulomas often displace and resorb teeth. The resorption of tooth roots is not a constant feature, but when it occurs, it may be profound and irregular in outline. The lamina dura of teeth within the lesion usually is missing. The

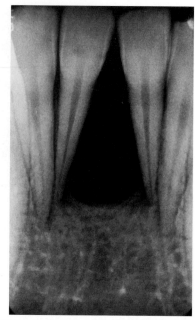

FIG. **23-21** A giant cell granuloma in the anterior mandible with no evidence of internal structure.

inferior alveolar canal may be displaced in an inferior direction. This lesion has a strong propensity to expand the cortical boundaries of the mandible and maxilla. The expansion usually is uneven or undulating in nature, which may give the appearance of a double boundary when the expansion is viewed using occlusal film. In some instances the outer cortical plate of bone is destroyed instead of expanded; this occurs more often in the maxilla, where the cortical bone destruction may give the lesion a malignant appearance.

Differential Diagnosis

If the internal structure of the CGCG contains septa, the differential diagnosis may include ameloblastoma, odontogenic myxoma, and aneurysmal bone cyst. If a granular internal structure is present, COF may be considered. Useful characteristics for differentiating an ameloblastoma include the following: ameloblastomas tend to occur in an older age group and more often in the posterior mandible, and ameloblastomas have coarse, curved, well-defined trabeculae, whereas giant cell granulomas have wispy, ill-defined trabeculae, some of which are at right angles to the periphery. Odontogenic myxomas occur in an older age group, may have sharper and straighter septa, and do not have the same propensity to expand as giant cell granulomas. It is interesting to note that aneurysmal bone cysts can appear radiographically identical to giant cell granulomas, especially in the appearance of the internal septa. However, aneurysmal bone cysts are comparatively rare

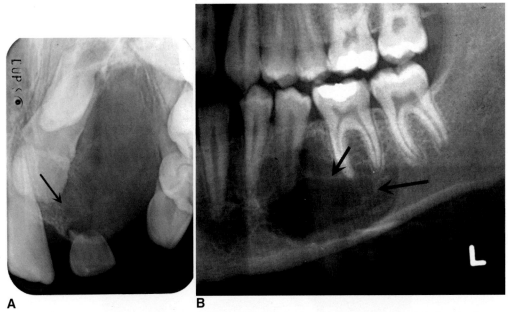

FIG. **23-22** Various internal patterns seen in giant cell granulomas. **A,** A lesion in the anterior maxilla with a very fine granular pattern *(arrow)*. **B,** A portion of a panoramic film showing wispy, ill-defined internal septa *(arrows)*.

lesions that occur more often in the posterior aspect of the jaws and usually cause profound expansion.

A small CGCG lesion with a totally radiolucent internal structure may be similar in appearance to a cyst, especially a simple bone cyst. Evidence of displacement or resorption of the adjacent teeth or expansion of the outer cortical bone is more characteristic of a giant cell granuloma. The radiographic image and histologic appearance of brown tumors of hyperparathyroidism may be identical to those of CGCG. Also the appearance may be identical to that seen in cherubism; however, the lesions in cherubism are multiple and have epicenters that are located in the most posterior aspect of the mandible and maxilla.

Management

If the lesion is in the maxilla, CT scans can be used to establish the exact extent and the involvement of surrounding structures, such as the maxillary antrum or nasal cavity. Also, CT imaging is required for large lesions, which pose the possibility of destruction of the outer cortical bone, to determine whether the adjacent soft tissue has been invaded. Occasionally this lesion behaves very aggressively. If CGCG occurs after the second decade of life, hyperparathyroidism should be considered and serum testing for elevated calcium or parathormone or full-body technetium bone scans can be ordered.

Treatment may include enucleation and curettage and in some instances resection of the jaw. The patient should be followed carefully to rule out recurrence, especially if conservative treatment is used. Recurrences are rare and are more common in the maxilla.

ANEURYSMAL BONE CYST

Definition

An aneurysmal bone cyst (ABC) usually is considered to be a reactive lesion of bone rather than a cyst or true neoplasm. Some believe that it represents an exaggerated, localized, proliferative response of vascular tissue in bone. This lesion may be related to the CGCG, because of similarities in both the radiographic and histologic appearance (presence of giant cells). ABCs occasionally develop in association with other primary lesions such as fibrous dysplasia, central hemangioma, giant cell granuloma, and osteosarcoma. Its etiology remains unclear.

Clinical Features

More than 90% of reported jaw lesions have occurred in individuals under 30 years of age. The condition appears to have a predilection for females. An ABC in the jaw usually manifests as a fairly rapid bony swelling (usually buccal or labial). Pain is an occasional complaint, and the involved area may be tender on palpation.

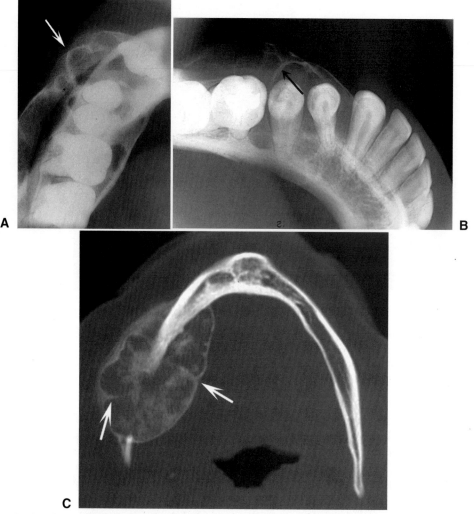

FIG. **23-23**   Characteristic expansion of the outer cortical plates caused by giant cell granulomas. Note the uneven expansion in **A** *(arrow)* and the indentation of the expansion with a right-angled septum in **B** *(arrow)*. **C,** An axial CT scan using bone algorithm revealing a giant cell granuloma within the mandible causing undulating expansion and contains two right-angled septa *(arrows)*.

Radiographic Features

Location. The mandible is involved more often than the maxilla (ratio of 3:2), and the molar and ramus regions are more involved than the anterior region (Fig. 23-24).

Periphery and shape. The periphery usually is well defined, and the shape is circular or "hydraulic."

Internal structure. Small initial lesions may show no evidence of an internal structure. Often the internal aspect has a multilocular appearance. The septa bear a striking resemblance to the wispy, ill-defined septa seen in giant cell granulomas (Fig. 23-25; see also Fig. 23-24). Another similar finding is septa positioned at right angles to the outer expanded border. In CT soft tissue algorithm images there may be more radiolucent regions, some of which have a roughly circular shape. These likely represent large vascular spaces.

Effects on surrounding structures. After an ABC becomes large, there is a strong propensity for extreme expansion of the outer cortical plates (see Figs. 23-24

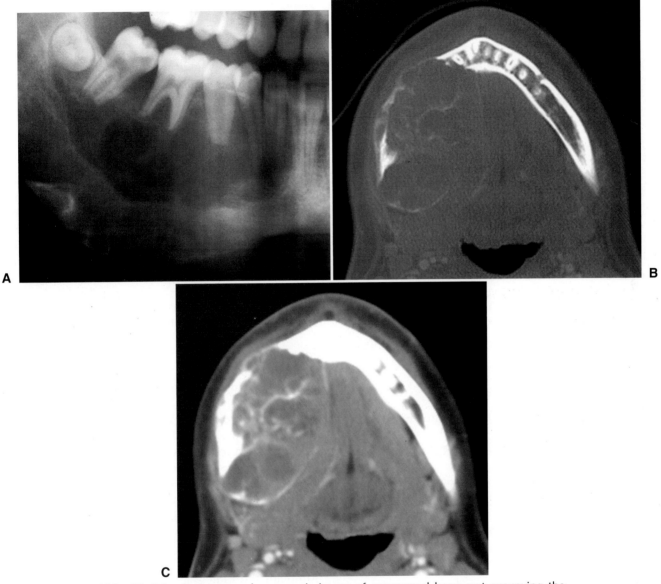

FIG. **23-24** **A,** A cropped panoramic image of aneurysmal bone cyst occupying the body of the right mandible. Two axial CT images at the same level of this case using bone algorithm (**B**) and soft tissue algorithm (**C**).

and 23-25). This characteristic is more dramatic in these cysts than in most other lesions. ABCs can displace and resorb teeth.

Differential Diagnosis

The multilocular appearance of ABCs most resembles that of giant cell granulomas; in fact, the radiographic appearance of the two lesions may be identical. However, ABCs may expand to a greater degree, and

they are more common in the posterior parts of the mandible, whereas giant cell granulomas are found more often anterior to the first molar. Ameloblastoma may be considered, but this lesion usually occurs in an older age group. ABCs may show a similarity to cherubism, which has giant cell–like features, but cherubism is a multifocal, bilateral disease.

The diagnosis is based on biopsy results. A hemorrhagic aspirate favors the diagnosis of ABC. A CT scan

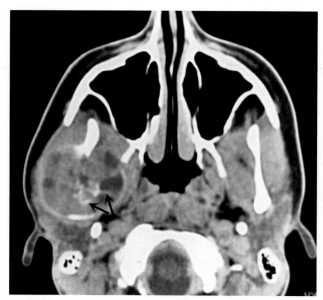

FIG. **23-25**   An axial CT scan using a soft tissue algorithm demonstrating the presence of an ABC of the left mandibular condyle. Note the severe expansion and the wispy ill-defined septa *(arrows)*.

also is recommended to better determine the extent of the lesion.

Management
Surgical curettage and partial resection are the primary means of treatment. The recurrence rate is fairly high, ranging from 19% to about 50% after curettage and approximately 11% after resection. This indicates a need for careful follow-up.

CHERUBISM

Synonym
Familial fibrous dysplasia

Definition
Cherubism is a rare, inherited developmental abnormality that causes bilateral enlargement of the jaws, giving the child a cherubic facial appearance. Rare unilateral lesions have been reported. The term *familial fibrous dysplasia* was an unfortunate choice of early terminology, because this lesion is not a bone dysplasia. It is composed of giant cell granuloma–like tissue and does not form a bone matrix. These lesions regress with age.

Clinical Features
Cherubism develops in early childhood between 2 and 6 years of age. The most common presenting sign is a painless, firm, bilateral enlargement of the lower face. Enlargement of the submandibular lymph nodes may occur, but no systemic abnormalities are involved. Because children's faces are rather chubby, mild cases may go undetected until the second decade. Profound swelling of the maxilla may result in stretching of the skin of the cheeks, which depresses the lower eyelids, exposing a thin line of sclera and causing an "eyes raised to heaven" appearance.

Radiographic Features
Location.   This lesion is bilateral and often affects both jaws. When it is present in only one jaw, the mandible is the most common location. The epicenter is always in the posterior aspect of the jaws, in the ramus of the mandible, or the tuberosity of the maxilla (Fig. 23-26). The lesion grows in an anterior direction and in severe cases can extend almost to the midline.

Periphery.   The periphery usually is well defined and in some instances corticated.

Internal structure.   The internal structure resembles that of CGCG, with fine, granular bone and wispy trabeculae forming a prominent multilocular pattern.

Effects on surrounding structures.   Expansion of the cortical boundaries of the maxilla and mandible by cherubism can result in severe enlargement of the jaws. Maxillary lesions enlarge into the maxillary sinuses. Because the epicenter is in the posterior aspect of the jaws, the teeth are displaced in an anterior direction. The degree of displacement can be severe, and with some lesions the tooth buds are destroyed.

Differential Diagnosis
Although the radiographic appearance of cherubism may be similar to that of giant cell granuloma, the fact that cherubism is bilateral with an epicenter in the ramus should provide a clear differentiation. The differentiation of cherubism from fibrous dysplasia should not present any difficulties, because fibrous dysplasia is more commonly a unilateral disease; also, the multilocular appearance and anterior displacement of teeth are more characteristic of cherubism. Cherubism may bear some similarity to multiple odontogenic keratocysts in basal cell nevus syndrome. The bilateral symmetry of cherubism, along with the anterior displacement of teeth and pronounced multilocular appearance, help with the differential diagnosis.

Management
The distinctive radiographic features of cherubism may be more diagnostic than the histopathologic findings;

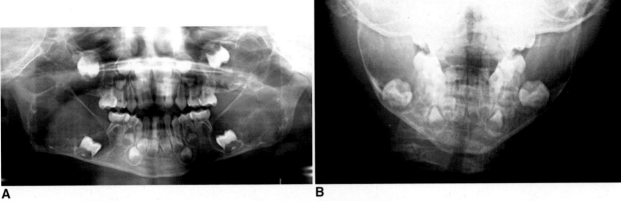

FIG. **23-26** A case of cherubism. **A,** A panoramic image showing four lesions in the maxilla and mandible. Note that the epicenters of the lesions are in the maxillary tuberosity and mandibular ramus; also note the anterior displacement of the unerupted maxillary first molars. The internal structure contains ill-defined septa. **B,** A portion of the posteroanterior skull view showing expansion of the mandible.

therefore the diagnosis can rely on the radiologic findings alone. Treatment can be delayed, because the cyst-like lesions usually become static and fill in with granular bone during adolescence and at the end of skeletal growth. After skeletal growth has stopped, conservative surgical procedures, if required, may be done for cosmetic problems. Surgery also may be required to uncover displaced teeth, and orthodontic treatment may be needed.

PAGET'S DISEASE

Synonym
Osteitis deformans

Definition
Paget's disease is a condition of abnormal resorption and apposition of osseous tissue in one or more bones. The disease may involve many bones simultaneously, but it is not a generalized skeletal disease. It is initiated by an intense wave of osteoclastic activity, with resorption of normal bone resulting in irregularly shaped resorption cavities. After a period of time, vigorous osteoblastic activity ensues, forming woven bone. Paget's disease is seen most frequently in Great Britain and Australia and somewhat less often in North America.

Clinical Features
Paget's disease is primarily a disease of later middle and old age, having an incidence of about 3.5% of individuals over 40 years of age. The incidence of involvement in males is approximately twice that of females at age 65 years.

Affected bone is enlarged and commonly deformed, resulting in bowing of the legs, curvature of the spine, and enlargement of the skull. The jaws also enlarge when affected. Separation and movement of teeth may occur, causing malocclusion. Dentures may be tight or may fit poorly in edentulous patients.

Bone pain is an inconsistent symptom, most often directed toward the weight-bearing bones; facial or jaw pain is uncommon. Patients with Paget's disease may also have ill-defined neurologic pain as the result of bone impingement on foramina and nerve canals. Patients with Paget's disease often have severely elevated levels of serum alkaline phosphatase (greater than with any other disorder) during osteoblastic phases of the disease. These patients also often have high levels of hydroxyproline in the urine.

Radiographic Features

Location. Paget's disease occurs most often in the pelvis, femur, skull, and vertebrae and infrequently in the jaws (Fig. 23-27). It affects the maxilla about twice as often as the mandible. Whenever the jaws are involved, it is important to note whether all of the mandible or maxilla is affected. Although this disease is bilateral, occasionally only one maxilla is involved or the involvement may be significantly greater on one side.

Internal structure. Generally the appearance of the internal structure depends on the developmental stage of the disease. Paget's disease has three radiographic stages, although these often overlap in the clinical

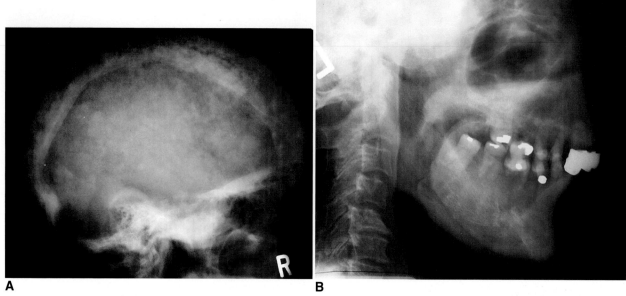

FIG. **23-27**   A case of Paget's disease involving the skull, maxilla, and mandible. **A,** A lateral view of the skull showing an increase in density and dimension between the internal and outer cortex of the skull. A cotton wool pattern can be seen. **B,** A lateral view of the jaws of the same patient showing the increase in jaw size and density. There is a subtle linear orientation of the trabeculae of the mandible.

setting: an early radiolucent resorptive stage; a granular or ground-glass–appearing second stage; and a denser, more radiopaque appositional late stage. These stages are less apparent in the jaws.

The trabeculae are altered in number and shape. Most often they increase in number, but in the early stage they may decrease. The trabeculae may be long and may align themselves in a horizontal linear pattern (Fig. 23-28), which is more common in the mandible. They also may be short, with random orientation, and may have a granular pattern similar to that of fibrous dysplasia. A third pattern occurs when the trabeculae may be organized into rounded, radiopaque patches of abnormal bone, creating a cotton-wool appearance (Fig. 23-29).

The overall density of the jaws may decrease (Fig. 23-30) or increase, depending on the number of trabeculae. Often the disease produces areas of bone that appear radiolucent (commonly the alveolar process) and regions of increased density in one bone.

Effects on surrounding structures. Paget's disease always enlarges an affected bone to some extent, even in the early stage. Often the bone enlargement is impressive. Prominent pagetoid skull bones may swell to three or four times their normal thickness. In enlarged jaws the outer cortex may be thinned but remains intact. The outer cortex may appear to be lam-

inated in occlusal projections (see Fig. 23-30). When the maxilla is involved, the disease invariably involves the sinus floor. However, the air space usually is not diminished to a great extent. Cortical boundaries such as the sinus floor may be more granular and less apparent as sharp boundaries. The lamina dura may become less evident and may be altered into the abnormal bone pattern. Often hypercementosis develops on a few or most of the teeth in the involved jaw. This hypercementosis may be exuberant and irregular, which is characteristic of Paget's disease (Fig. 23-31). As previously mentioned, the teeth may become spaced or displaced in the enlarging jaw.

Differential Diagnosis

Paget's disease may appear similar to fibrous dysplasia. However, Paget's disease occurs in an older age group and is almost always bilateral. In the maxilla, fibrous dysplasia has a tendency to encroach upon the antral air space, whereas Paget's disease does not. The linear trabeculae and cotton-wool appearance of Paget's disease are distinctive. FOD may have a cotton-wool pattern, but these lesions are centered above the inferior alveolar nerve canal and most commonly have a radiolucent capsule. The changes seen in FOD do not affect all of the jaw, unlike with Paget's disease. The bone pattern in Paget's disease may show some similarities to the bone pattern in metabolic bone diseases, and both conditions

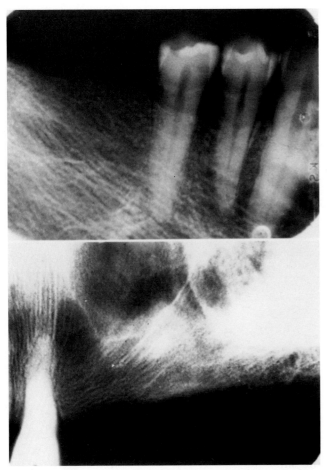

FIG. **23-28**   Paget's disease with an altered trabecular pattern. The trabeculae are aligned in linear striations, which follow an approximately horizontal direction in the mandible but are randomly oriented in the maxilla. (Courtesy Dr. H.G. Poyton, Toronto, Canada.)

may be bilateral. However, Paget's disease enlarges bone, whereas metabolic diseases do not.

The specific bone pattern changes, the late age of onset, the enlargement of the involved bone, and the extreme elevation of serum alkaline phosphatase aid in the differential diagnosis.

Management

Currently Paget's disease usually is managed medically, using either calcitonin or sodium etidronate. Calcitonin relieves pain and reduces the serum alkaline phosphatase levels and osteoclastic activity. Sodium etidronate covers bone surfaces and retards bone resorption and formation. Surgery may be required to correct deformities of the long bones and treat fractures.

There are complications of this disease that are of concern. Extraction sites heal slowly. The incidence of

jaw osteomyelitis is higher than for nonaffected individuals. About 10% of cases with polyostotic disease develop osteogenic sarcoma. Characteristics such as invasion and bone destruction, as described in Chapter 22, indicate the presence of a malignant neoplasm.

LANGERHANS' CELL HISTIOCYTOSIS

Synonyms
Histiocytosis X, idiopathic histiocytosis, and Langerhans' cell disease

Definition
The disorders included in the category of Langerhans' cell histiocytosis (LCH) are abnormalities that result from the abnormal proliferation of Langerhans' cells or their precursors. Langerhans' cells are specialized cells of the histiocytic cell line that normally are found in the skin. The abnormal proliferation of Langerhans' cells and eosinophils results in a spectrum of clinical diseases. Historically, histiocytosis X was classified into three distinct clinical forms: eosinophilic granuloma (solitary), Hand-Schüller-Christian disease (chronic disseminated), and Letterer-Siwe disease (acute disseminated).

A newly proposed LCH classification creates two categories: nonmalignant disorders, such as unifocal or multifocal eosinophilic granuloma, and malignant disorders, including Letterer-Siwe disease and variants of histiocytic lymphoma. Recent research has shown that all forms of LCH are clonal and thus may represent a form of malignancy.

Clinical Features
Head and neck lesions are common at initial presentation, and approximately 10% of all patients with LCH have oral lesions. Often the oral changes are the first clinical signs of the disease.

Eosinophilic granuloma (EG) usually appears in the skeleton (ribs, pelvis, long bones, skull, and jaws) and in rare cases in soft tissue. This condition occurs most often in older children and young adults but may develop later in life. The lesions often form quickly and may cause a dull, steady pain. In the jaws the disease may cause bony swelling, a soft tissue mass, gingivitis, bleeding gingiva, pain, and ulceration. Loosening or sloughing of the teeth often occurs after destruction of alveolar bone by one or more foci of EG. The sockets of teeth lost to the disease generally do not heal normally. EG may have a single focus or may develop into a multifocal, aggressive disease. The disseminated form may involve multiple bone lesions, diabetes insipidus, and exophthalmos, a condition previously defined as *Hand-Schüller-Christian disease.*

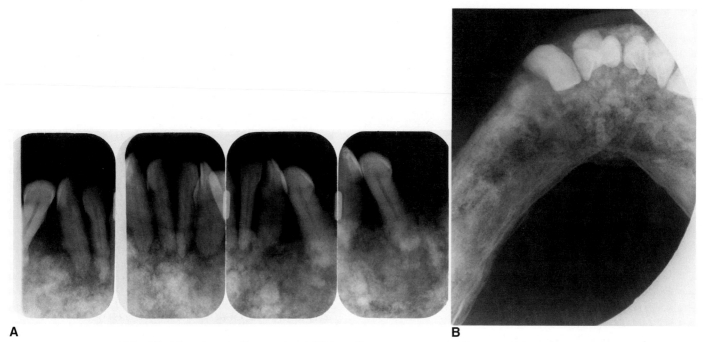

FIG. **23-29**   Paget's disease. **A,** Multiple radiopaque masses in the mandible that have a cotton-wool appearance. **B,** Note the expansion of the mandible and the maintenance of a thin outer cortical plate.

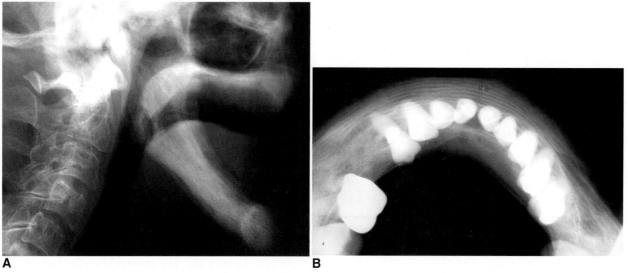

FIG. **23-30**   **A,** An edentulous mandible involved with Paget's disease. **B,** Occlusal film of another case of Paget's disease. Note the loss of normal outer cortex and the linear alignment of trabeculae. (**B,** Courtesy of Dr. Ross Macdonald, Adelaide, Australia.)

Letterer-Siwe disease is a malignant form of LCH that most often occurs in infants under 3 years of age. Soft tissue and bony granulomatous reactions disseminate throughout the body, and the condition is marked by intermittent fever, hepatosplenomegaly, anemia, lymph-adenopathy, hemorrhage, and failure to thrive.

Lesions in bone are rare. Death usually occurs within several weeks of the onset of the disease.

Radiographic Features

For ease of discussion, the author divides LCH jaw lesions into two groups: those that occur in the alveo-

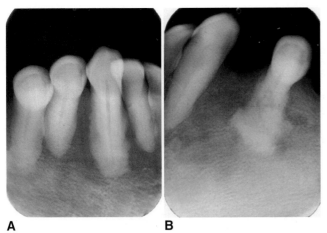

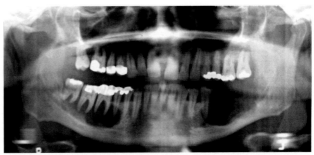

FIG. **23-32**   A panoramic film of multiple lesions of Langerhans' cell histiocytosis. Note the scooped-out shape of the bone destruction in the mandible. The floor of the right maxillary antrum has been destroyed.

A   B

FIG. **23-31**   A and B, Paget's disease showing exuberant irregular hypercementosis of the roots.

lar process and intraosseous lesions that occur elsewhere in the jaws. The radiographic features of this condition generally are similar to those of malignant neoplasms.

Location. The alveolar type of LCH lesions are commonly multiple, whereas the intraosseous type usually is solitary. The mandible is a more common site than the maxilla, and the posterior regions are more involved than the anterior regions (Fig. 23-32). The mandibular ramus is a common site of intraosseous lesions. Solitary lesions of the jaws may be accompanied by lesions in other bones.

Periphery and shape. The periphery of EG lesions varies from moderately to well defined but without cortication; the periphery sometimes appears punched out (Fig. 23-33). The margins may be smooth or somewhat irregular. The alveolar lesions commonly start in the midroot region of the teeth. The bone destruction progresses in a circular shape, and after it includes a portion of the superior border of the alveolar process, it may give the impression that a section of the alveolar process has been scooped out (Fig. 23-34; see also Fig. 23-32). The shape of intraosseous lesions may be irregular, oval, or round.

Internal structure. The internal structure usually is totally radiolucent.

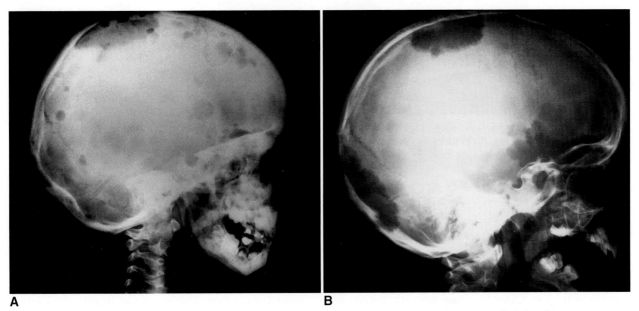

A   B

FIG. **23-33**   A and B, Skull lesions of Langerhans' cell histiocytosis, showing well-defined, punched-out lesions. (Courtesy Dr. H.G. Poyton, Toronto, Ontario.)

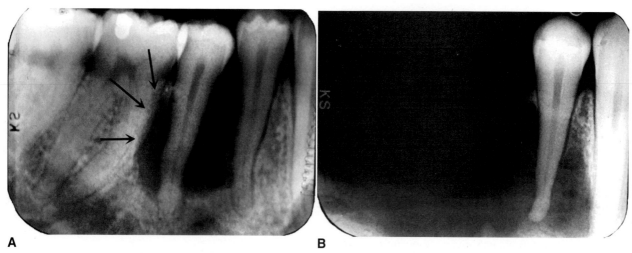

A   **B**

FIG. **23-34**   Two periapical films of the same area of the mandible taken approximately 1 year apart in a patient with Langerhans' cell histiocytosis. **A,** The earlier phase of the disease produces a scooped-out shape *(arrows),* which shows that the epicenter of the lesion is in the midroot area of the involved teeth, unlike in periodontal disease. **B,** One year later, bone destruction is extensive, resulting in loss of teeth. (Courtesy Dr. D. Stoneman, Toronto, Ontario, Canada.)

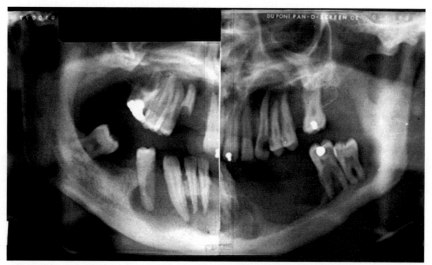

FIG. **23-35**   A panoramic film showing the bone destruction that can occur with Langerhans' cell histiocytosis. Note that the bone around many of the remaining mandibular teeth has been destroyed, leaving the teeth apparently unsupported. (Courtesy Dr. D. Stoneman.)

Effects on surrounding structures. LCH destroys bone. In alveolar lesions the bone around teeth, including the lamina dura, is destroyed; as a result, the teeth appear to be standing in space. The lesion does not displace teeth, although teeth may move because they are bereft of bone support (Fig. 23-35). Only minor root resorption has been reported. Of note is the ability of these lesions to stimulate periosteal new bone formation; this occurs more commonly with the intraosseous type of lesion (Fig. 23-36). The periosteal new bone formation is indistinguishable from the appearance seen in inflammatory lesions of the jaws. This lesion can destroy the outer cortical plate and in rare cases extends into the surrounding soft tissues in the CT examination.

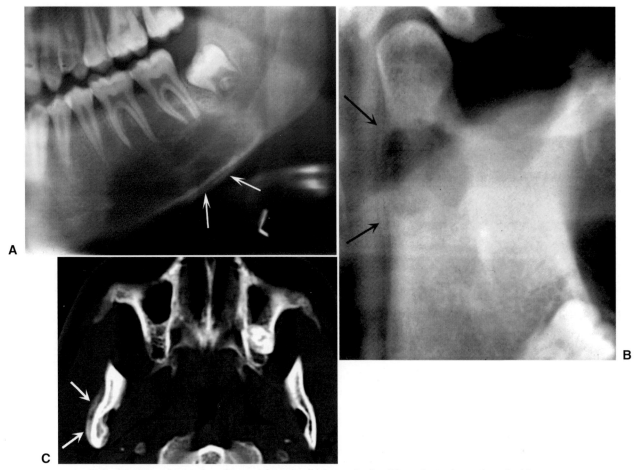

FIG. **23-36** Examples of Langerhans' cell histiocytosis with periosteal reaction. **A,** A large region of bone destruction in the body of the mandible with periosteal reaction along the inferior border *(arrows).* **B,** A lesion in the condylar neck with a faint periosteal reaction along the posterior border of the ramus *(arrows).* **C,** An axial CT scan of the lesion in **B,** showing a periosteal reaction *(arrows)* that extends to beyond the area of bone destruction.

Differential Diagnosis

The major differential diagnosis of alveolar-type lesions is periodontal disease and squamous cell carcinoma. An important characteristic in differentiation of periodontal disease is the fact that the epicenter of the bone destruction in LCH is approximately in the midroot region, resulting in a scooped-out appearance. In contrast, the bone destruction in periodontal disease starts at the alveolar crest and extends apically down the root surface. Differentiation of a squamous cell carcinoma may not be possible by radiographic characteristics alone, although the borders of an LCH lesion typically are better defined. Multiple lesions in a younger age group (usually the first 3 decades) are more likely to be

LCH than squamous cell carcinoma, which typically appears as a single lesion in middle or old age. LCH may bear a superficial resemblance to simple bone cysts, but the alveolar crest is maintained in simple bone cysts, and a partial cortex may be present.

The differential diagnosis of solitary intraosseous lesions includes metastatic malignant neoplasia and malignant tumors from adjacent soft tissues. However, the well-defined borders and the periosteal reaction seen in histiocytosis help in the differential diagnosis.

Patients suspected of having LCH should be referred to an oral and maxillofacial radiologist for a complete workup; this may include nuclear imaging to detect other possible bone lesions. The radiologic workup should be followed by a biopsy. The histologic appearance of histiocytosis may be hidden by changes caused by secondary infection from the oral cavity in alveolar lesions. Therefore it is important to correlate the radiographic findings with the histologic appearance of the biopsy.

Management

Treatment of localized lesions usually consists of surgical curettage or limited radiation therapy. Surgical management of jaw lesions usually is preferable because it has a low recurrence rate. The earlier EG of the mandible is diagnosed and controlled, the fewer teeth are lost to bone destruction. Disseminated disease is treated with chemotherapy.

SUGGESTED READINGS

FIBROUS DYSPLASIA

Ebata K et al: Chondrosarcoma and osteosarcoma arising in polyostotic fibrous dysplasia, J Oral Maxillofac Surg 50:761, 1992.

Eversole L et al: Fibrous dysplasia: a nosologic problem in the diagnosis of fibroosseous lesions of the jaws, J Oral Pathol 1:189, 1972.

Obisean A et al: The radiologic features of fibrous dysplasia of the craniofacial bones, Oral Surg 44:949, 1977.

Present D et al: Osteosarcoma of the mandible arising in fibrous dysplasia: a case report, Clin Orthop 204:238, 1986.

Tokano H et al: Sequential computed tomography images demonstrating characteristic changes in fibrous dysplasia, J of Laryngol Otol. 115:757, 2001.

Waldron C, Giansanti J: Benign fibroosseous lesions of the jaws: a clinical-radiologic-histologic review of sixty-five cases. I. Fibrous dysplasia of the jaws, Oral Surg 35:190, 1973.

PERIAPICAL CEMENTAL DYSPLASIA

Waldron C, Giansanti J: Benign fibroosseous lesions of the jaws: a clinical-radiologic-histologic review of sixty-five cases. II. Benign fibroosseous lesions of periodontal ligament origin, Oral Surg 35:340, 1973.

FLORID OSSEOUS DYSPLASIA

Fun-Chee L, Jinn-Fei Y: Florid osseous dysplasia in Orientals, Oral Surg Oral Med Oral Pathol 68:748, 1989.

MacDonald-Jankowski DS: Gigantiform cementoma occurring in two populations, London and Hong Kong, Clin Radiol 45:316, 1992.

Melrose RJ et al: Florid osseous dysplasia: a clinical-pathologic study of 34 cases, Oral Surg 41:62, 1976.

Thompson SH, Altini M: Gigantiform cementoma of the jaws, Head Neck 11:538, 1989.

CEMENTO-OSSIFYING FIBROMA

Eversole L et al: Radiographic characteristics of central ossifying fibroma, Oral Surg 59:522, 1985.

Hamner J et al: Benign fibroosseous jaw lesions of periodontal membrane origin: an analysis of 249 cases, Cancer 22:861, 1968.

Sciubba JJ, Younai F: Ossifying fibroma of the mandible and maxilla: review of 18 cases, J Oral Pathol Med 18:315, 1989.

GIANT CELL GRANULOMA

Cohen MA, Hertzanu Y: Radiologic features, including those seen with computed tomography, of central giant cell granuloma of the jaws, Oral Surg Oral Med Oral Pathol 65:255, 1988.

Horner K: Central giant cell granuloma of the jaws: a clinicoradiological study, Clin Radiol 40:622, 1989.

Waldron CA, Shafer WG: The central giant cell granuloma of the jaws: an analysis of 38 cases, Am J Clin Pathol 45:437, 1966.

ANEURYSMAL BONE CYST

Buraczewski J, Dabska P: Pathogenesis of aneurysmal bone cyst: relationship between the aneurysmal bone cyst and fibrous dysplasia of bone, Cancer 28:597, 1971.

Dahlin D, McLeod R: Aneurysmal bone cyst and other nonneoplastic conditions, Skeletal Radiol 8:243, 1982.

Giddings NA et al: Aneurysmal bone cyst of the mandible, Arch Otolaryngol Head Neck Surg 115:865, 1989.

Struthers P et al: Aneurysmal bone cyst of the jaws. I. Clinicopathological features, Int J Oral Surg 13:85, 1984.

Struthers P et al: Aneurysmal bone cyst of the jaws. II. Pathogenesis, Int J Oral Surg 13:92, 1984.

Tillman BP: Aneurysmal bone cyst: an analysis of 95 cases, Mayo Clin Proc 43:478, 1968.

CHERUBISM

Bianchi SD et al: The computed tomographic appearances of cherubism, Skeletal Radiol 16:6, 1987.

Faircloth WJ Jr et al: Cherubism involving a mother and daughter: case reports and review of the literature, J Oral Maxillofac Surg 49:535, 1991.

Katz JO et al: Cherubism: report of a case showing regression without treatment, J Oral Maxillofac Surg 50:301, 1992.

Reade P et al: Unilateral mandibular cherubism: brief review and case report, Br J Oral Maxillofac Surg 22:189, 1984.

PAGET'S DISEASE

Barker D: The epidemiology of Paget's disease, Metab Bone Dis Rel Res 3:231, 1981.

Kanis J et al: Paget's disease of bone: diagnosis and management, Metab Bone Dis Rel Res 3:219, 1981.

Rao V, Karasick D: Hypercementosis: an important clue to Paget's disease of the maxilla, Skeletal Radiol 9:126, 1982.

Singer F, Millo B: Evidence for a viral etiology of Paget's disease of bone, Clin Orthop 178:245, 1983.

Smith B, Eveson J: Paget's disease of bone with particular reference to dentistry, J Oral Pathol 10:233, 1981.

Sofaer J: Dental extractions in Paget's disease of bone, Int J Oral Surg 13:79, 1984.

LANGERHANS' CELL HISTIOCYTOSIS

Bottomley WK et al: Histiocytosis X: report of an oral soft tissue lesion without bony involvement, Oral Surg Oral Med Oral Pathol 63:228, 1987.

Cline MJ: Histiocytes and histiocytosis, Blood 84:2840, 1996.

Domboski M: Eosinophilic granuloma of bone manifesting mandibular involvement, Oral Surg Oral Med Oral Pathol 50:116, 1980.

Gorsky M et al: Histiocytosis X: occurrence and oral involvement in six adolescent and adult patients, Oral Surg Oral Med Oral Pathol 55:24, 1983.

Hartman KS: Histiocytosis X: a review of 114 cases with oral involvement, Oral Surg Oral Med Oral Pathol 49:38, 1980.

Wong GB et al: Eosinophilic granuloma of the mandibular condyle: report of three cases and review of the literature, J Oral Maxillofac Surg 55:870, 1997.

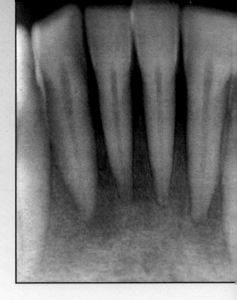

CHAPTER 24

Systemic Diseases Manifested in the Jaws

Definition

Disorders of the endocrine system, bone metabolism, and other systemic diseases may have an effect on the form and function of bone and teeth. The function of bone not only includes support, protection, and an environment for hemopoiesis but also serves as a major reserve of calcium for the body. More than 99% of the total body calcium is contained within the skeletal structure. When considering the influence of systemic conditions on the jaws, it is important to recognize that bone is constantly remodeling. Approximately 5% to 10% of the total bone mass is replaced each year. The turnover rate of trabecular bone is higher than for cortical bone; 20% of its mass is replaced per year, compared with 5% for cortical bone. The effects of systemic diseases of bone are brought about by changes in the number and activity of osteoclasts, osteoblasts, and osteocytes.

Radiographic Features

Because systemic disorders affect the entire body, the radiographic changes manifested in the jaws are generalized (Table 24-1). In most cases it is not possible to identify diseases based on radiographic characteristics. The general changes include the following:

1. A change in size and shape of the bone
2. A change in the number, size, and orientation of trabeculae
3. Altered thickness and density of cortical structures
4. An increase or decrease in overall bone density

Changes in the first three elements can result in a decrease or increase in bone density.

Because many parameters in the production of a radiograph influence the density of the image, it is difficult to detect genuine changes in the density of bone. Systemic conditions that result in a decrease in bone density do not affect the teeth; therefore the image of the teeth may stand out with normal density against a generally radiolucent jaw. In severe cases the teeth may appear to be bereft of any bony support. Also, cortical structures appear thin and less defined and occasionally disappear. On the other hand, a true increase in bone density may be detected by a loss of contrast of the inferior cortex of the mandible as the radiopacity of the cancellous bone approaches that of cortical bone. Often the inferior alveolar nerve canal appears more distinct in contrast to the surrounding dense bone.

Some systemic diseases that occur during tooth formation may result in dental alterations. Lamina dura is part of the bone structure of the alveolar process, but because it is usually examined in conjunction with the periodontal membrane space and roots of teeth, it is included with the description of the dental structures (Table 24-2). Changes to teeth and associated structures include the following:

1. Accelerated or delayed eruption
2. Hypoplasia
3. Hypocalcification
4. Loss of a distinct lamina dura

Often bone and teeth exhibit no detectable radiographic changes associated with systemic diseases.

TABLE **24-1**
Radiographic Changes in Bone Observed in Systemic Disease*

| | | | BONE | | |
| | | | | TRABECULAE | |
SYSTEMIC DISEASE	DENSITY	SIZE OF JAWS	INCREASE	DECREASE	GRANULAR
Hyperparathyroidism	Decrease	No	Yes	Yes	Yes
Hypoparathyroidism	Rare increase	No	No	No	No
Hyperpituitarism	No	Large	No	No	No
Hypopituitarism	No	Small	No	No	No
Hypothyroidism	Decrease	No	No	No	No
Hyperthyroidism	No	Small	No	No	No
Cushing's syndrome	Decrease	No	No	Yes	Yes
Osteoporosis	Decrease	No	No	Yes	No
Rickets	Decrease	No	No	Yes	No
Osteomalacia	Rare decrease	No	No	Rare decrease	No
Hypophosphatasia	Decrease	No	No	Yes	No
Renal osteodystrophy	Decrease; Rare increase	No	Rare	Yes	Yes
Hypophosphatemia	Decrease	No	No	Yes	Yes

*This table summarizes the major radiographic changes to bone with endocrine and metabolic bone diseases. It does not include all the possible variable appearances.

However, on occasion the first symptoms of a disease may present as a dental problem.

Endocrine Disorders

HYPERPARATHYROIDISM

Definition

Hyperparathyroidism is an endocrine abnormality in which there is an excess of circulating parathyroid hormone (PTH). An excess of serum PTH increases bone remodeling in preference of osteoclastic resorption, which mobilizes calcium from the skeleton. In addition, PTH increases renal tubular reabsorption of calcium and renal production of the active vitamin D metabolite $1,25(OH)_2D$. The net result of these functions is in an increase in serum calcium.

Primary hyperparathyroidism usually results from a benign tumor (adenoma) of one of the four parathyroid glands, which produces excess PTH. Less frequently, individuals may have hyperplastic parathyroid glands that secrete excess PTH. The combination of hypercalcemia and an elevated serum level of PTH is diagnostic of primary hyperparathyroidism. The incidence of primary hyperparathyroidism is about 0.1%.

Secondary hyperparathyroidism results from a compensatory increase in the output of PTH in response to hypocalcemia. The underlying hypocalcemia may result from an inadequate dietary intake or poor absorption of vitamin D or from deficient metabolism of vitamin D in the liver or kidney. This condition produces clinical and radiographic effects similar to those of primary hyperparathyroidism.

Clinical Features

Women are two to three times more commonly affected than men by primary hyperparathyroidism. The condition occurs mainly in those 30 to 60 years of age. Clinical manifestations of the disease cover a broad range, but most patients have renal calculi, peptic ulcers, psychiatric problems, or bone and joint pain. These clinical symptoms are mainly related to hypercalcemia. Gradual loosening, drifting, and loss of teeth may occur. Definite consistent hypercalcemia is virtually pathognomonic of primary hyperparathyroidism.

TABLE 24-2
Effects of Systemic Disease on Dental Structures*

SYSTEMIC DISEASE	EFFECTS ON TEETH AND ASSOCIATED STRUCTURES					
	HYPOCALCIFICATION	HYPOPLASIA	LARGE PULP CHAMBER	LOSS OF LAMINA DURA	LOSS OF TEETH	ERUPTION
Hyperparathyroidism	No	No	No	Yes	Rare	No
Hypoparathyroidism	No	Yes	No	No	No	Delayed
Hyperpituitarism	No	No	No	No	No	Supereruption
Hypopituitarism	No	No	No	No	No	Delayed
Hypothyroidism	No	No	No	No	Yes	Early
Hyperthyroidism	No	No	No	Thin	Yes	Delayed
Cushing's syndrome	No	No	No	Partial	No	Premature
Osteoporosis	No	No	No	Thin	No	No
Rickets	Yes—enamel	Yes—enamel	No	Thin	No	Delayed
Osteomalacia	No	No	No	No	No	No
Hypophosphatasia	Yes	Yes	Yes	Yes	Yes	No
Renal osteodystrophy	Yes	Yes	No	Yes	Yes	No
Hypophosphatemia	Yes	Yes	Yes	Yes	Yes	No
Osteopetrosis	No	rare	No	No	No	Delayed

*This table summarizes the major radiographic changes that can occur to teeth and associated structures with endocrine and metabolic bone diseases. It does not include all the possible variable appearances.

(Rarely, multiple myeloma and metastatic tumors may produce the same serum alterations.) Because of daily fluctuations, the serum calcium level should be tested at different intervals. The serum alkaline phosphatase level, a reliable indicator of bone turnover, may also be elevated in hyperparathyroidism.

Radiographic Features
Only about one in five patients with hyperparathyroidism has radiographically observable bone changes.

General radiographic features. The following are the major manifestations of hyperparathyroidism:
1. The earliest and most reliable changes of hyperparathyroidism are subtle erosions of bone from the subperiosteal surfaces of the phalanges of the hands.
2. Demineralization of the skeleton results in an unusual radiolucent appearance.
3. Osteitis fibrosa cystica are localized regions of bone loss produced by osteoclastic activity, resulting in a loss of all apparent bone structure.

4. Brown tumors occur late in the disease and in about 10% of cases. These peripheral or central tumors of bone are radiolucent. The gross specimen has a brown or reddish-brown color.
5. Pathologic calcifications in soft tissues have a punctate or nodular appearance and occur in the kidneys and joints.
6. In prominent hyperparathyroidism, the entire calvarium has a granular appearance caused by the loss of central (diploic) trabeculae and thinning of the cortical tables.

Radiographic features of the jaws. Demineralization and thinning of cortical boundaries often occur in the jaws in cortical boundaries such as the inferior border, mandibular canal, and the cortical outlines of the maxillary sinuses. The density of the jaws is decreased, resulting in a radiolucent appearance that contrasts with the density of the teeth. The teeth stand out in contrast to the radiolucent jaws (Fig. 24-1). A change in the normal trabecular pattern may occur, resulting in a

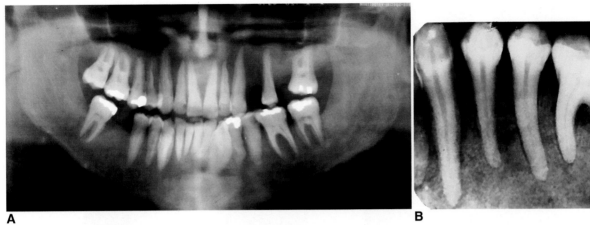

FIG. **24-1** **A,** In this panoramic image, the loss of bone in hyperparathyroidism results in the image of the radiopaque teeth standing out in contrast to the radiolucent jaws. **B,** Note the loss of a distinct lamina dura and the granular texture of the bone pattern. (**B,** Courtesy H.G. Poyton, DDS, Toronto, Ontario.)

ground-glass appearance of numerous, small, randomly oriented trabeculae.

Brown tumors of hyperparathyroidism may appear in any bone but are frequently found in the facial bones and jaws, particularly in long-standing cases of the disease. These lesions may be multiple within a single bone. They have variably defined margins and may produce cortical expansion (Fig. 24-2). If solitary, the tumor may resemble a central giant cell granuloma or an aneurysmal bone cyst. It is interesting to note that the histologic appearance of the brown tumor is identical to that of the giant cell granuloma. Therefore, if a giant cell granuloma occurs later than the second decade, the patient should be screened for an increase in serum calcium, PTH, and alkaline phosphatase.

Radiographic features of the teeth and associated structures. Occasionally periapical radiographs reveal loss of the lamina dura in patients (only about 10%) with hyperparathyroidism. Depending on the duration and severity of the disease, loss of the lamina dura may occur around one tooth or all the remaining teeth. The loss may be either complete or partial around a particular tooth. The result of lamina dura loss may give the root a tapered appearance because of decreased image contrast. Although PTH mobilizes minerals from the skeleton, mature teeth are immune to this systemic demineralizing process.

Management
After successful surgical removal of the causative parathyroid adenoma, almost all radiographic changes revert to normal. The only exception may be the site of a brown tumor, which often heals with bone that is radiographically more sclerotic than normal. Many people with this disease are being diagnosed earlier, resulting in fewer severe cases.

HYPOPARATHYROIDISM AND PSEUDOHYPOPARATHYROIDISM

Definition
Hypoparathyroidism is an uncommon condition in which insufficient secretion of PTH occurs. Several causes exist, but the most common is damage or removal of the parathyroid glands during thyroid surgery. In pseudohypoparathyroidism there is a defect in the response of the tissue target cells to normal levels of PTH.

Clinical Features
Both hypoparathyroidism and pseudohypoparathyroidism produce hypocalcemia, which has a variety of clinical manifestations. Most often this includes sharp flexion (tetany) of the wrist and ankle joints (carpopedal spasm). Some patients have sensory abnormalities consisting of paresthesia of the hands, feet, or area around the mouth. Neurologic changes may include anxiety and depression, epilepsy, parkinsonism, and chorea. Chronic forms may produce a reduction in intellectual capacity. Some patients show no changes at all. Patients with pseudohypoparathyroidism often have early closure of certain bony epiphyses and thus manifest short stature or extremity disproportions.

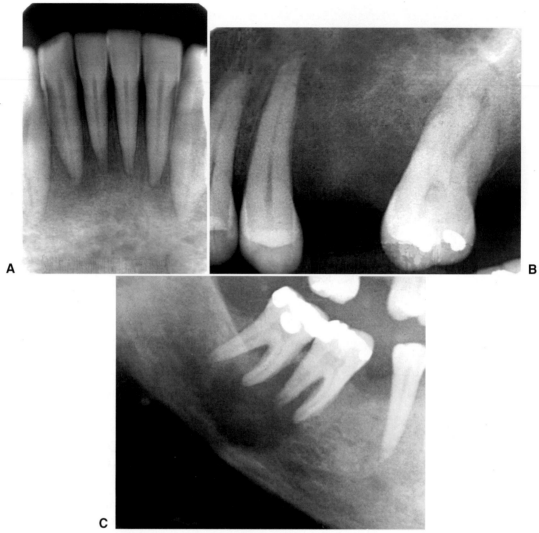

FIG. **24-2**   Hyperparathyroidism. **A** and **B** reveal a granular bone pattern that was characteristic in all intraoral films. Note the loss of a distinct lamina dura and floor of the maxillary antrum. **C,** This panoramic view of the same case reveals a brown tumor related to the apical region of the second and third molars.

Radiographic Features

The principal radiographic change is calcification of the basal ganglia. On skull radiographs this calcification appears flocculent and paired within the cerebral hemispheres on the posteroanterior view. Radiographic examination of the jaws may reveal dental enamel hypoplasia, external root resorption, delayed eruption, or root dilaceration (Fig. 24-3).

Treatment

These conditions are managed with orally administered supplemental calcium and vitamin D.

HYPERPITUITARISM

Synonyms

Acromegaly and giantism

Definition

Hyperpituitarism results from hyperfunction of the anterior lobe of the pituitary gland, which increases the production of growth hormone. An excess of growth hormone causes overgrowth of all tissues in the body still capable of growth. The usual cause of this problem is a benign, functioning tumor of the acidophilic cells in the anterior lobe of the pituitary gland.

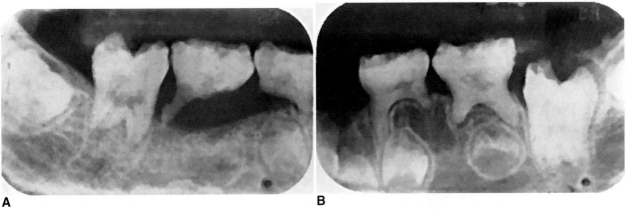

FIG. **24-3** Pseudohypoparathyroidism-induced dental anomalies. (Courtesy Dr. S. Bricker, San Antonio, Tex.)

Clinical Features

Hyperpituitarism in children involves generalized overgrowth of most hard and soft tissues, a condition termed *giantism.* Active growth occurs in those bones in which the epiphyses have not united with the bone shafts. Throughout adolescence, generalized skeletal growth is excessive and may be prolonged. Those affected may ultimately attain heights of 7 to 8 feet or more yet exhibit remarkably normal proportions. The eyes and other parts of the central nervous system do not enlarge, except in rare cases in which the condition is manifested in infancy.

Adult hyperpituitarism, called *acromegaly,* has an insidious clinical course, quite different from the clinical profile seen in the childhood disease. In adults the clinical effects of a pituitary adenoma develop quite slowly because many types of tissues have lost the capacity for growth. This is true of much of the skeleton; however, an excess of growth hormone can stimulate the mandible and the phalanges of the hand. Mandibular condylar growth may be very prominent. Also, the supraorbital ridges and the underlying frontal sinus may be enlarged. Excess growth hormone in adults may also produce hypertrophy of some soft tissues. The lips, tongue, nose, and soft tissues of the hands and feet typically overgrow in adults with acromegaly, sometimes to a striking degree.

Radiographic Features

General radiographic features. The pituitary tumor responsible for hyperpituitarism often produces enlargement ("ballooning") of the sella turcica (Fig. 24-4, *B*). It is important to note, however, that in some examples the sella may not expand at all. Skull radiographs characteristically reveal enlargement of the paranasal sinuses (especially the frontal sinus). These air sinuses

are more prominent in acromegaly than in pituitary giantism because sinus growth in giantism tends to be more in step with the generalized enlargement of the facial bones. Hyperpituitarism in adults also produces diffuse thickening of the outer table of the skull.

Radiographic features of the jaws. Hyperpituitarism causes enlargement of the jaws, most notably the mandible (Fig. 24-4, *A*). The increase in the length of the dental arches results in spacing of the teeth. In acromegaly the angle between the ramus and body of the mandible may increase. This, in combination with enlargement of the tongue (macroglossia), may result in anterior flaring of the teeth and the development of an anterior open bite. The sign of incisor flaring is a helpful point of differentiation between acromegalic prognathism and inherited prognathism. In acromegaly the most profound growth occurs in the condyle and ramus, often resulting in a class III skeletal relationship between the jaws. The thickness and height of the alveolar processes may also increase.

Radiographic changes associated with the teeth. The tooth crowns are usually normal in size, although the roots of posterior teeth often enlarge as a result of hypercementosis. This hypercementosis may be the result of functional and structural demands on teeth instead of a secondary hormonal effect. Supereruption of the posterior teeth may occur in an attempt to compensate for the growth of the mandible.

HYPOPITUITARISM

Definition

Hypopituitarism results from reduced secretion of pituitary hormones.

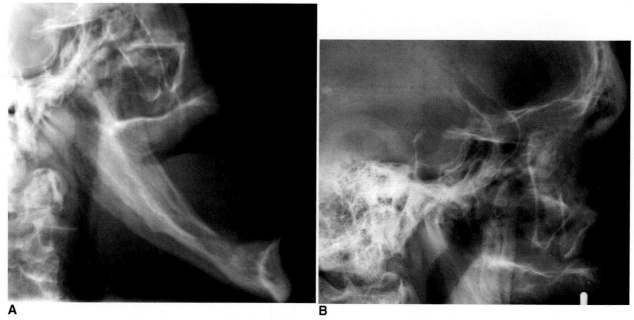

A   **B**

FIG. **24-4** **A,** An example of acromegaly manifesting as excessive growth of the mandible, resulting in a class III skeletal relationship of the jaws. **B,** A portion of a lateral skull view of the same patient demonstrating enlargement of the sella turcica.

Clinical Features
Individuals with this condition show dwarfism but have relatively well-proportioned bodies. One study reported a marked failure of development of the maxilla and the mandible. The dimensions of these bones in these adults were approximately the same as those of normal children 5 to 7 years of age.

Radiographic Features
Eruption of the primary dentition occurs at the normal time, but exfoliation is delayed by several years. The crowns of the permanent teeth form normally, but their eruption is delayed several years. The third molar buds may be completely absent. In hypopituitarism the jaws are small, especially the mandible; this results in crowding and malocclusion.

Treatment
Treatment is usually directed toward removal of the cause or replacement of the pituitary hormones or those of its target gland. The response of the dentition to treatment with growth hormone is variable but seems to parallel skeletal response.

HYPERTHYROIDISM
Synonyms
Thyrotoxicosis and Graves' disease

Definition
Hyperthyroidism is a syndrome that involves excessive production of thyroxin in the thyroid gland. This condition occurs most commonly with diffuse toxic goiter (Graves' disease) and less frequently with toxic nodular goiter or toxic adenoma, a benign tumor of the thyroid gland. Each of these conditions results in increased levels of circulating thyroxin. Excessive thyroxin causes a generalized increase in the metabolic rate of all body tissues, resulting in tachycardia, increased blood pressure, sensitivity to heat, and irritability. Hyperthyroidism is more common in females.

Radiographic Features
Hyperthyroidism results in an advanced rate of dental development and early eruption, with premature loss of the primary teeth. Adults may show a generalized decrease in bone density or loss of some areas of edentulous alveolar bone.

HYPOTHYROIDISM
Synonyms
Myxedema and cretinism

Definition
Hypothyroidism usually results from insufficient secretion of thyroxin by the thyroid glands, despite the presence of thyroid-stimulating hormone.

Clinical Features

In children, hypothyroidism may result in retarded mental and physical development. The base of the skull shows delayed ossification, and the paranasal sinuses only partially pneumatize. Dental development is delayed, and the primary teeth are slow to exfoliate.

Hypothyroidism in the adult results in myxedematous swelling but not the dental or skeletal changes seen in children. Adult symptoms may range from lethargy, poor memory, inability to concentrate, constipation, and cold intolerance to the more florid clinical picture of dull and expressionless face, periorbital edema, large tongue, sparse hair, and skin that feels "doughy" to the touch.

Radiographic Features

Radiographic features in children include delayed closing of the epiphyses and skull sutures with the production of numerous wormian bones (accessory bones in the sutures). Effects on the teeth include delayed eruption, short roots, and thinning of the lamina dura. The maxilla and mandible are relatively small. Patients with adult hypothyroidism may show periodontal disease, loss of teeth, separation of teeth as a result of enlargement of the tongue, and external root resorption.

DIABETES MELLITUS

Definition

Diabetes mellitus is a metabolic disorder that has two primary forms. Type 1, insulin-dependent diabetes mellitus (previously known as *juvenile-onset diabetes*), results from an absence or insufficiency of insulin, a hormone normally produced by the beta cells of the islets of Langerhans in the pancreas. Type 2, noninsulin-dependent diabetes mellitus, results from insulin resistance. Patients with type 1 diabetes have virtually no beta cells (in the islets), whereas patients with type 2 diabetes have approximately half the normal number. A shortage of insulin adversely affects carbohydrate metabolism. The principal clinical laboratory signs of the disease are hyperglycemia and glycosuria, both reflecting a complex biochemical imbalance between tissue demand for glucose and the release of this nutrient by the liver.

Clinical Features

Untreated diabetes may manifest classic symptoms and signs such as polydipsia (excessive intake of fluids), polyuria (excessive urination), and in more severe cases, acetone present in the urine and on the breath. This metabolic disorder, if not adequately treated, lowers the resistance of the body to infection. Diabetes may demonstrate a number of adverse effects in the oral cavity. Most prominently, uncontrolled diabetes acts as a continuing factor that predisposes to, aggravates, and accelerates periodontal disease. Patients with controlled diabetes do not appear to have more periodontal problems than do persons without diabetes. Some children with uncontrolled diabetes have an increased likelihood of caries activity because of a high-carbohydrate diet. Another occasional oral complication of diabetes mellitus is xerostomia resulting from a reduced salivary flow (about one third of normal).

Radiographic Features

Diabetes mellitus exhibits no characteristic radiographic features of the jaws or teeth. Periodontal disease associated with diabetes is indistinguishable radiographically from periodontal disease in patients without diabetes.

CUSHING'S SYNDROME

Definition

Cushing's syndrome arises from an excess of secretion of glucocorticoids by the adrenal glands. This may result from any of the following:
1. An adrenal adenoma
2. An adrenal carcinoma
3. Adrenal hyperplasia (usually bilateral)
4. A basophilic adenoma of the anterior lobe of the pituitary gland (Cushing's disease), producing excess adrenocorticotropic hormone (ACTH)
5. Medical therapy with exogenous corticosteroids

The increased level of glucocorticoid results in a loss of bone mass from reduced osteoblastic function and either directly or indirectly increased osteoclastic function.

Clinical Features

Patients with Cushing's syndrome often show obesity (which spares the extremities), kyphosis of the thoracic spine ("buffalo hump"), weakness, hypertension, striae, or concurrent diabetes. This condition affects females three to five times as frequently as males. Onset may occur at any age but is usually seen in the third or fourth decade.

Radiographic Features

The primary radiographic feature of Cushing's syndrome is generalized osteoporosis, which may have a granular bone pattern. This demineralization may result in pathologic fractures. The skull can show diffuse thinning accompanied by a mottled appearance. The teeth may erupt prematurely, and partial loss of the lamina dura may occur (Fig. 24-5).

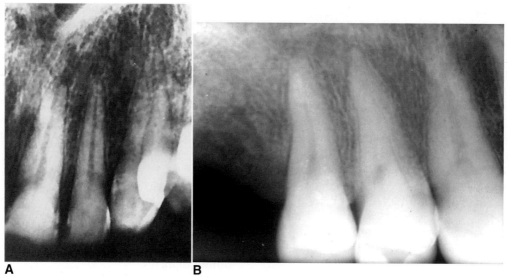

FIG. **24-5**   **A** and **B,** Cushing's syndrome manifested in the jaws as thinning of the lamina dura. (Courtesy H.G. Poyton, DDS, Toronto, Ontario.)

Metabolic Bone Diseases

OSTEOPOROSIS

Definition

Osteoporosis is a generalized decrease in bone mass in which the histologic appearance of bone is normal. An imbalance occurs in bone resorption and formation. Decrease in bone formation results in a lower trabecular bone volume and thinning of cortical bone and trabeculae.

Osteoporosis occurs with the aging process of bone and can be considered a variation of normal (primary osteoporosis). Bone mass normally increases from infancy to about 35 to 40 years of age. At this time there begins a gradual and progressive decline, occurring at the rate of about 8% per decade in women and 3% per decade in men. The loss of bone mass with age is so gradual that it is virtually imperceptible until it reaches significant proportions.

Secondary osteoporosis may result from nutritional deficiencies, hormonal imbalance, inactivity, or corticosteroid or heparin therapy.

Clinical Features

The most important clinical manifestation of osteoporosis is fracture. The most common locations are the distal radius, proximal femur, ribs, and vertebrae. Patients may suffer from bone pain. The population most at risk is postmenopausal women.

Radiographic Features

Osteoporosis results in an overall reduction in the density of bone. This reduction may be observed in the jaws by using the unaltered density of teeth as a comparison. There may be evidence of a reduced density and thinning of cortical boundaries such as the inferior mandibular cortex (Fig. 24-6). Reduction in the volume of cancellous bone is more difficult to assess. Reduction in the number of trabeculae is least evident in the alveolar process, possibly because of the constant stress applied to this region of bone by the teeth. On occasion the lamina dura may appear thinner than normal. In other regions of the mandible a reduction in the number of trabeculae may be evident. Accurate assessment of bone mass loss is difficult but may be done with sophisticated techniques such as dual energy photon absorption (DEXA) or quantitative computed tomography (QCT) programs.

Treatment

The administration of estrogens and calcium supplements after menopause helps to prevent further cortical and trabecular bone loss. Exercise programs are also effective.

RICKETS AND OSTEOMALACIA

Definition

Rickets and osteomalacia result from inadequate serum and extracellular levels of calcium and phosphate,

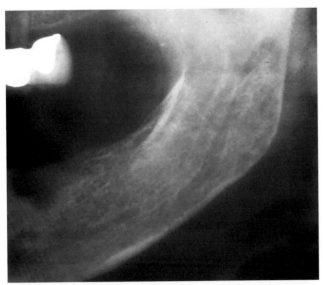

FIG. **24-6** Osteoporosis evident as a loss of the normal thickness and density of the inferior cortex of the mandible.

minerals required for the normal calcification of bone and teeth. Both abnormalities result from a defect in the normal activity of the metabolites of vitamin D, especially 1,25(OH)$_2$D, required for resorption of calcium in the intestine. Failure of normal mineralization is seen histologically as wide uncalcified osteoid (new bone matrix) seams. The term *rickets* is usually applied when the disease affects the growing skeleton in infants and children. The term *osteomalacia* is used when this disease affects the mature skeleton in adults.

Failure of normal activity of vitamin D may occur as a result of the following:
1. Lack of vitamin D in the diet
2. Lack of absorption of vitamin D resulting from various gastrointestinal malabsorption problems
3. Lack of metabolism of the active metabolite 1,25(OH)$_2$D that is required for intestinal absorption of calcium

Interference may occur anywhere along the metabolic pathway for 1,25(OH)$_2$D:
1. Lack of exposure to ultraviolet light required for conversion of provitamin D$_3$
2. Lack of conversion of vitamin D$_3$ to 25(OH)D in the liver because of liver disease
3. Lack of metabolism of 25(OH)D$_2$ to 1,25(OH)$_2$D by the kidney because of kidney diseases
4. A defect in the intestinal target cell response to 1,25(OH)$_2$D or inadequate calcium supply

Clinical Features

Rickets. In the first 6 months of life, tetany or convulsions are the most common clinical problems resulting from the hypocalcemia of rickets. Later in infancy the skeletal effects of the disease may be more clinically prominent. Craniotabes, a softening of the posterior of the parietal bones, may be the initial sign of the disease. The wrists and ankles typically swell. Children with rickets usually have short stature and deformity of the extremities. Development of the dentition is delayed, and the eruption rate of the teeth is retarded.

Osteomalacia. Most patients with osteomalacia have some degree of bone pain. The majority of patients with osteomalacia have muscle weakness of varying severity. Other clinical features include a peculiar waddling or "penguin" gait, tetany, and greenstick bone fractures.

Radiographic Features

General radiographic features. In rickets the earliest and most prominent radiographic manifestation is a widening and fraying of the epiphyses of the long bones. The soft weight-bearing bones such as the femur and tibia undergo a characteristic bowing. Greenstick fractures (an incomplete fracture) occur in many patients with rickets.

In osteomalacia the cortex of bone may be thin. Pseudofractures, which are poorly calcified, ribbonlike zones extending into bone at approximate right angles to the margin of the bone, may also be present. Pseudofractures occur most commonly in the ribs, pelvis, and weight-bearing bones and rarely in the mandible.

Radiographic features of the jaws. In rickets, jaw cortical structures, such as the inferior mandibular border or the walls of the mandibular canal, may thin. Changes in the jaws generally occur after changes in the ribs and long bones. Within the cancellous portion of the jaws, the trabeculae become reduced in density, number, and thickness. In severe cases, the jaws appear so radiolucent that the teeth appear to be bereft of bony support.

Most cases of osteomalacia produce no radiographic manifestations in the jaws. However, there may be an overall radiolucent appearance and sparse trabeculae.

Radiographic changes associated with the teeth. Rickets in infancy or early childhood may result in hypoplasia of developing dental enamel (Fig. 24-7). If the disease occurs before 3 years, such enamel hypoplasia is fairly common. Radiographs may reveal this early manifestation of rickets in unerupted and erupted teeth. Radiographs may also document retarded tooth eruption in early rickets. The lamina dura and the

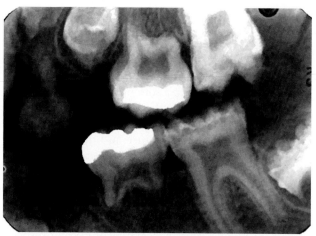

FIG. **24-7**   Rickets may cause thinning (hypoplasia) or decreased mineralization (hypocalcification) of the enamel as is seen in this bitewing view. (Courtesy H.G. Poyton, DDS, Toronto, Ontario.)

cortical boundary of tooth follicles may be thin or missing.

Osteomalacia does not alter the teeth because they are fully developed before the onset of the disease. The lamina dura may be especially thin in individuals with long-standing or severe osteomalacia.

HYPOPHOSPHATASIA

Definition
Hypophosphatasia is a rare inherited disorder that is caused by either a reduced production or a defective function of alkaline phosphatase. This enzyme is required for normal mineralization of osteoid. Patients have a low level of serum alkaline phosphatase activity and elevated urinary excretion of phospho-ethanolamine. The usual pattern of inheritance is an autosomal dominant mode of disease transmission.

Clinical Features
The disease in individuals with homozygous involvement usually begins in utero, and affected patients often die within the first year. These infants demonstrate bowed limb bones and a marked deficiency of skull ossification. Individuals with heterozygous disease show the biochemical defects but a milder disease clinically. These children show poor growth, fractures, and deformities similar to rickets. A history may exist of fractures, delayed walking, or rickets-like deformities that heal spontaneously. About 85% of these children show premature loss of the primary teeth, particularly the incisors, and delayed eruption of the permanent dentition. This is often the first clinical sign of hypophosphatasia.

Radiographic Features
General radiographic features. In young children with hypophosphatasia the long bones show irregular defects in the epiphysis, and the skull is poorly calcified. In older children with premature closure of the skull sutures, multiple lucent areas of the calvarium may exist, called *gyral* or *convolutional markings*. These markings resemble hammered copper. The skull may assume a brachycephalic shape. A generalized reduction in bone density may occur in adults.

Radiographic features of the jaws. A generalized radiolucency of the mandible and maxilla is evident. The cortical bone and lamina dura are thin, and the alveolar bone is poorly calcified and may appear deficient.

Radiographic changes associated with the teeth. Both primary and permanent teeth have a thin enamel layer and large pulp chambers and root canals (Fig. 24-8). The teeth may also be hypoplastic and may be lost prematurely.

RENAL OSTEODYSTROPHY

Synonym
Renal rickets

Definition
In renal osteodystrophy, bone changes result from chronic renal failure. The kidney disease interferes with the hydroxylation of $25(OH)D$ into $1,25(OH)_2D$, which normally occurs in the kidney. The vitamin D metabolite $1,25(OH)_2D$ is responsible for the active transport of calcium in the duodenum and upper jejunum. Affected patients often have hypocalcemia as a result of impaired calcium absorption and hyperphosphatemia resulting from reduction in renal phosphorus excretion. A prolonged low serum level of calcium stimulates the parathyroid glands to produce PTH. The result is a secondary hyperparathyroidism.

Clinical Features
The clinical features of renal osteodystrophy are those of chronic renal failure. In children, growth retardation and frequent bone fractures may occur. Adults may experience a gradual softening and bowing of the bones.

Radiographic Features
General radiographic features. The radiographic features of renal osteodystrophy are quite variable. Some changes of the skeleton resemble those seen in rickets, and other changes are consistent with hyperparathyroidism, including generalized loss of bone

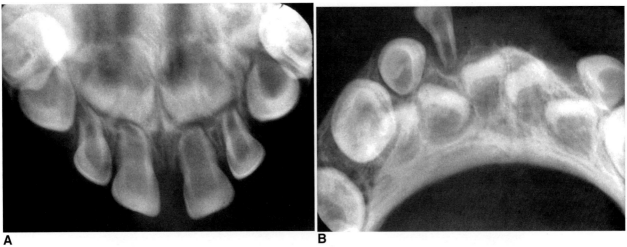

FIG. **24-8** **A** and **B,** An example of hypophosphatasia. Note the large pulp chambers in the deciduous dentition and the premature loss of the mandibular incisors. (Courtesy of H.G. Poyton, DDS, Toronto, Ontario.)

density and thinning of bony cortices. Of interest is the occasional finding of an increase in bone density (Fig. 24-9). There may be brown tumors, similar to those seen in primary hyperthyroidism, but these are less frequent.

Radiographic features of the jaws. In renal osteodystrophy the density of the mandible and maxilla may be less than normal and occasionally may be greater than normal. Manifestations include a decrease or an increase in the number of internal trabeculae, and the trabecular bone pattern may be granular. The cortical boundaries may be thinner or less apparent. It is important to note that these bone changes may persist after a successful renal transplant because of hyperplasia of the parathyroid glands, resulting in a continued elevation of PTH.

Radiographic changes associated with the teeth. Hypoplasia and hypocalcification of the teeth are possible, sometimes resulting in loss of any radiographic evidence of enamel. The lamina dura may be absent or less apparent in instances of bone sclerosis.

HYPOPHOSPHATEMIA

Synonym
Vitamin D–resistant rickets, hyposphosphatemic rickets

Definition
Hypophosphatemia represents a group of inherited conditions that produce renal tubular disorders,

resulting in excessive loss of phosphorus. There is a failure to reabsorb phosphorus in the distal renal tubules, which results in a decrease in serum phosphorus (hypophosphatemia). Normal calcification of the osseous structures requires the correct amount and ratio of serum calcium and phosphorus. Multiple myeloma may induce hypophosphatemia as a result of secondary damage to the kidneys.

Clinical Features
Children with hypophosphatemia show reduced growth and rickets-like bony changes. These include bowing of the legs, enlarged epiphyses, and skull changes. Adults have bone pain, muscle weakness, and vertebral fractures.

Radiographic Features
General radiographic features. In children with hypophosphatemia, radiographic findings are indistinguishable from those of rickets. In adults the long bones may show persistent deformity, fractures, or pseudofractures.

Radiographic features of the jaws. The jaws are usually osteoporotic and in extreme cases are remarkably radiolucent. Cortical boundaries may be unusually radiolucent or not apparent (Fig. 24-10). Other possibilities include fewer visible trabeculae and a granular trabecular pattern.

Radiographic features associated with the teeth. The teeth may be poorly formed, with thin enamel caps and

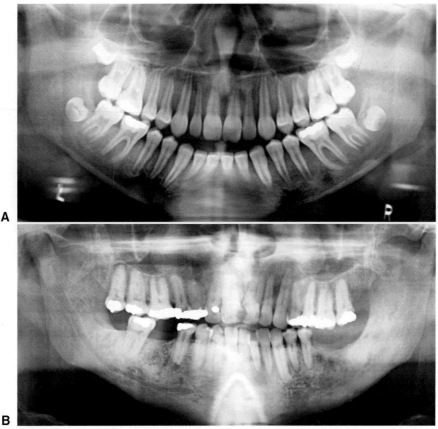

FIG. 24-9   Two cases of renal osteodystrophy. **A,** This panoramic image reveals areas of radiolucency corresponding to loss of bone mass, loss of distinct lamina dura, and a sclerotic bone pattern around the roots of the teeth. **B,** This panoramic image reveals a diffuse sclerotic (radiopaque) bone pattern throughout the jaws. Note the loss of a distinct inferior cortex of the mandible resulting from an increase in the radiopacity of the internal aspect of the bone.

large pulp chambers and root canals (see Fig. 24-10, *B* and *C*). In addition, periapical and periodontal abscesses occur frequently. The occurrence of periapical rarefying osteitis without an etiology may be a result of large pulp chambers and defects in the formation of dentin. This may allow for the ingress of oral microorganisms and subsequent pulp necrosis. If the disease is severe, the patient experiences premature loss of the teeth. The lamina dura may become sparse, and cortical boundaries around tooth crypts may be thin or entirely absent.

OSTEOPETROSIS

Synonyms
Albers-Schönberg and marble bone disease

Definition
Osteopetrosis is a disorder of bone that results from a defect in the differentiation and function of osteoclasts. The lack of normally functioning osteoclasts results in abnormal formation of the primary skeleton and a generalized increase in bone mass. The failure of normal bone remodeling results in dense, fragile bones that are susceptible to fracture and infection. Obliteration of the marrow compromises hematopoiesis and compresses cranial nerves. This disorder is inherited as an autosomal recessive type (osteopetrosis congenita) and autosomal dominant type (osteopetrosis tarda).

Clinical Features
The more severe, recessive form of osteopetrosis is seen in infants and young children, and the more benign,

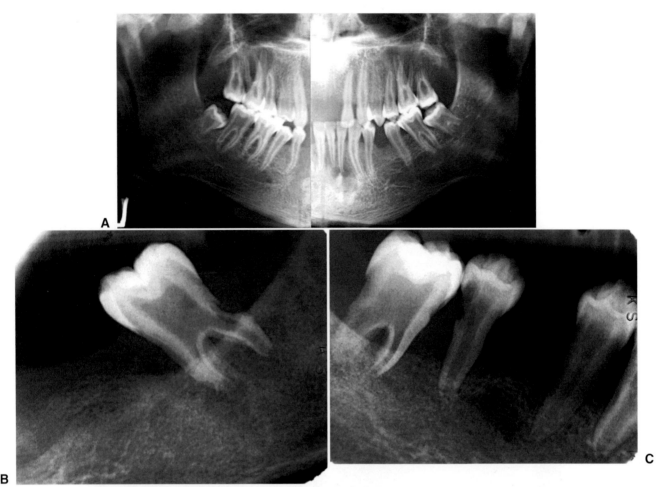

FIG. **24-10**   **A,** A panoramic image of hypophosphatemia. Note the radiolucent appearance of the jaws and hence the lack of bone density and the large pulp chambers. **B** and **C,** These periapical films of a case of hypophosphatemia demonstrate apparent bone loss around the teeth, a granular bone pattern, large pulp chambers, and external root resorption.

dominant form appears later. The severe form is invariably fatal early in life. The patient experiences progressive loss of the bone marrow and its cellular products and a severe increase in bone density. The narrowing of bony canals results in hydrocephalus, blindness, deafness, vestibular nerve dysfunction, and facial nerve paralysis. The benign, dominant form is milder and may be entirely asymptomatic. It may be discovered any time from childhood into adulthood. The disease may be found as an incidental finding or appear as a pathologic fracture of a bone. In some of the more chronic cases, bone pain and cranial nerve palsies caused by neural compression may be clinical problems. Osteomyelitis may complicate this disease because of the relative lack of vascularity of the dense bone. This problem is more

common in the mandible, whereas osteomyelitis is usually secondary to dental or periodontal disease.

Radiographic Features

General radiographic features. In the classic radiographic presentation of osteopetrosis, all bones show greatly increased density, which is bilaterally symmetric. The increased density throughout the skeleton is homogeneous and diffuse (Fig. 24-11). The internal aspect of the involved bone may be so dense or radiopaque that the trabecular patterns of the medullary cavity may not be visible. The internal radiopacity also reduces the contrast between the outer cortical border and the cancellous portion of the bone. The entire bone may be mildly enlarged.

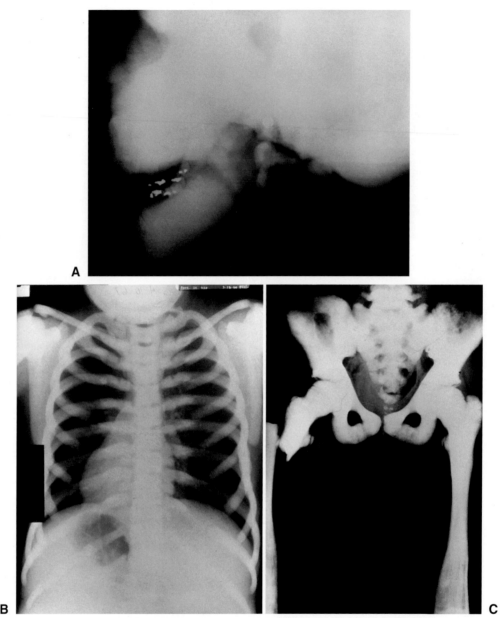

FIG. **24-11**   Osteopetrosis, showing dense calcification of all the bones. **A,** Skull and facial bones. **B,** Chest. **C,** Pelvis and femurs. Note the fracture of the proximal right femur.

Radiographic features of the jaws. The increased radiopacity of the jaws may be so great that the radiographic image may fail to reveal any internal structure and even the roots of the teeth may not be apparent. The increased bone density and relatively poor vascularity results in a susceptibility of the mandible to osteomyelitis, usually from odontogenic inflammatory lesions (Fig. 24-12).

Radiographic features associated with the teeth. Effects on teeth may include delayed eruption, early tooth loss, missing teeth, malformed roots and crowns, and teeth that are poorly calcified and prone to caries. The normal eruption pattern of the primary and secondary dentition may be delayed as a result of bone density or ankylosis. The lamina dura and cortical borders may appear thicker than normal.

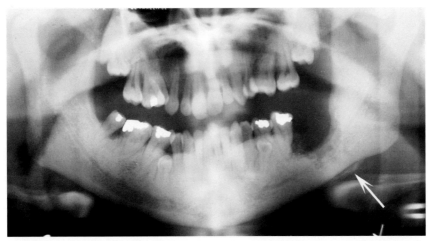

FIG. 24-12 A panoramic film of a patient with osteopetrosis. Note the increased density of the jaws, lack of eruption of the mandibular second bicuspids, narrow inferior alveolar nerve canal, and the development of osteomyelitis in the body of the left mandible with periostitis *(arrow)*.

Differential Diagnosis

The differential diagnosis includes other sclerosing bone dysplasias such as sclerosteosis, infantile cortical hyperostosis, pyknodysostosis, craniometaphyseal dysplasia, diaphyseal dysplasia, melorheostosis, and osteopathia striata. Osteosclerosis from fluoride poisoning and secondary hyperparathyroidism from renal disease also may produce a general sclerotic appearance.

Treatment

Treatment of osteopetrosis consists of bone marrow transplants to attempt to stimulate the formation of functional osteoclasts and systemic steroids for the hematologic component. The osteomyelitis is difficult to treat, and a combination of antibiotics and hyperbaric oxygen therapy is used. It is imperative that affected patients avoid odontogenic inflammatory disease.

Other Systemic Diseases

PROGRESSIVE SYSTEMIC SCLEROSIS

Synonym
Scleroderma

Definition

Progressive systemic sclerosis (PSS) is a generalized connective tissue disease that causes hardening (sclerosis) of the skin and other tissues. The involvement of the gastrointestinal tract, heart, lungs, and kidneys usually results in more serious complications. The cause of the disease is unknown.

Clinical Features

PSS is a disease of middle age, with the greatest incidence between the ages of 30 and 50 years. It is rarely seen in adolescents or older adults. Women are affected about three times as often as men.

In most patients with moderate to severe PSS, the involved skin has a thickened, leathery quality. The skin is not mobile over the underlying soft tissues, and involvement of the facial region may inhibit normal mandibular opening. Patients with diffuse disease are also likely to have xerostomia; increased numbers of decayed, missing, or filled teeth; and carious lesions. Furthermore, patients with systemic disease are more likely to have deeper periodontal pockets and higher gingivitis scores. Patients with cardiac and pulmonary problems may have varying degrees of heart failure and respiratory insufficiencies. Renal involvement usually leads to some degree of uremia, with or without hypertension.

Radiographic Features

Radiographic features of the jaws. A radiographic feature in some cases of PSS is an unusual pattern of mandibular erosions at regions of muscle attachment such as the angles, coronoid process, digastric region, or condyles (Fig. 24-13). This type of resorption is typically bilateral and fairly symmetric. Most of these erosive borders are smooth and sharply defined. This resorption may be progressive with the disease.

Radiographic changes associated with the teeth. The most common oral radiographic manifestation of PSS is an increase in the width of the periodontal ligament

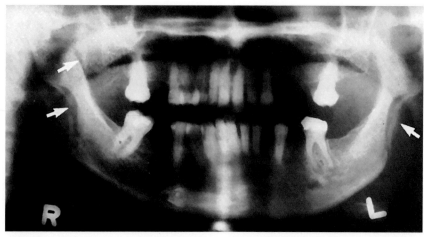

FIG. **24-13**   PSS, demonstrating a loss of bone in the region of the angle of the mandible *(arrows)* and at the right coronoid process *(arrow),* which are locations of muscle attachments.

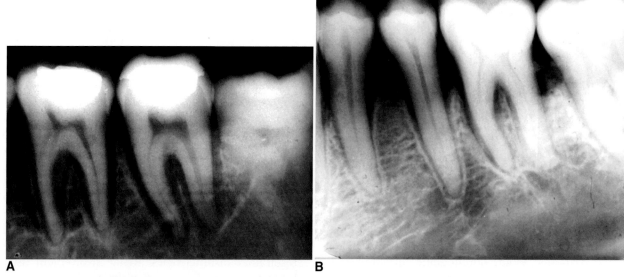

A   **B**

FIG. **24-14**   A and B, Two periapical films of two different patients with PSS. Note the widening of the periodontal membrane space around some of the teeth.

(PDL) spaces around the teeth (Fig. 24-14). Approximately two thirds of patients with PSS show this change. The PDL spaces affected by PSS usually are at least twice as thick as normal and both anterior and posterior teeth are affected, although it is more pronounced around the posterior teeth. The lamina dura remains normal. Despite the widening of the PDL spaces, the clinician finds that involved teeth are often not mobile and their gingival attachments are usually intact. Almost half of the patients with PDL space thickening also had some mandibular erosive bone changes.

Differential diagnosis. Other causes of widening of the periodontal membrane space include tooth mobility, orthodontic tooth movement, intermaxillary fixation with arch bars, and invasion of the PDL by malignant neoplasms. Widening of the PDL space with malignant neoplasia differs in destruction of the lamina dura and irregular widening.

Management. The aforementioned thickening of PDL spaces does not seem to present any clinical difficulties. The progressive loss of bone in the region of the mandibular angle, however, is more serious because of potential fracture. It is reasonable to obtain initial and periodic panoramic radiographs in all patients with PSS to assess mandibular integrity.

SICKLE CELL ANEMIA

Definition

Sickle cell anemia is an autosomal recessive, chronic, hemolytic blood disorder. Patients with this disorder have abnormal hemoglobin (deoxygenated hemoglobins), which under low oxygen tension results in sickling of the red blood cells. These blood cells have a reduced capacity to carry oxygen to the tissues and, because of damage to their membrane lipids and proteins, adhere to vascular endothelium and obstruct capillaries. The spleen traps and readily destroys these abnormal red cells. The hematopoietic system responds to the resultant anemia by increasing the production of red blood cells, which requires compensatory hyperplasia of the bone marrow.

Clinical Features

The homozygous form of sickle cell anemia occurs in approximately 1 of every 400 African-Americans. Although the gene is present in the heterozygous state in about 6% to 8% of African-Americans, those who manifest this form of the sickle cell trait do not show related clinical findings.

Although symptoms and signs vary considerably, most patients with the disease normally manifest mild, chronic features. Long, quiet spells of hemolytic latency occur, occasionally punctuated by exacerbations known as *sickle cell crises*. During the crisis state, patients often experience severe abdominal, muscle, and joint pain, have a high temperature, and may even undergo circulatory collapse. During milder periods the patient may complain of fatigability, weakness, shortness of breath, and muscle and joint pain. As in the other chronic anemias, the heart is usually enlarged and a murmur may be present. The disease occurs mostly in children and adolescents. It is compatible with a normal life span, although many patients die of complications of the disease before the age of 40 years.

Radiographic Features

The hyperplasia of the bone marrow at the expense of cancellous bone is the primary reason for the radiographic manifestations of sickle cell anemia. The extent of bone changes in sickle cell anemia relates to the degree of this hyperplasia.

General radiographic features. The thinning of individual cancellous trabeculae and cortices is most common in the vertebral bodies, long bones, skull, and jaws. The skull may have widening of the diploic space and thinning of the inner and outer tables (Fig. 24-15). In extreme cases (5%) the outer table of the skull will not be apparent and a hair-on-end appearance may occur. Small areas of infarction may be present within bones after blockage of the microvasculature; these are seen radiographically as areas of localized bone sclerosis. Osteomyelitis may complicate sickle cell anemia if infection begins in an area of pronounced hypovascularity. There may also be retardation of generalized bone growth.

Radiographic features of the jaws. The radiographic manifestations of sickle cell anemia in the jaws include general osteoporosis. This occurs because of a decrease in the volume of trabecular bone and, to a lesser extent, thinning of the cortical plates. In most cases the change is mild or moderate, with extreme radiographic manifestations being unusual. The bone pattern may be altered to one with fewer but coarser trabeculae. Radiographs of the jaws of children with sickle cell anemia have been reported to show a high frequency of severe osteoporosis. Rarely, bone marrow hyperplasia may cause enlargement and protrusion of the maxillary alveolar ridge.

THALASSEMIA

Synonyms

Cooley's anemia, Mediterranean anemia, and erythroblastic anemia

Definition

Thalassemia is a hereditary disorder that results in a defect in hemoglobin synthesis. This defect may involve either the alpha or beta globulin genes. The resultant red blood cells have reduced hemoglobin content, are thin, and have a shortened life span. The heterozygous form of the disease (thalassemia minor) is mild, whereas the homozygous form (thalassemia major) may be severe. A moderately severe form, thalassemia intermedia, also occurs.

Clinical Features

In the severe form of the disease, the onset is in infancy and the survival time may be short. The face develops prominent cheekbones and a protrusive premaxilla, resulting in a "rodent-like" face. The milder form of the disease occurs in adults.

Radiographic Features

General radiographic features. Similarly to sickle cell anemia, the radiographic features of thalassemia generally result from hyperplasia of the ineffective bone marrow and its subsequent failure to produce normal

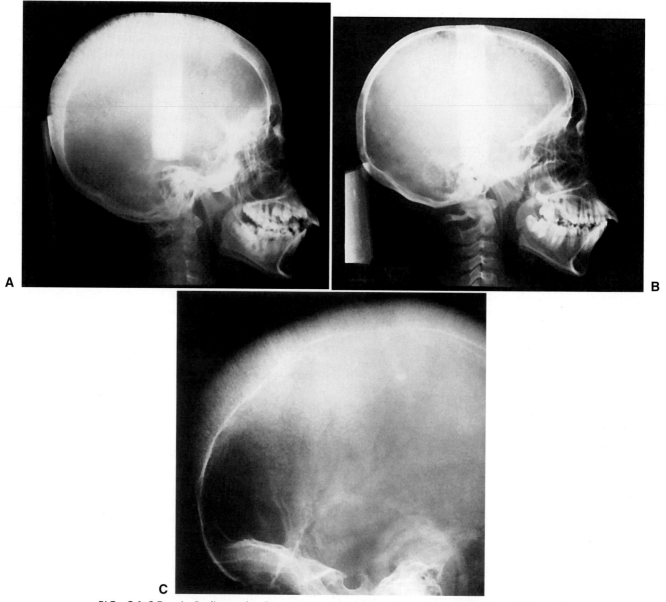

FIG. **24-15**   **A,** Radiograph of a patient with sickle cell anemia, showing a thickened diploic space and thinning of the skull cortex. **B,** Normal skull for comparison. **C,** Skull showing the hair-on-end bone pattern. **(B,** Courtesy Dr. B. Sarnat, Los Angeles; **C,** Courtesy H.G. Poyton, DDS, Toronto, Ontario.)

red cells. However, these changes are usually more severe than with other anemias. There is a generalized radiolucency of the long bones with cortical thinning. In the skull the diploic space exhibits marked thickening, especially in the frontal region. The skull shows a generalized granular appearance (Fig. 24-16), and occasionally a hair-on-end effect may develop.

Radiographic appearance of the jaws. Severe bone marrow hyperplasia prevents pneumatization of the paranasal sinuses, especially the maxillary sinus, and causes an expansion of the maxilla that results in malocclusion (Fig. 24-17, *A*). The jaws appear radiolucent, with thinning of the cortical borders and enlargement of the marrow spaces. The trabeculae are large and

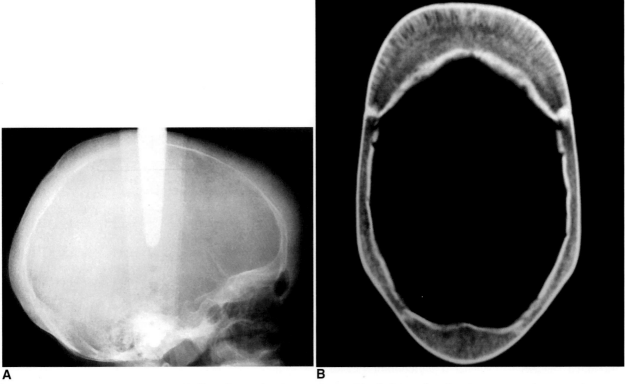

FIG. **24-16** **A,** Skull radiograph of a patient with thalassemia, showing a granular appearance of the skull and thickening of the diploic space. **B,** An axial CT image of the skull of a patient with thalassemia. Note the thickened diploic space and there is hint linear orientation of the trabeculae, especially in the frontal bone. (**A,** Courtesy H.G. Poyton, DDS, Toronto, Ontario.)

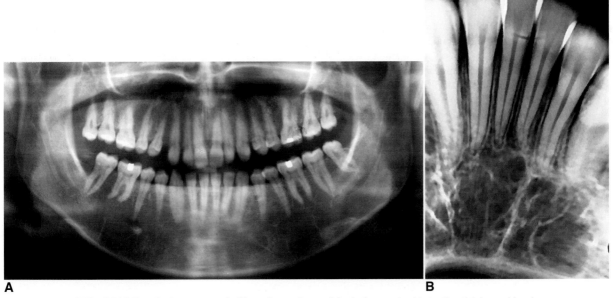

FIG. **24-17** **A,** A panoramic film of a patient with thalassemia. Note the thickened body of the mandible and the sparse trabeculae and lack of maxillary antra. **B,** Radiograph of a different patient with thalassemia with thick trabeculae and large bone marrow spaces. (Courtesy H.G. Poyton, DDS, Toronto, Ontario.)

coarse (Fig. 24-17, *B*). The lamina dura is thin, and the roots of the teeth may be short.

BIBLIOGRAPHY

Aegerter E, Kirkpatrick JA: Orthopedic diseases, ed 4, Philadelphia, 1975, WB Saunders.

Keller EE, Stafne EC, Gibilisco JA: Oral radiographic manifestations of systemic disease. In Gibilisco JA, Turlington EG, editors: Stafne's oral roentgenographic diagnosis, ed 5, Philadelphia, 1985, WB Saunders.

Paterson CR: Metabolic disorders of bone, Oxford, 1974, Blackwell Scientific.

Trapnell DH, Boweman JE: Dental manifestation of systemic disease, London, 1973, Butterworth.

DIABETES MELLITUS

Lamey PJ, Darwazeh AM, Frier BM: Oral disorders associated with diabetes mellitus, Diabet Med 9:410, 1992.

Mackenzie RS, Millard HD: Interrelated effects of diabetes, arteriosclerosis and calculus on alveolar bone loss, J Am Dent Assoc 54:191, 1963.

Murrah VA: Diabetes mellitus and associated oral manifestations: a review, J Oral Pathol 14:271, 1985.

Stahl SS: Roentgenographic and bacteriologic aspects of periodontal changes in diabetics, J Periodontol 19:130, 1948.

HYPERPARATHYROIDISM

Bilezikian JP: Hyper- and hypoparathyroidism. In Rakel R, editor: Conn's current therapy, Philadelphia, 1985, WB Saunders.

Boonstra CE, Jackson CE: Serum calcium survey for hyperparathyroidism: results in 50,000 clinic patients, Am J Clin Pathol 55:523, 1971.

Cooper D, Wood L: Hyperthyroidism. In Rakel R, editor: Conn's current therapy, Philadelphia, 1985, WB Saunders.

Rosenberg E, Guralnick W: Hyperparathyroidism: a review of 220 proved cases with special emphasis on findings in the jaws, Oral Surg Oral Med Oral Pathol 15(suppl 2):84, 1962.

Steinbach HL et al: Primary hyperparathyroidism: a correlation of roentgen, clinical and pathologic features, Am J Roentgenol 86:329, 1961.

HYPOPARATHYROIDISM

Frensilli J, Stoner R, Hinrichs E: Dental changes of idiopathic hypoparathyroidism, J Oral Surg 29:727, 1971.

Glynne A, Hunter I, Thomson J: Pseudohypoparathyroidism with paradoxical increase in hypocalcemic seizures due to long-term anticonvulsant therapy, Postgrad Med J 48:632, 1972.

Silverman S, Ware W, Gillody C: Dental aspects of hyperparathyroidism, Oral Surg Oral Med Oral Pathol 26:184, 1968.

HYPOPHOSPHATASIA

Eastman JR, Bixler D: Clinical, laboratory, and genetic investigations of hypophosphatasia: support for autosomal dominant inheritance with homozygous lethality, J Craniofac Genet Dev Biol 3:213, 1983.

Jedrychowski JR, Duperon D: Childhood hypophosphatasia with oral manifestations, J Oral Med 34:18, 1979.

Macfarland JD, Swart JGN: Developmental aspects of hypophosphatasia: a case report, family study, and literature review, Oral Surg Oral Med Oral Pathol 67:521, 1989.

HYPOPITUITARISM

Conley H et al: Clinical and histologic findings of the dentition in a hypopituitary patient: report of case, ASDC J Dent Child 57:376, 1990.

Edler RJ: Dental and skeletal ages in hypopituitary patients, J Dent Res 56:1145, 1977.

Kosowicz J, Rzymski K: Abnormalities of tooth development in pituitary dwarfism, Oral Surg Oral Med Oral Pathol 44:853, 1977.

Myllarniemi S, Lenko HL, Perheentupa J: Dental maturity in hypopituitarism, and dental response to substitution treatment, Scand J Dent Res 86:307, 1978.

OSTEOPOROSIS

Gallagher C: Osteoporosis. In Rakel R, editor: Conn's current therapy, Philadelphia, 1985, WB Saunders.

Garn S, Rohmann C, Wagner B: Bone loss as a general phenomenon in man, Fed Proc 26:1729, 1967.

Law AN, Bollen AM, Chen SK: Detecting osteoporosis using dental radiographs: a comparison of four methods, J Am Dent Assoc 127:1734, 1996.

Mohammad AR, Alder M, McNally MA: A pilot study of panoramic film density at selected sites in the mandible to predict osteoporosis, Int J Prosthodont 9:290, 1996.

Taguchi A et al: Oral signs as indicators of possible osteoporosis in elderly women, Oral Surg Oral Med Oral Pathol Oral Radiol Endod 80:612, 1995.

Taguchi A et al: Usefulness of panoramic radiography in the diagnosis of postmenopausal osteoporosis in women. Width and morphology of inferior cortex of the mandible, Dentomaxillofac Radiol 25:263, 1996.

OSTEOPETROSIS

Dick H, Simpson W: Dental changes in osteopetrosis, Oral Surg 34:408, 1972.

Ruprecht A, Wagner H, Engel H: Osteopetrosis: report of a case and discussion of the differential diagnosis, Oral Surg Oral Med Oral Pathol 66:674, 1988.

Steiner M, Gould A, Means W: Osteomyelitis of the mandible associated with osteopetrosis, J Oral Maxillofac Surg 41:395, 1983.

Younai F, Eisenbud L, Sciubba JJ: Osteopetrosis: a case report including gross and microscopic findings in the mandible at autopsy, Oral Surg Oral Med Oral Pathol 65:214, 1988.

PROGRESSIVE SYSTEMIC SCLEROSIS

Alexandridis C, White SC: Periodontal ligament changes in patients with progressive systemic sclerosis, Oral Med Oral Pathol 58:113, 1984.

Rout PG, Hamburger J, Potts AJ: Orofacial radiological manifestations of systemic sclerosis, Dentomaxillofac Radiol 25:193, 1996.

Ruprecht A, Dolan K, Lilly GE: Osteolysis of the mandible associated with progressive systemic sclerosis, Dentomaxillofac Radiol 19:31, 1990.

White SC, Frey NW, Blaschke DD et al: Oral radiographic changes in patients with progressive systemic sclerosis (scleroderma), J Am Dent Assoc 94:1178, 1977.

Wood RE, Lee P: Analysis of the oral manifestations of systemic sclerosis (scleroderma), Oral Med Oral Pathol 65:172, 1988.

RENAL OSTEODYSTROPHY

Bras J et al: Radiographic interpretation of the mandibular angular cortex: a diagnostic tool in metabolic bone loss. II, Renal osteodystrophy, Oral Surg 53:647, 1982.

Scutellari PN et al: Radiographic manifestations in teeth and jaws in chronic kidney insufficiency, Radiol Med (Torino) 92:415, 1996.

Syrjanen S, Lampainen E: Mandibular changes in panoramic radiographs of patients with end stage renal disease, Dentomaxillofac Radiol 12:51, 1983.

RICKETS

Harris R, Sullivan H: Dental sequelae in deciduous dentition in vitamin-D resistant rickets, Aust Dent J 5:200, 1960.

Marks SC, Lindahl RL, Bawden JW: Dental and cephalometric findings in vitamin D resistant rickets, J Dent Child 32:259, 1965.

SICKLE CELL ANEMIA

Brown DL, Sebes JI: Sickle cell gnathopathy: radiologic assessment, Oral Surg Oral Med Oral Pathol 61:653, 1986.

Halstead CL: Oral manifestations of hemoglobinopathies. A case of homozygous hemoglobin C disease diagnosed as a result of dental radiographic changes, Oral Surg Oral Med Oral Pathol 30:615, 1970.

Mourshed F, Tuckson C: A study of radiographic features of the jaws in sickle-cell anemia, Oral Surg Oral Med Oral Pathol 37:812, 1974.

Sanger RG, Bystrom EB: Radiographic bone changes in sickle cell anemia, J Oral Med 32:32, 1977.

Sanger RG, Greer R, Averbach R: Differential diagnosis of some simple osseous lesions associated with sickle-cell anemia, Oral Surg Oral Med Oral Pathol 43:538, 1977.

Sears RS, Nazif MM, Zullo T: The effects of sickle-cell disease on dental and skeletal maturation, ASDC J Dent Child 48:275, 1981.

THALASSEMIA

Caffey J: Cooley's anemia: a review of the roentgenographic findings in the skeleton, AJR Am J Roentgenol 78:381, 1957.

Poyton HG, Davey KW: Thalassemia: changes visible in radiographs used in dentistry, Oral Surg Oral Med Oral Pathol 25: 564, 1968.

Sommermater JI, Bacon W: Dentomaxillary and maxillofacial manifestations of thalassemia major apropos of a case, Actual Odontostomatol 35:489, 1981.

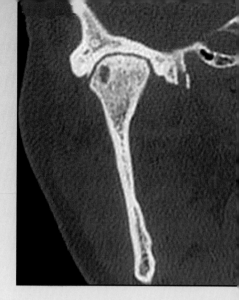

CHAPTER 25

Diagnostic Imaging of the Temporomandibular Joint

C. GRACE PETRIKOWSKI

Disorders of the temporomandibular joint are abnormalities that interfere with the normal form or function of the joint. These disorders include dysfunction of the articular disk and associated ligaments and muscles, joint arthritides, inflammatory lesions, neoplasms, and growth or developmental abnormalities.

Clinical Features

Temporomandibular joint (TMJ) dysfunction is the most common jaw disorder, with 28% to 86% of adults and adolescents showing one or more clinical signs or symptoms. A higher incidence of the disorder has been reported in females, although the reason for this preponderance is not clear. Signs and symptoms of dysfunction may include one or more of the following: pain in the TMJ or ear or both, headache, muscle tenderness, joint stiffness, clicking or other joint noises, reduced range of motion, locking, and subluxation. In most cases the clinical signs and symptoms are transitory, and treatment is not indicated. However, a small percentage of patients (5%) suffer severe dysfunction (e.g., severe pain, marked functional impairment, or both), which requires a thorough diagnostic workup,

including diagnostic imaging, before commencing treatment.

The clinical signs and symptoms of other disorders of the TMJ may include swelling in and around the joint, an elevated temperature, and redness of the overlying skin.

Application of Diagnostic Imaging

TMJ imaging may be necessary to supplement information obtained from the clinical examination, particularly when an osseous abnormality or infection is suspected, conservative treatment has failed, or symptoms are worsening. Diagnostic imaging also should be considered for patients with a history of trauma, significant dysfunction, alteration in range of motion, sensory or motor abnormalities, or significant changes in occlusion. TMJ imaging is not indicated for joint sounds if other signs or symptoms are absent or for asymptomatic children and adolescents before orthodontic treatment. The purposes of TMJ imaging are to evaluate the integrity and relationships of the hard and soft tissues, confirm the extent or stage of progression of known disease, and evaluate the effects of treatment. The clinician must correlate the radiographic information with the patient's history and clinical findings to arrive at a final diagnosis and plan the management of the underlying disease process.

Radiographic Anatomy of the TMJ

A thorough understanding of the anatomy and morphology of the TMJ is essential so that a normal variant is not mistaken for an abnormality. The TMJs are unique in that although they constitute two separate joints anatomically, they function together as a single unit. Each condyle articulates with the mandibular fossa of the temporal bone. A disk composed of fibrocartilage is interposed between the condyle and mandibular fossa. A fibrous capsule lined with synovial membrane surrounds and encloses the joint. Ligaments and muscles restrict or allow movement of the condyle.

CONDYLE

The condyle is a bony, ellipsoid structure connected to the mandibular ramus by a narrow neck (Fig. 25-1). The condyle is approximately 20 mm long mediolaterally and 8 to 10 mm thick anteroposteriorly. The shape of the condyle varies considerably; the superior aspect may be flattened, rounded, or markedly convex, whereas the mediolateral contour usually is slightly convex. These variations in shape may cause difficulty with radiographic interpretation; this underlines the

importance of understanding the range of normal appearance. The extreme aspects of the condyle are called the *medial pole* and *lateral poles*. The long axis of the condyle is slightly rotated on the condylar neck such that the medial pole is angled posteriorly, forming an angle of 15 to 33 degrees with the sagittal plane. The two condylar axes typically intersect near the anterior border of the foramen magnum in the submentovertex projection.

Most condyles have a pronounced ridge oriented mediolaterally on the anterior surface, marking the anteroinferior limit of the articulating area. This ridge is the upper limit of the pterygoid fovea, a small depression on the anterior surface at the junction of the condyle and neck. It is the attachment site of the superior head of the lateral pterygoid muscle and should not be mistaken for an osteophyte (spur), which indicates degenerative joint disease.

Although the mandibular and temporal components of the TMJ are calcified by 6 months of age, complete calcification of cortical borders may not be completed until 20 years of age. As a result, radiographs of condyles in children may show little or no evidence of a cortical border. In the absence of disease, the cortical borders in adults are visible radiographically. A layer of fibrocartilage covers the condyle but is not visible radiographically.

MANDIBULAR FOSSA

The glenoid (mandibular) fossa is located at the inferior aspect of the squamous part of the temporal bone and is composed of the glenoid fossa and articular eminence of the temporal bone (Fig. 25-2, *A*). It is some-

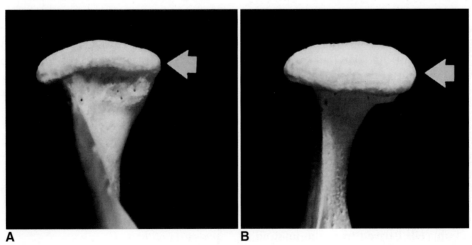

A   **B**

FIG. **25-1**   Mandibular condyle. The medial pole *(arrow)* is on the right in each case. **A,** Anterior aspect. **B,** Superior aspect.

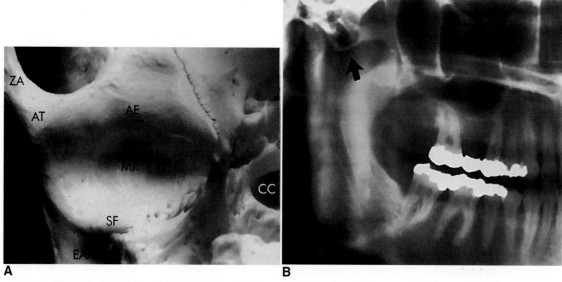

FIG. 25-2   **A,** Basal view of the skull showing the mandibular fossa. *AE,* Articular eminence; *AT,* articular tubercle; *CC,* carotid canal; *EAM,* external auditory meatus; *MF,* mandibular fossa; *SF,* squamotympanic fissure; *ZA,* zygomatic arch. **B,** Pneumatization of the articular eminence with a mastoid air cell (panoramic view) *(arrow).* (**B,** Courtesy Dr. D. Tyndall and Dr. S.R. Matteson, Chapel Hill, N.C.)

times described as the *temporal component* of the TMJ. The articular eminence forms the anterior limit of the glenoid fossa and is convex in shape. Its most inferior aspect is called the *summit* or *apex* of the eminence. In a normal TMJ, the roof of the fossa, the posterior slope of the articular eminence, and the eminence itself form an S shape when viewed in the sagittal plane. The most lateral aspect of the eminence consists of a protuberance, called the *articular tubercle,* which is a ligamentous attachment. The squamotympanic fissure and its medial extension, the petrotympanic fissure, form the posterior limit of the fossa. The middle portion of the roof of the fossa forms a small portion of the floor of the middle cranial fossa, and only a thin layer of cortical bone separates the joint cavity from the intracranial subdural space. The spine of the sphenoid forms the medial limit of the fossa. Fossa depth varies, and the development of the articular eminence relies on functional stimulus from the condyle. For example, the mandibular fossa is very flat and underdeveloped in patients with micrognathia or condylar agenesis. The fossa and articular eminence develop during the first 3 years and reach mature shape by the age of 4 years; young infants lack a definite fossa and articular eminence.

All aspects of the temporal component may be pneumatized with small air cells derived from the mastoid air cell complex (Fig. 25-2, *B*). Pneumatization of the articular eminence is seen radiographically in approximately 2% of patients. Like the condyle, the mandibular fossa is covered with a thin layer of fibrocartilage.

INTERARTICULAR DISK

The interarticular disk (meniscus), composed of fibrous connective tissue, is located between the condylar head and mandibular fossa. The disk divides the joint cavity into two compartments, called the inferior (lower) and superior (upper) joint spaces, which are located below and above the disk, respectively (Fig. 25-3). A normal disk has a biconcave shape with a thick anterior band, thicker posterior band, and a thin middle part. The disk also is thicker medially than laterally. The medial and lateral margins of the disk blend with the capsule. The thin central portion normally serves as an articulating cushion between the condyle and articular eminence. The anterior band is thought to be attached to the superior head of the lateral pterygoid muscle, and the posterior band attaches to the posterior retrodiskal tissues (also called the *posterior attachment*). The junction between the posterior band and posterior attachment usually lies within 10 degrees of vertical above the condylar head. The disk and posterior attachment are collectively called the *soft tissue component of the TMJ.*

During mandibular opening, as the condyle translates downward and forward, the disk also moves

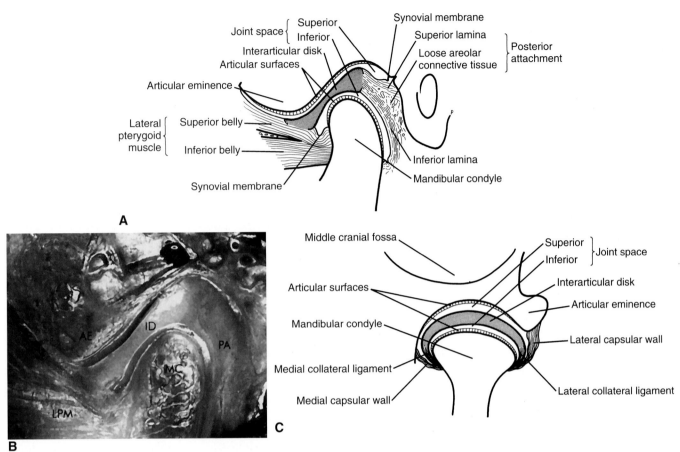

FIG. **25-3** TMJ anatomy. **A,** Lateral view. **B,** Sectioned cadaver specimen in the same orientation. *AE,* Articular eminence; *ID,* interarticular disk; *LPM,* lateral pterygoid muscle; *MC,* mandibular condyle; *PA,* posterior attachment. **C,** Coronal view. (Courtesy Dr. W.K. Solberg, Los Angeles, Calif.)

forward and rotates so that its thin central portion remains between the articulating convexities of the condylar head and articular eminence. Laterally and medially, the disk attaches to the condylar poles, helping to ensure passive movement of the disk with the condyle so that the condyle and disk translate forward together to the summit of the articular eminence. As the mandible opens, the condyle also rotates against the lower surface of the disk in the inferior joint space. On mandibular closing, this process reverses, with the disk moving back with the condyle into the mandibular fossa.

POSTERIOR ATTACHMENT (RETRODISKAL TISSUES)

The posterior attachment consists of a bilaminar zone of vascularized and innervated loose fibroelastic tissue. The superior lamina, which is rich in elastin, inserts into the posterior wall of the mandibular fossa. The superior lamina stretches and allows the disk to move forward with condylar translation. The inferior lamina attaches to the posterior surface of the condyle. The posterior attachment is covered with a synovial membrane that secretes synovial fluid, which lubricates the joint. As the condyle moves forward, tissues of the posterior attachment expand in volume, primarily as a result of venous distention, and as the disk moves forward, tension is produced in the elastic posterior attachment. This tension is thought to be responsible for the smooth recoil of the disk posteriorly as the mandible closes.

TMJ BONY RELATIONSHIPS

Radiographic joint space is a general term used to describe the radiolucent area between the condyle and temporal component (see Fig. 25-3). This general term should not be confused with the terms *superior joint space* and *inferior joint space* described earlier, which refer to soft tissue spaces above and below the disk. The radiographic joint space contains the soft tissue components of the joint. The left and right condylar positions within the fossa can be determined and compared by the dimensions of the radiographic joint space viewed on corrected lateral tomographs. A condyle is positioned concentrically when the anterior and posterior aspects of the radiolucent joint space are uniform in width. The condyle is retruded when the posterior joint space width is less than the anterior (Fig. 25-4) and protruded when the posterior joint space is wider than the anterior.

The diagnostic significance of mild or moderate condylar eccentricity is not clear; condylar eccentricity is seen in one third to one half of asymptomatic individuals and is not a reliable indicator of the soft tissue status of the joint, particularly because the shape of the condylar head is not concentric to the shape of the fossa. Markedly eccentric condylar positioning usually represents an abnormality. For example, inferior condylar positioning (widened joint space) may be seen in cases involving fluid or blood within the joint, and superior condylar positioning (decreased joint space or no joint space, with osseous contact of joint components) may indicate loss, displacement, or perforation of intracapsular soft tissue components. Marked posterior condylar positioning is seen in some cases of disk displacement, and marked anterior condylar positioning may be seen in juvenile rheumatoid arthritis.

CONDYLAR MOVEMENT

The condyle undergoes complex movement during mandibular opening. Downward and forward translation (sliding) of the condyle occurs, whereby the superior surface of the disk slides against the articular eminence; at the same time a hingelike, rotatory movement occurs with the superior surface of the condyle against the inferior surface of the disk. The extent of normal condylar translation varies considerably. In most individuals, at maximal opening the condyle moves down and forward to the summit of the articular eminence or slightly anterior to it (see Fig. 25-4). The condyle typically is found within a range of 2 to 5 mm posterior and 5 to 8 mm anterior to the crest of the eminence. Reduced condylar translation, in which the condyle has little or no downward and forward movement and does not leave the mandibular fossa, is seen in patients who clinically have a reduced degree of mouth opening. Hypermobility of the joint may be suspected if the condyle translates more than 5 mm anterior to the eminence. This may permit anterior locking or dislocation of the condyle if a superior movement also occurs above and anterior to the summit of the articular eminence.

Diagnostic Imaging of the TMJ

The type of imaging technique selected depends on the specific clinical problem, whether imaging of hard or soft tissues is desired, the amount of diagnostic information available from a particular imaging modality, the cost of the examination, and the radiation dose. In most cases the imaging protocol begins with hard tissue imaging to evaluate the osseous contours, the positional relationship of the condyle and fossa, and the range of motion, although a combination of imaging techniques may be indicated. Soft tissue imaging is indicated when information about disk position, morphology, or integrity is needed or to image abnormalities in the

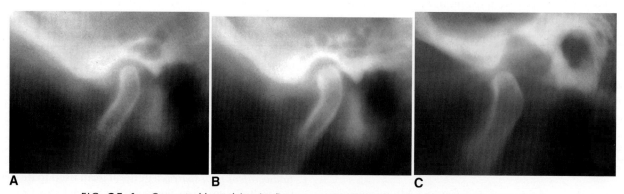

A   **B**   **C**

FIG. **25-4**   Corrected lateral (sagittal) tomograms. **A** represents a lateral image slice, and **B** represents a medial image slice of the same joint. Notice that the condyle appears centered in the lateral image and retruded in the medial image. **C,** Open view showing the degree of condyle translation during mandibular opening.

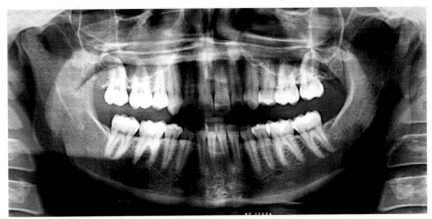

FIG. **25-5** Panoramic view. The right condyle is smaller than the left and is not smoothly corticated. Tomograms later showed marked erosive changes of the right condylar head.

muscles or surrounding tissues. A summary of the diagnostic information provided by each imaging technique is presented in Table 25-1.

HARD TISSUE IMAGING

Panoramic Projection

Because the panoramic projection provides an overall view of the teeth and jaws, it serves as a screening projection to identify odontogenic diseases and other disorders that may be the source of TMJ symptoms. Some panoramic machines have specific TMJ programs, but these are of limited usefulness because of thick image layers and the oblique, distorted view of the joint they provide, which severely limits image quality. Gross osseous changes in the condyles may be identified, such as asymmetries, extensive erosions, large osteophytes, or fractures (Fig. 25-5). However, no information about condylar position or function is provided because the mandible is partly opened and protruded when this radiograph is exposed. Also, mild osseous changes may be obscured, and only marked changes in articular eminence morphology can be seen as a result of superimposition by the skull base and zygomatic arch. For these reasons, the panoramic view does not provide an adequate examination of the hard tissues of the joints.

Transcranial Projection

The transcranial projection provides a sagittal view of the lateral aspects of the condyle and temporal component. The patient is positioned in a cephalostat; the x-ray beam is directed downward from the opposite side, through the cranium and above the petrous ridge of the temporal bone, at a 25-degree positive angle centered through the joint. The horizontal direction of the beam may be individually corrected for the condylar

long axis (see Conventional Tomography, Chapter 13), an average 20-degree anterior angle may be used. The film cassette is placed on the side to be imaged (Fig. 25-6). A routine transcranial series includes projections of both TMJs in the closed and maximally open positions (Fig. 25-7).

Because of the positive beam angulation, the central and medial aspects of the joint are projected inferiorly, and only lateral joint contours are visible in this pro-

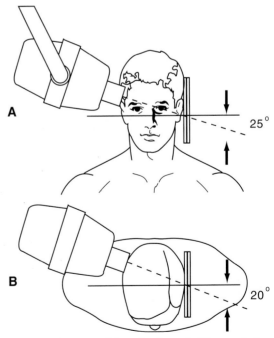

FIG. **25-6** Transcranial projection. **A,** The central ray is oriented at a 25-degree positive angle from the opposite side **(B)** and anteriorly 20 degrees, centered over the TMJ of interest.

TABLE 25-1
Diagnostic Information Provided by Various TMJ Imaging Techniques

	IMAGING TECHNIQUE*				
ABNORMALITY	PANORAMIC	TRANSCRANIAL	TRANSPHARYNGEAL	TRANSORBITAL	SUBMENTOVERTEX
Hard Tissue					
Bony ankylosis	−	−	−	−	−
Arthritides	+	++	+	+	−
Remodeling	+	++	+	+	−
Developmental abnormalities	++	+	+	+	+
Neoplasm	+	+	+	+	+
Trauma (fracture)	++	+	+	+++	++
Range of motion	−	+++	+	−	−
Asymmetry	++	+	+	+	++
Soft Tissue					
Disk position	−	−	−	−	−
Disk perforation	−	−	−	−	−
Fibrous ankylosis	−	−	−	−	−
Joint effusion	−	−	−	−	−
Inflammatory conditions	−	−	−	−	−
Joint space calcifications	−	+	+	−	−

Modified from Brooks SL et al: Imaging of the temporomandibular joint, position paper of the American Academy of Oral and Maxillofacial Radiology, Oral Surg Oral Pathol Oral Radiol Endod 83:609, 1997.
*−, Does not provide diagnostic information for the abnormality; +, only occasionally useful; ++, often useful; +++, almost always useful.
†When including arthrocentesis.

jection. The ipsilateral petrous ridge often is superimposed over the condylar neck, which may obscure osseous changes in the condyle or temporal component. The image of the condyle, temporal component, and joint space is distorted, and condylar position cannot be reliably determined, particularly if the horizontal beam angle is not individualized for each patient. The transcranial projection is useful for identifying gross osseous changes on the lateral aspect of the joint only, displaced condylar fractures, and range of motion (open views).

Transpharyngeal (Parma) Projection
The transpharyngeal (Parma) projection provides a sagittal view of the medial pole of the condyle. The x-ray beam is directed superiorly at −5 degrees through the sigmoid notch of the opposite side and 7 to 8 degrees from the anterior (Fig. 25-8); the film cassette is placed on the side being imaged. The patient opens the mouth maximally to avoid superimposition of the condyle on the temporal component. Because of the negative beam angulation, this view depicts the medial aspect of the condyle. The transpharyngeal view provides limited diagnostic information because the temporal component is not imaged well (Fig. 25-9). The transpharyngeal projection is effective for visualizing erosive changes of the condyle rather than more subtle changes.

Transorbital Projection
The transorbital projection is similar to the transmaxillary projection in that both provide an anterior view of the TMJ, perpendicular to transcranial and transpharyngeal projections. In the transorbital view, the

| | IMAGING TECHNIQUE* | | | |
SKULL VIEWS	CONVENTIONAL TOMOGRAPHY	COMPUTED TOMOGRAPHY	ARTHROGRAPHY	MAGNETIC RESONANCE IMAGING
−	++	+++	−	+
−	++	+++	−	+++
−	++	++	−	−
+	++	+++	−	+
+	++	+++	−	+++
++	++	+++	−	++
−	+++	−	+++	++
++	++	+	−	−
−	−	+	+++	+++
−	−	−	+++	−
−	−	−	+++	+++
−	−	−	+++	+++
−	−	−	++<+>	+++
−	++	+++	−	+

patient's head is tilted downward 10 degrees so that the canthomeatal line is horizontal (Fig. 25-10). The x-ray beam is directed from the front of the patient through the ipsilateral orbit and TMJ of interest. The film cassette is placed behind the patient's head, perpendicular to the x-ray beam. The patient opens maximally or, as an alternative, protrudes the mandible, thereby positioning the condyle at the summit of the articular eminence and avoiding superimposition of the articular eminence or skull base on the condyle.

The entire mediolateral dimension of the articular eminence, condylar head, and condylar neck is visible, which makes this view particularly useful for visualizing condylar neck fractures. The morphology of the convex surface of the condylar head can be evaluated, making this projection a useful adjunct to transcranial and transpharyngeal projections in the diagnosis of gross degenerative changes or other anomalies (Fig. 25-11). The usefulness of this projection is limited by the ability of the condyle to move to the summit of the articular eminence. If condylar motion is limited, only the condylar neck is visible because areas of the joint articulating surfaces are obscured by superimposition of the temporal component on the condylar head. A similar projection is the reverse open Towne's projection, which sometimes is used to image condylar neck fractures, particularly if medial displacement has occurred, because the condylar head and neck are visualized in the frontal plane.

Submentovertex (Basal) Projection

The submentovertex (SMV) projection provides a view of the skull base and condyles superimposed on the condylar necks and mandibular rami. For this reason

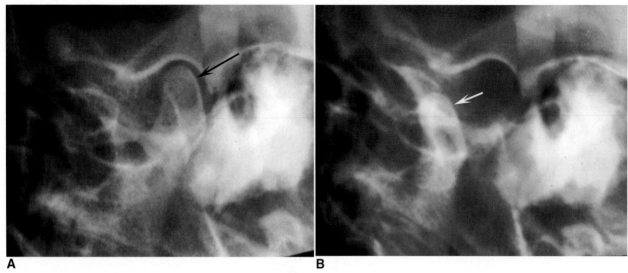

FIG. **25-7**   Transcranial projections of the left TMJ. The profile of the lateral aspect of the condylar head is indicated by an arrow. Note the degree of translatory movement between the closed view **(A)** and the open view **(B)**.

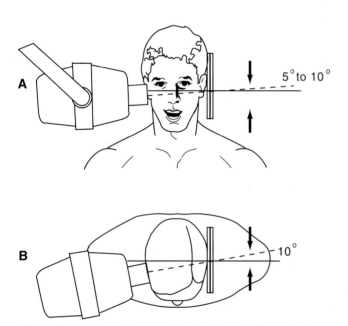

FIG. **25-8**   Transpharyngeal projection. **A,** The central ray is oriented superiorly 5 to 10 degrees and **(B)** posteriorly approximately 10 degrees, centered over the TMJ of interest. Note that the mandible is positioned at maximal opening.

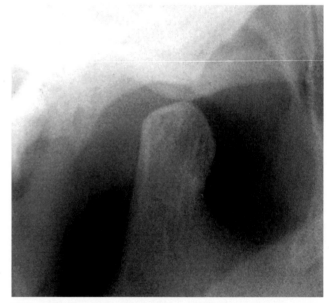

FIG. **25-9**   Transpharyngeal projection showing the condyle at the articular eminence. The zygomatic arch is superimposed over the glenoid fossa.

the SMV projection often is used to determine the angulations of the long axis of the condylar head for corrected tomography (see Chapter 11 for technique). This view may be used as an adjunct to views depicting the TMJs in the lateral plane and is particularly useful for evaluating facial asymmetries, condylar displacement, or rotation of the mandible in the horizontal plane associated with trauma or orthognathic surgery.

Conventional Tomography

Tomography is a radiographic technique that produces multiple thin image slices, permitting visualization of an anatomic structure essentially free of superimpositions of overlapping structures (see Chapter 13). Because this technique can provide multiple image

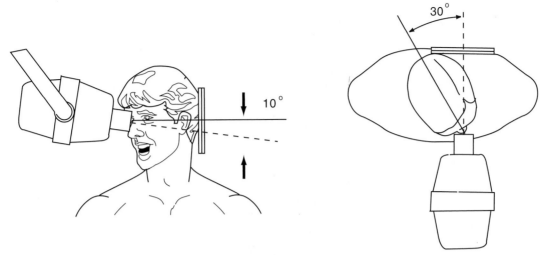

FIG. **25-10** Transorbital projection. The central ray is oriented downward approximately 10 degrees and laterally approximately 30 degrees through the ipsilateral orbit, centered over the TMJ of interest.

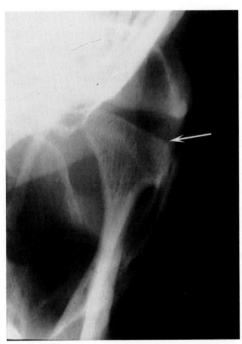

FIG. **25-11** Transorbital view showing the condyle *(arrow)* below the articular eminence. The mastoid process partly obscures the articulating surface on the most medial aspect.

slices at right angles through the joint, it is superior to the transcranial view in depicting true condylar position and revealing osseous changes. For these reasons, tomography is a valuable adjunct to plain film radiography and can provide information that may not be available with plain films alone.

Tomographs typically are exposed in the sagittal (lateral) plane with several image slices in the closed (maximal intercuspation) position and usually only one image in the maximal open position. In "corrected" sagittal tomography, the condylar long axis with respect to the midsagittal plane is determined using an SMV projection (Fig. 25-12). The patient's head is then rotated to this angle, permitting alignment of image slices perpendicular to the condylar long axis. This minimizes geometric distortion of the joint and allows accurate assessment of condylar position. Although a corrected tomographic technique is preferred, when not available, a 20-degree head rotation toward the side of interest is superior to image slices parallel to the midsagittal plane. To minimize patient movement in open views, a bite-block may be inserted between the patient's anterior teeth because it takes several seconds to complete each tomographic exposure.

It is desirable to supplement this examination with coronal (frontal) tomographs, particularly when morphologic abnormalities or erosive changes of the condylar head are suspected. For coronal tomographs, the patient is in a maximal open or protruded position, which brings the condyle to the summit of the articular eminence, free of superimposition of the posterior slope of the eminence. The entire condylar head is visible in the mediolateral plane (Fig. 25-13).

Computed Tomography

Computed tomography (CT) is indicated when more information is needed about the three-dimensional shape and internal structure of the osseous compo-

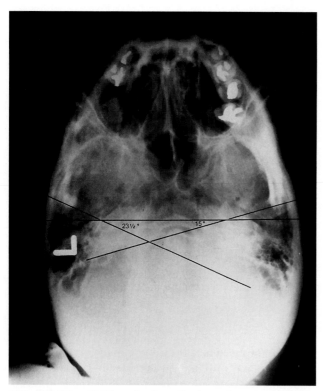

FIG. **25-12**   SMV projection. Tracing of angles between the long axis of each condyle and the midsagittal plane. For tomographic views the patient is rotated according to the measured angles to produce an undistorted radiographic view of each TMJ.

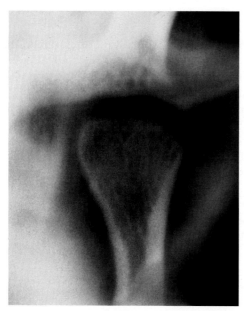

FIG. **25-13**   Frontal tomographic image of the mandibular condyle.

nents of the joint or if information regarding the surrounding soft tissues is required. CT produces digital image slices (see Chapter 13). Multiple image slices are made in both the axial and coronal planes, although the coronal images are the more useful. Data from axial and coronal scans can be manipulated to produce (reformat) images in the sagittal plane. Three-dimensional reformatted images also can be produced. These are useful for assessing osseous deformities of the jaws or surrounding structures. CT cannot produce accurate images of the articular disk.

CT may be considered for determining the presence and extent of ankylosis and neoplasms and the extent of bone involvement in some arthritides, imaging complex fractures, and evaluating complications from the use of polytetrafluoroethylene or silicon sheet implants such as erosions into the middle cranial fossa and heterotopic bone growth.

SOFT TISSUE IMAGING

The soft tissues of the joint can be imaged with magnetic resonance imaging (MRI) or arthrography. Conventional imaging techniques do not demonstrate disk position, morphology, or function. Soft tissue imaging is indicated when TMJ pain and dysfunction are present or when the clinical findings suggest disk displacement along with symptoms that are unresponsive to conservative therapy.

MRI and arthrography should be used only when information about the condition of the soft tissue components of the joint is required to formulate a treatment plan. The choice of technique depends on patient factors, such as allergy to contrast agents and claustrophobia, as well as on the cost, availability, and objectives of the imaging technique. Arthrography is superior for diagnosis of small disk perforations and joint adhesions. MRI can indicate a pathologic condition of the soft tissue through altered tissue signal, allowing evaluation of the disk and surrounding muscles, and can image joint effusion. The technique is noninvasive and does not use ionizing radiation. Arthrography with videofluoroscopy provides a superior motion study of the joint, although some MRI techniques can provide limited dynamic information.

Arthrography

Imaging of the hard tissues should be completed before arthrographic imaging is performed. Arthrography is a technique in which an indirect image of the disk is obtained by injecting a radiopaque contrast agent into one or both joint spaces under fluoroscopic guidance (Fig. 25-14). A perforation is detected by the flow of contrast agent into the superior joint space from the

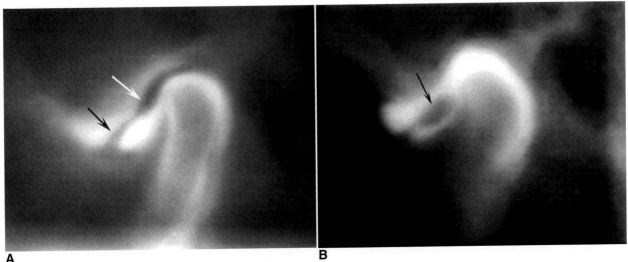

FIG. **25-14**   A and B, Arthrographs in which both the lower and upper joint spaces have been injected with contrast media *(spaces appear white)* that highlights the disc *(black)*. In both images the anterior aspect of the patient is on the left side of the image. In **A** the posterior band *(white arrow)* and the anterior band *(black arrow)* are evident. **B** reveals a disc with an enlarged posterior band *(arrow)*.

lower space, and adhesions are detected by the manner in which contrast agent fills the joint space. After both spaces are filled, disk function is studied using fluoroscopy during open and closing movements. The fluoroscopic study usually is supplemented with tomographs of the joint.

Arthrography is indicated when information about disk position, function, morphology, and the integrity of diskal attachments is required for treatment planning. The risks of this procedure include allergic reaction to the nonionic iodine contrast agent and infection. Drawbacks of this procedure are its invasive nature and its association with postoperative discomfort.

Magnetic Resonance Imaging

MRI uses a magnetic field and radiofrequency pulses rather than ionizing radiation to produce multiple digital image slices (see Chapter 13). Because MRI can provide superb images of soft tissues, this technique can be used for imaging the articular disk. MRI allows construction of images in the sagittal and coronal planes without repositioning the patient (Fig. 25-15). These

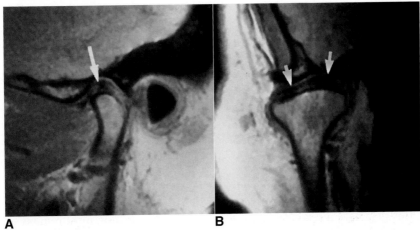

FIG. **25-15**   MRI of a normal TMJ. **A,** Closed view showing the condyle and temporal component. The biconcave disk is located with its posterior band *(arrow)* over the condyle. **B,** Coronal image showing the osseous components and disk *(arrows)* superior to the condyle. (Courtesy Dr. Per-Lennart Westesson, Rochester, N.Y.)

images usually are acquired in open and closed mandibular positions using surface coils to improve image resolution. Sagittal slices should be oriented perpendicular to the condylar long axis. The examinations usually are performed using T1-weighted, proton-weighted, or T2-weighted pulse sequences. T1-weighted or proton-weighted images best demonstrate osseous and diskal tissues, whereas T2-weighted images demonstrate inflammation and joint effusion. Motion MRI studies during opening and closing can be obtained by having the patient open in a series of stepped distances and using rapid image acquisition ("fast scan") techniques. Medial disk displacements are best detected using MRI. The change in tissue signal that results from tissue changes in the disk and retrodiskal tissue may make accurate identification of the disk difficult.

MRI does not have the morbidity associated with the introduction of needles into the joint (as occurs in arthrography), but MRI is a more expensive examination and is contraindicated in patients who are pregnant or who have pacemakers, intracranial vascular clips, or metal particles in vital structures. Some patients may not be able to tolerate the procedure because of claustrophobia or an inability to remain motionless.

Radiographic Abnormalities of the TMJ

DEVELOPMENTAL ABNORMALITIES

Developmental abnormalities may be broadly categorized as anomalies in the form and size of joint components. The most striking radiographic changes usually are seen in the condyle, although the temporal component also may be deformed, often remodeling to accommodate the abnormal condyle. Condylar articular cartilage is a mandibular growth site, and as a result, developmental abnormalities at this location may manifest as altered growth on the affected side of the condyle, mandibular ramus, mandibular body, and alveolar process on the affected side(s).

CONDYLAR HYPERPLASIA

Definition

Condylar hyperplasia is a developmental abnormality that results in enlargement and occasionally deformity of the condylar head; this may have a secondary effect on the mandibular fossa as it remodels to accommodate the abnormal condyle. The etiology may be overactive cartilage or persistent cartilaginous rests, increasing the thickness of the entire cartilaginous and precartilagi-

nous layers. This condition usually is unilateral and may be accompanied by varying degrees of hyperplasia of the ipsilateral mandible.

Clinical Features

Condylar hyperplasia is more common in males, and it usually is discovered before the age of 20 years. The condition is self-limiting and tends to arrest with termination of skeletal growth, although in a small number of cases continued growth and adult onset have been reported. The condition may progress slowly or rapidly. Patients have a mandibular asymmetry that varies in severity, depending on the degree of condylar enlargement. The chin may be deviated to the unaffected side, or it may remain unchanged but with an increase in the vertical dimension of the ramus, mandibular body, or alveolar process of the affected side. As a result of this growth pattern, patients may have a posterior open bite on the affected side. Patients may also have symptoms related to TMJ dysfunction and may complain of limited or deviated mandibular opening or both caused by restricted mobility of the enlarged condyle.

Radiographic Features

The condyle may appear relatively normal but symmetrically enlarged, or it may be altered in shape (e.g., conical, spherical, elongated, lobulated) or irregular in outline. It may be more radiopaque because of the additional bone present. A morphologic variation manifesting as elongation of the condylar head and neck with a compensating forward bend, forming an inverted L, may be seen. Also, the condylar neck may be elongated and thickened and may bend laterally when viewed in the coronal (anteroposterior) plane (Fig. 25-16). The cortical thickness and trabecular pattern of the enlarged condyle usually are normal, which helps to distinguish this condition from a condylar neoplasm. The glenoid fossa may be enlarged, usually at the expense of the posterior slope of the articular eminence. The ramus and mandibular body on the affected side also may be enlarged, resulting in a characteristic depression of the inferior mandibular border at the midline, where the enlarged side joins the contralateral normal mandible. The affected ramus may have increased vertical depth and may be thicker in the anteroposterior dimension.

Differential Diagnosis

A condylar tumor, most notably an osteochondroma, is included in the differential diagnosis. An osteochondroma usually is more irregular in shape compared with a hyperplastic condyle. Surface irregularities and continued growth after cessation of skeletal growth should

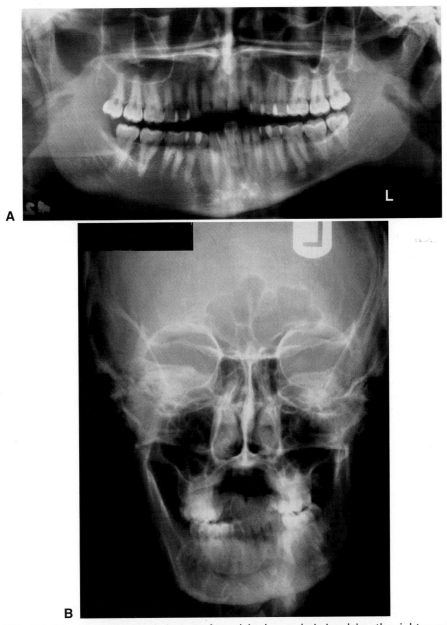

FIG. **25-16**   **A,** A panoramic image of condylar hyperplasia involving the right condyle. The resulting asymmetry of the mandible is apparent in the posterior-anterior skull view **(B).**

increase suspicion of this tumor. Occasionally a condylar osteoma or large osteophyte that occurs in chronic degenerative joint disease may simulate condylar hyperplasia.

Treatment

Treatment consisting of orthodontics combined with orthognathic surgery ideally should be attempted after condylar growth is complete. Determining when condylar growth has stopped may be difficult; imaging may include longitudinal radiographic studies to assess the dimensions of the condyle and mandible, nuclear imaging techniques, or both. A lack of unusual bone activity, demonstrated in a technetium bone scan, is a useful indication of arrested condylar growth.

CONDYLAR HYPOPLASIA

Definition

Condylar hypoplasia is failure of the condyle to attain normal size because of congenital and developmental abnormalities or acquired diseases that affect condylar growth. The condyle is small, but condylar morphology usually is normal. The condition may be inherited or may appear spontaneously. Some cases have been attributed to early injury or injury to the articular cartilage by birth trauma or intraarticular inflammatory lesions.

Clinical Features

Condylar hypoplasia usually is a component of a mandibular growth deficiency and therefore often is associated with an underdeveloped ramus and (occasionally) mandibular body. Congenital abnormalities may be unilateral or bilateral and usually are manifestations of a more generalized condition (e.g., micrognathia, Treacher Collins syndrome); they also may be associated with congenital defects of the ear and zygomatic arch. Developmental abnormalities that manifest during growth usually are unilateral. Acquired abnormalities are the result of damage during the growth period from sources such as therapeutic radiation or infection that diminish or prevent further condylar growth and development. Patients with condylar hypoplasia have mandibular asymmetry and may have symptoms of TMJ dysfunction. The chin commonly is deviated to the affected side, and the mandible deviates to the affected side during mandibular opening. Degenerative joint disease is a common long-term sequela.

Radiographic Features

The condyle may be normal in shape and structure but is diminished in size, and the mandibular fossa also is proportionally small. The condylar neck and coronoid process usually are very slender and in some cases are shortened or elongated. The posterior border of the ramus and condylar neck may have a dorsal (posterior) inclination. The ramus and mandibular body on the affected side may also be small, resulting in a mandibular asymmetry and occasional dental crowding, depending on the severity of mandibular underdevelopment. The antegonial notch is deepened. The associated mandibular hypoplasia is more pronounced if the effect takes place early in life (Fig. 25-17).

Differential Diagnosis

Condylar destruction from juvenile rheumatoid arthritis may appear similar to that of hypoplasia. A survey of other joints or testing for rheumatoid factor may be helpful. Changes in condylar morphology in severe degenerative joint disease or other arthritic conditions may have a similar appearance, although arthritic disease does not cause mandibular hypoplasia of the affected side unless it occurs during growth and other signs of arthritis are usually visible in the affected joint.

Treatment

Orthognathic surgery, bone grafts, and orthodontic therapy may be required.

JUVENILE ARTHROSIS

Synonyms

Boering's arthrosis and arthrosis deformans juvenilis

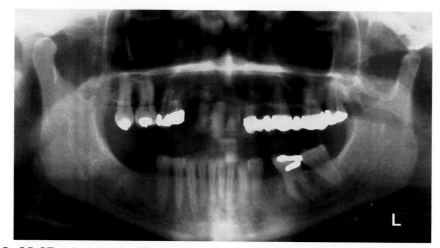

FIG. **25-17** A panoramic film revealing hypoplasia of the left condyle. In this case the hypoplasia is restricted to the condylar head and neck with minimum involvement of the mandibular ramus and body.

Definition

Juvenile arthrosis, a condylar growth disturbance first described by Boering, manifests as hypoplasia and characteristic morphologic abnormalities. This condition may be a form of condylar hypoplasia but is thought to differ in that the affected condyle at one time was normal and became abnormal during growth. Juvenile arthrosis may be unilateral or bilateral, and it predisposes the TMJ to secondary degenerative changes.

Clinical Features

Juvenile arthrosis affects children and adolescents during the period of mandibular growth. It is more common in females. It may be an incidental finding in a panoramic projection, or the patient may have mandibular asymmetry, signs and symptoms of TMJ dysfunction, or both.

Radiographic Features

The condylar head develops a characteristic "toadstool" appearance, with marked flattening and apparent elongation of the articulating condylar surface and dorsal (posterior) inclination of the condyle and neck. The condylar neck is shortened or even absent in some cases, with the condyle resting on the upper margin of the ramus (Fig. 25-18). The articulating surface of the temporal component often is flattened. Progressive shortening of the ramus occurs on the affected side, and the antegonial notch may be deepened, indicating mandibular hypoplasia. In long-standing cases, superimposed degenerative changes may be present.

Differential Diagnosis

The radiographic appearance of juvenile arthrosis may be very similar to, and in some cases is indistinguish-able from, developmental hypoplasia of the condyle. Destruction of the anterior aspect of the condylar head from rheumatoid arthritis and severe degenerative joint disease or severe condylar degeneration after orthognathic surgery or joint surgery also may simulate juvenile arthrosis.

Treatment

Orthognathic surgery and orthodontic therapy may be required to correct the mandibular asymmetry. Caution should be exercised in undertaking orthodontic therapy because stress on the joint may result in further degeneration and orthodontic relapse.

CORONOID HYPERPLASIA

Definition

Coronoid process hyperplasia may be acquired or developmental, resulting in elongation of the coronoid process. In the developmental variant, the condition usually is bilateral. Acquired types may be unilateral or bilateral and usually are a response to restricted condylar movement caused by abnormalities such as ankylosis.

Clinical Features

Bilateral developmental coronoid hyperplasia is more common in males, often commencing at the onset of puberty, although the condition was reported in a 3-year-old. Patients complain of a progressive inability to open the mouth and may have an apparent closed lock. The condition is painless.

Radiographic Features

Coronoid hyperplasia is best seen in panoramic, Waters', and lateral tomographic views and on CT

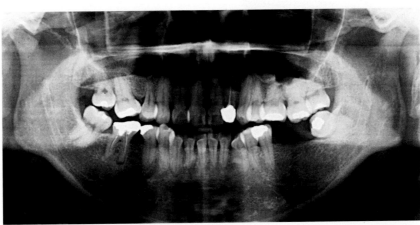

FIG. **25-18** Juvenile arthrosis. The condylar heads have a "toadstool" appearance and are posteriorly inclined. The condylar necks are absent.

scans. The coronoid processes are elongated, and the tips extend at least 1 cm above the inferior rim of the zygomatic arch (Fig. 25-19). As a result, the coronoid processes may impinge on the medial surface of the zygomatic arch during opening, restricting condylar translation. The coronoid processes may have a large but normal shape or may curve anteriorly and may appear very radiopaque. The posterior surface of the zygomatic process of the maxilla may be remodeled to accommodate the enlarged coronoid process during function. The radiographic appearance of the TMJs usually is normal.

Differential Diagnosis

Unilateral cases should be differentiated from a tumor of the coronoid process such as an osteochondroma or osteoma. Unlike coronoid hyperplasia, tumors usually have an irregular shape. The differential diagnosis also includes any cause of inability to open, such as soft tissue abnormalities and ankylosis, emphasizing the importance of including the coronoid process in images of the TMJs. An axial CT image with the patient in a wide-open position is useful in establishing coronoid interference to opening.

Treatment

Treatment consists of osteotomy or surgical removal of the coronoid process and postoperative physiotherapy.

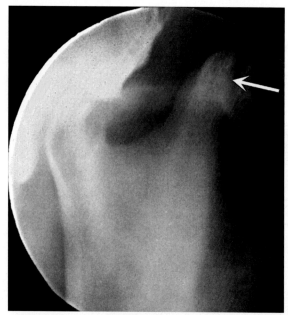

FIG. **25-19** Coronoid hyperplasia *(sagittal tomogram)*. The coronoid process is elongated and extends above the inferior rim of the zygomatic arch *(arrow)* but otherwise is shaped normally.

BIFID CONDYLE

Definition

A bifid condyle has a vertical depression, notch, or deep cleft in the center of the condylar head seen in the frontal or sagittal plane or an actual duplication of the condyle, resulting in the appearance of a "double" or "bifid" condylar head. This condition may be unilateral or bilateral. It may result from an obstructed blood supply or other embryopathy, although a traumatic cause has been postulated as a result of a longitudinal linear fracture of the condyle.

Clinical Features

Bifid condyle usually is an incidental finding in panoramic views or anteroposterior projections. Some patients have signs and symptoms of temporomandibular dysfunction, including joint noises and pain.

Radiographic Features

A depression or notch is present on the superior condylar surface, giving the anteroposterior silhouette a heart shape; in more severe cases a duplicate condylar head is present in the mediolateral plane (Fig. 25-20). The mandibular fossa may remodel to accommodate the altered condylar morphology.

Differential Diagnosis

A slight medial depression on the superior condylar surface may be considered a normal variation; the point at which the depth of the depression signifies a bifid condyle is unclear. The differential diagnosis also includes a vertical fracture through the condylar head.

Treatment

Treatment is not indicated unless pain or functional impairment is present.

Soft Tissue Abnormalities

INTERNAL DERANGEMENTS

Definition

An internal derangement is an abnormality in the position and sometimes the morphology of the articular disk that may interfere with normal function. The disk most often is displaced in an anterior direction, but it may be displaced anteromedially, medially, or anterolaterally. Lateral and posterior displacements are extremely rare. Some hypothesize that disk displacements may be considered a normal variation based on the frequency of this finding in asymptomatic patients. The cause of internal derangements is unknown,

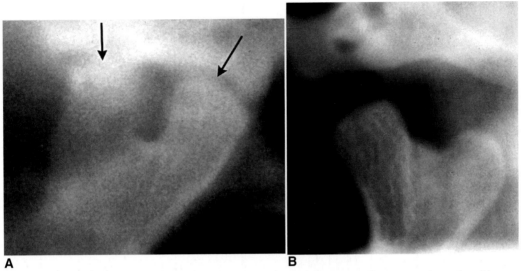

FIG. **25-20** Bifid condyle. **A,** Sagittal tomogram showing a deep central notch with duplication of the condylar head *(arrows)*. The glenoid fossa has remodeled (enlarged) to accommodate the abnormal condyle. **B,** Coronal tomogram. Another example showing a depression in the center of the condylar head.

although parafunction, jaw injuries (e.g., direct trauma), whiplash injury, and forced opening beyond the normal range have been implicated.

Internal derangements can be diagnosed using either arthrography or MRI. In some instances the disk may resume a normal position with respect to the condyle (called *reduction of the disk*) during mandibular opening; when the disk remains displaced throughout the entire range of mandibular movement, the term *nonreduction* is used (Fig. 25-21). A chronically displaced disk may become deformed, losing its normal biconcave shape, and it may become thickened and fibrotic. Possible complications in long-standing chronic disk displacement are degenerative joint disease and perforation through the disk or (more commonly) the posterior attachment.

Clinical Features

Disk displacement has been found both in symptomatic patients and in healthy volunteers, suggesting that it may be a normal variant and not necessarily a predisposing factor in TMJ dysfunction. It is not known why some disks remain displaced or why symptoms of pain and dysfunction are not found in all affected patients. Symptomatic patients may have a decreased range of mandibular motion. Internal derangements can be unilateral or bilateral; unilateral cases may manifest clinically as mandibular deviation to the affected side on opening. Joint noises are common and may manifest as a click as the disk reduces to a normal position during mandibular opening and occasionally as a softer click

as the disk becomes displaced again during mandibular closing. Noises may be absent in chronically displaced, nonreducing disks, or crepitus may be heard. Patients may complain of pain in the preauricular region or headaches and may have episodes of closed or open locking of the joint. Patients may have to manipulate the mandible to open it fully past an apparent closed lock by applying medially directed pressure to the affected joint or mandible with the hand.

Radiographic Features

The disk cannot be visualized with conventional radiography or tomography; arthrography and MRI are the techniques of choice. Although a retruded condylar position has been associated with disk displacement, condylar position in maximal intercuspation is not a reliable indicator of disk displacement. Likewise, diminished range of motion at maximal opening is not a reliable indication of a nonreducing disk.

Disk Displacement

Identifying the disk may be difficult in cases of gross deformation of the disk and other soft tissue components. Anterior displacement is the most common disk displacement. When the mandible is in maximal intercuspation, partial or full anterior disk displacement is indicated by anterior location of the posterior band of the disk from the normal position, which is directly superior to the condylar head. The normal articulating surface of the disk (thin intermediate zone) is somewhat anteriorly positioned, and as a result the osseous

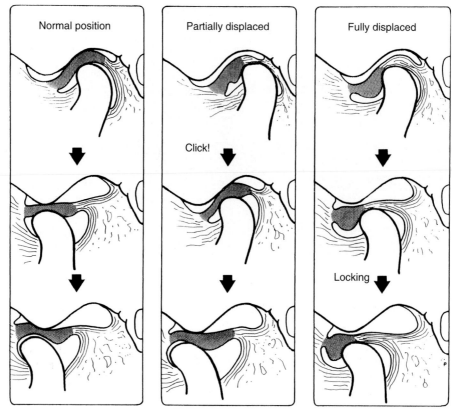

FIG. **25-21**   Position and movement of the disk during jaw opening. Normal position *(left)*; mildly displaced anteriorly *(with reduction, middle)*; severely displaced anteriorly *(without reduction, right).* (Courtesy Dr. W.K. Solberg, Los Angeles, Calif.)

structures of the joint articulate with the posterior band of the disk or the retrodiskal tissue. Anteromedial displacement is indicated in sagittal image slices when the disk is in a normal position in the medial images of the joint but anteriorly positioned in the lateral images of the same joint. Medial displacement is indicated in MRI coronal images when the body of the disk is positioned at the medial aspect of the condyle (Fig. 25-22).

Disk Reduction and Nonreduction

Arthrography allows a motion study of the condyle and disk during mandibular movement. Videofluoroscopy of mandibular movements during arthrography may show a sudden movement of the disk from an anterior displacement to a normal position during mandibular opening and back to the abnormal anterior (displaced) position during mandibular closing (Fig. 25-23). Often coinciding opening and closing (reciprocal) clicks are heard.

   If the disk remains anteriorly displaced (nonreduction) on opening, it may bend or deform as the condyle pushes against it (Fig. 25-24). The nonreduced disk is

readily seen on MRI scans, although fibrotic changes of the bilaminar zone may alter the signal to approximate the signal of the disk and thus make identification of the disk itself difficult. In such cases the disk may be erroneously interpreted as occupying a normal position at maximal opening.

Disk Perforation and Deformities

Arthrography can reveal a tear in the joint capsule or a perforation in the disk or posterior attachment by demonstrating the flow of contrast agent from the inferior to the superior joint space during the injection phase (Fig. 25-25). Disk perforations are not reliably detected with MRI. Both MRI and arthrography can indicate alteration in the normal biconcave outline of the disk, which may vary from enlargement of the posterior band to a bilinear or biconvex disk outline.

Fibrous Adhesions and Effusion

Fibrous adhesions are masses of fibrous tissue or scar tissue that form in the joint space, particularly after TMJ

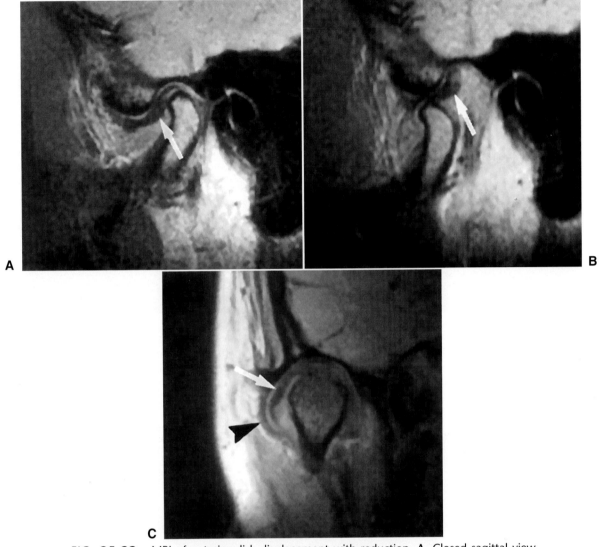

FIG. **25-22** MRI of anterior disk displacement with reduction. **A,** Closed sagittal view showing the disk with its posterior band *(arrow)* anterior to the condyle. **B,** Open view showing the normal relationship of the disk and condyle and the posterior band of the disk *(arrow)*. **C,** Coronal view showing the disk *(white arrow)* laterally displaced. The joint capsule *(black arrowhead)* bulges laterally. (Courtesy Dr. Per-Lennart Westesson, Rochester, N.Y.)

surgery. Adhesions are best identified with arthrography by resistance to injection of contrast agent or may be detected in MRI studies as tissue with low signal intensity. The pressure of injected contrast agent may tear some of these adhesions, resulting in increased joint mobility after the procedure. MRI can detect accumulation of fluid in joint spaces, which appears as a high signal in the joint spaces in T2-weighted images (Fig. 25-26).

Remodeling and Arthritic Conditions

REMODELING

Definition
Remodeling is an adaptive response of cartilage and osseous tissue to forces applied to the joint that may be excessive, resulting in alteration of the shape of

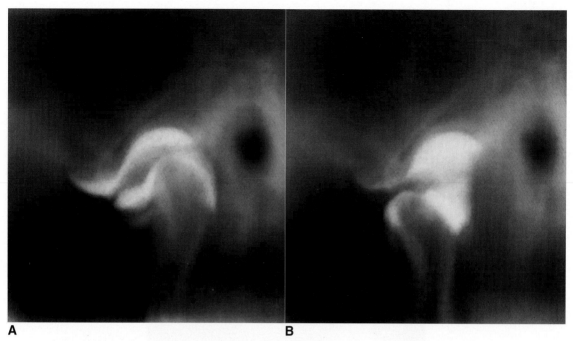

A   **B**

FIG. **25-23**   Arthrograms of a disk in closed position **(A)** and open position **(B)**. Contrast material can be seen redistributing between the compartments in the open and closed
images. The disk is displaced anteriorly in the closed position and reduces on opening.
(Courtesy Dr. Alan G. Lurie, Farmington, Conn.)

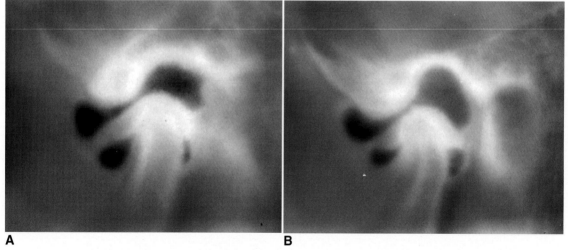

A   **B**

FIG. **25-24**   Examples of double contrast arthrography in which the contrast medium
is removed and replaced with air so that the joint spaces now appear radiolucent and the
disc is radiopaque. The disk is displaced anterior to the condylar head in the closed position **(A)** and remains displaced in the open position **(B)**.

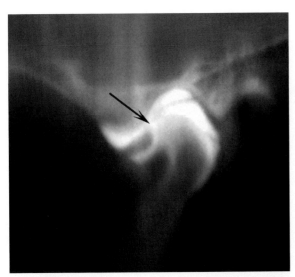

FIG. **25-25** A single contrast arthrogram demonstrating a perforation *(arrow)* immediately posterior to a deformed disc. Note that the contrast in the inferior joint space is continuous with the contrast in the superior space through the perforation.

the condyle and articular eminence. This adaptive response may result in flattening of curved joint surfaces, which effectively distributes forces over a greater surface area. The number of trabeculae also increases, increasing the density of subchondral cancellous bone (sclerosis) to better resist applied forces. No destruction or degeneration of articular soft tissues occurs. TMJ remodeling occurs throughout adult life and is considered abnormal only if accompanied by clinical signs and symptoms of pain or dysfunction or if the degree of remodeling seen radiographically is judged to be severe. Remodeling may be unilateral and does not invariably serve as a precursor to degenerative joint disease.

Clinical Features

Remodeling may be asymptomatic, or patients may have signs and symptoms of temporomandibular dysfunction that may be related to the soft tissue components, associated muscles, or ligaments. Accompanying internal derangement of the disk may be a factor.

Radiographic Features

Radiographic changes may affect the condyle, temporal component, or both; they first occur on the anterosuperior surface of the condyle and posterior slope of the articular eminence. The lateral aspect of the joint is affected in early stages, and the central and medial aspects become involved as remodeling progresses. The radiographic appearance may include one or a combination of the following: flattening, cortical thickening of articulating surfaces, and subchondral sclerosis (Fig. 25-27).

Differential Diagnosis

Severe joint flattening and subchondral sclerosis may be difficult to differentiate from early degenerative joint disease. It is known that the microscopic changes of degeneration occur before they can be detected radiographically. The radiographic appearance of bone erosions, osteophytes, and loss of joint space are signs signifying degenerative joint disease.

Treatment

When no clinical signs or symptoms are present, treatment is not indicated. Otherwise, treatment directed to relieve stress on the joint, such as splint therapy, may be considered. This should be preceded by an attempt to discover the cause of the joint stress.

DEGENERATIVE JOINT DISEASE

Synonym
Osteoarthritis

Definition

Degenerative joint disease (DJD) is a noninflammatory disorder of joints characterized by joint deterioration and proliferation. Joint deterioration is characterized by loss of articular cartilage and bone erosion. The proliferative component is characterized by new bone formation at the articular surface and in the subchondral region. Usually a variable combination of deterioration and proliferation occurs, but occasionally one aspect predominates; deterioration is more common in acute disease, and proliferation predominates in chronic disease. DJD is thought to occur when the ability of the joint to adapt to excessive forces (remodel) is exceeded. The etiology of DJD is unknown, although a number of factors may be important, including acute trauma, hypermobility, and loading of the joint such as occurs in parafunction. Internal derangements may be contributing etiologic factors, but this theory is controversial.

Clinical Features

DJD can occur at any age, although the incidence increases with age. DJD has a female preponderance. The disease may be asymptomatic, or patients may complain of signs and symptoms of TMJ dysfunction, including pain on palpation and movement, joint noises (crepitus), limited range of motion, and muscle spasm. The onset of symptoms may be sudden or gradual, and symptoms may disappear spontaneously, only to return

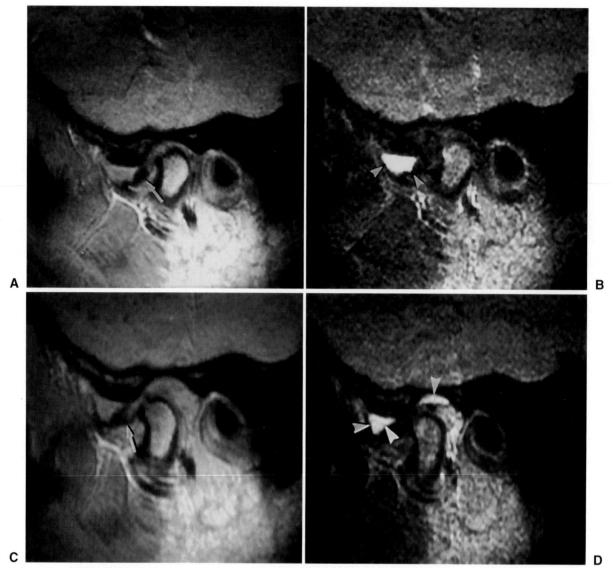

FIG. **25-26**   MRI of disk displacement without reduction in the presence of joint effusion. **A,** The disk *(arrow)* is anteriorly displaced in this closed T1-weighted image. **B,** A T2-weighted image of the same section shows the collection of joint effusion *(arrowheads)* in the anterior recess of the upper joint space. **C,** Open T1-weighted image showing the disk anterior to the condyle and the posterior band of the disk *(arrow).* **D,** This T2-weighted image is at the same level as **C.** Note the joint effusion *(arrowheads)* in the anterior and posterior recesses of the upper joint space. (Courtesy Dr. Per-Lennart Westesson, Rochester, N.Y.)

in recurring cycles. Some studies report that the disease eventually "burns out" and symptoms disappear or markedly decrease in severity in long-standing cases.

Radiographic Features

When the patient is in maximal intercuspation, the joint space may be narrow or absent, which often correlates with an internal derangement and frequently with a perforation of the disk or posterior attachment, resulting in bone-to-bone contact of the joint components. Signs of previous remodeling, such as flattening and subchondral sclerosis, may be evident, although degenerative changes may obscure these findings. Loss of cortex or erosions of the articulating surfaces of the

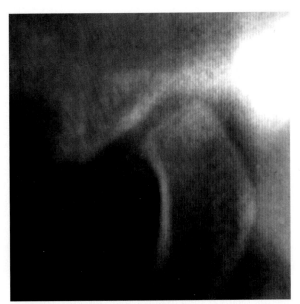

FIG. **25-27**   Remodeling. Flattening of the articulating surface of the condyle with flattening and subchondral sclerosis of the temporal component.

condyle or temporal component (or both) are characteristic of this disease (Fig. 25-28). In some cases small, round, radiolucent areas with irregular margins surrounded by a varying area of increased density are visible deep to the articulating surfaces. These lesions are called *Ely cysts* but are not true cysts; they are areas

of degeneration that contain fibrous tissue, granulation tissue, and osteoid (Fig. 25-29).

Later in the course of the disease, bony proliferation occurs at the periphery of the articulating surface, increasing the articulating surface area. This new bone is called an *osteophyte*, which typically appears on the anterosuperior surface of the condyle, lateral aspect of the temporal component, or both (Fig. 25-30). Osteophytes also may form on the lateral, medial, and posterosuperior aspect of the condyle. In severe cases, osteophyte formation originating in the glenoid fossa extends from the articular eminence to almost encase the condylar head. Osteophytes may break off and lie free within the joint space (these fragments are known as *joint mice*), and these must be differentiated from other conditions that cause joint space radiopacities (Fig. 25-31; see also Fig. 25-30).

In severe DJD, the glenoid fossa may appear grossly enlarged because of erosion of the posterior slope of the articular eminence, and the condyle may be markedly diminished in size and altered in shape because of destruction and erosion of the condylar head. This in turn may allow the condylar head to move forward and superiorly into an abnormal anterior position that may result in an anterior open bite.

Differential Diagnosis

DJD can have a spectrum of appearances ranging from substantial subchondral sclerosis and osteophyte formation (proliferative component) to extensive erosions

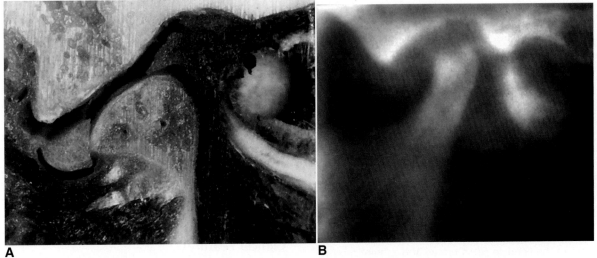

A   **B**

FIG. **25-28**   DJD. **A,** A cadaver specimen. Note the flattened temporal component and anterosuperior condylar surface, with destruction of the disk between the condyle and temporal component. **B,** A lateral tomograph of a joint with degenerative joint disease. Note the erosions of the superior aspect of the condylar head and flattening of the articular eminence.

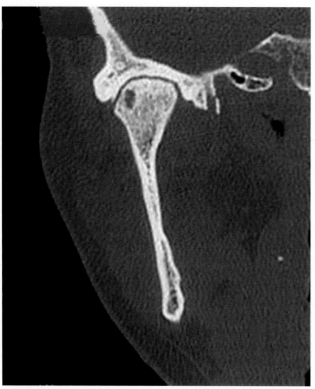

FIG. **25-29**   Pseudocyst (Ely cyst). Coronal CT image of a subchondral erosion that appears as a cystic radiolucency within the condylar head.

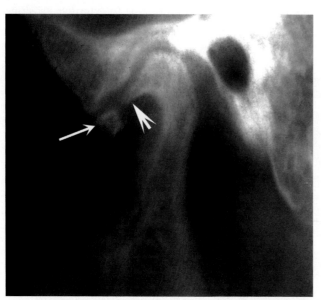

FIG. **25-30**   A large osteophyte eminating from the anterior aspect of the condyle *(short arrow)* and a "joint mouse" *(long arrow)* positioned anterior to the condyle in the joint space.

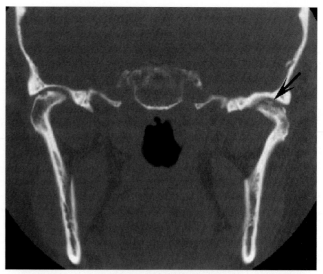

FIG. **25-31**   A coronal CT image using bone algorithm of a case of bilateral degenerative joint disease. There is an erosion of the superior aspect of the right condyle and "joint mice" *(arrow)* present within the left joint.

(degenerative component). A more erosive appearance may simulate inflammatory arthritides such as rheumatoid arthritis, whereas a more proliferative appearance with extensive osteophyte formation may simulate a benign tumor such as osteoma or osteochondroma.

Treatment
Treatment is directed toward relieving joint stress (e.g., splint therapy), relieving secondary inflammation with antiinflammatory drugs, and increasing joint mobility and function (e.g., physiotherapy).

RHEUMATOID ARTHRITIS

Definition
Rheumatoid arthritis (RA) is a heterogeneous group of systemic disorders that manifests mainly as synovial membrane inflammation in several joints. The TMJ becomes involved in approximately half of affected patients. The characteristic radiographic findings are a result of villous synovitis, which leads to formation of synovial granulomatous tissue (pannus) that grows into fibrocartilage and bone, releasing enzymes that destroy articular surfaces and underlying bone.

Clinical Features
RA is more common in females and can occur at any age but increases in incidence with increasing age. A juvenile variant is discussed separately. Usually the small joints of the hands, wrists, knees, and feet are affected in a bilateral, symmetric fashion, whereas TMJ involve-

ment varies. Patients with TMJ involvement complain of swelling, pain, tenderness, stiffness on opening, limited range of motion, and crepitus. The chin appears receded, and an anterior open bite is a common finding because of the bilateral destruction and anterosuperior positioning of the condyles. TMJ involvement usually is bilateral and symmetric.

Radiographic Features

The initial changes may be generalized osteopenia (decreased density) of the condyle and temporal component. The pannus may destroy the disk, resulting in diminished width of the joint space. Bone erosions by the pannus most often involve the articular eminence and the anterior aspect of the condylar head, which permits anterosuperior positioning of the condyle when the teeth are in maximal intercuspation and results in an anterior open bite (Fig. 25-32). Erosion of the anterior and posterior condylar surfaces at the attachment of the synovial lining may result in a "sharpened pencil" appearance of the condyle. Erosive changes may be so severe that the entire condylar head is destroyed, with only the neck remaining as the articulating surface. Similarly, the articular eminence may be destroyed to the extent that a concavity replaces the normally convex eminence. Joint destruction eventu-

ally leads to secondary DJD. Subchondral sclerosis and flattening of articulating surfaces may occur, as well as subchondral "cyst" and osteophyte formation. Fibrous ankylosis or, in rare cases, osseous ankylosis, may occur; reduced mobility is related to the duration and severity of the disease.

Differential Diagnosis

The differential diagnosis includes severe DJD and psoriatic arthritis. Osteopenia and severe erosions, particularly of the articular eminence, are more characteristic of RA. Psoriatic arthritis may be ruled out by the patient's history.

Treatment

Treatment is directed toward pain relief (analgesics), reduction or suppression of inflammation (nonsteroidal antiinflammatory drugs, gold salts, corticosteroids), and preservation of muscle and joint function (physiotherapy). Joint replacement surgery may be necessary in patients with severe joint destruction.

JUVENILE CHRONIC ARTHRITIS

Synonyms

Juvenile rheumatoid arthritis and Still's disease

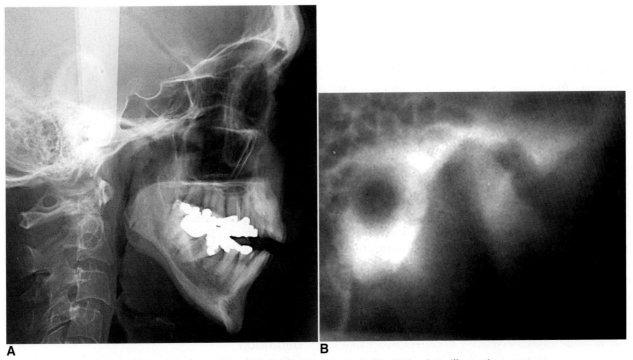

FIG. 25-32 Rheumatoid arthritis. **A,** Lateral cephalometric view illustrating a steep mandibular plane and anterior open bite. **B,** Lateral tomogram illustrating a large erosion of the anterosuperior condylar head accompanied by severe erosions of the temporal component, including the articular eminence.

Definition

Juvenile chronic arthritis (JCA), formerly called *juvenile rheumatoid arthritis*, is a chronic inflammatory disease that appears before the age of 16 years (the mean age is 5 years). It is characterized by chronic, intermittent synovial inflammation that results in synovial hypertrophy, joint effusion, and swollen, painful joints. As the disease progresses, cartilage and bone are destroyed. Rheumatoid factor may be absent, hence the preferred use of the term *JCA* rather than *juvenile rheumatoid arthritis*. JCA differs from adult RA in that it has an earlier onset, and systemic involvement usually is more severe. TMJ involvement occurs in approximately 40% of patients and may be unilateral or bilateral.

Clinical Features

The patient usually has pain and tenderness in the affected joint or joints, although the disease can be asymptomatic. Unilateral onset is common, but contralateral involvement may occur as the disease progresses. Severe TMJ involvement results in inhibition of mandibular growth. Affected patients may have micrognathia and posteroinferior chin rotation, resulting in a facial appearance known as *bird face*, which may also be accompanied by an anterior open bite. The degree of micrognathia is proportional to the severity of joint involvement and the early onset of disease. Additionally, when only one TMJ is involved or if one side is more severely affected, the patient may have a mandibular asymmetry with the chin deviated to the affected side.

Radiographic Features

Osteopenia (decreased density) of the affected TMJ components may be the only initial radiographic finding. Radiographic findings are similar to those for the adult form except for the addition of impaired mandibular growth. Erosions may extend to the mandibular fossa, and the articular eminence may be destroyed. Similarly, erosion of the anterior or superior aspect of the condyle may occur, and in more severe cases only a pencil-shaped small condyle remains; the condyle may be destroyed. Because the inflammation is intermittent, during quiescent periods the cortex of the joint surfaces may reappear, and the surfaces will appear flattened. As a result of bone destruction, the condylar head typically is positioned anterosuperiorly in the mandibular fossa (Fig. 25-33). Hypomobility at maximal opening is common, and fibrous ankylosis may occur in some cases. Secondary degenerative changes manifesting as sclerosis and osteophyte formation may be superimposed on the rheumatoid changes, and ankylosis may occur. Manifestations of inhibited mandibular growth, such as deepening of the antego-

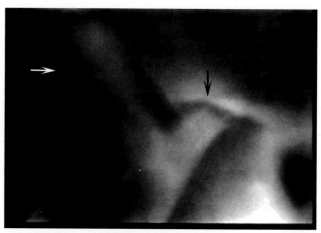

FIG. 25-33 Juvenile chronic arthritis. Sagittal tomogram (closed position) showing irregular erosions of the superior aspect of the condyle and erosion of all of the articular eminence and an anterior positioning of the condyle over the former position of the articular eminence *(black arrow)*. Note the secondary enlargement of the coronoid process *(white arrow)* as a result of fibrous ankylosis of the joint.

nial notch, diminished height of the ramus, and dorsal bending of the ramus and condylar neck, also may occur unilaterally or bilaterally, resulting in an obtuse angle between the mandibular body and ascending ramus.

PSORIATIC ARTHRITIS AND ANKYLOSING SPONDYLITIS

Psoriatic arthritis and ankylosing spondylitis are seronegative, systemic arthritides that may affect the TMJs. Psoriatic arthritis occurs in patients suffering from psoriasis of the skin, with inflammatory joint disease occurring in 7% of patients. Ankylosing spondylitis occurs predominantly in males, progressing to spinal fusion. TMJ radiographic changes seen in these disorders may be indistinguishable from those caused by RA, although occasionally a profound sclerotic change is seen in psoriatic arthritis.

SEPTIC ARTHRITIS

Synonym

Infectious arthritis

Definition

Septic arthritis is infection and inflammation of a joint that can result in joint destruction. It is rare in comparison with the incidence of degenerative joint disease and RA in the TMJ. Septic arthritis may be caused by direct spread of organisms from an adjacent cellulitis or from parotid, otic, or mastoid infections. It also may occur by direct extension of osteomyelitis of the mandibular body and ramus or spread from a middle ear infection, although hematogenous spread from a distant nidus has also been reported.

Clinical Features

Individuals can be affected at any age, and the condition shows no gender predilection. It usually occurs unilaterally. The patient may have redness and swelling over the joint; trismus; severe pain on opening; inability to occlude the teeth; large, tender cervical lymph nodes; fever; and malaise. The mandible may be deviated to the unaffected side as a result of joint effusion.

Radiographic Features

No radiographic signs may be present in early stages of the disease, although the space between the condyle and the roof of the mandibular fossa may be widened because of inflammatory exudate in the joint spaces. Osteopenic (radiolucent) changes of the joint components and mandibular ramus may be evident. More obvious bony changes are seen approximately 7 to 10 days after the onset of clinical symptoms. As a result of the osteolytic effects of inflammation, the condylar articular cortex may become slightly radiolucent, and discontinuity or subtle irregularity of the anterior cortical surface may be evident. As the disease progresses, the condyle and articular eminence, including the disk, may be destroyed. Osseous ankylosis may occur after the infection subsides. If the disease occurs during the period of mandibular growth, radiographic manifestations of inhibited mandibular growth may be evident.

Differential Diagnosis

The radiographic changes caused by septic arthritis may mimic those of severe DJD or RA, although septic arthritis usually occurs unilaterally, and the patient often has clinical signs and symptoms of infection. Inflammatory changes that may accompany septic arthritis may be seen in CT images, such as involvement of mastoid air cells, osteomyelitis of the mandible, and inflammation of surrounding soft tissue. MRI, using T2-weighted images, may also be helpful in diagnosis as well as scintigraphy using technetium bone scans followed by gallium scans.

Treatment

Treatment includes antimicrobial therapy, drainage of effusion, and joint rest. Physiotherapy to reestablish joint mobility is initiated after the acute phase of infection has passed.

Articular Loose Bodies

Articular loose bodies are radiopacities of varying origin located in the synovium, within the capsule in the joint spaces or outside the capsule in soft tissue. They appear radiographically as soft tissue calcifications positioned around the condylar head. The loose bodies may represent bone that has separated from joint components, as in DJD (joint mice), hyaline cartilage metaplasia (calcification) that occurs in synovial chondromatosis, crystals deposited in the joint space in crystal-associated arthropathy (pseudogout), or tumoral calcinosis associated with renal disease. In rare cases chondrosarcoma also may mimic the appearance of articular loose bodies.

SYNOVIAL CHONDROMATOSIS

Synonyms

Synovial chondrometaplasia and osteochondromatosis

Definition

Synovial chondromatosis is an uncommon disorder characterized by metaplastic formation of multiple cartilaginous and osteocartilaginous nodules within connective tissue of the synovial membrane of joints. Some of these nodules may detach and form loose bodies in the joint space, where they persist and may increase in size, being nourished by synovial fluid. This condition is more common in the axial skeleton than in the TMJ. When the cartilaginous nodules ossify, the term *synovial osteochondromatosis* may be used.

Clinical Features

Patients may be asymptomatic or may complain of preauricular swelling, pain, and decreased range of motion. Some patients have crepitus or other joint noises. The condition usually occurs unilaterally.

Radiographic Features

The osseous components may appear normal or may exhibit osseous changes similar to those in DJD. The joint space may be widened, and if ossification of the cartilaginous nodules has occurred, a radiopaque mass or several radiopaque loose bodies may be seen surrounding the condylar head (Fig. 25-34). CT imaging can identify the location of the calcifications. Occasionally erosion through the glenoid fossa into the middle cranial fossa may occur, which is best detected with CT imaging.

Differential Diagnosis

The appearance of synovial chondromatosis cannot always be differentiated from chondrocalcinosis. Con-

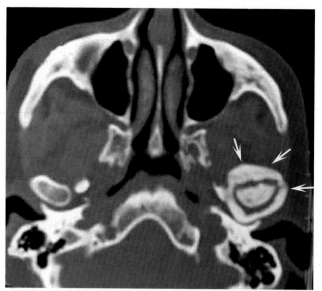

FIG. 25-34   An axial CT image using bone algorithm of synovial osteochondromatosis, note the ossification surrounding the condylar head *(arrows).*
(Courtesy Dr. Bernard Friedland, Harvard University.)

ditions that appear similar include DJD with joint mice or chondrosarcoma. Chondrosarcoma may be accompanied by severe bone destruction, which may help in differentiating the condition from synovial chondromatosis.

Treatment

Treatment consists of removal of the loose bodies and resection of abnormal synovial tissue in the joint by arthroscopic or open joint surgery.

CHONDROCALCINOSIS

Synonyms

Pseudogout and calcium pyrophosphate dihydrate deposition disease

Definition

Chondrocalcinosis is characterized by acute or chronic synovitis and precipitation of calcium pyrophosphate dihydrate crystals in the joint space. It differs from gout, in which urate crystals are precipitated; hence the term *pseudogout.*

Clinical Features

The joints more commonly affected are the knee, wrist, hip, shoulder, and elbow; TMJ involvement is uncommon. The condition occurs unilaterally and is more common in males. Patients may be asymptomatic or may complain of pain and joint swelling.

Radiographic Features

The radiographic appearance of chondrocalcinosis may simulate synovial chondromatosis, described above. Often the radiopacities within the joint space are finer and have a more even distribution than in osteochondromatosis (Fig. 25-35). Bone erosions as well as a severe increase in condylar bone density also have been described. Erosions of the glenoid fossa may be present, which require CT for detection.

Differential Diagnosis

The differential diagnosis is the same as for synovial chondromatosis.

Treatment

Treatment consists of surgical removal of the crystalline deposits. Steroids, aspirin, and nonsteroidal anti-inflammatory agents may provide relief. Colchicine may be used to alleviate acute symptoms and for prophylaxis.

Trauma

EFFUSION

Definition

Effusion is an influx of fluid into the joint, usually as a result of trauma (hemorrhage) or inflammation (exudate).

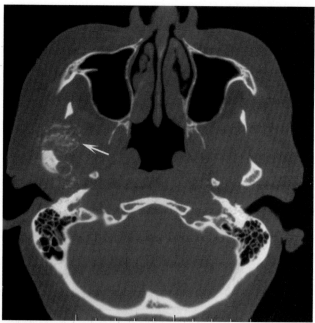

FIG. 25-35   An axial CT image using bone algorithm of chondrocalcinosis involving the right joint. Note the calcifications anterior to the condyle *(arrow)* and large erosion involving the medial pole of the condyle.

Clinical Features

The patient may have swelling over the affected joint; pain in the TMJ, preauricular region, or ear; and limited range of motion. Patients may also complain of the sensation of fluid in the ear, tinnitus, and hearing difficulties, as well as difficulty occluding the posterior teeth.

Radiographic Features

Joint effusion is more commonly seen in conjunction with internal derangements, although it has been described in normal joints. The joint space is widened, and T2-weighted MRI studies may show a bright signal (white), indicating fluid adjacent to the disk or posterior to the condyle (see Fig. 25-26).

Differential Diagnosis

Effusion must be differentiated from septic arthritis; in the latter case the accompanying signs and symptoms of infection are present.

Treatment

Treatment may include antiinflammatory drugs, although surgical drainage of the effusion occasionally is necessary.

DISLOCATION

Definition

Dislocation is abnormal positioning of the condyle out of the mandibular fossa but within the joint capsule. It usually occurs bilaterally and most commonly in an anterior direction. Dislocation may be caused by a failure of muscular coordination, subluxation, or external trauma and may be associated with a condylar fracture.

Clinical Features

Patients are unable to close the mandible to maximal intercuspation; some patients cannot reduce the dislocation, whereas others may be able to reduce the mandible by manipulation. In the former case associated pain and muscle spasm often are present.

Radiographic Features

In bilateral cases both condyles are located anterior and superior to the summits of the articular eminentia. Clinical information is important because the normal range of motion may extend anterior to the summit of the articular eminence.

Differential Diagnosis

The diagnosis is confirmed by the radiographic findings, although some fracture dislocations may be difficult to visualize, particularly if the dislocation is very slight.

Treatment

Treatment consists of manual manipulation of the mandible to reduce the dislocation. Surgery occasionally is necessary to reduce the condyle in the case of a fracture dislocation, although treatment may not be indicated for this type of dislocation if mandibular function is adequate.

FRACTURE

Definition

Fractures of the TMJ usually occur at the condylar neck and often are accompanied by dislocation of the condylar head. Fractures may be divided into those involving the condylar head and those involving the condylar neck, although occasionally both may be involved. On rare occasions the fracture may involve the temporal component.

Clinical Features

Unilateral fractures, which are more common than bilateral fractures, may be accompanied by a parasymphyseal or mandibular body fracture on the contralateral side. The patient may have swelling over the TMJ, pain, limited range of motion, and an anterior open bite. Some TMJ fractures are relatively asymptomatic and may not be discovered at the time of trauma; instead, these come to light as incidental findings at a later time when radiographs are taken for other reasons. Condylar fractures should be ruled out if the patient has a history of a blow to the mandible, especially to the anterior aspect.

Radiographic Features

In relatively recent condylar neck fractures, a radiolucent line limited to the outline of the neck is visible. This line may vary in width, depending on whether the bone fragments are still aligned (narrow line) or displacement/dislocation has occurred (wider line). If the bone fragments overlap, an area of apparent increase in radiopacity may be seen instead of a radiolucent line (Fig. 25-36). Also, the outer cortical boundary may have an irregular outline or a step defect. Approximately 60% of condylar fractures show evidence of fragment angulation and a variable degree of displacement (dislocation) of the fracture ends. Fractures of the condylar head are less common and may be of the vertical (responsible for the traumatic type of bifid condyle) or compressive type (Fig. 25-37). Multiple right-angle radiographic projections from the lateral, frontal, and basilar aspects are required to detect a fracture and to

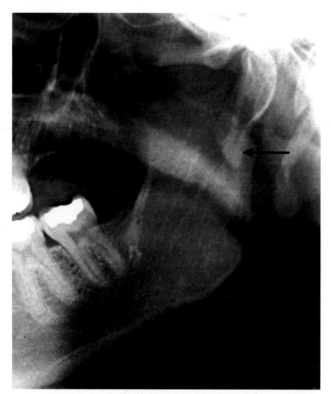

FIG. **25-36** Condylar neck fracture (panoramic view). The arrow points to overlapped fragments, as evidenced by increased radiopacity.

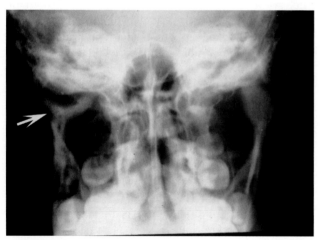

FIG **25-37**   Open Towne's view of a compression fracture of the right condylar head *(arrow)*.

determine fragment displacement. CT is also an excellent imaging modality for detecting condylar fractures.

The amount of remodeling seen in the TMJ after a condylar fracture with medial displacement varies considerably. In some cases the condyle remodels to a form that is essentially normal, whereas in other cases the condyle and mandibular fossa become flattened,

with loss of vertical height on the affected side. The condyle eventually may show degenerative changes, including flattening, erosion, and osteophytes, and ankylosis. These changes are more severe if the condyle is displaced.

Differential Diagnosis

Occasionally old fractures that have remodeled may be difficult to differentiate from developmental abnormalities of the condyle. The most common difficulty is in determining whether a fracture is indeed present. Transorbital or reverse Towne's views are particularly useful when there is minimal or medial displacement of the condylar head.

Treatment

Treatment may not be indicated if mandibular mobility is adequate; otherwise, the fracture is reduced surgically.

Trauma to the Developing Condyle

If a condylar fracture occurs during the period of mandibular growth, growth may be inhibited because of damage to the condylar growth center. The degree of subsequent hypoplasia is related to the stage of mandibular development at the time of injury (younger patients have more profound hypoplasia) and the severity of the injury. Injury to the joint may result in hemorrhage or effusion into the joint spaces that eventually may form bone during the healing process, which in turn may result in severe hypoplasia and limited joint function.

NEONATAL FRACTURES

The use of forceps during delivery of neonates may result in fracture and displacement of the rudimentary condyle, which later manifests as severe mandibular hypoplasia and lack of development of the glenoid fossa and articular eminence. Such cases have a characteristic radiographic appearance in the panoramic image, having the appearance of a partly opened pair of scissors in place of a normal condyle (Fig. 25-38). This presentation results from the overlapping images of the medially displaced "carrot-shaped" condyle and remnants of the condylar neck.

Differential Diagnosis

This condition often is not diagnosed until later in life, at which time a diagnosis of fracture may be made

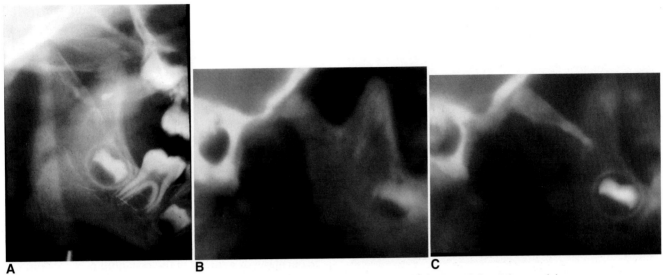

FIG **25-38** **A,** A cropped panoramic image of a neonatal fracture of the right condyle, note the unusual shape of the coronoid notch similar to a partially opened pair of scissors. **B,** A tomographic image slice of the lateral aspect of the same joint. Note the normal-appearing coronoid notch but a lack of formation of the glenoid fossa and eminence and the abnormal anterior position of the condyle. **C,** A medial tomographic slice of the same case disclosing the fractured segment.

without a history that the fracture occurred at the time of birth. The condition must be differentiated from a developmental hypoplasia of the mandible, which is unrelated to birth injury.

Treatment

The fracture usually is not treated, but the mandibular asymmetry may be corrected with a combination of orthodontics and orthognathic surgery.

ANKYLOSIS

Definition

Ankylosis is a condition in which condylar movement is limited by a mechanical problem in the joint ("true" ankylosis) or by a mechanical cause not related to joint components ("false" ankylosis). True ankylosis may be bony or fibrous. In bony ankylosis the condyle or ramus is attached to the temporal bone by an osseous bridge. In fibrous ankylosis a soft tissue (fibrous) union of joint components occurs; the bone components appear normal. False ankylosis may result from conditions that inhibit condylar movement such as muscle spasm, myositis ossificans, or coronoid process hyperplasia.

Clinical Features

Most unilateral cases are caused by mandibular trauma or infection. The most common cause of bilateral TMJ ankylosis is rheumatoid arthritis, although in rare cases

bilateral fractures may be the cause. Most if not all cases of TMJ ankylosis in infancy occur secondary to birth injury. Patients have a history of progressively restricted jaw opening, or they may have a long-standing history of limited opening. Some degree of mandibular opening usually is possible through flexing of the mandible, although opening may be restricted to only a few millimeters, particularly in the case of bony ankylosis.

Radiographic Features

In fibrous ankylosis the articulating surfaces are usually irregular because of erosions. The joint space is usually very narrow and the two irregular surfaces may appear to fit one another like a jigsaw puzzle. Little or no condylar movement is seen. Radiographic signs of remodeling occasionally are visible as the joint components adapt to repeated attempts at mandibular opening. In bony ankylosis the joint space may be partly or completely obliterated by the osseous bridge, which can vary from a slender segment of bone, which may be difficult to locate, to a large bony mass. This extensive new bone may fuse the condyle to the cranial base (Fig. 25-39). Secondary degenerative changes of the joint components are common. Often morphologic changes occur, such as compensatory progressive elongation of the coronoid processes and deepening of the antegonial notch in the mandibular ramus on the affected side as a result of muscle function during attempted

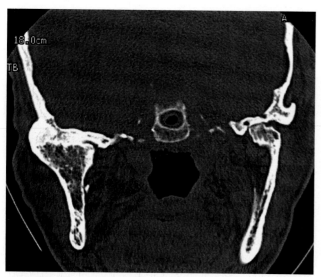

FIG. 25-39 Bony ankylosis (CT, coronal image slice). The right condyle and ramus are markedly enlarged. The articulating surface is irregular, and the central and lateral aspects are fused to the roof of the glenoid fossa, as evidenced by a lack of joint space. Note that the left condylar articulating surface is eroded, and the joint space is decreased on the medial aspect; these changes are consistent with DJD.

mandibular opening. If ankylosis occurs before mandibular growth is complete, growth of the affected side of the mandible is inhibited. Coronal CT images are the best diagnostic imaging method to evaluate ankylosis.

Differential Diagnosis

The major differential diagnosis is a condylar tumor. However, a history of trauma, infection, or other joint diseases should help rule out neoplastic disease. Detection of fibrous ankylosis is difficult because fibrous tissue is not visible in the radiographic image and therefore may be difficult to differentiate from false ankylosis.

Treatment

Joint mobility is improved by surgical removal of the osseous bridge or creation of a pseudarthrosis.

Tumors

Benign and malignant tumors originating in or involving the TMJ are rare. Tumors may be intrinsic or extrinsic (adjacent) to the TMJ. Intrinsic tumors may develop in the condyle, temporal bone, or coronoid process. Extrinsic tumors may affect the morphology, structure,

or function of the joint without invading the joint itself. They may cause indirect effects on growth, such as those seen with vascular lesions or from pressure, or they may influence mandibular positioning.

BENIGN TUMORS

The most common benign intrinsic tumors affecting the TMJ are osteomas, osteochondromas, Langerhans histiocytosis and osteoblastomas. Chondroblastomas, fibromyxomas, benign giant cell lesions, and aneurysmal bone cysts also occur. Benign tumors and cysts of the mandible (e.g., ameloblastomas, odontogenic keratocysts, simple bone cysts) may involve the entire ramus and in rare cases the condyle. In cases of false ankylosis in which the TMJs appear radiographically normal, hyperplasia or a tumor of the coronoid process must be ruled out.

Clinical Features

Condylar tumors grow slowly and may attain considerable size before becoming clinically noticeable. Patients may complain of TMJ swelling, which may be accompanied by pain and decreased range of motion. The clinical examination may reveal facial asymmetry, malocclusion, and deviation of the mandible to the unaffected side; these may be accompanied by symptoms of TMJ dysfunction. Tumors of the coronoid process typically are painless, but patients may complain of progressive limitation of motion.

Radiographic Features

Condylar tumors cause condylar enlargement that often is irregular in outline. The trabecular pattern may be altered, resulting in regions of destruction seen as radiolucencies or new abnormal bone formation, which may increase the radiopacity of the condyle with abnormal trabeculae. An osteoma or osteochondroma appears as an abnormal, pedunculated mass attached to the condyle (Fig. 25-40). Osteochondromas often extend from the anterior or superior surface of the condyle. Tumors of the coronoid process may affect TMJ function, which emphasizes the need to image and evaluate the coronoid process when evaluating joint abnormalities. The most common benign tumor is the osteochondroma. This tumor may interfere with joint function and erode adjacent osseous structures.

Differential Diagnosis

Condylar neoplasms may simulate unilateral condylar hyperplasia because of condylar enlargement, although osteomas and osteochondromas give an irregular appearance, such as bulbous or globular expansion of the condyle or, more commonly, a pedunculated

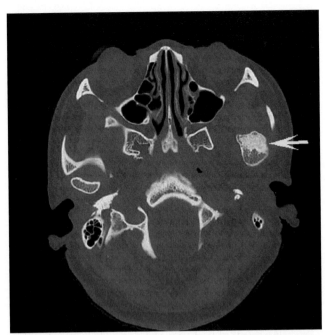

FIG. **25-40** An axial CT image using bone algorithm revealing an osteochondroma extending from the anterior surface of the left condylar head *(arrow)*. Note that the sclerotic internal structure of the osteochondroma is continuous with the remaining condylar head.

growth. Also, the characteristic condylar shape and proportions are better preserved in condylar hyperplasia. Coronoid tumors must be differentiated from coronoid hyperplasia, which differs from a condylar tumor in that the coronoid process remains regular in shape.

Treatment

Treatment consists of surgical excision of the tumor and occasionally excision of the condylar head or coronoid process.

MALIGNANT TUMORS

Malignant tumors of the jaws may be primary or, more commonly, metastatic. Primary intrinsic malignant tumors of the condyle are extremely rare and include chondrosarcoma, osteogenic sarcoma, synovial sarcoma, and fibrosarcoma of the joint capsule. Extrinsic malignant tumors may represent direct extension of adjacent parotid salivary gland malignancies, rhabdomyosarcoma (particularly in children), or other regional carcinomas from the skin, ear, and nasopharynx. The most common metastatic lesions include neoplasms originating in the breast, kidney, lung, colon, prostate, and thyroid gland.

Clinical Features

Malignant tumors (primary or metastatic) may be asymptomatic, or patients may have symptoms of TMJ dysfunction such as pain, limited mandibular opening, mandibular deviation, and swelling. Unfortunately, a patient occasionally is treated for TMJ dysfunction without recognition that the underlying condition is a malignancy.

Radiographic Features

Malignant primary and metastatic TMJ tumors appear as a variable degree of bone destruction with ill-defined, irregular margins. Most lack tumor bone formation, with the exception of osteogenic sarcoma. Chondrosarcoma may appear as an indistinct, essentially radiolucent destructive lesion of the condyle with surrounding discrete soft tissue calcifications that may simulate the appearance of the articular loose bodies seen in chondrocalcinosis or pseudogout (Fig. 25-41). In the case of metastatic tumors, the radiographic appearance usually is nonspecific condylar destruction (with a few exceptions, such as metastatic prostate carcinoma) and does not indicate the site of origin (Fig. 25-42).

Differential Diagnosis

Joint destruction caused by a malignant tumor must be differentiated from the osseous destruction seen in

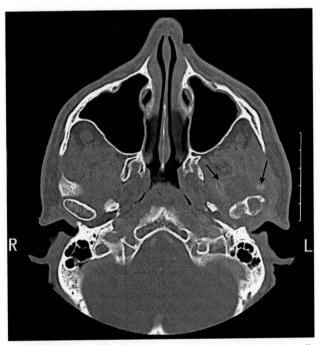

FIG. **25-41** Chondrosarcoma (CT, axial section). A radiolucent destructive lesion is present in the left condylar head, and faint radiopacities (soft tissue calcifications) are visible anterior to the condylar head *(arrows)*.

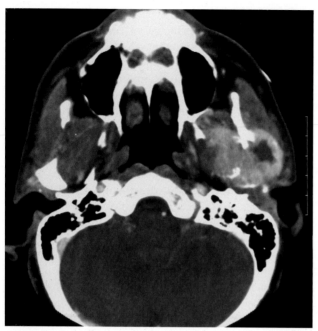

FIG. **25-42**   An axial CT image using soft tissue algorithm of a metastatic lesion from a carcinoma of the thyroid gland, which has destroyed all of the left mandibular condyle.

severe DJD. Malignant tumors cause profound central bone destruction, whereas DJD causes more peripheral bone destruction. Proliferative changes such as osteophyte formation may be seen in DJD, but unlike with a malignant tumor, no soft tissue mass or swelling is evident. Chondrosarcoma may simulate joint space calcifications (discussed earlier), but in the case of malignancy, severe bone destruction also occurs.

Treatment

In the case of primary malignant tumors, treatment consists of wide surgical removal of the tumor. Tumor extension to vital anatomic structures may compromise survival. Metastatic tumors of the TMJ rarely are treated surgically; treatment mainly is palliative and may include radiotherapy and chemotherapy.

BIBLIOGRAPHY

DISORDERS OF THE TEMPOROMANDIBULAR JOINT

Brooks SL et al: Imaging of the temporomandibular joint. Position paper of the American Academy of Oral and Maxillofacial Radiology, Oral Surg Oral Med Oral Pathol Oral Radiol Endod 83:609, 1997.

Helkimo M: Studies on function and dysfunction of the masticatory system. II. Index for anamnestic and clinical dysfunction and occlusal state, Swed Dent J 67:101, 1974.

McNeill C et al: Temporomandibular disorders: diagnosis, management, education, and research, J Am Dent Assoc 120:253, 1990.

Petrikowski CG, Grace MG: Temporomandibular joint radiographic findings in adolescents, J Craniomand Pract 14:30, 1996.

Rugh JD, Solberg WK: Oral health status in the United States: temporomandibular disorders, J Dent Educ 49:398, 1985.

Wänman A, Agerberg G: Mandibular dysfunction in adolescents. I. Prevalence of symptoms, Acta Odontol Scand 44:47, 1986.

ANATOMY OF THE TEMPOROMANDIBULAR JOINT

Blaschke DD, Blaschke TJ: A method for quantitatively determining temporomandibular joint bony relationships, J Dent Res 60:35, 1981.

Drace JE, Enzmann DR: Defining the normal temporomandibular joint: closed, partially open, and open mouth MR imaging of asymptomatic subjects, Radiology 177:67, 1990.

Hansson LG et al: A comparison between clinical and radiologic findings in 259 temporomandibular joint patients, J Prosthet Dent 50:89, 1983.

Ingervall B et al: Postnatal development of the human temporomandibular joint. II. A microradiographic study, Acta Odont Scand 34:133, 1976.

Larheim TA: Radiographic appearance of the normal temporomandibular joint in newborns and small children, Acta Radiol Diagn 22(5):593, 1981.

Pullinger AG et al: A tomographic study of mandibular condyle position in an asymptomatic population, J Prosthet Dent 53:706, 1985.

Taylor RC et al: A study of temporomandibular joint morphology and its relationship to the dentition, Oral Surg 33:1002, 1972.

Ten Cate AR: Gross and micro anatomy. In Zarb GA et al, editors: Temporomandibular joint and masticatory muscle disorders, ed 2, Copenhagen, 1994, Munksgaard.

Westesson P-L et al: Cryosectional observations of functional anatomy of the temporomandibular joint, Oral Surg Oral Med Oral Pathol 68:247, 1989.

Yale SH et al: An epidemiological assessment of mandibular condyle morphology, Oral Surg 21:169, 1966.

DIAGNOSTIC IMAGING OF THE TEMPOROMANDIBULAR JOINT

Brooks SL et al: Imaging of the temporomandibular joint, position paper of the American Academy of Oral and Maxillofacial Radiology, Oral Surg Oral Med Oral Pathol Oral Radiol Endod 83:609, 1997.

Helms CA, Kaplan P: Diagnostic imaging of the temporomandibular joint: recommendations for use of the various techniques, AJR Am J Roentgenol 154:319, 1990.

Katzberg RW: Temporomandibular joint imaging, Radiology 170:297, 1989.

Hard tissue imaging

Bean L et al: The transmaxillary projection in temporomandibular joint radiography, Dentomaxillofac Radiol 4:13, 1975.

Christiansen EL et al: Computed tomography of the normal temporomandibular joint, Scand J Dent Res 95:499, 1987.

Coin CG: Tomography of the temporomandibular joint, Dent Radiol Photogr 47:23, 1974.

Hansson L-G, Petersson A: Radiography of the temporomandibular joint using the transpharyngeal projection, Dentomaxillofac Radiol 7:69, 1987.

Mongini F: The importance of radiography in the diagnosis of TMJ dysfunctions: a comparative evaluation of transcranial radiographs and serial tomography, J Prosthet Dent 45:186, 1981.

Soft tissue imaging

Conway WF et al: Dynamic magnetic resonance imaging of the temporomandibular joint using FLASH sequences, J Oral Maxillofac Surg 46:930, 1988.

Hansson L-G et al: Comparison of tomography and midfield magnetic resonance imaging for osseous changes of the temporomandibular joint, Oral Surg Oral Med Oral Pathol Oral Radiol Endod 82:698, 1996.

Moses JJ et al: Magnetic resonance imaging or arthrographic diagnosis of internal derangement of the temporomandibular joint, Oral Surg Oral Med Oral Pathol 75:268, 1993.

Schellhas KP et al: The diagnosis of temporomandibular joint disease: two-compartment arthrography and MR, AJR Am J Roentgenol 151:341, 1988.

Westesson P-L: Double-contrast arthrography of the temporomandibular joint: introduction of an arthrographic technique for visualization of the disc and articular surfaces, J Oral Maxillofac Surg 41:163, 1983.

Westesson P-L, Bronstein SL: Temporomandibular joint: comparison of single- and double-contrast arthrography, Radiology 164:65, 1987.

RADIOGRAPHIC ABNORMALITIES OF THE TEMPOROMANDIBULAR JOINT

Condylar hyperplasia

Gray RJM et al: Histopathological and scintigraphic features of condylar hyperplasia, Int J Oral Maxillofac Surg 19:65, 1990.

Jonck LM: Facial asymmetry and condylar hyperplasia, Oral Surg 40:567, 1975.

Rubenstein LK, Campbell RL: Acquired unilateral condylar hyperplasia and facial asymmetry: report of a case, ASDC J Dent Child 52:114, 1985.

Condylar hypoplasia

Jerell RG et al: Acquired condylar hypoplasia: report of a case, ASDC J Dent Child 58:147, 1991.

Worth HM: Radiology of the temporomandibular joint. In Zarb GA, Carlsson GE, editors: Temporomandibular joint function and dysfunction, Copenhagen, 1979, Munksgaard.

Juvenile arthrosis

Boering G: Temporomandibular joint arthrosis and facial deformity, Trans Int Conf Oral Surg 258, 1967.

Worth HM: Radiology of the temporomandibular joint. In Zarb GA, Carlsson GE, editors: Temporomandibular joint function and dysfunction, Copenhagen, 1979, Munksgaard.

Coronoid hyperplasia

McLoughlin PM et al: Hyperplasia of the mandibular coronoid process: an analysis of 31 cases and a review of the literature, J Oral Maxillofac Surg 53:250, 1995.

Bifid condyle

Loh FC, Yeo JF: Bifid mandibular condyle, Oral Surg Oral Med Oral Pathol 69:24, 1990.

SOFT TISSUE ABNORMALITIES

Dolwick MF, Sanders B: TMJ internal derangement and arthrosis. In Surgical atlas, St. Louis, 1985, Mosby.

Helms CA et al: Temporomandibular joint: morphology and signal intensity characteristics of the disk at MR imaging, Radiology 172:817, 1989.

Katzberg RW: Temporomandibular joint imaging, Radiology 170:297, 1989.

Katzberg RW et al: Internal derangements of the temporomandibular joint: findings in the pediatric age group, Radiology 154:125, 1985.

Larheim TA: Current trends in temporomandibular joint imaging, Oral Surg Oral Med Oral Pathol Oral Radiol Endod 80:555, 1995.

Nuelle DG et al: Arthroscopic surgery of the temporomandibular joint, Angle Orthod 56:118, 1986.

Rammelsberg P et al: Variability of disk position in asymptomatic volunteers and patients with internal derangements of the TMJ, Oral Surg Oral Med Oral Pathol Oral Radiol Endod 83:393, 1997.

Sano T, Westesson P-L: Magnetic resonance imaging of the temporomandibular joint: increased T2 signal in the retrodiskal tissue of painful joints, Oral Surg Oral Med Oral Pathol Oral Radiol Endod 79:511, 1995.

Wilkes CH: Internal derangements of the temporomandibular joint: pathological variations, Arch Otolaryngol Head Neck Surg 115:469, 1989.

REMODELING AND ARTHRITIC CONDITIONS

Remodeling

Brooks SL et al: Prevalence of osseous changes in the temporomandibular joint of asymptomatic persons without internal derangement, Oral Surg Oral Med Oral Pathol 73:118, 1992.

Moffett BC et al: Articular remodeling in the adult human temporomandibular joint, Am J Anat 115:119, 1964.

Degenerative joint disease

deLeeuw R et al: Temporomandibular joint osteoarthrosis: clinical and radiographic characteristics 30 years after nonsurgical treatment—a preliminary report, J Craniomand Pract 11:15, 1993.

Mayne JG, Hatch GS: Arthritis of the temporomandibular joint, J Am Dent Assoc 79:125, 1969.

Radin EL et al: Role of mechanical factors in pathogenesis of primary osteoarthritis, Lancet 1(749):519, 1972.

Sato H et al: Temporomandibular joint osteoarthritis: a comparative clinical and tomographic study pre- and posttreatment, J Oral Rehab 21:383, 1994.

Rheumatoid arthritis

Gynther GW et al: Radiographic changes in the temporomandibular joint in patients with generalized osteoarthritis and rheumatoid arthritis, Oral Surg Oral Med Oral Pathol Oral Radiol Endod 81:613, 1996.

Larheim TA et al: Rheumatic disease of the temporomandibular joint: MR imaging and tomographic manifestations, Radiology 175:527, 1990.

Syrjänen SM: The temporomandibular joint in rheumatoid arthritis, Acta Radiologica Diagnosis 26(3):235, 1985.

Juvenile chronic arthritis

Ganik R, Williams FA: Diagnosis and management of juvenile rheumatoid arthritis with TMJ involvement, J Craniomandib Pract 4:255, 1986.

Hu Y-S, Schneiderman ED: The temporomandibular joint in juvenile rheumatoid arthritis. I. Computed tomographic findings, Pediatr Dent 17:46, 1995.

Hu Y-S et al: The temporomandibular joint in juvenile rheumatoid arthritis. II. Relationship between computed tomographic and clinical findings, Pediatr Dent 18:312, 1996.

Karhulahti T et al: Mandibular condyle lesions related to age at onset and subtypes of juvenile rheumatoid arthritis in 15-year-old children, Scand J Dent Res 101:332, 1993.

Psoriatic arthritis

Koorbusch GF et al: Psoriatic arthritis of the temporomandibular joints with ankylosis, Oral Surg Oral Med Oral Pathol 71:267, 1991.

Wilson AW et al: Psoriatic arthropathy of the temporomandibular joint, Oral Surg Oral Med Oral Pathol 70:555, 1990.

Ankylosing spondylitis

Locher MC et al: Involvement of the temporomandibular joints in ankylosing spondylitis (Bechterew's disease), J Craniomaxillofac Surg 24:205, 1996.

Ramos-Remus C et al: Temporomandibular joint osseous morphology in a consecutive sample of ankylosing spondylitis patients, Ann Rheum Dis 56(2):103, 1997.

Septic arthritis

Leighty SM et al: Septic arthritis of the temporomandibular joint: review of the literature and report of two cases in children, Int J Oral Maxillofac Surg 22:292, 1993.

ARTICULAR LOOSE BODIES

Carls FR et al: Loose bodies in the temporomandibular joint, J Craniomaxillofac Surg 23:215, 1995.

Chuong R, Piper MA: Bilateral pseudogout of the temporomandibular joint: report of a case and review of the literature, J Oral Maxillofac Surg 53:691, 1995.

Dijkgraaf LC et al: Calcium pyrophosphate dihydrate crystal deposition disease: a review of the literature and a light and electron microscopic study of a case of the temporomandibular joint with numerous intracellular crystals in the chondrocytes, Osteoarthritis Cartilage 3:35, 1995.

Lustmann J, Zeltser R: Synovial chondromatosis of the temporomandibular joint: review of the literature and case report, Int J Oral Maxillofac Surg 18:90, 1989.

Orden A et al: Chronic preauricular swelling, J Oral Maxillofac Surg 47:390, 1989.

Pynn BR et al: Calcium pyrophosphate dihydrate deposition disease of the temporomandibular joint: a case report and review of the literature, Oral Surg Oral Med Oral Pathol Oral Radiol Endod 79:278, 1995.

TRAUMA

Effusion

Schellhas KP, Wilkes CH: Temporomandibular joint inflammation: comparison of MR fast scanning with T1- and T2-weighted imaging techniques, AJNR 10:589, 1989.

Schellhas KP et al: Facial pain, headache, and temporomandibular joint inflammation, Headache 29:229, 1989.

Takaku S et al: Magnetic resonance images in patients with acute traumatic injury of the temporomandibular joint: a preliminary report, J Craniomaxillofac Surg 24:173, 1996.

Westesson P-L, Brooks SL: Temporomandibular joint: relationship between MR evidence of effusion and the presence of pain and disk displacement, AJR Am J Roentgenol 159:559, 1992.

Dislocation

Kai S et al: Clinical symptoms of open lock position of the condyle: relation to anterior dislocation of the temporomandibular joint, Oral Surg Oral Med Oral Pathol 74:143, 1992.

Kallal RH et al: Cranial dislocation of mandibular condyle, Oral Surg 43:2, 1977.

Wijmenga JP et al: Protracted dislocation of the temporomandibular joint, Int J Oral Maxillofac Surg 15:380, 1986.

Fracture

Dahlstrom L et al: 15 years follow-up on condylar fractures, Int J Oral Maxillofac Surg 18:18, 1989.

Horowitz I et al: Demonstration of condylar fractures of the mandible by computed tomography, Oral Surg 54:263, 1982.

Lindahl L, Hollender L: Condylar fractures of the mandible. II. A radiographic study of remodeling processes in the temporomandibular joint, Int J Oral Surg 6:153, 1977.

Raustia AM et al: Conventional radiographic and computed tomographic findings in cases of fracture of the mandibular condylar process, J Oral Maxillofac Surg 48:1258, 1990.

Schellhas KP: Temporomandibular joint injuries, Radiology 173:211, 1989.

TRAUMA TO THE DEVELOPING CONDYLE

Pharoah MJ: Radiology of the temporomandibular joint. In Zarb GA et al, editors: Temporomandibular joint and masticatory muscle disorders, ed 2, Copenhagen, 1994, Munksgaard.

Neonatal fractures

Pharoah MJ: Radiology of the temporomandibular joint. In Zarb GA et al, editors: Temporomandibular joint and masticatory muscle disorders, ed 2, Copenhagen, 1994, Munksgaard.

Worth HM: Radiology of the temporomandibular joint. In Zarb GA, Carlsson GE, editors: Temporomandibular joint function and dysfunction, Copenhagen, 1979, Munksgaard.

Ankylosis

Rowe NL: Ankylosis of the temporomandibular joint, J R Coll Surg Edinb 27:67, 1982.

Wood RE et al: The radiologic features of true ankylosis of the temporomandibular joint: an analysis of 25 cases, Dentomaxillofac Radiol 17:121, 1988.

TUMORS

Benign tumors

James RB et al: Osteochondroma of the mandibular coronoid process: report of a case, Oral Surg 37:189, 1974.

Nwoku ALN, Koch H: The temporomandibular joint: a rare localisation for bone tumors, J Maxillofac Surg 2:113, 1974.

Pharoah MJ: Radiology of the temporomandibular joint. In Zarb GA et al, editors: Temporomandibular joint and masticatory muscle disorders, ed 2, Copenhagen, 1994, Munksgaard.

Svensson B, Isacsson G: Benign osteoblastoma associated with an aneurysmal bone cyst of the mandibular ramus and condyle, Oral Surg Oral Med Oral Pathol 76:433, 1993.

Thoma KH: Tumors of the temporomandibular joint, J Oral Surg 22:157, 1964.

Worth HM: Radiology of the temporomandibular joint. In Zarb GA, Carlsson GE, editors: Temporomandibular joint function and dysfunction, Copenhagen, 1979, Munksgaard.

Malignant tumors

Morris MR et al: Chondrosarcoma of the temporomandibular joint: case report, Head Neck Surg 10:113, 1987.

Rubin MM et al: Metastatic carcinoma of the mandibular condyle presenting as temporomandibular joint syndrome, J Oral Maxillofac Surg 47:507, 1989.

CHAPTER 26

Paranasal Sinuses

AXEL RUPRECHT ■ ERNEST W.N. LAM

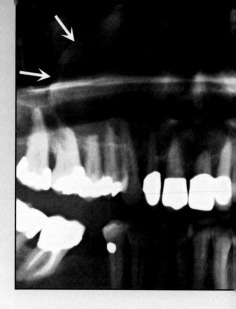

The paranasal sinuses are air-filled cavities of the craniofacial complex, comprising the maxillary, frontal, and sphenoid sinuses, and the ethmoid air cells. The maxillary sinuses are of particular importance to the dentist because of their proximity to the dental structures. Consequently, diseases of the sinuses may mimic odontogenic disease, and conversely, odontogenic disease may spread to the sinuses or mimic sinus disease. Part or all of the paranasal sinuses may appear on radiographs made for dental purposes, including maxillary periapical and panoramic radiographs. All of the paranasal sinuses can appear on lateral or posterior-anterior cephalometric skull radiographs made for orthodontic or orthognathic surgical purposes, although not necessarily in the most diagnostic fashion. Therefore the dentist should have some familiarity with the normal appearances and more common diseases of the paranasal sinuses.

Normal Development and Variations

The paranasal sinuses develop as invaginations from the nasal fossae into their respective bones (maxillary, frontal, sphenoid, and ethmoid). The maxillary sinuses (sometimes called the *maxillary antra* or *antra of Highmore*) are the first to develop, becoming apparent by day 17 *in utero*. These invaginations begin just above the inferior concha in the middle meatus, and grow laterally. At birth each sinus is quite small and slitlike, lying in the most medial aspect of the maxilla. Their greatest dimension in the anteroposterior direction is no more than 8mm. With growth, the sinuses enlarge laterally under the orbits, and by the second year, they reach lat-

erally to the infraorbital canals. By the ninth year, the maxillary sinuses extend to the zygomatic bones and to the level of the floor of the nasal fossae. Lateral growth usually ceases by the fifteenth year.

The average volume of the adult maxillary sinus is approximately 15ml but may continue to enlarge throughout life. In some cases, the maxillary sinus may extend into the zygomatic, alveolar, frontal, and occasionally, the palatal processes of the maxilla. Extensive enlargement of the maxillary and other paranasal sinuses is a well-known feature of acromegaly. Hypoplasia of the maxillary sinuses occurs unilaterally in about 1.7% of patients and bilaterally in 7.2%. In these patients, the radiographic images of the affected sinus may appear more radiopaque than normal because of the relatively large amount of surrounding maxillary bone. The configuration of the maxillary sinus walls frequently helps to distinguish between a hypoplastic sinus and one that is pathologically radiopaque. Hypoplasia may be evident in the occipitomental (Waters) view, with the appearance of an inward bowing of the sinus wall, resulting in a smaller-than-normal–sized air cavity.

The ethmoid sinuses, better known as the *ethmoid air cells,* consist of multiple interconnected, or sometimes separate, small chambers. Developing as outgrowths of the nasal fossae, the ethmoid air cells extend into the ethmoid bones during the fifth fetal month and continue to enlarge until the end of puberty. The number of ethmoid air cells varies considerably, with each ethmoid bone containing between 8 and 15 cells. In some cases, the ethmoid air cells may extend into the neighboring maxillary, lacrimal, frontal, sphenoid, and palatine bones.

The development of the frontal sinuses does not usually begin until the fifth or sixth year. The frontal sinuses may develop either directly as extensions from the nasal fossae or from anterior ethmoid air cells. In about 4% of the population, the frontal sinuses fail to develop. As with the other paranasal sinuses, the right and left frontal sinus cavities develop separately. As these cavities expand, they approach each other in the midline, where a thin bony septum separates them. In some individuals, the intersinus septum may be absent. In the adult, the frontal sinuses are usually seen as two asymmetric cavities located above the level of the supra-orbital ridges and the nasion. The sinuses may also extend posteriorly over the orbital roofs. The frontal sinuses drain directly into the nasal fossae via the frontonasal ducts (in about half the cases), or alternatively, through the anterior ethmoid air cells into the nasal fossae through the infundibula.

The sphenoid sinuses begin growth from the nasal cavities in the fourth fetal month as invaginations from the sphenoethmoid recesses of the nasal cavities. At birth, the sphenoid sinuses are minute cavities in the body of the sphenoid bone. Most of their development takes place after puberty. Like the frontal sinuses, the right and left sphenoid sinuses are separated by a bony septum and are usually asymmetric in size and shape. The overall size of the sinuses is quite variable. They may extend beyond the body of the sphenoid bone into the dorsum sellae, the clinoid processes, the greater or lesser wings, and the pterygoid processes. The sphenoid sinuses communicate with the nasal cavities through ostia (singular, ostium), which are usually 2 to 3 mm in diameter. This may explain why, as with the maxillary sinuses, mucoceles (destructive enlargements resulting from blockage of the drainage from the sinuses) are uncommon in the sphenoid sinuses (see the Mucocele section later in this chapter).

Various functions have been ascribed to these sinuses, including the following:
- Air conditioning (heating and humidification)
- Acting as an air reservoir
- Ventilation
- Aiding in olfaction
- Reduction in weight of the cranium
- Addition of resonance to the voice
- Protection
- Insulation of the cerebrum and orbits
- Participation in formation of the cranium

The paranasal sinuses may also have no function; that is, they may be evolutionary unwanted space. The maxillary and ethmoid sinuses may assist in respiration, with the growth of the maxillary sinuses also representing an adjustment to the changing size of the maxillofacial area. The frontal sinuses participate in the growth and development of the cerebral cranium, and

the sphenoid sinuses allow for adjustments of the buckling in the cranial base in evolution.

The mucosal lining of the paranasal sinuses is similar to that found in the nasal cavity, but with slightly fewer mucous glands. In the absence of disease, the epithelial cilia move mucous toward their respective communications with the nasal fossae.

Diseases Associated with the Paranasal Sinuses

Because the maxillary sinus is of most concern to the dentist, the following text will emphasize diseases related to the maxillary sinus.

DEFINITION

Diseases associated with the maxillary sinuses include both intrinsic diseases (originating primarily from within the sinus), and those that originate outside the sinus (most commonly odontogenic disease) that either impinge on or infiltrate the sinus. These types of abnormalities include inflammatory odontogenic disease, odontogenic cysts, benign odontogenic and malignant neoplasms, bone dysplasias, and trauma.

CLINICAL FEATURES

The clinical signs and symptoms of maxillary sinus disease include a feeling of pressure, altered voice characteristics, pain on movement of the head, percussion sensitivity of the teeth or cheek region, regional paresthesia or anesthesia, and swelling of the facial structures adjacent to the maxilla.

When the clinical signs indicate that maxillary sinus disease may be related to the alveolar process of the maxilla or teeth, it is reasonable for the dentist to proceed with the initial radiologic investigation. If there are positive findings, the patient should be referred to an oral and maxillofacial radiologist to complete the examination. The application of specific imaging modalities is reviewed in the following section.

APPLIED DIAGNOSTIC IMAGING

The intraoral periapical radiograph provides the most detailed, if limited view of the floor of the maxillary antrum (a description of the normal appearance is provided in Chapter 9). If during this examination the dental practitioner suspects an abnormality, the maxillary lateral occlusal projection may be used for a more extensive view of the antrum. The panoramic radiograph depicts both maxillary sinuses, revealing greater internal structure and parts of the inferior, posterior, and anteromedial walls. It is difficult to compare the internal radiopacities of the right and left sinus in the panoramic image because of variations that result from overlapping phantom images of other structures.

Specialized skull views are the next step in the investigation. The standard series of plain film views of the sinuses include the occipitomental (Waters), lateral, submentovertex and Caldwell (15° PA) skull views. The Waters projection is optimal for visualization of the maxillary sinuses, especially to compare internal radiopacities, as well as the frontal sinuses and ethmoid air cells. If the Waters view is made with the mouth open, the sphenoid sinuses may also be visualized. The submentovertex view may be useful in evaluating the lateral and posterior borders of the maxillary sinuses, as well as the ethmoid air cells. The Caldwell view is most useful in evaluating the frontal sinuses and ethmoid air cells. The lateral skull view allows examination of all four pairs of the paranasal sinuses but with each member of a pair superimposed on the other.

Computed tomography (CT) and magnetic resonance imaging (MRI) have become increasingly important for evaluation of sinus disease and have virtually replaced conventional tomography for investigations of these structures. Because CT and MRI provide multiple sections through the sinuses in different planes, they may contribute significantly to delineating the extent of disease and the final diagnosis. High-resolution axial and coronal CT and MRI examinations are the most revealing, noninvasive techniques for the paranasal sinuses and adjacent structures and areas. CT examination is appropriate to determine the extent of disease in patients who have chronic or recurrent sinusitis. Indeed coronal CT provides superior visualization of the ostiomeatal complex (the region of the ostium of the maxillary sinus and the ethmoidal ostium) and nasal cavities, as well as for demonstrating any reaction in the surrounding bone to sinus disease. MRI provides superior visualization of the soft tissues, especially the extension of infiltrating neoplasms into the sinuses or surrounding soft tissues, or the differentiation of retained fluid secretions from soft tissue masses in the sinuses.

Intrinsic Diseases of the Paranasal Sinuses

The following are disorders that originate from within the sinuses.

INFLAMMATORY DISEASE

Inflammation may result from a variety of causes, such as infections, chemical irritation, allergies, the introduction of a foreign body, or facial trauma. The radiographic changes associated with inflammation include thickened sinus mucosa, air-fluid levels in the sinuses, polyps, empyema, and retention pseudocysts. Viral infections may, however, not cause any radiographic change in a sinus.

MUCOSITIS

Synonym
Thickened mucous membrane

Definition
The mucosal lining of the paranasal sinuses is composed of respiratory epithelium, and is normally about 1 mm thick. Normal sinus mucosa is not visualized on a radiograph; however, when the mucosa becomes inflamed from either an infectious or allergic process, it may increase in thickness 10 to 15 times and may be seen radiographically. This inflammatory change is referred to as *mucositis*. Mucosal thickening greater than 3 mm is most likely pathologic.

Clinical Features
The thickness of sinus mucosa in an asymptomatic individual may vary considerably over a relatively short period of time. Consequently, the discovery of thickened mucosa in an individual who is otherwise asymptomatic does not necessarily imply that further investigations are warranted, or that treatment is required. Most of the inflammatory episodes that result in thickening of the mucosal lining of the sinus are unrecognized by the patient and are discovered only incidentally on a radiograph.

Radiographic Features
The image of thickened mucosa is readily detectable in the radiograph as a noncorticated band noticeably more radiopaque than the air-filled sinus, paralleling the bony wall of the sinus (Fig. 26-1).

SINUSITIS

Definition
Sinusitis is a condition involving generalized inflammation of the paranasal sinus mucosa. The etiologic agent may be an allergen, bacterial, or viral. Sinusitis may cause blockage of drainage from the ostiomeatal complex. Inflammatory changes may lead to ciliary dysfunction and retention of sinus secretions. Perhaps 10%

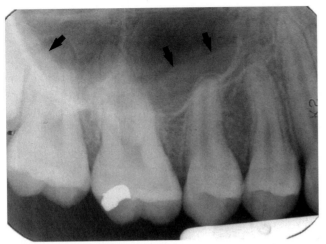

FIG. **26-1** *Mucositis.* Locally thickened mucosa is seen as a noncorticated, radiopaque band *(arrows)* that follows the contour of the sinus floor.

of inflammatory episodes of the maxillary sinuses are extensions of dental infections. Although not universally accepted, a classification is commonly used to divide sinusitis into three subtypes, based on length of time the disease has been present. *Acute sinusitis* refers to conditions present for less than 2 weeks; *subacute sinusitis,* to those present from 2 weeks to 3 months; and *chronic sinusitis,* to conditions that have been present for more than 3 months. The term *pansinusitis* describes sinusitis affecting all the paranasal sinuses. In children, pansinusitis may suggest the possibility of cystic fibrosis.

Clinical Features

Acute maxillary sinusitis is often a complication of the common cold and is accompanied by a clear nasal dis-

charge or pharyngeal drainage. After a few days, the stuffiness and nasal discharge increase, and the patient may complain of pain and tenderness to pressure or swelling over the involved sinus. The pain may also be referred to the premolar and molar teeth on the affected side, and these teeth may also be sensitive to percussion, although this is more commonly seen in bacterial sinusitis. Under these conditions, a green- or greenish-yellow–colored nasal discharge may also be appreciated. This finding requires that the teeth be ruled out as a possible source of the pain or infection. However, the key signs and symptoms are those of sepsis: fever, chills, malaise, and an elevated leukocyte count. Acute sinusitis is the most common of the sinus conditions that cause pain.

Chronic maxillary sinusitis is typically a sequela of an acute infection that fails to resolve by 3 months. In general, no external signs occur, except during periods of acute exacerbations when increased pain and discomfort are apparent. Chronic sinusitis is often associated with anatomic derangements that inhibit the outflow of mucus, including deviation of the nasal septum and presence of a concha bullosa (pneumatization of the middle concha). Chronic sinusitis is also often associated with allergic rhinitis, asthma, cystic fibrosis, and dental infections.

Radiographic Features

Thickening of sinus mucosa and the accumulation of secretions that accompany sinusitis reduce the air content of the sinus and cause it to become increasingly radiopaque (Fig. 26-2). The most common radiopaque patterns that occur in the Waters view are localized mucosal thickening along the sinus floor, generalized thickening of the mucosal lining around the entire wall

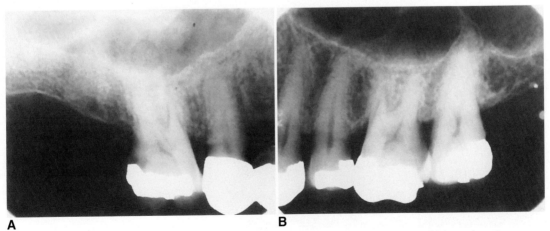

FIG. **26-2** Sinusitis results in generalized thickening of the mucosa, which makes the internal structure of the maxillary sinus more radiopaque. (Compare the internal radiopacity of the maxillary sinus **[A]** with the normal sinus, **B.**)

of the sinus, and near complete or complete radiopacification of the sinus.

Such changes are best seen in the maxillary sinuses, but the frontal and sphenoid sinuses may be similarly affected. Scrutinizing the area around the maxillary ostium on any of the views from Waters projections to CT images may reveal the presence of thickened mucosal tissue, which may cause blockage of the ostium. Mucosal thickening in just the base of the sinus may not represent sinusitis. Rather, it may represent the more localized thickening that can occur in association with rarefying osteitis from a tooth with a nonvital pulp. This may, however, progress to involve the entire sinus. The inability to perceive the delicate walls of the ethmoid air cells is a particularly sensitive sign of ethmoid sinusitis. The image of thickened sinus mucosa on the radiograph may be uniform or polypoid. In the case of an allergic reaction, the mucosa tends to be more lobulated. In contrast, in cases of infection, the thickened mucosal outline tends to be smoother, with its contour following that of the sinus wall.

An air-fluid level resulting from the accumulation of secretions may also be present. Because the radiopacities of transudates, exudates, blood, and pathologically altered mucosa are similar, the differentiation among them relies on their shape and distribution. When present, fluid appears radiopaque and occupies the inferior aspect of the sinus. The border between the radiopaque fluid and the relatively radiolucent antrum is horizontal and straight, with a meniscus (Fig. 26-3, *A* and *B*). It is possible to confirm that this is indeed an air-fluid interface by tilting the patient's head and making another radiograph. This changes the orientation of the fluid level, which eliminates any doubt as to its fluid nature. However, when attempting to verify this, sufficient time should be allowed between the first and second exposures for the fluid level to change. If a significant proportion of the fluid is mucus, some minutes may be required before it attains its new level. To demonstrate an air-fluid level, the central ray of the x-ray beam must be horizontal and at the level of the air-fluid interface. Chronic

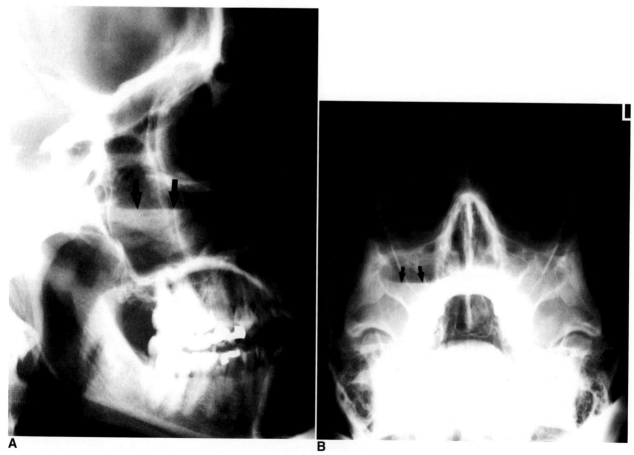

A   **B**

FIG. **26-3**   An air-fluid level in the maxillary sinus *(arrows)* on lateral skull **(A)** and occipitomental (Waters) **(B)** views.

sinusitis may result in persistent radiopacification of the sinus with sclerosis and/or thickening of the sinus wall (Fig. 26-4). Resorption of the bony border is unusual.

The resolution of acute sinusitis becomes apparent on the radiograph as a gradual increase in the radiolucency of the sinus. This can first be recognized when a small clear area appears in the interior of the sinus; the thickened mucous membrane gradually shrinks so that it begins to follow the outline of the bony wall. In time the mucous membrane again becomes radiographically invisible, and the sinus appears normal. In chronic sinusitis the inflammation may stimulate the sinus periosteum to produce bone, resulting in thick sclerotic borders of the maxillary antrum.

Management

The goals of treatment of sinusitis are to control the infection, promote drainage, and relieve pain. Acute sinusitis is usually treated medically with decongestants to reduce mucosal swelling and, in the case of a bacterial sinusitis, with antibiotics. Chronic sinusitis is primarily a disease of obstruction of the ostia; thus the goal is ventilation and drainage. This is often accomplished through endoscopic surgery to enlarge obstructed ostia or by establishing an alternate path of drainage.

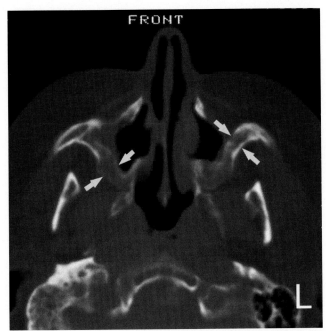

FIG. **26-4** *Chronic sinusitis.* Bone-window, axial CT image shows thickening of the posterolateral walls of the maxillary sinuses *(arrows)*. This thickening is the result of chronic inflammation in the sinuses.

EMPYEMA

Definition

An empyema is a cavity filled with pus. It may result as a possible sequela of a sinus ostium blocked by a thickened, inflamed mucous membrane or some other pathologic process, especially in the maxillary sinus. Empyema is probably a variant of a mucocele or pyocele.

RETENTION PSEUDOCYSTS

Synonyms

Antral pseudocyst, benign mucous cyst, mucous retention cyst, mesothelial cyst, pseudocyst, interstitial cyst, lymphangiectatic cyst, false cyst, retention cyst of the maxillary sinus, benign cyst of the antrum, benign mucosal cyst of the sinus, serous nonsecretory retention pseudocyst, and mucosal antral cyst

Definition

The term *retention pseudocyst* is used to describe several related conditions. The actual pathogenesis of these lesions is controversial; however, because their clinical and radiographic features are similar, no attempt is made here to distinguish them. One etiology suggests that blockage of the secretory ducts of seromucous glands in the sinus mucosa may result in a pathologic submucosal accumulation of secretions, resulting in swelling of the tissue. A second possibility suggests that the serous nonsecretory retention cyst arises as a result of cystic degeneration within an inflamed, thickened sinus lining. Both types of lesions are called *pseudocysts* because they are not lined with epithelium.

Clinical Features

Retention pseudocysts may be found in any of the sinuses at any time of the year, but they occur more often around April and November. This suggests that they might be related to changes in season or to heating or air conditioning in buildings. Most studies have found that the retention pseudocyst is more common in males.

The retention pseudocyst rarely causes any signs or symptoms, and thus the patient is usually unaware of the lesion. It often is noticed as an incidental finding on radiographs made for other purposes. However, when the pseudocyst completely fills the maxillary sinus cavity, it may prolapse (extrude) through the ostium and cause nasal obstruction and postnasal discharge. This may be the only clinical evidence of the presence of the pseudocyst. Because either type of retention pseudocyst may enlarge and fill a sinus cavity, it frequently ruptures as a result of abrupt pressure changes caused by sneezing or blowing of the nose. If this does not happen, the expanding pseudocyst may herniate through the ostium into the nasal cavity, where it subsequently ruptures. The pseudocyst may be present on radiographic examination of the maxillary sinus, perhaps absent only a few days later, only to reappear on subsequent examinations.

The maxillary sinus is the most common site of antral retention pseudocysts, although they are occasionally found in the frontal or sphenoid sinuses. Antral retention pseudocysts are not related to extractions or associated with periapical disease.

Radiographic Features

Location. Partial images of retention pseudocysts of the maxillary antrum may appear on maxillary posterior periapical radiographs (Fig. 26-5, *A*), but they are best demonstrated in panoramic radiographs (Fig. 26-5, *B*). Although pseudocysts may occur bilaterally, usually only a single pseudocyst develops. Occasionally more than one pseudocyst may form in a sinus. These pseudocysts usually project from the floor of the sinus, although some may form on the lateral walls. The size of retention pseudocysts may vary from that of a fingertip to a size large enough to completely fill the sinus and make it radiopaque.

Periphery and shape. Both varieties of pseudocysts usually appear as noncorticated, smooth, dome-shaped radiopaque masses. Because the lesion originates within the maxillary sinus, no osseous border surrounds it. The base of the lesions may be narrow or, more commonly, broad.

Internal structure. The internal aspect is homogeneous and more radiopaque than the surrounding air of the sinus cavity (Fig. 26-5, *C* to *E*). The radiopacity of the lesion is caused by the accumulation of fluid, and as such, normal osseous landmarks may often be seen through its image.

Effects on surrounding structures. Usually no effects are present on the surrounding structures, and thus it is of note that the sinus floor is intact.

Differential Diagnosis

It is important to distinguish retention pseudocysts from odontogenic cysts (for example, radicular or dentigerous cysts or keratocysts), antral polyps, or any rounded neoplastic mass. This can usually be done radiographically and by reviewing the patient's history. The retention pseudocyst is dome-shaped and does not have the thin marginal radiopaque line representing the corticated border characteristic of the odontogenic

cyst. The odontogenic cyst is also more rounded or tear drop–shaped. The lamina dura of the tooth or teeth associated with a radicular cyst is not intact in the apical area; it may be continuous with the corticated outline of the odontogenic cyst. In contrast, the roots of healthy teeth projecting over an area of an antral cavity occupied by a retention pseudocyst usually have the intact lamina dura apparent. Also, commonly the floor of the antrum is missing or displaced by the odontogenic cyst.

Antral polyps of infectious or allergic origin may be distinguished radiographically from a retention pseudocyst in that they are more often multiple. They are commonly associated with a thickened mucous membrane, which is less frequently observed with retention pseudocysts.

Neoplasms may also mimic retention pseudocysts. If benign and originating from outside the sinus, they are separated from the cavity of the sinus by a radiopaque border, similar to the odontogenic cysts. Malignant neoplasms may destroy the osseous border of the sinus, whether it arises from within the sinus, or from the alveolar process. The neoplasm is, however, less likely to be as dome-shaped as the retention pseudocyst.

Management

Retention pseudocysts in the maxillary sinus usually require no treatment because they customarily resolve spontaneously without any residual effect on the antral mucosa.

POLYPS

Definition

The thickened mucous membrane of a chronically inflamed sinus frequently forms into irregular folds called polyps. Polyposis of the sinus mucosa may develop in an isolated area or in a number of areas throughout the sinus.

Clinical Features

Polyps may cause displacement or destruction of bone. In the ethmoid air cells, polyps may cause destruction of the medial wall of the orbit (lamina papyracea of the ethmoid bone), and a unilateral proptosis may develop.

Radiographic Features

A polyp may be differentiated from a retention pseudocyst on a radiograph by noting that a polyp usually occurs with a thickened mucous membrane lining (Fig. 26-6) because the polypoid mass is no more than an accentuation of the mucosal thickening. In the case of a retention pseudocyst, however, the adjacent mucous membrane lining is not usually apparent. If multiple

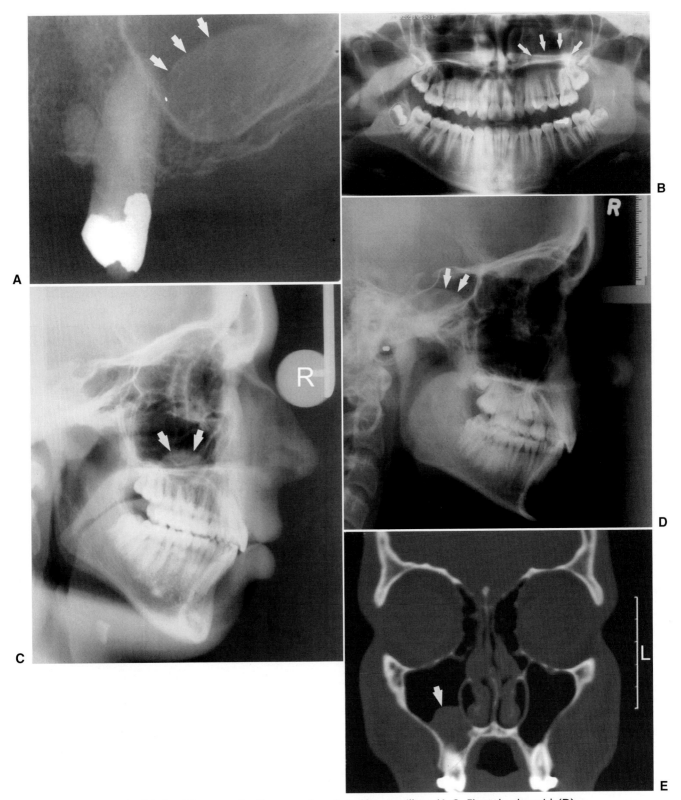

FIG. **26-5** Mucous retention pseudocysts in the maxillary (**A-C, E**) and sphenoid (**D**) sinuses *(arrows)* are seen as well-defined, noncorticated, circular, or "hydraulic" radiopaque areas within the sinus. The lack of a peripheral cortex surrounding the cyst indicates that it arose in the soft tissues within the sinus. **A,** periapical; **B,** panoramic; **C** and **D,** lateral skull; **E,** coronal bone-window CT images.

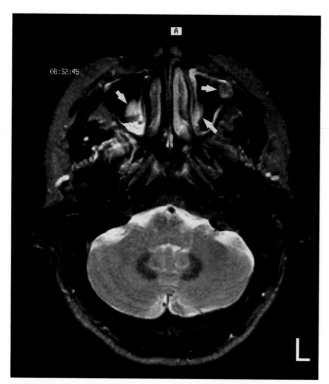

FIG. 26-6 A T2-weighted, axial MR image shows multiple areas of high signal intensity *(white)*, consistent with sinus polyps *(arrows)*.

retention pseudocysts are seen within a sinus, the possibility of sinus polyposis should be entertained.

The radiographic image of the bone displacement or destruction associated with polyps may mimic a benign or malignant neoplasm. Because many sinus neoplasms are asymptomatic, examination of a paranasal sinus that reveals bone destruction associated with radiopacification is an indication for biopsy, which should not be delayed by initial conservative treatment.

ANTROLITHS

Definition

Antroliths occur within the maxillary sinuses and are the result of deposition of mineral salts such as calcium phosphate, calcium carbonate, and magnesium around a nidus, which may be introduced into the sinus (extrinsic) or could be intrinsic, such as masses of stagnant mucous in sites of previous inflammation.

Clinical Features

The smaller antroliths are asymptomatic and usually are discovered as incidental findings on radiographic examination. If they continue to grow, the patient may experience an associated sinusitis, blood-stained nasal discharge, nasal obstruction, or facial pain.

Radiographic Features

Location. Antroliths occur within the maxillary sinus and thus are positioned above the floor of the maxillary antrum in periapical, occlusal, or panoramic radiographs.

Periphery and shape. Antroliths are well defined and may have a smooth or irregular shape (Fig. 26-7).

Internal structure. The internal aspect may vary in density from a barely perceptible radiopacity to an extremely radiopaque structure. The internal density may be homogenous or heterogeneous, and in some instances, alternating layers of radiolucency and radiopacity in the form of laminations may be seen.

Differential Diagnosis

Antroliths may be distinguished from root fragments in the sinus by inspection of the mass for the usual root anatomy, such as the presence of a pulp canal. A displaced root fragment in the sinus may move when radiography is performed with the head in different positions, unless it is lodged between the bone and the sinus lining. Rhinoliths are similar calcifications but are found within the nasal fossae. A posteroanterior skull view helps identify the location of a rhinolith.

Management

An otolaryngologist may need to remove symptomatic antroliths.

MUCOCELE

Synonyms

Pyocele and mucopyocele

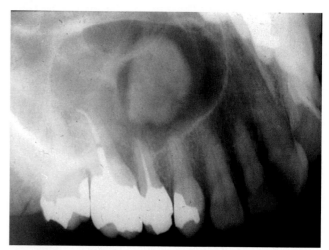

FIG. 26-7 A lateral maxillary occlusal film that reveals the presence of a radiopaque antrolith. Note that the antrolith is positioned above the sinus floor.

Definition

A mucocele is an expanding, destructive lesion that results from a blocked sinus ostium. The blockage may result from intraantral or intranasal inflammation, polyp, or neoplasm. The entire sinus thus becomes the pathologic cavity or cystlike lesion. As mucus is accumulated and the sinus cavity has filled, the increase in intraantral pressure results in a thinning, displacement and, in some cases, destruction of the sinus walls. If the mucocele becomes infected, it is called a *pyocele* or a *mucopyocele.*

Clinical Features

A mucocele in the maxillary sinus may exert pressure on the superior alveolar nerves and thus cause radiating pain. The patient may first complain of a sensation of fullness in the cheek, and the area may swell. This swelling may first become apparent over the anteroinferior aspect of the antrum, the area where the wall is thin or destroyed. If the lesion expands inferiorly, it may cause loosening of the posterior teeth in the area. If the medial wall of the sinus is expanded, the lateral wall of the nasal cavity will deform and the nasal airway may be obstructed. Should it expand into the orbit, it may cause diplopia (double vision) or proptosis (protrusion of the globe of the eye).

Radiographic Features

Location. About 90% of mucoceles occur in the ethmoidal and frontal sinuses and are rare in the maxillary and sphenoid sinuses.

Periphery and shape. The normal shape of the sinus is changed into a more circular shape as the mucocele enlarges.

Internal structure. The internal aspect of the sinus cavity is uniformly radiopaque.

Effects on surrounding structures. The shape of the sinus changes with the bony expansion. Septa and the bony walls may be thinned or destroyed (Fig. 26-8, *A*). When the mucocele is associated with the maxillary antrum, teeth may be displaced or roots resorbed. In the frontal sinus the usually scalloped border is smoothed by expansion, and the intersinus septum may be displaced (Fig. 26-8, *B*). The supramedial border of the orbit is displaced or destroyed. In the ethmoid air cells, displacement of the lamina papyracea may occur, displacing the contents of the orbit. In the sphenoid sinus the expansion may be in a superior direction, suggesting a pituitary neoplasm.

Differential Diagnosis

Although it may not be possible to distinguish between a mucocele in the maxillary antrum and a cyst or neoplasm, any suggestion that the lesion is associated with an occluded ostium should strengthen the likelihood of a mucocele. Blockage of the ostium is usually the result of a previous surgical procedure, although a deviated nasal septum or polyp may be a factor. A large odontogenic cyst displacing the maxillary antral floor may mimic a mucocele. Look for any remnants of the internal aspect of the antrum between the wall of the cyst and the wall of the antrum. CT is the imaging method of choice for making these distinctions.

Management

Treatment of the mucocele is usually surgical, using a Caldwell-Luc operation to allow excision of the lesion. The prognosis is excellent.

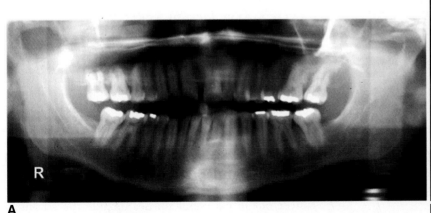
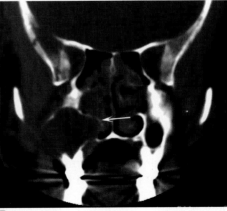

FIG. **26-8**　**A,** There is a mucocele involving the right maxillary sinus in this panoramic radiograph. Note the lack of distinct borders of the right sinus and a lack of a definite cortex of the zygomatic process. **B,** This CT coronal image slice through the maxillary mucocele in **A** shows expansion into the nasal fossa *(arrow)* and on the lateral aspect of the maxilla.

Neoplasms

Benign neoplasms of the paranasal sinuses, other than inflammatory polyps are rare. The radiographic images of such benign neoplasms are nonspecific. Usually the involved portion of the sinus appears radiopaque because of the presence of a mass, and they may cause displacement of adjacent sinus borders.

The most common malignant neoplasms of the paranasal sinuses are squamous cell carcinomas and, to a lesser extent, malignant salivary gland neoplasms. Of carcinomas of the paranasal sinuses, 74% originate in the maxillary sinus. Although radiopacification is a feature of both the inflammatory conditions and neoplasms, bone destruction is more common with malignant neoplasms.

BENIGN NEOPLASMS OF THE PARANASAL SINUSES

EPITHELIAL PAPILLOMA

Definition

The epithelial papilloma is a rare neoplasm of respiratory epithelium that occurs in the nasal cavity and paranasal sinuses. It occurs predominantly in men.

Clinical Features

Unilateral nasal obstruction, nasal discharge, pain, and epistaxis may occur. The patient may have complained of recurring sinusitis for years and a subsequent nasal obstruction on the same side as the sinusitis. The epithelial papilloma, although benign and relatively rare, has a 10% incidence of associated carcinoma.

Radiographic Features

The features may not be specific, and the diagnosis can be made only by histopathologic examination of the tissue.

Location. The epithelial papilloma is usually in the ethmoidal or maxillary sinus. It may also appear as an isolated polyp in the nose or sinus.

Internal structure. This neoplasm appears as a homogeneous radiopaque mass of soft tissue density.

Effects on surrounding structures. If bone destruction is apparent, it is the result of pressure erosion.

OSTEOMA

Definition

The osteoma is the most common of the mesenchymal neoplasms in the paranasal sinuses. For a detailed description, see Chapter 21.

Clinical Features

Osteomas are almost twice as common in males as females and are most common in the second, third, and fourth decades. Most are slow-growing and asymptomatic; thus they are usually detected as an incidental finding in an examination made for another purpose. When symptoms do occur, they are the result of obstruction of the sinus ostium or infundibulum or are secondary to erosion or deformity, orbital involvement, or intracranial extension. Those growing in the maxillary sinus may extend into the nose and cause nasal obstruction or a swelling of the side of the nose. They may expand the sinus and produce swelling of the cheek or hard palate. In cases extending to the orbit, the patient may have proptosis. In some cases, external fistulae have occurred. Osteomas of the maxillary sinus have been described after Caldwell-Luc operations.

Radiographic Features

Location. Although osteomas occasionally develop in the maxillary sinus, they more often occur in the frontal and ethmoidal sinuses. The incidence in the maxillary antrum varies between 3.9% and 28.5% of the incidence in all paranasal sinuses.

Periphery and shape. The osteoma is usually lobulated or rounded and has a sharply defined margin.

Internal structure. The internal aspect is homogeneous and extremely radiopaque (Fig. 26-9).

Differential Diagnosis

The differential diagnosis includes the antrolith, mycolith, teeth, or odontogenic neoplasms, including odontoma, although these are all usually not as homogeneous in appearance as the osteoma.

MALIGNANT NEOPLASMS OF THE PARANASAL SINUSES

Malignant neoplasms of the paranasal sinuses are rare, accounting for less than 1% of all malignancies in the body. Squamous cell carcinoma, comprising 80% to 90% of the cancers in this site, is by far the most common primary malignant neoplasm of the paranasal sinuses. Other primary neoplasms include adenocarcinoma, carcinomas of salivary gland origin, soft and hard tissue sarcomas, melanoma, and malignant lymphoma. Factors that contribute to a poor prognosis for cancer of the paranasal sinuses include the advanced stage of the disease when it is finally diagnosed and the close proximity of vital anatomic structures. The clinical signs and symptoms may masquerade as inflammatory sinusitis. The early primary lesions may only appear as a soft tissue mass in the sinus before they

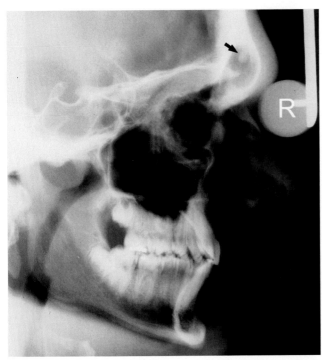

FIG. **26-9** A lateral cephalometric skull projection shows a frontal sinus osteoma as a well-defined, uniformly radiopaque mass *(arrow)*.

cause bone destruction. The lesion may become extensive, involving the entire sinus, with radiographic evidence of bone destruction before symptoms become apparent. Therefore any unexplained radiopacity in the maxillary sinus of an individual older than 40 years should be investigated thoroughly.

SQUAMOUS CELL CARCINOMA

Definition
Squamous cell carcinoma likely originates from metaplastic epithelium of the sinus mucosal lining.

Clinical Features
The most common symptoms of cancer in the maxillary sinus are facial pain or swelling, nasal obstruction, and a lesion in the oral cavity. The mean age of the patient is 60 years (range 25 to 89 years). Twice as many men as women are affected. Lymph nodes are involved in about 10% of cases, and the symptoms are present for about 5 months before diagnosis.

The symptoms produced by neoplasms in the maxillary sinus depend on which wall(s) of the sinus is/are involved. The medial wall is usually the first to become eroded, leading to such nasal signs and symptoms as obstruction, discharge, bleeding, and pain. These symptoms may appear trivial, and their significance may not be appreciated. Lesions that arise on the floor of the

sinus may first produce dental signs and symptoms, including expansion of the alveolar process, unexplained pain and numbness of the teeth, loose teeth, and swelling of the palate or alveolar ridge and ill-fitting dentures. The neoplasm may erode the floor and penetrate into the oral cavity. Such oral manifestations appear in 25% to 35% of patients with cancer in the maxillary sinus. When the lesion penetrates the lateral wall, facial and vestibular swelling becomes apparent and the patient may complain of pain and hyperesthesia of the maxillary teeth. Involvement of the sinus roof and the floor of the orbit cause symptoms related to the eye: diplopia, proptosis, pain, and hyperesthesia or anesthesia and pain over the cheek and upper teeth. Invasion and penetration of the posterior wall lead to invasion of the muscles of mastication, causing painful trismus, obstruction of the eustachian tube causing a stuffy ear, and referred pain and hyperesthesia over the distribution of the second and third divisions of the fifth nerve.

Radiographic Features
Sometimes the radiographic findings, especially in early malignant disease of the paranasal sinuses, are nonspecific. It may not be possible to differentiate the early manifestations in radiographs of the maxillary sinus from the radiopacity of the sinus that develops in sinusitis and polyp formation. Evidence relies on changes seen in the surrounding bone, the sinus walls, and the maxillary alveolar process.

Location. Most carcinomas occur in the maxillary sinuses, but involvement of the frontal and sphenoid sinuses is also comparatively common.

Internal structure. The internal aspect of the maxillary sinus has a soft tissue radiopaque appearance.

Effects on surrounding structures. As the lesion enlarges, it may destroy sinus walls and in general, cause irregular radiolucent areas in the surrounding bone. A detailed examination of the adjacent alveolar process may reveal bone destruction around the teeth or irregular widening of the periodontal ligament space. Frequently the medial wall of the maxillary sinus is thinned or destroyed, although there may also be destruction of the floor and anterior or posterior walls that may be detected in the panoramic film. The medial wall of the maxillary sinus is best seen on the Caldwell and Waters projections. In addition to loss of the medial wall, it may extend into the nasal cavity.

Additional Imaging
If a conventional radiograph of any radiopacified sinus reveals the slightest suggestion of bone destruction, advanced imaging is imperative (Fig. 26-10). On CT, the

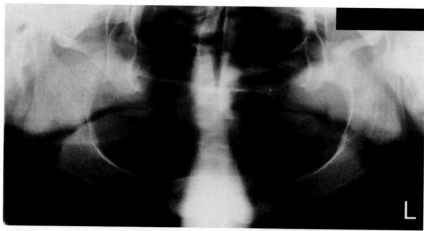

FIG. 26-10   In this panoramic image a squamous cell carcinoma has destroyed the floor of the left maxillary sinus as well as the left posterior maxillary alveolar process and tuberosity.

most characteristic sign of malignancy is invasion into the soft tissue facial planes beyond the sinus walls. Consequently CT is useful in revealing the extent of paranasal sinus neoplasms, especially when extension into the orbit, infratemporal fossa, or cranial cavity has occurred. MRI examinations are excellent for revealing the extent of soft tissue penetration into adjacent structures and in differentiating mucus accumulation from the soft tissue mass of the neoplasm.

Differential Diagnosis

The differential includes all the conditions that may cause radiopacity of the antrum, such as sinusitis, large retention pseudocysts, and odontogenic cysts. It is important to note that bone destruction may also occur in infectious and benign as well as malignant conditions. Neoplasms should be suspected in any older patient in whom chronic sinusitis develops for the first time without obvious cause.

Management

Treatment of squamous cell carcinoma in the paranasal sinuses generally combines surgery and radiation therapy. Malignant neoplasms in the paranasal sinuses usually have a poor prognosis because they are usually well advanced by the time of diagnosis. Other factors contributing to the poor prognosis include frequently inaccurate preoperative staging and the complex anatomy of the region.

PSEUDOTUMOR

Synonyms

Invasive fungal sinusitis, inflammatory pseudotumor, fibroinflammatory pseudotumor, plasma cell granuloma, sinonasal fungal disease, mucormycosis, aspergillosis, zygomycosis of the paranasal sinuses, and Rhizopus sinusitis

Definition

Pseudotumor is a descriptive name for a group of apparently related diseases of fungal origin that occur in the paranasal sinuses, as well as other parts of the head and neck.

Clinical Features

Pseudotumor often occurs after a series of recurrent infections. The symptoms may not be very specific. There may be recurring pain, as well as a mass simulating a neoplasm. The latter may cause erosion of the walls of the involved sinus and proptosis if the orbit is involved. Altered nerve function resulting from involvement of the nerve or occlusion of blood vessels by the mass has also been reported. Although cases have been reported in otherwise healthy individuals, many cases appear in patients who are immunocompromised or have systemic diseases such as diabetes mellitus, von Willebrand disease, or myelodysplasia.

Radiographic Features

The radiographic findings in pseudotumor include masses simulating malignant neoplasms that cause erosion of bony walls of the involved sinuses.

Differential Diagnosis

The differential includes benign and malignant neoplasms.

Management

The treatment of pseudotumor, which can include debridement of the sinuses and administration of antifungal medication, a Caldwell-Luc surgical approach, and therapy, reflects the differences in the specific lesions included under the term *pseudotumor of the sinuses*, the exact location of the disease, the organism involved, and the medical status of the patient.

Extrinsic Diseases Involving the Paranasal Sinuses

INFLAMMATORY DISEASE

Dental inflammatory lesions such as periodontal disease or periapical disease may cause a localized mucositis in the adjacent floor of the maxillary antrum. This is a result of the diffusion of inflammatory exudate (mediators) beyond the cortical floor of the antrum and into the periosteum and the mucosal lining of the sinus. The localized type of mucositis related to dental inflammatory disease usually resolves in days or weeks after successful treatment of the underlying cause.

Radiographic Features

The involved mucosa presents as a homogeneous radiopaque, ribbon-shaped shadow that follows the contour of the floor of the maxillary sinus. The enlarged mucosa is usually centered directly above the inflammatory lesion.

PERIOSTITIS

Definition

As described above, the exudate from dental inflammatory lesions can diffuse through the cortical boundary of the antral floor. These products can strip and

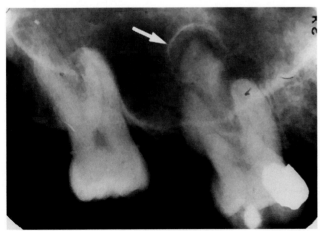

FIG. **26-11** *Periostitis.* The halo-like appearance of bone *(arrow)* surrounding the palatal root of the first molar is the result of periosteal new bone formation.

elevate the periosteal lining of the cortical bone of the floor of the maxillary antrum, stimulating the periosteum to produce a thin elevated layer of new bone adjacent to the root apex of the involved tooth (Fig. 26-11), the presence of a halo-like layer of new bone indicates inflammation of the periosteum.

Radiographic Features

Although the periosteal tissue is not visible on the radiograph, this is referred to as *periosteal new bone formation.* This new bone may take the form of one thin radiopaque line, or it may be very thick or, rarely, laminated (similar to onion skin). This new bone should be centered directly above the inflammatory lesion.

BENIGN ODONTOGENIC CYSTS AND TUMORS

ODONTOGENIC CYSTS

Odontogenic cysts are the most common group of extrinsic lesions that encroach on the maxillary sinuses. These cysts comprise almost half of the lesions involving the maxillary sinuses. Most are radicular cysts, followed by dentigerous cysts and odontogenic keratocysts (see Chapter 20 for detailed descriptions). These cysts that originate outside the maxillary sinuses encroach on the space of the sinuses by displacing the sinus borders. The cyst cortex and the sinus wall may be indistinguishable from one another, and thus as the cyst enlarges, the sinus decreases in size (Fig. 26-12). The result is a radiopaque line between the cyst and the air space of the sinus; dividing the contents of the cyst from the internal aspect of the sinus. This appearance is in contrast to a retention pseudocyst, which, being inside the sinus, does not have a cortex around its periphery.

Radicular cysts commonly encroaching upon the space of the maxillary sinus arise from the first molar and lateral incisor (Fig. 26-13). Dentigerous cysts most commonly are related to the third molar. Large cysts can displace third molars as far as the floor of the orbit. It may not be possible to differentiate a dentigerous cyst from an odontogenic keratocyst that has a pericoronal relationship to the third molar if only plain film radiographs are used.

Radiographic Features

Periphery and shape. The invaginating cyst has a curved or oval shape defined by a corticated border.

Internal structure. The internal structure of the cyst is homogeneous and radiopaque relative to the sinus cavity. The degree of radiopacity may appear to be that of bone resulting from the extreme contrast to the radiolucent air within the sinus.

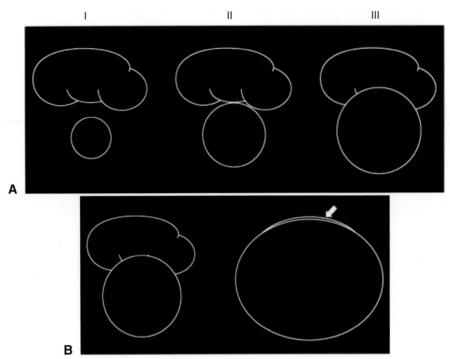

FIG. **26-12**   **A,** The odontogenic cyst starts near the sinus *(I).* As it enlarges, the cyst encroaches on the border of the maxillary sinus *(II)* and displaces the sinus border as it continues to enlarge *(III).* **B,** The odontogenic cyst, as it continues to enlarge, may encroach on almost all the space of the sinus, leaving a small saddle-like air space over the cyst *(arrow).* The appearance may mimic sinusitis.

Effects on surrounding structures. The cyst may displace the floor of the maxillary antrum. In some cases the cyst may enlarge to the point that it has encroached on almost the entire sinus, and the residual sinus space may appear as a thin saddle over the cyst (see Fig. 26-12, *B*).

Differential Diagnosis
A common lesion to differentiate is the retention pseudocyst, which can have the same shape but does not have a cortex at the periphery. If the odontogenic cyst were to become infected, the cortex may be lost. At this point it may become difficult to determine whether the lesion arises from outside or from within the sinus. However, in most cases careful scrutiny of the lesion will reveal some remaining cyst cortex. Also, the relationship to neighboring teeth may help to make this decision. This is true for all odontogenic cysts, including radicular cysts, dentigerous cysts, and keratocysts. Very large cysts may completely efface the sinus cavity. When this occurs, no radiographic evidence may exist of the air space left, and it may appear as if the cyst is the sinus.

In this case, because of the radiopacity of the cyst, the appearance may resemble sinusitis with radiopacification of the sinus. Evaluation of such conditions is aided by noting that the wall of the cyst is often thicker and more regular than that of a sinus. In addition, the normal vascular markings on the wall of the maxillary sinus are not present on the walls of a cyst. A cyst that occupies the entire sinus usually causes expansion of the medial wall (middle meatus) of the sinus and will alter the sigmoid contour of the posterior-lateral wall of the sinus as viewed in axial CT images.

An antral loculation may occasionally have a round shape and sometimes appear to have a cortex. However, because the loculation contains air, which is more radiolucent than the fluid within a cyst, the loculation appears more radiolucent than the surrounding antrum.

ODONTOGENIC TUMORS

Generally benign odontogenic tumors can cause facial deformity, nasal obstruction, and displacement or loosening of teeth. For detailed descriptions of specific

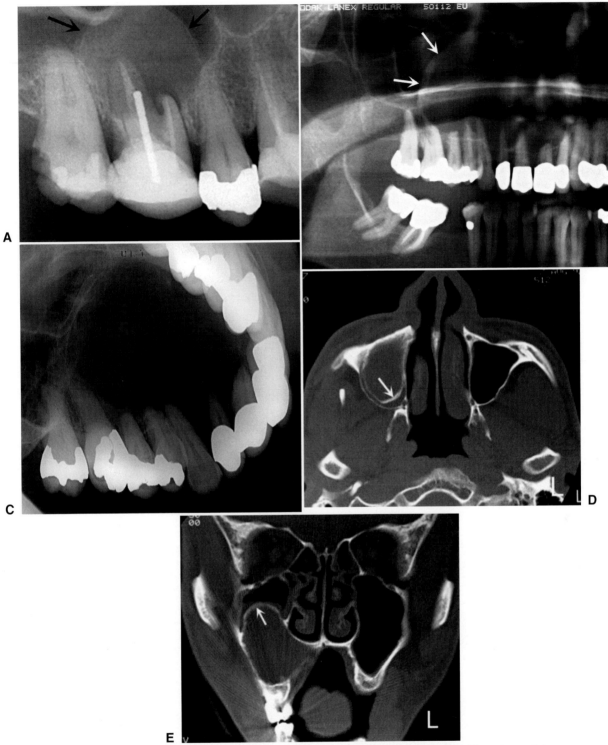

FIG. **26-13** *Three examples of radicular cysts encroaching on the maxillary sinus.* **A** is associated with the apices of the maxillary first molar. Note the presence of a thin cortex between the cyst and the sinus. **B** and **C** are panoramic and lateral occlusal projections of a large radicular cyst, respectively, involving the lateral incisor encroaching on the anterior aspect of the maxillary sinus. **D** and **E** are axial and coronal bone-window CT images of a radicular cyst encroaching on a large volume of the maxillary sinus cavity. Again, note the presence of a cortex between the sinus and cyst *(arrows).*

tumors, see Chapter 21. The nature of bony barriers in this region of the face, and the relatively good blood supply are probably also responsible for efficient local spread. The aggressive growth pattern of some tumors such as ameloblastomas, may directly invade into adjacent vital anatomic structures, including the skull base, and compromise patients. Therefore, management is often more aggressive than in cases involving the mandible.

Radiographic Features
Periphery and shape. The invaginating tumor may have a curved, oval, or multilocular shape that may be defined by a thin, cortical border. More aggressively growing tumors may even lack a border.

Internal structure. The internal structure of the tumor may have coarse or fine septae, or regions of dystrophic calcification depending on the histopathologic nature of the tumor.

Effects on surrounding structures. The tumor may displace the floor of the maxillary antrum and cause thinning of the peripheral cortex. As with odontogenic cysts, in some cases, the tumor may enlarge to the point where it has almost completely encroached on the sinus space (Fig. 26-14), and the residual sinus space may appear as a thin saddle over the tumor. The bony walls of the sinus may be thinned or eroded, and adjacent structures may be displaced. A tooth or part of a tooth may be embedded in the neoplasm.

FIBROUS DYSPLASIA

Craniofacial fibrous dysplasia may arise in the maxillary, sphenoid, frontal, ethmoid, and temporal bones, causing displacement of sinus borders and resulting in a smaller sinus on the affected side. For a detailed description of fibrous dysplasia, see Chapter 23.

CRANIOFACIAL FIBROUS DYSPLASIA
Clinical Features
The involvement of the facial skeleton with fibrous dysplasia can result in facial asymmetry, nasal obstruction, proptosis, pituitary gland compression, impingement on cranial nerves, or sinus obliteration. The sinus obliteration results when the expanding lesion of dysplastic bone encroaches on it. The lesion may displace the roots of teeth and cause teeth to separate or migrate, but it usually does not cause root resorption. Fibrous dysplasia is more common in children and young adults and tends to stop growing when skeletal growth ceases, although cases in adults are found.

Radiographic Features
Location. The posterior maxilla is the most common location for fibrous dysplasia.

Periphery. The lesion itself is usually not well defined, tending to blend into the surrounding bone. The external cortex of the bone is, however, maintained intact, although it may be displaced.

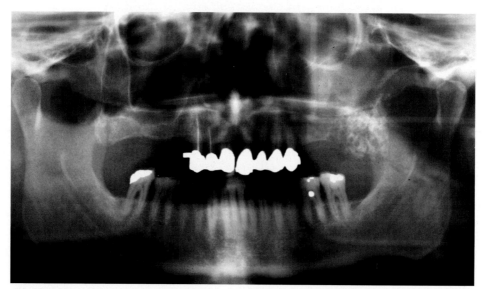

FIG. **26-14**   A panoramic view shows an ameloblastoma extending from the left tuberosity region (note the multilocular appearance) and encroaching upon the sinus, resulting in a more radiopaque sinus compared to the right side.

Internal structure. The normal radiolucent maxillary antrum may be partially or totally replaced by the increased radiopacity of this lesion. The degree of radiopacity depends on its stage of development and the relative amounts of bone present. Usually the radiopaque areas have the characteristic "ground glass" appearance on extraoral radiographs or an "orange peel" appearance on intraoral views (Fig. 26-15).

Effects on surrounding structures. Fibrous dysplasia may replace most of the sinus by encroaching on and displacing the antral walls, elevating the orbital floor or obstructing the nasal fossa.

Differential Diagnosis

The diagnosis of fibrous dysplasia in a relatively young person is usually not difficult. Paget's disease of bone does not usually obliterate the sinus, as does fibrous dysplasia. A complex odontoma is usually associated with one or more unerupted teeth and is surrounded by a radiolucent line (soft tissue capsule), in turn surrounded by a radiopaque line. An ossifying fibroma similar to fibrous dysplasia may have a uniform radiopaque appearance but usually has a definite border. However, in some cases the differential diagnosis of ossifying fibroma involving the antrum and fibrous dysplasia can be extremely difficult. The shape of the new bone encroaching on the internal aspect of the antrum often parallels the original shape of the external walls of the antrum in fibrous dysplasia.

Traumatic Injuries to the Paranasal Sinuses

DENTAL STRUCTURES DISPLACED INTO THE SINUS

Definition

Tooth roots may be fractured as a result of various forms of trauma, including iatrogenic causes. Fractured roots may be forced into the sinus during extraction or subsequent attempts to retrieve them.

Clinical Features

No specific features may be visible if the root was displaced into the sinus recently. However, the dentist may note the absence of the root fragment on examining the extracted tooth and be unable to locate it anywhere else. Sometimes asking the patient to hold his or her nose while attempting to breathe out through it, similar to a Valsalva maneuver, will cause bubbles to appear within the blood contained within the fresh extraction socket.

If the patient has had the root or tooth in the sinus for a number of days, he or she may present with sinusitis (see the previous discussion on Sinusitis).

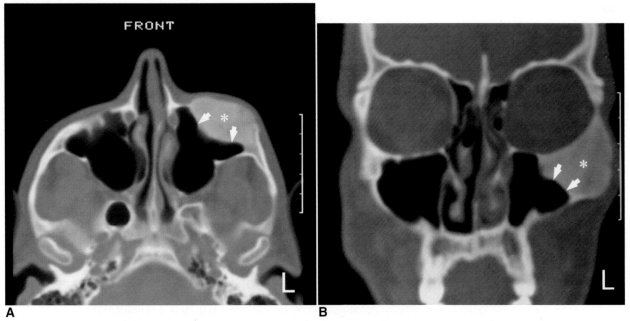

FIG. 26-15 *Fibrous dysplasia.* Axial **(A)** and coronal **(B)** bone-window CT images show a "ground glass" pattern in the enlarged frontal and lateral walls of the maxilla (*). The abnormal bone encroaches on the anterior and lateral walls of the maxillary sinus *(arrows)*.

Radiographic Features

Location. Roots or teeth in the sinus are associated with premolars and molars because the sinus is often in close proximity to the roots. These may be found anywhere within the sinus, but more often they are located near the floor of the sinus because of gravity. Sometimes the displaced structure may be submucosal, between the osseous wall of the sinus and the periosteum.

Lateral maxillary occlusal views are useful for examining root tips in the maxillary sinus. Other films in a different anatomic plane, such as a Waters projection, may help in the three-dimensional localization.

Periphery and shape. No immediate evidence may be present of any change in the sinus, even when an oroantral fistula has been created. The disruption of the sinus wall may be difficult or impossible to see on periapical or occlusal radiographs if it is not in the mesial, distal, or superior (apical) part of the alveolar process.

Internal structure. In the early stages no internal structural changes are present, except that the dental fragment may appear as a radiopaque mass of a size corresponding to the missing dental fragment. The tooth structure may have a layer of enamel or a pulp canal.

Effects on surrounding structures. The dental fragment usually has no effect on surrounding structures; however, a sinusitis may result (see changes described previously under Sinusitis). The floor of the maxillary sinus may break as a result of the displacement of the tooth or fragment into the sinus.

Differential Diagnosis

Bony masses, such as exostoses of the sinus wall or floor and septa within the sinus, may mimic dental root fragments or even whole teeth. Antroliths may also present a similar appearance. The shape of the radiopacity, or the presence of a pulp canal or a layer of enamel may help in the differential diagnosis. Also it may be possible to cause the tooth fragment to move by having the patient move the head abruptly between views. If the root tip remains in its socket, it may be superimposed radiographically over the maxillary sinus, but the presence of a lamina dura and periodontal ligament space indicate a position within the alveolar process.

The root may be subperiosteal, and thus within the osseous cavity of the sinus, but not within the antral lumen. Alternatively, the root may have been forced out of the socket, into the surrounding bone, or even through the bone to lie between the soft tissue of the oral mucosa and the bone of the alveolar process. Also, the fragment may be forced into surrounding structures such as the infratemporal space. Another possible result is that the fragment may have been displaced into a cyst that was preoperatively mistaken for a loculus of the sinus cavity. Use of radiographs at different angles should help to localize the dental structure.

Management

Management ranges from following the patient to see whether a small root tip will be removed from the sinus via the ostium by ciliary action to surgically entering the sinus via a Caldwell-Luc procedure to remove the dental structure. Sinusitis may develop and should be managed with the appropriate treatment.

For other trauma involving the paranasal sinuses, see Chapter 28.

SUGGESTED READINGS

NORMAL DEVELOPMENT AND VARIATIONS

Dodd GD, Jing BS: Radiology of the nose, paranasal sinus and nasopharynx, Baltimore, 1977, Williams & Wilkins.

DuBrul EL: Sicher's oral anatomy, ed 7, St. Louis, 1980, Mosby.

Grant JCB: A method of anatomy, Baltimore, 1958, Williams & Wilkins.

Hengerer AS: Embryonic development of the sinuses, Ear Nose Throat J 63:134, 1984.

Karmody CS, Carter B, Vincent ME: Developmental anomalies of the maxillary sinus, Trans Am Acad Ophthalmol Otolaryngol 84:723, 1977.

Lusted LB, Keats TE: Atlas of roentgenographic measurement, ed 3, Chicago, 1972, Year Book Medical Publishers.

Ritter FN: The paranasal sinuses: anatomy and surgical technique, St. Louis, 1973, Mosby.

Shapiro R: Radiology of the normal skull, Chicago, 1981, Year Book Medical Publishers.

Som PM: The paranasal sinuses. In Som PM, Curtin HD editors: Head and neck imaging, ed 4, St. Louis, 2003, Mosby.

Takahashi R: The formation of the human paranasal sinuses, Acta Otolaryngol Suppl (Stockh) 408:1, 1984.

APPLIED DIAGNOSTIC IMAGING

Lloyd GA: Diagnostic imaging of the nose and paranasal sinuses, J Laryngol Otol 103:453, 1989.

Zinreich SJ: Imaging of chronic sinusitis in adults: x-ray, computed tomography, and magnetic resonance imaging, J Allergy Clin Immunol 90:445, 1992.

INFLAMMATORY CHANGES

Robinson K: Roentgenographic manifestations of benign paranasal sinus disease, Ear Nose Throat J 63:144, 1984.

THICKENED MUCOUS MEMBRANE

Mucositis

Dolan K, Smoker W: Paranasal sinus radiology: part 4A, maxillary sinuses, Head Neck Surg 5:345, 1983.

Killey HC, Kay LA: The maxillary sinus and its dental implications, Bristol, 1975, John Wright.

PERIOSTITIS

Sinusitis

Druce HM: Diagnosis and medical management of recurrent and chronic sinusitis in adults. In Gershwin ME, Incaudo GA, editors: Diseases of the sinuses, Ottawa, Canada, 1996, Humana Press.

Fireman P: Diagnosis of sinusitis in children: emphasis on the history and physical examination, J Allergy Clin Immunol 90:433, 1992.

Incaudo G, Gershwin ME, Nagy SM: The pathophysiology and treatment of sinusitis, Allergol Immunopathol (Madr) 14:423, 1986.

Kennedy DW: Surgical update, Otolaryngol Head Neck Surg 103:884, 1990.

Killey HC, Kay LA: The maxillary sinus and its dental implications, Bristol, 1975, John Wright.

Palaceos E, Valvassori G: Computed axial tomography in otorhinolaryngology, Adv Otorhinolaryngol 24:1, 1978.

Paparella MM: Mucosal cyst of the maxillary sinus, Arch Otolaryngol 77:650, 1963.

Poyton H: Maxillary sinuses and the oral radiologist, Dent Radiol Photogr 45:43, 1972.

Reilly JS: The sinusitis cycle, Otolaryngol Head Neck Surg 103:856, 1990.

Shapiro GG, Rachelefsky GS: Introduction and definition of sinusitis, J Allergy Clin Immunol 90:417, 1992.

Zinreich SJ: Imaging of chronic sinusitis in adults: x-ray, computed tomography, and magnetic resonance imaging, J Allergy Clin Immunol 90:445, 1992.

EMPYEMA

Ash JE, Raum M: An atlas of otolaryngic pathology, New York, 1956, American Registry of Pathology.

Groves J, Gray RF: A synopsis of otolaryngology, Bristol, 1985, John Wright.

POLYPS

Potter GD: Inflammatory disease of the paranasal sinuses. In Valvassori GE, Potter GD, Hanefee WN, editors: Radiology of the ear, nose and throat, Philadelphia, 1982, WB Saunders.

RETENTION PSEUDOCYSTS

Allard RHB, Van der Kwast WAM, Van der Wall JI: Mucosal antral cysts: review of the literature and report of a radiographic survey, Oral Surg 51:2, 1981.

Dolan K, Smoker W: Paranasal sinus radiology: part 4A, maxillary sinuses, Head Neck Surg 5:345, 1983.

Gothberg K et al: A clinical study of cysts arising from mucosa of the maxillary sinus, Oral Surg 41:52, 1976.

Hardy G: Benign cysts of the antrum, Ann Otol Rhinol Laryngol 48: 649, 1939.

Kadymova MI: Lymphangietctatic (false) cysts of the maxillary sinuses and their relation with allergy, Vestn Otorinolaringol 28:58, 1966.

Kaffe I, Littner MM, Moskona D: Mucosal-antral cysts: radiographic appearance and differential diagnosis, Clin Prev Dent 10:3, 1988.

McGregor GW: Formation and histologic structure of cysts of the maxillary sinus, Arch Otolaryngol 8:505, 1928.

Mills CP: Secretory cysts of the maxillary antrum and their relationship to the development of antrochoanal polypi, J Laryngol Otol 73:324, 1959.

Neville B, Damm DD, Allen CM, Bouquot J: Oral and Maxillofacial Pathology, ed 4, Philadelphia, 2002, WB Saunders.

Poyton HG: Oral radiology, Baltimore, 1982, Williams & Wilkins.

Ruprecht A, Batniji S, El-Neweihi E: Mucous retention cyst of the maxillary sinus, Oral Surg Oral Med Oral Pathol 62:728, 1986.

Van Norstrand AWP, Goodman WS: Pathologic aspects of mucosal lesions of the maxillary sinus, Otolaryngol Clin North Am 9:21, 1976.

MUCOCELE

Atherino C, Atherino T: Maxillary sinus mucopyoceles, Arch Otolaryngol 110:200, 1984.

Jones JL, Kaufman PW: Mucopyocele of the maxillary sinus, J Oral Surg 39:948, 1981.

Zizmor JK, Noyek AM: The radiologic diagnosis of maxillary sinus disease, Otolaryngol Clin North Am 9:93, 1976.

ODONTOGENIC CYSTS

Killey HC, Kay LA: The maxillary sinus and its dental implications, Bristol, 1975, John Wright.

Poyton H: Maxillary sinuses and the oral radiologist, Dent Radiol Photogr 45:43, 1972.

Van Alyea OE: Nasal sinuses, Baltimore, 1951, Williams & Wilkins.

ODONTOGENIC KERATOCYSTS

MacDonald-Jankowski DS: The involvement of the maxillary antrum by odontogenic keratocysts, Clin Radiol 45:31, 1992.

NEOPLASMS

Goepfert H et al: Malignant salivary gland tumors of the paranasal sinuses and nasal cavity, Arch Otolaryngol 109:662, 1983.

St-Pierre S, Baker S: Squamous cell carcinoma of the maxillary sinus: analysis of 66 cases, Head Neck Surg 5:508, 1983.

EPITHELIAL PAPILLOMA

Rogers JH, Fredrickson JM, Noyek AM: Management of cysts, benign tumors, and bony dysplasia of the maxillary sinus, Otolaryngol Clin North Am 9:233, 1976.

OSTEOMA

Dolan K, Smoker W: Paranasal sinus radiology: part 4B, maxillary sinuses, Head Neck Surg 5:428, 1983.

Goodnight J, Dulguerov P, Abemayor E: Calcified mucor fungus ball of the maxillary sinus, Am J Otolaryngol 14:209, 1993.

Reuben B: Odontoma of the maxillary sinus: a case report, Quint Int 14:287, 1983.

Samy LL, Mostofa H: Osteoma of the nose and paranasal sinuses with a report of twenty-one cases, J Laryngol Otol 85:449, 1971.

AMELOBLASTOMA

Hames RS, Rakoff SJ: Diseases of the maxillary sinus, J Oral Med 27:90, 1972.

Reanue C et al: Ameloblastoma of the maxillary sinus, J Oral Surg 38:520, 1980.

MALIGNANT NEOPLASMS OF THE PARANASAL SINUSES

Batsakis JG: Tumors of the head and neck, ed 2, Baltimore, 1979, Williams & Wilkins.

St-Pierre S, Baker S: Squamous cell carcinoma of the maxillary sinus: analysis of 66 cases, Head Neck Surg 5:508, 1983.

Tsaknis PJ, Nelson JF: The maxillary ameloblastoma: an analysis of 24 cases, J Oral Surg 38:336, 1980.

Zizmor J, Noyek AM: Cysts, benign tumors and malignant tumors of the paranasal sinuses, Otolaryngol Clin North Am 6:487, 1973.

SQUAMOUS CELL CARCINOMA

Batsakis JG, Rice DH, Solomon AR: The pathology of head and neck tumors: squamous and mucous-gland carcinomas of the nasal cavity, paranasal sinuses and larynx: part 6, Head Neck Surg 2:497, 1980.

Boone MLM, Harle TS: Malignant tumors of the paranasal sinuses, Semin Roentgenol 3:202, 1968.

Bridger M, Beale F, Bryce D: Carcinoma of the paranasal sinuses: a review of 158 cases, J Otolaryngol 7:379, 1978.

Eddleston B, Johnson R: A comparison of conventional radiographic imaging and computed tomography in malignant disease of the paranasal sinuses and the post-nasal space, Clin Radiol 56:161, 1983.

Haso A: CT of tumors and tumor-like conditions of the paranasal sinuses, Radiol Clin North Am 22:119, 1984.

Larheim T, Kolbenstvdt A, Lien H: Carcinoma of maxillary sinus, palate and maxillary gingiva, occurrence of jaw destruction, Scand J Dent Res 92:235, 1984.

Lund V, Howard D, Lloyd G: CT evaluation of paranasal sinus tumors for cranio-facial resection, Br J Radiol 56:439, 1983.

Mancuso A et al: Extensions of paranasal sinus tumors and inflammatory disease: an evaluation by CT and pluri-directional tomography, Neuroradiology 16:449, 1978.

St-Pierre S, Baker S: Squamous cell carcinoma of the maxillary sinus: analysis of 66 cases, Head Neck Surg 5:508, 1983.

Webeer A et al: Malignant tumors of the sinuses: radiologic evaluation, including CT scanning, with clinical and pathologic correlation, Neuroradiology 16:443, 1978.

PSEUDOTUMOR

Butugan O et al: Rhinocerebral mucormycosis: predisposing factors, diagnosis, therapy, complications and survival, Rev Laryngol Otol Rhinol (Bord) 117:53, 1996.

Del Valle Zapico A et al: Mucormycosis of the sphenoid sinus in an otherwise healthy patient. Case report and literature review, J Laryngol Otol 110:471, 1996.

Ishida M et al: Five cases of mucormycosis in paranasal sinuses, Acta Oto-Laryngologica 501(suppl):92, 1993.

Lee BL, Holland GN, Glasgow BJ: Chiasmal infarction and sudden blindness caused by mucormycosis in AIDS and diabetes mellitus, Am J Ophthalmol 122:895, 1996.

Muzaffar M, Hussain SI, Chughtai A: Plasma cell granuloma: maxillary sinuses, J Laryngol Otol 108:357, 1994.

Ng TT et al: Successful treatment of sinusitis caused by Cunninghamella bertholetiae, Clin Infect Dis 19:313, 1994.

Ozhan S et al: Pseudotumor of the maxillary sinus in a patient with von Willebrand's disease, AJR Am J Roentgenol 166:950, 1996.

Perolada Valmana JM et al: Mucormycosis of the paranasal sinuses, Rev Laryngol Otol Rhinol (Bord) 117:51, 1996.

Som PM et al: Inflammatory pseudotumor of the maxillary sinus: CT and MR findings in six cases, AJR Am J Roentgenol 163:689, 1994.

Tkatch LS, Kusne S, Eibling D: Successful treatment of zygomycosis of the paranasal sinuses with surgical debridement and amphotericin B colloidal dispersion, Am J Otolaryngol 14:249, 1993.

Utas C et al: Acute renal failure associated with rhinosinuso-orbital mucormycosis infection in a patient with diabetic nephropathy [letter], Nephron 71:235, 1995.

Zapater E et al: Invasive fungal sinusitis in immunosuppressed patients. Report of three cases, Acta Oto-Rhino-Laryngologica Belgica 50:137, 1996.

FIBROUS DYSPLASIA

Malcolmson KG: Ossifying fibroma of the sphenoid, J Laryngol 81:87, 1967.

Thomas GK, Kasper KA: Ossifying fibroma of the frontal bone, Arch Otolaryngol 83:43, 1966.

Wong A, Vaughan CW, Strong MS: Fibrous dysplasia of temporal bone, Arch Otolaryngol 81:131, 1965.

CHAPTER 27

Soft Tissue Calcification and Ossification

LAURIE CARTER

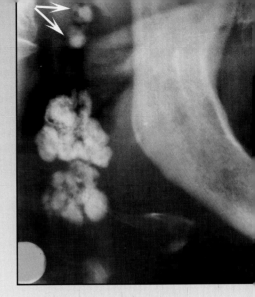

The deposition of calcium salts, primarily calcium phosphate, usually occurs in the skeleton. When it occurs in an unorganized fashion in soft tissue, it is referred to as *heterotopic calcification*. This soft tissue mineralization may develop in a wide variety of unrelated disorders and degenerative processes. Heterotopic calcifications may be divided into three categories:

- Dystrophic calcification
- Idiopathic calcification
- Metastatic calcification

Dystrophic calcification refers to calcification that forms in degenerating, diseased, and dead tissue despite normal serum calcium and phosphate levels. The soft tissue may be damaged by blunt trauma, inflammation, injections, the presence of parasites, soft tissue changes arising from disease, and many other causes. This calcification usually is localized to the site of injury. Idiopathic calcification (or calcinosis) results from deposition of calcium in normal tissue despite normal serum calcium and phosphate levels. Examples include chondrocalcinosis and phleboliths. Metastatic calcification results when minerals precipitate into normal tissue as a result of higher than normal serum levels of calcium (e.g., hyperparathyroidism, hypercalcemia of malignancy) or phosphate (e.g., chronic renal failure). Metastatic calcification usually occurs bilaterally and symmetrically.

When the mineral is deposited in soft tissue as organized, well-formed bone, the process is known as *heterotopic ossification*. The term *heterotopic* indicates that bone has formed in an abnormal (extraskeletal) location. The heterotopic bone may be all compact bone, or it may show some trabeculae and fatty marrow. The deposits may range from 1 mm to several centimeters in diameter, and one or more may be present. The causes range from posttraumatic ossification, bone produced by tumors, and ossification caused by diseases such as progressive myositis ossificans and ankylosing spondylitis.

Clinical Features

Sites of heterotopic calcification or ossification may not cause significant signs or symptoms; they most often are detected as incidental findings during radiographic examination.

Radiographic Features

Soft tissue opacities are fairly common, present on about 4% of panoramic radiographs. In most cases the goal is to identify the calcification correctly to determine whether treatment or further investigation is required. Some soft tissue calcifications require no intervention or long-term surveillance, whereas others may be life-threatening and the underlying cause requires treatment. When the soft tissue calcification is adjacent to bone, it sometimes is difficult to determine whether the calcification is within bone or soft tissue. Another radiographic view at right angles is useful. These important criteria must be considered in arriving at the correct interpretation: the anatomic location, number, distribution, and shape of the calcifications. Analysis of the location requires knowledge of soft tissue anatomy, such as the position of lymph nodes, stylohyoid ligaments, blood vessels, laryngeal cartilages, and the major ducts of the salivary glands.

Dystrophic Calcification

GENERAL DYSTROPHIC CALCIFICATION OF THE ORAL REGIONS

Definition
Dystrophic calcification is the precipitation of calcium salts into primary sites of chronic inflammation or dead and dying tissue. This process is usually associated with a high local concentration of phosphatase, as in normal bone calcification, an increase in local alkalinity, and anoxic conditions within the inactive or devitalized tissue. A long-standing, chronically inflamed cyst is a common location of dystrophic calcification.

Clinical Features
Common soft tissue sites include the gingiva, tongue, lymph nodes, and cheek. Dystrophic calcifications may produce no signs or symptoms, although occasionally enlargement and ulceration of overlying soft tissues may occur, and a solid mass of calcium salts sometimes can be palpated.

Radiographic Features
The radiographic appearance of dystrophic calcification varies from barely perceptible, fine grains of radiopacities to larger, irregular radiopaque particles that rarely exceed 0.5 cm in diameter. One or more of these radiopacities may be seen, and the calcification may be homogeneous or may contain punctate areas. The outline of the calcified area usually is irregular or indistinct. Common sites are long-standing, chronically inflamed cysts (Fig. 27-1) and polyps (Fig. 27-2).

CALCIFIED LYMPH NODES

Definition
Dystrophic calcification occurs in lymph nodes that have been chronically inflamed because of various diseases, frequently granulomatous disorders. The lymphoid tissue becomes replaced by hydroxyapatite-like calcium salts nearly effacing all of nodal architecture. In the past, tuberculosis was the most common disease causing calcified lymph nodes (scrofula or cervical tuberculous adenitis). Other well-know causes of lymph node calcification include BCG vaccination, sarcoidosis, cat-scratch disease, lymphoma previously treated with radiation therapy, fungal infections, and metastases from distant calcifying neoplasms.

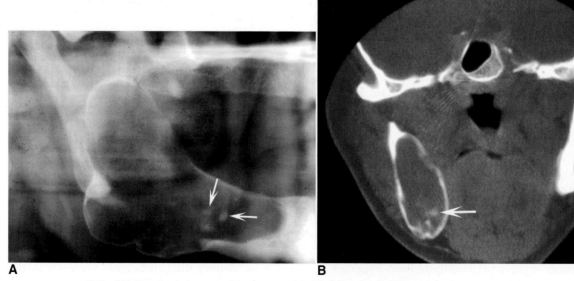

A   **B**

FIG. **27-1**   **A,** A large residual cyst with ill-defined calcifications seen in a panoramic image *(arrows)*. **B,** A coronal CT image using bone algorithm of the same case that demonstrates the dystrophic calcification within the cyst *(arrow)*.

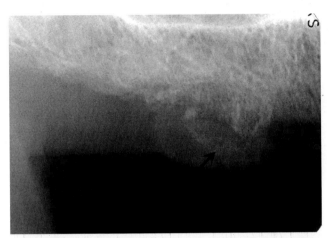

FIG. **27-2** A periapical film showing the soft tissue mass, inflammatory fibrous hyperplasia, emanating from the edentulous ridge. This soft tissue mass contains a dystrophic calcification (arrow).

Clinical Features

Calcified lymph nodes are generally asymptomatic, and these nodes are first discovered as an incidental finding on a panoramic radiograph. The most commonly involved nodes are the submandibular and cervical nodes (superficial and deep) and less commonly, the preauricular and submental nodes. When these nodes can be palpated, they are hard round or oblong masses.

Radiographic Features

Location. The most common location is the submandibular region, either at or below the inferior border of the mandible near the angle, or between the posterior border of the ramus and cervical spine. The image of the calcified node sometimes overlaps the inferior aspect of the ramus. Lymph node calcifications may affect a single node or a linear series of nodes, in a phenomenon known as lymph node chaining (Fig. 27-3).

Periphery. The periphery is well defined and usually irregular, occasionally having a lobulated appearance similar to the outer shape of cauliflower. This irregularity of shape is of great significance in distinguishing node calcifications from other potential soft tissue calcifications in the area.

Internal structure. The internal aspect is without pattern but may vary in the degree of radiopacity, giving the impression of a collection of spherical or irregular masses. Occasionally the lesion has a laminated appearance.

Differential Diagnosis

Differentiation between a single calcified lymph node and a sialolith in the hilar region of the submandibular gland may be difficult. Usually a sialolith has a smooth outline, whereas a calcified lymph node is usually irregular and sometimes lobulated. The differentiation can be made if the patient has symptoms related to the submandibular salivary gland (see Chapter 30). Occasionally sialography may be necessary to make the differentiation. Another calcification that may have a similar appearance in this region is a phlebolith; however, phleboliths are usually smaller and multiple, with concentric radiopaque and radiolucent rings, and its shape may mimic a portion of a blood vessel.

Management

Calcified lymph nodes usually do not require treatment; however, the underlying cause should be established in case treatment is required, such as in the case of a lymphoma.

DYSTROPHIC CALCIFICATION IN THE TONSILS

Synonyms

Tonsillar calculi, tonsil concretions, and tonsilloliths

Definition

Tonsillar calculi are formed when repeated bouts of inflammation enlarge the tonsillar crypts. Incomplete resolution of dead bacteria and pus serve as the nidus for dystrophic calcification.

Clinical Features

Tonsilloliths usually present as hard, round, white or yellow objects projecting from the tonsillar crypts. Small calcifications usually produce no clinical signs or symptoms. However, pain, swelling, fetor orisdysphagia, and a foreign body sensation on swallowing have been reported with larger calcifications. Giant tonsilloliths stretching lymphoid tissue and resulting in ulceration and extrusion are much less common. These calcifications have been reported to occur between 20 and 68 years of age; they are found more often in older age groups.

Radiographic Features

Location. In the panoramic film, tonsilloliths appear as single or multiple radiopacities that overlap the midportion of the mandibular ramus in the region where the image of the dorsal surface of the tongue crosses the ramus in the palatoglossal or glossopharyngeal air spaces (Fig. 27-4).

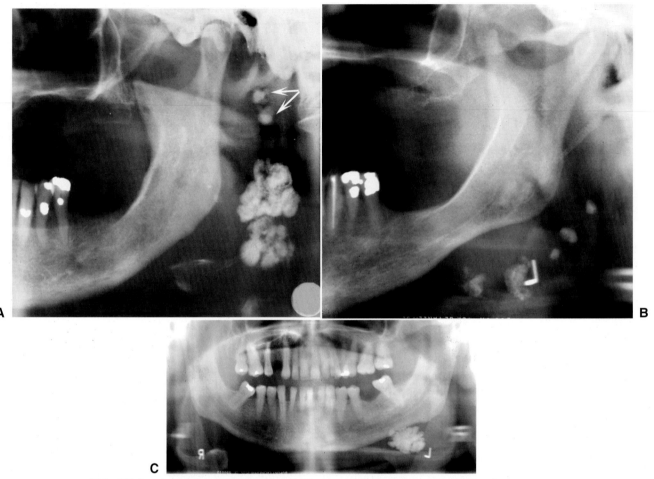

FIG. **27-3**   *Examples of dystrophic calcification in the lymph nodes.* **A,** Two large examples positioned behind the ramus, both with a cauliflower-like shape, and two smaller examples in a more superior position *(arrows).* **B,** Several smaller examples positioned below the lower border of the mandible. **C,** A larger example.

Periphery. The most common appearance of tonsilloliths is a cluster of multiple small, ill-defined radiopacities. Rarely this calcification may attain a large size.

Internal structure. These calcifications appear slightly more radiopaque than cancellous bone and approximately the same as cortical bone.

Differential Diagnosis

The clinical differential diagnosis includes calcified granulomatous disease, syphilis, mycosis, or lymphoma, which may produce a firm tonsillar mass. The essential radiographic differential diagnosis is a radiopaque lesion within the mandibular ramus, such as a dense bone island. When in doubt, a right-angle view such as a posteroanterior skull view or an open Towne's view

may show that the calcification lies to the medial aspect of the ramus.

Treatment

No treatment is required for most tonsillar calcifications. However, large calcifications with associated symptoms are removed surgically. Treatment of asymptomatic tonsilloliths may be considered in elderly patients with mechanical deglutition disorders and in immunocompromised patients because of the risk for aspiration pneumonia.

CYSTICERCOSIS

Definition

When humans ingest eggs or gravid proglottids from *Taenia solium* (pork tapeworm), the covering of the

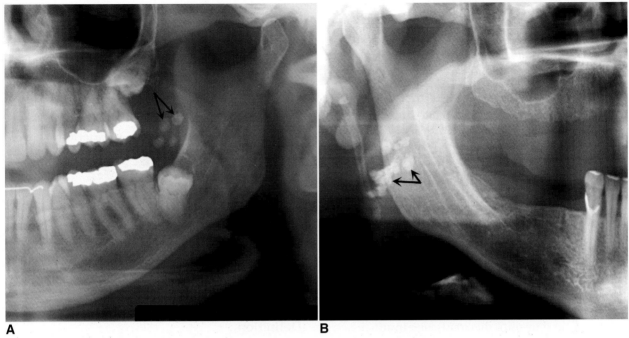

FIG. **27-4** *Dystrophic calcification of the tonsils.* These two examples show positions anterior to the ramus **(A)** and overlapping the posterior aspect of the ramus **(B)** *(arrows).* Note the calcified stylohyoid ligament.

eggs is digested in the stomach and the larval form *(Cysticercus cellulosae)* of the parasite is hatched. The larvae penetrate the mucosa, enter the blood vessels and lymphatics, and are distributed in the tissues all over the body, but preferentially locate to brain, muscle, skin, and heart. They are also found in the oral and perioral tissues, especially the muscles of mastication. In tissues other than the intestinal mucosa, the larvae eventually die and are treated as foreign bodies causing granuloma formation, scarring and calcification approximately 3 months later. These areas in the tissues are called *cysticerci.* There is currently an increased incidence of cysticercosis in the American Southwest and urban Northeast, especially among Koreans and Hispanics. The problem is much worse in underdeveloped countries such as Mexico, where fecal contamination of agricultural soil is common and pork is a valued food.

Clinical Features
Mild cases of cysticercosis are completely asymptomatic. More severe cases have symptoms that range from mild to severe gastrointestinal upset with epigastric pain and severe nausea and vomiting. Invasion of the brain may result in seizures, headache, visual disturbances, acute obstructive hydrocephalus, irritability, and loss of consciousness. Examination of the head and neck may disclose palpable, well-circumscribed soft fluctuant swellings, which resemble a mucocele. Multiple small nodules may be felt in the region of the masseter and suprahyoid muscles and in the buccal mucosa and lip.

Radiographic Features
While alive, larvae are not visible radiographically.

Location. The locations of calcified cysticerci include the muscles of mastication and facial expression, the suprahyoid muscle, and the postcervical musculature.

Periphery and shape. Multiple, well-defined, elliptical radiopacities are viewed, resembling grains of rice.

Internal structure. The internal aspect is homogeneous and radiopaque.

Differential Diagnosis
Cysticercus may appear similar to a sialolith. However, the small size of the calcified nodules of cysticerci and their widespread dissemination, particularly in brain and muscles, are highly suggestive of the diagnosis.

Management
Although prevention is the best treatment (proper preparation of pork and avoiding fecal contamination), the symptoms that accompany the initial infestation are best treated by a physician using an antihelminthic. After the larvae have settled and calcified in the oral tissues, however, they are harmless.

Arterial Calcification

Two distinct patterns of arterial calcification can be identified both radiographically and histologically: Monckeberg's medial calcinosis and calcified atherosclerotic plaque.

MONCKEBERG'S MEDIAL CALCINOSIS (ARTERIOSCLEROSIS)

Definition

The hallmark of arteriosclerosis is the fragmentation, degeneration, and eventual loss of elastic fibers followed by the deposition of calcium within the medial coat of the vessel.

Clinical Features

Most patients are asymptomatic initially, although late in the course of the disease clinical pathosis may develop, such as cutaneous gangrene, peripheral vascular disease, and myositis due to vascular insufficiency. Patients with Sturge-Weber syndrome also develop intracranial arterial calcifications.

Radiographic Features

Location. Medial calcinosis involving the facial artery or, less commonly, the carotid artery, may be viewed on panoramic radiographs.

Periphery and shape. The calcific deposits in the wall of the artery outline an image of the artery. From the side, the calcified vessel appears as a parallel pair of thin, radiopaque lines (Fig. 27-5) that may have a straight course or a tortuous path; this is described as a *pipe stem*

or *tram-track appearance.* In cross-section, involved vessels will display a circular or ring-like pattern.

Internal structure. There is no internal structure because the diffuse, finely divided calcium deposits occur solely in the medial wall of the vessels.

Differential Diagnosis

The radiographic appearance of arteriosclerosis is so distinctive as to be pathognomonic of the condition.

Management

Evaluation of the patient for occlusive arterial disease as well as peripheral vascular disease may be appropriate. In addition, hyperparathyroidism may be considered as medial calcinosis frequently develops as a metastatic calcification in patients with this condition.

CALCIFIED ATHEROSCLEROTIC PLAQUE

Definition

Atheromatous plaque in the extracranial carotid vasculature is the major contributing source of cerebrovascular embolic and occlusive disease. Dystrophic calcification can occur in the evolution of plaque within the intima of the involved vessel.

Radiographic Features

Location. Atherosclerosis first develops at arterial bifurcations as a result of increased endothelial damage at these sites. When calcification has occurred, these lesions may be visible in the panoramic radiograph in the soft tissues of the neck adjacent to the greater cornu of the hyoid bone and the cervical vertebrae C3, C4, or the intervertebral space between them (Fig. 27-6).

Periphery and shape. These soft tissue calcifications are usually multiple and irregular in shape; they are usually sharply defined from the surrounding soft tissues and have a vertical linear distribution.

Internal structure. The internal aspect is composed of a heterogeneous radiopacity.

Differential Diagnosis

Calcified triticeous cartilage may be mistaken for atheromatous plaque, although the uniform size, shape, and location of calcified triticeous cartilage in the laryngeal cartilage generally aids in identification of this condition.

Management

Patients with atherosclerosis should be referred to their physician for cerebrovascular and cardiovascular workup.

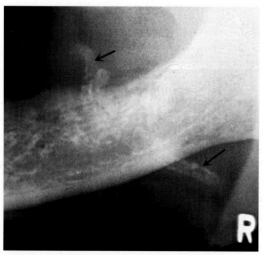

Fig. 27-5   A section of a panoramic image showing calcification of a blood vessel, probably the facial vein *(arrows)*.

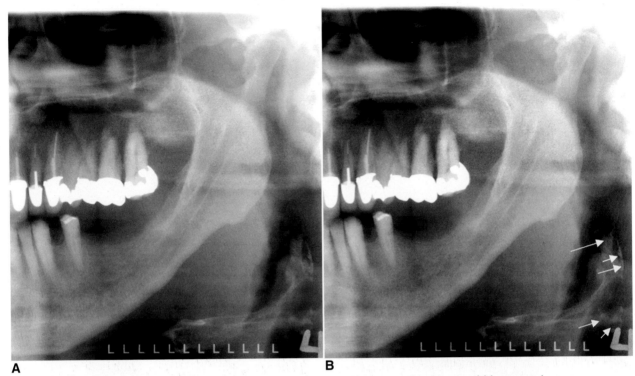

A B

Fig. **27-6** **A** and **B**, Identical cropped panoramic images of a 64-year-old hypertensive male, demonstrating multiple heterogeneous radiopacities in a vertical linear distribution in the soft tissues of the left side of the neck adjacent to the epiglottis (*arrows* in **B**).

Idiopathic Calcification

SIALOLITH

Definition
Sialoliths are stones found within the ducts of salivary glands (see Chapter 30). Mechanical conditions contributing to a slow flow rate and physiochemical characteristics of the gland secretion both contribute to the formation of a nidus and subsequent precipitation of calcium and phosphate salts.

Clinical Features
Sialoliths are most common in the submandibular glands of men in their middle and later years. They usually occur singly (70% to 80%) but may occur multiply. Patients with salivary stones may be asymptomatic, but they usually have a history of pain and swelling in the floor of the mouth and in the involved gland. This discomfort may intensify at mealtimes, when salivary flow is stimulated. Because the stone usually does not block the flow of saliva completely, the pain and swelling gradually subside. As many as 9% of patients have recurrent sialolithiasis, and about 10% of patients with sialolithiasis also suffer nephrolithiasis.

Radiographic Features
Location. The submandibular gland is involved more often (83% to 94% of cases) than the parotid gland (4% to 10%) or sublingual gland (1% to 7%), probably because the submandibular gland has a longer and more tortuous duct, an uphill flow in the proximal portion, and more viscous saliva with a higher mineral content. About half of submandibular stones lie in the distal portion of Wharton's duct, 20% in the proximal portion, and 30% in the gland.

Periphery and shape. Sialoliths located in the duct of the submandibular gland usually are cylindric. Stones that form in the hilus of a submandibular gland tend to be larger and more irregularly-shaped (Fig. 27-7).

Internal structure. Some stones are homogeneously radiopaque, and others show evidence of multiple layers of calcification. Less than 20% of submandibular gland sialoliths and 40% of those in the parotid gland are radiolucent because of the low mineral content of the parotid secretions.

Applied Radiology
Salivary stones occasionally are seen on periapical views superimposed over the mandibular premolar and

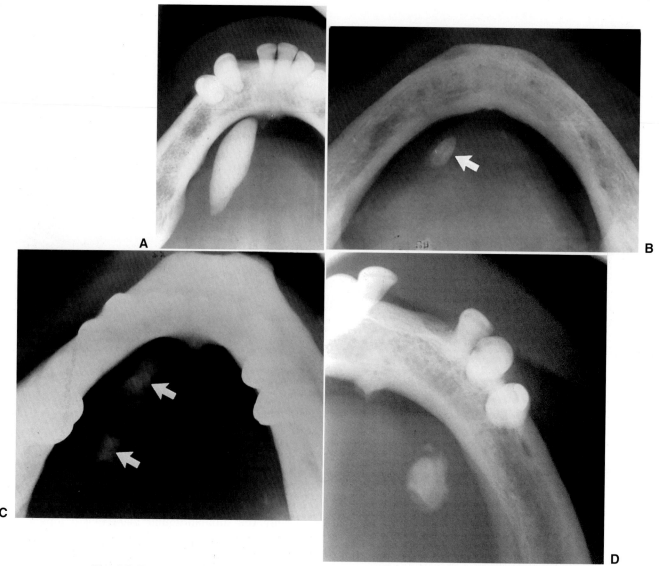

Fig. **27-7**   **A** to **D,** Standard occlusal projections of various shapes and sizes of calcified sialoliths *(arrows)* in the duct of a submandibular gland. Exposure times have been reduced to better demonstrate these calcifications, which are less calcified than the mandible.

molar apices (Fig. 27-8). The best view for visualizing stones in the distal portion of Wharton's duct is a standard mandibular occlusal view using half the usual exposure time, which displays the floor of the mouth without overlap from the mandible. Stones in a more posterior location are best visualized on lateral oblique views of the mandible or on a panoramic film. To demonstrate stones in the parotid gland duct, the clinician places a periapical film in the buccal vestibule, reduces the exposure time and orients x-ray beam through the cheek. Also, stones in the parotid duct can be seen if the patient "blows out" the cheek as an

anteroposterior skull view is exposed. An open-mouth lateral skull projection can be used. When producing radiographs to detect sialoliths, the exposure time should be reduced to about half of normal. This helps in detecting stones that are lightly calcified. If a noncalcified stone is suspected, sialography is used (see Chapter 30).

Differential Diagnosis
Sialoliths can be distinguished from other soft tissue calcifications because they usually are associated with pain or swelling of the involved salivary gland. Other calcifi-

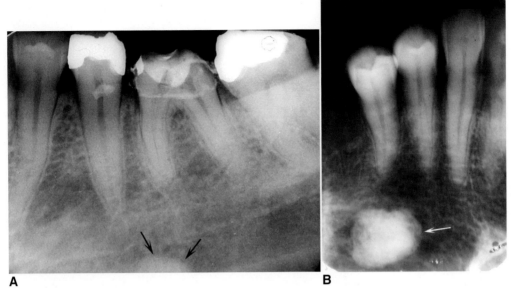

FIG. **27-8** Submandibular sialoliths are usually superimposed on the mandible and may be difficult to differentiate from a dense bone island without an occlusal film. **A,** Periapical film just reveals the superior aspect of a sialolith. **B,** The sialolith is superimposed over the anterior aspect of the mandible.

cations (e.g., lymph nodes) are asymptomatic. If the diagnosis is unclear, the clinician can prescribe a sialogram.

Management

Small stones often may be "milked out" through the duct orifice using bimanual palpation. If the stone is too large or located in the proximal duct, piezoelectric extracorporeal shock wave lithotripsy or surgical removal of the stone or gland may be required.

PHLEBOLITHS

Definition

Intravascular thrombi, which arise secondary to venous stagnation, sometimes become organized or even mineralized. Such mineralization begins in the core of the thrombus and consists of crystals of apatite with calcium phosphate and calcium carbonate. Phleboliths are calcified thrombi found in veins, venulae, or the sinusoidal vessels of hemangiomas (especially the cavernous type).

Clinical Features

In the head and neck, phleboliths nearly always signal the presence of a hemangioma. In an adult, phleboliths may be the sole residua of a childhood hemangioma that has long since regressed. The involved soft tissue may be swollen, throbbing, or discolored by the presence of veins or a soft tissue heman-gioma. Hemangiomas often fluctuate in size, associated with changes in body position or during a Valsalva maneuver. Applying pressure to the involved tissue should cause a blanching or change in color if the lesion is vascular in nature. Auscultation may reveal a bruit in cases of cavernous hemangioma, but not in the capillary type.

Radiographic Features

Location. Phleboliths most commonly are found in hemangiomas (see Chapter 21).

Periphery and shape. In cross-section the shape is round or oval, up to 6mm in diameter with a smooth periphery. If the involved blood vessel is viewed from the side, the phlebolith may resemble a straight or slightly curved sausage.

Internal structure. The internal aspect may be homogeneously radiopaque but more commonly has the appearance of laminations, giving phleboliths a "bull's-eye" or target appearance. A radiolucent center may be seen, which may represent the remaining patent portion of the vessel (Fig. 27-9).

Differential Diagnosis

A phlebolith may have a shape similar to that of a sialolith. Sialoliths usually occur singly; if multiple sialoliths are present, they usually are oriented in a single line, whereas phleboliths are usually multiple

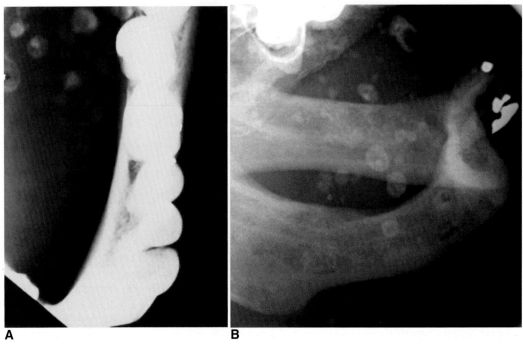

FIG. **27-9**　**A** and **B,** Phleboliths are soft tissue dystrophic calcifications found in veins. They are usually associated with hemangiomas.

and have a more random, clustered, distribution. The importance of correctly identifying phleboliths lies in the identification of a possible vascular lesion such as a hemangioma. This is critical if surgical procedures are contemplated.

LARYNGEAL CARTILAGE CALCIFICATIONS

Definition
The small, paired triticeous cartilages are found within the lateral thyrohyoid ligaments. Both the thyroid and triticeous cartilages consist of hyaline cartilage, which has a tendency to calcify or ossify with advancing age.

Clinical Features
Calcification of tracheal cartilages is an incidental radiographic finding with no clinical features.

Radiographic Features
Location. The calcified triticeous cartilage is located on a lateral view within the pharyngeal airspace inferior to the greater cornu of the hyoid bone and adjacent to the superior border of C4. The superior cornu of a calcified thyroid cartilage appears medial to C4 and is superimposed on the prevertebral soft tissue (Fig. 27-10).

Periphery and shape. The word *triticeous* means "grain of wheat," and the cartilage measures 7 to 9 mm in

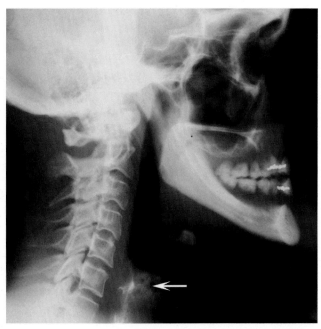

FIG. **27-10**　Lateral cephalometric film revealing calcification of the thyroid cartilage *(arrow).*

length and 2 to 4 mm in width. The periphery of the calcified triticeous cartilage is well-defined and smooth. Usually only the top 2 to 3 mm of a calcified thyroid cartilage will be visible at the lower edge of a panoramic radiograph.

Internal structure. Calcified tracheal cartilages generally present a homogeneous radiopacity but may occasionally demonstrate an outer cortex.

Differential Diagnosis

Calcified triticeous cartilage may be confused with calcified atheromatous plaque in the carotid bifurcation, but the solitary nature and extremely uniform size and shape of the former should be discriminatory.

Management

No treatment is needed for calcified tracheal cartilages, but careful attention to the differences in morphology and location enable the clinician to distinguish between calcified triticeous cartilage and calcified carotid atheromata.

RHINOLITH/ANTROLITH

Definition

Hard calcified bodies or stones that occur in the nose (rhinoliths) or the antrum of the maxillary sinus (antroliths) arise from the deposition of mineral salts such as calcium phosphate, calcium carbonate, and magnesium around a nidus. In cases of rhinolith, the nidus is usually an exogenous foreign body (coins, beads, etc.), whereas the nidus for an antrolith is usually endogenous (root tip, bone fragment, inspissated mucus, etc.)

Clinical Features

The patient may be asymptomatic for extended periods of time, but the expanding mass may impinge on the mucosa, producing pain, congestion, and ulceration. The patient may develop a unilateral purulent rhinorrhea, sinusitis, headache, epistaxis, anosmia, fetor, and fever.

Radiographic Features

Location. Rhinoliths develop in the nose (Fig. 27-11), whereas antroliths develop in the antrum of the maxillary sinus (see Fig. 26-7).

Periphery and shape. These stones have a variety of shapes and sizes.

Internal structure. They may present as homogeneous or heterogeneous radiopacities, depending on the nature of the nidus and sometimes have laminations. Occasionally the density will exceed the surrounding bone.

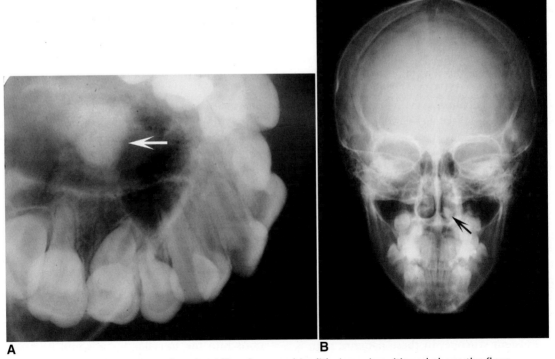

A　　　　　　　　　　　　　　　　　　　**B**

FIG. **27-11** **A,** Lateral occlusal film shows a rhinolith *(arrow)* positioned above the floor of the nose. **B,** Posterior-anterior skull film of the same case demonstrating that the rhinolith is positioned within the nasal fossa *(arrow).*

Differential Diagnosis

The differential diagnosis includes osteoma, healing odontogenic cyst and mycolith.

Management

Patients should be referred to an otorhinolaryngologist for removal of the mass.

Metastatic Calcification

Calcification of the soft tissues in the oral region caused by conditions involving elevated serum calcium and phosphate, such as hyperparathyroidism (see Chapter 24) or hypercalcemia of malignancy, are extremely rare.

Heterotopic Bone

OSSIFICATION OF THE STYLOHYOID LIGAMENT

Definition

Ossification of the stylohyoid ligament usually extends downward from the base of the skull and commonly occurs bilaterally. However, in rare cases the ossification begins at the lesser horn of the hyoid and in fewer still in a central area of the ligament. Conditions associated with ossification of the stylohyoid ligament include Eagle's syndrome, stylohyoid syndrome, and stylohyoid chain ossification.

Clinical Features

Even when extensive ossification of one or both stylohyoid ligaments is seen, more than 50% of patients are clinically asymptomatic. The ossified ligament usually can be detected by palpation over the tonsil as a hard, pointed structure. Very little correlation exists between the extent of ossification and the intensity of the accompanying symptoms. One symptom is vague, nagging to intense pain in the pharynx on swallowing, turning the head, or opening the mouth, especially on yawning. When this entity is associated with discomfort and the patient has a recent history of neck trauma (e.g., tonsillectomy), the condition is called *Eagle's syndrome*. The elongated styloid process and local scar tissue probably causes symptoms by impinging on the glossopharyngeal nerve. Similar clinical findings without a history of neck trauma constitute stylohyoid (carotid artery) syndrome. The patient may describe attacks of otalgia, tinnitus, temporal headache, and vertigo or transient syncope. In these patients, pain is produced by mechanical irritation of sympathetic nerve tissue in the arterial wall, producing regional carotidynia. These individuals usually are over 40 years

of age. This condition is more prevalent than Eagle's syndrome.

Radiographic Features

Ossification of the stylohyoid ligament is detected fairly commonly as an incidental feature on panoramic radiographs. In one study, approximately 18% of a population examined showed ossification of more than 30 mm of the stylohyoid ligament. The ligament may have at least some calcification in individuals of any age.

Location. In a panoramic image the linear ossification extends forward from the region of the mastoid process and crosses the posterior-inferior aspect of the ramus toward the hyoid bone. The hyoid bone is positioned roughly parallel to or superimposed on the posterior aspect of the inferior cortex of the mandible.

Shape. The styloid process appears as a long, tapering, thin, radiopaque process that is thicker at its base and projects downward and forward (Fig. 27-12). It normally varies from about 0.5 to 2.5 cm in length. The ossified ligament has roughly a straight outline, but in some cases irregularity may be seen in the outer surface. The farther the radiopaque ossified ligament extends toward the hyoid bone, the more likely it is that it will be interrupted by radiolucent, joint-like junctions (pseudoarticulations).

Internal structure. Small ossifications of the stylohyoid ligament appear homogeneously radiopaque. As the ossification increases in length and girth, the outer cortex of this bone becomes evident as a radiopaque band at the periphery.

Differential Diagnosis

The symptoms accompanying stylohyoid ligament ossification and Eagle's syndrome or stylohyoid syndrome generally are vague; however, when they occur with the distinctive radiographic evidence of ligament ossification, little chance exists that the complaint will be confused with another entity. Occasionally, though, the symptoms may be similar to those seen in temporomandibular joint dysfunction.

Management

Most patients with ossification of the stylohyoid ligament are asymptomatic, and no treatment is required. For patients with vague symptoms, a conservative approach of reassurance and steroid or lidocaine injections into the tonsillar fossa would be recommended initially. However, for patients with persistent or intense symptoms, the recommended treatment is amputation of the stylohyoid process.

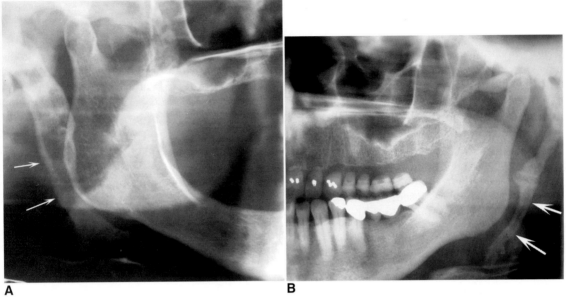

FIG. **27-12** **A** and **B**, Examples of prominent ossification of the stylohyoid ligament *(arrows)*; these individuals did not have any symptoms.

OSTEOMA CUTIS

Definition

Osteoma cutis is a rare soft tissue ossification in the skin. Approximately 85% of cases occur secondary to acne of long duration, developing in a scar or chronic inflammatory dermatosis. Histologically these lesions are areas of dense viable bone in the dermis or subcutaneous tissue. They occasionally are found in diffuse scleroderma, replacing the altered collagen in the dermis and subcutaneous septa.

Clinical Features

Osteoma cutis can occur anywhere, but the face is the most common site. The tongue is the most common intraoral site (osteoma mucosae or osseous choristoma). Osteoma cutis does not cause any visible change in the overlying skin other than an occasional color change that may appear yellowish white. If the lesion is large, the individual osteoma may be palpated. A needle inserted into one of the papules is met with stonelike resistance. Some patients develop numerous lesions (dozens to hundreds), usually on the face in females and on the scalp or chest in males. This form is known as *multiple miliary osteoma cutis.*

Radiographic Features

Location. Radiographically, osteoma cutis most commonly appears in the cheek and lip regions (Fig. 27-13). In this location the image can be superimposed over a tooth root or alveolar process, giving the appearance of

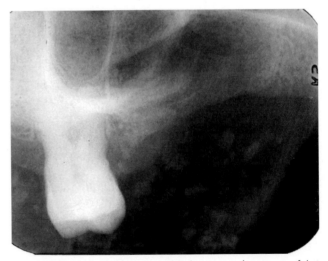

FIG. **27-13** Osteoma cutis is seen here as faint radiopaque calcifications in the cheek.

an area of dense bone. Accurate localization can be achieved by placing an intraoral film between the cheek and alveolar process to image the cheek alone. As an alternative, a posteroanterior skull view with the cheek blown outward using a soft tissue technique of 60 kVp helps localize osteomas in the skin.

Periphery and shape. Osteoma cutis appears as smoothly outlined, radiopaque, washer-shaped images. These single or multiple radiopacities usually are very small, although the size can range from 0.1 to 5 cm.

Internal structure. The internal aspect may be homogeneously radiopaque but usually has a radiolucent center that represents normal fatty marrow, giving the lesion a donut appearance radiographically. Trabeculae occasionally develop in the marrow cavity of larger osteomas. Individual lesions of calcified cystic acne resemble a snowflake-like radiopacity, which corresponds to the clinical location of the scar.

Differential Diagnosis

The differential diagnosis should include myositis ossificans, calcinosis cutis, and osteoma mucosae. If the blown-out cheek technique is used, the lesions of osteoma cutis appear much more superficial than mucosal lesions. Myositis ossificans is of greater proportions, in some cases causing noticeable deformity of the facial contour.

Management

No treatment is required, but these osteomas occasionally are removed for cosmetic reasons. Although an osteoma cutis usually is quite small, it cannot be removed with a needle and must be excised. Recently, resurfacing of the skin with erbium:YAG laser using tretinoin cream has been successful in treating multiple miliary osteoma cutis.

MYOSITIS OSSIFICANS

Definition

In myositis ossificans fibrous tissue and heterotopic bone form within the interstitial tissue of muscle and associated tendons and ligaments. Secondary destruction and atrophy of the muscle occur as this fibrous tissue and bone interdigitate and separate the muscle fibers. There are two principal forms: localized and progressive.

LOCALIZED (TRAUMATIC) MYOSITIS OSSIFICANS

Synonyms

Posttraumatic myositis ossificans and solitary myositis

Definition

Localized myositis ossificans results from acute or chronic trauma or from heavy muscular strain caused by certain occupations and sports. Muscle injury from multiple injections (occasionally from dental anesthetic) also may be a cause. The injury leads to considerable hemorrhage into the muscle or associated tendons or fascia. This hemorrhage organizes and undergoes progressive scarring. During the healing process, heterotopic bone and in some cases cartilage is formed. The term *myositis* is misleading because no

inflammation is involved. The fibrous tissue and bone form within the interstitial tissue of the muscle; no actual ossification of the muscle fibers occurs.

Clinical Features

Localized myositis ossificans can develop at any age in either gender, but it occurs most often in young men who engage in vigorous activity. The site of the precipitating trauma remains swollen, tender, and painful much longer than expected. The overlying skin may be red and inflamed, and when the lesion involves a muscle of mastication, opening the jaws may be difficult. After about 2 or 3 weeks, the area of ossification becomes apparent in the tissues; a firm, intramuscular mass can be palpated. The localized lesion may enlarge slowly, but eventually it stops growing. The lesion may appear fixed, or it may be freely movable on palpation.

Radiographic Features

Location. The most commonly involved muscles of the head and neck are the masseter and sternocleidomastoid. However, other muscles of mastication may be involved, such as the lateral pterygoid muscle. Usually a radiolucent band can be seen between the area of ossification and adjacent bone, and the heterotopic bone may lie along the long axis of the muscle (Fig. 27-14).

Periphery and shape. The periphery commonly is more radiopaque than the internal structure. There is a variation in shape from irregular, oval to linear streaks (pseudotrabeculae) running in the same direction as the normal muscle fibers. These pseudotrabeculae are characteristic of myositis ossificans and strongly imply a diagnosis.

Internal structure. The internal structure varies with time. Within the third or fourth week after injury, the radiographic appearance is a faintly homogeneous radiopacity. This organizes further, and by 2 months a delicate lacy or feathery radiopaque internal structure develops. These changes indicate the formation of bone; however, this bone does not have a normal-appearing trabecular pattern. Gradually the image becomes denser and better defined, maturing fully in about 5 to 6 months. After this period the lesion may shrink.

Differential Diagnosis

The differential diagnosis of localized myositis ossificans includes ossification of the stylohyoid ligament and other soft tissue calcifications. However, both the form and location of myositis ossificans often are

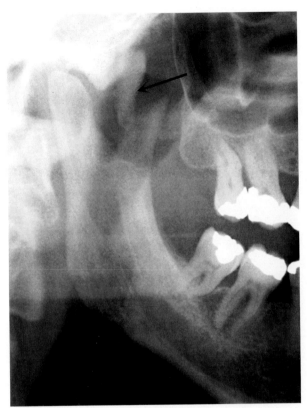

FIG. **27-14** Soft tissue ossification extending from the coronoid process in a superior direction, following the anatomy of the temporalis muscle *(arrow)*. This condition arose after several attempts were made to provide a sub-mandibular nerve block, leaving the patient unable to open the mandible.

enough to make the differential diagnosis. Other lesions to consider are bone-forming tumors. Although tumors such as osteogenic sarcoma can form a linear bone pattern (see Chapter 22), the tumor is contiguous with the adjacent bone, and signs of bone destruction often are present.

Management

Rest and limitation of use are recommended to diminish the extent of the calcific deposit. Early surgical removal of the lesion usually stimulates rapid (within 1 month) and extensive recurrence (from origin to insertion of the affected muscle). Recurrence is not likely if removal of the involved area of muscle is postponed until the process has become stationary.

PROGRESSIVE MYOSITIS OSSIFICANS

Definition

Progressive myositis ossificans is a rare disease of unknown cause that usually affects children before 6 years of age, occasionally as early as infancy. It is more common in males. Progressive formation of heterotopic bone occurs within the interstitial tissue of muscles, tendons, ligaments, and fascia, and the involved muscle atrophies. This condition may be inherited or may be a spontaneous mutation affecting the mesenchyma.

Clinical Features

In most cases the heterotopic ossification starts in the muscles of the neck and upper back and moves to the extremities. The disease commences with soft tissue swelling that is tender and painful and may show redness and heat, indicating the presence of inflammation. The acute symptoms subside, and a firm mass remains in the tissues. This condition may affect any of the striated muscles, including the heart and diaphragm. In some cases the spread of ossification is limited; in others it becomes extensive, affecting almost all the large muscles of the body. Stiffness and limitation of motion of the neck, chest, back, and extremities (especially the shoulders) gradually increase. Advanced stages of the disease result in the "petrified man" condition. During the third decade the process may spontaneously arrest; however, most patients die during the third or fourth decade. Premature death usually results from respiratory embarrassment or from inanition through the involvement of the muscles of mastication.

Radiographic Features

The radiographic appearance of progressive myositis ossificans is similar to that described for the limited form. The heterotopic bone more commonly is oriented along the long axis of the involved muscle (Fig. 27-15). Osseous malformation of the regions of muscle attachment, such as the mandibular condyles, also may be seen.

Differential Diagnosis

In the initial stages of the disease, distinguishing between progressive myositis ossificans and rheumatoid arthritis may be difficult. However, the presence of specific anomalies suggests the diagnosis. In the case of calcinosis, the deposits of amorphous calcium salts frequently resorb, but in progressive myositis ossificans, the bone never disappears.

Management

No effective treatment exists for progressive myositis ossificans. Nodules that are traumatized and that ulcerate frequently should be excised. If interference with respiration or respiratory infection occurs in the later stages of the disease, supportive therapy may be required.

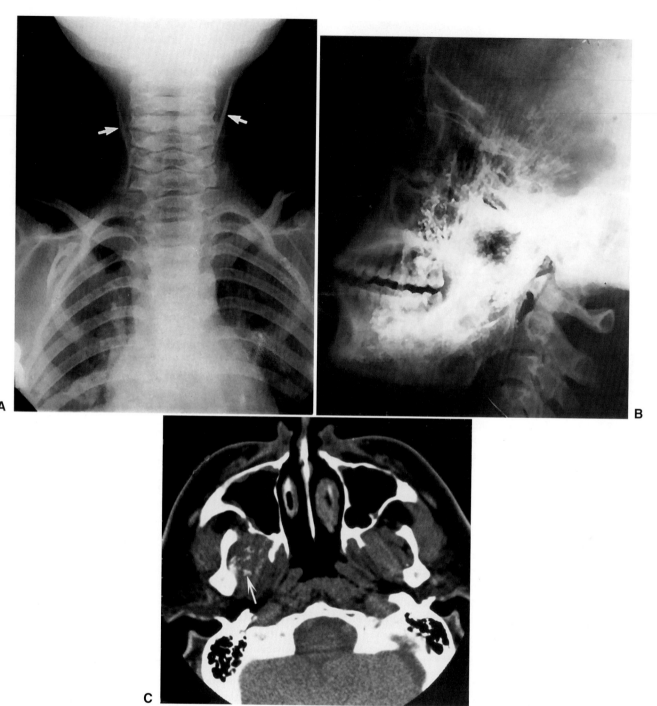

FIG. **27-15**   **A,** Myositis ossificans, seen as bilateral linear calcifications *(arrows)* of the sternohyoid muscle. **B,** Extensive ossification of the masseter and temporalis muscles. **C,** Axial CT scan using soft tissue algorithm, demonstrating calcifications in the lateral pterygoid muscle. (**A,** Courtesy Dr. H. Worth, Vancouver, British Columbia; **B,** From Shawkut AH: Oral Surg 23:751, 1967.)

BIBLIOGRAPHY

Allen AC: Skin. In Kissane JM, editor: Anderson's pathology, ed 8, vol 2, St. Louis, 1985, Mosby.

Connor JM: Soft tissue ossification, Berlin, 1983, Springer-Verlag.

Monsour PA et al: Soft tissue calcifications in the differential diagnosis of opacities superimposed over the mandible by dental panoramic radiography, Aust Dent J 36:94, 1991.

Worth HM: Principles and practice of oral radiologic interpretation, St. Louis, 1963, Mosby.

CALCIFIED LYMPH NODES

Muto T, Michiya H, Kanazawa M, Sato K: Pathological calcification of the cervico-facial region. Br J Oral Maxillofac Surg 29:120-122, 1991.

DYSTROPHIC CALCIFICATION IN THE TONSILS

Espe BT, Newmark H: A tonsillolith seen on CT. Comput Med Imaging Graph 16:59-61, 1992.

Pruet CW, Duplan DA: Tonsil concretions and tonsilloliths, Otolaryngol Clin North Am 20(2):305, 1987.

CYSTICERCOSIS

Hulbert TV, Larsen RA: Seizures and soft tissue calcifications in a Hispanic woman. Chest 101:1125-1127, 1992.

Romero De Leon E, Aguirre A: Oral cysticercosis Oral Surg Oral Med Oral Pathol Oral Radiol Endod 79:572-577, 1995.

CALCIFIED BLOOD VESSEL

Carter LC et al: Carotid calcifications on panoramic radiography identify an asymptomatic male patient at risk for stroke: a case report, Oral Surg Oral Med Oral Pathol Oral Radiol Endod 85:119, 1998.

Friedlander AH, Altman L: Carotid artery atheromas in postmenopausal women. Their prevalence on panoramic radiographs and their relationship to atherogenic risk. J Am Dent Assoc 132:1130-1136, 2001.

Miles DA, Craig RM, Langlais RP, Wadsworth WC: Facial artery calcification: a case report of its clinical significance. J Can Dent Assoc 49:200-202, 1983.

Hayes JB et al: Calcification of vessels in cheek of patient with medial atherosclerosis, Oral Surg 21:299, 1966.

RHINOLITH/ANTROLITH

Cohen MA, Packota GV, Hall MJ, Steinberg J: Large asymptomatic antrolith of the maxillary sinus. Report of a case. Oral Surg Oral Med Oral Pathol 71:155-157, 1991.

Ishiyama T: Maxillary antrolith: report of a case. Aurus Nasis Larynx 15:185-189, 1988.

Munoz A, Pedrosa I, Villafruela M: "Eraseroma" as a cause of rhinolith: CT and MRI in a child, Neuroradiol 39:824-826, 1997.

Royal SA, Gardner RE: Rhinolithiasis: an unusual pediatric nasal mass. Pediatr Radiol 28:54-55, 1998.

SIALOLITH

Ho V et al: Sialolithiasis of minor salivary glands, Br J Oral Maxillofac Surg 30:273, 1992.

Iro H et al: Shockwave lithotripsy of salivary duct stones, Lancet 339:1333, 1992.

Jensen J et al: Minor salivary gland calculi: a clinicopathologic study of forty-seven new cases, Oral Surg 47:44, 1979.

Kulkens C, Quetz JU, Lippert BM, Folz BJ, Werner JA: Ultrasound-guided piezoelectric extracorporeal shock wave lithotripsy of parotid gland calculi. J Clin Ultrasound 29:389-394, 2001.

Lustmann J et al: Sialolithiasis: a survey on 245 patients and a review of the literature, Int J Oral Maxillofac Surg 19:135, 1990.

Mandel ID, Thompson RH Jr: The chemistry of parotid and submaxillary saliva in heavy calculus formers and nonformers, J Periodontol 38:310, 1967.

Williams MF. Sialolithiasis. Otolaryngol Clin North Am 32:819-834, 1999.

PHLEBOLITHS

McMenamin M, Quinn A, Barry H, Sleeman D, Wilson G, Toner M: Cavernous hemangioma in the submandibular gland masquerading as sialadenitis. Oral Surg Oral Med Oral Pathol Oral Radiol Endod 84:146-148, 1997.

Zachariades N, Rallis G, Papademetriou J, Konsolaki E, Markaki S, Mezitis M. Phleboliths: A report of three unusual cases. Br J Oral Maxillofac Surg 29:117-119, 1991.

CALCIFIED TRACHEAL CARTILAGES

Carter L: Discrimination between calcified triticeous cartilage and calcified carotid atheroma on panoramic radiography. Oral Surg, Oral Med, Oral Pathol, Oral Radiol, Endod 90:108-110, 2000.

Talmi Y, Bedrin L, Ofer A, Kronenberg J: Prevertebral calcification masquerading as a hypopharyngeal foreign body. Ann Otol Rhinol Laryngol 106:435-436, 1997.

OSSIFIED STYLOHYOID LIGAMENT

Bafaqeeh SA: Eagle syndrome: classic and carotid artery types. J Otolaryngol 29:88-94, 2000.

Balbuena L, Hayes D, Ramirez SG, Johnson R: Eagle's syndrome (elongated styloid process) South Med J 90:331-334, 1997.

Camarda AJ et al: Stylohyoid chain ossification: a discussion of etiology, Oral Surg 67:508, 1989.

Eagle W: Elongated styloid process, symptoms and treatment, Arch Otolaryngol 67:172, 1958.

OSTEOMA CUTIS

Farhood V et al: Osteoma cutis: cutaneous ossification with oral manifestations, Oral Surg 45:98, 1978.

Goldstein B et al: Dystrophic calcification in the tongue: a late sequel to radiation therapy, Oral Surg 46:12, 1978.

Hughes PS: Multiple miliary osteomas of the face ablated with the erbium:YAG laser. Arch Dermatol 135:378-380, 1999.

Krolls SO et al: Osseous choristomas of intraoral soft tissue, Oral Surg 32:588, 1971.

Peterson WC Jr, Mandel SL: Primary osteomas of the skin, Arch Dermatol 87:626, 1963.

Shigehara H et al: Radiographic and morphologic studies of multiple miliary osteomas of cadaver skin, Oral Surg Oral Med Oral Pathol Oral Radiol Endod 86:121, 1998.

MYOSITIS OSSIFICANS

Buhain WJ et al: Pulmonary function in myositis ossificans progressiva, Am Rev Respir Dis 110:333, 1974.

Mevio E, Rizzi L, Bernasconi G: Myositis ossificans traumatica of the temporal muscle: a case report. Aurus Nasus Larynx 28:345-347, 2001.

Sarac S, Snnaroglu L, Hosal AS, Sozeri B: Myositis ossificans in the neck. Eur Arch Otorhinolaryngol 256:199-201, 1999.

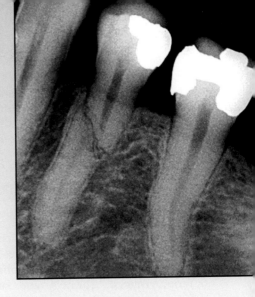

CHAPTER 28

Trauma to Teeth and Facial Structures

Radiologic examination is essential for evaluating the sequelae of trauma, including displacement and fracture of teeth and bone, and localizing foreign objects within the soft tissues. Radiology aids in identifying the location and orientation of fractures and indicates the degree of separation or displacement of fracture margins. Follow-up radiographs are useful in evaluating the extent of healing after an injury and the development of long-term changes resulting from the trauma.

Applied Radiology

The prescription of appropriate films can be made only after a careful clinical examination. Multiple projections at differing angles, including at least two views at right angles to each other, are necessary. The application of ideal radiography may be difficult at times because of the nature of the injury and patient discomfort. The most common imaging procedures applied in various forms of trauma follow.

TRAUMA TO TEETH

The investigation of dental trauma always requires intraoral periapical films to obtain adequate image detail. It is important to radiograph not only the involved teeth but also the teeth of the opposing arch. Depending on the severity of the trauma and the ability of the patient to open the mouth, a bisecting-angle technique instead of paralleling technique for intraoral radiography, including occlusal views, may be necessary.

Tooth Fracture

Intraoral periapical films (a minimum of two) should be taken at differing horizontal angulations of the x-ray beam. A panoramic film may serve as a survey film, but it may not have the image detail to reveal a nondisplaced root fracture.

Tooth Avulsion or Fractured Crown

If a tooth or a large fragment of a tooth is missing, a chest film may be considered to rule out aspiration of the tooth. If there are lacerations in the lips or cheek, a soft tissue image may be obtained by placing an intraoral film in the mouth adjacent to the traumatized soft tissue and then exposing it. If the laceration is in the tongue, a standard mandibular occlusal film may be exposed or the tongue can be protruded and then imaged.

Mandibular Fracture

The panoramic film is a good initial survey film for assessing mandibular fracture, but it must not be used alone. The standard occlusal film provides a good right-angle image. Other images that may be used include a posteroanterior skull view and a submentovertex skull view. If panoramic images are not available, lateral oblique views of the mandible are useful.

Trauma to the Mandibular Condyle

The panoramic view should be supplemented with either a transorbital view or an open Towne's skull view in cases of suspected trauma to the mandibular condyle. These anteroposterior views are important to supplement lateral views of the joint, especially in cases of nondisplaced greenstick fractures of the condylar neck.

These views may be supplemented with tomographic views and a submentovertex skull view. If the fracture of the condyle is complex, computed tomography (CT) imaging may be required to locate fracture fragments anatomically. Soft tissue injury to the joint capsule or articular disk warrants consideration of arthrography or magnetic resonance imaging (MRI).

Maxillary Fracture

CT is the imaging method of choice to identify the number and location of fractures of the fine structure of the maxilla. Plain radiographs include posteroanterior, Waters', Towne's, and submentovertex skull views.

RADIOGRAPHIC SIGNS OF FRACTURE

The following are general signs that may indicate the presence of a fracture of bone or tooth:

1. The presence of a radiolucent line (usually sharply defined) within the anatomic boundaries of the structure—If the line extends beyond the boundaries of the mandible, for instance, it is more likely to represent an overlapping structure.
2. A change in the normal anatomic outline or shape of the structure—For instance, a mandible that is noticeably asymmetric between the left and right sides may indicate a fracture. A fracture of the mandible often shows a sharp change in the occlusal plane at the location of the fracture.
3. A defect in the outer cortical boundary, which may appear as a deviation in the smooth outline, a gap in the outer cortical bone, or a steplike defect.
4. An increase in the density of the bone, which may be caused by the overlapping of two fragments of bone.

A fracture may be missed if the plane of the fracture is not in the same direction as the x-ray beam. For this reason, multiple films at different angulations should be used.

Traumatic Injuries of the Teeth

CONCUSSION

Definition

The term *concussion* indicates a crushing injury to the vascular structures at the tooth apex and to the periodontal ligament, resulting in inflammatory edema. Only minimal loosening or displacement of the tooth occurs. The injury frequently results in the elevation of the tooth out of the socket so that its occlusal surface makes premature contact on mandibular closing.

Clinical Features

The patient usually complains that the traumatized tooth is painful. On examination, the tooth is sensitive to both horizontal and vertical percussion. It may also be sensitive to biting forces, but patients usually try to modify their occlusion to reduce pressure on the tooth or teeth.

Radiographic Features

The radiographic appearance of a dental concussion is widening of the periodontal ligament space. This widening usually occurs only in the apical portion of the periodontal ligament space because the raising of the tooth out of the socket results in an essentially parallel movement of the coronal two thirds of the root surface with the lamina dura (Fig. 28-1). Reduction in the size of the pulp chamber and pulp canals may develop in the months and years after such traumatic injury (Fig. 28-2). A slow-developing pulp necrosis may result in an increase in the width of the pulp chamber and canals compared with the adjacent teeth because of the death of odontoblasts responsible for laying down secondary dentin. Pulpal necrosis may occur, resulting in the development of a periapical lesion. In rare cases internal root resorption may occur (see Fig. 28-2).

Management

Because displacement of the tooth or teeth does not occur, the appropriate treatment is conservative and may include slight adjustment of the opposing teeth (if necessary), repeated vitality tests, and radiographic examination during the period after the injury.

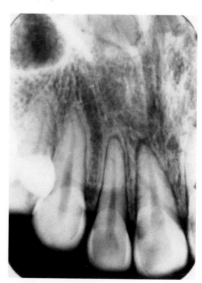

FIG. **28-1**　Dental concussion has resulted in widening of the periodontal ligament spaces of the incisors.

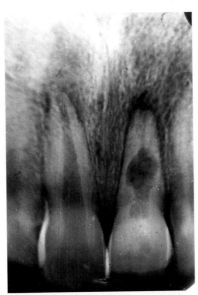

FIG. **28-2** Dental concussion has resulted in obliteration of the pulp chamber but not the pulp canal; internal root resorption and an incisal fracture of the left central incisor and necrosis of the pulp of the right central incisor resulting in a wide pulp chamber and canal extending to the apex of the tooth.

LUXATION

Definition

Luxation of teeth is dislocation of the articulation (represented by the periodontal attachment) of the tooth. Such teeth are both abnormally mobile and displaced. Subluxation of the tooth denotes an injury to the supporting structures of the tooth that results in abnormal loosening of the tooth without frank dislocation.

Traumatic forces, depending on their nature and orientation, can cause intrusive luxation (displacement of teeth into the alveolar bone), extrusive luxation (partial displacement of teeth out of the sockets), or lateral displacement (movement of teeth other than axial displacement). In intrusive and lateral luxation, comminution (crushing) or fracture of the supporting alveolar bone accompanies dislocation of the tooth.

The movement of the apex and disruption of the circulation to the traumatized tooth that accompanies luxation usually induce temporary or permanent pulpal changes, which may result in complete or partial pulpal necrosis. If the pulp survives, the rate of hard tissue formation by the pulp accelerates and continues until it obliterates the pulp chamber and canal. This may take place in permanent and deciduous teeth.

Clinical Features

An adequate history is helpful in identifying luxation and ordering the appropriate radiographs. Subluxated teeth are in their normal location but are abnormally mobile. There may be some blood flowing from the gingival crevice, indicating periodontal ligament damage. Subluxated teeth are extremely sensitive to percussion and masticatory forces. The clinical crowns of intruded teeth may appear shortened. Maxillary incisors may be driven so deeply into the alveolar ridge that they appear to be avulsed (lost). The displaced tooth may cause some damage to adjacent teeth, including any developing succedaneous teeth. Depending on the orientation and magnitude of the force and the shape of the root, the root may be pushed through the buccal or, less commonly, the lingual alveolar plate, where it can be seen and palpated. On repeated vitality testing, the sensitivity of a luxated tooth may be temporarily decreased or nondetectable, especially shortly after the accident. Vitality may return, however, after weeks or even several months.

The teeth most frequently subjected to luxation are the maxillary incisors in both the deciduous and permanent dentitions. The mandibular teeth are seldom involved. The type of luxation varies with age, possibly as an expression of change in the nature of maturing bone. Intrusions and extrusions are the primary dislocations found in the deciduous teeth. In the permanent dentition, the intrusive type of luxation is seen less frequently. When teeth are luxated, in either dentition, usually two or more are involved, and seldom just a single tooth.

Radiographic Features

Radiographic examinations of luxated teeth may demonstrate the extent of the injury to the root, periodontal ligament, and alveolar bone. A radiograph made at the time of injury serves as a valuable reference point for comparison with subsequent radiographs. As with dental concussion, the minor damage associated with subluxation may be limited to elevation of the tooth out of the socket. The sole radiographic finding may be a widening of the apical portion of the periodontal ligament space. Slight elevation of the tooth may not be radiographically apparent.

The identification and evaluation of dislocated teeth may require multiple radiographic projections. The depressed position of the crown of an intruded tooth is often apparent on a radiograph (Fig. 28-3), although a minimally intruded tooth may be difficult to demonstrate radiographically. Intrusion may result in partial or total obliteration of the periodontal ligament space. Multiple radiographic projections, including occlusal views, may show the direction of displacement and its relationship to the outer cortical bone and developing teeth.

An extrusively luxated tooth results in increased width of the periodontal ligament space. The widening

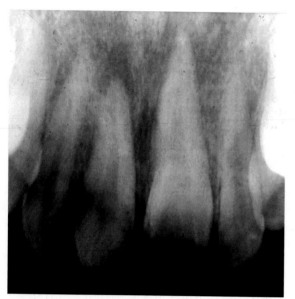

FIG. 28-3   Intruded maxillary central incisor after trauma. Note the fractured incisal edges of both central incisors.

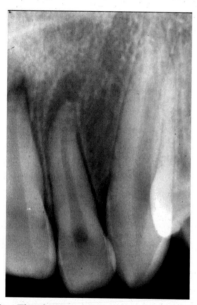

FIG. 28-4   The lateral incisor has been extruded after trauma. Note the increased radiolucency about the apical portion of the tooth caused by an increased width of the periodontal ligament space.

may be accentuated in the apical region (Fig. 28-4), whereas in a more severely extruded tooth all the periodontal ligament space may be increased. A laterally luxated tooth may show a widened periodontal ligament space, with greater width on the side of impact. Often these teeth are somewhat extruded.

Management

A subluxated permanent tooth may be restored to its normal position by digital pressure shortly after the accident. If swelling precludes repositioning, minimal reduction of antagonists to relieve discomfort may be necessary. Stabilize teeth by splinting to prevent further damage to the pulp and periodontal ligament. However, remove a dislocated tooth if its apex is near its succedaneous tooth. If the alveolar bone over the root of a luxated tooth has been fragmented and displaced, reposition the fragments by digital pressure. Periodically examine a subluxated primary tooth after the injury. If it causes some discomfort as the result of extrusion, the tooth can be removed without undue concern for occlusal problems.

AVULSION

Definition

Avulsion (or *exarticulation*) is the term used to describe the complete displacement of a tooth from the alveolar process. Teeth may be avulsed by direct trauma when the force is applied directly to the tooth, or by indirect trauma (e.g., when indirect force is applied to teeth as the result of the jaws striking together). Avulsion occurs in about 15% of traumatic injuries to the teeth. Fights are responsible for the avulsion of most permanent teeth, whereas accidental falls account for the traumatic loss of most deciduous teeth.

Clinical Features

Maxillary central incisors are the teeth most often avulsed from both dentitions. The appearance of the alveolar process around the missing tooth depends on the time between its loss and the clinical examination. Typically this injury occurs in a relatively young age group, when the permanent central incisors are just erupting and the periodontal ligament is immature. Most often only a single tooth is lost, and fractures of the alveolar wall and lip injuries are frequently seen.

Radiographic Features

In a recent avulsion the lamina dura of the empty socket is apparent and usually persists for several months. The replacement of the socket site with new bone requires months and, in some cases, years. As new bone forms, the opposite walls of the healing socket approach each other, reducing the socket width. Time passes, and only a thin vertical radiolucent shadow remains and may have a similar appearance to a pulp canal. In some instances the new bone replacing the socket is very dense and radiopaque and may appear similar to a retained root (Fig. 28-5).

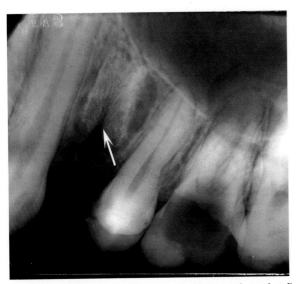

FIG. **28-5** Bone formation in a healing socket of a first bicuspid develops from the lateral walls and may leave a central radiolucent line *(arrow)* that has an appearance similar to that of a pulp canal and falsely give the impression of a retained tooth fragment.

The missing tooth may be in adjacent soft tissue, and its image may project on radiographs and over the alveolar process, giving the false impression that it lies within the bone. Therefore, to differentiate between an intruded tooth and an avulsed tooth lying within the soft tissues, a radiograph of the lacerated lip or tongue should be produced.

Management

If the avulsed tooth is not found by clinical or radiographic examination, a chest radiograph may be considered to rule out aspiration of the tooth. Reimplanting permanent teeth after avulsion often restores function. If the tooth is intact and without extensive caries or periodontal disease, and the length of time that the tooth is outside the oral cavity has not been extensive, success is possible. The less time that elapses between avulsion and reimplantation, the better the prognosis. Other factors, such as keeping the tooth moist, improve prognosis as well. Successful reimplantation depends largely on the viability of the residual periodontal ligament fibers. If the apical foramen is open, endodontic therapy may not be required. Endodontic therapy can be delayed until the first signs of apical resorption are radiographically detected (usually 2 or 3 weeks after reimplantation). If the apical foramen is closed, endodontic treatment is required, but it should be delayed 1 or 2 weeks. External root resorption may occur in the months and years after reimplantation, and the resorption may progress to complete the destruction of the root. Reimplanting avulsed deciduous teeth carries the danger of interfering with the developing succedaneous teeth.

FRACTURES OF THE TEETH

DENTAL CROWN FRACTURES

Definition

Fractures of the dental crown account for about 25% of traumatic injuries to the permanent teeth and 40% of injuries to the deciduous teeth. The most common event responsible for the fracture of permanent teeth is a fall, followed by accidents involving vehicles (e.g., bicycles, automobiles) and blows from foreign bodies striking the teeth. Fractures involving only the crown normally fall into three categories:

1. Fractures that involve only the enamel without the loss of enamel substance (infraction of the crown or crack)
2. Fractures that involve enamel or enamel and dentin with loss of tooth substance but without pulpal involvement (uncomplicated fracture)
3. Fractures that pass through enamel, dentin, and pulp with loss of tooth substance (complicated fracture)

Clinical Features

Fracture of the dental crowns most frequently involves anterior teeth. Infractions, or cracks in the enamel, are quite common but frequently are not readily detectable. Illuminating crowns with indirect light (directing the beam in the long axis of the tooth) causes cracks to appear distinctly in the enamel. Histologic studies show that the cracks pass through the enamel but not into the dentin. The pattern and distribution of these cracks are unpredictable and apparently relate to the trauma.

Uncomplicated fractures do not involve the pulp. Uncomplicated crown fractures that do not involve the dentin usually occur at the mesial or distal corner of the maxillary central incisor. Loss of the central portion of the incisal edge is also common. Fractures that involve dentin can be recognized by the contrast in color between dentin and the peripheral layer of enamel. The exposed dentin is usually sensitive to chemical, thermal, and mechanical stimulation. In deep fractures, the pink image of the pulp may shine through the thin remaining dentinal wall.

Uncomplicated fractures that involve both the enamel and the dentin of permanent teeth are more common than complicated fractures. In contrast, the incidence of complicated and uncomplicated fractures is about equal in the deciduous teeth.

Complicated crown fractures are distinguishable by bleeding from the exposed pulp or by droplets of blood forming from pinpoint exposures. The pulp is visible and may extrude from the open pulp chamber if the fracture is old. The exposed pulp is sensitive to most forms of stimulation.

Radiographic Features

The radiograph provides information regarding the location and extent of the fracture and the relationship to the pulp chamber, as well as the stage of root development of the involved tooth (Fig. 28-6). This initial film also provides a means of comparison for follow-up studies of the involved teeth.

Management

Although crown infractions do not require treatment, the vitality of the tooth should be questioned and determined. The sharp edges of enamel that result from an uncomplicated fracture may be smoothed by grinding and may require restoration for cosmetic reasons. It is reasonable to delay this procedure for a number of weeks until the pulp has recovered and is starting to lay down secondary dentin. The prognosis for teeth with fractures limited to the enamel is quite good, and pulpal necrosis develops in fewer than 2% of such cases. If a fracture involves both dentin and enamel, the frequency of pulpal necrosis is about 3%. Oblique fractures have a worse prognosis than horizontal fractures

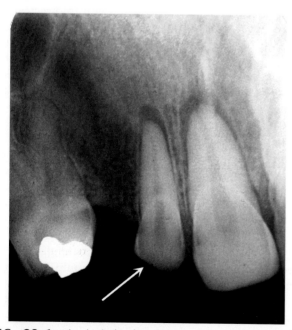

FIG. **28-6** An incisal edge fracture involving the right maxillary lateral incisor (arrow) and subluxation of both the central and lateral incisors.

because a greater amount of dentin is exposed. The frequency of pulpal necrosis increases greatly with concussion and mobility of the tooth.

Treatment of complicated crown fractures of permanent teeth may involve pulp capping, pulpotomy, or pulpectomy, depending on the stage of root formation. If a coronal fracture of a deciduous tooth involves the pulp, it is usually best treated by extraction.

DENTAL ROOT FRACTURES

Definition

Fractures of tooth roots are uncommon and account for 7% or fewer of traumatic injuries to permanent teeth and for about half that many in deciduous teeth. This difference probably results from the fact that the deciduous teeth are less firmly anchored in the alveolus.

Clinical Features

Most root fractures occur in maxillary central incisors. The coronal fragments are usually displaced lingually and slightly extruded. The degree of mobility of the crown relates to the level of the fracture: the closer the fracture is to the apex, the more stable the tooth is. When testing the mobility of a traumatized tooth, place a finger over the alveolar bone. If movement of only the crown can be detected, root fracture is likely. Fractures of the root may occur with fractures of the alveolar bone, which are commonly not detected. This is most often observed in the anterior region of the mandible, where root fractures are infrequent. Although root fracture is usually associated with temporary loss of sensitivity (by all usual criteria), the sensitivity of most teeth returns to normal within about 6 months.

Radiographic Features

Fractures of the dental root may occur at any level and involve one (Fig. 28-7) or all the roots of multirooted teeth. Most of the fractures confined to the root occur in the middle third of the root. The ability of the film to reveal the presence of a root fracture depends on the degree of distraction of the fragments and whether the x-ray beam is in alignment with the plane of the fracture. When visible, the fracture appears as a sharply defined radiolucent line confined to the anatomic limits of the root. If, however, the orientation of the beam is not directly through the plane of the fracture, the image of the fracture appears as a more poorly defined gray shadow. Most nondisplaced root fractures are usually difficult to demonstrate radiographically, and several views at differing angles may be necessary. In some instances when the fracture line is not visible, the only evidence of a fracture may be a localized

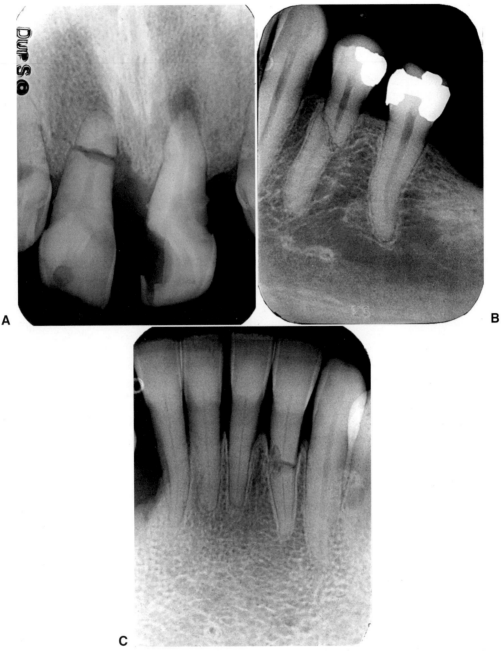

FIG. **28**-7   **A,** A recent horizontal fracture of the right maxillary central incisor and apical rarefying osteitis related to the left central incisor. **B,** A healed fracture with slight displacement of the fragments. **C,** A healed fracture with an increase in the distance between the fracture segments due to root resorption.

increase in the periodontal ligament space adjacent to the fracture site (Fig. 28-8).

Most fractures are transverse and oblique, and the shadow of the fracture line at the buccal and lingual surfaces may suggest the presence of more than one (comminuted) fracture. Longitudinal root fractures are relatively uncommon but are most likely in teeth with posts that have been subjected to trauma. The width of fractures tends to increase with time, probably because of resorption of the fractured surfaces. Over time, calcification and obliteration of the pulp chamber and canal may be seen.

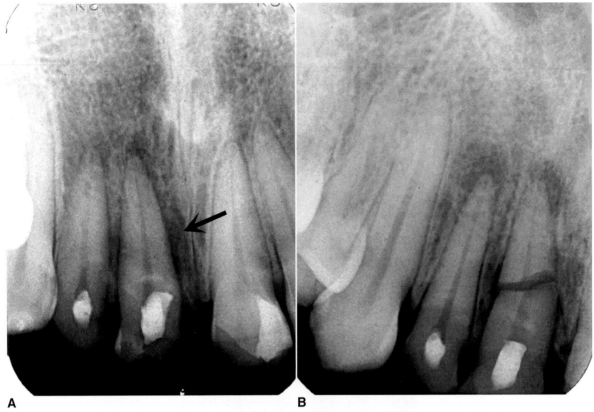

FIG. 28-8   Incisal fractures involving the maxillary central incisors and the right lateral incisor. In addition, there is subtle evidence of a root fracture involving the distal aspect of the root of the right central incisor (**A**). The fracture line is not apparent on the mesial aspect of the root because the plane of fracture is not in alignment with the x-ray beam. However, there is widening of the periodontal membrane space on the mesial surface *(arrow)* at the site of the fracture. **B,** Later dislocation of the root fragments.

Differential Diagnosis

The superimposition of soft tissue structures such as the lip, ala of the nose, and nasolabial fold over the image of a root may suggest a root fracture. To avoid this diagnostic error, note that the soft tissue image of the lip line usually extends beyond the tooth margins. Fractures of the alveolar process may also overlap the root and suggest a root fracture.

Management

Fractures in the middle or apical third of the root of permanent teeth can be manually reduced to the proper position and immobilized. Prognosis is generally favorable; the incidence of pulpal necrosis is about 20% to 24%. The more apical the fracture is, the better the prognosis. Perform endodontic therapy only when evidence exists of pulpal necrosis. It is common for bone resorption to occur at the site of the fracture rather than at the apex. When the fracture occurs in the coronal third of the root, the prognosis is poor and

extraction is indicated unless the apical portion of the root fragment can be extruded orthodontically and restored. The roots of fractured deciduous teeth that are not badly dislocated may be retained with the expectation that they will be normally resorbed. Attempts at removal may result in damage to the developing succedaneous tooth.

VERTICAL ROOT FRACTURES

Definition

Vertical root fractures run lengthwise from the crown toward the apex of the tooth. Usually both sides of a root are involved. The crack is usually oriented in the facial-lingual plane in both anterior and posterior teeth. These fractures usually occur in the posterior teeth in adults, especially in mandibular molars. They are usually iatrogenic, following insertion of retention screws or pins into vital or nonvital teeth. Uncrowned posterior teeth that have been treated endodontically are most at risk. Large occlusal forces are another etiology for vertical root fracture, particularly in restored teeth.

Clinical Features

Patients with vertical root fractures complain of persistent dull pain (cracked tooth syndrome), often of long duration. This pain may be elicited by applying pressure to the involved tooth. Pain may be nonexistent or mild. The patient may have a periodontal lesion resembling a chronic abscess or a history of repeated failed endodontic therapy. Occasionally, definitive diagnosis can be made only by inspection after surgical exposure.

Radiographic Features

If the central ray of the x-ray beam lies in the plane of the fracture, the fracture may be visible as a radiolucent line on the radiograph. Usually, however, radiographs are not useful in identifying vertical root fractures in their early stages. Later, after the development of an inflammatory lesion, there will be evidence of bone loss (Fig. 28-9). The widening of the periodontal membrane space and this bone loss may not be centered at the apex but often positioned more coronally towards the alveolar crest. Lesions may also extend apically from the alveolar crest and resemble periodontal lesions.

Management

Single-rooted teeth with vertical root fractures must be extracted. Multirooted teeth may be hemisected and

the intact remaining half of the tooth restored with endodontic therapy and a crown.

CROWN-ROOT FRACTURES

Definition

Crown-root fractures involve both the crown and roots. Although uncomplicated fractures may occur, crown-root fractures usually involve the pulp. About twice as many affect the permanent as the deciduous teeth. Most crown-root fractures of the anterior teeth are the result of direct trauma. Many posterior teeth are predisposed to such fractures by large restorations or extensive caries.

Clinical Features

The typical crown-root fracture of an anterior tooth has a labial margin in the gingival third of the crown and courses obliquely to exit below the gingival attachment on the lingual surface. Displacement of the fragments is usually minimal. Crown-root fractures occasionally present with bleeding from the pulp. The patient with a crown-root fracture usually complains of pain during mastication. The teeth are sensitive to occlusal forces, which cause separation of the fragments.

Radiographic Features

These fractures are often not visible in the radiographic image because the x-ray beam is rarely aligned with the plane of the fracture. Also, distraction of the fragments is usually not present. The vertical fractures of crown

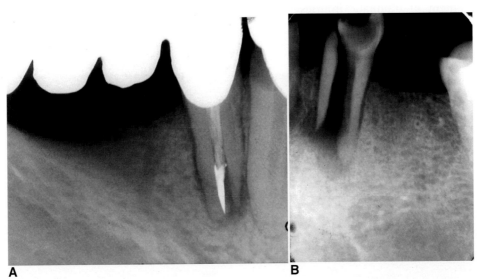

A **B**

FIG. **28-9** **A**, A vertical fracture through the root of a mandibular first bicuspid with endodontic treatment. Note that the fracture extends through the pulp canal and that there is more displacement between the root fragments at the apex of the root. **B**, A vertical root fracture through the root of a mandibular cuspid; significant displacement of the fragments aids in detection.

and root that are mainly tangential to the direction of the radiographic beam are readily apparent on the radiograph. Unfortunately, this is not common.

Management

Removal of the coronal fragment permits the evaluation of the extent of the fracture. If the coronal fragment includes as much as 3 to 4 mm of clinical root, successful restoration of the tooth is doubtful and removal of the residual root is recommended. Also, if the crown-root fracture is vertical, prognosis is poor regardless of treatment. If the pulp is not exposed and the fracture does not extend more than 3 to 4 mm below the epithelial attachment, conservative treatment is likely to be successful. Uncomplicated crown-root fractures are frequently encountered in posterior teeth, and with the appropriate crown-lengthening procedures (gingivectomy and ostectomy), the tooth is likely to be amenable to successful restoration. If only a small amount of root is lost with the coronal fragment but the pulp has been compromised, it is likely that the tooth can be restored after endodontic treatment.

Traumatic Injuries to the Facial Bones

Injury to the facial bones may occur in one or more of the bones. Facial fractures most frequently occur in the zygoma or mandible and, to a lesser extent, in the maxilla. Radiography plays a crucial role in the diagnosis and management of traumatic injuries to the facial bones. The appropriate radiologic investigation is prescribed only after a thorough examination of the teeth and facial bones. Obtaining the history of the trauma also contributes to the selection of the appropriate radiographs. Obtaining multiple views (at least two at right angles) aids in assessing the location, extent, and displacement of fractures. Some fractures are not readily apparent when the x-ray beam is not oriented parallel to the plane of the fracture.

MANDIBULAR FRACTURES

The most common mandibular fracture sites are the condyle, body, and angle, followed less frequently by the parasymphyseal region, ramus, coronoid process, and alveolus. The most common cause of mandibular fractures is assault, followed by automobile accidents, falls, and sports injuries. About half of all mandibular fractures occur in individuals between 16 and 35 years of age, and fractures are more likely on Fridays and Saturdays than on other days of the week. Males are affected about three times as frequently as females. Trauma to the mandible is often associated with other injuries, most commonly concussion (loss of consciousness) and other fractures, usually of the maxilla, zygoma, and skull.

MANDIBULAR BODY FRACTURES

Definition

The mandible is the most commonly fractured facial bone. It is important to realize that a fracture of the mandibular body on one side is frequently accompanied by a fracture of the condylar process on the opposite side (Fig. 28-10). Trauma to the anterior mandible

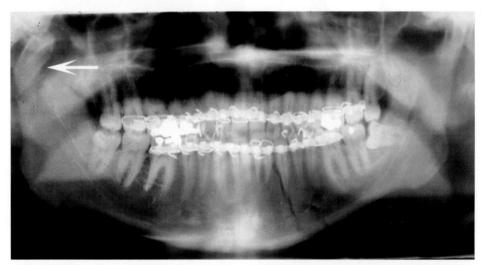

FIG. **28-10** This panoramic film reveals a fracture through the left parasymphyseal region and also a fracture through the right condylar neck and displacement of the condylar head *(arrow)*.

may result in a unilateral or bilateral fracture of the condylar processes. When a heavy force strikes a small area laterally, fracture of the angle, ramus, or even the coronoid process may result. In children, fractures of the mandibular body usually occur in the anterior region. Mandibular fractures are classified as favorable or unfavorable, depending on their orientation. Unfavorable fractures are those in which the action of muscles attached to the mandible are likely to displace the fracture margins. For instance if a fracture site in the body of the mandible slants posteriorly and inferiorly such that the masseter and internal pterygoid muscles pull the ramus segment away from the body of the mandible, the fracture is unfavorable. In favorable fractures, muscle action tends to reduce the fracture.

Clinical Features

A history of injury is typical, substantiated by some evidence of the trauma that caused the fracture, such as contusions or wounds in the skin. Frequently the patient experiences swelling and a deformity that is accentuated when the patient opens the mouth. A discrepancy is often present in the occlusal plane, and manipulation may produce crepitus or abnormal mobility. Intraoral examination may reveal ecchymosis in the floor of the mouth. In the case of bilateral fractures to the mandible, a risk exists that the digastric and mylohyoid muscles will pull the mandible against the pharynx and compromise the airway.

Radiographic Features

The radiographic examination of a suspected fracture should include a panoramic view; however, it is important to supplement this film with right-angle views. These include occlusal and extraoral views such as the posteroanterior and submentovertex skull views. Frequently such supplemental views disclose fractures not evident on panoramic projections; for instance, intraoral periapical films have greater resolution (Fig. 28-11, A and B). The margins of fractures usually appear as sharply defined radiolucent (dark) lines of separation that are confined to the structure of the mandible. They are best visualized when the x-ray beam is oriented in the plane of the fracture.

Displacement of the fragments results in a cortical discontinuity or "step" (Fig. 28-11, C). An irregularity in the occlusal plane is often apparent, indicating the fracture site. Occasionally, the margins of the fracture overlap each other, resulting in an area of increased radiopacity at the fracture site. Nondisplaced mandibular fractures may involve both buccal and lingual cortical plates or only one cortical plate. An incomplete fracture involving only one cortical plate is often called a *greenstick fracture*. Such fractures usually occur in children. An oblique fracture that involves both cortical plates may cause some diagnostic difficulties if the fracture lines in the buccal and lingual plates are not superimposed (Fig. 28-12). In this case, two fracture lines are apparent, suggesting two distinct fractures when in reality only one exists. A right-angle view such as an occlusal view and the fact that the two fracture lines join at the same point on the inferior border of the mandible help with the correct diagnosis.

Differential Diagnosis

The superimposition of soft tissue shadows on the image of the mandible may simulate fractures. A narrow air space between the dorsal surface of the tongue and the soft palate superimposed across the angle of the mandible in a panoramic image may appear as a fracture. The air space between the dorsal surface of the tongue and the posterior pharyngeal wall can appear similar to a fracture on lateral views of the mandible. Similar appearances can occur in the region of soft palate superimposition on the ramus.

Management

The management of a fracture of the mandible presents a variety of surgical problems that involve the proper reduction, fixation, and immobilization of the fractured bone. Minimally displaced fractures are managed by closed reduction and intermaxillary fixation, whereas fractures with more severely displaced fragments may require open reduction. Treatment for fractures of the body often includes antibiotic therapy because a tooth root may be in the line of the fracture. When the fracture line involves third molars, severely mobile teeth, or teeth with at least half their roots exposed in the fracture line, the involved teeth are often extracted to reduce the risk for infection and problems with fixation.

MANDIBULAR CONDYLE FRACTURES

Definition

Fractures in the region of the condyle can be divided into condylar neck fractures and condylar head fractures. Condylar neck fractures are more common and are located below the condylar head. When a condylar neck fracture occurs, the head is usually displaced medially, inferiorly, and anteriorly (as a result of pull from the lateral pterygoid muscle). Severe trauma may displace the condylar head into the skull or sinuses. Fractures of the condylar head are fissure-like, with a vertical cleft dividing the head; they may result in multiple fragments in a compression-like fracture. Almost half the patients with condylar fractures also have fractures in the mandibular body.

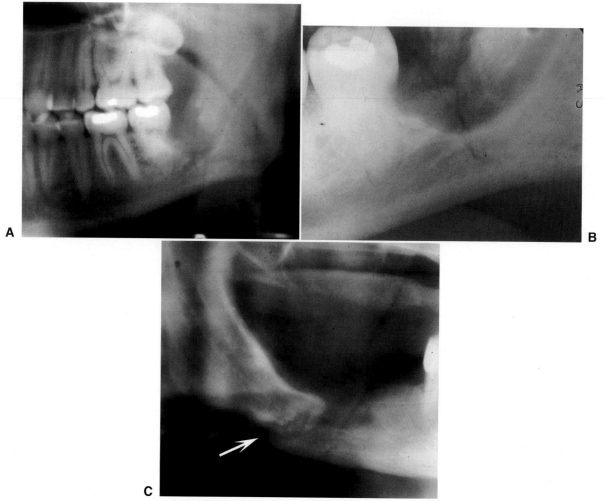

FIG. 28-11   A, This panoramic image was taken subsequent to the removal of the third molar. Although a nondisplaced mandibular fracture was suspected, only the intraoral film (B) has the required resolution to clearly demonstrate the fracture. C reveals a fracture of the edentulous body of this mandible. Note the step defect (arrow).

Clinical Features

The clinical symptoms of a fractured condylar process are not always apparent, so the preauricular area must be carefully examined and palpated. A condylar fracture may be suspected when the clinician cannot palpate the condyle in the external ear canal when the jaw is closed. Movement of the jaw may cause crepitus. The patient may have pain on opening or closing the mouth, but so much swelling and trismus may exist that the patient is unable to move the jaw. Usually an anterior open bite is present, with the last molars in contact. Also, the mandible may be displaced forward or, in the case of a unilateral fracture, deviated toward the side of the fracture, especially on opening. A significant feature is the inability of the patient to bring the jaw

forward because the external pterygoid muscle is attached to the condyle.

Radiographic Features

Radiographic examination of the condyles should always include lateral and anteroposterior views of each condyle. Appropriate lateral projections include panoramic, Parma, and lateral oblique views of the ramus and condylar regions. Frontal views include reverse-Towne's and transorbital projections (Fig. 28-13). Nondisplaced fractures of the condylar process may be difficult to detect on lateral views and are best demonstrated on anteroposterior views. Careful tracing of the outer cortical plate of the posterior border of the ramus, the condylar head, and the condylar notch on

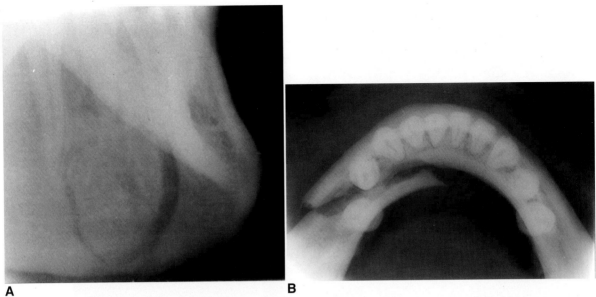

FIG. **28-12** **A,** A lateral oblique image of the right mandible in the region of the bicuspids. Note the two fracture lines that appear to meet at the inferior cortex and the occlusal film of the same case **(B),** demonstrating only one fracture; therefore the two fracture lines in A represent fractures of the buccal and lingual plates.

the lateral and posteroanterior projections may reveal the presence of fractures.

Studies of remodeling of fractured condyles show that young persons have much greater remodeling potential than do adults. In children younger than 12 years, most fractured condyles show a radiographic return to normal morphology after healing, whereas in teenagers the remodeling is less complete, and in adults only minor remodeling is observed. The extent of remodeling is also greater with fractures of the condylar head than with condylar neck fractures with displacement of the condylar head. The most common deformities are medial inclination of the condyle, abnormal shape of the condyle, shortening of the neck, erosion, and flattening. Early condylar fractures commonly result in hypoplasia of the ipsilateral side of the mandible.

Management

The technical details of treating condylar fractures vary according to whether one or both condyles are involved, the extent of displacement, and the occurrence and severity of concomitant fractures. The treatment is directed to relieve acute symptoms, restore proper anatomic relationships, and prevent bony ankylosis. If a malocclusion develops, intermaxillary fixation may be provided in an attempt to restore proper occlusion. Often fractures are not reduced because of the morbidity of the procedure and the size and position of the fracture fragments.

FRACTURES OF THE ALVEOLAR PROCESS

Definition

Simple fractures of the alveolar process may involve the buccal or lingual cortical plates of the alveolar process of the maxilla or mandible. Commonly these fractures are associated with traumatic injuries to teeth that are luxated with or without dislocation. Several teeth are usually affected, and the fracture line is most often horizontal. The labial plate of the alveolar process is more prone to fracture than the palatal plate.

Some fractures extend through the entire alveolar process (in contrast to the simple fracture that involves only one cortical plate) and may be apical to the teeth or involve the tooth socket. These are also commonly associated with dental injuries and extrusive luxations with or without root fractures.

Clinical Features

A common location of alveolar fractures is the anterior aspect of the maxilla. Simple alveolar fractures are relatively rare in the posterior segments of the arches. In this location, fracture of the buccal plate usually occurs during removal of a maxillary posterior tooth. Fractures of the entire alveolar process occur in the anterior and premolar regions and in an older age group.

A characteristic feature of alveolar process fracture is marked malocclusion with displacement and mobility of the fragment. The attached gingiva may have lacerations. When the practitioner tests the mobility of a

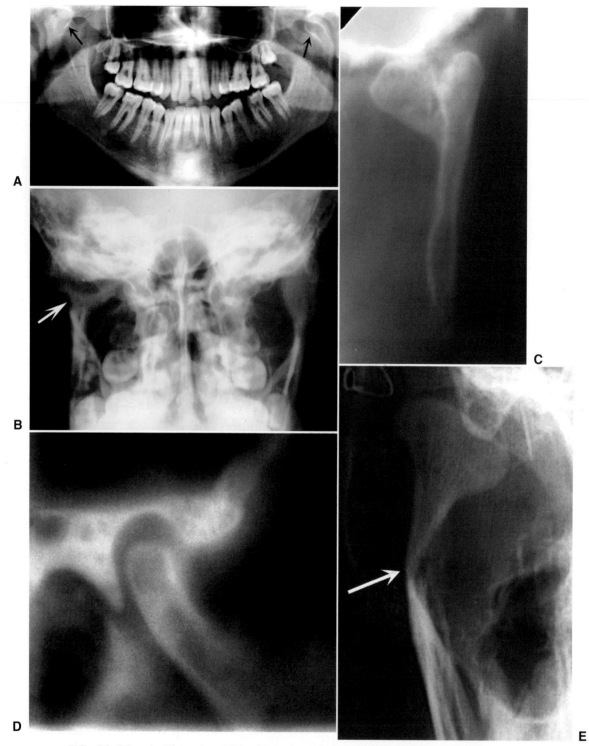

FIG. **28-13**   **A,** Bilateral condylar fractures with forward displacement of the condylar head fragments (arrows) and an anterior open bite. **B,** An open Towne's view revealing a compression fracture of the right condyle *(arrow).* **C,** An anterior-posterior tomograph of a fissural fracture of the condylar head, leaving the lateral pole still attached to the condylar neck. **D,** A lateral tomograph failed to reveal a condylar neck fracture. **E,** A periorbital view of the same condyle showing a greenstick condylar neck fracture.

single tooth, the entire fragment of bone moves. The teeth in the fragment also have a recognizable dull sound when percussed. The detached bone may include the floor of the maxillary sinus, which may cause bleeding from the nose on the involved side. Ecchymosis of the buccal vestibule is usually evident.

Radiographic Features

Intraoral radiographs often do not reveal fractures of a single cortical wall of the alveolar process, although evidence exists that the teeth have been luxated. However, a fracture of the anterior labial cortical plate may be apparent on a lateral extraoral radiograph if some bone displacement occurs and if the direction of the x-ray beam profiles the fracture site. Fractures of both cortical plates of the alveolar process are usually apparent (Fig. 28-14). The closer the fracture is to the alveolar crest, the greater the possibility that root fractures are present. It may be difficult to differentiate a root fracture from an overlapping fracture line of the alveolar bone. Several films produced with different projection angles help with this differentiation. If the fracture line is truly associated with the tooth, the line does not move relative to the tooth structure. Fractures of the posterior alveolar process may involve the floor of the maxillary sinus and result in abnormal thickening of the sinus mucosa.

Management

Fractures of the alveolar process are treated by repositioning the displaced teeth and associated bone fragments with digital pressure. Gingival lacerations are sutured. If the luxated permanent teeth are splinted and stable, intermaxillary fixation is not necessary. Permanent teeth are splinted for about 6 weeks. The faster healing in children permits their removal in about half that time. A soft diet for 10 to 14 days is recommended. Antibiotic coverage is provided because of communication with tooth sockets. Teeth that have lost their vascular supply may eventually require endodontic treatment.

MAXILLARY FRACTURES

MIDFACE FRACTURES

Definition

Fractures of the midfacial region may be limited to the maxilla alone or may involve other bones, including the frontal, nasal, lacrimal, zygoma, vomer, ethmoid, and sphenoid. Such complex fractures may be quite variable but often follow general patterns classified by Léon Le Fort: zygomatic (complex), horizontal, pyramidal, and craniofacial disjunction fractures. These fractures may be evident clinically or radiographically. They are rare in children.

The radiographic interpretation of fractures of the midface is difficult because of the complex anatomy in this region and the multiple superimpositions of structures. A plain film examination should include posteroanterior, Waters', reverse Towne's, lateral skull, and submentovertex projections. Each film should be searched systematically for fractures in the frontal bone, nasion, orbital walls, zygomatic arches, and maxillary antrum. Fractures may appear as linear radiolucencies that are usually widest at discontinuities in the cortical margins of bone, alterations of normal skeletal contour, displaced fragments of bone, and separated bony sutures. Some fractures are not apparent because of minimal separation of the bony margins, orientation of the fracture at an oblique angle to the x-ray beam, or superimposition of fracture lines over other complex anatomic structures. Abnormal soft tissue densities may both help and hinder the examination of facial trauma. When the fracture tears the antral or nasal mucosa, radiographs reveal densities associated with edema and bleeding in those areas and thus help to identify regions of fracture. However, facial edema detracts from the clarity of the radiographs, and preexisting inflammatory or allergic paranasal sinus disease may be misleading.

CT is the diagnostic imaging method of choice for maxillary fractures. It provides image slices (axial and coronal images using bone algorithm) through the maxilla, allowing for the display of osseous structures without the images of overlapping anatomy. This provides suitable image detail to detect bony fractures and changes in the soft tissues, such as herniation of orbital fat and extraocular muscle and tissue swelling. As an aid

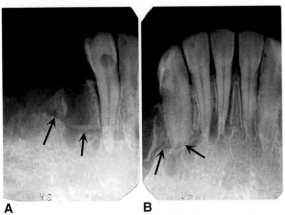

A   **B**

FIG. 28-14 These two images demonstrate an alveolar fracture extending from the distal aspect of the mandibular right cuspid in an anterior direction *(arrows)* and through the tooth socket of the right central incisor.

in determining the spatial orientation of fractures or bone fragments, the CT images may be reformatted in three-dimensional images.

HORIZONTAL FRACTURE (LE FORT I)

Definition

The Le Fort I fracture is a relatively horizontal fracture in the body of the maxilla that results in detachment of the alveolar process of the maxilla from the middle face. It is the result of a traumatic force directed to the lower maxillary region. The fracture line passes above the teeth, below the zygomatic process, and through the maxillary sinuses and tuberosities to the inferior portion of the pterygoid processes (Fig. 28-15). It may be unilateral or bilateral. In the unilateral fracture, an auxiliary fracture exists in the midline of the palate. The unilateral fracture must be distinguished from a fracture within the alveolar process (as discussed previously), which does not extend to the midline. Fractures of the mandible (54%) and zygoma (23%) may also be found in these patients.

Clinical Features

If the fragment is not distally impacted, it can be manipulated by holding on to the teeth. If the fracture line is at a high level, the fragment may include the pterygoid muscle attachments, which pull the fragment posteriorly and inferiorly. As a result, the posterior maxillary teeth contact the mandibular teeth first, resulting in an anterior open bite, retruded chin, and long face, an appearance characteristic of this type of fracture. If the fracture is at a low level, no displacement may occur. Other symptoms may include an associated swelling and bruising about both eyes, pain over the nose and face, deformity of the nose, and flattening of the middle of the face. Epistaxis is inevitable, and occasionally double vision and varying degrees of paresthesia over the distribution of the infraorbital nerve occur. Manipulation may reveal a mobile maxilla and crepitation.

Radiographic Features

This fracture may be difficult to detect. The views to use are the posteroanterior, lateral skull, and Waters' projections and CT scans. Both maxillary sinuses are usually radiopaque and may show air-fluid levels. The lateral view may disclose a slight posterior displacement of the fragment (the inferior portion of the maxilla below the fracture line) and, if present, the fracture line through the pterygoid bones. The intervertebral spaces of the cervical spine may simulate fracture lines in the

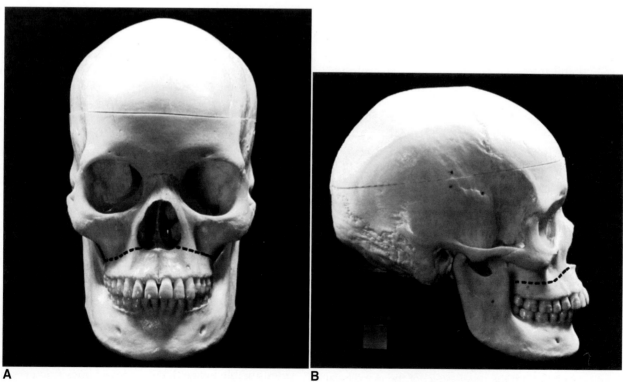

A   **B**

FIG. **28-15**   Usual position of the Le Fort I horizontal fracture on a frontal **(A)** and lateral **(B)** view.

posteroanterior skull views. This type of fracture unites rapidly, so if a few days lapse between injury and radiographic examination, the fracture may not be detectable radiographically.

Management

If the fracture is not displaced and is at a relatively low level in the maxilla, it can be treated by intermaxillary fixation. Those that are high, with the fragment displaced posteriorly or with pronounced separation, require craniomaxillary fixation in addition to intermaxillary fixation. A unilateral horizontal fracture is usually immobilized by intermaxillary fixation. However, if it cannot be reduced manually, elastic traction in the required direction (across the palate or between the arches) is employed. Antibiotics are usually administered because the fracture line involves the maxillary sinuses.

PYRAMIDAL FRACTURE (LE FORT II)

Definition

The Le Fort II fracture has a pyramidal appearance on the posteroanterior skull radiograph—hence the name *pyramidal fracture*. The fracture results from a violent force applied to the central region of the middle third of the facial skeleton. This force separates the maxilla from the base of the skull by causing fractures of the nasal bones and frontal processes of the maxilla (Fig. 28-16). The fractures extend laterally through the lacrimal bones and floors of the orbits and inferiorly through the zygomaticomaxillary sutures (Fig. 28-17). Frequently, on one side the fracture passes through the suture or through the zygomatic complex, and on the other side it passes around and beneath the base of the zygomatic process of the maxilla. From this area, the fracture then passes posteriorly along the lateral wall of the maxilla, across the pterygomaxillary fossa, and through the pterygoid plates. It usually extends through the maxillary sinuses. The frontal and ethmoid sinuses are involved in about 10% of cases, especially in severe comminuted fractures.

Clinical Features

In contrast to the Le Fort I (horizontal) fracture, characterized by only slight swelling about the upper lips, the Le Fort II injury results in massive edema and marked swelling of the middle third of the face. Typically, an ecchymosis around the eyes develops within minutes of the injury. The edema about the eyes is likely

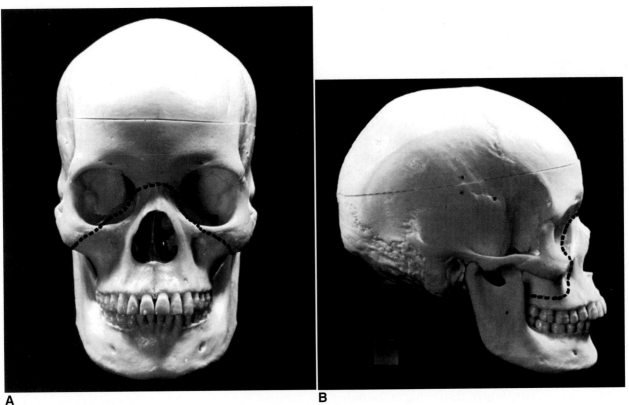

A   **B**

FIG. **28-16** Usual position of the Le Fort II pyramidal fracture on a frontal (**A**) and lateral (**B**) view.

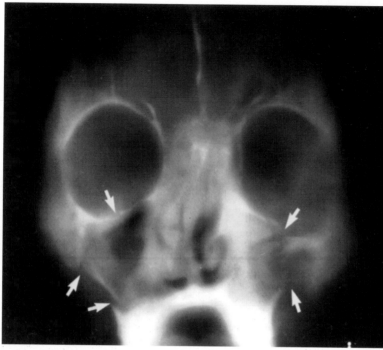

FIG. **28-17**   Tomographic view of multiple facial fractures, including a Le Fort II fracture and fractures through the ethmoid bone, infraorbital rims *(arrows)* and lateral wall of the maxilla *(arrows).* (Courtesy Dr. C. Schow, Galveston, Texas.)

to be so severe that it is impossible to see the eyes without prying the lids open. The conjunctivas over the inner quadrants of the eyes are bloodshot, and if the zygomatic bones are involved, this ecchymosis extends to the outer quadrant. The broken nose is displaced, and because the face has fallen, the nose and face are lengthened. An anterior open bite occurs (with molars in contact). Epistaxis is inevitable, and a cerebrospinal fluid rhinorrhea may also result. Palpation reveals the discontinuity of the lower borders of the orbits. By applying pressure between the bridge of the nose and the palate, the "pyramid" of bone can be moved. Other common symptoms include double vision and variable degrees of paresthesia over the distribution of the infra-orbital nerve.

Radiographic Features

The radiographic examination reveals fractures of the nasal bones, both frontal processes of the maxilla (and ethmoid and frontal sinuses, if involved), and the infra-orbital rims on both sides (and the floor of both orbits). Fractures in the zygoma or zygomatic process of the maxilla, separation of the zygomaticomaxillary sutures on both sides, deformity and discontinuity of the lateral walls of both maxillary sinuses, thickening of the lining mucosa or increased radiopacity of the maxillary sinus and sometimes the frontal and ethmoid sinuses, and

fractures through both pterygoid plates also occur. CT examination is required to supplement plain views of the skull because of multiple superimpositions of structures.

Examining the floor of the orbit in Waters' projections of the skull may be difficult because two different radiopaque lines often represent the lower limit of the orbit. One is the actual floor of the orbit, which is often thin and difficult to discern. The other is the inferior rim of the orbit, which is usually thicker bone and appears above the floor of the orbit. The presence of a less distinct orbital floor may suggest a blowout fracture of the orbital floor. The presence of herniated orbital contents through the floor and into the maxillary sinus is a useful sign of a blowout fracture. However, orbital floor fractures do not always have associated soft tissue herniation. CT imaging is useful in arriving at an accurate diagnosis.

Management

The treatment of this fracture is accomplished by reduction of the downward displacement of the maxilla. The maxilla is fixed in place by intermaxillary wires or arch bars. Usually treatment includes open reduction and interosseous wiring of the infraorbital rims. The accompanying fractures of the nose, nasal septum, orbital floor, and detached medial canthal ligaments also require repair. Leakage of cerebrospinal fluid requires the attention of a neurosurgeon. Antibiotics are required because of communication of the fractures with the paranasal sinuses.

CRANIOFACIAL DISJUNCTION (LE FORT III)

Definition

A Le Fort III midface fracture results when the traumatic force is of sufficient magnitude to completely separate the middle third of the facial skeleton from the cranium. The fracture line usually extends through the nasal bones and the frontal processes of the maxilla or nasofrontal and maxillofrontal sutures, across the floors of the orbits, and through the ethmoid and sphenoid sinuses and the zygomaticofrontal sutures (Fig. 28-18). It passes across both pterygomaxillary fissures and separates the pterygoid plates where they arise from the sphenoid bone (at their roots). If the maxilla is displaced and freely movable, a fracture must also have occurred in the area of the zygomaticotemporal suture. Because the zygoma or zygomatic arch is involved, these injuries are as a rule associated with multiple other maxillary fractures. Mandibular fractures are also observed in half the cases.

Clinical Features

Craniofacial disjunction produces a clinical appearance similar to pyramidal fracture. However, this injury is considerably more extensive. The soft tissue injuries are severe, with massive edema. The nose may be blocked with a blood clot, or blood, serum, or cerebrospinal fluid rhinorrhea may be present. Bleeding may occur into the periorbital tissues and all quadrants of the conjunctiva; a number of eye signs of neurologic importance are likely to be present. A "dish face" deformity is characteristic of these fractures, as is an anterior open bite (because of retro position of the maxillary incisors) with the posterior teeth in occlusion. Although the mandible is wide open, the patient is unable to separate the molars. Intraoral and extraoral palpation reveals irregular contours and step deformities, and crepitation is also apparent when the fragments are moved.

Radiographic Features

The radiographic projections of Le Fort III fractures usually are hazy because of extensive soft tissue swelling. The main radiographic findings are separated nasofrontal, maxillofrontal, zygomaticofrontal, and zygomaticotemporal sutures (Fig. 28-19). The nasal bones, frontal processes of the maxilla, both orbital

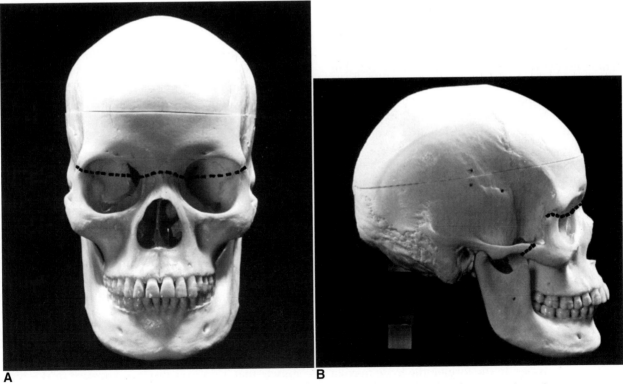

FIG. 28-18 Usual position of the Le Fort III craniofacial disjunction fracture on a frontal (**A**) and lateral (**B**) view.

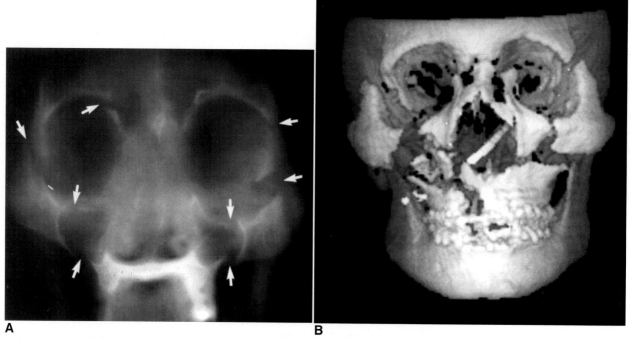

FIG. **28-19**   **A,** Tomographic view of multiple facial fractures, including a Le Fort III, through the ethmoid bones, lateral walls of the orbits *(arrows),* infraorbital rims *(arrows),* and lateral walls of the maxilla *(arrows).* **B,** Three-dimensional reformatted CT image of another patient with comparable facial fractures. Note the separation of each zygomati-cofrontal suture as well as fractures of the ethmoid bone, each anterior maxilla inferior to the orbit, and the maxillary alveolar ridge from the midface. (**A,** Courtesy C. Schow, DDS, Galveston, Texas; **B,** Courtesy M. Alder, DDS, San Antonio, Texas.)

floors, and pterygoid plates are likely to show radiolucent lines and discontinuity in some of these areas. The ethmoid and sphenoid sinuses are radiopaque, indicating the presence of fractures; the frontal sinus is also frequently involved. Associated fractures of the walls of the maxillary sinuses also result in a radiopaque appearance.

It is extremely difficult to document these multiple fractures with plain films alone; therefore CT images in concert with the clinical information are required.

Management

The associated severe soft tissue injury necessitates initial hemorrhage control, airway maintenance, and repair of lacerations. Surgery may be delayed until the edema has sufficiently resolved. The treatment of transverse fractures is complicated; fixation of the loose middle third of the facial skeleton is difficult because fractures of the zygomatic arch often occur. The only possibilities are external immobilization or immobilization within the tissues. In the former, the loose maxilla is suspended by wires through the cheeks from a metal head frame (halo) or fixed by using external pins

anchored in bone. The other possibility is immobilization within the tissues by using internal wiring to the closest solid bone superior to the fracture. A number of complications may develop during or after this treatment.

ZYGOMATIC FRACTURES

Definition

Unilateral fractures involving the zygoma are of two types: zygomatic arch fractures, in which just the arch is fractured, and zygomatic complex fractures, in which the zygomatic bone is separated from its frontal, maxillary, and temporal connections. Bilateral zygomatic fractures occur in association with Le Fort II and III fractures, described previously. Injuries to the zygomatic arch usually result from a forceful blow to the side of the face. Although the blow may displace the fragment medially, the arch is so well supported superiorly by the temporalis muscle and inferiorly by the masseter muscle that it is rarely displaced upward or downward. The arch may fracture at its center, resulting in a V-shaped medial displacement, or near its articulation with the zygomatic process of the maxilla, resulting in medial displacement of the anterior end of the zygomatic bone.

Clinical Features

Flattening of the upper cheek with tenderness and dimpling of the skin over the zygomatic arch and zygomaticofrontal suture and a fullness of the lower cheek may occur after zygomatic complex fracture. Step defects may be palpated in the zygomaticofrontal area and along the infraorbital rim. Some of the clinical characteristics of a zygomatic fracture may not be apparent much longer than an hour after trauma. Subsequently, they are masked by edema for about a week. In most cases, circumorbital ecchymosis and hemorrhage into the sclera (near the outer canthus) occur. Additional symptoms include unilateral epistaxis (for a short time after the accident), anesthesia or paresthesia of the cheek, and an altered level of the eye. The presence of diplopia suggests a significant injury to the floor of the orbit. Mandibular movement may be limited if the displaced zygomatic bone impinges on the coronoid process.

Radiographic Features

Because of edema obscuring the clinical features, the radiographic examination may provide the only means of determining the presence and extent of the injury. The occipitomental (Waters') radiograph provides an image of the whole zygoma and maxillary sinus. The submentovertex projection provides a good view of the zygomatic arch (Fig. 28-20). CT images can provide valuable three-dimensional information.

The zygomatic arch may fracture at its weakest point, about 1 cm posterior to the zygomaticotemporal suture. Separation or fracture of the frontozygomatic suture may occur. Fractures do not usually occur through the zygomaticomaxillary suture, but medially within the thin bone comprising the lateral wall of the antrum. As a result of this type of fracture, in some cases the maxillary antrum may become radiopaque and demonstrate a fluid level resulting from bleeding into the sinus.

Panoramic views of the zygomatic arch often reveal the zygomaticotemporal suture as a radiolucent line, which may even have the appearance of a discontinuity in the inferior border. This is a variation of normal anatomy and should not be misinterpreted as a fracture.

Management

When symptoms include minimal displacement of the zygomatic arch and no cosmetic deformity or impairment of eye movement, no treatment may be required. Otherwise, reduction is usually indicated. Fractures of the arch may be reduced through an intraoral or extraoral approach. If a fractured zygoma is treated within 5 days, the bones frequently snap into place and do not require fixation. When treatment has been delayed more than 5 days, the fragments can usually be reduced, but they do not remain in place. In such delayed treatment cases, the zygoma is fixed in place by elastic traction anchored to a headcap. If the fracture is left untreated for several months, it is almost impossible to reduce. In this case, treatment is not generally undertaken for the fracture itself, but rather focused on the associated structures with the objective of restoring function and appearance.

Monitoring the Healing of Fractures

Radiographic examination of the facial bones after trauma is usually necessary to measure the degree of reduction from treatment and to monitor the continued immobilization of the fracture site during repair. The monitoring of fracture repair should include examination of both the alignment of the cortical plates of the involved bone and remodeling and remineralization of the fracture site. During normal healing the fracture line increases in width about 2 weeks after reduction of the fracture. This results from the resorption of the fractured ends and small sequestered fragments of bone. Evidence of remineralization usually occurs 5 to 6 weeks after treatment. Unlike the long

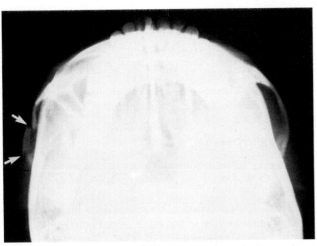

FIG. **28-20** Fractures of the zygomatic arch (arrows) are demonstrated on this submentovertex projection with reduced exposure time.

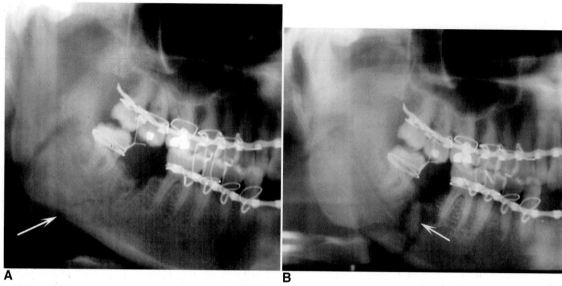

FIG. **28-21**   **A,** An example of a fracture through the tooth socket of the mandibular second molar (removed at the time of treatment), extending through the body of the mandible. The fracture line is barely perceptible, extending to the inferior cortex, where there is a small step defect *(arrow).* **B,** The same case after 6 months (the patient did not return for continued care); there are now signs of nonunion, including rounding of the edges of the fracture segments and an increase in the width of fracture line, as well as also signs of osteomyelitis with the presence of sequestra *(arrow).*

bones of the skeleton, rarely is a callus formed in healing jaw fractures. The complete remodeling of the fracture site with obliteration of the fracture line may take several months. On rare occasions, fracture lines may persist for years, even when the patient has made a clinically complete recovery. Possible complications of healing include malalignment of the fracture segments and inflammatory lesions related to nonvital teeth near or in the line of the fracture. Other complications include nonunion of the fractured segments seen as increased width of fracture line, cortication of the fractured surfaces and rounding of the sharp edges of the segments. The development of osteomyelitis of the fracture site (Fig. 28-21) will appear as an increase in sclerosis of the surrounding bone, inflammatory periosteal new bone, and development of sequestra.

BIBLIOGRAPHY

Brook IW, Wood N: Aetiology and incidence of facial fractures in adults, Int J Oral Surg 12:293, 1983.

Daffner RH: Imaging of facial trauma, Curr Probl Diagn Radiol 26:153, 1997.

Dingman TM, Natvig AC: Surgery of facial fractures, Philadelphia, 1967, WB Saunders.

Gerlock AJ Jr, Sinn DP, McBride KL: Clinical and radiographic interpretation of facial fractures, Boston, 1981, Little, Brown.

Hunter JG: Pediatric maxillofacial trauma, Pediatr Clin North Am 39:1127, 1992.

Kaban LB: Diagnosis and treatment of fractures of the facial bones in children 1943-1993, J Oral Maxillofac Surg 51:722, 1993.

Koltai PJ, Rabkin D: Management of facial trauma in children, Pediatr Clin North Am 43:1253, 1996.

Laine FJ, Conway WF, Laskin DM: Radiology of maxillofacial trauma, Curr Probl Diagn Radiol 22:145, 1993.

Matteson SR et al: Advanced imaging methods, Crit Rev Oral Biol Med 7:346, 1996.

Matteson S, Tyndall D: Pantomographic radiology: II, pantomography of trauma and inflammation of the jaws, Dent Radiol Photogr 56:21, 1982.

Newman J: Medical imaging of facial and mandibular fractures, Radiol Technol 69(5):417, 1998.

Shumrick KA: Recent advances and trends in the management of maxillofacial and frontal trauma, Facial Plast Surg 9(1):16, 1993.

TRAUMA TO TEETH

Andreasen JO, Andreasen FM: Essentials of traumatic injuries to the teeth: a step-by-step treatment guide, St. Louis, 2000, Mosby.

Andreasen JO et al: Effect of treatment delay upon pulp and periodontal healing of traumatic dental injuries—a review article, Dent Traumatol 18:116, 2002.

Josell SD, Abrams RG: Traumatic injuries to the dentition and its supporting structures, Pediatr Clin North Am 29:717, 1982.

LUXATION

Andreasen JO: Luxation of permanent teeth due to trauma: a clinical and radiographic follow-up study of 189 injured teeth, Scand J Dent Res 78:273, 1970.

AVULSION

Donaldson M, Kinirons MJ: Factors affecting the time of onset of resorption in avulsed and replanted incisor teeth in children, Dent Traumatol 17:205, 2001.

TOOTH CROWN FRACTURE

Ravn JJ: Follow-up study of permanent incisors with enamel fractures as a result of acute trauma, Scand J Dent Res 89:213, 1981.

Ravn JJ: Follow-up study of permanent incisors with enamel-dentin fracture after acute trauma, Scand J Dent Res 89:355, 1981.

Stockton LW, Suzuki M: Management of accidental and iatrogenic injuries to the dentition, J Can Dent Assoc 64:378, 1998.

CRACKED TOOTH SYNDROME

Fox K, Youngson CC: Diagnosis and treatment of the cracked tooth, Prim Dent Care 4:109, 1997.

Turp JC, Gobetti JP: The cracked tooth syndrome: an elusive diagnosis, J Am Dent Assoc 127:1502, 1996.

TOOTH ROOT FRACTURE

Cvek M, Mejare I, Andreason JO: Healing and prognosis of teeth with intra-alveolar fractures involving the cervical part of the root, Dent Traumatol 18:57, 2002.

Hovland EJ: Horizontal root fractures: treatment and repair, Dent Clin North Am 36:509, 1992.

Luebke RG: Vertical crown-root fractures in posterior teeth, Dent Clin North Am 28:883, 1984.

Majorana A et al: Clinical and epidemiological study of traumatic root fractures, Dent Traumatol 18:77, 2002.

Schetritt A, Steffensen B: Diagnosis and management of vertical root fractures, J Can Dent Assoc 61:607, 1995.

Schmidt BL, Stern M: Diagnosis and management of root fractures and periodontal ligament injury, J Calif Dent Assoc 24:51, 1996.

Walton RE, Michelich RJ, Smith GN: The histopathogenesis of vertical root fractures, J Endodont 10:48, 1984.

Wright EF: Diagnosis, treatment, and prevention of incomplete tooth fractures, Gen Dent 40:390, 1992.

COMPUTED TOMOGRAPHY OF JAW FRACTURES

Creasman CN et al: Computed tomography versus standard radiography in the assessment of fractures of the mandible, Ann Plast Surg 29:109, 1992.

Johnson DH: CT of maxillofacial trauma, Radiol Clin North Am 22:131, 1984.

Kassel EE, Noyek AM, Cooper PW: CT in facial trauma, J Otolaryngol 12:2, 1983.

Marsh JL et al: In vivo delineation of facial fractures: the application of advanced medical imaging technology, Ann Plast Surg 17:364, 1986.

Raustia AM et al: Conventional radiographic and computed tomographic findings in cases of fracture of the mandibular condylar process, J Oral Maxillofac Surg 48:1258, 1990.

TRAUMA TO THE MANDIBLE

Bailey BJ, Clark WD: Management of mandibular fractures, Ear Nose Throat J 62:371, 1983.

Chayra GA, Meador LR, Laskin DM: Comparison of panoramic and standard radiographs for the diagnosis of mandibular fractures, J Oral Maxillofac Surg 44:677, 1986.

Clark WD: Management of mandibular fractures, Am J Otolaryngol 13:125, 1992.

Ellis E, Moos KF, El-Attar A: Ten years of mandibular fractures: an analysis of 2,137 cases, Oral Surg 59:120, 1985.

Olson RA et al: Fractures of the mandible: a review of 580 cases, J Oral Maxillofac Surg 40:23, 1982.

Reiner SA et al: Accurate radiographic evaluation of mandibular fractures, Arch Otolaryngol Head Neck Surg 115:1083, 1989.

Winstanley RP: The management of fractures of the mandible, Br J Oral Maxillofac Surg 22:170, 1984.

CONDYLAR FRACTURES

Consensus Conference on Open or Closed Management of Condylar Fractures. 12th ICOMS. Budapest, 1995, Int J Oral Maxillofac Surg 27:243, 1998.

Dahlstrauom L, Kahnberg KE, Lindahl L: 15-year follow-up on condylar fractures, Int J Oral Maxillofac Surg 18:18, 1989.

Dimitroulis G: Condylar injuries in growing patients, Aust Dent J 42:367, 1997.

Hall MB: Condylar fractures: surgical management, J Oral Maxillofac Surg 52:1189, 1994.

Hayward JR, Scott RF: Fractures of the mandibular condyle, J Oral Maxillofac Surg 51:57, 1993.

Sahm G, Witt E: Long-term results after childhood condylar fractures: a computer-tomographic study, Eur J Orthod 11:154, 1989.

Silvennoinen U et al: Different patterns of condylar fractures: an analysis of 382 patients in a 3-year period, J Oral Maxillofac Surg 50:1032, 1992.

Walker RV: Condylar fractures: nonsurgical management, J Oral Maxillofac Surg 52:1185, 1994.

FRACTURES OF THE ALVEOLAR PROCESS

Andreasen JO: Fractures of the alveolar process of the jaw: a clinical and radiographic follow-up study, Scand J Dent Res 78:263, 1970.

Giovannini UM, Goudot P: Radiologic evaluation of mandibular and dentoalveolar fractures, Plast Reconstr Surg 109:2165, 2002.

TRAUMA TO THE MAXILLA

Banks P: Kiley's fractures of the middle third of the facial skeleton, Bristol, UK, 1981, Wright.

Close LG: Fractures of the maxilla, Ear Nose Throat J 62:365, 1983.

Luce EA: Developing concepts and treatment of complex maxillary fractures, Clin Plast Surg 19:125, 1992.

Marciani RD: Management of midface fractures: fifty years later, J Oral Maxillofac Surg 51:960, 1993.

Teichgraeber JF, Rappaport NJ, Harris JH Jr: The radiology of upper airway obstruction in maxillofacial trauma, Ann Plast Surg 27:103, 1991.

Tung TC et al: Dislocation of anatomic structures into the maxillary sinus after craniofacial trauma, Plast Reconstr Surg 101:1904, 1998.

ZYGOMATIC COMPLEX FRACTURES

Fuji N: Classification of malar complex fractures using computed tomography, J Oral Maxillofac Surg 41:562, 1983.

McLoughlin P, Gilhooly M, Wood G: The management of zygomatic complex fractures—results of a survey, Br J Oral Maxillofac Surg 32:284, 1994.

Prendergast ML, Wildes TO: Evaluation of the orbital floor in zygoma fractures, Arch Otolaryngol Head Neck Surg 114:446, 1988.

Sands T et al: Fractures of the zygomatic complex: a case report and review, J Can Dent Assoc 59:749, 1993.

Winstanley RP: The management of fractures of the zygoma, Int J Oral Surg 10(suppl 1):235, 1981.

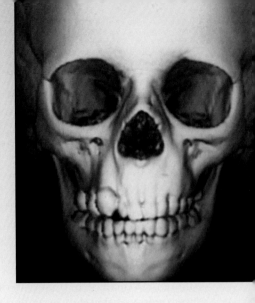

CHAPTER 29

Developmental Disturbances of the Face and Jaws

CAROL ANNE MURDOCH-KINCH

Developmental disturbances affect the normal growth and differentiation of craniofacial structures. As a consequence, they are usually first discovered in infancy or childhood. Many of the conditions discussed in this chapter have an unknown etiology. Some are caused by known and recently discovered genetic mutations, whereas others result from environmental factors. These conditions result in a variety of abnormalities of the face and jaws, including abnormalities of structure, shape, organization, and function of hard and soft tissues.

A multitude of conditions exist that affect the morphogenesis of the face and jaws, many of which are rare syndromes. This chapter briefly reviews the more common developmental abnormalities that may be encountered in dental practice.

Cleft Lip and Palate

Definition

A failure of fusion of the developmental processes of the face during fetal development may result in a variety of facial clefts. Cleft lip and cleft palate are the most common developmental craniofacial anomalies. Cleft lip with or without cleft palate (CL/P) and cleft palate (CP) are two different conditions with different etiologies. CL/P results from a failure of fusion of the medial nasal process and the maxillary process. This condition can range in severity from a unilateral cleft lip to bilateral complete clefting through the lip, alveolus, hard

and soft palate in the most severe cases. CP develops from a failure of fusion of the lateral palatal shelves. The minimal manifestation of cleft palate is a submucous cleft. Here, the palate appears to be intact, except for notching of the uvula (bifid uvula) or notching in the posterior border of the hard palate detectable by palpation. The most severe presentation is complete clefting of the hard and soft palate. The precise etiology of orofacial clefting is not completely understood. However, most cases of CL/P and CP are considered to be multifactorial with a strong genetic component. CL/P and CP can each be associated with other abnormalities, as part of a genetic malformation syndrome such as velocardiofacial syndrome (del 22q.11 syndrome—cleft palate, facial and cardiac abnormalities) or van der Woude syndrome (cleft lip and/or cleft palate and lip pits). Other factors that are implicated in the development of orofacial clefts include nutritional disturbances (prenatal folate deficiency); environmental teratogenic agents (maternal smoking, *in utero* exposure to anticonvulsants); stress, which results in increased secretion of hydrocortisone; defects of vascular supply to the involved region; and mechanical interference with the closure of the embryonic processes (cleft palate in Pierre Robin sequence). Clefts involving the lower lip and mandible are extremely rare.

Clinical Features

The frequency of CL/P and CP varies with gender and race, but in general CL/P is most common in males, whereas CP is more common in females. Both conditions are more common in Asians and Hispanics than African-Americans or Caucasians. The severity of CL/P varies from a notch in the upper lip to a cleft involving only the lip to extension into the nostril, resulting in deformity of the ala of the nose. As CL/P increases in severity, the cleft will include the alveolar process and palate. Bilateral cleft lip is more frequently associated with cleft palate. CP also varies in severity, ranging from involvement of only the uvula or soft palate to extension all the way through the palate to include the alveolar process in the region of the lateral incisor on one or both sides. With involvement of the alveolar process, there is an increase in frequency of dental anomalies in the region of the cleft including missing, hypoplastic, and supernumerary teeth, and enamel hypoplasia. Dental anomalies are also more prevalent in the mandible in these patients. In both CL/P and CP the palatal defects interfere with speech and swallowing. Affected individuals with palatal clefts are also at increased risk for recurrent middle ear infections because of the abnormal anatomy and function of the eustachian tube.

Radiographic Features

The typical appearance is a well-defined vertical radiolucent defect in the alveolar bone, as well as numerous associated dental anomalies (Fig. 29-1). These may include the absence of the maxillary lateral incisor and the presence of supernumerary teeth in this region. Often the involved teeth are malformed and poorly positioned. In patients with cleft lip and palate, there may be a mild delay in the development of maxillary and mandibular teeth, and an increased incidence of hypodontia in both arches. The osseous defect may extend to include the floor of the nasal cavity. In patients with a repaired cleft, a well-defined osseous defect may not be apparent but only a vertically short alveolar process at the cleft site.

Management

Management of CL/P and CP is complex, requiring the coordinated efforts of a multidisciplinary team know as a *Cleft Palate Team*. This team usually includes a plastic and reconstructive surgeon, oral and maxillofacial surgeon, ENT surgeon, orthodontist, dentist, speech therapist, psychologist, nutritionist, and social worker. Clefts of the palate are usually surgically repaired within the first year, whereas clefts of the lip are usually repaired within the first 3 months to aid in feeding and maternal/infant bonding. The bone in the cleft site is often augmented with bone grafting prior to replacement of missing teeth with either fixed or removable prosthodontics or dental implants. Orthodontic treatment is usually necessary to

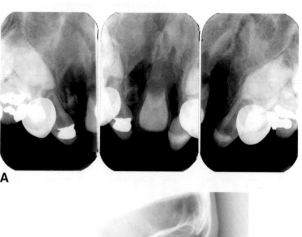

A

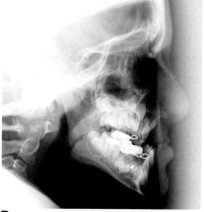

B

FIG. **29-1**   Cleft palate results in defects in the alveolar ridge and abnormalities of the dentition. **A,** Bilateral clefts of the maxilla in the lateral incisor regions and defects of the dentition. **B,** Lateral cephalometric view showing underdevelopment of the maxilla.

recreate a normal arch form and functional occlusion.

Crouzon Syndrome

Synonyms

Craniofacial dysostosis, syndromic craniosynostosis, premature craniosynostosis

Definition

Crouzon syndrome (CS) is an autosomal-dominant skeletal dysplasia characterized by variable expressivity and almost complete penetrance. It is one of many diseases characterized by premature craniosynostosis (closure of cranial sutures). Its incidence is estimated at 1/25,000 births. Of these cases, 33% to 56% may arise as a consequence of spontaneous mutations, with the remaining being familial. CS is caused by a mutation in fibroblast growth factor receptor II on chromosome 10. Mutations at this site are also responsible for other craniosynostosis syndromes with similar facial features but clinically visible limb abnormalities. In patients with CS the coronal suture usually closes first, and eventually all cranial sutures close early. Premature fusion of the synchondroses of the cranial base also occurs. The subsequent lack of bone growth perpendicular to the synchondroses and cranial coronal sutures produces the characteristic cranial shape and facial features.

Clinical Features

Patients characteristically have brachycephaly (short anterior-posterior skull length), hypertelorism (increased distance between eyes), and orbital proptosis (protruding eyes) (Fig. 29-2, *A* and *B*). In familial cases, the minimal criteria for diagnosis are hypertelorism and orbital proptosis. Patients may become blind as a result of early suture closure and increased intracranial pressure. The nose often appears prominent and pointed because the maxilla is narrow and short in a vertical and an anterior-posterior dimension. The anterior nasal spine is hypoplastic and retruded, failing to provide adequate support to the soft tissue of the nose. The palatal vault is high and the maxillary arch narrow and retruded, resulting in crowding of the dentition.

Radiographic Features

General radiographic features. The earliest radiographic signs of cranial suture synostosis are sclerosis and overlapping edges. Sutures that normally should look radiolucent on the skull film will not be detectable or will show sclerotic changes. Interestingly, on rare occasions the facial features may present prior to radiographic evidence of sutural synostosis. Premature fusion of the cranial base leads to diminished facial growth. In some cases, prominent cranial markings are noted, which are also seen in normal-growing patients, but they are more prominent because of an increase in intracranial pressure from the growing brain. These markings may be seen as multiple radiolucencies appearing as depressions (so-called *digital impressions*) of the inner surface of the cranial vault, which results in a beaten-metal appearance (Fig. 29-2, *C-E*).

Radiographic features of the jaws. The lack of growth in an anterior-posterior direction at the cranial base results in maxillary hypoplasia, creating a class III malocclusion in some patients. The maxillary hypoplasia contributes to the characteristic orbital proptosis because the maxilla forms part of the inferior orbital rim and, if severely hypoplastic, fails to adequately support the orbital contents. The mandible is typically smaller than normal but appears prognathic in relation to the severely hypoplastic maxilla.

Differential Diagnosis

Premature craniosynostosis, either isolated or part of a genetic syndrome, is a fairly common disorder. Its incidence is reported to range from 1/2100 to 1/2500 births. Other causes of craniosynostosis must be differentiated from Crouzon syndrome, including other syndromic forms of craniosynostosis and nonsyndromic coronal craniosynostosis. The characteristic facial features must be present to suggest Crouzon syndrome.

Management

The craniofacial features of Crouzon syndrome worsen over time because of the abnormal craniofacial growth. Early diagnosis permits surgical and orthodontic treatment from infancy through adolescence, coordinated by a Craniofacial Team. The objectives of these treatments are to allow normal brain growth and development by preventing increased intracranial pressure, to protect the eyes by providing adequate bony support, to provide an adequate airway, and to improve facial aesthetics and occlusal function. Because of early diagnosis and improvements in medical and dental care, most patients have normal intelligence and can expect a normal lifespan.

Hemifacial Microsomia

Synonyms

Hemifacial hypoplasia, craniofacial microsomia, lateral facial dysplasia, Goldenhar syndrome, oculo-auriculo-vertebral dysplasia

Definition

Hemifacial microsomia (HFM), the second most common developmental craniofacial anomaly after cleft lip and palate, affects 1/5600 live births. Patients with HFM display reduced growth and development of half of the face because of abnormal development of the first and second branchial arches. This malformation sequence is usually unilateral but occasionally may involve both sides (*craniofacial microsomia*). When the whole side of the face is involved, the mandible, maxilla, zygoma, external and middle ear, hyoid bone, parotid gland, fifth and seventh cranial nerves, musculature, and other soft tissues are diminished in size and sometimes fail to develop. Most cases occur spontaneously, but familial cases have been reported. There is a male predominance of 3:2 and a right side predominance of 3:2. Cases with vertebral abnormalities and

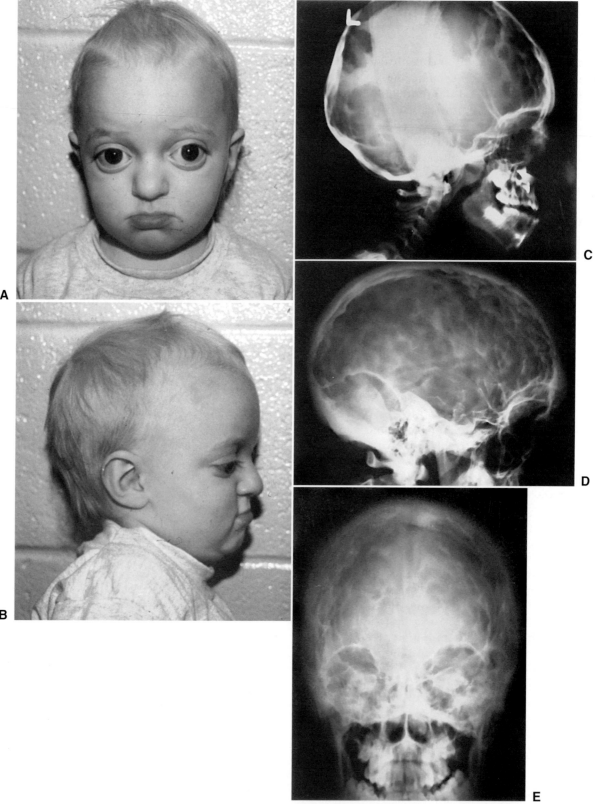

FIG. **29-2**   **A** and **B,** Characteristic facial features of Crouzon syndrome in this 2-year-old boy include orbital proptosis, hypertelorism, and midfacial hypoplasia. Rarely, they may precede the radiographic features of sutural synostosis. **C,** Crouzon syndrome results in early closure of the cranial sutures and depressions (digital impressions) on the inner surface of the calvarium from growth of the brain. **D** and **E,** Closure of the cranial sutures in another patient. Note also the prominent digital markings. (**D** and **E,** Courtesy Department of Radiology, Baylor University Hospital, Dallas, Texas.)

epibulbar dermoids have been considered to form a separate category within this condition, known as *Goldenhar syndrome* or *oculo-auriculo-vertebral dysplasia*.

Clinical Features

Hemifacial microsomia is usually apparent at birth. Patients with this condition have a striking appearance caused by progressive failure of the affected side to grow, which gives the involved side of the face a reduced dimension. In addition, aplasia or hypoplasia of the external ear (microtia) is common, and the ear canal often is missing. In some patients the skull is diminished in size. In about 90% of cases, there is malocclusion on the affected side. The midsagittal plane of the patient's face is curved toward the affected side. The occlusal plane will often be canted up to the affected side.

Radiographic Features

The primary radiographic finding is a reduction in the size of the bones on the affected side. This change is clearest in the mandible, which may show a reduction in the size of—or in severe cases, lack of *any* development of—the condyle, coronoid process, or ramus. The body is reduced in size, and a portion of the distal aspect may be missing (Fig. 29-3). The dentition on the affected side may show a reduction in the number or size of the teeth. CT examination shows a reduction in the size of the muscles of mastication and muscles of facial expression, and hypoplasia or atresia of the auditory canal and ossicles of the middle ear. The course of the facial nerve is often shown to be abnormal on CT examination of the temporal bone.

Differential Diagnosis

The features of hemifacial microsomia are characteristic. Condylar hypoplasia, especially that caused by a fracture at birth or by juvenile arthrosis (Boering's arthrosis), may be similar, but it does not produce the ear changes (see Chapter 25). Exposure of the face of a child to radiation therapy during growth also may result in underdevelopment of the irradiated tissues. In progressive hemifacial atrophy (Parry-Romberg syndrome), changes will become more severe over time but are generally not present at birth, and the ears are normal.

Management

The mandibular abnormalities may be corrected by conventional orthognathic surgery and/or distraction osteogenesis to lengthen the ramus on the affected side. Orthodontic intervention may correct or prevent malocclusion. The ear abnormalities may be repaired by plastic surgery or corrected with maxillofacial pros-

thetics, and the hearing loss may be partly corrected by hearing aids.

Treacher Collins Syndrome

Synonym

Mandibulofacial dysostosis

Definition

Treacher Collins syndrome (TCS) is an autosomal-dominant disorder of craniofacial development. It is the most common type of mandibulofacial dysostosis, with an incidence of 1/50,000. TCS has variable expressivity and complete penetrance. Approximately half of cases arise as the result of sporadic mutation; the rest are familial. TCS is caused by a mutation in the TCOF1 gene on chromosome 5.

Clinical Features

Individuals with Treacher Collins syndrome have a wide range of anomalies, depending on the severity of the condition. The most common clinical findings are relative underdevelopment or absence of the zygomatic bones, resulting in a small narrow face; a downward inclination of the palpebral fissures; underdevelopment of the mandible, resulting in a down-turned, wide mouth; malformation of the external ears; absence of the external auditory canal; and occasional facial clefts (Fig. 29-4, *A* and *B*). The palate develops with a high arch or cleft in 30% of cases. Hypoplasia of the mandible and a steep mandibular angle results in an Angle class II anterior open-bite malocclusion. Hypoplasia or atresia of the external ear, auditory canal, and ossicles of the middle ear may result in partial or complete deafness.

Radiographic Features

A striking finding is the hypoplastic or missing zygomatic bones, and hypoplasia of the lateral aspects of the orbits. The auditory canal, mastoid air cells, and articular eminence often are smaller than normal or absent. The maxilla and especially the mandible are hypoplastic, showing accentuation of the antegonial notch and a steep mandibular angle, which gives the impression that the body of the mandible is bending in an inferior and posterior direction (Fig. 29-4, *C-F*). The ramus is especially short, and the condyles are positioned posteriorly and inferiorly. The maxillary sinuses may be underdeveloped or absent.

Differential Diagnosis

Other disorders that may result in severe hypoplasia of the entire mandible include condylar agenesis,

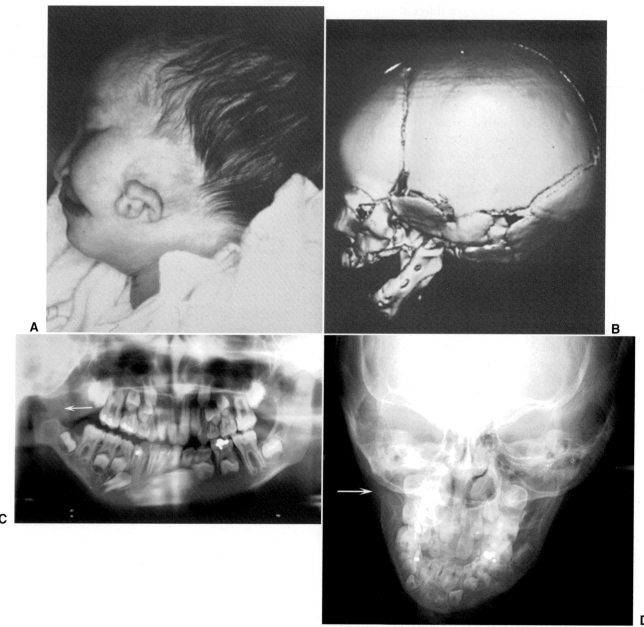

FIG. 29-3   A and B, Hemifacial microsomia, showing reduced size and malformation of the left ear and left side of the mandible. A, Clinical photograph of infant with hemifacial microsomia. B, Three-dimensional CT image of the affected side shows the extent of the bony malformation. Note the complete absence of the TMJ and coronoid process, as well as auditory canal atresia. A panoramic image (C) and a posterior-anterior skull view (D) of other cases showing lack of development of ramus, coronoid process, and condyle (arrows). (A and B, Courtesy Dr. Arlene Rozzelle, Children's Hospital of Michigan, Detroit, Mich.)

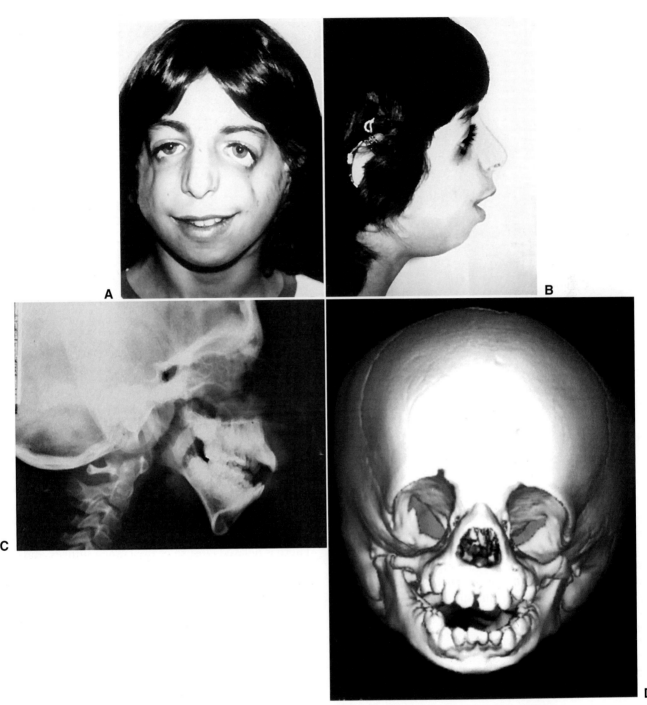

FIG. **29-4** **A** and **B,** Treacher Collins syndrome. Note the characteristic facies: downward-sloping palpebral fissures, colobomas of the outer third of the lower lids, depressed cheekbones, receding chin, little if any nasofrontal angle, and a nose that appears relatively large. **C,** Correlation of radiographic features with clinical features: short mandibular rami, steep mandibular angle, and an anterior open bite. The zygomas are poorly formed. **D-F,** Three-dimensional CT images of young child with Treacher Collins syndrome show the extent of the bony abnormalities, including the bilateral auditory canal atresia, aplasia of the zygomatic arch, and hypoplasia of the mandibular ramus with characteristic "curved" shape of the mandibular body and pronounced antegonial notching. (**F,** Courtesy Dr. Arlene Rozzelle, Children's Hospital of Michigan, Detroit, Mich.)

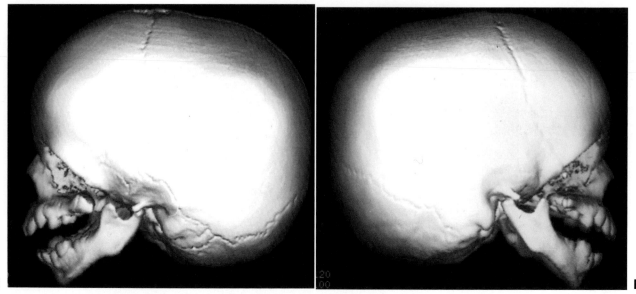

FIG. **29-4**—*cont'd*

Hallermann-Streiff syndrome, Nager syndrome, and Pierre Robin sequence, which can be a part of several other genetic syndromes.

Management

Comprehensive treatment of patients with Treacher Collins syndrome is optimally provided by a multidisciplinary Craniofacial Team. Growth of the facial bones during adolescence results in some cosmetic improvement. Surgical intervention, including bilateral distraction osteogenesis of the mandible, may be used to improve the osseous defects. Treatment of the external ear defects may involve plastic and reconstructive surgery and/or maxillofacial prosthetics. Coordinated orthodontics and orthognathic surgery are often used to treat the malocclusion and improve function and esthetics.

Cleidocranial Dysplasia

Synonym

Cleidocranial dysostosis

Definition

Cleidocranial dysplasia (CCD) is an autosomal-dominant malformation syndrome affecting bones and teeth; it affects both sexes equally. Its prevalence is estimated at 1 per 1 million. It can be inherited, or it may arise as a result of sporadic mutation. CCD is caused by a mutation in the RUNX2 gene on chromosome 6. It has variable expressivity and almost complete penetrance.

Clinical Features

Although the disease affects the entire skeleton, CCD primarily affects the skull, clavicles, and dentition. Affected individuals have been shown to be of shorter stature than unaffected relatives but not short enough for this to be considered a form of dwarfism. The face appears small in contrast to the cranium because of hypoplasia of the maxilla, a brachycephalic skull (reduced anteroposterior dimension with increased skull width), and the presence of frontal and parietal bossing. The paranasal sinuses may be underdeveloped. There is delayed closure of the cranial sutures, and the fontanels may remain patent years beyond the normal time of closure. The bridge of the nose may be broad and depressed, with hypertelorism (excessive distance between the eyes). The complete absence (aplasia) or reduced size (hypoplasia) of the clavicles allows excessive mobility of the shoulder girdle (Fig. 29-5, *A* and *B*).

The dental abnormalities produce most of the morbidity associated with cleidocranial dysplasia and are often the reason for diagnosis in mildly affected individuals. Characteristically, patients with this disease show prolonged retention of the primary dentition and delayed eruption of the permanent dentition. Extraction of primary teeth does not adequately stimulate eruption of underlying permanent teeth. A study of teeth from patients with cleidocranial dysplasia revealed a paucity or complete absence of cellular cementum on both erupted and unerupted teeth. Often unerupted supernumerary teeth are present, and considerable crowding and disorganization of the developing permanent dentition may occur. Recently

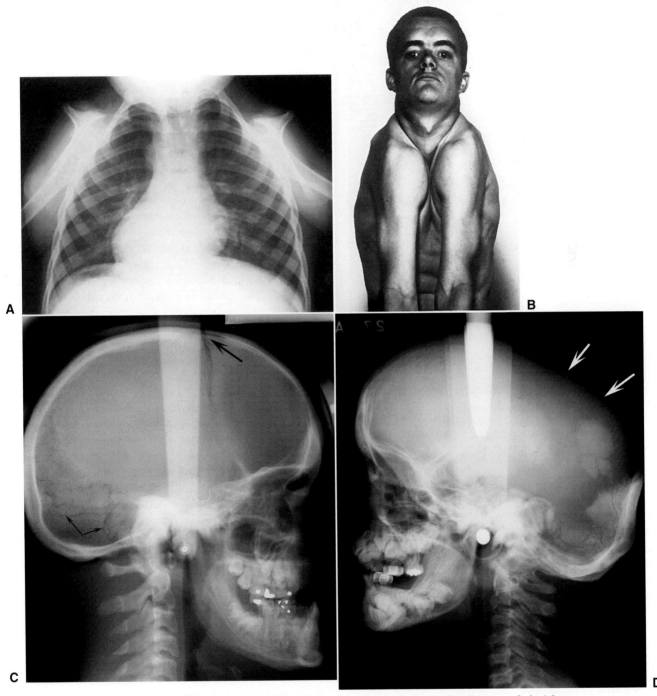

FIG. **29-5** Cleidocranial dysplasia. **A,** Chest radiograph. Note the absence of clavicles. **B,** The result is excessive mobility of the shoulders. Note also the frontal bossing and underdeveloped maxilla. **C,** On a lateral radiograph, note the wormian (sutural) bones in the occipital region *(arrows)* and the open fontanel *(large arrow)*. **D,** A lateral skull film showing a lack of development of the parietal bones *(arrows)*. (**A,** Courtesy Department of Radiology, Baylor University Hospital, Dallas, Tex.)

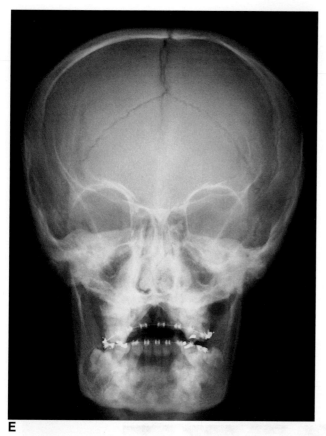

E

FIG. **29-5**—*cont'd* **E**, A posterior-anterior skull film. The brachycephaly results in a light-bulb–like shape to the silhouette of the skull and mandible.

the number of supernumerary teeth has been correlated with a reduction in skeletal height in these patients.

Radiographic Features

General radiographic features. The characteristic skull findings are brachycephaly, delayed or failed closure of the fontanels, open skull sutures, and multiple wormian bones (small, irregular bones in the sutures of the skull that are formed by secondary centers of ossification in the suture lines) (Fig. 29-5, *C-E*). In the most severe cases, very little formation of the parietal and frontal bones may occur. Typically the clavicles are underdeveloped to varying degrees, and in approximately 10% of cases, they are completely absent. Other bones also may be affected, including the long bones, vertebral column, pelvis, and bones of the hands and feet.

Radiographic features of the jaws. In cleidocranial dysplasia the maxilla and paranasal sinuses characteristically are underdeveloped, resulting in maxillary micrognathia. The mandible is usually normal in size.

A patent (open) mandibular symphysis has been reported in 3% of adults and 64% of children. Several investigators have described the alveolar bone overlying unerupted teeth as being denser than usual, with a coarse trabecular pattern in the mandible. This correlates to the histologic findings of decreased resorption and multiple reversal lines. It may account for the delayed eruption in teeth not mechanically obstructed by supernumerary and other unerupted teeth.

Radiographic features associated with the teeth. Characteristic features include prolonged retention of the primary dentition and multiple unerupted permanent and supernumerary teeth (Fig. 29-6). The number of supernumerary teeth varies; as many as 63 in one individual have been reported. The unerupted teeth develop most commonly in the anterior maxilla and bicuspid regions of the jaws. Many resemble bicuspids, and these unerupted teeth may develop dentigerous cysts. The supernumerary teeth develop, on average, 4 years later than the corresponding normal teeth. Because of this it has been proposed that the supernumerary teeth represent a third dentition.

Differential Diagnosis

Cleidocranial dysplasia may be identified by the family history, excessive mobility of the shoulders, clinical examination of the skull, and pathognomonic radiographic findings of prolonged retention of the primary teeth with multiple unerupted supernumerary teeth. Other conditions associated with multiple unerupted and supernumerary teeth, such as Gardner's syndrome and pycnodysostosis, must be considered in the differential diagnosis.

Management

In cleidocranial dysplasia dental care should include the removal of primary and supernumerary teeth to improve the possibility of spontaneous eruption of the permanent teeth. In order to aid the eruption of normal permanent teeth, the overlying bone should be removed to expose the crown when half of the root is formed to aid their eruption. Autotransplantation of teeth has been shown to be a successful strategy in treating older patients. Ideally, patients should be identified early, before 5 years of age, in order to take advantage of combined orthodontic/surgical treatment. Prosthodontic rehabilitation with dental implants has been used in some cases. Patients should be monitored for development of distal molars and cysts until late adolescence.

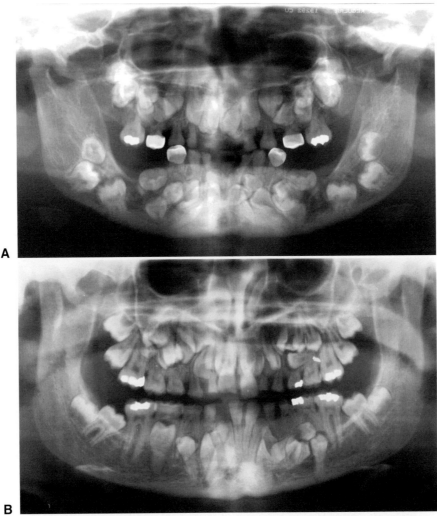

FIG. **29-6** A and B, Panoramic images of cleidocranial dysplasia. Note the prolonged retention of the primary dentition and multiple unerupted supernumerary teeth and lack of normal coronoid notches.

Hemifacial Hyperplasia

Synonyms
Hemifacial hypertrophy, hemihyperplasia

Definition
Hemifacial hyperplasia is a condition in which half of the face—the maxilla alone, the maxilla with the mandible, or half of the faces in concert with other parts of the body—grows to unusual proportions. The cause of this condition is unknown. Some cases are associated with genetic diseases such as Beckwith-Weidemann syndrome.

Clinical Features
Hemifacial hyperplasia begins at birth and usually continues throughout the growing years. In some cases it may not be recognized at birth but becomes more apparent with growth. It often occurs with other abnormalities, including mental deficiency, skin abnormalities, compensatory scoliosis, genitourinary tract anomalies, and various neoplasms, including Wilms' tumor of the kidney, adrenocortical tumor, and hepatoblastoma (Beckwith-Weidemann syndrome). Females and males are affected with approximately equal frequency. The dentition of affected individuals may show unilateral enlargement, accelerated development, and

premature loss of primary teeth. The tongue and alveolar bone enlarge on the involved side.

Radiographic Features

Radiographic examination of the skulls of these patients reveals, on the affected side, enlargement of the bones, including the mandible (Fig. 29-7), maxilla, zygoma, and frontal and temporal bones. There have been a few cases reported involving only one side of the maxilla or one side of the mandible.

Differential Diagnosis

The differential diagnosis should consider hemifacial hypoplasia of the opposite side, arteriovenous aneurysms, hemangioma, and congenital lymphedema. Also, severe condylar hyperplasia that may involve half of the mandible should be considered (see Chapter 25). The presence of enlarged teeth together with rapid eruption of the dentition suggests hemifacial hyperplasia. Cases limited to one side of the maxilla must be differentiated from monostotic fibrous dyspla-

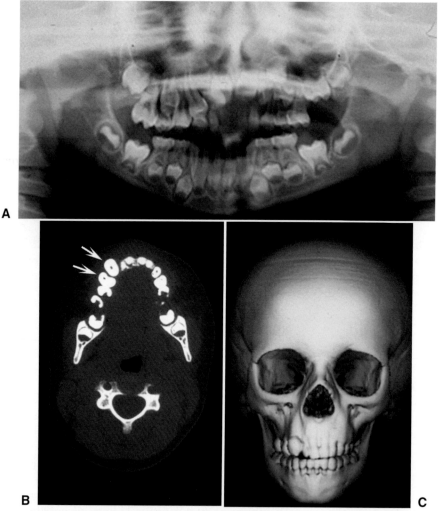

FIG. **29-7**   Hemifacial hyperplasia, revealing enlargement of the right maxilla only. **A,** Panoramic radiograph shows accelerated dental development limited to the right maxilla in a 5-year-old male. **B,** A CT axial image using bone algorithm of the same patient, demonstrating enlargement of the maxillary cuspid and first bicuspid *(arrows)* as compared with the contralateral side. **C,** Three-dimensional CT scan shows the subtle bony enlargement of the right maxilla and the right cuspid.

sia and segmental odontomaxillary dysplasia, both of which have characteristic changes in the radiographic appearance of the alveolar bone, not present in hemifacial hyperplasia.

Management

There have not been a significant number of cases of hemifacial hyperplasia reported with long-term follow-up to make definitive recommendations for treatment. Although most cases are isolated, a child with suspected hemifacial hyperplasia should be referred to a medical geneticist for diagnosis and early detection of one of several genetic syndromes that can be associated with this condition.

Segmental Odontomaxillary Dysplasia

Synonym

Hemimaxillofacial dysplasia

Definition

Segmental odontomaxillary dysplasia (SOD) is a developmental abnormality of unknown etiology that affects the posterior alveolar process of one side of one maxilla, including the teeth and attached gingiva.

Clinical Features

The abnormality is always unilateral and results in enlargement of the alveolar process, gingiva, and teeth. Frequently teeth are missing (most commonly the bicuspids), and some of the teeth that remain are unerupted. Unilateral hypertrichosis and mild facial enlargement have been reported in a few cases. Most cases are detected in childhood because a parent notices the lack of tooth eruption or mild facial asymmetry, or the dentist notices missing premolars radiographically.

Radiographic Features

The density of the maxillary alveolar process is increased, with a greater number of thick trabeculae that appear to be aligned in a vertical orientation (Fig. 29-8). The roots of the deciduous teeth are larger than on the unaffected side and usually are splayed in shape. The crowns of the deciduous teeth and sometimes the permanent teeth are enlarged. Enlargement of pulp chambers and irregular resorption of the roots of deciduous teeth also may be seen. The maxillary sinus does not pneumatize the alveolar process and thus appears smaller than on the contralateral side. There is often delayed eruption of the first and second permanent molars.

Differential Diagnosis

Other conditions that must be differentiated from SOD include segmental hemifacial hyperplasia, monostotic fibrous dysplasia, and regional odontodysplasia. Hemifacial hyperplasia is not associated with coarse vertically oriented trabeculae in the bone; monostotic fibrous dysplasia is not typically associated with missing teeth and unlike SOD, will continue to show disproportionate growth of the affected side; and regional odontodysplasia typically is associated with ghost teeth and is not associated with expansion and alteration in trabecular pattern in the alveolar bone.

Lingual Salivary Gland Depression

Synonyms

Lingual mandibular bone depression, developmental salivary gland defect, Stafne defect, Stafne bone cyst, static bone cavity, and latent bone cyst

Definition

Lingual mandibular bone depressions represent a group of concavities in the lingual surface of the mandible, where the depression is lined with an intact outer cortex. Historically they were referred to as *pseudocysts* because they resemble cysts radiographically, but they are not true cysts because no epithelial lining is present. The most common location is within the submandibular gland fossa and often close to the inferior border of the mandible. This lingual posterior variant (LP) of these depressions was first described by Stafne in 1942. This well-defined deep depression is thought to result from or be associated with growth of the salivary gland adjacent to the lingual surface of the mandible. Similar defects have also been described in the anterior region near the apical region of the bicuspids, associated with the sublingual glands (lingual anterior variant, or LA), and very rarely on the medial surface of the ascending ramus, associated with the parotid gland (medial ramus variant, or MR). In LP developmental bone defects investigated surgically, an aberrant lobe of the submandibular gland has been described to extend into the bony depression; however, CT imaging of some of these defects reveals fat tissue and no evidence of gland. The etiology remains unknown, but the condition is a developmental anomaly that has been documented to develop in patients as old as 30 years and as young as 11 years. These defects may continue to slowly grow in size.

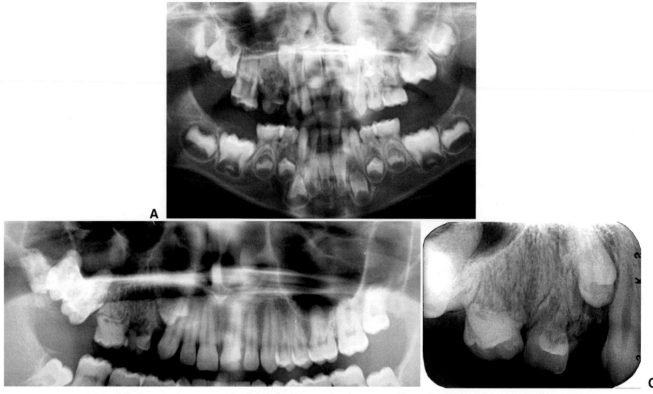

FIG. **29-8**   **A,** A panoramic view of segmental odontomaxillary dysplasia. Note the large left maxillary deciduous molars compared with the right side and the lack of formation of the bicuspids, delayed eruption of the first molar, and the dense bone pattern of the left maxillary alveolar process. **B** and **C,** A second case demonstrating the coarse trabecular pattern of the right maxillary alveolar process and delayed eruption of the maxillary right first bicuspid and molars.

Clinical Features

Although lingual mandibular bone depressions appear to be relatively rare, with an incidence of LP of about 0.10%-0.48%, it is likely that many go unreported. LA incidence is even less, at 0.009%. These concavities are asymptomatic and almost impossible to palpate; generally they are discovered only incidentally during radiographic examination of the area. In a recent review of a large number of cases, males predominated females at 6.1:1 with a peak incidence in the fifth and sixth decades.

Radiographic Features

A lingual mandibular bone depression is a well-defined round, ovoid, or occasionally, lobulated radiolucency that ranges in diameter from 1 to 3 cm (Fig. 29-9). The LP defect is located below the inferior alveolar nerve canal and anterior to the angle of the mandible, in the region of the antegonial notch and submandibular gland fossa. Rare LA examples are located in the apical region of the mandibular premolars or cuspids and are related to the sublingual gland fossa, above the mylohyoid muscle. The margins of the radiolucent defect are well defined by a dense sclerotic radiopaque margin of variable width, which is usually thicker on the superior aspect. This appearance is the result of the x rays passing tangentially through the relatively thick walls of the depression. This cortical outline is often less distinct in the LA variant. The LP defect may involve the inferior border of the mandible. Computed tomography (CT) images reportedly reveal tissue, with the same density as fat within the defect (Fig. 29-10), or in some cases, there is continuity of the tissue within the defect with the adjacent salivary gland.

Differential Diagnosis

The appearance and location of the radiographic image of this developmental bone defect are characteristic and

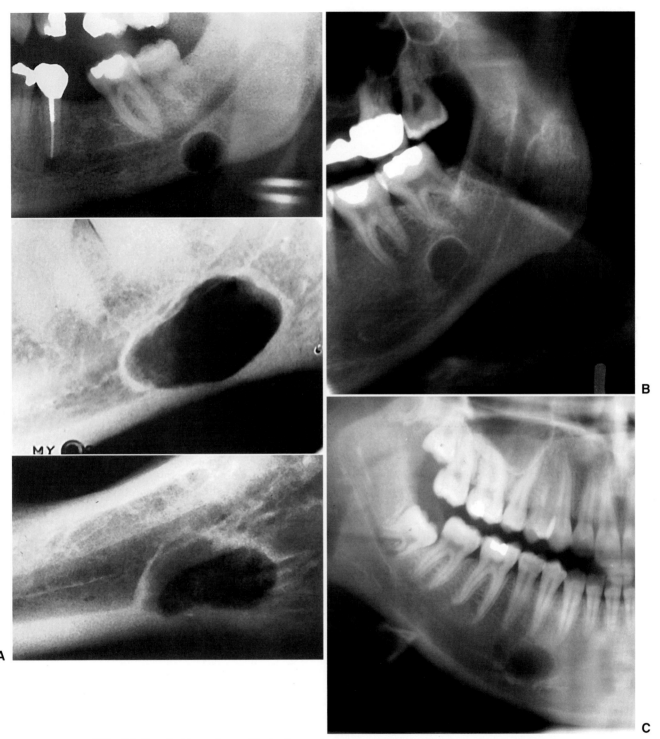

FIG. **29-9**   **A,** Lingual mandibular bone depressions of the posterior variant usually are seen as sharply defined radiolucencies beneath the mandibular canal in the region of the submandibular gland fossa. These defects can erode the inferior border of the mandible. **B,** An unusual variant with a superior position above the inferior alveolar canal. **C,** An anterior variant within the sublingual gland fossa.

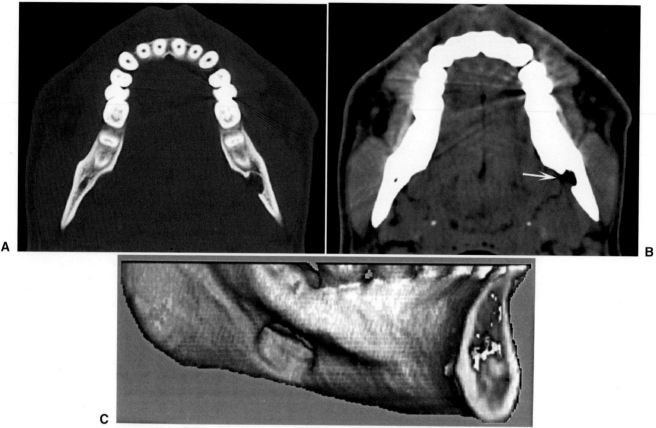

FIG. 29-10   CT scans of lingual mandibular bone depressions, posterior variant. **A** and **B** are axial bone and soft tissue windows of the same case. Note the well-defined defect extending from the medial surface of the mandible and the corresponding soft tissue image, which shows radiolucent tissue within the defect that has the density equivalent of fat tissue *(arrow)*. **C**, A three-dimensional, reformatted CT image revealing a defect extending from the medial surface of the mandible.

easily identified. Lingual mandibular bone depressions can be readily differentiated from odontogenic lesions such as cysts because the epicenter of odontogenic lesions is located above the inferior alveolar canal. However, when the defect is related to the sublingual gland and appears above the canal, odontogenic lesions should be considered in the differential diagnosis.

Management
Recognition of the lesion should preclude any treatment or surgical exploration or the need for advanced imaging such as CT. The defect may increase in size with time. There are rare reports of salivary gland neoplasms developing in the soft tissue within the defect. Destruction of the well-defined cortex of the defect may indicate the presence of a neoplasm.

Focal Osteoporotic Bone Marrow

Synonym
Marrow space

Definition
Focal osteoporotic bone marrow is a radiologic term indicating the presence of radiolucent defects within the cancellous portion of the jaws. Histologic examination reveals normal areas of hematopoietic or fatty marrow. The etiology is unknown but has been postulated to be (1) bone marrow hyperplasia, (2) persistent embryologic marrow remnants, or (3) sites of abnormal healing following extraction, trauma, or local inflammation. This entity is a variation of normal anatomy.

Clinical Features

Focal osteoporotic bone marrow defects are usually clinically asymptomatic and are commonly an incidental radiographic finding. These marrow spaces are more common in middle-aged women.

Radiographic Features

A common site for focal osteoporotic bone marrow is the mandibular molar-premolar region. Other sites include the maxillary tuberosity region, mandibular retromolar area, edentulous locations, occasionally the furcation region of mandibular molars, and rarely the area near the apex of teeth. The radiographic appearance of focal osteoporotic bone marrow space is quite variable. The internal aspect is radiolucent because of the presence of fewer trabeculae in comparison with the surrounding bone. The periphery may be ill-defined and blending or may appear to be corticated.

The immediate surrounding bone is normal, without any sign of a bone reaction (Fig. 29-11).

Differential Diagnosis

A small simple bone cyst may have a similar appearance because there is usually no bone reaction at the periphery of a simple bone cyst. When the osteoporotic bone marrow occurs in the furcation region or at the apex of a tooth, the differential diagnosis includes the presence of an inflammatory lesion. If the area is normal bone marrow, the lamina dura should be intact. Very early inflammatory lesions that have not yet stimulated a visible osteoblastic response may appear similar.

Management

No treatment is required for the osteoporotic bone marrow space. Prior radiographs of the region should always be obtained if available. When doubt exists about

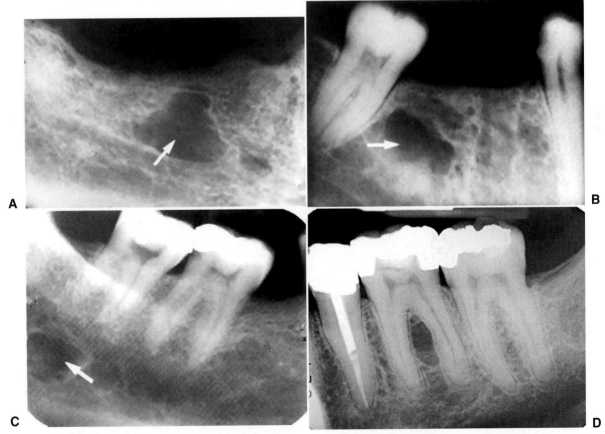

FIG. **29-11** A–C, Focal osteoporotic bone marrow defect, seen as a radiolucency (*arrow*). A few internal trabeculae may be present, and the periphery varies from well defined to ill defined. **D,** An example located in the furcation of a mandibular first molar. Note that the periodontal ligament space and lamina dura are intact.

the true nature of the radiolucency, a longitudinal study with films at 3-month intervals may be prescribed. The marrow space should not increase in size.

BIBLIOGRAPHY

Cohen MM Jr., McLean RE: Craniosynostosis: diagnosis, evaluation, and management, ed 2, New York, 2000, Oxford University Press.

Elmslie FV, Reardon W: Craniofacial developmental abnormalities, Curr Opin Neurol 11:103, 1998.

Friede H: Abnormal craniofacial growth, Acta Odontol Scand 53:203, 1995.

Goodman RM, Gorlin RJ: Atlas of the face in genetic disorders, ed 2, St. Louis, 1977, Mosby.

Gorlin RJ, Cohen MM Jr., Hennekam RCM: Syndromes of the head and neck, ed 4, New York, 2001, Oxford University Press.

Neville BW, Damm DD, Allen CM, and Bouquot JE: Oral and Maxillofacial Pathology, ed 2, Philadelphia, 2002, WB Saunders.

Worth HM: Principles and practice of oral radiologic interpretation, Chicago, 1963, Year Book.

Zarb GA et al: Temporomandibular joint and masticatory muscle disorders, Copenhagen, 1994, Munksgaard.

CLEFT LIP AND CLEFT PALATE

Brouwers HJ, Kuijpers-Jagtman AM: Development of permanent tooth length in patients with unilateral cleft lip and palate, Am J Orthod Dentofacial Orthop 99:543, 1991.

Derijcke A et al: The incidence of oral clefts: a review, Br J Oral Maxillofac Surg 34:488, 1996.

Habel A et al: Management of cleft lip and palate, Arch Dis Child 74:360, 1996.

Harris EF, Hullings JG: Delayed dental development in children with isolated cleft lip and palate, Arch Oral Biol 35:469, 1990.

Hibbert SA, Field JK: Molecular basis of familial cleft lip and palate, Oral Dis 2:238, 1996.

Koch H et al: Cleft malformation of lip, alveolus, hard and soft palate, and nose (LAHSN): a critical view of the terminology, the diagnosis and gradation as a basis for documentation and therapy, Br J Oral Maxillofac Surg 33:51, 1995.

Pham AND, Seow WK, Shusterman S: Developmental dental changes in isolated cleft lip and palate. Pediatr Dent 19(2):109-113, 1997.

Shapira Y, Lubit E, Kuftinec MM: Hypodontia in children with various types of clefts, Angle Ortho 70(1):16-21, 2000.

Smahel Z, Mullerova Z: Craniofacial growth and development in unilateral cleft lip and palate: clinical implications (a review), Acta Chir Plast 37:29, 1995.

Wyszynski DF et al: Genetics of nonsyndromic oral clefts revisited, Cleft Palate Craniofac J 33:406, 1996.

CROUZON SYNDROME

Bruce DA: Consensus: craniofacial synostoses: Apert and Crouzon syndromes, Childs Nerv Syst 12:734, 1996.

Murdoch-Kinch CA, Bixler D, and Ward RE: Cephalometric analysis of families with dominantly inherited Crouzon syndrome: an aid to diagnosis in family studies. Am J Med Genet 77:405-411, 1998.

Tuite GF, Evanson J, Chong WK, Thompson DNP, Harkness WF, Jones BM, and Hayward RD: The beaten copper cranium: a correlation between intracranial pressure, cranial radiographs, and computed tomographic scans in children with craniosynostosis. Neurosurgery 39:691-699, 1996.

HEMIFACIAL MICROSOMIA

Figueroa AA, Fields H: Craniovertebral malformation in hemifacial microsomia, J Cranio Genet Dev Biol 1(suppl): 167, 1985.

Finegold M: Hemifacial microsomia. In Bergsma D, editor: Birth defects compendium, ed 2, New York, 1973, Alan R Liss.

Marsh JL et al: Facial musculoskeletal asymmetry in hemifacial microsomia, Cleft Palate J 26:292, 1989.

Maruko E, Hayes C, Evans CA, Padwa B, Mulliken JB: Hypodontia in Hemifacial microsomia, Cleft Palate Craniofac J38(1):15-19, 2001.

Mazzeo N et al: Progressive hemifacial atrophy (Parry-Romberg syndrome): case report, Oral Surg Oral Med Oral Pathol Oral Radiol Endod 79:30, 1995.

Monahan R, Seder K, Patel P, Alder M, Grud S, and O'Gara M: Hemifacial microsomia. Etiology, diagnosis and treatment, JADA 132:1402-1408, 2001.

Sze RW, Paladin AM, Lee S, Cunningham ML: Hemifacial microsomia in pediatric patients: asymmetric abnormal development of the first and second branchial arches, AJR 178:1523-1530, 2002.

TREACHER COLLINS SYNDROME

Dixon MJ: Treacher Collins syndrome, J Med Genet 32:806, 1995.

Herman TE, Siegel MJ: Special imaging casebook: Treacher Collins syndrome, J Perinatol 16:413, 1996.

Marres HA et al: The Treacher Collins syndrome: a clinical, radiological, and genetic linkage study on two pedigrees, Arch Otolaryngol Head Neck Surg 121:509, 1995.

Posnick JC: Treacher Collins syndrome: perspectives in evaluation and treatment, J Oral Maxillofac Surg 55:1120, 1997.

CLEIDOCRANIAL DYSPLASIA

Ishii K et al: Characteristics of jaw growth in cleidocranial dysplasia, Cleft Palate Craniofac J 35:161, 1998.

Jensen BL, Kreiborg S: Craniofacial growth in cleidocranial dysplasia: a roentgencephalometric study, J Craniofac Genet Dev Biol 15:35, 1995.

Jensen BL, Kreiborg S: Development of the dentition in cleidocranial dysplasia, J Oral Pathol Med 19:89, 1990.

Rushton MA: Anomaly of cementum in cleidocranial dysostosis, Br Dent J 100:81, 1956.

Seow WK, Hertzberg J: Dental development and molar root length in children with cleidocranial dysplasia, Pediatr Dent 17:101, 1995.

Yamamoto H et al: Cleidocranial dysplasia: a light microscope, electron microscope, and crystallographic study, Oral Surg Oral Med Oral Pathol 68:195, 1989.

Yoshida T, Kanegane H, Osata M, Yanagida M, Miyawaki T, Ito Y, Shigesada K: Functional analysis of RUNX2 mutations in Japanese patients with Cleidocranial dysplasia demonstrates novel genotype-phenotype correlations, Am J Hum Genet 71:724-738, 2002.

HEMIFACIAL HYPERPLASIA

Fraumeni JF et al: Wilms' tumor and congenital hemihypertrophy: report of five new cases and review of the literature, Pediatrics 40:886, 1967.

Golnaz K, LaPointe HJ, Armstrong JEA, Wysocki GP: Idiopathic noncondylar hemimandibular hyperplasia, Int J Paediatr Dent 11:298-303, 2001.

Hoyme HE, Seaver LH, Procopio F, Crooks W, Feingold M: Isolated hemihyperplasia (hemihypertrophy): report of a prospective multicenter study of the incidence of neoplasia and review. Am J Med Genet 79(2):274-278, 1998.

Kogon SL, Jarvis AM, Daley TD, Kane MF: Hemifacial hypertrophy affecting the maxillary dentition: report of a case, Oral Surg Oral Med Oral Pathol 58(5):549-553, 1984.

SEGMENTAL ODONTOMAXILLARY DYSPLASIA

Danforth RA et al: Segmental odontomaxillary dysplasia: report of eight cases and comparison with hemimaxillofacial dysplasia, Oral Surg Oral Med Oral Pathol 70:81, 1990.

DeSalvo MS et al: Segmental odontomaxillary dysplasia (hemimaxillofacial dysplasia): case report, Pediatr Dent 18:154, 1996.

Miles DA et al: Hemimaxillofacial dysplasia: a newly recognized disorder of facial asymmetry, hypertrichosis of the facial skin, unilateral enlargement of the maxilla, and hypoplastic teeth in two patients, Oral Surg Oral Med Oral Pathol 64:445, 1987.

Packota GV et al: Radiographic features of segmental odontomaxillary dysplasia: a study of 12 cases, Oral Surg Oral Med Oral Pathol Oral Radiol Endod 82:577, 1996.

Prusack N, Pringle G. Scotti V, Chen S-Y: Segmental odontomaxillary dysplasia: a case report and review of the literature, Oral Surg Oral Med Oral Pathol Oral Radiol Endod 90:483-8, 2000.

LINGUAL MANDIBULAR BONE DEPRESSION

Hansson L: Development of a lingual mandibular bone cavity in an 11-year-old boy, Oral Surg 49:376, 1980.

Karmiol M, Walsh R: Incidence of static bone defect of the mandible, Oral Surg 26:225, 1968.

Parvizi F, Rout PG: An ossifying fibroma presenting as Stafne's idiopathic bone cavity, Dentomaxillofac Radiol 26(6):361, 1997.

Philipsen HP, Takata T, Reichart PA, Sato S, Suei Y: Lingual and buccal mandibular bone depressions: a review based on 583 cases from a world-wide literature survey, including 69 new cases from Japan, Dentomaxillofac Radiol 31:281-290, 2002.

Tolman DE, Stafne EC: Developmental bone defects of the mandible, Oral Surg 24:488, 1967.

FOCAL OSTEOPOROTIC BONE MARROW

Barker B et al: Focal osteoporotic bone marrow defects of the jaws, Oral Surg 38:404, 1974.

Crawford B, Weathers D: Osteoporotic marrow defects of the jaws, J Oral Surg 28:600, 1970.

Schneider LC et al: Osteoporotic bone marrow defect: radiographic features and pathogenic factors, Oral Surg 65:127, 1988.

Standish S, Shafer W: Focal osteoporotic bone marrow defects of the jaws, J Oral Surg 20:123, 1997.

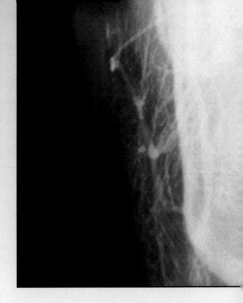

CHAPTER 30

Salivary Gland Radiology

BYRON W. BENSON

Definition of Salivary Gland Disease

Dental diagnosticians are responsible for detecting disorders of the salivary glands. A familiarity with salivary gland disorders and applicable current imaging techniques is an essential element of the clinician's armamentarium. Both major and minor salivary glands may be involved pathologically; however, this chapter deals only with the major glands. Salivary gland disease processes may be divided into the following clinical categories: inflammatory disorders, noninflammatory disorders, and space-occupying masses. Inflammatory disorders are acute or chronic and may be secondary to ductal obstruction by sialoliths, trauma, infection, or space-occupying lesions such as neoplasia. Noninflammatory disorders are metabolic and secretory abnormalities associated with diseases of nearly all the endocrine glands, malnutrition, and neurologic disorders. Space-occupying masses are cystic or neoplastic; the neoplasms are benign or malignant.

Clinical Signs and Symptoms

Diseases of the major salivary glands may have single or multiple clinical features. Unilateral or bilateral swellings in the areas of the parotid and submandibular glands should create a clinical suspicion of salivary gland disease. Pain and altered salivary flow may be present. Because the periodicity and longevity of these symptoms are important in the differential diagnosis, a review of the medical history and physical condition of the patient may provide important information. A history of skin, endocrine, or swallowing abnormalities may suggest a systemic collagen disease or metabolic disorder.

Differential Diagnosis of Salivary Enlargements

ENLARGEMENTS OF THE PAROTID AREA

Unilateral enlargements of the parotid area are categorized by the presence of a discrete, palpable mass or a diffuse swelling. If no mass is apparent, sialadenitis should be considered. Sialadenitis may be primary or secondary to ductal obstruction (retrograde). A mass superficial to the gland suggests lymphadenitis, an infected preauricular cyst, an infected sebaceous cyst, benign lymphoid hyperplasia, or an extraparotid tumor. A mass intrinsic to the gland suggests a neoplasm (benign or malignant), intraglandular lymph node, or hamartoma. Rapid growth, facial nerve paralysis, rock-hard texture, pain, and older age of occurrence are clinically suggestive of malignant neoplasms.

The differential diagnosis of asymptomatic bilateral enlargements of the parotid area may include benign lymphoepithelial lesion, Sjögren syndrome, alcoholism, medication (iodine and certain heavy metals), and Warthin tumor. Painful bilateral enlargement may occur after radiation treatment or secondary to bacterial or viral sialadenitis (including mumps) when accompanied by systemic symptoms.

A differential diagnosis of diffuse facial swelling in the parotid region, but not related to abnormalities of the gland, includes hypertrophy of the masseter muscle, accessory parotid gland, lesions related to the temporomandibular joint, and osteomyelitis of the ramus of the mandible. A palpable mass superficial to the gland suggests lymphadenitis, an infected preauricular or sebaceous cyst, benign lymphoid hyperplasia, or extraparotid tumor (Box 30-1).

BOX 30-1
Differential Diagnosis of Enlargements in the Salivary Gland Areas

Parotid Gland Area
UNILATERAL
- Bacterial sialadenitis
- Sialodochitis
- Cyst
- Benign neoplasm
- Malignant neoplasm
- Intraglandular lymph node
- Masseter muscle hypertrophy
- Lesions of adjacent osseous structures

BILATERAL
- Bacterial sialadenitis
- Viral sialadenitis (mumps)
- Sjögren syndrome
- Warthin tumor
- Alcoholic hypertrophy
- Medication-induced hypertrophy (iodine, heavy metals)
- HIV-associated multicentric cysts
- Masseter muscle hypertrophy
- Accessory salivary glands
- TMJ-related lesions

Submandibular Gland Area
UNILATERAL
- Bacterial sialadenitis
- Sialodochitis
- Fibrosis
- Cyst
- Benign neoplasm
- Malignant neoplasm

BILATERAL
- Bacterial sialadenitis
- Sjögren syndrome
- Lymphadenitis
- Branchial cleft cyst
- Submandibular space infection

ENLARGEMENTS OF THE SUBMANDIBULAR AREA

Unilateral enlargement of the submandibular area associated with tender lymph nodes is suggestive of sialadenitis, which may be primary or secondary to ductal obstruction or decreased salivary flow (retrograde). Unilateral enlargement without tender lymph nodes suggests a neoplasm, cyst, lymphoepithelial lesion, or fibrosis. An intraglandular mass may be neoplastic or cystic. Neoplasms of the submandibular gland have a greater chance of being malignant than do those of the parotid gland. In turn, sublingual gland neoplasms have a still greater chance of being malignant than do those of the submandibular glands. As with parotid neoplasms, rapid growth, rock-hard texture, pain, and older age of occurrence are clinically suggestive of malignancy. Masses superficial or adjacent to the submandibular gland are assumed to be lymph nodes or extraglandular neoplasms.

Bilateral enlargement of the submandibular gland area suggests bacterial or viral sialadenitis. Although mumps is primarily a viral infection of the parotid glands, it may also occur in the submandibular glands. Other causes of swelling in the submandibular region include Sjögren syndrome, enlarged lymph nodes, submandibular space infection, and branchial cleft cyst (see Box 30-1).

Applied Diagnostic Imaging of the Salivary Glands

Diagnostic imaging of salivary gland disease may be undertaken to differentiate inflammatory processes from neoplastic disease, distinguish diffuse disease from focal suppurative disease, identify and localize sialoliths, and demonstrate ductal morphology. In addition, diagnostic imaging attempts to determine the anatomic location of a tumor, differentiate benign from malignant disease, demonstrate the relationship between a mass and adjacent anatomic structures, and aid in the selection of biopsy sites.

ALGORITHM FOR DIAGNOSTIC IMAGING

Plain film radiography is typically the appropriate starting point for imaging the major salivary glands from a cost-benefit point of view. It can demonstrate sialoliths and the possible involvement of adjacent osseous structures. Because obstructive and associated inflammatory conditions are the most common disorders and primarily involve the ductal system, conventional sialography is the most appropriate imaging modality. If the patient is allergic to the iodine contrast agent used in sialography, magnetic resonance imaging (MRI), computed tomography (CT), or ultrasonography (US) may be selected as an alternative imaging modality. Recent studies comparing the diagnostic yield of MRI with sialography suggest that MRI might replace sialography in the future as the imaging modality of choice for ductal pathosis. Sialography or CT is the best imaging modality for the detection of sialoliths (sialolithiasis). If sialography eliminates inflammatory disorders or suggests the presence of a space-occupying mass (either cystic or solid), then contrast-enhanced (CT) or MRI is appropriate for evaluation. US is an alternative technique to differentiate cystic lesions from solid masses, as well as for identifying advanced autoimmune lesions. Functional disorders such as xerostomia are appropriately imaged with sialography or scintigraphy. Scintigraphy can provide important physiologic information that may be helpful in forming the differential diagnosis.

PLAIN FILM RADIOGRAPHY

Plain film radiography is a fundamental part of the examination of the salivary glands and may provide sufficient information to preclude the use of more sophisticated and expensive imaging techniques. It has the potential to identify unrelated pathoses in the areas of the salivary glands that may be mistakenly identified as salivary gland disease, such as resorptive or osteoblastic changes in adjacent bone causing periauricular swelling mimicking a parotid tumor. Panoramic and conventional posteroanterior (PA) skull radiographs may demonstrate bony lesions, thus eliminating salivary pathosis from the differential diagnosis. Unilateral or bilateral functional or congenital hypertrophy of the masseter muscle may clinically mimic a salivary tumor. A plain film extraoral radiograph may demonstrate a deep antegonial notch, overdeveloped mandibular angle, and exostosis on the outer surface of the angle in cases of masseter hypertrophy.

Plain film radiographs are useful when the clinical impression, supported by a compatible history, suggests the presence of sialoliths (stones or calculi). Such an examination should include both intraoral and extraoral images to demonstrate the entire region of the gland. Several sialoliths may be present at different locations. It is expedient to use about half the usual exposure to avoid overexposure of the sialoliths. However, this technique is limited by the fact that 20% of the sialoliths of the submandibular gland and 40% of those of the parotid gland are not well calcified and therefore are radiolucent and not visible in plain films.

Radiolucent sialoliths are rarely found in the sublingual glands.

INTRAORAL RADIOGRAPHY

Sialoliths in the anterior two thirds of the submandibular duct are typically imaged with a cross-sectional mandibular occlusal projection as described in Chapter 8 (Fig. 30-1). The posterior part of the duct is demonstrated with a posterior oblique view, wherein the head of the patient is tilted back and maximally inclined toward the unaffected side. The central ray is directed parallel with the mandible in the area of the submandibular fossa and into the posterior part of the floor of the mouth.

Parotid sialoliths are more difficult to demonstrate than the submandibular variety as a result of the tortuous course of Stensen duct around the anterior border of the masseter and through the buccinator muscle. As a rule, only sialoliths in the anterior part of the duct, anterior to the masseter muscle, can be imaged on an intraoral film. To demonstrate sialoliths in the anterior part of the duct, an intraoral film packet is held with a hemostat inside the cheek, as high as possible in the buccal sulcus and over the parotid papilla. The central ray is directed perpendicular to the center of the film.

EXTRAORAL RADIOGRAPHY

A panoramic projection frequently demonstrates sialoliths in the posterior duct or reveals intraglandular sialoliths in the submandibular gland if they are within the image layer (Fig. 30-2). The image of most parotid sialoliths is superimposed over the ramus and body of the mandible, making lateral radiographs of limited value. To demonstrate sialoliths in the submandibular gland, the lateral projection is modified by opening the mouth, extending the chin, and depressing the tongue with the index finger. This improves the image of the sialolith by moving it inferior to the mandibular border.

Sialoliths in the distal portion of Stensen duct or in the parotid gland are difficult to demonstrate by intraoral or lateral extraoral views. However, a PA skull projection with the cheeks puffed out may move the image of the sialolith free of the bone, rendering it visible on the projected image. This technique may also demonstrate interglandular sialoliths that may be obscured during sialography. Less mineralized sialoliths may be obscured by the radiopaque soft tissue shadow in the PA skull view.

CONVENTIONAL SIALOGRAPHY

First performed in 1902, sialography is a radiographic technique wherein a radiopaque contrast agent is

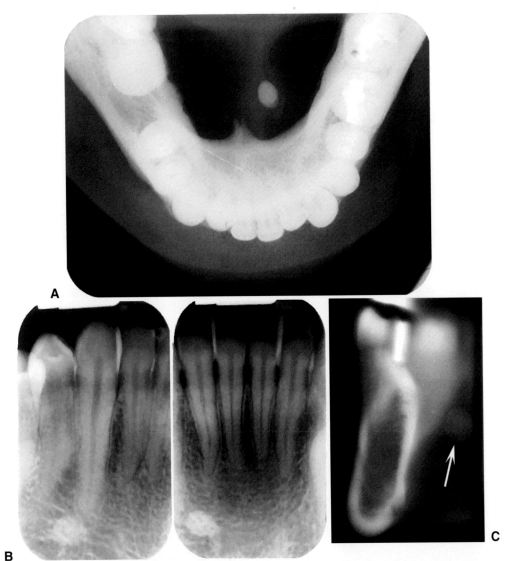

FIG. **30-1**   **A,** Underexposed mandibular occlusal radiograph demonstrating radiopaque sialolith in Wharton duct. Note the classic laminated appearance. **B,** Periapical radiographs of the same case. The radiopaque calculus can be localized lingual to the teeth by applying appropriate object localization rules. **C,** A cross-sectional tomogram of another case demonstrating concentric laminations of a submandibular sialolith *(arrow).*

infused into the ductal system of a salivary gland before imaging with plain films, fluoroscopy, panoramic radiography, conventional tomography, or CT. Sialography remains the most detailed way to image the ductal system (Fig. 30-3). The parotid and submandibular glands are more readily studied with this technique. Although the sublingual gland is difficult to infuse intentionally, it may be fortuitously opacified while infusing Wharton duct to image the submandibular gland.

A survey or "scout" film is usually made before the infusion of the contrast solution into the ductal system as an aid in verifying the optimal exposure factors and patient positioning parameters and for detecting radiopaque sialoliths or extraglandular pathosis.

With this technique, a lacrimal or periodontal probe is used to dilate the sphincter at the ductal orifice before the passage of a cannula (blunt needle or catheter) connected by extension tubing to a syringe containing contrast agent. Lipid-soluble (e.g.,

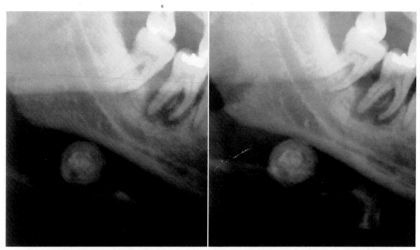

FIG. **30**-**2**   *Stereoscopic panoramic plain film projections.* Note the laminated appearance of this sialolith in the submandibular gland. The image of the sialolith is magnified because of its relatively lingual placement in the image layer. Taken from slightly different horizontal angles, a three-dimensional appearance can be obtained when viewed with stereobinoculars.

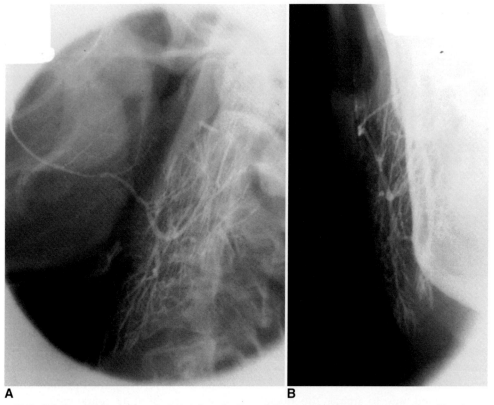

A   **B**

FIG. **30**-**3**   *Sialography.* **A,** Lateral projection of the parotid demonstrating opacification all the way to the terminal ducts and acini. **B,** Anterior-posterior projection of the same gland demonstrating "parenchymal blushing" from acinar opacification. (Courtesy Oral & Maxillofacial Imaging Center, Baylor College of Dentistry, Dallas, Texas.)

Ethiodol) or non–lipid-soluble (e.g., Sinografin) contrast solution is then slowly infused until the patient feels discomfort (usually between 0.2 and 1.5 ml, depending on the gland being studied). These iodine-containing agents render the ductal system radiopaque. The filling phase can be monitored by fluoroscopy or with static films. The intent is to opacify the ductal system all the way to the acini. The image of the ductal system appears as "tree limbs," with no area of the gland devoid of ducts. With acinar filling, the "tree" comes into "bloom," which is the typical appearance of the parenchymal opacification phase (Fig. 30-4). The gland is allowed to empty for 5 minutes without stimulation. If postevacuation images suggest contrast retention, a sialogogue such as lemon juice or 2% citric acid may be administered to augment evacuation by stimulating secretion. Non–lipid-soluble contrast agents are preferred because of reports of inflammatory reactions subsequent to inadvertent extravasation of lipid-soluble agents.

Sialography is indicated for the evaluation of chronic inflammatory diseases and ductal pathoses. Contraindications include acute infection, known sensitivity to iodine-containing compounds, and immediately anticipated thyroid function tests.

COMPUTED TOMOGRAPHY

CT is useful in evaluating structures in and adjacent to salivary glands; it displays both soft and hard tissues, as well as minute differences in soft tissue densities. Thin axial and coronal images are typically acquired (Fig. 30-5). (See Chapter 13 for a description of the CT process.) Glandular tissues are usually easily discernible from surrounding fat and muscle. The parotid glands are more radiopaque than the surrounding fat but less opaque than adjacent muscles. Although the submandibular and sublingual glands are similar in density to adjacent muscles, they are readily identified on the basis of shape and location. The submandibular and sublingual glands are most easily identified on directly acquired contrast-enhanced coronal CT scans. CT is useful in assessing acute inflammatory processes and abscesses, as well as

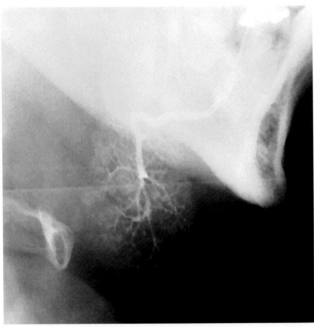

FIG. **30-4** *Sialogram of normal submandibular gland.* This lateral view demonstrates parenchymal blushing. Normal fine branching is visible. Lack of parenchymal blushing at the anteroinferior margin is caused by radiographic burnout.

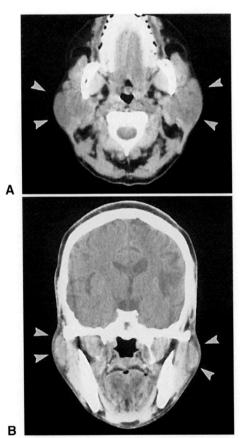

FIG. **30-5** *CT images.* **A,** Axial view demonstrating bilateral enlargement of the parotid glands (*arrowheads*). **B,** Coronal view of the same patient. The clinical/histopathologic diagnosis was autoimmune parotitis. (Courtesy Department of Radiology, Baylor University Medical Center, Dallas, Texas.)

cysts, mucoceles, and neoplasia. Calcifications, such as sialoliths are also well depicted with CT.

MAGNETIC RESONANCE IMAGING

MRI typically provides better images of soft tissue structures than does CT; it also results in fewer problems with streak artifacts from metallic dental restorative materials (Fig. 30-6). (See Chapter 13 for a description of the basic concepts and principles of MRI.) Axial views are acquired for all sequences, with coronal and sagittal views taken as needed. Noncontrast T1- and T2-weighted sequences are obtained followed by T1-weighted postcontrast, fat-suppressed images. Fast-spin echo T2-weighted images may also require fat suppression.

Although indications for CT and MRI occasionally overlap, MRI demonstrates as well as or better than CT the margins of salivary gland masses, internal structures, and regional extension of the lesions into adjacent tissues or spaces, as occurs with some lesions of the deep lobe of the parotid. MRI also discloses the major vessels, identified as areas of no tissue signal (dark) without the use of contrast medium. The use of intravenous contrast is helpful in distinguishing between cystic and solid masses and in the evaluation of per-

ineural spread of malignant tumors. Recent studies have shown MRI to accurately reveal ductal morphology, but it may not be sufficiently sensitive to identify small sialoliths.

SCINTIGRAPHY (NUCLEAR MEDICINE, POSITRON EMISSION COMPUTED TOMOGRAPHY)

Nuclear medicine, or scintigraphy, provides a functional study of the salivary glands, taking advantage of the selective concentration of specific radiopharmaceuticals in the glands. (See Chapter 13 for a description of the nuclear medicine procedures used to acquire images.) When ^{99m}Tc-pertechnetate is injected intravenously, it is concentrated in and excreted by glandular structures, including the salivary, thyroid, and mammary glands. The radionuclide appears in the ducts of the salivary glands within minutes and reaches maximal concentration within 30 to 45 minutes. A sialogogue is then administered to evaluate secretory capacity. All major salivary glands can be studied at once.

Although this technique has high diagnostic sensitivity, it lacks specificity and demonstrates little morphology. Pathosis may be demonstrated by an increased,

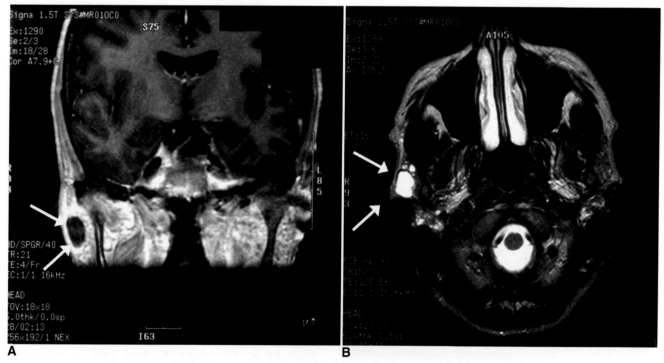

FIG. 30-6 *MRI study.* A well-defined mass in the deep lobe of the right parotid gland as imaged with coronal T1-weighted format (**A**) and axial T2-weighted format (**B**). The tumor *(arrows)* is low-signal on the T1-weighted image and high-signal on T2-weighted images. Histopathologic diagnosis was benign mixed tumor. (Courtesy Salivary Dysfunction Center, Baylor College of Dentistry, Dallas, Texas.)

decreased, or absent radionuclide uptake (Fig. 30-7). Lesions that concentrate ^{99m}Tc-pertechnetate are Warthin tumor and oncocytoma. The diagnosis of salivary gland tumors from nuclear medicine scans is not completely reliable. Because of low image resolution, CT and MRI are preferred for the evaluation of salivary masses. A recent advance in nuclear medicine is positron emission computed tomography (PET). In spite of a much greater resolution than scintigraphy, PET has not been useful classifying salivary tumors as benign or malignant.

ULTRASONOGRAPHY

Compared with CT and MRI, US has the advantages of being relatively inexpensive, widely available, painless, easy to perform, and noninvasive. (For a full descrip-

tion of US, see Chapter 13) The primary application of US is the differentiation of solid masses from cystic ones (Fig. 30-8). Recent studies suggest that this technique may also be helpful in detecting sialoliths and diagnosing advanced autoimmune lesions (Sjögren syndrome).

Image Interpretation of Salivary Gland Disorders

OBSTRUCTIVE AND INFLAMMATORY DISORDERS

SIALOLITHIASIS

Synonyms
Calculus and salivary stone

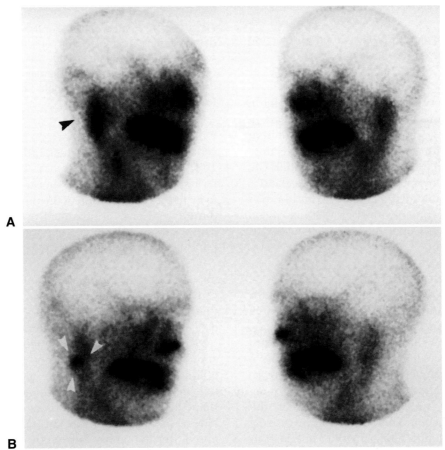

FIG. **30-7** *Scintigraphy.* **A,** ^{99m}Tc-pertechnetate scan of the salivary glands (right and left anterior oblique views) demonstrates increased uptake of radioisotope in the right parotid gland *(black arrowhead)*. **B,** Scintigram taken after administration of a sialogogue (lemon juice) demonstrates retention of isotope in right parotid gland *(white arrowheads)*. This is a typical presentation of salivary stasis, Warthin tumor, or oncocytoma.

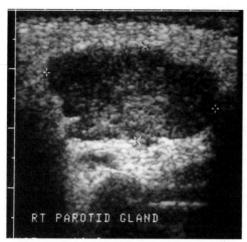

FIG. **30-8**　*Ultrasound image of right parotid gland.* A well-delineated, solid mass is suggested by echo returns within the lesion. Ultrasound appearance is typical of a benign salivary tumor. (Courtesy Department of Radiology, Baylor University Medical Center, Dallas, Texas.)

Definition

Sialolithiasis is the formation of a calcified obstruction within the salivary duct.

Clinical Features

Sialoliths can obstruct the secretory ducts, resulting in chronic retrograde infections because of a decrease in salivary flow. Clinical symptoms include intermittent swelling and pain with eating and signs of infection. Sialoliths may form in any of the major or minor salivary glands or their ducts, but usually only one gland is involved. The submandibular gland and Wharton duct are by far the most frequently involved (83% of cases). If one stone is found, at least a one-in-four chance exists that others are present.

Radiographic Features

Depending on their degree of calcification, sialoliths may appear either radiopaque or radiolucent on radiographic examinations (20% to 40% of cases) (see Fig. 30-1). Sialoliths vary in shape from long cigar shapes to oval or round shapes. When visible, they usually have a homogeneous radiopaque internal structure. Sialography is helpful in locating obstructions that are undetectable with plain radiography, especially if the sialoliths are radiolucent. The contrast agent usually flows around the sialolith, filling the duct proximal to the obstruction (Fig. 30-9). The ductal system is frequently dilated proximal to the obstruction and infers the presence of an obstruction even when it is not visible. The contrast agent that flows around the sialolith is more radiopaque and may obscure small sialoliths. Radiolu-

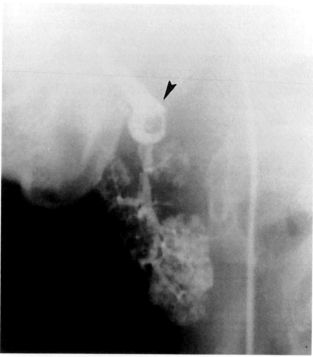

FIG. **30-9**　*Sialography.* Slightly oblique lateral view demonstrating parenchymal opacification of the submandibular gland. *Arrowhead* points to an obstruction (radiolucent sialolith) within the main duct. Opacification of the parenchyma is patchy resulting from fibrosis secondary to chronic obstruction.

cent sialoliths appear as ductal filling defects (Fig. 30-10). Sialography should not be performed if a radiopaque stone has been shown by plain radiography to be in the distal portion of the duct, because the procedure may displace it proximally into the ductal system, complicating subsequent removal. CT may also detect minimally calcified sialoliths not visible on plain films.

US is of limited value in the diagnosis of inflammatory and obstructive diseases, but recent studies indicate it is fairly reliable in demonstrating sialoliths. More than 90% of stones larger than 2 mm are detected as echo-dense spots with a characteristic acoustic shadow.

Sialoliths must be differentiated from phleboliths and dystrophic calcification of lymph nodes. Phleboliths typically demonstrate a radiolucent center. Calcified lymph nodes usually appear to be "cauliflower-shaped." In the panoramic image palatine tonsilliths have a similar location as parotid sialoliths, superimposed over the ramus, but can be differentiated in that they are typically multiple and punctate.

Treatment

Treatment of sialolithiasis may consist of encouragement of spontaneous discharge through the use of

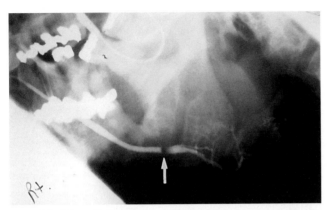

FIG. **30-10** *Sialography.* Lateral view of submandibular glands demonstrating a radiolucent sialolith in the main duct. This is to be differentiated from inclusion air bubbles, in which the interface with the contrast media is convex.

sialogogues to stimulate secretion. Sialography may also stimulate discharge, especially if an oil-based contrast agent is used. If discharge does not occur, surgical removal of the sialolith or even the involved salivary gland may be indicated.

BACTERIAL SIALADENITIS

Synonyms
Parotitis and submandibulitis

Definition
Bacterial sialadenitis is an acute or chronic bacterial infection of the terminal acini or parenchyma of the salivary glands.

Clinical Features
Acute bacterial infections most commonly affect the parotid gland, but the submandibular gland may also be involved. Most cases are unilateral and may occur at any age. The typical clinical presentation is swelling, redness, tenderness, and malaise. Enlarged regional lymph nodes and suppuration may also be noted. Those most commonly afflicted are older adults, postoperative patients, and debilitated patients who have poor hygiene as a result of reduced salivary secretion and retrograde infection by the oral flora (usually *Staphylococcus aureus* and *S. viridans*). Reduced salivary secretion may also be drug-related or secondary to occlusion of a major duct. Untreated acute suppurative infections typically form abscesses. Diagnosis is based on clinical observation, systemic symptoms, and the expression of pus from the duct.

Chronic inflammation may affect any of the major salivary glands, causing extensive swelling and culminating in fibrosis. This may be a consequence of an untreated acute sialadenitis or associated with some type of obstruction resulting from sialolithiasis, noncalcified organic debris, or stricture (scar or fibrosis) formation in the excretory ducts. Bacteria or viruses may not be detected in the gland or saliva. The parotid is most often involved. During periods of painful swelling, pus may be expressed from the ductal orifice and salivary stimulation may cause pain. Episodic in nature, signs of generalized sepsis are seldom present. The obstruction may be congenital or secondary to sialolithiasis, trauma, infection, or neoplasia. Typical clinical symptoms are intermittent swelling, pain when eating, and superimposed infection resulting from salivary stasis.

Radiographic Features
Sialography is contraindicated in acute infections because disrupted ductal epithelium may allow extravasation of contrast agent, resulting in a foreign body reaction and severe pain. This technique is appropriate for use in cases of suspected chronic infections. Epithelial flattening may lead to mildly dilated terminal ducts and saclike acini, which is demonstrable with sialography. The saclike acinar areas are referred to as *sialectasia*. An even distribution throughout the gland is seen in recurrent parotitis and autoimmune disorders. If connected to the ductal system, abscess cavities may fill with contrast media during sialography. Abscess cavities appear on CT as walled-off areas of lower attenuation within an enlarged gland. US may distinguish between diffuse inflammation (echo-free, light image) and suppuration (less echo-free, darker image) and may detect sialoliths greater than 2 mm in diameter. US examination may also demonstrate abscess cavities, if present, and may be the study of choice for recurrent parotitis, especially in children. Contrast-enhanced CT may demonstrate glandular enlargement (Fig. 30-11). However, MRI is an appropriate alternative examination in cases in which sialography is contraindicated or not technically possible. On MRI, inflamed glands are usually enlarged and demonstrate a lower tissue signal on T1-weighted images and higher signal on T2-weighted images than that of the surrounding muscle. Advanced sialadenitis may present in combination with sialolithiasis, sialodochitis, abscess formation, and fistulas.

Treatment
Treatment of bacterial sialadenitis typically begins conservatively with attention to oral hygiene, local massage, increased fluid intake, and the use of oral sialogogues (sour citrus fruit wedges or salivary stimulants). An appropriate antibiotic regimen may also be

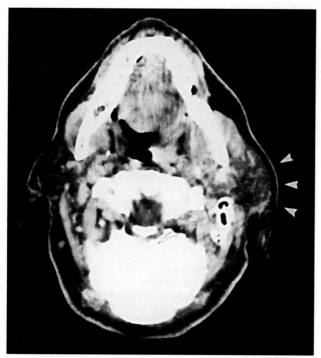

FIG. **30-11** *Contrast-enhanced CT image.* The left parotid gland *(arrowheads)* is larger than the right, with no suggestion of abscess formation. This appearance is consistent with diffuse parotitis and cellulitis. (Courtesy Department of Radiology, Baylor University Medical Center, Dallas, Texas.)

indicated. If symptoms continue, surgical remedies ranging from partial to total excision of the gland may be considered.

SIALODOCHITIS

Synonym
Ductal sialadenitis

Definition
Sialodochitis is an inflammation of the ductal system of the salivary glands.

Clinical Features
Dilation of the ductal system is a prominent sialographic presentation of sialodochitis. It is common in both the submandibular (Fig. 30-12) and parotid glands. If interstitial fibrosis develops, it is apparent in sialograms as a sausage-string appearance of the main duct and its major branches produced by alternate strictures and dilations. Recently these changes have been seen with the use of thin-section MRI. Scintigraphy and CT are not typically indicated in the diagnosis of inflammatory ductal diseases of the salivary glands.

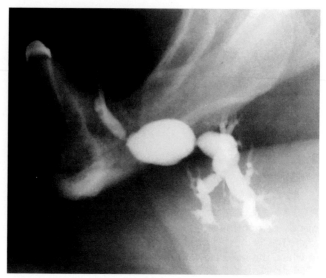

FIG. **30-12** *Sialography.* Lateral view of the submandibular gland shows prominent intermittent stricture and dilation of the main and secondary ducts, which is typical of advanced sialodochitis.

They are costly nonspecific, and typically do not provide any more useful information than sialography.

Treatment
The management of sialodochitis is similar to that described for sialadenitis.

AUTOIMMUNE SIALADENITIS

Synonyms
Myoepithelial sialadenitis, Sjögren syndrome, benign lymphoepithelial lesion, Mikulicz disease, sicca syndrome, and autoimmune sialosis

Definition
Autoimmune sialadenitis represents a group of disorders that affect the salivary glands and share an autosensitivity. The range of clinical and histopathologic manifestations suggests that these disorders represent different developmental stages of the same immunologic mechanisms, differing only in the extent and intensity of tissue reaction. Different forms may share a common etiology.

Clinical Features
The clinical manifestations range from recurrent painless swelling of the salivary glands (usually the parotid gland) to a stage that includes enlargement of the lacrimal glands. Glandular swelling may be accompanied by xerostomia and xerophthalmia (primary Sjögren syndrome) and subsequently by a

connective tissue disease such as rheumatoid arthritis, progressive systemic sclerosis, systemic lupus erythematosus, or polymyositis (secondary Sjögren syndrome). The process may progress to benign lymphoepithelial lesions that can assume the proportions of a tumor. A presumptive diagnosis can be made on the basis of any two of the following three features: dry mouth, dry eyes, and rheumatoid disease. The disease is most common in adults, occurring primarily in the 40- to 60-year age group, with a 90% to 95% female prevalence. The childhood form is only one-tenth as common as the adult form, and there is much less chance of advanced parotid disease. Studies have shown a risk for developing non-Hodgkin lymphoma 44 times greater than in control subjects.

Radiographic Features

Sialography is helpful in the diagnosis and staging of autoimmune disorders. The early stages of disease are witness to the initiation of punctate (less than 1 mm) and globular (1 to 2 mm) spherical collections of contrast agent evenly distributed throughout the glands. These collections are referred to as *sialectases* (Fig. 30-13). At this stage, the main duct may appear to be normal, but the intraglandular ducts may be narrowed or not even evident. Sialectasia typically remains after the administration of a sialogogue, which is an indication that contrast agent is pooled extraductally.

As the disease progresses, the collections of contrast agent increase in size (greater than 2 mm in diameter) and are irregular in shape. These pools of contrast agent are termed *cavitary sialectases*. These larger sialectases are fewer in number and less uniformly distributed throughout the glands than are punctate or globular sialectases (Fig. 30-14). Progressively larger cavities of contrast agent and dilation of the main ductal system may also be present. At the endpoint of this disorder, complete destruction of the gland occurs. Cavitation and glandular fibrosis are the result of recurrent inflammation. The differential diagnosis of this appearance would include chronic bacterial or granulomatous infections and multiple parotid cysts associated with HIV infection. However, diffuse cervical lymphadenopathy is common in HIV disease and uncommon in Sjögren syndrome. Recently, thin-section MRI has been shown to be reliable in depicting sialodochitis and sialectasia, especially when globular changes are present.

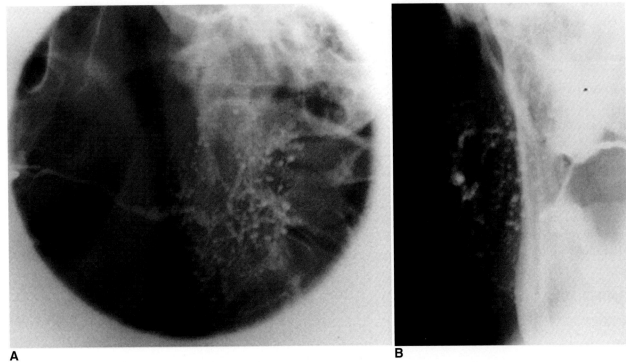

A   **B**

FIG. **30-13** *Conventional sialography of left parotid gland.* **A,** Lateral projection demonstrates punctate sialectases distributed throughout the gland, which is suggestive of autoimmune sialadenitis. The "sausage-link" appearance of the main duct indicates that sialodochitis is present. Clinical/histopathologic diagnosis was Sjögren's syndrome. **B,** AP projection of the same gland. (Courtesy Oral & Maxillofacial Imaging Center, Baylor College of Dentistry, Dallas, Texas.)

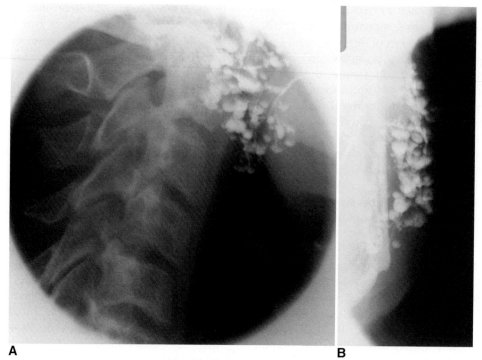

A   **B**

FIG. **30-14** *Sialography of the left parotid gland.* Punctate (small spherical), globular (larger spherical), and cavitary (larger, irregular) sialectases with some dilation of the main duct are suggestive of advanced autoimmune disease with parenchymal destruction with retrograde infection in lateral **(A)** and AP **(B)** projections. Clinical/ histopathologic diagnosis was Sjögren's syndrome. (Courtesy Oral and Maxillofacial Imaging Center, Baylor College of Dentistry, Dallas, Texas.)

Treatment

The management of autoimmune disorders of the salivary glands is directed toward relief of symptoms. Underlying rheumatoid conditions are systemic and typically treated with antiinflammatory agents, corticosteroids, and immunosuppressive therapeutic agents. Salivary stimulants, increased fluid intake, and artificial saliva and tears are symptomatic treatment regimens for the eyes and mouth. More advanced inflammatory changes may be treated surgically by local or total excision of the symptomatic gland.

NONINFLAMMATORY DISORDERS

SIALADENOSIS

Synonym
Sialosis

Definition
Sialadenosis is a nonneoplastic, noninflammatory enlargement of primarily the parotid salivary glands. It is usually related to metabolic and secretory disorders

of the parenchyma associated with diseases of nearly all the endocrine glands (hormonal sialadenoses), protein deficiencies, malnutrition in alcoholics (dystrophic-metabolic sialadenoses), vitamin deficiencies, and neurologic disorders (neurogenic sialadenoses).

Clinical Features
Affected glands are typically enlarged.

Radiographic Features
Sialography may demonstrate enlargement of the affected glands or a normal appearance. In enlarged glands, the ducts will be splayed. CT and MRI provide a more straightforward depiction of the glands, but are nonspecific and require correlation with the clinical findings and history.

Treatment
The management of sialadenosis hinges on identifying the etiology of the metabolic or secretory disorder. Conservative treatment, including local massage, increased fluid intake, and the use of oral sialogogues (sour citrus fruit wedges or salivary stimulants), is appropriate.

CYSTIC LESIONS

Definition

Cysts of the salivary glands are rare (less than 5% of all salivary gland masses) and most commonly occur unilaterally in the parotid gland. They may be congenital (branchial), lymphoepithelial, dermoid, or acquired, including mucus-retention cysts (obstructions with any etiology). Cystic salivary lesions may be intraglandular or extraglandular in nature and may progress to such proportions that they are clinically palpable and must be distinguished from neoplasia. Cystic neoplasms do occur, but they are discussed separately in this chapter. Mucus-extravasation pseudocysts lack an epithelial lining and result from ductal rupture. Ranulas are retention cysts that usually occur secondary to obstruction of the sublingual duct. Benign lymphoepithelial cysts are thought to be sequelae of cystic degeneration of salivary inclusions within lymph nodes. Multicentric parotid cysts associated with HIV have been reported. These lesions are accompanied by cervical lymphadenopathy, occur bilaterally, and are usually in the superficial portion of the parotid gland (Fig. 30-15). A secondary parotitis may develop.

Radiographic Features

On sialographic examination, cystic masses are indirectly visualized only by the displacement of the ducts arching around them. Cystic lesions typically appear as well-circumscribed, nonenhancing (with contrast), low-density areas when examined on CT. Cysts appear as well-circumscribed, high-signal areas on T2-weighted MRI, but they do not enhance after gadolinium contrast as do benign mixed tumors. When imaged with US, cysts are sharply marginated and echo-free (represented as a dark area) (Fig. 30-16).

Treatment

Management of cystic lesions is typically surgical, involving local or total excision of the gland.

BENIGN TUMORS

Salivary gland tumors are relatively uncommon and occur in less than 0.003% of the population. They account for about 3% of all tumors. Some 80% of the salivary tumors arise in the parotid, 5% in the submandibular, 1% in the sublingual, and 10% to 15% in the minor salivary glands. The majority (70% to 80%) of these tumors occur in the superficial lobe of the parotid gland. Most are benign or low-grade malignancies. High-grade malignancies are uncommon. The chance of neoplasia of major salivary glands being benign varies directly with the size of the gland.

Radiographic Features

Benign tumors and low-grade malignancies typically have well-defined margins, which are most apparent on CT or MRI examinations. Because of the higher density of the submandibular gland, which can equal that of

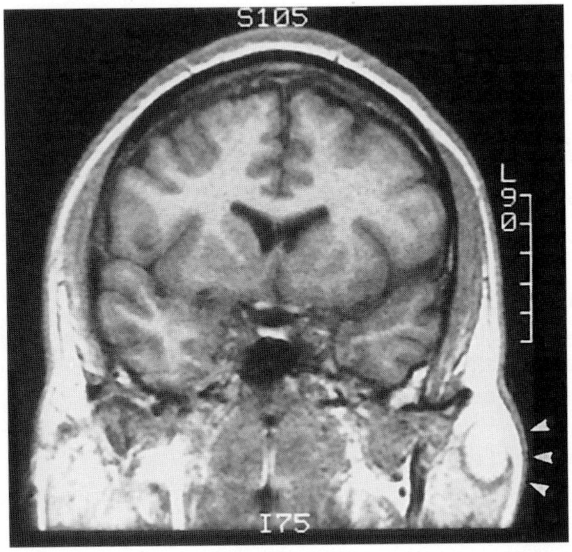

FIG. 30-15 *Coronal section MRI.* The high-signal mass *(arrowheads)* in the left parotid gland was diagnosed as a cyst. This patient was found to be HIV-positive. (Courtesy Department of Radiology, Baylor University Medical Center, Dallas, Texas.)

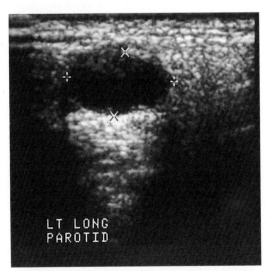

FIG. 30-16 *Ultrasound image of the parotid gland.* Echo-free mass with well-defined margins presents a typical cystic appearance. (Courtesy Department of Radiology, Baylor University Medical Center, Dallas, Texas.)

the neoplasm and obscure the tumor, intravenous contrast enhancement is required during the CT examination. This causes the tumor to appear more radiopaque because the vascularity of the tumor is greater than the adjacent salivary gland tissue. In the US examination, benign masses are typically sharply defined, less echogenic than parenchyma, and of essentially homogeneous echo strength and density. Benign tumors may present as low-intensity (dark) or high-intensity (light) tissue signals on MRI, although the relative intensity of the signal may indicate the presence of lipid, vascular, or fibrous tissues. Some consider MRI to be superior to CT for salivary masses. Sialography may suggest a space-occupying mass when the ducts are compressed or smoothly displaced around the lesion (the "ball-in-hand" appearance) (Fig. 30-17).

Treatment

The management of benign tumors of the major salivary glands is typically surgical. Benign tumors of the parotid gland may be either partially or totally excised. Submandibular and sublingual glands are invariably totally excised.

BENIGN MIXED TUMOR

Synonym
Pleomorphic adenoma

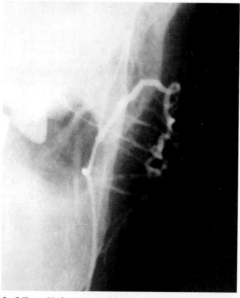

FIG. **30-17** *Sialogram of left parotid gland (AP view).* A mass within the gland is inferred by the appearance of the ducts displaced around the lesion. This is referred to as the "ball-in-hand" appearance, which is suggestive of a space-occupying mass. (Courtesy Department of Radiology, Baylor University Medical Center, Dallas, Texas.)

Definition
The benign mixed tumor is a neoplasm arising from the ductal epithelium of major and minor salivary glands exhibiting epithelial and mesenchymal components.

Clinical Features
The benign mixed tumor accounts for 75% of all salivary gland tumors; 80% are found in the parotid gland, 4% in the submandibular gland, 1% in the sublingual gland, and 10% in the minor salivary glands. This tumor typically occurs in the fifth decade of life as a slow-growing, unilateral, encapsulated, asymptomatic mass. A slight female predilection exists. Recurrence occurs in 50% of cases after excision.

Radiographic Features
The CT presentation of the benign mixed tumor is a sharply circumscribed, infrequently lobulated, and essentially round homogeneous lesion that has a higher density than the adjacent glandular tissue. Calcifications within the tumor are commonly seen and are well depicted on CT. This tumor has various tissue signals in different MRI techniques—for example, relatively low (dark) in T1-weighted images, intermediate on proton density–weightedimages, and homogeneous high-intensity (bright) on T2-weighted images (see Fig. 30-6). Foci of low signal intensity (dark areas) usually represent areas of fibrosis or dystrophic calcifications. If a calcification is present (signal void), the diagnosis favors a benign mixed tumor; otherwise, it is difficult to differentiate this tumor from other parotid masses.

A benign mixed tumor does not usually concentrate ^{99m}Tc-pertechnetate. Therefore the tumor appears as a cold spot when examined by scintigraphy. Solid tumors larger than 5 mm are usually well visualized.

WARTHIN TUMOR

Synonym
Papillary cystadenoma lymphomatosum

Definition
Warthin tumor is a benign tumor arising from proliferating salivary ducts trapped in lymph nodes during embryogenesis of the salivary glands.

Clinical Features
Warthin tumor is the second most common benign neoplasm of the salivary glands, accounting for 2% to 6% of the parotid tumors. In the parotid, it is usually found in the inferior lobe of the gland. This unusual type of tumor is slow growing, painless, and frequently bilateral. Warthin tumor typically afflicts males over the age of 40 years.

Radiographic Features

CT and MRI are the preferred techniques for imaging Warthin tumor. The CT and MRI appearance of this tumor is not specific and is typical of benign salivary tumors, as described for the benign mixed tumor. On CT, this tumor may be of either soft tissue or cystic density. On MRI, it is heterogeneous and may demonstrate hemorrhagic foci. Warthin tumor is characteristically intensely hot on ^{99m}Tc-pertechnetate scans. Oncocytoma (oxyphilic adenoma) may also accumulate the ^{99m}Tc-pertechnetate but are uncommon and less likely to be bilateral (see Fig. 30-7). Oncocytoma has been reported to be present in essentially everyone over the age of 70 years. The US presentation of Warthin tumor is that of a solid mass (hypoechoic), unless, the tumor mass happens to be cystic in nature (see Fig. 30-8).

HEMANGIOMA

Synonym
Vascular nevus

Definition

Hemangioma is a benign neoplasm of proliferating endothelial cells (congenital hemangioma) and vascular malformations, including lesions resulting from abnormal vessel morphogenesis.

Clinical Features

Hemangioma is the most frequently occurring nonepithelial salivary neoplasm, accounting for 50% of the cases. As many as 85% arise in the parotid gland. It is the most common salivary gland tumor during infancy and childhood. The average age at diagnosis is 10 years, with 65% occurring in the first two decades of life. Hemangiomas are frequently unilateral and asymptomatic. A 2:1 female-to-male predilection exists. Treatment is by local excision for those that do not undergo spontaneous remission.

Radiographic Features

Phleboliths are common in this tumor. They appear as calculi with a radiolucent center and are best identified on plain films and CT. Displaced ducts curving about the mass may also be apparent on sialography. The CT presentation of hemangioma is a soft tissue mass that is well distinguished from surrounding tissue, especially when intravenous contrast enhancement is used. On MRI, the tumor has a similar signal as adjacent muscle on T1-weighted images and a very high signal on T2-weighted images. Although US usually demonstrates well-defined margins in the hemangioma, ill-defined margins may also be noted. Strongly hypoechoic hemangiomas may have a complex US appearance, resulting from the multiple interfaces in the lesion. Phleboliths image as multiple hyperechoic areas within the body of the gland itself.

MALIGNANT TUMORS

About 20% of tumors in the parotid are malignant, compared with 50% to 60% of submandibular tumors, 90% of sublingual tumors, and 60% to 75% of minor salivary gland tumors.

Radiographic Features

The radiographic presentation of malignant tumors is variable and is related to the grade, aggressiveness, location, and type of tumor. However, features such as ill-defined margins, invasion of adjacent soft tissues (such as fat spaces), and destruction of adjacent osseous structures, are considered to be typical indicators of malignancy.

Treatment

The management of malignant tumors of the major salivary glands is typically surgical. Low-grade malignant tumors of the parotid gland may be either partially or totally excised. Submandibular and sublingual glands are invariably totally excised. High-grade tumors may require radical neck dissection. Combinations of surgery, therapeutic radiation, and chemotherapy may also be used.

MUCOEPIDERMOID CARCINOMA

Definition

Mucoepidermoid carcinoma is a malignant tumor of epidermoid, intermediate, and mucous cells of the salivary glands.

Clinical Features

This is the most common malignant salivary gland tumor (35%). Just over half of these tumors occur in the major salivary glands, most commonly the parotid gland; the rest are found in the minor glands, with the palate being the most frequent location. The aggressiveness of the lesion varies with its histologic grade. A wide age range exists, with the highest prevalence in the fifth decade of life. A slight predilection for females exists. The low-grade variety rarely metastasizes. Clinically, this tumor appears as a movable, slowly growing, painless nodule not unlike a benign mixed tumor. It is usually only 1 to 4 cm in diameter. The prognosis is good; the 5-year survival rate is greater than 95%.

In contrast to low-grade mucoepidermoid carcinomas, high-grade tumors often cause facial pain and paralysis, have ill-defined margins, and are relatively immobile. Metastasis by blood and lymph are common, with recurrence in half the patients after excision. The prognosis is poor and varies with the histologic grade; the 5-year survival rate may be as low as 25%.

Radiographic Features

Low-grade mucoepidermoid carcinomas are typically not apparent on plain films unless destructive changes to adjacent osseous structures have occurred. The sialographic, CT, MRI, US, and scintigraphic presentations of this tumor are similar to those previously described for benign salivary tumors. However, low-grade mucoepidermoid carcinoma may present a lobulated or irregularly sharply circumscribed appearance on CT or MRI (Fig. 30-18). Cystic areas may present, and rarely, calcifications may be seen.

The radiographic diagnosis of high-grade mucoepidermoid carcinoma typically relies on the appearance of irregular margins and ill-defined form when the mass is examined with CT or MRI. The CT section shows the tumor as an irregular homogeneous mass, not much more dense than the parenchyma. A CT with intravenous contrast enhancement shows the tumor as a sharply defined homogeneous mass that is considerably more opaque than on the CT images without contrast. CT is also a reliable technique for the detection of bony invasion.

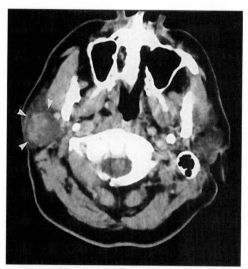

FIG. **30-18** *Contrast-enhanced CT image.* Mass in right parotid gland demonstrates a poorly marginated, heterogeneous, slightly lobulated appearance *(white arrowheads).* Poorly defined margins suggest a low-grade malignancy rather than a benign tumor, even though the CT appearance of both is similar. Histopathologic diagnosis was low-grade mucoepidermoid carcinoma. (Courtesy Department of Radiology, Baylor University Medical Center, Dallas, Texas.)

In contrast to the low-grade malignancies and benign neoplasms, high-grade mucoepidermoid carcinomas, like most high-grade malignancies, have low signal intensity on T1-weighted and T2-weighted MRIs. The T1-weighted images have lower intensity (are darker) than the surrounding structures and are relatively homogeneous. T2-weighted images of the tumor are more heterogeneous and intense (brighter) than T1-weighted images and are just slightly darker than the surrounding tissues. Regardless of clinical presentation and margins, low signal intensity is suggestive of a high-grade malignancy. Cavitary sialectasia and ductal displacement may be noted on sialographic images of this tumor.

MALIGNANT MIXED TUMOR

Synonyms

Carcinoma ex mixed tumor, carcinoma ex pleomorphic adenoma, and malignant pleomorphic adenoma

Definition

There are three distinct types of malignant mixed tumors. The most common is carcinoma ex mixed tumor, which arises from the epithelial components of a preexisting benign mixed tumor. The other two types are extremely rare: a true malignant mixed tumor (from both epithelial and mesenchymal components of a mixed tumor) and the metastasizing mixed tumor that appears histologically benign but behaves in a malignant fashion.

Clinical Features

The malignant mixed tumor typically begins as a slowly growing mass that suddenly undergoes rapid proliferation, often accompanied by pain and facial paralysis. Metastasis is early and the prognosis is unfavorable.

Radiographic Features

The presentation of this tumor is similar to that of the high-grade mucoepidermoid carcinoma previously described. MRI is usually superior to CT for tumor definition.

OTHER MALIGNANT AND METASTATIC TUMORS

Although the incidence of other malignant tumors of the major salivary glands is low, a significant variety exists in their histogenesis. Of all malignant salivary gland tumors, 23% are adenoid cystic carcinomas; however, the majority of these neoplasms develop in the minor salivary glands.

Adenocarcinoma accounts for 6.4% of all salivary gland malignancies, with acinic cell carcinoma, primary lymphoma, and squamous cell carcinoma occurring with even less frequency. Pain, paresthesia, and even paralysis may be present, especially in high-grade tumors. It is interesting to note that the pain associated with acinic cell carcinoma is not considered to be as grave a sign as in other malignant salivary tumors. Tumor spread may be by direct invasion or metastasis. Adenoid cystic carcinoma also spreads along nerve sheaths and is best demonstrated on postcontrast MRI, where nerve enhancement and enlargement is present. Metastasis of tumors of the salivary glands is not unusual. Metastatic lesions in the parotid gland are more common than in the other salivary glands because of the extensive lymphatic and circulatory components of the parotid gland. Most metastatic lesions of the parotid gland are via the lymphatic system and include squamous cell carcinoma, lymphoma, and melanoma. Although considerably fewer lesions are the result of hematogenous dissemination, metastasis from the lung, breast, kidney, and gastrointestinal tract has been reported.

Radiographic Features

The presentation of these tumors is nonspecific and similar to that of the high-grade mucoepidermoid carcinoma previously described. US may demonstrate echo-free cystic areas in adenoid cystic carcinomas (Fig. 30-19).

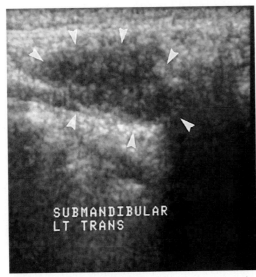

FIG. **30-19** *Ultrasonography.* The mass in the submandibular gland *(arrowheads)* demonstrates a heterogeneous hypoechoic pattern compared with the adjacent tissue. The histopathologic diagnosis was adenoid cystic carcinoma. (Courtesy Department of Radiology, Baylor University Medical Center, Dallas, Texas.)

BIBLIOGRAPHY

Del Balso AM et al: Diagnostic imaging of the salivary glands and periglandular regions. In Del Balso AM, editor: Maxillofacial imaging, Philadelphia, 1990, WB Saunders.

Freling NJM: Imaging of salivary gland disease. Seminars in Roentgenology 35:12, 2000.

Lufkin RB, Hanafee WN: MRI of the head and neck, New York, 1992, Raven Press.

Rabinov K, Weber AL: Radiology of the salivary glands, Boston, 1985, GK Hall Medical Publishers.

Rankow RM, Polayes IM: Diseases of the salivary glands, Philadelphia, 1976, WB Saunders.

Rice DH, Becker TS: The salivary glands. In Hanafee WN, Ward PH, editors: Clinical correlations in the head and neck, vol 2, New York, 1994, Thieme Medical Publishers, Inc.

Seifert G et al: Diseases of the salivary glands, Stuttgart, Germany, 1986, George Thieme Verlag.

Van den Akker HP: Diagnostic imaging in salivary gland disease, Oral Surg 66:625, 1988.

Watson MG: Investigation of salivary gland disease, Ear Nose Throat J 68:84, 1989.

PLAIN FILM RADIOGRAPHY

Ollerenshaw R, Ross SS: Radiological diagnosis of salivary gland disease, Br J Radiol 24:538, 1951.

Silvers AR, Som PM: Salivary glands, Radiol Clin North Am 36:941, 1998.

Weissman JL: Imaging of the salivary glands, Semin Ultrasound CT MR 16:546, 1995.

Yousem DM, Kraut MA, Chalian AA: Major salivary gland imaging, Radiology 216:19, 2000.

CONVENTIONAL SIALOGRAPHY

Drag NA, Brown JE, Wilson RF: Pain and swelling after sialography: is it a significant problem? Oral Surg Oral Med Oral Pathol Oral Radiol Endodont 90:385, 2000.

Eisenbud L, Cranin N: The role of sialography in the diagnosis and therapy of chronic obstructive sialadenitis, Oral Surg 16:1181, 1961.

Manashil GB: Clinical sialography, Springfield, 1978, Charles C Thomas.

Varghese JC, Thornton F, Lucey BC, Walsh M, Farrell MA, Lee MJ: A prospective comparative study of MR sialography and conventional sialography of salivary duct disease, AJR 173:1497, 1999.

Whaley K et al: Sialographic abnormalities in Sjögren's syndrome, rheumatoid arthritis, and other arthritides and connective tissue diseases: a clinical and radiological investigation using hydrostatic sialography, Clin Radiol 23:474, 1972.

Yune HY, Klatte EC: Current status of sialography, Am J Roent Rad Ther Nuc Med 115:420, 1972.

COMPUTED TOMOGRAPHY OF THE MAJOR SALIVARY GLANDS

Bryan RN et al: Computed tomography of the major salivary glands, AJR 139:547, 1982.

Casselman JW, Mancuso AA: Major salivary gland masses: comparison of MR imaging and CT, Radiology 165:183, 1987.

Kosaka M, Kamiishi H: New strategy for the diagnosis of parotid gland lesions utilizing three-dimensional sialography, Computer Aided Surgery 5:42, 2000.

Lloyd RE, Ho KH: Combined CT scanning and sialography in the management of parotid tumors, Oral Surg Oral Med Oral Pathol 65:142, 1988.

MAGNETIC RESONANCE IMAGING OF THE MAJOR SALIVARY GLANDS

Jager L, Menauer F, Holzknecht N, Scholz V, Grevers G, Reiser M. Sialolithiasis: MR sialography of the submandibular duct—an alternative to conventional sialography and US? Radiology 216:665, 2000.

Jungehulsing M, Fischbach R, Schroder U, Kugel H, Damm M, Eckel HE: Magnetic resonance sialography, Otolaryngol Head and Neck Surgery 121:488, 1999.

Kaneda T et al: MR of the submandibular gland: normal and pathologic states, AJNR 17:1575, 1996.

Mendelblatt S et al: Parotid masses: MR imaging, Radiology 163:411, 1987.

Som PM, Biller HF: High-grade malignancies of the parotid gland; identification with MR imaging, Radiology 173:823, 1989.

Swartz et al: MR imaging of parotid mass lesions: attempts at histopathologic differentiation, J Comput Assist Tomogr 13:789, 1989.

NUCLEAR MEDICINE (SCINTIGRAPHY) OF THE MAJOR SALIVARY GLANDS

Chaudhuri TK, Stadalnik RC: Salivary gland imaging, Sem Nucl Med 10:400, 1980.

Garcia RR: Differential diagnosis of tumors of the salivary glands with radioactive isotopes, Int J Oral Surg 3:330, 1974.

Greyson ND, Nikko AM: Radionuclide salivary scanning, J Otolaryngol 11:3, 1982.

Keyes JW Jr, Harkness BA, Greven KM, Williams DW 3rd, Watson NE Jr, McGuirt WF: Salivary gland tumors: pretherapy evaluation with PET, Radiology 192:99, 1994.

Mishkin FS: Radionuclide salivary gland imaging, Sem Nucl Med 11:258, 1981.

Van den Akker HP, Busemann-Sokole E: Absolute indications for salivary gland scintigraphy with ^{99m}Tc-pertechnetate, Oral Surg 60:440, 1985.

ULTRASONOGRAPHY OF THE MAJOR SALIVARY GLANDS

Gooding GAW: Gray scale ultrasound of the parotid gland, AJR 134:469, 1980.

Gritzman G: Sonography of the salivary glands, AJR 153:161, 1989.

Martinoli C et al: Color Doppler sonography of salivary glands, AJR 163:933, 1994.

Rothberg R et al: Diagnostic ultrasound imaging of parotid disease—a contemporary clinical perspective, J Otolaryngol 13:232, 1984.

Shimizu M, Ussmuller J, Donath K, Toshiura K, Ban S, Kanda S, Ozeki S, Shinohara M: Sonographic analysis of recurrent parotitis in children: a comparative study with sialographic findings, Oral Surg Oral Med Oral Pathol Oral Radiol Endodont 86:606, 1998.

OBSTRUCTIVE AND INFLAMMATORY DISORDERS

Aung W, Yamada I, Umehara I, Ohbayashi N, Yoshimo N. Shibuya H: Sjögren's syndrome: comparison of assessments with quantitative salivary gland scintigraphy and contrast sialography, Journal of Nuclear Medicine 41:257, 2000.

Gonzales L, Mackenzie AH, Tarar RA: Parotid sialography in Sjögren's syndrome, Radiology 97:91, 1970.

Hughes M et al: Scintigraphic evaluation of sialadenitis, Brit J Radiol 67:328, 1994.

Langlais RP, Kasle MJ: Sialolithiasis: the radiolucent stones, Oral Surg Oral Med Oral Pathol 40:686, 1975.

Scully C: Sjögren's syndrome: clinical and laboratory features, immunopathogenesis, and management, Oral Surg 62:510, 1986.

Som PM et al: Manifestations of parotid gland enlargement: radiographic, pathologic, and clinical correlation—part 1, the autoimmune pseudosialectasias, Radiology 141:415, 1981.

NONINFLAMMATORY DISORDERS

Chilla R: Sialadenosis of the salivary glands of the head, Acta Otorhinolaryngolgica 26:1, 1981.

CYSTS AND NEOPLASMS

Boles R et al: Malignant tumors of salivary glands: a university experience, Laryngoscope 60:729, 1980.

Byrne MN et al: Preoperative assessment of parotid masses: a comparative evaluation of radiographic techniques to histologic diagnosis, Laryngoscope 99:284, 1989.

Del Balso AM, Williams E, Tane TT: Parotid masses: current modes of diagnostic imaging, Oral Surg 54:360, 1982.

Eneroth CM: Salivary gland tumors in the parotid gland and the palate region, Cancer 27:1415, 1971.

Gottesman RI, Som PM, Mester J, Silvers A: Observations on two cases of apparent submandibular gland cysts in HIV positive patients: MR and CT findings, J Comput Assist Tomogr 20:444, 1996.

Mirich DR, McArdle CB, Kulkarni MV: Benign pleomorphic adenomas of the salivary glands: surface coil MR imaging versus CT, J Comp Assist Tomogr 11:620, 1987.

Thawley SE, Panbje WR: Comprehensive management of head and neck tumors, Philadelphia, 1987, WB Saunders.

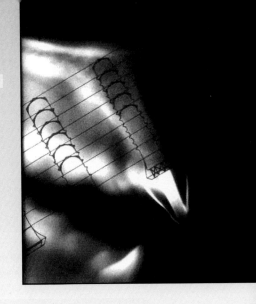

CHAPTER 31

Orofacial Implants

VIVEK SHETTY ■ BYRON W. BENSON

Few advances in dentistry have been as remarkable as the use of dental implants (Fig. 31-1) to restore orofacial form and function. Implant technology has enabled the dentist to help affected patients regain the ability to chew normally and function without embarrassment. With the application of precise surgical and prosthodontic techniques, implant-facilitated restorations allow for a very predictable prosthodontic successful rehabilitation of a broad spectrum of patients with very challenging needs. The reliability of contemporary implant systems derive, in part, from the increasingly sophisticated imaging techniques used in all phases of implant treatment. These imaging modalities contribute information for every stage of the treatment, extending from presurgical diagnosis and treatment planning, through surgical placement and postoperative assessment of the implant, into the prosthetic restoration and long-term surveillance phase.

Acceptance of dental implantology as an integral part of conventional practice makes it necessary for the general dentist to be knowledgeable of implant imaging techniques and their clinical application. With the exception of the occasional subperiosteal, blade implant, and transosteal implant systems (Figs. 31-2 and 31-3), dental implants used today are almost exclusively root-form devices (see Fig. 31-1) embedded within the jaw bone (endosseous implants). The focus of this chapter is to provide information about the various imaging technologies available, their specific applications, and the potential information that each can provide to facilitate the placement of endosseous implant restorations.

Diagnostic Imaging for Dental Implants

Conventional imaging, such as panoramic and periapical radiographs, are generally useful and cost-effective but cannot provide the cross-sectional visualization or interactive image analysis that can be obtained with more sophisticated imaging techniques. The various imaging techniques can be applied to various phases of the surgical and restorative procedures (Table 31-1). The selection of specific imaging technique should be based on the technique best suited to provide the information required by the implant team—the restorative dentist, surgeon, and radiologist (Table 31-2).

Imaging Techniques

The ideal imaging technique should have several essential characteristics, including the ability to visualize the implant site in the mesial-distal, facial-lingual, and superior-inferior dimensions; the ability to allow reliable, accurate measurements; a capacity to evaluate the density of trabecular bone and cortical thickness; a capacity to correlate the imaged site with the clinical site; reasonable access and cost to the patient; and minimal radiation dose. Usually a combination of radiographs is used. Available radiographic techniques include intraoral radiography (film and digital), cephalometric radiography, panoramic radiography, conventional tomography and computed tomography (CT). The following is a review of these imaging

677

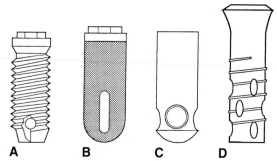

FIG. **31-1**   Four common types of root-form implant fixtures. **A,** Brånemark. **B,** IMZ. **C,** Integral. **D,** ITI.

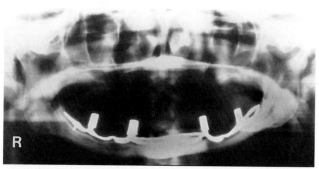

FIG. **31-3**   Subperiosteal implant used for aiding denture support.

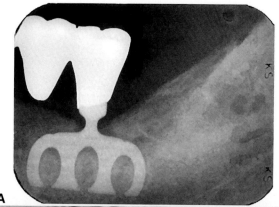

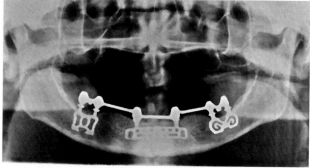

FIG. **31-2**   **A,** Blade implant integrated with bone to support a fixed bridge (periapical radiograph of a mandibular molar). **B,** Three blade implants integrated with bone using common abutments to support a mandibular denture region. (**A,** Courtesy Krishan Kapur, DDS, Los Angeles, Calif.)

techniques applicable to dental implant case management.

INTRAORAL RADIOGRAPHY

Intraoral images may be acquired on film or as direct digital images. Periapical and occlusal radiographic films provide images with superior resolution and sharpness. Maxillary and mandibular periapical radiographs commonly are used to evaluate the status of adjoining teeth and remaining alveolar bone in the mesial-distal dimension. They may also be used for determining vertical height, architecture, and bone quality (bone

TABLE **31-1**		
Commonly Used Radiographic Procedures With Time Intervals for Treatment Planning and Assessment of Dental Implants		
STAGE OF TREATMENT	TIME (MONTHS)	RADIOGRAPHIC PROCEDURES
Treatment planning	−1	PA, pan, tomo, CT, ceph
Surgery (placement)	0	PA, pan, tomo, CT, ceph for correction of problems
Healing	0 to 3	PA, pan, tomo, CT, ceph for correction of problems
Remodeling	4 to 12	PA, pan
Maintenance (without problems)	13+	PA, pan, (follow up approximately every 3 years)
Complications	Anytime	PA, pan, CT (as indicated)

PA, Periapical; *pan,* panoramic radiography; *tomo,* conventional tomography; *CT,* reformatted computed tomography; *ceph,* lateral or lateral-oblique cephalometric radiography.

density, amount of cortical bone, and amount of trabecular bone). Although readily available and relatively inexpensive, periapical radiography has geometric and anatomic limitations. Periapical radiographs, made on a dentate arch, typically are exposed using the paralleling technique, resulting in an image with minimal foreshortening and elongation (Fig. 31-4). Because of variations in the morphology of the residual edentulous alveolar ridge (Fig. 31-5), the ridge may not have the same "long axis" as a tooth, and positioning the film may not result in an accurate display of the height of the alveolar ridge due to image foreshortening and elongation. Also, it frequently is not possible to place the film either superior or inferior enough to capture an image of the entire maxillary or mandibular ridge. It is reported that 25% of mandibular periapical radiographs do not

TABLE 31-2
Summary of Techniques for Implant Imaging

IMAGING TECHNIQUE	APPLICATIONS	ADVANTAGES	DISADVANTAGES
Intraoral periapical radiography	S, M, E, A	Readily available High image definition Minimal distortion Least cost and radiation exposure	Limited imaging area No facial-lingual dimension Limited reproducibility Image elongation and foreshortening
Intraoral occlusal radiography	S, M, A	Readily available High image definition Gross facial-lingual dimension Relatively large imaging area Least cost and radiation exposure	No detailed facial-lingual dimension Limited reproducibility Not as applicable for maxilla Image superimposition
Panoramic radiography	S, M, E, A	Readily available Large imaging area Minimal cost and radiation exposure	No facial-lingual dimension Image distortion Technique errors common Inconsistent magnification Geometric distortion
Conventional tomography	S, M, E, A	Minimal superimposition Facial-lingual dimension Uniform magnification Measurements accurate within about 1 mm Moderate cost Simulates placement with software	Less image definition than plain films Somewhat limited availability Special training for interpretation Sensitive to technique errors Greater radiation exposure for multiple sites
Reformatted computed tomography	M, E, A	Allows evaluation of all possible sites No superimposition Uniform magnification Measurements accurate within about 1 mm timates internal bone density Simulates placement with software	Limited availability Sensitive to technique errors Metallic image artifacts Special training for interpretation Higher cost and radiation exposure Volume averaging contributes to measurement error

S, Single implant; *M*, multiple implants (2 to 5); *E*, edentulous (6+); *A*, augmentation.

demonstrate the mandibular canal. In cases when the canal was identifiable, only 53% of measurements from the alveolar crest to the superior wall of the mandibular canal were accurate within 1 mm.

Because periapical radiographs are unable to provide any cross-sectional information, occlusal radiographs sometimes are used to determine the facial-lingual dimensions of the mandibular alveolar ridge. Although somewhat useful, the occlusal image records only the widest portion of the mandible, which typically is located inferior to the alveolar ridge. This may give the clinician the impression that more bone is available in the cross-sectional (facial-lingual) dimension than actually exists. The occlusal technique is not useful in imaging the maxillary arch because of anatomic limitations.

LATERAL AND LATERAL-OBLIQUE CEPHALOMETRIC RADIOGRAPHY

Lateral cephalometric radiography provides an image of known magnification (usually 7% to 12%) that documents axial tooth inclinations and the dentoalveolar ridge relationships in the midline of the jaws. The soft tissue profile also is apparent on this film and can be used to evaluate profile alterations after prosthodontic rehabilitation. This projection can provide a cross-sectional view of only the maxillary and mandibular midline. The images of structures not in the midline are superimposed on the contralateral side, complicating the evaluation of other implant sites. Occasionally, lateral-oblique cephalometric radiography is used with one side of the body of the mandible positioned paral-lel to the film cassette. Image magnification on these views is not predictable, because the body of the mandible is not the same distance from the film as is the rotation center of the cephalostat (used to calculate object-film distance for image magnification values). Thus measurements made from these films are not reliable. In general, cephalometric radiographs have significant limitations but may be useful in placement of implants near the midline for overdentures.

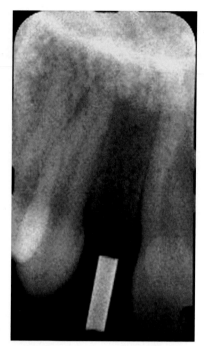

FIG. **31-4**   An intraoral periapical radiograph of a potential implant site. An imaging stent in place indicates the desired axis of insertion.

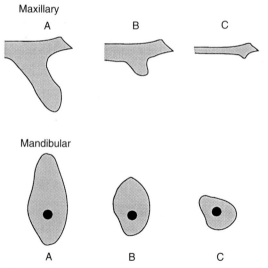

Maxillary

A   B   C

Mandibular

A   B   C

FIG. **31-5**   Patterns of bone morphology in the anterior maxilla *(above)* and posterior mandible *(below)* in potential implant therapy patients. Minimal resorption **(A)**, moderate resorption **(B)**, and severe resorption **(C)** of alveolar bone. (Modified from Brånemark P-I et al: Tissue integrated prostheses, Chicago, 1985, Quintessence.)

PANORAMIC RADIOGRAPHY

Although the resolution and sharpness of panoramic radiographs are less than those of intraoral films, panoramic projections provide a broader visualization of the jaws and adjoining anatomic structures.

Panoramic radiography units are widely available, making this imaging technique very useful as a screening and assessment instrument. Panoramic radiographs are useful in making preliminary estimations of crestal alveolar bone and cortical boundaries of the mandibular canal, maxillary sinus, and nasal fossa (Fig. 31-6).

Information acquired from panoramic radiographs must be applied judiciously because this technique has significant limitations as a definitive presurgical planning tool. Angular measurements on panoramic radiographs tend to be accurate, but linear measurements are not. Image size distortion (magnification) varies significantly among films from different panoramic units and even within different areas of the same film. Vertical measurements are unreliable because of foreshortening and elongation of the anatomic structures, since the x-ray beam is not perpendicular to the long axis of the anatomic structures or to the film plane. The negative vertical angulation of the x-ray beam also may cause lingually positioned objects such as mandibular tori to be projected superiorly on the film, which may result in an overestimation of vertical bone height. Furthermore, the anatomic vertical axis varies within the film image, particularly in nonmidline areas. Compared with contact radiographs of dissected anatomic specimens, only 17% of panoramic measurements between the alveolar crest and superior wall of the mandibular canal were found to be accurate within 1 mm.

Similarly, dimensional accuracy in the horizontal plane of panoramic radiographs is highly dependent on the position of the structures of interest relative to the central plane of the image layer. The horizontal dimension of images of structures located facial or lingual to the central plane but still within the image layer tends to be minified or magnified. The degree of horizontal size distortion is difficult to ascertain on panoramic

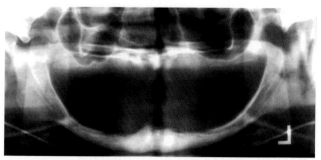

FIG. **31-6** Evaluation of potential implant sites by panoramic radiograph. Note the severe atrophy of the maxillary and mandibular alveolar process.

radiographs because the shape of the image layer is configured to a population average and the anatomic morphology of only a few individuals conforms totally to that image layer. In summary, horizontal image magnification with panoramic radiographs varies from 0.70 to 2.2 times actual size, although some manufacturers still claim a 1.25 average magnification (at the central plane of the image layer). Errors in patient positioning can further exacerbate measurement error in the horizontal dimension. Finally, panoramic radiographs provide a two-dimensional image with no cross-sectional information.

CONVENTIONAL TOMOGRAPHY

Used as an adjunct to screening films, cross-sectional tomograms enhance visualization of the available bone by providing reliable dimensional measurements at proposed implant sites, including the cross-sectional (facial-lingual) dimension. It also is widely available. This technique produces a cross-sectional, flat-plane image layer that is perpendicular to the x-ray beam. Images of anatomic structures of interest are relatively sharp, and images of structures outside the image layer are blurred beyond recognition by the motion of the x-ray tube and film. The thickness, orientation, and anatomic location of the image layer can be predetermined and manipulated. To obtain reliable measurements, it is imperative that the image layer be a true cross-section of the curve of the alveolar process, rather than oblique. Scout films (usually a submentovertex, occlusal or panoramic projection) or wax bite registrations or dental models commonly are used to determine the appropriate cross-sectional angulation. The complex (multidirectional) tube motion of current conventional tomographic units minimizes image superimposition and provides fixed, uniform image magnification, allowing for accurate measurements. Complex tube motion also permits use of a thicker image layer while retaining diagnostic quality. A thicker image layer is desirable to maximize image contrast, making the identification of structures such as the mandibular canal more predictable.

The dimensional accuracy of cross-sectional tomograms is particularly useful in measuring the distance between the alveolar crest and adjacent structures, such as the floor of the nasal fossa, maxillary sinus floor, mandibular canal, mental canal, and inferior mandibular cortex. The appropriate buccal-lingual axis of insertion of the implant may also be predicted. Measurements are directly acquired from the films and subsequently corrected by the magnification factor used. As an alternative, acetate overlays with appropriately magnified 1 mm grids may be used (Fig. 31-7).

Published research suggests a measurement error of less than 1 mm in optimal images. Typically, two to three cross-sectional tomographic slices are required to adequately image each intended implant site. Conventional tomography is especially convenient in the planning of single implants or multiple implants within a quadrant (Fig. 31-8).

REFORMATTED COMPUTED TOMOGRAPHY

Patients who are edentulous or who are being considered for multiple implants and augmentation procedures may be best imaged with CT in order to investigate all possible implant sites. A lateral scout image of the selected jaw with the necessary alignment corrections for the mandible or maxilla is an essential initial step for the CT study. The jaws are aligned so that the acquired axial CT images are parallel to the occlusal plane. These axial images are thin (1–2 mm) and overlapping, resulting in approximately 30 axial image slices per jaw. The image information of these sequential axial images can be manipulated to produce multiple two-dimensional images in various planes, using a computer-based process called *multiplanar reformatting (MPR)*. The CT analysis results in three basic image types: axial images with a superimposed curve, reformatted cross-sectional images, and panoramic-like images. An axial scan including the full contour of the mandible (or maxilla) at a level corresponding to the dental roots is selected as a reference for the reformatting process. The computer places a series of sequential dots on the selected scan and connects them to develop a customized arch or curve unique for each jaw. The computer program then generates a series of lines perpendicular to the curve of the individual arch (Fig. 31-9, *A*). These lines are made at constant intervals (usually 1 to 2 mm) and numbered sequentially on the axial image to indicate the position at which each cross-sectional slice will be reconstructed (Figs. 31-9, *B*, and 31-10). Cross-sectional reconstructions are made perpendicular to the curve, and panoramic (curved linear) reconstructions are made parallel with the curve. Three-dimensional representations may also be constructed in various orientations.

These reformatted images provide the clinician with two-dimensional diagnostic information in all three dimensions. Typical studies provide information on the continuity of the cortical bone plates, residual bone in the mandible and maxilla, the relative location of adjoining vital structures, and the contour of soft tissues covering the osseous structures. Studies have reported that 94% of CT measurements between the alveolar crest and wall of the mandibular canal were accurate

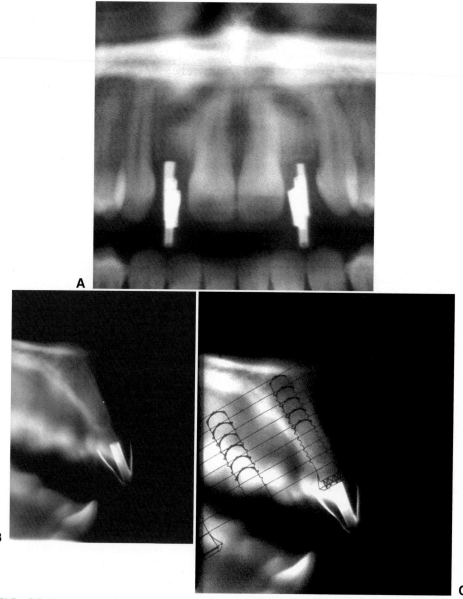

FIG. **31-7**   Conventional tomographic series of the maxilla using Scanora integrated imaging system (Orion Corporation/Soredex, Helsinki, Finland). Metal cylinders retained within an acrylic imaging stent are used to indicate the planned implant sites. Foil strips have been placed on the stent to indicate desired buccal and lingual contours of the restoration. **A,** Scout panoramic radiograph used to orient subsequent tomograms. **B,** Cross-sectional tomograms appropriate for measuring the height and width of the alveolar ridge, as well as the axial orientation of the proposed implant. **C,** A clear plastic overlay is placed over the tomogram to visualize implant placement and determine desired length. The overlay is the same magnification as the tomographic image. (Courtesy Oral and Maxillofacial Imaging Center, Baylor College of Dentistry, Dallas, Texas.)

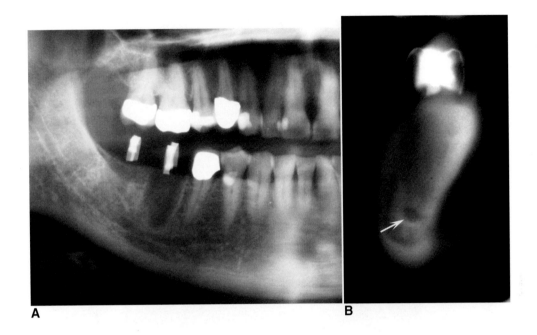

FIG. **31-8** Conventional tomographic series of the mandible using Scanora integrated imaging system (Orion Corporation/Soredex, Helsinki, Finland). Metal cylinders retained within an acrylic imaging stent have been used to indicate the planned implant sites. **A,** Scout panoramic radiograph used to orient the subsequent tomograms. **B,** Cross-sectional tomograms appropriate for measuring the height and width of the alveolar ridge and the axial orientation of the proposed implant. Note the mandibular canal *(arrow)*. (Courtesy Oral and Maxillofacial Imaging Center, Baylor College of Dentistry, Dallas, Texas.)

within 1 mm. Three-dimensional reformations are particularly useful in the planning of augmentation procedures such as a sinus lift and can provide an estimate of the internal density.

The reformatted images typically are presented life-size on photographic prints or radiographic film. The panoramic (curved linear) images are helpful in identifying mesial-distal relationships and noncorticated mandibular canals. However, the quality of the reformatted CT study depends on the ability of the patient to remain still during image acquisition, because movement may produce geometric image distortion. Metallic restorations can cause streak image artifacts, but this can be avoided by aligning the jaws so that the acquired axial scans are parallel to the occlusal plane; thereby allowing the axial images including metallic restorations to be excluded from the study.

Preoperative Planning

Radiographic visualization of potential implant sites is an important extension of clinical examination and assessment. Radiographs help the clinician visualize the alveolar ridges and adjacent structures in all three dimensions and guide the choice of site, number, size, and axial orientation of the implants. Site selection includes consideration of adjacent anatomic structures, such as the incisive and mental foramina, inferior alveolar canal, existing teeth, nasal fossae, and maxillary sinuses. Conditions including retained root fragments, impacted teeth, and any osseous pathology that could compromise the outcome must be identified and located relative to the site of the proposed implant.

Diagnostic images of potential implant sites can provide information about the quality and quantity of bone that would be adequate to support the implant fixture. The quality of bone includes assessment of the cortical bone since it is best suited to withstand the functional loading forces of dental implants. In general, the thicker the cortical bone, the greater the likelihood of successful osseous integration. A greater number of internal trabeculae per unit area is also advantageous.

Bone quantity is assessed by documenting the height and width of available alveolar bone, as well as the morphology of the ridge. The chances of a successful

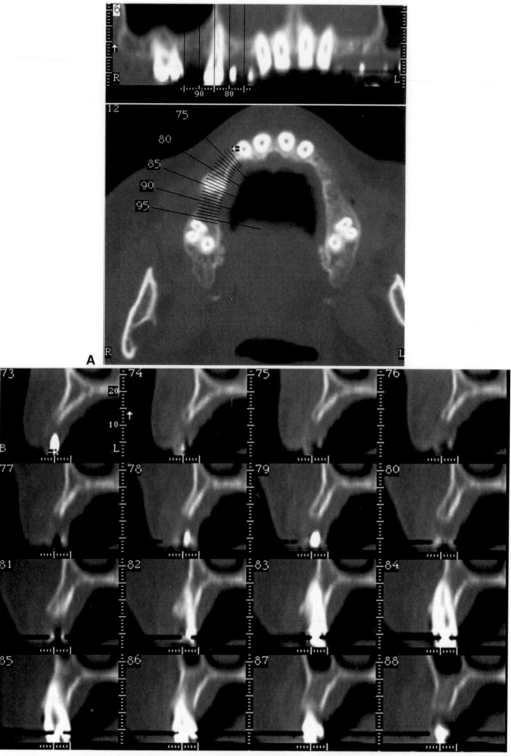

FIG. **31-9**   Reformatted CT study of the maxilla using 3-D Dental software (Columbia Scientific, Inc., Columbia, Md.). **A,** Axial and panoramic-like curved linear reconstructed images using an imaging stent incorporating gutta-percha markers. **B,** Cross-sectional images that correlate with the images in **A.** These images typically are printed life-size for ease of evaluation. (Courtesy Oral and Maxillofacial Imaging Center, Baylor College of Dentistry, Dallas, Texas.)

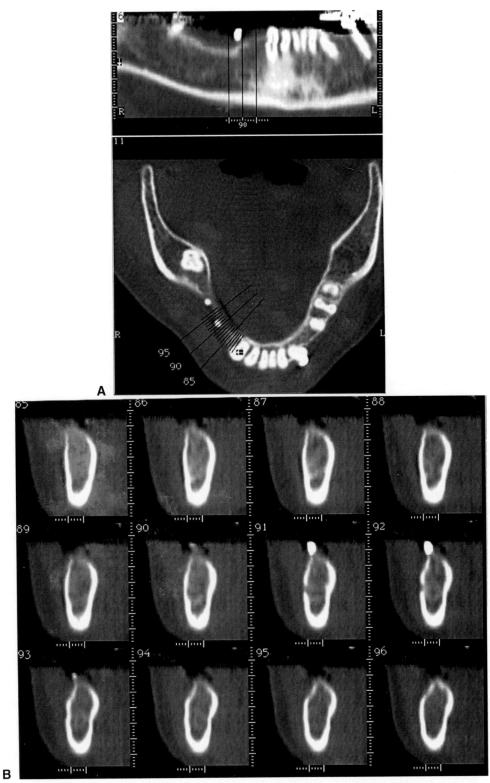

FIG. **31-10** Reformatted CT study of the mandible using 3-D Dental software (Columbia Scientific, Inc., Columbia, Md.). **A,** Axial and panoramic-like curved linear reconstructed images. An imaging stent with gutta-percha markers was used in this case. **B,** Correlating cross-sectional images. These images typically are printed life-size for ease of evaluation. (Courtesy Oral and Maxillofacial Imaging Center, Baylor College of Dentistry, Dallas, Texas.)

outcome will increase with a greater amount of bone available for anchorage. A cross-sectional image to document the facial-lingual width and height of the ridge, along with the inclination of the bone contours, is especially useful in the preoperative planning phase. Ridge width measurements aid in selecting the implant diameter and implant placement to maximal engagement of cortical bone, and ridge height measurements help select the longest appropriate fixture to maximize anchorage and distribution of masticatory forces. Frequently, morphologic features such as osseous undercuts and ridge concavities that are not immediately apparent on clinical examination become evident with cross-sectional imaging.

Accurate bone measurements are essential for determining the optimal size, length, and orientation of the proposed implants. When making measurements on any image, one should be aware that the magnification factor of the image may vary with the imaging technique used. Except for specialized reformatted CT implant programs, all other radiographic images have a magnification factor, which must be taken into account when calculating the dimensions of the bone. The measurements obtained from the images (usually in millimeters) are divided by the magnification factor for that particular imaging technique. Unfortunately the magnification factor of some techniques may be variable (periapical, panoramic), and thus a constant magnification factor cannot be applied. With dental implant CT reformatting software, the image is reproduced in the actual size of the jaw without magnification. If the magnification factor is constant, clear plastic overlays with 1 mm grids or diagrams of available implant sizes already corrected for the specific magnification factor can be used directly on the image.

IMAGING STENTS

The clinical utility of presurgical imaging can be enhanced by the use of an imaging stent that helps relate the radiographic image and its information to a precise anatomic location or potential surgical site. In the case of conventional and computed tomography, an imaging stent also facilitates association of the individual image slices to an anatomic location in the scout films. The intended implant sites are identified by markers made of radiopaque spheres or rods (metal, composite resin, or gutta-percha) retained within an acrylic stent (Fig. 31-11; see also Fig. 31-7), which the patient wears during the imaging procedure so that images of the markers will be created in the diagnostic images. The imaging stent subsequently may be used as

a surgical guide to orient the insertion angle of the guide bur and ultimately the angle of the implant. For optimal visualization, the width of the markers should be less than the thickness of the conventional tomographic image layer. Diagnostic dentures coated with barium paste may be used during imaging for localization and can also establish the spatial relationships between the anticipated prosthesis and implant fixtures. Only nonmetallic radiopaque markers (gutta-percha, composite resin) should be used in CT imaging because metal markers produce image artifacts.

INTERACTIVE DIAGNOSTIC SOFTWARE

Several different interactive software packages have been developed to allow presurgical simulation of implant orientation and placement on a computer screen. Designed for use on personal computers the software is available for both conventional tomography (SURGPlan®, Imaging Sciences International, Hatfield, Penn.) and reformatted computed tomography (SIMPlant®; Materialise Medical, Glen Burnie, Md). These programs provide an interactive platform, permitting analysis of potential implant sites for bone quantity, quality, and morphology, as well as simulating the surgical placement of the implant in real time. Visualization of anatomic structures, volumetric analysis for bone grafts, and mechanical analysis of structural forces during restoration are also within the capability of the software packages (Fig. 31-12).

SELECTING DIAGNOSTIC IMAGING FOR PREOPERATIVE PLANNING

A good starting point is to begin with a panoramic image and supplement it with intraoral films if greater image detail is required of any particular region of interest. These survey films would help to indicate whether the patient is a good candidate for implant procedures. For instance, if there is a pathologic lesion in the planned implant site or if there is obviously inadequate vertical dimension due to severe atrophy of the alveolar ridges, it is futile to proceed with more expensive imaging procedures such as conventional or computed tomography. If the initial scout films reveal reasonable potential implant sites, either conventional tomography or CT can be employed to obtain image slices of these sites (see Table 30-2). Ideally, if images were required of all of the maxilla and mandible to evaluate possible implant sites, CT would be the best modality, and if potential sites were restricted to a few selected regions, conventional tomography would be a suitable choice.

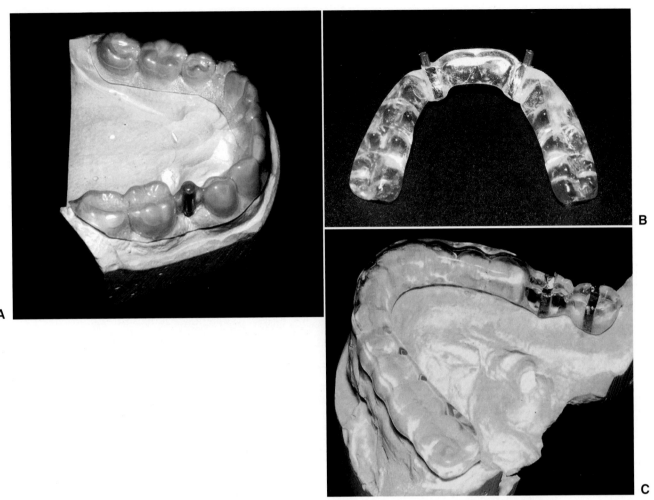

FIG. **31-11** Three examples of imaging stents. **A,** Vacuum-formed imaging stent with a metal rod to indicate desired axis of insertion. **B,** Processed stent with metal cylinders marking the implant sites. This can also be used as a surgical stent by inserting the guide bur through the cylinders. **C,** Processed stent with insertion axis markers, along with a radiopaque strip outlining the buccal and lingual contours of the planned restoration. This provides an image of the emergence profile of the restored implant. This stent can also be used as a surgical guide.

Intraoperative and Postoperative Assessments

Intraoral and panoramic radiographs usually are adequate for both intraoperative and postoperative assessments. Intraoperative films may be required to confirm correct placement of the implant or to locate a lost implant (Fig. 31-13). The two aspects that are usually assessed with time after implant placement are the alveolar bone height around the implant and the appearance of the bone immediately adjacent and surrounding the implant. If threaded root-form fixtures have been placed, the optimal radiographic image must separate the threads for best visualization. This may not always be a predictable procedure because the exact angulation of the implant is not known. The angulation of the x-ray beam must be within 9 degrees of the long axis of the fixture to open the threads on the image on most threaded fixtures (Fig. 31-14). Angular deviations of 13 degrees or more result in complete overlap of the threads. In general, periapical radiographs are appro-

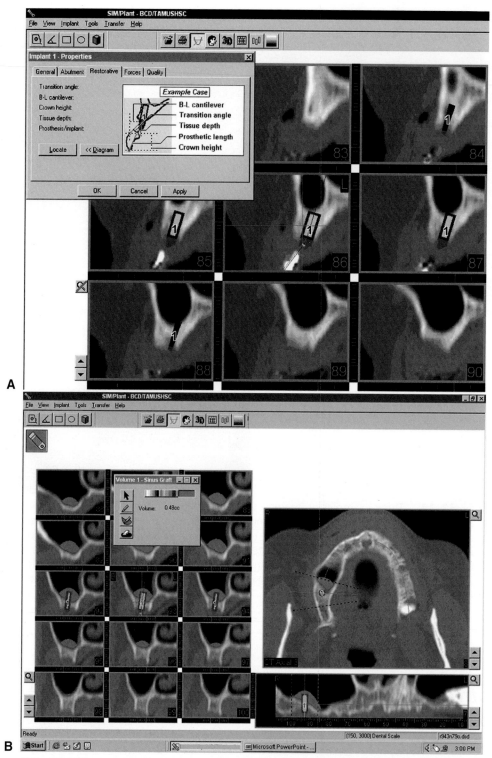

FIG. **31-12**　Images from a computer monitor using SIMPlant® (Materialise Medical, Glen Burnie, Md.) interactive software with reformatted CT images. **A,** Simulation of implant placement and predicted restorative dimensions are displayed on cross-sectional images. **B,** The volume of bone grafting material for a sinus lift procedure is predicted in a case with inadequate alveolar ridge height.

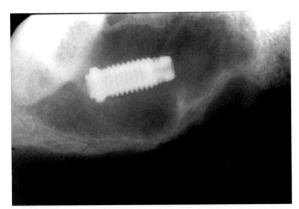

FIG. **31-13** A periapical film revealing an implant loose within the maxillary sinus.

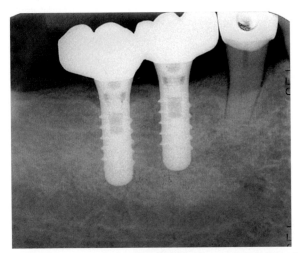

FIG. **31-14** A periapical radiograph of two successful dental implants. Note the close apposition of the bone to the surface of each implant. A minor amount of saucerization is present at the alveolar crest adjacent to the distal fixture.

evidenced by apical migration of the alveolar bone or indistinct osseous margins. These adverse changes are progressive and should be differentiated from the initial circumscribed resorptive osseous changes around the cervical area of the fixture during the first 6 months induced by the surgical procedure itself (Fig. 31-15). Studies suggest that the rate of marginal bone loss after successful implantation is approximately 1.2 mm in the first year, subsequently tapering off to about 0.1 mm in succeeding years. Subtle areas of bone resorption adjacent to the fixture may be made more evident with intraoral digital images by evaluating a density profile graph of radiographic density values, a feature available on most digital imaging units. If intraoral digital images are acquired at the time of surgery, they may be compared with subsequent digital images either by subjective visualization or digital subtraction. Digital subtraction of sequential films is a computerized process that may reveal areas of bone resorption not apparent visually, but it requires that the image geometry be reproduced between radiographic examinations. Areas of marginal bone gain also may be noted occasionally.

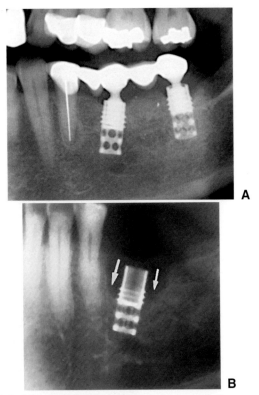

FIG. **31-15** **A,** Marginal bone loss around the cervical region of a root-form dental implant (portion of a panoramic radiograph). **B,** Periapical radiograph of moderate bone loss ("saucerization" type) around the cervical region of a root-form dental implant *(arrows)*.

priate for longitudinal assessments; however, in evaluating the bone height around an implant, an effort should be made to reproduce the vertical angulation of the central ray of the x-ray beam as closely as possible between films in order to closely duplicate the image geometry. Mesial and distal marginal bone height is measured from a standard landmark at the collar of the implant or, if it is a threaded type, using known interthread measurements and compared with bone levels in previous periapical radiographs. The presence of relatively distinct bone margins with a constant height relative to the implant suggests successful osseous integration. Any resorptive changes, if present, are

The success of an implant can also be evaluated by the appearance of normal bone surrounding and right up to the surface of the body of the implant. The development of a thin radiolucent area that closely follows the outline of the implant usually correlates to clinically detectable implant mobility and is an important indicator of failed osseointegration (Fig. 31-16). Also, changes in the periodontal ligament space of associated teeth (natural abutment) are useful in monitoring the functional competence of the implant-prostheses composite. Any widening of the periodontal ligament space compared with preoperative radiographs indicates poor stress distribution and forecasts implant failure (Table 31-3). After successful implantation, radiographs may be made at regular intervals to assess the success or failure of the implant fixture. Advanced imaging studies may be necessary for adequate assessment in some cases (Fig. 31-17).

In summary, diagnostic imaging is an integral part of dental implant therapy for presurgical planning, intraoperative assessment, and postoperative assessment by employing a variety of imaging techniques. Cross-sectional imaging is increasingly considered essential for optimal implant placement, especially in the case of complex reconstructions.

TABLE 31-3
Radiographic Signs Associated With Failing Endosseous Implants

RADIOGRAPHIC APPEARANCE	CLINICAL IMPLICATIONS
Thin radiolucent area that closely follows the entire outline of the implant	Failure of the implant to integrate with the adjoining bone
Crestal bone loss around the coronal portion of the implant	Osteitis resulting from poor plaque control, adverse loading, or both
Apical migration of alveolar bone on one side of the implant	Nonaxial loading resulting from improper angulation of the implant
Widening of the periodontal ligament space of the nearest natural (tooth) abutment	Poor stress distribution resulting from biomechanical inadequate prosthesis-implant system
Fracture of the implant fixture	Unfavorable stress distribution during function

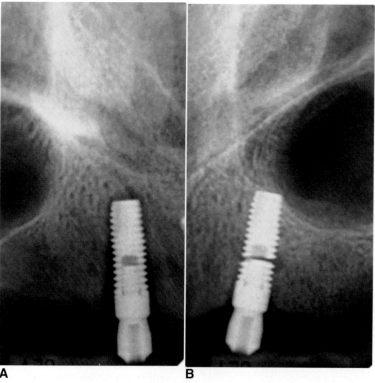

A   **B**

FIG. **31-16**   **A,** Periapical radiograph of bone loss around a root-form dental implant (thin radiolucent band surrounding the implant), indicating failure of osseous integration. **B,** Periapical view of a fractured endosseous implant.

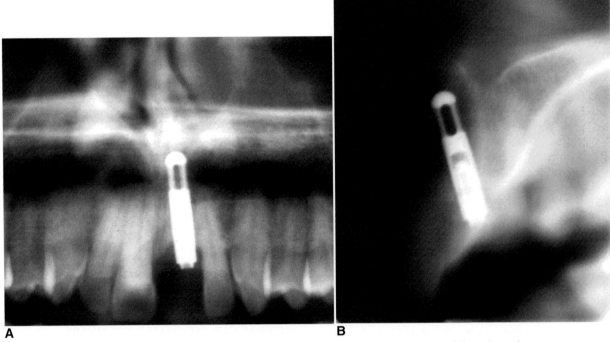

FIG. **31-17** **A,** Panoramic image demonstrating an apparently successful implant placement. **B,** Conventional cross-sectional tomogram reveals that the implant perforated the facial cortex in an attempt to avoid the nasopalatine canal. The angle of this implant also created a restorative dilemma.

BIBLIOGRAPHY

COMPARATIVE DOSIMETRY

Avendanio B et al: Estimate of radiation detriment: scanography and intraoral radiology, Oral Surg Oral Med Oral Pathol Oral Radiol Endod 82:713, 1996.

Frederiksen NL et al: Effective dose and risk assessment from computed tomography of the maxillofacial complex, Dentomaxillofac Radiol 24:55, 1995.

Frederiksen NL et al: Risk assessment from film tomography used for dental implant diagnostics, Dentomaxillofac Radiol 23:123, 1994.

Lecomber AR, Yoneyama Y, Lovelock DJ, Hosoi T, Adams AM: Comparison of patient dose from imaging protocols for dental implant planning suing conventional radiography and computed tomography, Dentomaxillofac Radiol 30:255, 2001.

Scaf G et al: Dosimetry and cost of imaging for osseointegrated implants with film-based and computed tomography, Oral Surg Oral Med Oral Pathol Oral Radiol Endod 83:41, 1997.

COMPUTED TOMOGRAPHY

Kraut RA: Utilization of 3D/DENTAL software for precise implant site selection: clinical reports, Implant Dent 1:134, 1992.

McGivney GP et al: A comparison of computer-assisted tomography and data-gathering modalities in prosthodontics, Int J Oral Maxillofac Implants 1:55, 1986.

Schwarz MS et al: Computed tomography. I. Preoperative assessment of the mandible for endosseous implant surgery, Int J Oral Maxillofac Implants 2:137, 1987.

Schwarz MS et al: Computed tomography. II. Preoperative assessment of the maxilla for endosseous implant surgery, Int J Oral Maxillofac Implants 2:143, 1987.

Wishan MS et al: Computed tomography as an adjunct in dental implant surgery, Int J Oral Maxillofac Implants 8:31, 1988.

CONVENTIONAL TOMOGRAPHY

Ekestubbe A et al: The use of tomography for dental implant planning, Dentomaxillofac Radiol 26:206, 1997.

Gröndahl K et al: Reliability of hypocycloidal tomography for the evaluation of the distance from the alveolar crest to the mandibular canal, Dentomaxillofac Radiol 20:200, 1991.

Kassebaum DK et al: Cross-sectional radiography for implant site assessment, Oral Surg Oral Med Oral Pathol 70:674, 1990.

Stella JP, Tharanon W: A precise radiographic method to determine the location of the inferior alveolar canal in the posterior edentulous mandible: implications for dental implants. I. Technique, Int J Oral Maxillofac Implants 5:15, 1990.

Stella JP, Tharanon W: A precise radiographic method to determine the location of the inferior alveolar canal in the posterior edentulous mandible: implications for dental implants. II. Clinical application, Int J Oral Maxillofac Implants 5:23, 1990.

GENERAL IMAGING TECHNIQUES

Benson BW: Presurgical radiographic planning for dental implants, Oral Maxillofac Surg Clin North Am 13:751, 2001.

Benson BW: Diagnostic imaging for dental implant assessment, Texas Dent J 112:37, 1995.

DeSmet E, Jacobs R, Gijbels F, Naert I: The accuracy and reliability of radiographic methods for the assessment of marginal bone level around oral implants, Dentomaxillofac Radiol 31:176, 2002.

Frederiksen NL: Diagnostic imaging in dental implantology, Oral Surg Oral Med Oral Pathol Oral Radiol Endod 80:540, 1995.

Hollender L, Rockler B: Radiographic evaluation of osseointegrated implants of the jaws, Dentomaxillofac Radiol 9:91, 1980.

Klinge B et al: Location of the mandibular canal: comparison of macroscopic findings, conventional radiography, and computed tomography, Int J Oral Maxillofac Implants 4:327, 1989.

Milgrom P, Getz T: Implants: growing concern, Dental Claims and Insurance News 8:1, 1994 [newsletter].

Pharoah MJ: Imaging techniques and their clinical significance, Int J Prosthodont 6:176, 1993.

Reisken AB: Implant imaging: status, controversies, and new developments, Dent Clin North Am 2:47, 1998.

Sahiwal IG, Woody RD, Benson BW, Guillen GE: Radiographic identification of threaded endosseous dental implants, J Prosthet Dent 87:563, 2002.

Sahiwal IG, Woody RD, Benson BW, Guillen GE: Radiographic identification of nonthreaded endosseous dental implants, J Prosthet Dent 87:552, 2002.

Tyndall DA, Brooks SL: Selection criteria for dental implant site imaging: a position paper of the American Academy of Oral and Maxillofacial Radiology, Oral Surg Oral Med Oral Pathol Oral Radiol Endod 89:630, 2000.

GENERAL IMPLANTOLOGY

Block MA et al, editors: Implants in dentistry, Philadelphia, 1997, WB Saunders.

Brånemark P-I et al, editors: Tissue integrated prostheses, Chicago, 1985, Quintessence.

Cranin AM et al: A statistical evaluation of 952 endosteal implants in humans, J Am Dent Assoc 94:315, 1977.

Sahiwal I, Woody RD, Benson BW, Guillen GE: Macro design morphology of endosseous dental implants, J Prosthet Dent 87:543, 2002.

IMAGING TECHNIQUES (IMAGING STENTS)

Cehreli MC, Aslan Y, Sahin S: Bilaminar dual-purpose stent for placement of dental implants, J Prosthet Dent 84:55, 2000.

Israelson H et al: Barium-coated surgical stents and computer-assisted tomography in the preoperative assessment of dental implant patients, Int J Periodont Restorative Dent 12:53, 1992.

Ku YC, Shen YF: Fabrication of a radiographic and surgical stent for implants with a vacuum former, J Prosthet Dent 83:252, 2000.

INTERACTIVE COMPUTER SOFTWARE

Cucchiara R, Franchini F, Lamma A, Lamma E, Sansoni T, Sarti E: Enhancing implant surgery planning via computerized image processing, Int J of Comput Dent 4:9, 2001.

Rosenfeld AL, Mecall RA: The use of interactive computed tomography to predict the esthetic and functional demands of implant-supported prostheses, Compend Contin Educ Dent 17:1125, 1996.

PANORAMIC RADIOGRAPHY

Lindh C, Petersson AR: Radiologic examination of the mandibular canal: a comparison between panoramic radiography and conventional tomography, Int J Oral Maxillofac Implants 4:249, 1989.

Tal H, Moses O: A comparison of panoramic radiography with computed tomography in the planning of implant surgery, Dentomaxillofac Radiol 20:40, 1991.

Truhlar RS et al: A review of panoramic radiography and its potential use in implant dentistry, Implant Dent 2:122, 1993.

Index

A

A-V aneurysm, 449
A-V defect, 449
A-V malformation, 449
A-V shunt, 449
ABC. *See* Aneurysmal bone cysts (ABC)
Abrasion
  overview of, 355
  secondary dentin and, 360
Abscess formation, periodontitis and, 314
Abscesses. *See also* Acute dentoalveolar
    abscess
  CT and, 664
Absorbed dose, rad and, 21
Acentric fragment, chromosome
    aberrations and, 28f
Acetone, diabetes mellitus and, 523
Acid, erosion and, 356
Acidifiers, fixing solution and, 98
Acidophilic cells, hyperpituitarism and,
    521
Acinic cell carcinoma, minor salivary
    glands and, 675
Acquired concrescence, 337
Acquired cysts, 671
Acromegalic prognathism, inherited
    prognathism v., 521
Acromegaly, 520
  excessive growth of mandible in, 522f
  hypercementosis and, 362
  hyperpituitarism v., 521
  paranasal sinus and, 576
Activator, overview of, 97
Acute apical periodontitis, 367
Acute dentoalveolar abscess, nasopalatine
    duct cysts v., 403
Acute inflammatory processes, CT and,
    663
Acute leukemias, 481
Acute lymphoblastic leukemia, 481
Acute myelogenous leukemia, 481
Acute osteomyelitis
  clinical features of, 374
  definition of, 374
  radiologic examination and features of,
    374-375
  synonyms for, 374
Acute radiation syndrome, overview of, 37,
    37t
Acute sinusitis
  overview of, 579
  radiograph and, 581
Acute suppurative osteomyelitis, 374
ADA. *See* American Dental Association
    (ADA)
Adenoameloblastoma, 431

Adenocarcinoma, minor salivary glands
    and, 675
Adenoid cystic carcinoma
  nerve sheath metastasis and, 675
  ultrasonography of, 675f
Adenoma, primary hyperparathyroidism
    and, 517
Adenomatoid odontogenic tumors
  calcification in, 433f
  calcifying epithelial odontogenic tumors
    v., 423
  calcifying odontogenic cyst v., 400
  cementoossifying fibroma v., 501
  clinical features of, 431
  differential diagnosis and, 433
  overview of, 431
  radiographic features of, 431-432
  synonyms for, 431
  treatment of, 433
Adhesions, overview of, 557
Administrative radiographs, overview of, 272
Adolescents
  carious lesions in, 301
  central giant cell granuloma and, 502
  TMJ dysfunction and, 538
Adrenal adenoma, Cushing's syndrome
    and, 523
Adrenal carcinoma, Cushing's syndrome
    and, 523
Adrenal glands, Cushing's syndrome and,
    523
Adrenal hyperplasia, Cushing's syndrome
    and, 523
Adrenocorticotropic hormone (ACTH),
    basophilic adenoma and, 523
Adults, cortical borders in, 539
African jaw lymphoma, children and, 478
Agenesis, basal cell nevus syndrome and,
    397
Aggressive fibromatosis, 454
Aggressive periodontitis
  clinical presentation of, 322, 323
  radiographic appearance of, 324
  treatment of, 324
Aging
  cemento-osseous dysplasia and, 405
  mandibular symphysis and, 181
  nasolabial fold and, 181
  nutrient canals and, 185
  periodontitis and, 267, 314
  pulpal sclerosis and, 362
  secondary dentin and, 360
AIDS
  infection control and, 115
  osteomyelitis and, 374
  periodontal disease and, 327

Aiming cylinder
  central ray and, 164
  horizontal bitewing films and, 148, 149
Air, subject density and, 78
Air kerma, exposure and, 21
Airway, lateral cephalometric projection
    and, 219f, 220
Ala-tragus line, lateral mandibular occlusal
    projection and, 159
ALARA, radiation and, 52, 61
Alcohol, maternal, prenatal irradiation *vs.*,
    39, 40t
Alcoholism
  parotid area v., 658
  sialadenosis and, 670
Alkali compounds, developers and, 97
Alkaline pH values, developers and, 97
Alkaline phosphatase, hypophosphatasia
    and, 526
Allergen, sinusitis and, 578
Allergic reaction, arthrography v., 548,
    549f
Allergic rhinitis, chronic sinusitis and, 579
Allogeneic bone marrow transplantation,
    leukemia and, 482
Alpha goblin genes, thalassemia and, 533
Alpha particles, 5
Aluminum filtration, patient exposure
    and, 60
Aluminum step wedge, 78f
  x-ray beam and, 79, 80f
Alveolar bone
  eosinophilic granuloma and, 509
  hemifacial hyperplasia and, 650
  lateral cephalometric projection and,
    219f, 220
  loss of height in, 282-283
  malignancy and, 459
  periodontal diseases and, 267, 315,
    315b, 316
  sinus and, 177
Alveolar bone crest, 172, 172f
  bitewing examinations and, 148
  overview of, 169, 169f
  periodontal disease and, 317, 317f, 366
Alveolar bone fracture, dislocation of
    tooth and, 617
Alveolar bone loss, vertical bitewing films
    and, 149, 149f
Alveolar crest
  interproximal radiographs (bitewings)
    and, 271
  small bone loss at, 318f
Alveolar lesions, Langerhans' cell
    histiocytosis and, 514
Alveolar margin, clinical features of, 339

Alveolar process, 282
  ameloblastic fibromas and, 428, 430f
  arteriovenous (A-V) fistula and, 449
  avulsion and, 618
  condylar hyperplasia and, 550
  eosinophilic granuloma and, 512f
  external oblique ridge v., 186, 186f
  fibrosarcoma and, 475
  film placement and, 140, 146
  foramen and, 183
  horizontal fracture and, 630
  monostotic fibrous dysplasia and, 485
  sinuses and, 177
  squamous cell carcinoma and, 464
Alveolar process fractures, dental root
    fractures v, 622
Alveolar ridges
  cemental dysplasia and, 495
  composition of teeth and, 166, 167f
  edentulous patients and, 165
Amalgam restoration
  base material in, 188f
  stainless steel pins and, 188f
Ameloblastic adenomatoid tumor, 431
Ameloblastic carcinoma, overview of, 466
Ameloblastic fibromas
  ameloblastic fibro-odontoma v., 429
  clinical features of, 428, 431
  dentigerous cyst v., 392
  differential diagnosis of, 429, 431
  overview of, 428
  radiographic features of, 428-429, 431
  synonyms for, 428
  third molar and, 430f
  treatment of, 431
  unilocular outgrowth of follicle and,
    430f
Ameloblastic fibroodontomas
  adenomatoid odontogenic tumor v., 433
  ameloblastic fibroma v., 431
  calcifying epithelial odontogenic tumors
    v., 423
  calcifying odontogenic cyst v., 400
  examples of, 432f
  overview of, 429-430
Ameloblastic myxomas, ameloblastic
    fibromas v., 429
Ameloblastomas
  additional imaging in, 420
  adenomatoid odontogenic tumor v., 431
  ameloblastic fibromas v., 429
  aneurysmal bone cyst v., 505
  benign neoplasm v., 411, 412
  calcifying epithelial odontogenic tumors
    v., 423
  calcifying odontogenic cyst and, 399
  central giant cell granuloma v., 502
  central mucoepidermoid carcinoma v.,
    465
  clinical features of, 419
  cropped panoramic image of, 423f
  dentigerous cyst and, 392
  differential diagnosis, 420
  lateral periodontal cyst v., 399
  odontogenic keratocyst v., 395
  odontogenic myxoma v., 434
  overview of, 419
  radiographic features of, 419-420
  radiopaque sinus in, 592f
  recurrent, 420, 424f
  root resorption and, 422f
  septa and, 291

Ameloblastomas (Continued)
  synonyms for, 419
  treatment of, 422
  of unusual type, 422
Ameloblasts
  ameloblastic fibroma and, 428
  hypoplasia and, 345
  jaw tumors and, 410
Amelogenesis imperfecta
  clinical features of, 345
  definition of, 344
  differential diagnosis of, 346
  film of cropped enamel in, 345f
  management of, 346
  panoramic film of, 345, 345f, 346f
  radiographic features of, 346
American Academy of Orthodontics,
    radiographic examination and, 274
American College of Radiology (ACR),
    digital imaging and, 241
American Dental Association (ADA)
  cross-contamination and, 115
  DICOM compliance and, 199
  film mount and, 108
  filtration recommendations from, 60
  radiographic examination and, 266
  radiographic guidelines and, 272
  radiologic process and, 55
  surface cleaners and, 116
Amorphous masses
  calcifying odontogenic cyst and, 400,
    400f
  vertical osseous defects and, 320, 322f
Amorphous radiopacities,
    cementoossifying fibroma and, 499f,
    500
Amperes, current flow and, 9
Amputation neuroma, 440
Amyloidosis, multiple myeloma and, 475
Analgesics, rheumatoid arthritis and, 563
Analog imaging, digital imaging v., 225-226
Analog to digital conversion (ADC),
    overview of, 226
Analog voltage signal, x-rays and, 226, 227f
Analog voltages, exposure latitudes and,
    223f
Anatomic structures
  conventional tomography and, 546
  extraoral images and, 218
  image analysis and, 282
  lateral cephalometric projections of,
    211f
  mandibular body and, 218f
  panoramic images on, 201-209
  posteroanterior cephalometric
    projection and, 216f
  radiographic examination, 270, 270t
  radiographic images and, 218
  reverse-Towne projection and, 217f
  submentovertex projection and, 214f
  TMJ dysfunction and, 539
  waters projection and, 215f
Anemia
  multiple myeloma and, 475
  radiation injury and, 38
Anesthesia, squamous cell carcinoma and,
    461
Aneurysmal bone cysts (ABC)
  central giant cell granuloma v., 502
  clinical features of, 503
  definition of, 503
  differential diagnosis of, 505-506

Aneurysmal bone cysts (ABC) (Continued)
  fibrous dysplasia v., 489, 491
  management of, 506
  radiographic features of, 504-505
  right mandible panoramic image of,
    505f
  TMJ tumors and, 570
Anger scintillation camera, tracers and,
    262
Angular distortion, radicular dilaceration
    and, 340
Angulation. See Horizontal angulation;
    Vertical angulation; Angulation
    guidelines; Bisecting-angle projections
Angulation guidelines, bisecting-angle
    projections and, 148b
Ankylosing spondylitis
  spinal irradiation for, 40
  TMJ and, 564
Ankylosis
  clinical features of, 569
  computed tomography (CT), 548
  coronoid hyperplasia v., 553, 554
  definition of, 569
  fracture and, 568
  radiographic features of, 569-570
Annual E, 50, 51
Anodes
  components of, 8-9, 9f
  cooling characteristics of, 12
Anodontia
  ectodermal dysplasia and, 333, 334f
  synonyms for, 332
Anosmia
  monostotic fibrous dysplasia and, 485
  rhinoliths and, 607
Antegonial notch, juvenile chronic
    arthritis and, 364
Anterior aspect of maxilla, fractures of
    alveolar process and, 627
Anterior disk displacement, MRI and,
    557f
Anterior loop of mandibular canal, mental
    foramina and, 203
Anterior mandible, trabeculae in, 170
Anterior mandibular occlusal projection
  film placement of, 157
  image field of, 157
  point of entry in, 157
  projection of central ray in, 157
Anterior maxilla
  compound odontomas and, 425
  image field of, 154
  neuromas and, 440
Anterior maxillary occlusal projection
  film placement in, 154
  image field in, 154
  point of entry in, 154
  projection of central ray in, 154
Anterior nasal spine, 173
  position of, 172, 172f
Anterior occlusal films, primary dentition
    and, 161, 161f
Anterior open bite
  dentinogenesis imperfecta and, 346
  rheumatoid arthritis and, 563
Anterior sextants, panoramic images and,
    201
Anteroposterior projections
  bifid condyle and, 554
  errors in, 198
  patient positioning and, 198

Anteroposterior views of condyles, mandibular condyle fractures and, 626
Anthelmintic, *cysticercus* and, 601
Antibiotics. *See* Drugs, antibiotics
Antiinflammatory agents. *See* Drugs, antiinflammatory
Antimicrobial therapy
    osteomyelitis and, 377
    septic arthritis and, 565
Antorlith, osteoma v., 586
Antoroliths, dental root fragments v., 594
Antra of Highmore, 576
Antral floor, periostitis and, 589
Antral polyps, retention pseudocysts v., 582
Antral pseudocyst, 581
Antroliths
    clinical features of, 584
    definition of, 584
    differential diagnosis of, 584
    lateral maxillary occlusal film of, 584f
    management of, 584
    maxillary sinus and, 607
    osteoma v., 586
    radiographic features of, 584
Antrum
    fibrous dysplasia and, 489
    image field, 155, 156
Apex of eminence, TMJ and, 540
Apex of tooth, periapical cemental dysplasia and, 492, 492f
Apical foramen
    composition of teeth and, 166, 167f
    dens in dente and, 342
Apical granuloma, radicular cyst v., 386
Apical periodontal cyst, 385
Apical periodontitis, inflammatory reaction and, 368
Apical rarefying osteitis
    dens evaginates and, 344f
    non-Hodgkin's lymphoma v., 478
Aplasia, odontomas and, 425
Apron, disinfecting, 115, 117f
Arc path, image layer and, 194
Arch aesthetics, gemination and, 338
Arterial bifurcations, calcified atherosclerotic plaque v., 602
Arteriosclerosis
    arterial calcification and, 602
    clinical features of, 602
    definition of, 602
    differential diagnosis of, 602
    management of, 602
    radiographic features of, 602, 602f
Arteriovenous aneurysms, hemifacial hyperplasia v., 650
Arteriovenous (A-V) fistula
    additional imaging of, 450
    clinical features of, 449-450
    neurilemmoma v., 440
    overview of, 449
    radiographic features of, 450
    treatment of, 450
Arthritidis, TMJ and, 269
Arthritis, condylar hypoplasia and, 552
Arthrogram
    adhesions and, 557
    deformed disk and, 559f
    disk in open v. closed position and, 558f
    perforation and, 559f

Arthrography
    internal derangement and, 555
    joint spaces and, 549f
    overview of, 548-549
    soft tissue imaging and, 548
    TMJ and, 269
Arthrosis deformans juvenilis, 552
Articular cartilage, joint proliferation, 559
Articular disk
    computed tomography (CT) and, 548
    internal derangement of, 554
    MRI and, 549-550
    TMJ dysfunction and, 538
Articular eminence
    condyle and, 540
    neonatal fractures and, 568
    panoramic projection and, 543, 543f
    pneumatization of, 540
    remodeling and, 559
    transpharyngeal projection, 546f
Articular loose bodies, overview of, 565
Articular tubercle, sagittal plane and, 540
Artifacts
    images and, 201
    panoramic film and, 200, 200f
    panoramic radiograph, 271
Artificial radiation
    distribution of, 49f
    three groups of, 50
Artificial radionuclides, nuclear weapons testing and, 51
Aspergillosis, 588
Aspiration, hemangioma and, 446
Aspiration pneumonia, dystrophic calcification in tonsils and, 599
Aspirin, chondrocalcinosis and, 566
Asthma, chronic sinusitis and, 579
Asymmetries, panoramic projection and, 543, 543f
Atheromatous plaque, calcified atherosclerotic plaque and, 602
Atomic bombs
    leukemia and, 41
    prenatal irradiation and, 39
Atomic number
    restorative materials and, 187
    target with, 8
Atoms
    MRI and, 255-260
    structure of, 3-4
Atoms, hydrogen, 259
Atrophy, muscle, progressive myositis ossificans and, 611
Attrition, 354
    clinical features of, 354
    definition of, 354
    differential diagnosis of, 355
    radiographic features of, 354-355
    secondary dentin and, 360
Auditory canals
    submentovertex projection and, 220, 220f
    Treacher Collins syndrome and, 643
Aunt Minnie analyzing method
    lesions and, 283
    limitations of, 283
Aurora borealis, cosmic ray dose and, 48
Autoclave, instruments and, 117
Autoimmune disorders, staging of, 669
Autoimmune lesions, ultrasonography, 665

Autoimmune sialadenitis
    clinical features of, 668-669
    definition of, 668
    radiographic features of, 669
    relief of symptoms in, 670
    synonyms for, 668
    three features of, 669
    treatment of, 670
Autoimmune sialosis, 668
Autologous bone marrow transplantation, leukemia and, 482
Automatic film processors, 100, 103f
    contamination and, 119-120
    temperature and, 111
Automatic replenishing system, 104
Autosomal dominant type (osteopetrosis tarda), osteopetrosis and, 528
Autosomal recessive type (osteopetrosis congenita), osteopetrosis and, 528
Autotransformer, 7f, 9-10
Autotransplantation of teeth, cleidocranial dysplasia and, 648
Avulsion
    clinical features of, 618
    definition of, 618
    management of, 619
    radiographic features of, 618-619, 619f
    reimplantation v., 619
Axial CT image
    fibrous dysplasia and, 488f
    history of, 251
    MRI and, 664
    nasolabial cyst and, 404f
Axial skeleton, synovial chondromatosis and, 565
Axons, neurofibroma and, 440

B

B cell lymphoma, Burkitt's lymphoma and, 478
Backscatter, lead foil and, 73
Backup, digital imaging and, 240f
Bacteria, gram-negative, periodontitis and, 314
Bacteria plaque (biofilm), dental caries and, 297
Bacterial sialadenitis
    clinical features of, 667
    definition of, 667
    radiographic features of, 667
    submandibular gland and, 659
    treatment of, 667-668
BAI bite-blocks
    children and, 162
    deciduous mandibular molar projection and, 162
    deciduous maxillary molar periapical projection and, 161
Ball in hand appearance, parotid gland sialogram with, 672, 672f
Barium fluorohalide, radiographic imaging and, 230
Barium glass, composite with, 189f
Barrier-protected film. *See* Film, barrier protected
Barriers, surface cleaners and, 116
Basal cell carcinomas, basal cell nevus syndrome and, 397
Basal cell nevus syndrome
    cherubism v., 506
    clinical features of, 397
    definition of, 397

Basal cell nevus syndrome *(Continued)*
management of, 398
odontogenic keratocyst v., 396, 398, 398f
radiographic features of, 398
synonyms for, 397
Base
amalgam restoration v., 188f
intensifying screen and, 76
radiolucent silicate restorations and, 189f
Baseline images
digital subtraction radiography and, 238, 238f
image contrast between, 238
Basophilic adenoma, Cushing's syndrome and, 523
Beam alignment device
calibration and, 113
disinfection of, 115
Beam attenuation, x-ray beam and, 19
Beam energy
overview of, 114
subject contrast and, 79
Beam quality, x-ray and, 14
Beckwith-Weidemann syndrome, hemifacial hyperplasia and, 649
Bence Jones protein, multiple myeloma and, 475
Benign ameloblastomas, malignant ameloblastoma v., 466
Benign cementoblastoma
clinical features of, 435
enostoses v., 416
mixed and late cemental dysplasia v., 495
osteoid osteoma v., 454
overview of, 435
radiographic features of, 436
synonyms for, 434
Benign cyst of antrum, 581
Benign fibroosseous lesion
osteosarcoma v., 469
radicular cyst v., 387
Benign lymphoepithelial cysts, lymph nodes and, 671
Benign lymphoepithelial lesion, 668
parotid area v., 658
Benign lymphoid hyperplasia, parotid v., 659
Benign mixed tumor
clinical features of, 672
definition of, 672
radiographic features of, 672
Benign mucosal cyst of sinus, 581
Benign mucous cyst, 581
Benign neoplasm, Warthin tumor as, 672
Benign tumors. *See* Tumors, benign
Benzotriazole, developing solution and, 97
Beta globulin genes, thalassemia, 533
Beta particles, 5
Bicuspids, developing, dentigerous cyst and, 392
Bifed rib, basal cell nevus syndrome and, 397
Bifid condyle
clinical features of, 554
definition of, 554
differential diagnosis of, 554
radiographic features of, 554
sagittal tomogram showing, 555f
treatment of, 554
Bifid crown, fusion of teeth and, 336

Bilaminar zone, posterior attachment (retrodiskal tissues) and, 541
Bilateral abnormality, normal anatomy and, 283
Bilateral fibrous dysplasia, 485, 486f
Bimanual palpation, stones and, 605
Bimodal age distribution, acute leukemias and, 481
Binding energies, atoms and, 4
Biochemical alteration, radionuclide imaging and, 260, 262f
Biologic effects, direct effects and, 25
Biologic molecules, changes in, 26-27
Biopsy
aneurysmal bone cyst and, 505
benign tumors and, 410
cemental dysplasia and, 495
diagnostic imaging and, 282
fibrous dysplasia and, 489
Langerhans' cell histiocytosis and, 514
lateral periodontal cyst v., 399
polyps and, 584
salivary gland disease and, 659
squamous cell carcinoma and, 461
Bird face, juvenile chronic arthritis v., 364
Birth
hemifacial hyperplasia and, 649
hemifacial microsomia and, 643
paranasal sinuses and, 576
Birth injury, neonatal fractures and, 568, 569
Bisecting-angle instrument, 125
Bisecting-angle projections, angulation guidelines and, 148b
Bisecting-angle technique
mental tubercle, 183
overview of, 90, 90f, 125f
parallel technique *vs.*, 62
periapical radiography and, 121-122
Bit depths, digital detector characteristics and, 232, 232f
Bite-block
conventional tomography and, 547
film placement and, 132, 138, 142, 144
hemostat and, 164
patient examination and, 123
projection of central ray and, 135
universal precautions and, 116
Bite-block, XCP, deciduous mandibular molar projection and, 162
Bitewing examinations, 299f
overview of, 148
periodontitis and, 267
problems associated with, 299
Bitewing projections, 282
ameloblastic fibroma and, 430f
child and, 161
dental caries and, 298, 299f
fate of incident photons in, 17t
lesions and, 304f
overview of, 121, 122f
purposes for, 73-74
rare-earth screens and, 198
value of, 148
Bitewing tab (loop), horizontal bitewing films and, 149, 149f
Blade implant, fixed bridge with, 678f
Bleeding
complicated crown fractures and, 620
craniofacial disjunction and, 633
crown-root fractures and, 623
gingivitis and, 314

Bleeding *(Continued)*
hemangioma and, 446
inferior condylar positioning (widened joint space) and, 542
paper film packets and, 118
periodontal disease and, 327
Blindness, monostotic fibrous dysplasia and, 485
Blood cells
radiation effects on, 38f
sickle cell anemia and, 533
Blood count, irradiation and, 37
Blood pressure, high, nutrient canals and, 185
Blood vessels
metastatic tumors and, 466
neurofibromatosis and, 441
Blue sclera, osteogenesis imperfecta and, 347
Blurring
conditions for, 245-245
faulty radiographs and, 107b
film based tomography and, 245
linear tomogram and, 247
Body section radiography, overview of, 245
Boering, juvenile arthrosis and, 553
Boering's arthrosis, 552
hemifacial microsomia v., 643
Bone(s)
arteriovenous (A-V) fistula and, 449
calcium reserve in, 516
central mucoepidermoid carcinoma from, 465
cleidocranial dysplasia and, 646
condylar hyperplasia and, 550-551
disorders of endocrine system and, 516
Ewing's sarcoma and, 473
external resorption and, 358, 359f
focal osteoporotic bone marrow and, 655
image field and, 136
implants and, 269
irradiated, 380
malignant ameloblastoma and, 466
mixed density lesions v., 290
moderate periodontitis and, 320, 321f
nasopalatine duct cyst and, 403, 404f
neurofibromatosis and, 441
non-Hodgkin's lymphoma and, 477
osteomas and, 443
Paget's disease and, 508
periodontal disease and, 326
radiation damage to, 36
radiolucent v.radiopaque materials and, 289
squamous cell carcinoma and, 462f
subject density and, 78
Bone, destruction, malignant neoplasms and, 586
Bone algorithm, aneurysmal bone cyst and, 505f
Bone cysts
desmoplastic fibromas of bone v., 454
fibrous dysplasia and, 489
florid osseous dysplasia and, 496, 498, 498f
multiple myeloma v., 477
odontogenic keratocyst v., 396
periapical cemental dysplasia v., 492, 495f

Bone density
  acute osteomyelitis and, 375, 376f
  osteopetrosis and, 529, 530f
  osteoporosis and, 524
  radiographic changes and, 516
  renal osteodystrophy and, 526, 528f
Bone destruction
  Langerhans' cell histiocytosis and, 512, 512f
  osteoradionecrosis and, 382
Bone dysplasias
  benign neoplasm v., 412
  maxillary sinuses and, 577
  overview of, 485
Bone erosions
  chondrocalcinosis and, 566
  joint proliferation and, 559
  rheumatoid arthritis and, 563, 563f
Bone exposure, osteoradionecrosis and, 380
Bone formation
  acute osteomyelitis and, 375
  inflammatory lesions and, 367
  joint proliferation and, 559
  osteoradionecrosis and, 380, 382
Bone fracture
  mandibular body fractures and, 625
  radiographic signs of, 616
Bone grafts, condylar hypoplasia and, 552
Bone island
  dystrophic calcification in tonsils v., 599
  mature cemental dysplasia v., 495
Bone loss
  furcations of multirooted teeth and, 321
  juvenile periodontitis and, 324f
  periapical radiograph of, 689f
  periodontal diseases and, 325
Bone marrow
  gastrointestinal syndrome and, 38-39
  leukemia, 481
Bone marrow transplant
  multiple myeloma v., 477
  osteopetrosis and, 531
Bone mass, osteoporosis and, 524
Bone measurements, dental implants and, 686
Bone metabolism
  fibrous dysplasia and, 485
  inflammatory lesions and, 367
  jaws and, 366
  periapical cemental dysplasia, 492
  simple bone cyst and, 405
Bone resorption
  acute osteomyelitis and, 375
  benign neoplasm and, 411
  inflammatory disease and, 291
Bone structure, periodontal disease and, 317
Bone trabeculae
  chronic osteomyelitis and, 379, 379f
  enlarging radiolucency in, 289
Bony ankylosis, 569
  CT scan of, 570f
  etiology of, 569, 570f
  mandibular condyle fractures and, 627
  secondary degenerative changes in, 569
Bony hyperplasias. See Hyperplasia
Bony investment, periodontal disease and, 326
Bony lesions
  image layer and, 194
  occult disease and, 268
  submandibular gland fossa and, 186

Bony pockets
  aggressive periodontitis and, 324
  stereoscopy technique and, 249, 249f
Bony proliferation, degenerative joint disease and, 561, 562f
Bony swelling
  eosinophilic granuloma and, 509
  florid osseous dysplasia and, 496
Bony tissues, MRI and, 255-260
Botryoid odontogenic cysts, lateral periodontal cyst and, 398
Brachycephalic skull, cleidocranial dysplasia and, 646
Brachycephaly
  cleidocranial dysplasia and, 648
  crouzon syndrome and, 641
Brain, *cysticercus cellulosae* and, 601
Branchial cleft cysts
  dermoid cysts v., 404
  submandibular gland and, 659
Brazil nut, radionuclides and, 50
Breast metastasis, osteosarcoma v., 469
Breathing, mouth, gag reflex and, 163
Bremsstrahlung interactions, electrons and, 12
Brightness, digital radiographs and, 235
Bromide ions, 94
  in emulsion, 95f
Bruit
  cavernous hemangioma and, 605
  hemangioma and, 445
Bruxism
  attrition and, 354
  PDL and, 170
Buccal bifurcation cyst (BBC)
  clinical features of, 392
  definition of, 392
  differential diagnosis of, 393
  effects on surrounding structures of, 392-393, 393f
  location of, 392
  management of, 393
  paradental cysts v., 392
  radiographic features of, 392
  synonyms for, 392
Buccal carious lesions
  enamel pits and, 303
  lingual caries v., 303
Buccal cortex, buccal bifurcation cyst and, 393
Buccal cortical plates, fractures of alveolar process and, 627
Buccal cusps, buccal bifurcation cyst and, 392
Buccal object rule, 91
  periodontal disease and, 321
Buccal pit, dentinal occlusal lesions and, 302
Buccal plate, moderate periodontitis and, 318-319, 318f
Buccal roots, 178
  central ray and, 89
Buccinator muscle, external oblique ridge v., 186, 186f
Bucky, grid and, 85
Burkitt's lymphoma
  clinical features of, 478
  definition of, 478
  differential diagnosis of, 480
  management of, 480-481
  radiographic features of, 480
Burkitt's tumor, extranodal disease and, 480

C

Café-au-lait spots, neurofibromatosis and, 442
Calcification(s)
  adenomatoid odontogenic tumor and, 431, 433f
  articular loose bodies and, 565
  blood vessel, 602f
  central odontogenic fibroma and, 438
  CT and, 664
  hypophosphatemia and, 527
  irradiation of teeth and, 34
  Monckeberg's medial calcinosis and, 602
  overview of, 602
  pulpal sclerosis and, 362
  reverse-Towne projection, 222, 223f
  salivary gland tumors and, 672
  sialoliths and, 666
  TMJ and, 539
  Turner's hypoplasia and, 352
  Waters projection and, 221
Calcifications, intracranial, stereoscopy technique and, 248
Calcified atheromatous plaque, calcified triticeous cartilage v., 607
Calcified atherosclerotic plaque
  definition of, 602
  differential diagnosis of, 602
  management of, 602
  radiographic features of, 602
Calcified carotid atheromata, calcified triticeous cartilage v., 607
Calcified cysticerci, locations of, 601
Calcified granulomatous disease, dystrophic calcification in tonsils v., 599
Calcified lymph nodes, 666
  clinical features of, 599
  definition of, 598
  differential diagnosis of, 599
  management of, 599
  radiographic features of, 599
Calcified material, cementoossifying fibroma and, 500
Calcified mixed odontoma, 424
Calcified sialoliths, occlusal projections of, 604f
Calcified structures
  ameloblastic fibroma and, 431, 432f
  radiopaque (mixed density) and, 289
Calcified triticeous cartilage
  calcified atherosclerotic plaque v., 602
  location of, 606
Calcifying epithelial odontogenic tumor (CEOT)
  adenomatoid odontogenic tumor v., 433
  ameloblastoma v., 422
  calcifying odontogenic cyst v., 400
  cementoossifying fibroma v., 501
  clinical features of, 422
  differential diagnosis for, 424
  radiographic features of, 422
  synonyms for, 422
Calcifying odontogenic cysts
  adenomatoid odontogenic tumor v., 433
  calcifying epithelial odontogenic tumors v., 423
  cementoossifying fibroma, 501
  clinical features of, 399

Calcifying odontogenic cysts *(Continued)*
  definition of, 399
  dentigerous cyst v., 392
  differential diagnosis of, 400
  management of, 400
  radiographic features of, 400, 400f
  synonyms for, 399
Calcinosis, 597
  osteoma cutis v., 610
Calcitonin, Paget's disease and, 509
Calcium
  arteriosclerosis and, 602, 602f
  metastatic calcification and, 597
  pseudohypoparathyroidism and, 520
  Strontium-90 v., 51
Calcium carbonate
  nidus and, 607
  rhinoliths and, 607
Calcium hydroxide, radiodensity and, 305
Calcium hydroxide base, restorative
    materials as, 187, 188f
Calcium phosphate
  nidus and, 607
  soft tissue and, 597
Calcium pyrophosphate dihydrate
    deposition disease, 566
Calcium salts
  dystrophic calcification and, 598
  soft tissue and, 597
Calcium serum
  osteomalacia and, 524
  parathyroid hormone and, 517
Calcium supplements, osteoporosis and,
    524
Calcium tungstate screens, rare earth
    screens *vs.*, 57-58
Calculus, 665
  enamel pearl v., 350
  periodontitis and, 267
Calculus deposits
  bitewing exam and, 148
  periodontal diseases and, 325
Caldwell-Luc operations
  mucocele and, 585
  osteoma and, 586
  pseudotumor and, 588
Caldwell projections, squamous cell
    carcinoma and, 587
Caldwell view
  maxillary sinus disease and, 578
  osteomas in, 443, 443f
Calibration, x-ray machine and, 113
Calvarium
  lateral cephalometric projection and,
    218-220, 219f
  posteroanterior cephalometric
    projection and, 221-222, 222f
  reverse-Towne projection, 222, 223f
  submentovertex projection and, 220,
    220f
  Waters projection and, 221
Cancellous bone
  anatomy of, 170
  fibrous dysplasia and, 485
  florid osseous dysplasia and, 495
  inflammatory lesions and, 367
Cancellous osteomas, 443
Cancer(s)
  causes of, 458
  radiation induced, 39, 40
  stomchastic effects and, 25, 51
Cancer, brain, radiation exposure and, 41

Cancer, esophageal, radiation exposure
    and, 41
Cancer, intestine, enostoses v., 416
Cancer, jaw, classifications of, 458
Cancer, salivary gland, radiation exposure
    and, 41
Cancer, thyroid, radiation exposure and,
    41
Cancer survivor, dental radiology and,
    482
Cancers, oral, overview of, 458
Candida albicans, oral mucous membrane
    and, 33
Canine(s)
  anterior mandibular occlusal projection
    and, 157
  compound odontomas and, 425
  digital imaging and, 241
  external resorption and, 358
  film placement and, 130, 132, 140, 142
  image field and, 130, 132, 142
  image field of, 154
  projection of central ray and, 129, 141
  toothbrush injury and, 355
Canine fossa, cementoossifying fibroma
    and, 498
Canine periapical projection, mixed
    dentition and, 162
Canine region, adenomatoid odontogenic
    tumor and, 431
Canthomeatal line
  extraoral radiographic examinations
    and, 210
  reverse-Towne projection (open mouth),
    213
  submentovertex (base) projection and,
    213
Capillary bed, arteriovenous (A-V) fistula
    and, 449
Carbohydrates, fermentable, dental caries
    and, 297
Carcinogenesis, overview of, 39-41
Carcinoma arising in dental cyst,
    malignant ameloblastoma v., 466
Carcinoma ex mixed tumor, 674
Carcinoma ex odontogenic cyst, 464
Carcinoma ex pleomorphic adenoma,
    674
Carcinomas
  alveolar bone and, 283
  primary osseous carcinoma v., 464
Cardiovascular system syndrome, overview
    of, 39
Caries. *See* Dental caries
Carious lesions. *See also* Dental caries
  arrested, 297
  behaviors of, 266
  dental floss injury and, 356
  initial, 297
  occult disease and, 268
  penetration depth of, 300
  periapical inflammatory lesions and,
    371
  posterior bitewing and, 299f
  recurrent, 310
  tooth surface with, 297
  treatment considerations for, 311-313
  Turner's hypoplasia and, 352
Caronal caries, 266
Carotid artery
  medial calcinosis and, 602
  panoramic radiographs and, 268

Carpopedal spasm
  hypoparathyroidism and, 519
  pseudohypoparathyroidism and, 519
Cartilage
  condylar hyperplasia and, 550
  osteomas and, 443
  remodeling and, 557
Cartilaginous lesions, jaws and, 285, 411
Cataracts, radiation in atomic bombs and,
    41
Cathode, overview of, 7, 8
Cathode ray tube (CRT) designs,
    computer monitors and, 233
Cathode rays, 5
Cavernous hemangioma, bruit and, 605
Cavitary sialectasis, 669
  contrast agent and, 669
Cavitated lesions
  operative treatment for, 301
  removal of, 312
Cavitation
  dentin and, 297
  radiographic accuracy of, 300
CBCT (cone-beam computed
    tomography), 256f
  flat panel detectors and, 232
  overview of, 255
Cell cycle, 27f
Cell death, mitotic delay and, 29
Cell kinetics, radiation effects on, 29
Cell recovery, process of, 29-30
Cells
  categories according to cell death of, 30
  irradiation modifying factors on, 31-32
Cellulitis
  periapical inflammatory lesions and, 371
  septic arthritis, 565
Cemental dysplasia, 492, 493f
  cementoossifying fibroma v., 501
  osteoblastomas and, 452
  osteoid osteoma v., 454
Cemental lesions, periapical cemental
    dysplasia v., 492
Cemental tissue, florid osseous dysplasia
    and, 498
Cementicles, periapical cemental dysplasia,
    492
Cementifying fibroma, 498
Cemento-osseous dysplasias
  jaw involvement and, 492
  simple bone cyst and, 405
Cemento-osseous tissue, florid osseous
    dysplasia and, 495
Cemento-ossifying fibromas (COF)
  bone patterns in, 500f
  cemental dysplasia v., 501
  clinical features of, 499
  complex odontomas v., 427
  definition of, 498
  differential diagnosis of, 500-501
  fibrous dysplasia v., 489, 500
  internal structure of, 500
  management of, 501
  osteoid osteoma v., 454
  periphery of, 499, 499f
  radiographic features of, 499-500
  synonyms for, 498
Cementoblastomas, 434
  panoramic radiograph of, 438f
  radiopaque lesion and, 288
Cementoblasts, benign cementoblastoma
    v., 435

Cementoenamal junction (CEJ), moderate periodontitis and, 318
Cementoenamel junction (CEJ)
  alveolar crest and, 169
  bone level measurement at, 315
  dentigerous cyst and, 388
  enamel pearl and, 350
  periodontal disease and, 316
  root surface lesions and, 304
  taurodontism and, 339
  toothbrush injury and, 355
Cementoma, 492
Cementum
  appearance of, 284f, 291
  benign cementoblastoma and, 435
  cleidocranial dysplasia and, 646
  composition of teeth and, 166
  concrescence and, 337, 337f
  dens in dente and, 340
  hypercementosis and, 362
  root surface lesions and, 303-304
  subject density and, 78
Cementum caries, root surface and, 309f
Central beam, tooth root and, 125
Central bone cyst, central giant cell granuloma v., 503
Central bone lesions, benign tumors and, 410
Central desmoplastic fibroma, CT image of, 455f
Central giant cell granuloma (CGCG)
  ameloblastic fibromas v., 429
  ameloblastoma v., 420
  aneurysmal bone cyst v., 504, 505, 505f, 506f
  benign neoplasm v., 412
  central mucoepidermoid carcinoma v., 465
  central odontogenic fibroma v., 439
  cherubism v., 506
  clinical features of, 502
  definition of, 501-502
  differential diagnosis of, 502-503
  expansion of cortical plates in, 504f
  fibrous dysplasia v., 489, 491
  malignant ameloblastoma v., 466
  management of, 502-503
  odontogenic myxoma v., 434
  radiographic features of, 502
  synonyms for, 501
Central hemangioma. *See also* Hemangioma
  odontogenic myxoma v., 434
  overview of, 445
Central incisor projections, 173
Central incisor roots, 174
Central incisors, 174, 175f
  central ray and, 127
  external resorption and, 358
  film and, 148
  film placement and, 138
  fusion of teeth and, 336, 336f
  image field and, 126, 128
  incisive foramen and, 175f
  internal resorption and, 356
  nasopalatine duct cyst and, 401
  projection of central ray and, 139
  regional odontodysplasia and, 349
Central incisors projection, edentulous patients and, 165
Central lesions, follicular type of, 431

Central mandibular carcinoma, 463
Central mucoepidermoid carcinoma
  clinical features of, 465
  differential diagnosis of, 465
  effects on surrounding structures by, 465
  management of, 465
  overview of, 465
  periphery and shape of, 465
  radiographic features of, 465
Central mucoepidermoid tumor, malignant ameloblastoma v., 466
Central nervous system, hyperpituitarism and, 521
Central nervous system syndrome, overview of, 39
Central neuromas. *See* Neuromas
Central odontogenic fibroma
  clinical features of, 438
  differential diagnosis of, 438-439
  overview of, 438
  radiographic features of, 438
  synonyms for, 438
  types of, 438
Central ray, 90
  anterior mandibular occlusal projection of, 157
  anterior maxillary occlusal projection and, 154
  cross-sectional mandibular occlusal projection, 158
  horizontal angulation and, 148
  horizontal bitewing films and, 149
  lateral mandibular occlusal projection and, 159
  lateral maxillary occlusal projection and, 156
  molar bitewing projection and, 153
  point of entry and, 153
  premolar bitewing projection and, 151
  projection of, 127, 129, 131, 133, 135, 137, 139, 141, 143, 145, 147
  tooth and, 89, 89f
  vertical angulation and, 148
Central squamous cell carcinomas, 463
  non-Hodgkin's lymphoma v., 478
Central tumors, adenomatoid odontogenic tumor and, 431
Central x-ray beam. *See also* X-ray beam
  lateral cephalometric projections and, 211, 212t
  posteroanterior cephalometric projection and, 213
  reverse-Towne projection and, 213, 218
  submentovertex (base) projection and, 213
  waters projection and, 213
CEOT. *See* Calcifying epithelial odontogenic tumor (CEOT)
Cephalometric, extraoral projections as, 74
Cephalometric film, 100
Cephalometric imaging, 223
  CCDs and, 228
  dental implants and, 677, 678b
  extraoral radiographic examinations and, 210, 283
  rare earth screens and, 48
Cephalometry, extraoral radiographic examinations and, 210
Cephalostat, extraoral radiograph and, 223
Cerebral cranium, frontal sinuses and, 577

Cerebrospinal fluid rhinorrhea, pyramidal fracture and, 632
Cerebrovascular accident, panoramic radiographs and, 268
Cervical burnout
  carious lesion v., 300
  composition of teeth and, 166, 167f
Cervical carious lesions, 312f
Cervical lymph nodes
  calcified lymph nodes and, 599, 600f
  malignant ameloblastoma and, 466
  septic arthritis and, 565
Cervical lymphadenopathy
  Ewing's sarcoma and, 473
  HIV disease and, 669
Cervical spine
  lateral cephalometric projection and, 219f, 220
  posteroanterior cephalometric projection and, 221-222, 222f
  radiographic examination and, 53
Cervical spine injuries, 3D CT and, 254
Cervical spine region, opacity and, 204
Cervical vertebrae
  mandibular ramal area and, 202
  panoramic film and, 200, 200f
Cesium, flat panel detectors and, 232
Cesium-137, Nevada test site and, 51
Cesium iodide, x-ray absorption and, 228
CGCG. *See* Central giant cell granuloma (CGCG)
Chair, disinfection of, 115
Characteristic curves
  films and, 79, 80f
  inherent latitude of film and, 82f
  InSight and, 81
  optical density v., 77, 78f
Characteristic radiation, overview of, 13, 13f
Charge packets, 227
Charged-coupled device (CCD) sensors, 228
Charged-coupled devices (CCD)
  digital detectors and, 226-229
  exposure latitudes and, 223f
  image and, 192
  image receptors and, 198
  structure of, 228f
Chédiak-Higashi syndrome, periodontal disease and, 327
Cheek, osteoma cutis and, 609, 609f
Chemical action, erosion and, 356
Chemical fogging, 96f
Chemical processing, digital imaging and, 225
Chemicals, rapid-processing, 102
Chemotherapy
  Burkitt's lymphoma v., 480
  Ewing's sarcoma and, 474
  fibrosarcoma v., 475
  leukemia and, 482
  malignant tumors and, 572, 673
  multiple myeloma v., 477
  non-Hodgkin's lymphoma v., 478
  primary osseous carcinoma and, 464
  squamous cell carcinoma and, 463
Chernobyl, radiation from, 51
Cherubism
  aneurysmal bone cyst v., 505
  basal cell nevus syndrome v., 398
  Burkitt's lymphoma v., 480
  central giant cell granuloma v., 503

Cherubism (Continued)
  clinical features of, 506
  definition of, 506
  differential diagnosis, 506
  jaw abnormalities and, 285f
  lesions in ramus and, 292
  management of, 506-507
  radiographic features of, 506
Chest, radiographic examination and, 53
Chest radiograph
  avulsed tooth and, 619
  mouth survey vs., 53
Chewing, secondary dentin and, 360
Child, initial dental visit, 273
Children
  African Burkitt's lymphoma and, 478
  carious lesions in, 301
  cherubism and, 506
  chronic osteomyelitis and, 379
  cleidocranial dysplasia and, 648
  condyles in, 539
  cortical borders in, 539
  craniofacial fibrous dysplasia and, 593
  deciduous mandibular molar projection
    and, 162
  electrical conductance measurements
    (ECM), 311
  eosinophilic granuloma and, 509
  examination coverage in, 161
  exposure factors and, 78
  fibrous dysplasia and, 375
  fractures of alveolar process and, 629
  greenstick fractures and, 625
  hemangiomas and, 673
  hemifacial microsomia and, 643
  hyperpituitarism and, 521
  hypophosphatasia and, 526
  hypophosphatemia and, 527
  hypothyroidism and, 523
  juvenile arthrosis and, 553
  mandibular condyle fractures and, 627
  maxillary anterior occlusal projection
    and, 161
  metastatic tumors and, 466
  occlusal radiographs and, 271
  orthodontic elastics and, 301
  osteopetrosis and, 528
  panoramic examination and, 267
  pansinusitis and, 579
  patient management with, 160-161
  periapical and, 267
  polyostotic fibrous dysplasia and, 485
  positioning, 197-198
  progressive myositis ossificans and, 611
  proliferative periostitis and, 375, 377f
  radiation therapy and, 34
  radiographic examination of, 160-162
  rampant caries and, 308f
  renal osteodystrophy and, 526
  rhabdomyosarcoma in, 571
  rickets in, 525
  thyroid cancer in, 41
  TMJ dysfunction and, 538
  trabeculation of mandible and, 202
Chin
  anteroposterior position radiograph
    and, 198
  lateral mandibular occlusal projection
    and, 159
Chin rotation, juvenile chronic arthritis v.,
  364
Chlorines, surface cleaners and, 116

Chondroblastic osteosarcoma, 469
Chondroblastomas, TMJ tumors and, 570
Chondrocalcinosis, 597
  clinical features of, 566
  CT image of, 566f
  definition of, 566
  differential diagnosis of, 566
  radiographic features of, 566
  synonyms for, 566
  synovial chondromatosis v., 565
  treatment of, 566
Chondrosarcoma
  articular loose bodies and, 565
  clinical features of, 471
  CT image of, 571f
  differential diagnosis of, 472
  Ewing's sarcoma v., 474
  histologic subtypes of, 471
  osteosarcoma v., 469, 472
  overview of, 471
  primary intrinsic malignant tumors and,
    571
  radiographic features of, 471-472, 571
  synovial chondromatosis v., 566
Chromatid aberration, DNA and, 27
Chromosome aberrations, 27f
  discussion of, 27, 28f
  overview of, 27, 27f
Chromosome abnormalities, leukemia, 482
Chronic abscess, vertical root fractures
    and, 623
Chronic apical periodontitis, 367
Chronic diffuse sclerosing osteomyelitis,
  377
Chronic inflammatory diseases,
    sialography and, 663
Chronic lymphocytic leukemia, 481
Chronic myelogenous leukemia, 481
Chronic osteomyelitis
  differential diagnosis of, 379-380
  effects on surrounding structures in,
    379
  internal structure and, 378-379, 378f
  management of, 380
Chronic renal failure, renal osteodystrophy
    and, 526
Chronic retrograde infections, salivary
    flow and, 666
Chronic sclerosing osteomyelitis, florid
    osseous dysplasia v., 496
Chronic sinusitis
  CT image of, 581, 581f
  overview of, 579
Ciliary dysfunction, sinusitis and, 578
Cingulum, dens in dente and, 342
Circular tomography, 246, 246f
Circumorbital ecchymosis, zygomatic arch
    fractures and, 635
Clark's rule, 91
Claustrophobia, MRI and, 260, 550
Clavicles, cleidocranial dysplasia and, 646,
    647f, 648
Clearing agents, fixing solution and, 98
Cleft lip, overview of, 639
Cleft palate
  alveolar ridge defects and, 640f
  craniofacial anomalies and, 639
  etiology of, 639
  mandibular symphysis and, 181
Cleft palate syndromes, talon cusp and,
  351
Cleft Palate Team, cleft palate and, 640

Cleidocranial dysostosis, 646
Cleidocranial dysplasia (CCD)
  clinical features of, 646, 648
  definition of, 646
  differential diagnosis of, 648
  management of, 648
  panoramic images of, 649f
  radiographic features of, 647f, 648, 648f
Clinical cavity
  dentin and, 301
  treatment for, 307f
Clinical crown, periodontal disease and,
  326
Clinical examination
  periodontal radiographic assessment v.,
    315, 315b
  radiographs and, 281
Clinoid processes, lateral cephalometric
    projection and, 218-220, 219f
Clivus sinuses
  lateral cephalometric projection and,
    218-220, 219f
  submentovertex projection and, 220,
    220f
CMOS (complementary metal oxide
    semiconductors) technology
  digital image receptors and, 299
  overview of, 229
Coating weight, film slide and, 72t
Cobalt, gamma radiation and, 33
Codman's triangle
  Ewing's sarcoma and, 473
  fibrosarcoma and, 475
  osteosarcoma and, 460f-461f, 469
Cof, central giant cell granuloma v., 502
Coherent scattering (Classical; Elastic;
    Thompson), overview of, 16-17, 17f
Colchicine, chondrocalcinosis and, 566
Collagen, 170
Collagen fibers, desmoplastic fibroma of
    bone and, 454
Collapsing radicular cysts, CT images of,
  387f
Collars, ADA recommendations for, 61
Collimation
  ADA on, 59
  calibration and, 113, 114f
  tissue irradiation effects of, 58f
  x-ray beam and, 15-16, 15f
  x-ray beam modification and, 13
Collimator, image layer and, 194
Color phosphors, cathode ray tube (CRT)
    designs and, 234
CommCAT, facial skeletal images and, 197,
    198f
Common cold, acute sinusitis and, 579
Complete twinning, supernumerary tooth
    and, 338
Complex composite odontoma, 424
Complex odontoma, 424
  ameloblastic fibroma v., 431
Composite
  barium glass and, 189f
  dentin and, 189f
  restorative materials as; 187, 188f
Compound odontomas, 424, 425, 426f
  ameloblastic fibroma v., 431
  examples of, 427f
Compounds, overview of, 3
Compression fracture, Town's view of, 568f
Compton interactions, 94
  x-ray beam and, 83

Compton scattering
  overview of, 17-18, 18f
  photons and, 16f
Computed tomography (CT). *See also* Axial
      CT image
  acute osteomyelitis and, 374, 375f
  advanced imaging procedures and, 271
  ameloblastoma and, 420, 422, 424f
  aneurysmal bone cyst and, 505
  benign tumors on, 410, 672
  bone algorithm of maxillary lesion in,
      491f
  cementifying fibroma in, 499f
  cementoossifying fibroma v., 501
  central giant cell granuloma v., 503
  chondrocalcinosis and, 566, 566f
  chronic osteomyelitis and, 380
  chronic sclerosing osteomyelitis and, 496
  condyle and, 542f
  craniofacial disjunction and, 634
  dental implants and, 677, 678b, 681, 683
  dermoid cysts and, 404, 405f
  desmoplastic fibromas of bone and, 454,
      455f
  diffuse sclerosing osteomyelitis and,
      375f, 378, 378f
  Ewing's sarcoma involving left
      mandibular condyle and, 473f
  fibrous desplasia maxillary lesion in,
      491f
  fibrous dysplasia and, 488f, 489, 491f
  formation of, 253f
  fracture and, 568
  hemangiomas and, 673
  hemifacial microsomia and, 643
  horizontal fracture and, 631
  Langerhans' cell histiocytosis and, 512
  lingual salivary gland depression and,
      651, 652, 654f
  mandibular condyle and, 616
  maxillary fractures and, 616, 629-630
  maxillary sinus disease and, 578
  mucocele and, 585
  mucosa thickening and, 580
  nasopalatine duct cyst and, 403
  neurofibromatosis and, 442f, 443
  odontogenic keratocyst and, 396, 397f
  odontogenic myxoma and, 434
  osteochondromatosis and, 566, 566f
  of osteomas, 445f
  osteosarcoma of maxilla and, 470f
  overview of, 251, 547-548
  panoramic units and, 246f
  parotid glands and, 663, 663f
  problems of, 200
  pterygomaxillary fissure and, 205, 207f
  purpose and uses of, 663
  pyramidal fracture and, 632
  radiation with, 55
  salivary gland disease and, 660
  septic arthritis and, 565
  simple bone cyst and, 407f, 408f
  skeletal fractures and, 163
  soft tissue infection and, 381f
  soft tissue infections v. neoplasia and, 380
  squamous cell carcinoma v., 588
  straight septa and, 455f
  synovial chondromatosis and, 565
  synovial osteochondromatosis in, 566f
  TMJ and, 269, 548
  Warthin tumor and, 673
  zygomatic arch fractures and, 635

Computed tomography (CT), reformatted
  edentulous patients and, 681
  multiple dental implants and, 681
Computed tomography (CT) movements,
      types of, 246-247
Computed tomography (CT) scanners
  conventional film v., 252
  mechanical geometry of, 251f
  principles of helical, 252f
Computed tomography (CT) soft tissue
      algorithm images, aneurysmal bone
      cyst and, 504
Computed tomography (CT) with contrast
      injection, arteriovenous (A-V) fistula
      and, 449
Computer monitors, cathode ray tube
      (CRT) designs and, 233
Computerized axial transverse scanning,
      Godfrey Hounsfield and, 250
Computers
  computed tomography (CT) image and,
      251
  digital imaging and, 225
  periodontal disease and, 316
COMS receptors, comparison of physical
      properties of, 243t
Concavities, dental anomalies and, 300
Conchae, 205
Concrescence
  clinical features of, 337
  definition of, 337
  differential diagnosis of, 338
  management of, 338
  radiographic features of, 337-338, 337f
Concussion. *See* Dental Concussion
Condensing osteitis, dilaceration v., 340
Condylar agenesis
  mandibular fossa v., 540
  Treacher Collins syndrome v., 643
Condylar degeneration, juvenile arthrosis
      v., 553
Condylar displacement, submentovertex
      (SMV) projection and, 546
Condylar head
  bifid condyle and, 554
  condylar hyperplasia and, 550
  degenerative joint disease and, 561,
      562f
  fracture and, 568
  juvenile arthrosis and, 553, 553f
  submentovertex projection and, 215
Condylar head fractures, 567
  mandibular growth and, 568
  overview of, 625
Condylar head fragments, mandibular
      condyle fractures and, 627, 628f
Condylar hyperplasia
  benign tumors v., 571
  clinical features of, 550
  definition of, 550
  differential diagnosis of, 550-551
  hemifacial hyperplasia v., 650
  osteomas v., 444
  panoramic image of, 551f
  radiographic features of, 550
  treatment of, 551
Condylar hypoplasia
  clinical features of, 552
  definition of, 552
  differential diagnosis of, 552
  hemifacial microsomia v., 643
  juvenile arthrosis v., 553

Condylar hypoplasia (*Continued*)
  panoramic film of, 552
  radiographic features of, 552
Condylar movement, ankylosis and, 569
Condylar neck
  condylar hypoplasia and, 552
  juvenile chronic arthritis and, 364
Condylar neck fractures
  overview of, 625
  panoramic view of, 568f
  radiographic features of, 567-568
  transorbital projection and, 545
Condylar neoplasms
  benign tumors v., 570
  condylar hyperplasia v., 550
Condylar osteoma, condylar hyperplasia v.,
      551
Condylar positioning, juvenile rheumatoid
      arthritis and, 542
Condylar process
  mandibular body fractures, 624, 624f
  panoramic image and, 201
  reverse-Towne projection, 222, 223f
Condylar translation
  movement during mandibular opening
      of, 542
  summit of articular eminence and, 542,
      542f
Condylar tumors
  condylar hyperplasia v., 550
  radiographic features of, 570
Condyles
  acromegaly v., 521
  anatomic structure of, 539f
  calcification and, 539
  corrected lateral CT of, 542f
  developmental abnormalities in, 550
  joint effusion and, 567
  mandibular fractures of, 624
  mandibular opening and, 540-541
  mandibular ramus projection of, 215
  remodeling and, 557
  reverse-Towne projection (open mouth),
      213
  rheumatoid arthritis and, 563, 563f
  submentovertex (SMV) projection and,
      545
  TMJ dysfunction and, 539
  transcarnial projection and, 543, 543f
  transpharyngeal (Parma) projection
      and, 544, 546f
Cone, focal spot to object and, 90
Cone-beam computed tomography. *See*
  CBCT (cone-beam computed
      tomography)
Cone-cut images, 125
  single size 3 film and, 298
Cone-cutting, horizontal bitewing films
      and, 149, 149f
Congenital cysts, 671
Congenital development, condylar
      hypoplasia and, 552
Congenital heart disease, microdontia and,
      335
Congenital hemangioma, 673
Congenital lymphedema, hemifacial
      hyperplasia v., 650
Congenital syphilis
  clinical features of, 353
  management of, 353-354
  overview of, 353
  radiologic features of, 353

Connective tissue
  osteoid osteoma and, 452
  simple bone cyst, 405
  synovial chondromatosis and, 565
Constant potential x-ray units, radiation and, 62
Constant tube voltage (kVp), spectrum of photons and, 13
Contamination
  barrier protected film and, 117, 118f
  digital imaging and, 118
Contrast agent(s)
  adhesions and, 557
  arthrography v., 548, 549f
  autoimmune sialadenitis and, 669
  CT images of soft tissue infection using, 381f
  decrease in, 237f
  digital radiographs and, 235
  insufficient, 106b
  panoramic images and, 281
  progression of autoimmune sialadenitis and, 669
Contrast-enhanced CT image, parotid gland and, 668f
Contrast enhancement, diagnostic value and, 236
Contrast resolution
  digital detector characteristics and, 232, 232f
  T1 weighted images and, 260
Conventional dental radiography, image dimensions of, 282
Conventional film, computed tomography scanners v., 252
Conventional radiograph, squamous cell carcinoma v., 587
Conventional tomography
  dental implants and, 677, 678b, 681, 682f
  internal derangement and, 555
  overview of, 546-547
  TMJ and, 269
Convolutional markings, hypophosphatasia and, 526
Cooley's anemia, 533
Coolidge tubes, medical usage and, 7
Copper, heat and, 8
Coronal dentin dysplasia (type 2), dentin dysplasia and, 347, 348, 348f
Coronal fragment, crown-root fractures and, 624
Coronal image, fibrous dysplasia and, 488f
Coronal invagination, dental papilla and, 340, 341
Coronal planes, MRI and, 549-550
Coronal tomography, conventional tomography v., 547
Coronoid hyperplasia
  clinical features of, 553
  definition of, 553
  differential diagnosis of, 554
  radiographic features of, 553-554
  sagittal tomogram of, 554, 554f
  treatment of, 554
Coronoid process
  anatomical overview of, 186-187
  bony ankylosis and, 569
  condylar hypoplasia and, 552
  coronoid hyperplasia and, 553, 554f
  osteomas v., 444

Coronoid process (Continued)
  panoramic image and, 201
  reverse-Towne projection, 222, 223f
Coronoid process hyperplasia, false ankylosis and, 569
Coronoid processes of mandible, Waters projection and, 221
Cortical bone, 168, 169-170
  expansile lesion and, 203
  response to lesion in, 293
Cortical border, condyles and, 539
Cortical boundary
  malignant ameloblastoma and, 466
  odontogenic keratocyst and, 394, 394f
  radicular cyst and, 386f
Cortical osteomas, 443
Cortical plates
  buccal bifurcation cyst and, 392, 393f
  calcifying odontogenic cyst and, 399, 400
  cementoossifying fibroma and, 500
  central mucoepidermoid carcinoma and, 465
  mandibular body fractures and, 625
  periodontal disease and, 315, 321
  rapidly growing lesion and, 293
Corticated margins, cysts and, 286f, 288
Corticated periphery, radiopaque lesion and, 288
Corticosteroids. See Drugs, corticosteroids
Cosmetic surgery, fibrous dysplasia and, 490f
Cosmic radiation
  external exposure and, 48
  overview of, 48
Cosmic radiation E rate, airline travel and, 48
Cracked tooth syndrome, vertical root fractures and, 623
Cranial bone disorders, TMJ and, 269
Cranial fossa, 540
  submentovertex projection and, 220, 220f
Cranial nerves, craniofacial fibrous dysplasia and, 593
Cranial plane, 540
Cranial suture synostosis, crouzon syndrome and, 641
Craniofacial complex, paranasal sinuses and, 576
Craniofacial disjunction (Le Fort III)
  clinical features of, 633
  definition of, 633
  management of, 634
  radiographic features of, 633-634, 634f
Craniofacial dysjunction fractures, 629
Craniofacial dysostosis, 640
Craniofacial fibrous dysplasia
  clinical features of, 592
  CT images of, 593f
  differential diagnosis of, 593
  radiographic features of, 592-593
Craniofacial lesions, monostotic fibrous dysplasia and, 485
Craniofacial microsomia, 641
  overview of, 641
Craniofacial reconstructive surgery, 3D CT and, 254
Craniofacial structures, developmental disturbances of, 639

Craniofacial team
  crouzon syndrome and, 641
  Treacher Collins syndrome and, 646
Craniometaphyseal dysplasia, osteopetrosis v., 531
Craniosynostosis, crouzon syndrome v., 64, 641
Cranium, craniofacial disjunction and, 633
Crepitans, synovial chondromatosis and, 565
Crepitation, craniofacial disjunction and, 633
Crepitus
  degenerative joint disease and, 559
  mandibular condyle fractures and, 626
  rheumatoid arthritis and, 563
Crestal bone, periodontal disease and, 321
Cretinism, 522
Cross-contamination, radiography and, 115
Cross-sectional imaging, implants and, 269
Cross-sectional mandibular occlusal projection
  buccal bifurcation cyst and, 392-393
  film placement in, 158
  image field in, 158
  point of entry and, 158
  projection of central ray in, 158
  sialoliths and, 660, 661f
Cross-sectional maxillary occlusal projection
  film placement in, 155
  image field in, 155
  point of entry in, 155
  projection of central ray in, 155
Crossover, image degradation and, 58
Crouzon syndrome (CS)
  characteristic facial features of, 641f
  clinical features of, 641
  definition of, 640-641
  differential diagnosis of, 641
  management of, 641
  radiographic features of, 641
Crown, tooth
  amelogenesis imperfecta and, 346
  dens in dente and, 340
  dentin dysplasia and, 349
  dislocated teeth and, 617
  fusion of teeth and, 336
  gemination and, 338
  hypocalcification and, 345
Crown-root fractures
  clinical features of, 623
  definition of, 623
  management of, 623
  radiographic features of, 623-624
  vertical fractures in, 623-624
Crown-to-tooth ratio, periodontal disease and, 326
Crowns, stainless steel, radiopaque, 190f
Crystalline lattice atoms, 94
CT. See Computed tomography (CT)
Cuboid voxels, 253
Curettage
  ameloblastic fibromas v., 429
  aneurysmal bone cyst and, 506
  buccal bifurcation cyst v., 393
  calcifying odontogenic cyst and, 400
  central giant cell granuloma v., 503
  Langerhans' cell histiocytosis and, 514
  odontogenic keratocyst and, 396
  osteoblastomas and, 452
  simple bone cyst and, 407-408

Curie (Ci), unit of measurement and, 21
Cushing's syndrome
    clinical features of, 523
    definition of, 523
    radiographic features of, 523, 524f
Cuspids, calcifying odontogenic cyst and, 400
Cutaneous gangrene, arteriosclerosis and, 602
Cutaneous neurofibromas, neurofibromatosis and, 442
Cutaneous pigmentation, McCune-Albright syndrome and, 485
Cutaneous sebaceous cysts, Gardner's syndrome and, 445
Cyclotron, PET and, 262
Cyst(s), 385. *See also specific cysts*
    ameloblastic fibromas and, 429
    ameloblastoma v., 419
    calcifications in, 598f
    cleidocranial dysplasia and, 648
    cortical bone and, 203
    corticated margin and, 286f, 288
    CT and, 664
    dystrophic calcification and, 598, 598f
    effects on surrounding structures, 384385
    external resorption and, 358
    internal structure of, 384
    lingual salivary gland depression v., 654
    location of, 384
    normal sinus v., 179
    occult disease and, 268
    peripheral cortex on, 287f
    periphery of, 384
    radicular dentin dysplasia (type 1) and, 348
    resorption and, 356
    totally radiolucent interior of, 286f, 289
Cyst(s), benign, central mucoepidermoid carcinoma v., 465
Cyst formation, incisive foramen and, 174
Cyst lining, central mucoepidermoid carcinoma from, 465
Cystic ameloblastoma
    dentigerous cyst v., 392
    panoramic image of, 286f
Cystic fibrosis
    chronic sinusitis and, 579
    pansinusitis and, 579
Cystic fluid, nasopalatine duct cyst and, 401
Cystic hygromas, dermoid cysts v., 404
Cystic lesions
    definition of, 671
    radiographic appearance of, 671, 671f
    radiographic features of, 671
    treatment of, 671
Cystic neoplasms, cystic salivary lesions vs, 671
Cystic odontoma, 424
Cystic salivary adenoma, nasopalatine duct cysts v., 403-404
Cystic salivary lesions
    extraglandular and, 671
    intraglandular and, 671
    neoplasms v., 671
Cysticerci, 601
Cysticercosis
    clinical features of, 601
    definition of, 600
    differential diagnosis of, 601

Cysticercosis *(Continued)*
    management of, 601
    radiographic features of, 601
Cysticercus cellulosae, cysticercosis and, 601
Cytoplasm, radiation effects on, 29

D
Dark spots, 106b
Darkroom, 99f
    contamination and, 118
    equipment for, 98-101
    film processing and, 104
    mounting film in, 101
    panoramic film and, 200
    safelight filters in, 112
Davidson, J. MacKenzie, stereoscopy technique and, 248
Daylight loading
    contamination and, 120
    film processing and, 103-104, 103f
Deafness, monostotic fibrous dysplasia and, 485
Death, central nervous system syndrome and, 39
Decalcification, irregular shapes of, 300, 303f
Decay, amelogenesis imperfecta and, 345
Deciduous central incisors, newborn and, 181, 182f
Deciduous dentition
    dental root fractures and, 620
    fractures of dental crown in, 619
    fused, 337
    fusion of teeth and, 336
    hypocalcification/hypocalcification, 345
Deciduous lateral incisor, gemination and, 338, 338f
Deciduous mandibular molar projection, children and, 162
Deciduous molar periapical projection
    child and, 161
    mixed dentition and, 162
Decongestants, acute sinusitis, 581
Decortication, osteomyelitis and, 380
Deformed disk, arthrogram and, 558, 559f
Deformities, CT and, 254
Degenerative changes, transorbital projection and, 545, 547f
Degenerative joint disease (DJD)
    characteristics of, 561, 561f
    clinical features of, 559-560
    condylar hyperplasia v., 551
    condylar hypoplasia v., 552
    coronal CT image of, 562f
    definition of, 559
    differential diagnosis of, 561-562
    internal derangement and, 555
    juvenile arthrosis v., 553
    lateral tomography of, 561f
    malignant tumors v., 572
    radiographic features of, 560-561
    remodeling v., 559
    septic arthritis v., 565
    synovial chondromatosis v., 566
    treatment of, 562
Demineralization process, radiograph of, 311
Dens evaginates
    clinical features of, 343
    definition of, 343
    differential diagnosis of, 344
    management of, 344
    radiographic features of, 343, 344f

Dens in dente
    clinical features of, 342
    definition for, 340
    demographic information on, 342
    differential diagnosis of, 343
    enfolding of enamel and, 341f
    management of, 343
    necrosis of pulp in, 343f
    radiographic features of, 342
    severe malformations of, 343f
    synonyms for, 340
Dens invaginates, 340
Dense bone island, 414
    dilaceration v., 340
Densitometers, digital imaging software and, 239, 239f
Density, changing solutions and, 103
Dental abnormalities
    defining, 285
    generalizing, 283
    localizing, 283
Dental anomalies
    acquired, 330
    developmental, 330
    Treacher Collins syndrome and, 643
Dental arch
    external resorption and, 358
    occlusal radiography and, 160
Dental caries. *See also* Carious lesions; Cavitated lesions; Cavitation; Clinical cavity; Demineralization process; Dentinal lesions; Occlusal caries; Radiation caries
    cancer and, 458
    child and, 273
    composite restorations and, 189f
    dens in dente and, 342
    diagnostic detection tools for, 305, 311
    external resorption v., 358
    file compression rate and, 240
    gemination and, 338
    ink-jet technology and, 235
    interaction factors in, 297
    internal resorption v., 358
    jaws and, 366
    occult disease and, 268
    progression of, 266-267
    radicular cyst and, 385
    radiographic examination and, 55, 266, 297
    talon cusp and, 351
Dental caries diagnosis, effect of kilovoltage on, 63
Dental caries history, monitoring lesions and, 297
Dental Concussion
    clinical features of, 616
    definition of, 616
    incisor periodontal ligament spaces and, 616f
    management of, 616
    pulp chamber obliteration and, 617f
    radiographic features of, 616
Dental crown fractures
    clinical features of, 619-620
    definition of, 619
    management of, 620
    radiographic features of, 620
Dental cyst. *See* Cyst(s)
Dental development, hyperthyroidism and, 522

Dental examination, ameloblastoma and, 419

Dental film processing, machines for, 64

Dental floss, abrasion and, 355

Dental floss injury
clinical features of, 355, 355f
differential diagnosis of, 355-356
management of, 355-356
radiographic features of, 355

Dental hypoplasia, congenital syphilis and, 353

Dental implants. *See* Implants, dental

Dental lamina
ameloblastoma and, 419
odontogenic keratocyst, 394

Dental papilla, ameloblastic fibroma and, 428

Dental Patient Selection Criteria Panel
oral radiographic examinations and, 61
selection criteria for oral radiography and, 56

Dental proximal caries, 303f

Dental pulp, pulp stones and, 361

Dental radiography
ameloblastic fibromas and, 428
patient dose and, 52
radiation-induced cancer and, 53

Dental radiologist, fibrous dysplasia v., 489

Dental radiology, cancer survivor and, 482

Dental root fractures. *See* Fractures, tooth root

Dental treatment, cancer survivor and, 482

Dental viewbox, photostimulable phosphor plates (PSP) and, 231

Dentigerous cyst(s)
ameloblastic fibromas v., 429
ameloblastoma and, 420, 424f
buccal bifurcation cyst v., 393
calcifying epithelial odontogenic tumors v., 423
calcifying odontogenic cyst v., 400
cleidocranial dysplasia and, 648
clinical features of, 388
definition of, 388
differential diagnosis of, 388
internal structure of, 388
odontogenic cysts and, 589
odontogenic keratocyst v., 395
periphery and shape of, 388
radiographic features of, 388
supplemental teeth and, 331

Dentin
clinical cavity and, 297, 301
composite and, 189f
composition of teeth and, 166
concrescence and, 338
demineralization progression and, 297
dentinogenesis imperfecta and, 346, 347
hypocalcification and, 345
lesion in, 305f
occlusal caries and, 302
optical density of, 63
radiolucencies within, 307f
regional odontodysplasia, 349
root surface lesions and, 303-304
subject density and, 78
tooth crown fractures and, 619

Dentin dysplasia
clinical features of, 348
definition of, 347-348
dentinogenesis imperfecta and, 347
differential diagnosis for, 349

Dentin dysplasia *(Continued)*
management of, 349
radiographic features of, 348
two types of, 347-348

Dentinal lesions, 300
operative treatment for, 301

Dentinal tubules, 300

Dentinoenamel junction (DEJ)
demineralizing front and, 299
occlusal lesion and, 301

Dentinogenesis imperfecta
amelogenesis imperfecta v., 346
clinical features of, 346
constriction of root, 347, 347f
definition of, 346
dentin dysplasia v., 347, 349
management of, 347
radiographic features of, 346-347
regional odontodysplasia v., 349
types of, 346

Dentition
abnormalities of, 209
aggressive periodontitis and, 324
cleidocranial dysplasia and, 646
examination process and, 283
fibrous dysplasia and, 489
hemifacial hyperplasia and, 649
hypophosphatasia and, 526
panoramic imaging and, 208-209

Deoxyribonucleic acid (DNA) molecule, altercations to, 26

Dermoid cysts, 404, 671
clinical features of, 404
differential diagnosis of, 404
management of, 404
nasopalatine duct cyst, 400
radiographic features of, 404

Desmoplastic fibroma, central odontogenic fibroma v., 438

Desmoplastic fibroma of bone
clinical features of, 454
differential diagnosis of, 454, 456
overview of, 454
radiographic features of, 454
synonyms for, 454
treatment of, 456

Despeckling filters, high frequency noise and, 236

Destines, 330

Detective quantum efficiency (DQE), imaging system and, 83

Detector latitude, digital detector characteristics and, 232

Deterministic effects, 51
radiation and, 25

Developer replenisher, overview of, 97

Developer solution, 100, 104
constituents of, 104
contamination and, 120
exhaustion of, 102
four components of, 97
overview of, 96-97, 97
rinsing and, 97
temperature of, 100

Development, film
manual tank processing and, 102
rinsing of, 97

Developmental anomaly
arteriovenous (A-V) fistula and, 449
dilaceration and, 340
summary of, 330

Developmental salivary gland defect, 651

Deviated nasal septum, mucocele v, 585

Diabetes, periodontitis and, 314

Diabetes insipidus, eosinophilic granuloma and, 509

Diabetes mellitus
clinical features of, 523
definition of, 523
periodontal disease and, 327
pseudotumor and, 588
radiographic features of, 523

Diagnodent laser-light, carious lesions and, 305

Diagnosis
file compression rate and, 240
image analysis and, 239
radiographic guidelines and, 272

Diagnostic density, 63
guidelines in, 63

Diagnostic images
acquiring appropriate, 281
osteoradionecrosis and, 380
quality of, 281
staging of cancer in, 458

Diagnostic radiology
dose reduction in, 55
exposure reduction in, 55
salivary gland disease and, 659
selection for preoperative planning, 686

Diagnostics, oral, CBCT and, 255

Diaphyseal dysplasia, osteopetrosis v., 531

Diastema, odontomas and, 425

DICOM. *See* Digital Imaging and Communications in Medicine (DICOM), .

Diet
attrition and, 354
dental caries and, 297
erosion and, 356
monitoring lesions and, 297

Differential absorption, overview of, 19

Differentiating intermitotic cells, radiosensitivity and, 30

Diffuse sclerosing osteomyelitis, 374
bone formation and, 377

Digital detectors
characteristics of, 232-233
charge-coupled device (CCD) and, 226-229
imaging and, 226

Digital image printing, diagnostic efficacy of, 234

Digital image receptors, solid-state sensors and, 299

Digital imaging, 100, 241
backup considerations in, 240b
characteristics of, 225
clinical considerations of, 241
computed tomography (CT) image and, 251, 253f
conclusions regarding, 241, 242f, 243, 244
contamination and, 118
crouzon syndrome and, 641
electronic devices and, 234
image resolution with, 58
overview of, 225
pixels and, 226f
subtraction image and, 301

Digital Imaging and Communications in Medicine (DICOM)
digital imaging and, 199, 241
file compression and, 240

Digital imaging software, image analysis and, 239
Digital intraoral radiography, film speed and, 57
Digital pressure, fractures of alveolar process and, 629
Digital receptors, clinical handling of, 241
Digital rulers, digital imaging software and, 239, 239f
Digital subtraction radiography (DSR)
    overview of, 238-239, 238f
    strengths of, 238-239, 238f
Digital video interface (DVI), digital-to-analog conversion and, 234
Digora system, photostimulable phosphor plates (PSP) and, 231
Dilacerated roots
    hypercementosis v., 363
    occult disease and, 268
Dilaceration. See also Radicular dilaceration
    clinical features of, 340, 340f
    definition of, 340
    differential diagnosis of, 340
    management of, 340
    radiographic features of, 340, 340f
Dilated odontoma, 340, 425
    panoramic film and, 343f
    radiographic features of, 342
    structure of, 427, 428f
Dimensional distortion, panoramic images and, 201
Diploic space, posteroanterior cephalometric projection and, 221-222, 222f
Diplopia
    mucocele and, 585
    zygomatic arch fractures and, 635
Dipoles
    MRI and, 256, 256f
    sonography and, 263
Direct digital image receptor, charge-coupled device and, 226-229
Direct effect, biologic macromolecules and, 25
Direct exposure film, 71
    characteristic curve of, 78f
    dental, 80
Disease
    maxillary sinus and, 177
    occlusal radiography and, 160
    panoramic imaging and, 191
    radiation therapy and, 275
    radiographic examination and, 265
    radiographic recognition of, 166
    trabeculae and, 171
Diseases, acquired, condylar hypoplasia and, 552
Diseases, infectious. See Infectious diseases
Disk displacement
    internal derangement and, 555
    MRI of, 560f
    soft tissue imaging and, 548
Disk herniation, 3D CT and, 254, 255f
Disk perforations, arthrography, 548
Disk tissue, MRI and, 550
Dislocation
    clinical features of, 567
    definition of, 567
    differential diagnosis of, 568
    radiographic features of, 567-568
    treatment of, 568

Disposable containers, contamination and, 117
Dissolution (demineralization), dental caries and, 297
Distal molars, cleidocranial dysplasia and, 648
Distal oblique projection, image field and, 144, 146
Distomolar teeth, 330, 331f
Distortion, 281
    anteroposterior position radiograph and, 198
    linear tomogram and, 247
    radiographs and, 121
    reverse-Towne projection and, 218
DNA
    cell cycle and, 27, 27f
    radiation and, 39-40
Dose
    fetus and, 61
    irradiated tissues and, 31
Dose limits, 52
Dose rate, irradiated tissues and, 31, 32f
Dose reduction, diagnostic radiology and, 55
Dose thresholds, stochastic effects and, 25
Dosimetry
    overview of, 20-21
    report sample of, 66f
Dot. See Identification dot
Dot pitch, CRT and, 234
Dots per inch (DPI), image quality and, 235
Double contrast arthrography, disk in open v. closed position and, 558f
Double emulsion film, image on, 83
Double vision, pyramidal fracture and, 632
Doubling dose, genetic exposure risk and, 42
Down syndrome, periodontal disease and, 327
Drainage, osteomyelitis and, 377
Drugs, antibiotics
    acute radiation syndrome and, 39
    acute sinusitis, 581
    aggressive periodontitis and, 324
    horizontal fracture and, 631
    mandibular body fractures and, 625
    osteomyelitis and, 374, 380
    osteopetrosis and, 531
    osteoradionecrosis and, 382
    pericoronitis and, 373
    pyramidal fracture and, 632
Drugs, antiinflammatory. See also Antimicrobial therapy
    autoimmune sialadenitis and, 670
    benign cementoblastoma and, 436
    degenerative joint disease and, 562
    joint effusion and, 567
    osteoid osteoma and, 452
    rheumatoid arthritis and, 563
Drugs, corticosteroids
    autoimmune sialadenitis and, 670
    rheumatoid arthritis and, 563
    secondary osteoporosis and, 524
Drying racks, overview of, 101
Dual energy photon absorption (DEXA), osteoporosis and, 524
Ductal filling defects, sialoliths and, 666
Ductal pathosis, sialography and, 663

Ductal system
    sialodochitis and, 668
    sialography and, 661
Duplicating film, 108
Duty cycle, tube rating and, 11-12
Dwarfism, hypopituitarism and, 522
Dye-sublimation printers, image quality with, 235
Dysesthesia, squamous cell carcinoma and, 461
Dysplastic dentin, calcifying odontogenic cyst and, 399
Dystrophic calcification in tonsils
    clinical features of, 599
    definition of, 599
    differential diagnosis of, 599
    examples of, 600f
    radiographic features of, 599
    synonyms for, 599
Dystrophic calcifications
    atherosclerotic plaque and, 602
    clinical features of, 598
    definition of, 598
    lymph nodes and, 291
    overview of, 597
    radicular cyst and, 386f
    radiographic features of, 598
    residual cyst and, 388
    sialoliths v., 666
Dystrophic metabolic sialadenoses, 670

E

E-speed film
    dental x-ray and, 57
    rare-earth screens and, 198
Eagle's syndrome, ossification of stylohyoid ligament, 609
Ear, joint effusion and, 567
Ear canal, hemifacial microsomia and, 643
Ear infections
    cleft palate and, 639
    diffuse sclerosing osteomyelitis and, 378
Ear lobe, mandibular ramal area and, 202
Ecchymosis
    fractures of alveolar process and, 627
    mandibular body fractures and, 625
Echo pattern, sonography and, 263
ECM. See Electrical conductance measurements (ECM)
Ectodermal dysplasia
    anodontia and, 333
    missing teeth, 334f
Edema. See also Swelling
    exposure time and, 163
    gingivitis and, 314
    midface fractures and, 629
    pyramidal fracture and, 631
    special patient considerations and, 162
    zygomatic arch fractures and, 635
Edentulous alveolar bone, hyperthyroidism and, 522
Edentulous patients. See Patients, edentulous
Edtavision G film, spectral sensitivities of, 100f
Education, radiation safety issues and, 66
Education, continuing, 67
Effective dose (E), 47
    overview of, 21
    x-ray examinations and, 54t
Effective focal spot, 8

Effusion, joint
  clinical features of, 567
  definition of, 566
  differential diagnosis of, 567
  radiographic features of, 567
  treatment of, 567
EG. *See* Eosinophilic granuloma (EG)
Ektavision film systems, crossover and, 58
Ektavision G film, spectral sensitivities of, 100f
Elastic fibers, arteriosclerosis and, 602
Elastic traction
  horizontal fracture and, 631
  zygomatic arch fractures and, 635
Electric current, 9
Electrical conductance measurements
    (ECM), carious lesions and, 311
Electromagnetic radiation, 4, 5-6, 5f
Electromagnetic spectrum, 6f
Electromagnetic wave, radio frequency
    and, 258, 258f
Electron beam, CRT hues and, 233
Electron binding energy, 4
Electron density, compton scattering and,
    18, 18f
Electron guns, cathode ray tube (CRT)
    designs and, 233
Electron hole pairs, silicon atoms and,
    227, 228f
Electron scan, cathode ray tube (CRT)
    designs and, 233
Electron volt, 6
Electrons
  atom structure and, 3
  cathode ray tube (CRT) designs and,
    233
  photostimulable phosphor plates (PSP)
    and, 231
  x-rays relationship to, 12
Electroplating methods, environmental
    damage and, 105
Elements, overview of, 3
Elliptical tomography, 246, 246f
Elongation. *See* Image elongation
Ely cysts, degenerative joint disease and,
    561, 562f
Embryo-fetus exposure, NCRP
    recommendations for, 61
Embryonal periosteum, osteomas and, 443
Embryopathy, bifid condyle and, 554
Embryos, radiation effects on, 39
Emotional tension, attrition and, 354
Empyema
  inflammatory disease and, 578
  overview of, 581
Emulsion
  changes in, 96f
  components of, 71
  film mount and, 108
  film processing and, 96f
  scanning electron micrographs of, 72f
En bloc surgical resection, malignant
    ameloblastoma and, 466
Enamel, tooth
  carious lesions and, 266
  congenital syphilis and, 353
  demineralization of, 298f
  demineralization progression and, 297
  dens evaginates and, 343
  dens in dente and, 342
  digital detector characteristics and, 232,
    233f

Enamel, tooth *(Continued)*
  hypocalcification and, 345
  hypomaturation and, 345
  hypoplasia and, 345
  internal resorption and, 356
  lesions and, 300
  occlusal lesion and, 301
  optical density of, 63
  radiolucency in, 308f
  radiolucent v. radiopaque materials and,
    289
  regional odontodysplasia, 349
  renal osteodystrophy and, 527
  subject density and, 78
  talon cusp and, 351
  tooth crown fractures and, 619
  toothbrush injury and, 355
Enamel cap, composition of teeth and,
    166
Enamel density, amelogenesis imperfecta
    and, 346, 346f
Enamel drop, 349
Enamel formation, amelogenesis
    imperfecta and, 344
Enamel fracture, dentinogenesis
    imperfecta and, 346
Enamel hypoplasia. *See also* Dental
    hypoplasia
  pseudohypoparathyroidism and, 520
  Turner's hypoplasia and, 352
Enamel matrix, adenomatoid odontogenic
    tumor and, 431
Enamel nodule, 349
Enamel pearl
  clinical features of, 350, 351f
  definition of, 349-350
  differential diagnosis of, 350
  management of, 350-351
  radiographic features of, 350, 351f, 352f
  synonyms for, 349
Enamel pits
  amelogenesis imperfecta and, 346
  buccal carious lesions and, 303
  lingual carious lesions and, 303
Enamel rods, 303
  radiolucent lesions and, 299, 302f
Enamelodentinal junction, composition of
    teeth and, 166
Enameloma, 349
Endocrine glands, sialadenosis and, 670
Endocrine system
  disorders of, 516
  neurofibromatosis and, 441
Endodontic therapy
  fused teeth and, 337
  gutta-percha and, 188f
  radicular cyst and, 387, 387f
  silver points and, 187, 188f
  stereoscopy technique and, 249, 249f
  vertical root fractures and, 623
Endodontics
  crown-root fractures and, 624
  radiographic techniques for, 164
Endoray film holder, endodontic
    radiographs and, 164f
Endothelial cells, hemangioma and, 673
Endothelial myeloma, 473
Energy states, external magnetic field and,
    257-258
Enostosis
  benign cementoblastoma v., 436
  differential diagnosis of, 416

Enostosis *(Continued)*
  exostoses v., 416
  first bicuspid and, 418f
  Gardner's syndrome and, 445
  hypercementosis v., 363
  osteoid osteoma v., 454
  periapical inflammatory lesions v., 370
  in periapical positions, 372f
  pericoronitis v., 373
  radiographic features of, 416
  synonyms for, 414
  treatment of, 416
Enucleation
  ameloblastic fibromas v., 429, 431
  benign cementoblastoma and, 436
  calcifying odontogenic cyst and, 400
  cementoossifying fibroma v., 501
  central giant cell granuloma v., 503
  lateral periodontal cyst v., 399
  nasopalatine duct cyst and, 401
Environment
  maxillary sinuses and, 177
  periodontal diseases and, 325
  torus palatinus and, 412
Environment, damage. *See* Wastes,
    radiographic
Environmental Protection Agency (EPA),
    surface cleaners and, 116
Environmental teratogenic agents,
    orofacial clefts and, 639
Eosinophilic granuloma (EG)
  Langerhans' cell histiocytosis and, 509
  Langerhans' X and, 509
  lesion periphery in, 511f
Eosinophilic granuloma of jaw, Ewing's
    sarcoma v., 474
Epidermoid carcinoma, 459, 464
Epistaxis
  epithelial papilloma and, 586
  osteosarcoma and, 469
  pyramidal fracture and, 632
Epithelial papilloma
  clinical features of, 586
  definition of, 586
  radiographic features of, 586
Epithelium
  odontogenic keratocyst and, 394
  squamous cell carcinoma and, 459,
    461
Equipment, dental
  CBCT and, 255
  choice of, 56
  cleaning of, 111
  disinfection of, 116
  film based tomography and, 245
  operation of, 62-63
  radiographic examination and choice
    of, 56
Equivalent dose, radiation and, 21
erbium:YAG laser, osteoma cutis and,
    610
Erosion
  clinical features of, 356
  definition of, 356
  differential diagnosis of, 356
  fibrous ankylosis and, 569
  juvenile chronic arthritis and, 364
  management of, 356
  osteoma and, 586
  panoramic projection and, 543, 543f
  radiographic features of, 356
  secondary dentin and, 360

Erupted teeth, 336
  amelogenesis imperfecta and, 345
  Burkitt's tumor and, 480
  hyperthyroidism and, 522
  odontomas and, 425
  osteopetrosis and, 530
  regional odontodysplasia and, 349
  rickets and, 525
Erupted teeth, accelerated, systemic
    disorders and, 516
Erupted teeth, delayed, systemic disorders
    and, 516
Eruption cysts, dentigerous cyst v., 388
Erythema, gingivitis and, 314
Erythroblastic anemia, 533
Estrogens, osteoporosis and, 524
Ethmoid air cells
  overview of, 576
  polyps and, 582
Ethmoid bone
  mid-facial area and, 204
  midface fractures and, 629
Ethmoid sinuses
  development of, 576
  pyramidal fracture and, 631
Ethylene oxide gas, instruments and, 117
Europium barium fluorohalide
  photostimulable phosphor plates (PSP)
    and, 230
  radiographic imaging and, 230
Eustachian tube
  cleft palate and, 640
  squamous cell carcinoma and, 461
Ewing's sarcoma
  clinical features of, 473
  definition of, 473
  differential diagnosis of, 474
  management of, 474
  non-Hodgkin's lymphoma v., 478
  osteosarcoma v., 469
  radiographic features of, 473-474
Ewing's tumor, Burkitt's lymphoma v.,
    480
Excision, surgical
  adenomatoid odontogenic tumor v.,
    433
  benign cementoblastoma and, 436
  benign tumors and, 571, 672
  central odontogenic fibroma v., 439
  neurilemmoma v., 440
  neurofibroma and, 441
  neuromas and, 440
  odontogenic keratocyst and, 396
  odontomas and, 428
  osteoblastomas and, 452
  osteoid osteoma v., 454
Exercise, osteoporosis and, 524
Exophthalmos
  eosinophilic granuloma and, 509
  osteosarcoma and, 469
Exostosis, 412
  clinical features of, 414
  enostoses v., 416
  radiographic features of, 414
Exponential absorption, 19, 19f
Exposure charts, checking of, 113
Exposure cycle, panoramic machine and,
    193
Exposure latitudes
  CCD and, 223f
  F speed film and, 223f
  PSP and, 223f

Exposure output, device for measuring,
    114f
Exposure parameters, extraoral
    radiographic examinations and, 210
Exposure reduction, film and, 57
Exposure time, 79
  cross-sectional mandibular occlusal
    projection, 158
  edema and, 163
  rare earth filtration and, 61
  x-ray spectrum and, 13, 14f
Exposures, radiographic
  children and, 161
  digital subtraction radiography and,
    238
  emulsion changes during, 96f
  film density and, 78
  film processing and, 63
  image quality and, 63
  intraoral radiographs and, 270
  milliampere-seconds and, 63, 63t
  patient examination and, 123
  slower film-screen and, 82
  standard conditions of temperature and
    pressure and, 20
  steps for making, 122-123
  stereoscopy technique and, 249
  units of measurement and, 21
External auditory meatus (EAM)
  lateral cephalometric projections and,
    211, 212t
  posteroanterior cephalometric
    projection and, 221-222, 222f
External exposure, cosmic radiation and,
    48
External magnetic field, hydrogen nuclei
    in, 256, 257f, 258f
External oblique ridges
  anatomical overview of, 186, 186f
  periodontal disease and, 322f
External pterygoid muscle, mandibular
    condyle fractures and, 626
External root resorption, 356
  clinical features of, 358
  definition of, 358
  differential diagnosis of, 358-359
  internal resorption v., 358
  management of, 360
  radiographic features of, 358
  reimplantation and, 619
Extraction, tooth
  benign cementoblastoma and, 436
  concrescence and, 337
  dentinogenesis imperfecta and, 347
  dilaceration and, 340
  florid osseous dysplasia and, 496
  fused teeth and, 337
  hypercementosis v., 363
  internal resorption and, 358
  mandibular body fractures and, 625
  osteomyelitis and, 377
  Paget's disease and, 509
  periapical cemental dysplasia and, 492,
    493f
  periapical inflammatory lesions and,
    371
  pericoronitis and, 373
  peripheral nerve damage and, 440
  radicular cyst and, 387
  regional odontodysplasia and, 349
  tooth crown fractures and, 620
  vertical root fractures and, 623

Extraoral film. See Film, extraoral
Extraoral radiographic examinations
  gag reflex and, 163
  overview of, 210
  panoramic images and, 283
  purpose of, 271
  technique in, 210
Extraoral radiographic projections, 239
  evaluation of, 218-224
  image field and, 134, 144
  intraglandular sialoliths and, 660
  resultant images of, 212t
  selection criteria for, 223-224
  technical aspects of, 212t
  usefulness of, 224f
Extraosseous soft tissue, arteriovenous
    (A-V) fistula and, 449
Extraparotid tumor, parotid v., 659
Extravasation cysts, 405
Extrinsic tumors of TMJ, locations of, 570
Extrusive luxation, trauma and, 617
Exudate, purulent, gingivitis and, 314

F
F-centers, europium barium fluorohalide
    and, 230
Face
  cherubism and, 506
  lower
    lateral cephalometric projection and,
      219f, 220
    posteroanterior cephalometric
      projection and, 221-222, 222f
  middle
    posteroanterior cephalometric
      projection and, 221-222, 222f
    submentovertex projection and, 220,
      220f
  upper
    posteroanterior cephalometric
      projection and, 221-222, 222f
    submentovertex projection and, 220,
      220f
Face shield, film placement and, 134
Facial artery, medial calcinosis and, 602
Facial asymmetries, submentovertex (SMV)
    projection and, 546
Facial bones
  cementoossifying fibroma and, 499
  traumatic injuries to, 624
Facial clefts
  dental anomalies and, 640
  lip and palate, 639
Facial deformity, odontogenic tumors and,
    590
Facial fractures. See Fractures, facial
Facial nerve, hemifacial microsomia and,
    643
Facial region
  grids and, 85
  wide latitude films and, 81
Facial skeleton, odontogenic myxoma and,
    434
False ankylosis, 569
False cyst, 581
False images, linear tomogram and, 247
Familial fibrous dysplasia, cherubism v.,
    506
Familial multiple cementomas, 495
Familial multiple polyposis, 444
  enostosis and, 445, 447f
  film of, 447f

Familial syndromes
 crouzon syndrome and, 64
 Treacher Collins syndrome as, 643
Fast intensifying screens
 characteristics of, 77
 mottle and, 82
Fast scan direction, photostimulable
 phosphor plates (PSP) and, 231
Fast speed films
 dental x-ray and, 57
 exposure latitudes and, 223f
 rare-earth screens and, 198
Fast-spin echo T2-weighted images, MRI
 and, 664
Fat images
 MRI and, 664
 relaxation time and, 259
 subject density and, 78
Fatigue, multiple myeloma and, 475
Favorable fractures, mandibular body
 fractures as, 625
Feature extraction, image analysis and, 239
Femur, Paget's disease in, 507
Ferromagnetic metals, MRI and, 260
Fetor, rhinoliths and, 607
Fetus
 full mouth examination and, 274
 radiation effects on, 39
Fever
 acute leukemias and, 481
 inflammation and, 366
 rhinoliths and, 607
 septic arthritis and, 565
Fibre-optic transillumination (FOTI),
 carious lesions and, 305, 311
Fibroadamantoblastoma, 428
Fibroatrophy, irradiated tissue and, 331
Fibroblastic osteosarcoma, 469
Fibrocartilage, condyle and, 540
Fibrocementoma, 492
Fibroinflammatory pseudotumor, 588
Fibromyxomas, 433
 TMJ tumors and, 570
Fibroosseous diseases, imaging for jaw
 pathology in, 268
Fibroosseous lesion, fibrous dysplasia and,
 485
Fibrosarcoma
 clinical features of, 474
 definition of, 474
 desmoplastic fibromas of bone v., 454
 Ewing's sarcoma v., 474
 osteosarcoma v., 469
 primary osseous carcinoma v., 464
 radiographic features of, 474-475
 right maxillary sinus and, 474, 474f
Fibrosarcoma of joint capsule, primary
 intrinsic malignant tumors and, 571
Fibrous adhesions, internal derangement
 and, 555-556
Fibrous ankylosis
 ankylosis v., 569
 erosions and, 569
 rheumatoid arthritis v., 563
 soft tissue and, 569
Fibrous connective tissue, florid osseous
 dysplasia and, 495
Fibrous dysplasia, 290, 291f
 abnormality and, 285
 baseline with CT scan in, 491, 491f
 benign neoplasm v., 412
 cementoossifying fibroma v., 500

Fibrous dysplasia (Continued)
 cherubism v, 506
 children and, 380
 chondrosarcoma v., 472, 473
 chronic osteomyelitis v., 379
 clinical features of, 485
 cyst-like radiolucent lesion in, 490f
 definition of, 485
 differential diagnosis of, 489
 early radiolucent lesions in, 487, 487f
 expansion of mandible caused by, 491f
 ill-defined borders in, 288, 289f
 inferior alveolar nerve canal and, 293
 internal patterns of, 490f
 juvenile ossifying fibroma v., 501, 501f
 management of, 489, 491
 osteomyelitis v., 375
 osteosarcoma v., 469
 overview of, 592
 Paget's disease v., 508
 pericoronitis v., 373
 periphery of, 487
 posterior maxilla and, 487, 487f
 radiographic features of, 485-489
 simple bone cyst v., 405, 407
Fibrous dysplasia granular pattern,
 cementoossifying fibroma and, 500f
Filament, x-ray tube with, 7, 7f, 8f
Filament step-down transformer, tube
 current and, 7f, 9
File compression, methods of, 240
File size, digital imaging and, 239
Film. *See also* Panoramic film
Film, dental
 barrier protected, contamination and,
 117, 118f
 comparison of physical properties of, 243t
 development of, common probems in,
 105b-107b
 factors affecting diagnostic quality of,
 57t
 improper handling of, 80
 mounting, manual tank processing and,
 101
 opaque, 97
 panoramic machine and, 192, 192f
 placement of, 125, 126, 128, 130, 132,
 134, 136, 138, 140, 142, 144, 146
 plastic barrier, 118f
 projections and, 164
 types of, 56
 washing of, 98
Film, extraoral, 100
 film processing and, 104
 screens and, 58
Film, x-ray. *See* X-ray film
Film badges, occupational exposure and,
 66
Film base, composition of, 72
Film clips, mounting film on, 102f
Film contrast
 overview of, 79-80
 processing and, 80
Film darkening, factors in, 77
Film density
 development time v., 96
 increasing, 78
Film emulsion
 contents of, 94
 photomicrograph of, 97, 98f
 sensitivity of, 71
 silver grains and, 82

Film exposure, 114
 characteristic curve of, 78
 common problems in, 105b-107b
Film fog, 106b
 darkroom and, 98, 99f
Film graininess, mottle and, 82
Film holding instruments, 91
 bitewing exam and, 148
 bitewing projection and, 161, 298
 edentulous patients and, 165
 film placement and, 134, 136, 146
 horizontal angulation and, 148
 overview of, 125
 patient examination and, 123-124
 periapical films and, 61
 projection of central ray and, 131, 135,
 143, 145, 147
 sterilizing, 117
Film images, monitor and, 234
Film latitude, overview of, 81
Film mount, radiographs in, 108, 108f
Film optical density. *See* Optical density
Film orientation, positioning in, 72
Film packets
 contamination and, 117, 118f, 120
 cross-contamination with, 115
 environmental damage and, 104
 film placement and, 130, 132
Film placement
 anterior mandibular occlusal projection
 of, 157
 anterior maxillary occlusal projection
 and, 154
 cross-sectional mandibular occlusal
 projection and, 158
 lateral mandibular occlusal projection
 and, 159
 lateral maxillary occlusal projection and,
 156
 molar bitewing projection and, 152
 patient examination and, 122-123
 periodontal disease and, 316
 premolar bitewing projection with,
 150
Film printers, radiologists and, 235
Film processing, 94
 contrast and, 80
 darkening and, 77
 emulsion and, 71
 emulsion changes during, 96f
 equipment for, 103-104, 103f
 faulty radiographs and, 105
 manual procedures for, 101-102, 101f
 mechanism of, 103, 104f
 overview of, 63
 procedures for, 96
 stereoscopy technique and, 249, 249f
Film speed, developer replenisher and,
 97
Film stock, rotation of, 113
Films
 contamination of, 118, 119f
 TMJ and, 269
Films,underexposed, periodontal disease
 and, 326
Filter, aluminum, energy distribution of
 beam and, 15, 15f
Filtration, 14-15, 15f
 ADA recommendations for, 60
 equipment choice of, 56
 external, 15
 total, 15

First molar
    aggressive periodontitis and, 324
    calcifying odontogenic cyst and, 400
    central giant cell granuloma and, 502
    central ray projection and, 153
    congenital syphilis and, 353
    film placement and, 126
    image field and, 132, 142
First premolar
    premolar bitewing projection and, 150
    projection of central ray and, 133
Fissures
    buccal carious lesions and, 303
    lingual carious lesions and, 303
Fistula (parulis). See also Arteriovenous
        (A-V) fistula
    periapical inflammatory lesion and, 368
    squamous cell carcinoma originating in
        cyst and, 464
Fistula tract, chronic osteomyelitis and, 379f
Fixed postmitotic cells, radiosensitivity
        and, 30
Fixer, 94, 98, 100
    constituents of, 104
    environmental damage and, 104
Fixing film, manual tank processing and,
        102
Fixing solution
    components of, 98
    function of, 96f, 97-98
    temperature of, 100
Fixing tank, 99, 104
Flat panel detectors, extraoral imaging
        devices and, 231
Flip angle of 90 degrees, 259
Flocculent pattern, cementoossifying
        fibroma and, 500, 500f
Floor of maxillary sinus, bone and, 179
Florid cemento-osseous dysplasia, 495
Florid osseous dysplasia (FOD)
    clinical features of, 496
    definition of, 495
    differential diagnosis of, 496
    management of, 496, 498
    Paget's disease v., 508
    periapical cemental dysplasia v., 496
    radiographic features of, 496
    synonyms for, 495
Fluid intake, autoimmune sialadenitis and,
        670
Fluids
    acute radiation syndrome and, 39
    adhesions and, 557
    inferior condylar positioning (widened
        joint space) and, 542
Fluoride
    caries and, 266
    demineralization process and, 311
    radiation caries and, 305
    remineralization and, 297
Fluoride, topical, radiation caries and, 35
Fluoride exposure, monitoring lesions
        and, 297
Fluoride rinse, erosion and, 356
Fluorine, PET and, 262
Focal osteoporotic bone marrow
    clinical features of, 655
    definition of, 654
    differential diagnosis of, 655
    management of, 655-656
    postulated etiology of, 654
    radiographic features of, 655, 655f

Focal plane
    film based tomography and, 245
    linear tomogram and, 247
Focal sclerosing osteitis, radiopaque
        presentations of, 367
Focal spot, 8, 9f
    film density and, 78
    size of, 115
    target size and, 8, 9f
    x-ray tube and, 86
Focal spot-to-object distance, 86, 88f, 89
    cone and, 90
Focal spot-to-spot distance (FSFDs)
    ADA and, 58
    effect of on tissue, 58f
Focal trough, 194f
    mandible in, 195f
    panoramic image and, 193
Focused grids, x-ray and, 84
Focusing cup, 8, 8f
FOD. See Florid osseous dysplasia (FOD)
Fogging, 99. See also Film fog
    safelight filters and, 112
    x-ray film and, 80
Follicular cyst, 388
    adenomaoid odontogenic tumor and,
        433
Food, radionuclides and, 49
Food and Drug Administration (FDA),
        radiographic guidelines by, 272, 274t
Foreshortened, tooth image being, 90
Forme fruste manifestations,
        neurofibromatosis and, 441, 442f
Fourier transform, roles of, 259
Fractionation, x-ray dose and, 33
Fracture line, horizontal fracture and,
        631
Fractures, crown fractures. See Dental
        crown fractures
Fractures, dental. See also Pathologic
        fracture
    airspace and, 207
    bifid condyle v., 554
    bilateral, TMJ ankylosis v., 569
    complex, computed tomography (CT)
        and, 548
    crown, radiograph appropriate for, 615
    divisions of, 567
    hypocalcification and, 345
    internal resorption and, 356
    mandibular symphysis and, 181
    monitoring healing of, 635-636, 636f
    neonatal
        condyle and, 569f
        rudimentary condyle and, 568
    occlusal radiography and, 160
    osteoporosis and, 524
    panoramic projection and, 543, 543f
    periapical inflammatory lesions and,
        366
    periapical radiographs and, 163
    peripheral nerve damage and, 440
    radiographic signs of, 616
    renal osteodystrophy and, 526
    squamous cell carcinoma and, 461
    tooth root, sinus and, 593
    unilateral, 567
Fractures, facial, radiography and, 624
Fractures, tooth crown
    prognosis for, 620
    pulp and, 619
    three categories of, 619

Fractures, tooth root
    clinical features of, 620
    definition of, 620
    differential diagnosis of, 621
    intraoral periapical films and, 615
    management of, 621
    radiographic features of, 620-621, 621f
    radiographic signs of, 616
Fractures of alveolar process
    clinical features of, 627, 629
    definition of, 627
    management of, 629
    radiographic features of, 629, 629f
Fractures of teeth, complicated,
        uncomplicated v., 619-620
Fragmentation, arteriosclerosis and, 602
Free induction decay (FID), resonant RF
        pulse and, 259
Free radicals, direct effect and, 25
Free silver ions, 94
Frequency, 5
Frontal bones
    Gardner's syndrome and, 445
    hemifacial hyperplasia and, 650
    mid-facial area and, 204
    midface fractures and, 629
Frontal sinuses
    craniofacial disjunction and, 634
    development of, 576-577
    osteomas of, 443, 443f, 444
    pyramidal fracture and, 631
    Waters projection and, 221
Frontal view, horizontal fracture and, 630f
Frontal views of condyles, mandibular
        condyle fractures and, 626
Full-mouth examination (FMX), 121, 122
    intraoral radiographs and, 270
Fundamental particles, radiology and, 3
Furcations, periodontal disease and, 321,
        322
Fused roots, dilaceration v., 340
Fusion, gemination v., 338
Fusion of teeth
    clinical features of, 336
    definition of, 336
    differential diagnosis of, 337
    management of, 337
    radiographic features of, 336

G

Gadolinium, flat panel detectors and, 232
Gadolinium contrast, cystic lesions and,
        671, 671f
Gadolinium oxybromide compounds, x-ray
        absorption and, 228
Gag reflex
    film placement and, 134
    radiographic examination and, 163
Gallium scans, septic arthritis and, 565
Gamma, decrease in, 237f
Gamma-emitting isotopes, radionuclide-
        labeled tracers and, 260
Gamma scintillation camera, tracers and,
        262
Gamma value, digital imaging and, 236
Gardner's syndrome
    cleidocranial dysplasia v., 648
    desmoplastic fibroma of bone and, 454
    enostosis v., 416, 445
    osteomas with, 446f
    overview of, 444-445
    treatment of, 445

Garrés chronic nonsupppurative sclerosing osteitis, 377
Garré's osteomyelitis, 374
Gastric reflux, erosion and, 356
Gastrointestinal disorders, erosion and, 356
Gastrointestinal syndrome, radiation injury and, 38-39
Gastrointestinal tract, progressive systemic sclerosis and, 531
Gaucher's disease, multiple myeloma v., 477
GBX-2 filter, spectral sensitivities of, 100, 100f
Gemination (Twinning)
    clinical features of, 338
    definition of, 338
    differential diagnosis of, 338
    management of, 338-339
    radiographic features of, 338
Gendex #2 CCD sensor, 229f
Gendex #2 PSP plate, 229f
Gendex Denoptix system, plate reading and, 231
Gene mutations
    radiation and, 42
    supernumerary teeth and, 330
Genetic diseases, neurofibromatosis and, 441
Genetic effect, stomchastic effect and, 51
Genetics
    complete twinning and, 338
    fusion of teeth and, 336
    periodontitis and, 314
    torus palatinus and, 412
Genial tubercles (mental spine)
    mandible and, 182
    overview of, 181-182
Genioglossus muscles, genial tubercles and, 181-182
Geniohyoid muscles, genial tubercles and, 181-182
Geometric blurring, 83
Germination, fusion of teeth and, 337
Gestant odontome, 340
Gestation, prenatal irradiation and, 39
Ghost images
    photostimulable phosphor plates (PSP) and, 231
    x-ray beams and, 207
Giant cell granulomas. *See* Central giant cell granulomas (CGCG)
Giant cell lesions, 501
    TMJ tumors and, 570
Giant cell reparative granuloma, 501
Giant cell tumor, 501
Giant cell tumor, benign, central giant cell granuloma v., 501, 502
Giant osteoid osteoma
    clinical features of, 450
    differential diagnosis of, 450-452
    overview of, 450
    radiographic features of, 450
Giantism, 520
    hypercementosis and, 362
    hyperpituitarism and, 521
Gigantiform cementoma, 495
Gingiva
    acute leukemias and, 481
    digital detector characteristics and, 232, 233f
    dystrophic calcification and, 598

Gingiva *(Continued)*
    film placement and, 142, 152
    fractures of alveolar process and, 627
    pericoronitis and, 373
    primary carcinomas and, 459
    segmental odontomaxillary dysplasia and, 651
Gingival cyst, lateral periodontal cyst v., 398
Gingival margin, 314
    lesion in proximal surfaces and, 300
Gingival recession
    root exposure in, 309f
    root surface lesions and, 303-304
Gingivectomy, crown-root fractures and, 624
Gingivitis, 267
    chronic infectious diseases and, 314
    eosinophilic granuloma and, 509
    periodontitis v., 314
Gingivitis scores, progressive systemic sclerosis and, 531
Glandular fibrosis, autoimmune sialadenitis and, 669
Glandular swelling, xerostomia and, 669
Glenoid fossa
    anatomical relationship of, 539
    chondrocalcinosis and, 566
    mastoid air cells, 207
    neonatal fractures and, 568
    TMJ and, 202
    transpharyngeal projection, 546f
Glenoid fossa. *See* Mandibular fossa
Globular sialectasis, sialectasis v., 669, 670f
Globulomaxillary cysts, former cysts and, 405
Glossopharyngeal nerve, ossification of stylohyoid ligament and, 609
Gloves
    contamination and, 120
    cross-contamination and, 115
Glucocorticoid, Cushing's syndrome and, 523
Gold, restorative materials as, 187, 187f
Gold salts, rheumatoid arthritis and, 563
Goldenhar syndrome, 641
Gonad dose
    abdomen and, 53
    dental radiography and, 52
    males and, 42
    oral radiography and, 61
Gorlin-Goltz syndrome, 397
Granular cell ameloblastic fibroma, 428
Granular sclerotic bone, chronic osteomyelitis and, 379
Granulomas
    nasopalatine duct cyst v., 401
    primary osseous carcinoma v., 463
    radicular dentin dysplasia (type 1) and, 348
Graves' disease, 522
Gray levels, digital detector characteristics and, 232, 232f
Greenstick bone fractures
    cortical plate and, 625
    osteomalacia and, 525
    rickets and, 525
Grid ratio, 84
Grids. *See* Radiographic grids
Grids, x-ray, 84, 84f
Gross caries, positioning patient and, 208

Growth, radiation in atomic bombs and, 41
Growth hormone, hyperpituitarism and, 521
Gutta-percha markers
    CT study using, 685f, 686
    endodontic therapy and, 188f
Gutta-percha point, vertical osseous defects and, 320, 321f
Gyral markings, hypophosphatasia and, 526

H
Half-value layer (HVL)
    exponential absorption and, 19, 19f, 20
    minimum, 60t
    x-ray and, 14
Half-wave rectified, x-ray and, 11
Halide ions, changing solutions and, 102
Hallermann-Streiff syndrome, Treacher Collins syndrome v., 646
Halo shadow, lesions and, 370, 371f
Hamartomas
    hemangioma v., 445
    jaw tumors and, 410
    osteomas and, 443
Hamular process, trabeculae and, 181, 181f
Hand-Schüller-Christian disease, Langerhans' X and, 509
Hand washing, patient procedure and, 122
Hangers, manual tank processing and, 101, 101f
Hard palate, lateral cephalometric projection and, 219f, 220
Hard tissue imaging
    panoramic projection of, 543, 543f
    transcranial projection and, 543, 543f
Hardeners, fixing solution and, 98
Head
    reverse-Towne projection (open mouth), 213
    x-ray machine and, 9
Head alignment
    panoramic radiographs and, 199f
    patient positioning and, 197-198
Head lesions, Langerhans' cell histiocytosis and, 509
Headache, rhinoliths and, 607
Healing
    fractures and, 635-636
    simple bone cyst and, 407, 408f
Healing odontogenic cyst, rhinoliths v., 608
Heart
    cysticercus cellulosae and, 601
    progressive systemic sclerosis and, 531
Heart failure, progressive systemic sclerosis and, 531
Helium, atomic structures of, 4f
Hemangiomas
    clinical features of, 445-446, 673
    definition of, 673
    developing dentition and, 449f
    differential diagnosis of, 448
    hemifacial hyperplasia v., 650
    neurilemmoma v., 440
    phleboliths and, 605, 606, 606f
    radiographic features of, 447, 673
    treatment of, 448-449
Hematologic disorders, periodontal disease and, 327

Hematopoietic marrow, focal osteoporotic bone marrow and, 654
Hematopoietic stem cells
    acute radiation syndrome and, 37-38
    leukemia and, 482
Hematopoietic syndrome, acute radiation syndrome and, 37-38
Hematopoietic system, malignancies of, 475-482, 475-484
Hemifacial hyperplasia, 649
    clinical features of, 649-650
    definition of, 649
    differential diagnosis of, 650-651
    management of, 651
    mandible and, 203
    radiographic features of, 650, 650f
Hemifacial hypertrophy, 649
Hemifacial hypoplasia, 641
Hemifacial microsomia (HFM)
    clinical features of, 643
    definition of, 641, 643
    differential diagnosis of, 643
    infant with, 644f
    management of, 643
    radiographic features of, 643
Hemimaxillofacial dysplasia, 651
Hemoglobin, sickle cell anemia and, 533
Hemophilia, periodontal disease and, 327
Hemorrhage
    arteriovenous (A-V) fistula and, 449
    localized (traumatic) myositis ossificans and, 610
    metastatic tumors and, 467
    squamous cell carcinoma and, 461
    zygomatic arch fractures and, 635
Hemorrhage, spontaneous, acute leukemias and, 481
Hemorrhagic aspirate, aneurysmal bone cyst and, 505
Hemorrhagic bone cyst, 405
Hemostat, mandibular projections and, 164
Heparin therapy, secondary osteoporosis and, 524
Hepatitis strains, 115
Hepatomegaly, acute leukemias and, 481
Hereditary opalescent dentin, 346
Hertwig's epithelial root sheath
    dens in dente and, 340
    enamel pearl, 350
Heterogeneous radiopacities, antroliths and, 607
Heterotopic bone
    overview of, 597
    progressive myostis ossificans and, 611
Heterotopic calcification
    degenerative processes and, 597
    three categories of, 597
Heterotopic ossification, soft tissue and, 597
Heterozygous diseases
    hypophosphatasia and, 526
    thalassemia and, 533
High contrast
    image and, 79
    radiograph showing, 79f
High contrast anatomy, film based tomography and, 245
High voltage transformer, 7f, 10
Histogram equalization, 236
Histopathology, cancer classification and, 458

HIV infection
    autoimmune sialadenitis v., 669
    multicentric parotid cysts and, 671
    universal precautions and, 115
Holding instrument. See Film holding instruments
Homozygous diseases, sickle cell anemia and, 533
Horizontal angle, bitewing examinations and, 148, 161
Horizontal angulation
    film placement and, 132
    horizontal bitewing films and, 148
    molar bitewing projection and, 152
    projection of central ray and, 127, 133, 145
    torus palatinus and, 412, 413f
    tube head and, 148
Horizontal beam angle, transcranial projection and, 544
Horizontal bitewing films, overview of, 148-149
Horizontal bone loss, moderate periodontitis and, 319, 319f, 320f
Horizontal distortion, image layer and, 194
Horizontal fracture, 629
    clinical features of, 630
    definition of, 630
    management of, 631
    radiographic features of, 630-631
Horizontal overlapping, central ray and, 125, 125f
Horizontal tooth crown fractures, prognosis for, 620
Hormonal sialadenoses, 670
Hormone changes
    fibrous dysplasia and, 491
    periodontal disease and, 327
Hormone treatment, metastatic tumors and, 467
Host bone, non-Hodgkin's lymphoma and, 477
Hounsfield units, computed tomography (CT) scanners and, 252f
Hutchinson's teeth, congenital syphilis and, 353
HVL. See Half-value layer (HVL)
Hyaline cartilage, calcification and, 606
Hydraulics, cysts and, 286f, 289
Hydrogen
    atomic structures of, 4f
    MRI and, 256
Hydrogen nuclei, 259
    external magnetic field and, 256, 257f, 258f
    MRI and, 256, 256f, 257f
Hydrogen peroxide, biologic molecules and, 26
Hydroquinone, radiology and, 97
Hydroxyl free radicals, molecules and, 26
Hygiene program
    florid osseous dysplasia and, 496
    rampant caries and, 302
Hyoid bone, ossification of stylohyoid ligament and, 609
Hyperbaric oxygen therapy
    osteopetrosis and, 531
    osteoradionecrosis and, 382
Hypercalcemia
    multiple myeloma and, 475
    primary hyperparathyroidism and, 517

Hypercalcemia of malignancy, metastatic calcification and, 608
Hypercementosis
    acromegaly v., 521
    attrition and, 355
    benign cementoblastoma v., 436
    definition of, 362
    differential diagnosis of, 363
    enostoses v., 416
    hyperpituitarism and, 521, 522f
    management of, 363
    occult disease and, 268
    Paget's disease and, 508, 511f
    radiographic features of, 362-363
Hypermobility, degenerative joint disease and, 559
Hypermobility of TMJ, mouth opening and, 542
Hyperocclusional teeth, hypercementosis and, 362
Hyperostosis (exostosis), 412, 414
    osteomas v., 444
    periapical film of, 417f
Hyperparathyroidism, 520f
    calcification of tissues and, 608
    central giant cell granuloma v., 503
    definition of, 517
    fibrous dysplasia and, 489
    medial calcinosis and, 602
    multiple myeloma v., 475, 477
Hyperphosphatemia, renal osteodystrophy and, 526
Hyperpituitarism
    clinical features of, 521
    definition of, 520
    hypercementosis and, 362
    radiographic features of, 521
    synonyms for, 520
Hyperplasia of bone marrow, sickle cell anemia and, 533
Hyperplasias
    false ankylosis and, 570
    hamartoma v., 410
    jaw tumors and, 410
    overview of, 412
    thalassemia and, 534, 535f
Hyperplastic follicle
    ameloblastic fibromas v., 429
    dentigerous cyst v., 390
Hyperplastic parathyroid glands, excess PTH and, 517
Hypertelorism
    basal cell nevus syndrome and, 397
    crouzon syndrome and, 641, 641f
Hyperthyroidism
    cortical bone and, 203
    definition of, 522
    radiographic features of, 522
    synonyms for, 522
Hypocalcemia
    hypoparathyroidism and, 519
    pseudohypoparathyroidism and, 519
    renal osteodystrophy and, 526
    secondary hyperparathyroidism v., 517
Hypocalcification
    amelogenesis imperfecta and, 345
    systemic disorders and, 516
Hypocalcified enamel, gemination and, 338
Hypocycloidal tomography, 246, 246f
    facial skeletal images and, 197

Hypodontia, 330
  clinical features of, 332
  psychological distress, 333
  synonyms for, 332
  transposition and, 336
Hypoechoic, Warthin tumor and, 673
Hypoesthesia, neurovascular canals and, 469
Hypomaturation, amelogenesis imperfecta and, 345
Hypomineralization, Turner's hypoplasia and, 352
Hypoparathyroidism
  clinical features of, 519-520
  hypocalcemia and, 519
  radiographic features of, 520
Hypophosphatasia
  clinical features of, 526
  definition of, 526
  radiographic features of, 526
Hypophosphatemia
  children v. adults with, 527
  clinical features of, 527
  definition of, 527
  periodontal disease and, 327
  radiographic features of, 527-528
  synonyms of, 527
Hypopituitarism
  clinical features of, 522
  definition of, 521
  radiographic features of, 522
  treatment of, 522
Hypoplasia
  amelogenesis imperfecta and, 345
  condylar fractures and, 568
  mandible and, 203
  overview, 576
  rickets and, 526f
  systemic disorders and, 516
Hypoplasia of external ear, Treacher Collins syndrome and, 643
Hypoplasia of microtia, hemifacial microsomia, 643
Hypoplastic dentin, regional odontodysplasia and, 349, 350f
Hypoplastic enamel
  gemination and, 338
  regional odontodysplasia and, 349, 350f
  rickets and, 525, 526f
Hypoplastic maxilla, crouzon syndrome and, 641
Hypoplastic pits, dental anomalies and, 300
Hyposphosphatemic rickets, 527
Hypothyroidism
  children and, 523
  synonyms for, 522

I

Identification dot, film processing and, 108
Idiopathic calcification, 603-608
  overview of, 597
Image, subject thickness and, 78
Image, panoramic. See Panoramic images; Panoramic imaging
Image analysis, 282
  diagnosis and, 239
  overview of, 281
  three steps of, 239
Image archiving, digital imaging and, 239

Image clarity
  focal spot and, 86
  methods for minimizing loss of, 86-87, 87f
  sharpness and, 86
Image compression. See also File compression
  digital imaging and, 240
Image contrast
  changing solutions and, 103
  digital subtraction radiography and, 238
  reference film and, 110
Image degradation, reasons for, 58
Image density, milliampere-seconds and, 63
Image elongation
  image and, 89f
  vertical angulation and, 148, 148b
Image enhancement, overview of, 235
Image field
  anterior mandibular occlusal projection in, 157
  anterior maxillary occlusal projection and, 154
  central incisors in, 126
  cross-sectional mandibular occlusal projection in, 158
  lateral mandibular occlusal projection and, 159
  lateral maxillary occlusal projection and, 156
  molar bitewing projection and, 152
  periapical areas in, 126
  premolar bitewing projection and, 150
Image formats, digital imaging and, 240
Image histogram, gray values and, 235, 236f
Image layer
  overview of, 193-194, 193f, 195
  panoramic imaging and, 191
  patient positioning in, 197-198
Image management software, 235
Image processing, dental radiography and, 235
Image quality
  collimators and, 15
  factors in, 63, 83
  film speed and, 57
  lead foil and, 73
  overview of, 83-84
  processing solutions and, 63
  reference film and, 110
  sharpening filters and, 236
  smoothing filters and, 236
Image receptor
  equipment choice of, 56
  extraoral radiographic examinations and, 210
  lateral cephalometric projections and, 211, 212t
  submentovertex (base) projection and, 213
Image receptor blurring
  overview of, 82-83
  silver grains and, 82
Image receptors
  overview of, 198-200
  quality assurance program and, 110
  radiography and, 94
Image resolution
  digital imaging and, 58
  photostimulable phosphor plates (PSP) and, 231

Image restoration, pixels and, 235
Image shape distortion, 89-90
Image sharpness
  intensifying screens and, 83
  light and, 83
Image sites, developing process and, 97
Image size distortion. See Magnification
Image spatial resolution, 86
Image transformation graphs, effect of brightness on, 237f
Images, number and type of, 281-282
Images, panoramic, neck area and, 208f
Imaging chain, 226
Imaging stents
  dental implants and, 686
  examples of, 687f
  purpose of, 686
Imaging system, selecting, 243
Imaging techniques
  diagnostic information provided by, 543, 544t-545t
  restorative procedures and, 677, 678b
Imatron, CT technology and, 255
Immobilization
  craniofacial disjunction and, 634
  hemangioma and, 448
Immune status, periodontitis and, 314
Immunosuppressive disorders, osteomyelitis and, 374
Immunosuppressive therapeutic agents, autoimmune sialadenitis and, 670
Immunotherapy, metastatic tumors and, 467
Impacted molars, osteogenesis imperfecta and, 347
Impacted teeth, 92
  adenomaoid odontogenic tumor and, 431
  adenomaoid odontogenic tumor v., 433
  ameloblastic fibroma and, 431
  calcifying epithelial odontogenic tumors and, 423
  external resorption and, 358
  image field and, 136, 144, 146
  microdontia and, 335f
  multiple myeloma and, 475
  occlusal radiography and, 160
  odontogenic myxoma and, 434
  radiographs and, 91
Impacted third molars, panoramic images and, 209
Impaction, odontomas and, 425
Implant imaging, summary of techniques for, 679t
Implant imaging techniques, endosseous implants and, 677, 678f, 679t
Implants. See also Osseointegrated implants
Implants, blade, fixed bridge with, 678f
Implants, dental
  cleidocranial dysplasia and, 648
  clinical considerations for, 269
  3D CT and, 255
  film based tomography and, 245
  hypodontia and, 333
  image of successful, 691f
  imaging for, 677
  overview of, 677, 678f
  patterns of bone morphology in, 680f
  periapical film and, 689f
  peripheral nerve damage and, 440
  preoperative planning with, 269

Implants, dental *(Continued)*
  radiographic visualization of potential sites for, 683
  stereoscopy technique and, 249
  success factors of, 690
  wide-angle tomography and, 247, 248f
Implants, endosseous, radiographic signs associated with failing, 690t
Implants, root-form, types of, 678f
Implants, subperiosteal, denture support and, 678f
Incident beam, differential absorption and, 19
Incident photon, 17
Incipient caries, resolution of image and, 72
Incipient proximal enamel lesions, 302f
Incisal edge fracture
  right maxillary central incisor and, 622f
  right maxillary lateral incisor and, 620f
Incisive canal cyst, 400
Incisive foramen
  central incisors and, 175f
  nasopalatine duct cyst v., 401
  overview of, 174
Incisive sutures, 174
Incisocervical groove, fusion of teeth and, 336
Incisor crowns, congenital syphilis and, 353
Incisor periapical films, children and, 162
Incisors
  aggressive periodontitis and, 324
  calcifying odontogenic cyst and, 400
  erosion and, 356
  image field and, 138
  root canals at, 167f
  toothbrush injury and, 355
Incremental scanners, computed tomography (CT) and, 251
Indirect effects, overview of, 26
Industrial products, annual E and, 50
Infantile cortical hyperostosis, osteopetrosis v., 531
Infants
  Letterer-Siwe disease in, 510
  mandibular symphysis in, 181
  osteopetrosis and, 528
  progressive myositis ossificans and, 611
  rickets in, 525
Infection, secondary, cemental dysplasia and, 495
Infection control
  dental personnel and, 115-120
  film processing and, 104
  purpose of, 110
  steps in, 115b
Infections, bacterial, autoimmune sialadenitis v., 669
Infections, dental
  ankylosis and, 569
  chronic sinusitis and, 579
  concrescence and, 337
  condylar hypoplasia and, 552
  diabetes mellitus and, 523
  florid osseous dysplasia and, 495
  joint effusion and, 567
  orofacial structures and, 162
  osteoradionecrosis and, 380
  pseudotumor and, 588
  radiation injury and, 38

Infections, dental *(Continued)*
  resorption and, 356
  septic arthritis, 565
  sinusitis and, 579
Infections, viral
  autoimmune sialadenitis v., 669
  inflammatory disease and, 578
Infectious arthritis, 564
Infectious diseases, surface cleaners and, 116
Inferior alveolar nerve canal (IAC), 285
  bone density and, 516
  cementoossifying fibroma and, 499
  central giant cell granuloma and, 502
  cysts and, 384
  dentigerous cyst and, 390
  fibrous dysplasia and, 293
  florid osseous dysplasia and, 496
  hemangioma and, 448, 448f
  jaw abnormalities and, 285
  neurilemmoma and, 439, 439f
  odontogenic keratocyst and, 395
  osteoblastomas and, 451f
  residual infected cyst, 388, 388f
Inferior border of jaw, fibrosarcoma and, 475
Inferior condylar positioning (widened joint space), fluid in joint and, 542
Inferior dental nerve, neurofibroma and, 441, 441f
Inferior joint space
  interarticular disk and, 540
  radiographic joint space v., 541, 541f
Inferior lamina, condyle and, 541
Inferior mandibular border, periapical projections and, 186, 186f
Inflammation
  aggressive periodontitis and, 322, 323
  buccal bifurcation cyst and, 392
  four signs of, 366
  hypercementosis and, 362
  juvenile chronic arthritis and, 364
  periodontitis and, 314
  of sinus, 178
  T2-weighted pulse sequences and, 550
Inflammation, chronic
  dystrophic calcification and, 598
  resorption of teeth and, 286f, 292
Inflammatory arthritidis, degenerative joint disease v., 562
Inflammatory collateral dental cyst, 392
Inflammatory disease
  bone resorption and, 291
  causes of, 578
  overview of, 588-589
  squamous cell carcinoma v., 461
  TMJ and, 269
Inflammatory exudate, acute osteomyelitis and, 375
Inflammatory host response, bacteria and, 314
Inflammatory infections, multiple myeloma v., 477
Inflammatory joint disease, psoriatic arthritis and, 564
Inflammatory lesions
  effects on surrounding structures, 367
  Ewing's sarcoma v., 474
  external resorption and, 358
  internal structure of, 367
  jaws and, 366
  multiple myeloma v., 477

Inflammatory lesions *(Continued)*
  periphery of, 367
  radiographic features of, 366-367
  reaction in bone of, 320
Inflammatory lesions of jaws, Langerhans' cell histiocytosis v., 512
Inflammatory odontogenic disease, maxillary sinuses and, 577
Inflammatory periapical disease, multiple myeloma and, 475
Inflammatory periapical keratocysts, squamous cell carcinoma originating in cyst and, 464
Inflammatory pseudotumor, 588
Inflammatory residual keratocysts, squamous cell carcinoma originating in cyst and, 464
Inflammatory response
  aggressive periodontitis and, 324
  oral radiation therapy and, 33
Inflammatory sinusitis, malignant neoplasms v., 586
Infrabony defect, vertical osseous defects and, 319
Infractions, dental crowns and, 619
Inherent filtration, 15
Inherited disorders, hypophosphatasia and, 526
Inital periodontal disease, cortical density and, 318f
Initial visit, child and, 273
Injuries, jaw, internal derangement and, 554
Injury, follow-up radiographs for, 615
Injury, whiplash, internal derangement and, 555
Inkjet printers, 235
Input values, output values v., 236, 237f
InSight film
  characteristic curves and, 81f
  composition of, 71
  electron micrograph of, 72f, 73f
  spectral sensitivities of, 100f
Instruments, dental, maxillary projections and, 164
Instruments, film holding. *See* Film holding instruments
Intensifying cassette
  purpose of, 75, 76f
  screen phosphors and, 75
Intensifying screens, 71, 82
  cleaning of, 112
  composition of, 75
  factors affecting resolution of, 76-77
  films with, 80
  flat panel detectors and, 231
  function of, 74, 75, 75f
  image sharpness and, 83
  panoramic radiography and, 198
  phosphors fluoresce in, 76t
  rare earth elements used in, 76t
  rare earth phosphors in, 57
Intensity
  subject contrast and, 79
  x-ray beam and, 16f
Interactive diagnostic hardware
  dental implant sites and, 686
  overview of, 686
Interanl trabeculation, coronoid process and, 187
Interarticular disk (meniscus), anatomical relationship with, 540

Interdental bone, moderate periodontitis and, 318
Intermaxillary fixation, horizontal fracture and, 631
Intermaxillary suture (median suture), periapical radiographs of, 172, 172f
Internal density, tooth structure and, 288, 291
Internal derangement
  adhesions in, 556-557
  clinical features of, 555
  definition of, 554-555
  degenerative joint disease and, 560
  disk displacement and, 555-556
  disk perforation and deformities in, 556
  disk reduction and, 556
  joint effusion and, 567
  nonreduction and, 556
  radiographic features of, 555
  TMJ dysfunction and, 555
Internal radiation, sources of, 49
Internal resorption, 356
  definition of, 356
  differential diagnosis of, 358
  external resorption v., 358
  management of, 358
  radiographic features of, 357-358
Internal root resorption, crown and, 357f
Internal structure
  aneurysmal bone cyst and, 504
  central giant cell granuloma and, 502, 502f
Internal trabecular bone, sarcomas and, 459
International Commission on Radiological Protection (ICRP)
  dose limits and, 52
  tissue weighting factors and, 47
International Organization for Standardization (ISO), intraoral film sensitivity and, 233
Interpolation, three-dimensional reformatting and, 252, 253f
Interproximal areas
  bitewing exam and, 148
  projection of central ray and, 133
Interproximal caries, 266
Interproximal cortex, periodontal disease and, 326
Interproximal crater, vertical osseous defects and, 319, 320f
Interproximal decay, radiographic examination and, 273
Interproximal examinations. See Bitewing examinations
Interproximal films, film mount for, 108
Interproximal radiographs (bitewings)
  child and, 273
  periodontium and, 316
  purpose of, 271
Interproximal space
  bitewing examinations and, 148
  projection of central ray and, 139
Interproximal views, periodontal disease and, 316
Interradicular bone
  furcation defects and, 321, 322
  periodontal disease and, 321
Interstitial cyst, 581
Interstitial fibrosis, sialodochitis and, 668
Interval timer, temperature of developer and, 101

Interval timer. See Timer, interval
Intestinal cancer, Gardner's syndrome and, 445
Intraalveolar carcinoma, 463
Intraarticular inflammatory lesions, condylar hypoplasia and, 552
Intracellular structures, radiation on, 27
Intracranial arterial calcifications, arteriosclerosis and, 602
Intracranial extension, osteoma and, 586
Intramandibular carcinoma, 463
Intraoperative assessments, radiographs and, 687-691
Intraoperative films, dental implants and, 687, 689f
Intraoral dental film, 100
  benefits of full mouth series in, 281
  extraoral films v., 223
  mottle and, 82
  panoramic film v., 200
  panoramic imaging and, 191
  speed classification of, 81t
Intraoral image receptors, overview of, 56
Intraoral imaging, 239
  benign tumors and, 410
  clinical comparison of alternatives in, 242t
  dentition and, 209
  digital image receptors and, 299
  fractures of alveolar process and, 629
  maxillary antrum and, 577
  overview of, 270-271
  parallax unsharpness and, 83, 83f
  potential implant site and, 678f
  procedure for, 270
  treatment planning and, 282-283
Intraoral mass, metastatic tumors and, 467, 468f
Intraoral periapical films
  dental trauma and, 615
  mandibular body fractures and, 625, 626f
  rotational scanography v., 250
Intraoral procedures, panoramic imaging and, 191
Intraoral radiographic examinations, categories of, 121
Intraoral radiographic technique, choice of, 62-64
Intraoral radiography
  dental implants and, 677, 678, 678b
  infection and, 162
  photostimulable phosphor plates (PSP) and, 231
  sialoliths and, 660
Intraoral technique, choice of, 61
Intraoral x-ray film, overview of, 72-73
Intraoral x-ray film packets, contents of, 73, 73f
Intraosseous lesions
  analysis of, 283-296, 295b
  radiographic examination and, 274
Intraosseous neoplasms, odontogenic myxoma and, 434
Intravascular thrombi, phleboliths and, 605
Intrinsic tumors of TMJ, locations of, 570
Introsseous nerve tumor, neurilemoma and, 439
Intruded maxillary central incisor, trauma and, 618f
Intrusive luxation, trauma and, 617

Invasive fungal sinusitis, 588
Invasive margins, metastatic tumors and, 467
Inverse square law, overview of, 16
Inverse voltage, x-ray and, 11
Iodine
  Nevada test site and, 51
  radionuclide-labeled tracers and, 260
  Ultra-speed film and, 71
Iodine-containing compounds, sialography and, 663
Iodine contrast agent, salivary gland disease and, 660
Iodophors, surface cleaners and, 116
Ionization, 4
Ionization chambers, computed tomography (CT) and, 251
Ionizing radiation
  annual effective dose of, 48t
  annual limits for human exposure of, 50t
  arthrography, 548
  biologic effects of, 25
  estimates of risk with, 53, 55
  induction of cancer by, 41
  MRI and, 260
  radiographic examination and, 265
  water and, 26
Ipsilateral petrous ridge, osseous changes and, 544
Irradiation, children and, 160

J
J shadow, bone destruction and, 323f
Jaw
  abnormality position in, 285
  adenomatoid odontogenic tumor and, 432
  arteriovenous (A-V) fistula and, 449
  cherubism and, 506
  cysts
    basal cell nevus syndrome and, 397
    nasopalatine duct cyst and, 401
  cysts of, 384
  dentigerous cyst and, 388
  diabetes mellitus and, 523
  diseases of, radiographic examination and, 266
  disorders, TMJ dysfunction and, 538
  enlargement of, hyperpituitarism and, 521, 522f
  Ewing's sarcoma and, 473
  expansion
    calcifying epithelial odontogenic tumor and, 422, 424
    periapical cemental dysplasia and, 495
  florid osseous dysplasia and, 495, 496, 497f
  focal osteoporotic bone marrow and, 654
  giant osteoid osteoma v., 450
  hypopituitarism and, 522
  inflammatory lesions of, 366
  lesions
    aneurysmal bone cyst and, 503
    imaging of, 268-269
    symtoms of, 469
  malignant tumors of, 571
  mandibular condyle fractures and, 626
  metastatic tumors and, 466
  missing teeth and, 333
  monostotic fibrous dysplasia and, 485

Jaw *(Continued)*
  multiple myeloma and, 475
  neurofibromatosis and, 442
  occlusal radiography and, 160
  occult disease of, 267-268
  odontogenic keratocyst and, 394
  odontogenic myxoma and, 434
  odontomas and, 425
  osseous deformities of, computed
      tomography (CT) and, 548
  osteomas and, 443, 443f
  osteoporosis and, 524, 525f
  other exostoses of, 414
  Paget's disease in, 507, 508f
  panoramic imaging and, 191
  position and movement of disk in, 556f
  primary carcinomas and, 459
  primary interosseous carcinoma and,
      463
  radicular cyst in, 385
  radiographic features in
      hyperparathyroidism of, 518
  rickets and, 525
  sickle cell anemia and, 533
  trabeculae in, 171, 172
  tumors, Burkitt's lymphoma and, 478
  tumors and, 410
Jaw osteomyelitis, Paget's disease and, 509
Jawbone, fibrosarcoma and, 475
Joint capsule, MRI and, 616
Joint destruction, septic arthritis and, 564
Joint effusion
  juvenile chronic arthritis v., 364
  MRI of, 560f
  septic arthritis and, 565
  T2-weighted pulse sequences and, 550
Joint mobility, ankylosis v., 569
Joint pain, primary hyperparathyroidism
      and, 517
Joint space
  adhesions and, 557
  arthrographs of, 549f
  chondrocalcinosis and, 566
  remodeling v., 559
  synovial chondromatosis and, 565
Joint space calcifications, malignant
      tumors v., 572
Joint space radiopacities, degenerative
      joint disease and, 561, 562f
Joint swelling, chondrocalcinosis and,
      566
Joints
  computed tomography (CT) and, 548
  condylar fractures and, 568
  degenerative joint disease and, 559
  rheumatoid arthritis and, 563
Joule (energy), SI system and, 21
JPEG (Joint Photographic Experts Group),
      file compression and, 240
Juvenile arthrosis
  clinical features of, 553
  definition of, 553
  differential diagnosis of, 553
  radiographic features of, 553
  synonyms for, 552
  treatment for, 553
Juvenile chronic arthritis (JCA)
  clinical features of, 363
  definition of, 363
  radiographic features of, 363
  sagittal tomogram of, 364f
  synonyms for, 363

Juvenile ossifying fibroma
  fibrous dysplasia v., 501
  jaw deformity in, 499
  radiologic findings in, 498
Juvenile rheumatoid arthritis
  condylar hypoplasia and, 552
  condylar positioning in, 542
  juvenile chronic arthritis v., 364

K

K-edge absorption, 20
K shell, atom structure and, 3, 4
K-shell electrons, 20
Keratin, odontogenic keratocyst and, 394
Kerma. *See* Air kerma
Kidney disease, renal osteodystrophy and,
      526
Kidneys, progressive systemic sclerosis and,
      531
Kilovoltages, 60, 63
  overview of, 62
Kilovolts peak (kVp) selector dial, 7f, 10
Kodak #2 film, 229f
Kodak GBX-2 filter, panoramic film and,
      200
kVp meter, plastic wrap and, 116
Kyphoscoliosis, basal cell nevus syndrome
      and, 397
Kyphosis, Cushing's syndrome and, 523

L

L-shell electrons, 20
Labial cortex, nasopalatine duct cyst and,
      401, 403f
Labial enamel, erosion and, 356
Labial plates, fractures of alveolar process
      and, 627
Lacrimal bone, midface fractures and, 629
Lacrimal glands, autoimmune sialadenitis
      and, 669
Lamina dura
  alveolar bone and, 283
  cementoossifying fibroma and, 500
  central giant cell granuloma and, 502
  central mucoepidermoid carcinoma
      and, 465
  Cushing's syndrome and, 523, 524f
  as diagnostic feature, 169
  external resorption and, 358
  fibrous dysplasia and, 490f
  malignant lesions and, 292, 292f
  mental foramen and, 184
  metastatic tumors and, 467
  multiple myeloma and, 475
  Paget's disease and, 508
  periapical cemental dysplasia, 492
  periapical inflammatory lesion and, 370
  periodontal disease and, 317, 317f
  primary hyperparathyroidism and, 519
  renal osteodystrophy and, 527
  sarcomas and, 459, 460f
  simple bone cyst and, 406f
  systemic disorders and, 516
  teeth and, 168, 168f
Laminar periosteal bone formation,
      Ewing's sarcoma v., 474
Langerhans cell histiocytosis (LCH)
  alveolar type of, 511
  buccal bifurcation cyst v., 393
  chronic osteomyelitis v., 380
  clinical features of, 509-510
  definition of, 509

Langerhans cell histiocytosis (LCH)
      (Continued)
  differential diagnosis of, 513-514
  Intraosseous type of, 511
  management of, 514
  non-Hodgkin's lymphoma v., 478
  osteomyelitis v., 377
  periodontal disease v., 327
  periosteal reaction in, 513f
  radiographic features of, 509-512
  skull lesions in, 511, 511f
  synonyms for, 509
  TMJ tumors and, 570
Langerhans cell histiocytosis (LCH) jaw
      lesions, two types of, 510-511
Langerhans cells, Langerhans' cell
      histiocytosis and, 509
Langerhans' X, three clinical forms of, 509
Large occlusal forces, vertical root
      fractures and, 623
Large retention pseudocysts, squamous
      cell carcinoma v., 588
Larmor frequency
  electromagnetic waves and, 258
  MR image and, 260
  precession and, 257
Laryngeal cartilage calcifications
  clinical features of, 606
  definition of, 606
  differential diagnosis of, 606
  management of, 606
  radiographic features of, 606
Laser beam, photostimulable phosphor
      plates (PSP) and, 231
Latent bone cyst, 651
Latent image sites, 96. *See also* Image sites
Latent images, 94, 96
  charge packets and, 227, 229f
  formation of, 94
  photostimulable phosphor plates (PSP)
      and, 231
Latent period, acute radiation syndrome
      and, 37
Lateral canine, adenomaoid odontogenic
      tumor and, 433f
Lateral-canine projections, edentulous
      patients and, 165
Lateral cephalometric examinations, grid
      and, 85
Lateral cephalometric projections (lateral
      skull projections)
  anatomic landmarks in, 211f
  central x-ray beam and, 211, 212t
  horizontal fracture and, 630f, 631
  image receptor and, 211, 212t
  overview of, 211, 212t
  patient placement and, 211, 212t
  steps in interpretation of, 218-220, 219f
Lateral cephalometric radiography, dental
      implants and, 680
Lateral displacement, trauma and, 617
Lateral facial dysplasia, 641
Lateral fossa (incisive fossa), overview of,
      174-175
Lateral incisors
  calcifying odontogenic cyst and, 400f
  film placement and, 130, 138
  image field and, 128, 156
  lateral fossa and, 176f
  microdontia in, 335
  projection of central ray and, 129
  supplemental teeth and, 332f

Lateral linear scanogram
  image contrast and, 250.250f
  maxillofacial complex and, 250, 250f
Lateral mandibular occlusal projection
  film placement in, 159
  image field in, 159
  point of entry in, 159
  projection of central ray in, 159
Lateral maxillary occlusal projection
  film placement in, 156
  image field in, 156
  point of entry in, 156
  projection of central ray in, 156
Lateral-oblique cephalometric
  radiography, dental implants and, 680
Lateral periodontal abscess, lateral
  periodontal cyst v., 398
Lateral periodontal cysts
  clinical features of, 398
  definition of, 398
  differential diagnosis of, 399
  management of, 399
  mandibular premolar region of, 399f
  radicular cyst v., 385f, 386
  radiographic features of, 398-399
Lateral pole, condyle and, 539
Lateral pterygoid muscle, localized
  (traumatic) myositis ossifcans and,
  610
Lateral skull projections. See Lateral
  cephalometric projections (lateral
  skull projections)
Lateral thyrohyoid ligaments, laryngeal
  cartilage calcifications within, 606
Lateral tomographic views
  coronoid hyperplasia and, 553
  degenerative joint disease in, 561f
Lateral views of condyles, mandibular
  condyle fractures and, 626
Latitude, digital detector characteristics
  and, 232, 233f
Lead
  disposing of, 105
  grid composition and, 84, 84f
Lead collimators
  movement of film and, 193f
  panoramic machine and, 192, 192f
Lead foil
  digital imaging and, 225
  environmental damage and, 104, 105
  purposes for, 73
Lead zirconate titanate (PZT), sonography
  and, 263
Leaded apron, 62f
  equipment choice of, 56
  pregnancy and, 275
Leaded thyroid collars, ADA and, 61
Lefort fractures, maxilla and, 205
Left mandibular condyle, thyroid
  metastatic lesion in, 468f
Left maxilla, fibrous dysplasia and, 488f
Left maxillary cuspid, dentigerous cyst of,
  390f
Leon de Fort's fracture pattern
  classifications, midface fractures and,
  629
Leong's premolar, 343
Lesions
  abnormalities and, 285
  coronal epicenter of, 286f
  cortical bone and, 203
  defined borders in, 288, 288f

Lesions (Continued)
  displacement of teeth and, 291
  effects on surrounding structures, 291
  general locations of, 285
  image layer and, 196
  inferior alveolar canal and, 287f
  internal appearance of, 289-291
  moderate periodontitis and, 320, 321f
  panoramic imaging and, 191
  periphery of, 285, 288
  shape of, 289
  size of, 285
  specific locations for, 285
  trabecular spaces and, 171
LET. See Linear energy transfer (LET)
Letterer-Siwe disease
  Langerhans' cell histiocytosis and, 510
  Langerhans' X and, 509
Leukemia
  chronic osteomyelitis v., 380
  clinical features of, 481
  definition for, 481
  differential diagnosis for, 482
  management of, 482
  mean active bone marrow dose and,
    52-53
  non-Hodgkin's lymphoma v., 478
  osteomyelitis v., 377
  periapical inflammatory lesions v., 370,
    372f
  radiation exposure and, 41
  radiographic features of, 481
  synonyms for, 481
Leukocytosis, acute osteomyelitis and, 374
Leukopenia, radiation injury and, 38
Light (phosphorescence)
  film opacity and, 77
  photostimulable phosphor plates, 230f
Light emission, intensifying screens and,
  76
Light fluorescence (QLF), carious lesions
  and, 305, 311
Light levels, film images and, 235
Line pair (lp), 82
  digital detector characteristics and, 232,
    233f
Linear energy transfer (LET)
  overview of, 32
  particulate radiation and, 5
Linear tomography
  executing, 246
  image quality of, 247
Lingual anterior variant (LA), lingual
  salivary gland depression and, 651,
  652
Lingual caries, buccal carious lesions v.,
  303
Lingual carious lesions, enamel pits and,
  303
Lingual cortical bone, imaging for jaw
  pathology and, 268
Lingual cortical plates
  fractures of alveolar process and, 627
  lateral mandibular occlusal projection
    and, 159
Lingual cusp tips, buccal bifurcation cyst
  and, 392
Lingual foramen, genial tubercles and,
  182, 182f
Lingual mandibular bone depression, 651
Lingual plate loss, moderate periodontitis
  and, 318-319

Lingual posterior variant (LP), lingual
  salivary gland depression and, 651,
  652, 653f
Lingual salivary gland depression
  clinical features of, 652
  definition of, 651
  differential diagnosis of, 653, 654
  management of, 654
  mandible and, 204, 205f
  radiographic features of, 652, 653f, 654f
  synonyms for, 651
Lip
  osteoma cutis and, 609
  primary carcinomas and, 459
Lip paresthesia, neoplasms and, 463
Lipoma, dermoid cysts v., 404
Liposarcoma, dermoid cysts v., 404
Liquid crystal display (LCD), transistor
  voltage and, 234
Lithium, atomic structures of, 4f
Localized (traumatic) myositis ossifcans
  clinical features of, 610
  definition of, 610
  differential diagnosis of, 610-611
  management of, 611
  radiographic features of, 610
Loculus of sinus cavity, dental root
  fragments v., 594
Long gray scale of contrast, image and, 79,
  79f
Longitudinal radiographic studies,
  condylar hyperplasia and, 551
Longitudinal root fractures, trauma and,
  621
Longitudinal study, focal osteoporotic
  bone marrow and, 655
Lossless compression, file compression
  and, 240
Lossy compression, file compression and, 240
Low contrast, radiograph showing, 79f
Low energy photons, filtration and, 60
Luminance (brightness), digital detector
  characteristics and, 232
Lungs
  malignant ameloblastoma and, 466
  progressive systemic sclerosis and, 531
Luxation of teeth
  clinical features of, 617
  definition of, 617
  management of, 617
  radiographic features of, 617
Lymph node chaining, calcified lymph
  nodes and, 599, 600f
Lymph nodes
  cancer and, 458
  central mucoepidermoid carcinoma
    and, 465
  dystrophic calcification and, 598
  non-Hodgkin's lymphoma and, 477
  submandibular area and, 659
  submandibular gland and, 659
Lymph nodes, calcified, granulomatous
  disorders and, 598
Lymphadenitis, parotid v., 658, 659
Lymphadenopathy
  acute leukemias and, 481
  acute osteomyelitis and, 374
  diffuse sclerosing osteomyelitis and, 378
  neoplasms and, 463
  non-Hodgkin's lymphoma and, 477
  periapical inflammatory lesion and, 368
  squamous cell carcinoma and, 459

Lymphangiectatic cyst, 581
Lymphoepithelial cysts, 671
Lymphoma
  calcified lymph nodes v., 599
  chronic osteomyelitis v., 380
  dystrophic calcification in tonsils v., 599
  Langerhans' cell histiocytosis and, 509
  leukemia v., 482
  metastatic lesions of parotid gland and, 675
  osteomyelitis v., 377
  panoramic image of, 478f
  widening of periodontal ligament space and, 480f
Lymphosarcoma, 477

M

mA, children and, 161
mA control, 114
Mach band, 301
Macrodont central incisor, dimension of, 334f
Macrodont molar, mesiodistal dimension of, 334f
Macrodontia
  definition of, 334, 334f
  differential diagnosis for, 335
  fusion of teeth and, 337
  management of, 335
  radiographic features of, 335
Magnesium, nidus and, 607
Magnetic dipoles, MRI and, 256
Magnetic field, MRI and, 256, 257f
Magnetic gradient, voxels and, 260
Magnetic resonance (MR) angiography, arteriovenous fistula and, 449
Magnetic resonance imaging (MRI), 550
  acute osteomyelitis and, 374
  advanced imaging procedures and, 271
  advantages of, 260
  ameloblastoma and, 420, 422, 424f
  anterior disk displacement and, 557f
  benign tumors and, 410
  benign tumors presenting on, 672
  computed tomography scanners v., 252
  dermoid cysts and, 404
  desmoplastic fibromas of bone in, 454, 455f
  disadvantages of, 260
  ductal morphology and, 664
  hemangiomas and, 673
  internal derangement and, 555
  maxillary sinus disease and, 578
  medial disk displacement and, 556
  nasopalatine duct cyst and, 403
  non-Hodgkin's lymphoma and, 478
  normal TMJ and, 549f
  odontogenic myxoma and, 434
  overview of, 255-260, 549-550, 664
  periapical film of, 437f
  radiographic examination and, 274
  salivary gland applications with, 664
  salivary gland disease and, 660
  septic arthritis and, 565
  sialectasia and, 669
  sialodochitis and, 668, 669
  soft tissue imaging and, 548-550
  soft tissue infections v. neoplasia, 380
  soft tissue injury, 615
  squamous cell carcinoma v., 588
  TMJ and, 202, 269
  Warthin tumor and, 673

Magnetic resonance imaging (MRI) studies
  adhesions and, 557
  joint effusion and, 567
  parotid gland and, 664f
Magnification, image size and, 87, 88f
Magnifying glass
  carious lesions and, 300f
  dental caries and, 298, 300f
Maintenance, guide for establishing, 67b
Malignancy
  ameloblastoma and, 419
  computed tomography (CT) and, 269
  osseous destruction and, 459, 461f
  periapical inflammatory lesions v., 370, 372f
  periodontal disease v., 327
  radiation therapy and, 275
Malignant ameloblastoma
  clinical features of, 466
  definition of, 466
  differential diagnosis of, 466
  radiographic features of, 466
Malignant change, neurofibroma and, 441
Malignant conversion, neurofibromatosis and, 443
Malignant cyst, squamous cell carcinoma originating in cyst v., 464
Malignant disorders, Langerhans' cell histiocytosis and, 509
Malignant lesions
  invasive border in, 289
  neurilemoma v., 440
  simple bone cyst v., 407
Malignant lymphoma, 477
Malignant mixed tumors
  clinical features of, 674
  definition of, 674
  radiographic features of, 674
  types of, 674
Malignant neoplasia, osteomyelitis v., 375
Malignant neoplasms
  desmoplastic fibromas of bone v., 454
  irregular widening of alveolar canal and, 293
  malignant ameloblastoma v., 466
  maxillary sinuses and, 577
  osteoradionecrosis v., 382
  poorly defined border of, 288f
  progressive systemic sclerosis v., 532
Malignant pleomorphic adenoma, 674
Malignant stroma, osteosarcoma and, 469
Malignant tumors
  benign neoplasm v., 412
  chronic osteomyelitis v., 380
  clinical features of, 458, 571
  desmoplastic fibromas of bone in, 454
  differential diagnosis of, 571-572
  features suggesting, 459
  hemangioma and, 446
  Langerhans' cell histiocytosis v., 513
  metastasis of, 675
  occult disease and, 268
  overview of, 458, 571, 673
  radiographic features of, 459, 571, 673
  treatment of, 572, 673
Malocclusion
  fractures of alveolar process and, 627
  gemination and, 338
  hemifacial microsomia and, 643
  mandibular condyle fractures and, 627
  microdontia and, 335f

Mammary glands, tc-pertechnetate and, 664
Management system, digital imaging and, 239
Mandible
  acute osteomyelitis and, 374, 375
  ameloblastic fibromas and, 428
  ameloblastoma and, 419
  aneurysmal bone cyst and, 504, 505f
  anterior mandibular occlusal projection and, 157
  arteriovenous (A-V) fistula and, 449
  asymmetry of size of, 203
  benign cementoblastoma in, 436
  calcifying epithelial odontogenic tumors and, 423
  cementoossifying fibroma and, 499
  central giant cell granuloma and, 502
  central mucoepidermoid carcinoma and, 465
  central odontogenic fibroma and, 438
  computed tomography (CT) scanners and, 252
  condylar hypoplasia and, 552
  condyle and, 541
  cross-sectional mandibular occlusal projection, 158
  cyst border in, 288f
  cysts and, 384
  dens evaginates and, 343
  desmoplastic fibromas of bone in, 454
  Ewing's sarcoma and, 473
  facial fractures in, 624
  fibrosarcoma and, 475
  fibrous dysplasia of, 490f
  film placement and, 142
  florid osseous dysplasia (FOD) and, 496, 497f
  Gardner's syndrome and, 445
  genial tubercles and, 182
  hemangioma and, 446
  hemifacial hyperplasia and, 650, 651
  hemifacial microsomia and, 643
  horizontal fracture and, 630f
  hyperpituitarism and, 521, 522f
  hypopituitarism and, 522
  image field and, 144, 146
  Langerhans' cell histiocytosis and, 511, 511f, 512
  lateral periodontal cyst, 398
  lingual salivary gland depression and, 651
  major areas of, 201-202
  malignant ameloblastoma and, 466
  mandibular oblique lateral projections, 215
  metastatic tumors and, 467, 468f
  multiple myeloma and, 475, 476f
  neurilemoma and, 439
  neurofibromatosis and, 442
  NewTom Plus and, 255, 256f
  non-Hodgkin's lymphoma and, 478
  odontogenic keratocyst and, 394, 395
  odontogenic myxoma and, 434
  osteoid osteoma and, 452
  osteomas and, 443
  osteoporosis and, 525f
  osteoradionecrosis and, 380, 382
  osteosarcoma and, 469, 470f
  overview of, 181-187
  periodontal disease and, 321-322
  renal osteodystrophy and, 527

Mandible *(Continued)*
    right angle technique and, 91
    simple bone cyst and, 405
    squamous cell carcinoma originating in
        cyst and, 464
    submentovertex projection and, 221
    supernumerary teeth and, 330
    Treacher Collins syndrome and, 643,
        645f
    wide-angle tomography and, 247, 248f
Mandible bone, mid-facial area and, 204
Mandible disorders, TMJ and, 269
Mandibular alveolar nerve canal, radicular
    cyst and, 386
Mandibular alveolar process,
    developmental abnormalities in,
    550
Mandibular anterior occlusal projection,
    child and, 161
Mandibular anterior periapical projection,
    mixed dentition and, 162
Mandibular arches, horizontal bitewing
    films and, 148
Mandibular body
    developmental abnormalities in, 550
    oblique lateral projection of, 218f
Mandibular body fractures
    clinical features of, 625
    definition of, 624-625
    differential diagnosis of of, 625
    favorable v. nonfavorable, 625
    management of, 625
    radiographic features of, 625
Mandibular body projection, 215
Mandibular bony structures, panoramic
    image and, 203f
Mandibular canals
    arteriovenous (A-V) fistula and, 449
    central mucoepidermoid carcinoma
        and, 465, 465f
    mandible v., 203
    neurofibroma and, 441
    neurofibromatosis and, 442-443
    neuromas and, 440
    overview of, 184, 184f
    stereoscopy technique and, 249
Mandibular canine
    horizontal bitewing films and, 149
    image field and, 140
    premolar bitewing projection and, 150
Mandibular canine projection, paralleling
    technique and, 140
Mandibular central incisors, image field
    and, 138
Mandibular centrolateral projection,
    paralleling technique and, 138
Mandibular condyle
    cartilaginous tumors, 411
    position of, 202
    radiologic examination of, 615-616
    trauma to, 615-616
Mandibular condyle fractures
    clinical features of, 625
    definition of, 625
    management of, 627
    radiographic features of, 626-627, 626f,
        627f
Mandibular deciduous molars, dentigerous
    cyst and, 392
Mandibular distal oblique molar
    projection, paralleling technique and,
    144

Mandibular first bicuspid, vertical root
    fractures of, 623f
Mandibular first molar
    buccal bifurcation cyst and, 392
    compound odontomas and, 425
    nutrient canals and, 185f
    periapical inflammatory lesion and, 369f
Mandibular first molar roots, double
    lamina dura and, 169, 169f
Mandibular first premolar, dilaceration of
    root in, 342
Mandibular foramen, neurilemoma and,
    439, 439f
Mandibular foramina, neurofibromatosis
    and, 443
Mandibular fossa
    condylar hyperplasia and, 550
    condylar hypoplasia and, 552
    condyle and, 541
    juvenile chronic arthritis and, 364
Mandibular fractures
    overview of, 624
    panoramic film of, 615
    trauma and, 269
Mandibular growth, juvenile chronic
    arthritis v., 364
Mandibular hemangiomas, hemangioma
    v., 445
Mandibular hypoplasia
    juvenile arthrosis v., 553
    neonatal fractures and, 568
Mandibular incisor radiographs, genial
    tubercles and, 182, 182f
Mandibular incisors
    attrition and, 354
    cross-sectional mandibular occlusal
        projection, 158
    gemination and, 338, 338f
    talon cusp and, 351
Mandibular infected buccal cyst, 392
Mandibular lateral incisors, image field
    and, 138
Mandibular lesions, osteosarcoma and, 469
Mandibular molar-premolar region, focal
    osteoporotic bone marrow and, 655
Mandibular molar projection, paralleling
    technique and, 144
Mandibular molars
    enamel pearl and, 350
    molar bitewing projection and, 152
    vertical root fractures and, 622
Mandibular nerve, neurofibroma and, 440
Mandibular neurovascular canal
    malignant ameloblastoma and, 466
    multiple myeloma and, 475
Mandibular oblique lateral projections
    central x-ray beam, 215
    image receptor and, 215
    patient placement and, 215
    resultant image for, 215
Mandibular occlusal radiographs, genial
    tubercles and, 182, 182f
Mandibular opening, condylar movement
    in, 542
Mandibular periapical radiographs, torus
    mandibularis and, 413
Mandibular permanent molars, image
    field and, 144
Mandibular premolar projection,
    paralleling technique and, 142
Mandibular premolar region, calcifying
    odontogenic cyst in, 399f

Mandibular premolars
    dens evaginatus and, 343, 344f
    image field and, 150
    Turner's hypoplasia and, 352
Mandibular projections
    hemostat and, 164
    patient examination and, 124
Mandibular radiolucency, bilateral, normal
    anatomy and, 283-284
Mandibular ramal area, shadows of
    structures and, 202
Mandibular ramus
    developmental abnormalities in, 550
    external oblique ridge v., 186, 186f
    film placement and, 155
    oblique lateral projection of, 219f
    submentovertex (SMV) projection and,
        545
Mandibular ramus projection
    image receptor and, 215
    patient placement and, 215
Mandibular retromolar area, focal
    osteoporotic bone marrow and, 655
Mandibular second molars
    compound odontomas and, 425
    horizontal bitewing films and, 148
Mandibular teeth
    bitewing exam and, 148
    central ray projection and, 153
    external resorption and, 358
Mandibular third molars
    dilaceration of root in, 341f
    pericoronitis and, 373, 373f
Mandibulofacial dysostosis, 643
    Treacher Collins syndrome as, 643
Mandibutal teeth, mandibular anterior
    occlusal projection and, 161
Manual film processing, procedures for,
    101-102
Manual processing tanks, 99
    film and, 101f
Manufacturers, noncompliant, Digital
    Imaging and Communications in
    Medicine (DICOM) standard and, 241
Marrow spaces, 654
    permeative borders and, 289, 290f
Marsupialization
    dentigerous cyst and, 392
    nasopalatine duct cyst and, 401
    odontogenic keratocyst and, 396
    residual cyst v., 388
Mass, fibrosarcoma and, 474
Masseter, localized (traumatic) myositis
    ossifcans and, 610
Masticatory stress, torus mandibularis and,
    413
Mastoid air cell infection, diffuse
    sclerosing osteomyelitis and, 378
Mastoid air cells, 540, 540f
    lateral cephalometric projection and,
        218-220, 219f
    panoramic image and, 207
    reverse-Towne projection, 222, 223f
    submentovertex projection and, 220,
        220f
    Treacher Collins syndrome and, 643
Matrix formation, Turner's hypoplasia
    and, 352
Matter
    composition of, 3-4
    interactions of x-rays with, 16-20
    penetration of, 14

Mature cemental dysplasia,
    hypercementosis v., 363
Maxilla
    adenomaoid odontogenic tumor and,
        431, 433f
    ameloblastoma and, 419
    central odontogenic fibroma and, 438
    cysts and, 384
    desmoplastic fibromas of bone in, 454
    fibrous dysplasia and, 485
    film placement in, 154
    Gardner's syndrome and, 445
    hemangioma and, 446
    hemifacial hyperplasia and, 649, 650
    hypopituitarism and, 522
    image field, 155, 156
    lateral fossa and, 176f
    metastatic tumors and, 459
    mid-facial area and, 204
    midface fractures and, 629
    NewTom Plus and, 255, 256f
    odontogenic myxoma and, 434
    osteoradionecrosis v., 382
    overview of, 172-181
    Paget's disease in, 507, 508f
    panoramic image and, 206f
    radicular cyst and, 385
    renal osteodystrophy and, 527
    simple bone cyst and, 405
    sites for examination of, 204-205
    Treacher Collins syndrome and, 643
    wide-angle tomography and, 247, 248f
Maxillary alveolar process
    exostoses and, 414
    segmental odontomaxillary dysplasia
        and, 651
    squamous cell carcinoma and, 587
Maxillary anterior occlusal projection,
    children and, 161
Maxillary anterior periapical projection,
    mixed dentition and, 162
Maxillary antra, 576
Maxillary antrum
    apical inflammatory lesions and, 371f
    dentigerous cyst and, 390
    intraoral periapical radiograph of, 577
    jaw abnormalities and, 285
    juvenile ossifying fibroma v., 501
    odontogenic cysts and, 589, 590f
    periapical cemental dysplasia and, 495
    residual cyst and, 388
    zygomatic process and, 180
Maxillary arches, horizontal bitewing films
    and, 148
Maxillary bones, 176
Maxillary canine
    dentigerous cyst of, 388, 389f
    radiograph of, 173, 173f
Maxillary canine projection, paralleling
    technique and, 130
Maxillary central incisor projection,
    paralleling technique and, 126
Maxillary central incisors
    anterior nasal spine relative to, 172
    avulsion and, 618
    congenital syphilis and, 353, 354f
    dens in dente and, 342
    dental root fractures and, 620
    film placement and, 126
Maxillary dentition, 205
Maxillary distal oblique molar projection,
    paralleling technique and, 136

Maxillary fracture, radiologic examination
    of, 616
Maxillary incisors
    hypodontia and, 333
    luxation and, 617
    projection of central ray and, 127
    talon cusp and, 351, 352f
Maxillary lateral incisors
    congenital syphilis and, 353
    dilaceration of root in, 341f
    film placement and, 128
    microdontia and, 335f
Maxillary lateral projection, paralleling
    technique and, 128
Maxillary lesions
    central giant cell granuloma and, 502
    multiple myeloma and, 475
Maxillary micrognathia, cleidocranial
    dysplasia and, 648
Maxillary molar projection, paralleling
    technique and, 134
Maxillary molars
    concrescence and, 338
    enamel pearl and, 350
    furcation defects and, 321, 322
    molar bitewing projection and, 152
    torus palatinus and, 412, 413f
Maxillary occlusal projections,
    nasolacrimal canals and, 176, 177f
Maxillary permanent molars, image field
    and, 134
Maxillary posterior periapical radiographs,
    retention pseudocysts and, 582, 583f
Maxillary premolar segment, horizontal
    bitewing films and, 148
Maxillary premolars
    radicular dilaceration and, 340
    toothbrush injury and, 355
Maxillary projections
    patient examination and, 124
    technique for, 164
Maxillary sinus disease, signs and
    symptoms of, 577
Maxillary sinuses, 205, 206, 282
    anatomical overview of, 177-179
    antroliths and, 584, 607
    cementoossifying fibroma and, 500, 501f
    cherubism and, 506
    craniofacial fibrous dysplasia and, 593,
        593f
    developmental stages of, 576
    diseases of, 577
    fibrosarcoma and, 475
    floor of nasal fossa v., 174f, 177, 178,
        178f
    fractures of alveolar process and, 629
    horizontal fracture and, 631
    imaging for jaw pathology and, 269
    inferior border of, 177f
    lamina dura and, 169
    mucocele in, 585, 585f
    non-Hodgkin's lymphoma and, 477
    occlusal radiography and, 160
    odontogenic cysts and, 589
    odontogenic myxoma and, 434
    osteoblastomas in, 450
    paranasal sinuses and, 576
    periapical radiographs of, 177
    radiolucent lines in, 178f
    retention pseudocysts and, 582, 583
    segmental odontomaxillary dysplasia
        and, 651

Maxillary sinuses (Continued)
    septa and, 179, 179f
    squamous cell carcinoma and, 587
    Treacher Collins syndrome and, 643,
        645f
    vertical osseous defects and, 320
    Waters projection and, 213, 221
Maxillary teeth, 173
    aggressive periodontitis and, 324
    bitewing exam and, 148
    maxillary anterior occlusal projection
        and, 161
    periapical cemental dysplasia and, 492,
        493f
    sinus pain and, 178
Maxillary third molars
    dentigerous cyst of, 388, 389f, 391f
    microdontia and, 335f
Maxillary tuberosity
    image field and, 136
    pterygoid plates and, 181f
Maxillofacial complex
    computed tomography (CT) scanners
        and, 252, 254f
    lateral linear scanning of, 250, 250f
Maxillofacial complex, malignant lesions,
    3D CT and, 254
Maxillofacial radiologist, Langerhans' cell
    histiocytosis and, 513
Maxillozygomatic suture, maxillary antrum
    and, 180
Maximal intercuspation, degenerative joint
    disease and, 560
McCune-Albright syndrome
    fibrous dysplasia and, 485
    hyperfunction of endocrine glands and,
        485
Mean active bone marrow dose, overview
    of, 52-53
Medial mandibular cysts, former cysts and,
    405
Medial palatal cysts, former cysts and,
    405
Median anterior maxillary cyst, 400
Median nasopalatine cyst, 400
Median pole, condyle and, 539
Medical geneticist, hemifacial hyperplasia
    and, 651
Medication, parotid area v., 658
Mediolateral plane, bifid condyle and, 554,
    555f
Mediterranean anemia, 533
Melanoma, metastatic lesions of parotid
    gland and, 675
Melorheostosis, osteopetrosis v., 531
Melting point, target with, 8
Memory, digital imaging and, 225
Mental foramen
    lateral periodontal cyst v., 399
    neurilemoma and, 439, 439f
    neuromas and, 440
    overview of, 183, 183f
    periapical disease and, 184, 184f
Mental foramina
    mandible v., 203
    neurofibromatosis and, 443
Mental fossa, overview of, 183, 183f
Mental retardation, radiation in atomic
    bombs and, 41
Mental ridge (protuberance), periapical
    radiographs and, 182, 183f
Mental tubercle, mental ridge and, 183

Mentally disabled patients. *See* Patients, mentally disabled
Mercator projection, panoramic images and, 201
Mesenchymal neoplasms, osteoma and, 586
Mesenchymal tumors (odontogenic ectomesenchyme), overview of, 433-439
Mesial contact area, image field and, 130, 140
Mesial interproximal area, image field and, 128
Mesiodens, 330
  dental anomalies and, 2667
  impaction of permanent teeth and, 332f
  supernumerary teeth and, 330, 331f
Message, sialadenosis and, 670
Metabolic bone diseases
  fibrous dysplasia and, 489
  Paget's disease v., 508
Metabolic disorders, leukemia v., 482
Metabolic rate, hyperthyroidism and, 522
Metal markers, extraoral radiographic examinations and, 210
Metalic objects, subject density and, 78
Metalic replacement, environmental damage and, 105
Metastasis
  ameloblastic carcinoma v., 466
  malignant mixed tumors and, 674
  minor salivary glands and, 675
  mucoepidermoid carcinoma and, 673
  primary introsseous carcinoma v., 463
Metastatic breast carcinoma, 468f
Metastatic calcification, overview of, 597
Metastatic carcinoma(s), 468f
  metastatic tumors and, 466-467
  multiple myeloma v., 477
  non-Hodgkin's lymphoma v., 478
  osteosarcoma v., 469
Metastatic disease, squamous cell carcinoma originating in cyst v., 464
Metastatic lesions
  CT image of, 572f
  malignant ameloblastoma v., 466
  osteoradionecrosis and, 380
  periapical inflammatory lesions v., 370, 372f
  primary osseous carcinoma v., 464
Metastatic malignancy, 458
Metastatic malignant neoplasia, Langerhans' cell histiocytosis v., 513
Metastatic neuroblastoma, Burkitt's lymphoma v., 480
Microdontia
  altered morphology and, 335
  clinical features of, 335
  definition of, 335
  differential diagnosis of, 335
  management of, 335
  maxillary third molars and, 335f
  radiographic features of, 335
Micrognathia, juvenile chronic arthritis v., 364
Microradiography, inactive carious lesion and, 298
Middle cranial fossa
  osteoblastomas in, 450
  reverse-Towne projection, 222, 223f

Midface fractures
  de Fort's pattern classification of, 629
  needed projections for, 629
  overview of, 629-630
Midfacial hypoplasia, crouzon syndrome and, 641f
Midfacial region
  examining, 205
  lateral cephalometric projection and, 219f, 220
  overview of, 204-207, 204f, 206f
Midsagittal plane
  lateral cephalometric projections and, 211, 212
  posteroanterior cephalometric projection, 213
  submentovertex (base) projection and, 213
Mikulicz disease, 668
Mild periodontitis, etiology of, 317-318
Milliamperage (mA), exposure and, 78
Milliampere-seconds
  diagnostic density and, 63, 63t
  image density and, 63
  overview of, 62, 63t
Mineral loss
  factors in, 297
  light fluorescence (QLF), 305, 311
Mineral salts, rhinoliths and, 607
Minimum half-value layer, 61t
Missing teeth, synonyms for, 332
Missing teeth, developmentally
  clinical features, 332
  differential diagnosis in, 332
  management of, 333
  maxillary premolars and, 333, 333f
  pathologic mechanisms for, 332
  radiologic features of, 332
Mitosis, radiation induced break and, 27
Mitotic delay
  overview of, 29
  radiation-induced, 29f
Mixed dentition
  overview of, 162
  panoramic imaging and, 191
Mixed odontogenic tumor, 428
Mixed radiolucent, lesion classification as, 289
Mixed tumors, 424-439
  adenomaoid odontogenic tumor and, 431
ML-2 filters, 100
  panoramic film and, 200
Moderate periodontitis
  buccal plate loss and, 318-319, 318f
  horizontal bone loss and, 319, 319f
  internal bone changes, 320, 321f
  lingual plate loss and, 318-319
  vertical osseous defects and, 319-320
Molar areas
  film placement and, 134
  image field and, 144
Molar bitewing projection
  film placement in, 152
  image field in, 152
Molar projection, edentulous patients and, 165
Molar region, primary osseous carcinoma in, 463, 463f
Molar roots
  enamel pearl, 350
  mylohyoid ridge and, 185

Molars
  cementoossifying fibroma and, 499
  film placement and, 136, 146
  molar bitewing projection and, 152
  odontogenic myxoma and, 434
  projection of central ray and, 135, 145
  pulp stones and, 361
  root position of, 177
  stereoscopy technique and, 249
  supplemental teeth and, 332f
  taurodontism and, 339
  torus mandibularis and, 413
Monckeberg's medial calcinosis. *See* Arteriosclerosis
Monostotic fibrous dysplasia
  hemifacial hyperplasia v., 650
  jaws and, 485
  segmental odontomaxillary dysplasia v., 651
Morphologic imaging techniques, image receptor and, 260
Motion blurring, overview of, 83
Mouth
  bisection examination technique and, 62
  film holding instruments and, 124-125
  film placement and, 132, 140, 142
  primary carcinomas and, 459
  reverse-Towne projection (open mouth), 213
Mouth, floor of
  cross-sectional mandibular occlusal projection and, 158
  lateral mandibular occlusal projection and, 159
  occlusal radiography and, 160
Mucoceles
  clinical features of, 585
  CT and, 664
  definition of, 585
  differential diagnosis of, 585
  management of, 585
  radiographic features of, 585
  synonyms for, 584
Mucoepidermoid carcinoma, 465
  clinical features of, 673-674
  malignant mixed tumors v., 674
  radiographic features of, 674, 674f
Mucoepidermoid tumor, central mucoepidermoid carcinoma v., 465
Mucopyocele, mucocele as, 584, 585
Mucormycosis, 588
Mucosal antral cyst, 581
Mucosal covering, osteoradionecrosis and, 380
Mucositis, 579f
  clinical features of, 578
  definition of, 578
  dental inflammatory lesions and, 588
  radiographic features of, 578
Mucous-extravasation cyst, nasopalatine duct cysts v., 403
Mucous retention cyst, 581
Mucueepidermoid carcinoma, dentigerous cyst and, 392
Mucus-extravasation pseudocysts, ductal rupture and, 671
Mucus-retaining cysts, 671
Mucus retention pseudocysts, maxillary and, 583f
Mulberry molars, congenital syphilis and, 353

Multicentric lesions, Ewing's sarcoma and, 473
Multicentric parotid cysts, HIV and, 671
Multidirectional tomographic motion, 247, 247f
Multifocal, abnormalities as, 285
Multilocular, 289, 290f
    septa as, 291
Multiocular ameloblastoma, 421f
Multiocular appearance, central giant cell granuloma and, 502
Multiocular expansion mass, central mucoepidermoid carcinoma and, 465, 465f
Multiocular lesions
    hemangioma and, 448
    malignant ameloblastoma and, 466
Multiocular pattern
    central odontogenic fibroma with, 438
    cherubism and, 506
Multiplanar CT imaging
    diagnosis and, 252
    MRI and, 260
Multiplanar reformatted imaging, computed tomography (CT) scanners and, 252
Multiple bone lesions, eosinophilic granuloma and, 509
Multiple dentigerous cysts, basal cell nevus syndrome v., 398
Multiple miliary osteoma cutis, 609
Multiple myeloma, 475
    basal cell nevus syndrome v., 398
    clinical features of, 475
    differential diagnosis of, 477
    film of, 287f
    management of, 477
    metastatic tumors v., 467, 468f
    non-Hodgkin's lymphoma v., 478
    primary osseous carcinoma v., 464
    punched hole border and, 287f, 288
    punched out lesions in, 477f
    radiographic features of, 475-477
    squamous cell carcinoma originating in cyst v., 464
    synonyms for, 475
Multiple myeloma lesions, periphery and shape of, 475
Multiple odontogenic keratocysts, cherubism v., 506
Multiple osteomas, Gardner's disease v., 445
Multiple parotid cysts, autoimmune sialadenitis v., 669
Multipotential connective tissue cells, radiosensitivity and, 30
Mumps, submandibular gland and, 659
Mural ameloblastoma, ameloblastoma v., 419, 419f
Muscle
    myositis ossificans and, 610
    progressive myositis ossificans and, 611
    subject density and, 78
Muscle fiber, localized (traumatic) myositis ossificans and, 610
Muscle injury, localized (traumatic) myositis ossificans and, 610
Muscle spasm
    degenerative joint disease and, 559
    false ankylosis and, 569
Mycolith
    osteoma v., 586
    rhinoliths v., 608

Mycosis, dystrophic calcification in tonsils v., 599
Myelodysplasia, pseudotumor and, 588
Myelogenous leukemia, periodontal disease and, 327
Mylohyoid muscle, anatomic position of, 185
Mylohyoid ridges
    mandible and, 200
    overview of, 185
Myoepithelial sialadenitis, 668
Myositis ossificans
    arteriosclerosis and, 602
    bilateral linear calcifications of sternohyoid muscle in, 612f
    definition of, 610
    false ankylosis and, 569
    lateral pterygoid muscle and, 612f
    masseter and temporalis muscles and, 612f
    osteoma cutis v., 610
Myxedema, 522
Myxofibroma, 433
Myxoid tumor, odontogenic myxoma and, 434
Myxoma, 433

N
Nagar syndrome, Treacher Collins syndrome v., 646
Narrow-angle tomography, overview of, 248, 249f
Nasal bones, 176
    mid-facial area and, 204
Nasal cavity (turbinates), 173, 176, 177, 205
    epithelial papilloma and, 586
    lateral cephalometric projection and, 219f, 220
    nasolabial cyst, 401
    nasopalatine canal and, 174
    nasopalatine duct cyst and, 401
    reverse-Towne projection, 222, 223f
    Waters projection and, 221
Nasal conchae, panoramic film and, 200, 200f
Nasal floor, fibrosarcoma and, 475
Nasal fossa, 172
    floor of, 174f
    image field of, 154
    nasopalatine canal and, 175f
    overview of, 173, 173f
Nasal furuncle, nasopalatine duct cysts v., 403
Nasal obstruction
    epithelial papilloma and, 586
    odontogenic tumors and, 590
    osteosarcoma and, 469
Nasal septum, 172, 173f
    image field of, 155
    radiograph of, 173
Nasoalveolar cyst, 401
Nasolabial cyst
    axial CT image and, 404f
    clinical features of, 401-402
    nasopalatine duct cyst and, 400
    occlusal view of, 404f
    radiographic features of, 402
Nasolabial fold, anatomical overview of, 180-181, 181f
Nasolacrimal canals
    canine and, 176
    image field of, 155
    overview of, 176

Nasopalatine canal cyst, 400
    external root resorption and, 403f
    nasopalatine duct cyst and, 400
    occlusal view and lateral aspect of, 403f
Nasopalatine canals, 174
    anatomy of, 174
    lateral walls of, 175f
    nasopalatine duct cyst and, 400
Nasopalatine duct cysts
    clinical features of, 401
    dermoid cysts and, 400
    differential diagnosis and, 401, 403-404
    management of, 401
    nasolabial cysts and, 400
    nonodontogenic cysts and, 400
    periodontal membrane space and, 402f
    radiographic features of, 401
    synonyms for, 400
Nasopalatine nerves, 174
Nasopalatine vessels, 174
Nasopharynx
    mandibular ramal area and, 202
    multiple myeloma and, 475
    squamous cell carcinoma and, 461
National Council on Radiation Protection and Measurements (NCRP), dose limits and, 52, 65
National Electrical Manufacturerers Association (NEMA), digital imaging and, 241
Natural exposure, x-ray examinations and, 54t
Natural radiation
    distribution of, 49f
    sources of, 47-48
Neck
    lateral cephalometric projection and, 219f, 220
    submentovertex (base) projection and, 213
Neck dissection, central mucoepidermoid carcinoma and, 465
Neck extension, anteroposterior position radiograph and, 198
Neck lesions, Langerhans' cell histiocytosis and, 509
Neck structures, panoramic image and, 204f
Neck trauma, ossification of stylohyoid ligament, 609
Neonatal fractures. See Fractures, neonatal
Neoplasia, CT and, 664
Neoplasm, benign bone, cementoossifying fibroma v., 498
Neoplasm, malignant, polyps and, 584
Neoplasms
    ameloblastoma and, 419
    benign cementoblastoma and, 435
    benign paranasal sinus, 586
    calcifying odontogenic cyst v., 399
    central odontogenic fibroma and, 438
    clinical features of, 463
    computed tomography (CT), 548
    desmoplastic fibroma of bone and, 454
    fibrous dysplasia and, 489
    Gardner's syndrome, 444-445
    hemangioma v., 445
    lingual salivary gland depression and, 654
    malignant paranasal sinus, 586
    pericoronitis v., 373
    retention pseudocysts v., 582
    submandibular area and, 659

Neoplasms, benign
  effects on surrounding structures of, 411-412
  features of, 410-412
  internal structure of, 411
  location of, 411
  malignant tumors v., 458
  osteomas and, 443
  periphery and shape of, 411
Neoplasms, odontogenic, osteoma v., 586
Neoplasms, teeth, osteoma v., 586
Neoplastic diseases
  ankylosis v., 569
  imaging for jaw pathology in, 268
Nephrolithiasis, sialolithiasis and, 603
Nerve fibers
  neurofibroma and, 440
  neuroma, 440
Nervous system, neurofibromatosis and, 441
Nervous system cancer, radiation exposure and, 41
Net spins, MRI and, 256, 256f
Neural lesions, mandibular canal and, 411
Neural tissue, jaw abnormalities and, 285
Neural tumors, neurilemoma v., 440
Neurilemoma (Schwannoma)
  differential diagnosis of, 440
  expanding, 439, 439f
  overview of, 439
  treatment of, 440
Neurinoma, 440
Neuroblastoma
  leukemia v., 482
  metastatic tumors and, 466
Neurofibroma
  clinical features of, 440-441
  differential diagnosis of, 441
  inferior dental nerve and, 441, 441f
  lateral periodontal cyst v., 399
  neurofibromatosis and, 441
  overview of, 440
  radiographic features of, 441
  treatment of, 441
Neurofibromatosis
  classifications of, 441
  clinical features of, 441
  overview of, 441
  radiographic features of, 442
  treatment of, 443
Neurogenic sialadenoses, 670
Neurologic disorders, sialadenosis and, 670
Neuromas
  clinical features of, 440
  overview of, 440
  radiographic features of, 440
  synonyms for, 440
  treatment of, 440
Neurosurgeon, pyramidal fracture and, 632
Neurovascular bundle, nutrient canals and, 184-185
Neurovascular canal, fibrosarcoma and, 475
Neutrons, atom structure and, 3, 4
Neutropenia
  cancer and, 458
  periodontal disease and, 327
Neutrophils
  inflammatory reaction and, 368
  periodontitis and, 314

Nevada test site, artificial radionuclides, 51
Nevoid basal cell carcinoma syndrome, 397
  multiple OKCs and, 398f
NewTom Plus, CBCT and, 255
Newton (force), SI system and, 21
NF-1, neurofibromatosis and, 441
NF-2, neurofibromatosis and, 441
Nidus, 603
  antroliths and, 607
  rhinoliths and, 607
Night sweats, non-Hodgkin's lymphoma and, 477
90 degree RF pulse, 259
^{99m}Tc-pertechnetate scans, Warthin tumor and, 673
No. 2 film, 148
Nodules, cartilaginous
  ossification of, 565, 566f
  synovial chondromatosis and, 565
Nodules, osteocartilaginous, synovial chondromatosis and, 565
Noise
  digital detector characteristics and, 232, 232f
  sharpening and, 236
Non-Hodgkin's lymphoma
  autoimmune sialadenitis and, 669
  Burkitt's lymphoma v., 480
  classification of tumors in, 477
  clinical features of, 477
  overview of, 477
  radiographic features of, 477
  synonyms for, 477
Non-lipid-soluble contrast agents, ductal system and, 663
Noncarious teeth, radicular dentin dysplasia (type 1) and, 348
Noncontrast T2-weighted images, MRI and, 664
Nonepithelial salivary neoplasm, 673
Nonhemophilic polycythemia vera, periodontal disease and, 327
Nonionic iodine contrast agent, arthrography v., 548, 549f
Nonionizing radiation, MRI and, 255-260
Nonmaligant disorders, Langerhans' cell histiocytosis and, 509
Nonodontogenic cysts, nasopalatine duct cyst and, 400
Nonreduction, mandibular movement and, 555, 556f
Nonsteroidal antiinflammatory agents, chondrocalcinosis and, 566
Nonvital teeth, radicular cyst and, 385
Normal anatomy, periodontal disease and, 316-317, 317f
Nose
  anterior maxilla and, 176f
  overview of, 176
  point of entry in, 155
  rhinoliths and, 607
Nuclear imaging
  condylar hyperplasia and, 551
  Langerhans' cell histiocytosis and, 513
Nuclear medicine
  acute osteomyelitis and, 374
  advanced imaging procedures and, 271
  metastatic tumors and, 467
Nuclear power, annual E and, 51
Nuclei, MRI and, 255-260
Nucleic acids, cellular functions and, 26

Nucleus
  atom structure and, 3
  radiation effects on, 27
Numata, panoramic radiography principles and, 192
Nutrient canals
  etiology of population with, 185
  overview of, 184-185
Nutrition, rampant caries and, 302
Nutritional deficiencies, secondary osteoporosis and, 524

O
Obesity, Cushing's syndrome and, 523
Object classification, image analysis and, 239
Object to film distance, 86-87, 88f
Oblique lateral jaw view, image field and, 134
Oblique lateral projections
  extraoral radiographic examinations and, 210
  mandibular body and, 218f
  mandibular ramus and, 219f
Oblique tooth crown fractures, prognosis for, 620
Occlusal caries, radiographic appearance of, 302
Occlusal dentinoenamel junction (DEJ), horizontal bitewing films and, 148
Occlusal films
  film mount for, 108
  mandibular fracture and, 615
  squamous cell carcinoma and, 290f
  treatment and, 91
Occlusal forces
  concrescence and, 337
  crown-root fractures and, 623
Occlusal image, fibrous dysplasia and, 488f
Occlusal lesions
  false-negative, 301
  metamorphosis of, 301
  radiographic change and, 306f
Occlusal plane
  horizontal bitewing films and, 148
  point of entry and, 153
  projection of central ray and, 143
Occlusal projections
  overview of, 121
  Paget's disease and, 508, 510f
Occlusal radiographs
  benign tumors and, 410
  periapical radiographs and, 163
  purpose of, 271
  torus mandibularis in, 416f
Occlusal radiography, overview of, 160
Occlusal surface enamel, attrition and, 354, 354f
Occlusal surfaces
  attrition and, 354
  Diagnodent laser-light and, 305
  electrical conductance measurements and, 311
  hypoplasia and, 345
Occlusal trauma
  periodontal diseases and, 325
  periodontitis and, 314
Occlusal views, 74
  fibrous dysplasia and, 491f
  lymphoma in, 290f
  nasolabial cyst and, 404f
Occlusion, film placement and, 144

Occlusive arterial disease, evaluation of, 602
Occult disease, overview of, 267-268
Occupational exposure, radiation safety procedures for, 64
Occupational hazards, abrasion and, 355
Oculo-auriculovertebral dysplasia, 641
Odontoblasts, secondary dentin and, 360
Odontoclasts
  external resorption and, 358
  resorption and, 356
Odontogenesis, fusion of teeth and, 336
Odontogenesis imperfecta, 349
Odontogenic carcinoma, 463
Odontogenic cysts
  development of, 590f
  differential diagnosis of, 589-590
  maxillary antrum and, 384
  maxillary sinuses and, 577
  metastatic tumors v., 467
  mucocele v, 585
  overview of, 589
  primary introsseous carcinoma v., 463
  primary osseous carcinoma v., 463
  radiographic features of, 589
  retention pseudocysts v., 582
  squamous cell carcinoma v., 588
Odontogenic diseases
  diseases of sinus v., 576
  panoramic projection and, 543, 543f
Odontogenic epithelial tumors, types of, 419-424
Odontogenic epithelium, jaw abnormalities and, 285, 286f
Odontogenic fibroma, 438
Odontogenic hamartoma, 424
Odontogenic inflammatory lesions, osteopetrosis and, 530, 531f
Odontogenic keratocysts (OKC)
  ameloblastoma v., 420
  basal cell nevus syndrome v., 398, 398f
  definition of, 394
  dentigerous cyst v., 392
  differential diagnosis of, 395
  lateral periodontal cyst v., 399
  malignant ameloblastoma v., 466
  management of, 396-397
  mandible and, 396f
  odontogenic cysts and, 589
  panoramic film of, 290f
  radicular cyst v., 386
  radiographic features of, 394
  residual cyst v., 388
  simple bone cyst and, 407
  squamous cell carcinoma originating in cyst and, 464
  synonym for, 393
Odontogenic lesions, 287f
  alveolar processes and, 411
  lingual salivary gland depression v., 654
Odontogenic myxomas
  additional imaging for, 434
  ameloblastic fibromas v., 429
  ameloblastoma v., 420
  central giant cell granuloma v., 502
  central mucoepidermoid carcinoma v., 465
  central odontogenic fibroma v., 438, 439
  clinical features of, 434
  differential diagnosis of, 434
  lateral oblique film of, 435f
  malignant ameloblastoma v., 466

Odontogenic myxomas (Continued)
  odontogenic keratocyst v., 396
  overview of, 433-434
  periapical film of, 437f
  radiographic features of, 434
  septa and, 291
  synonyms for, 433
  treatment for, 434
Odontogenic tissue, jaw abnormalities and, 285, 286f
Odontogenic tumors
  calcifying odontogenic cyst v., 399
  central mucoepidermoid carcinoma v., 465
  classification of, 418-419
  odontomas v., 425
Odontogentic epithelium, adenomaoid odontogenic tumor and, 431
Odontogentic lesions, lingual salivary gland depression v., 654
Odontomas
  ameloblastic fibroma v., 431
  border comparision in, 288f
  calcifying odontogenic cyst and, 399
  clinical features of, 424
  craniofacial fibrous dysplasia v., 593
  differential diagnosis of, 425-426
  mixed and late cemental dysplasia v., 495
  osteoma v., 586
  overview of, 424-425
  radiographic features of, 424-425
  radiopaque lesion and, 288, 288f
  synonyms for, 424
  tooth displacement and, 292
  treatment for, 428
Ohm's law
  conductor and, 9
  units of, 9
OKC. See Odontogenic keratocysts (OKC)
Oligodontia, synonyms for, 332
One Tesla, 257
One-walled, vertical osseous defects as, 319
Onocologist, metastatic tumors and, 467
Onocytoma (oxyphilic adenoma), ^{99m}Tc-pertechnetate and, 673
Opacity
  cervical spine region and, 204
  coronoid process and, 187
Open contacts, periodontal diseases and, 325
Open-mouth reverse-towne projection. See Reverse-town projection (open mouth)
Operculitis, 371
Optical density
  film and, 80
  graph of, 78
  x-ray film and, 77
Optimal image density, 63
Oral cavity, 173
  dermoid cysts and, 404
  diabetes mellitus and, 523
  examination of, 122
  film placement and, 128
  radiation effects on, 32
Oral contraceptives, fibrous dysplasia and, 491
Oral diagnostics. See Diagnostics, oral
Oral disease, panoramic radiograph, 271

Oral hygiene
  dental caries and, 297
  periodontal diseases and, 325
  periodontitis and, 314
Oral lesions, Langerhans' cell histiocytosis and, 509
Oral malignancy, central mucoepidermoid carcinoma and, 465
Oral mucous membrane, overview of, 33
Oral radiologist, Langerhans' cell histiocytosis and, 513
Oral sialogogues, sialadenosis and, 670
Oral tissues, radiation effect on, 33-37
Oral tumors, adenomaoid odontogenic tumor and, 431
Oral ulcer, squamous cell carcinoma and, 376, 377
Orange-peel pattern, fibrous dysplasia and, 490f
Orbital nerve, pyramidal fracture and, 632
Orbital proptosis, crouzon syndrome and, 641, 641f
Orbital rims, panoramic film and, 200, 200f
Orbits
  ameloblastoma and, 419
  Waters projection and, 221
Orex Paxorama Xi system, plate reading and, 231
Organic free radicals, 26
Organogenesis, prenatal irradiation and, 39
Organs
  dental radiography and, 52
  radiation effects on, 30-32
  radiation exposure and, 41
  relative radiosensitivity of, 31b
Orofacial lesions, MRI and, 260, 261f
Orofacial region, extraoral radiographs and, 271
Orofacial structures, infection and, 162
Orofaciodigital syndrome, missing teeth and, 333
Orthgnathic surgery, submentovertex projection and, 546
Orthodontic appliances, radiopaque appearance of, 190
Orthodontic elastics, cavitation and, 301
Orthodontic patients, radiograph algorithim for, 268f
Orthodontics
  cherubism and, 507
  cleft palate and, 640
  condylar hyperplasia and, 551
  condylar hypoplasia and, 552
  Crouzon syndrome and, 641
  dental anomalies and, 267, 268f
  hemifacial microsomia and, 643
  juvenile arthrosis v., 553
  neonatal fractures and, 568, 569
  radiographic examination and, 274
  Treacher Collins syndrome and, 646
Orthognathic surgery
  hemifacial microsomia and, 643
  peripheral nerve damage and, 440
  Treacher Collins syndrome and, 646
Orthopantomograph 100, panoramic machines and, 196, 196f
Orthophos Plus, panoramic machines and, 197
Orthoralix S, panoramic machines and, 197

Oseoclasts, jaws and, 366
Osseointegrated implants, missing teeth
    and, 269
Osseous ankylosis
    rheumatoid arthritis v., 563
    septic arthritis and, 565
Osseous changes, panoramic projection
    and, 543, 543f
Osseous contours, imaging of, 542
Osseous defect, cleft lip and, 640
Osseous deformities, furcations of
    multirooted teeth and, 321
Osseous fractures, osteogenesis imperfecta
    and, 347
Osseous structures, wide latitude films
    and, 81
Osseous tissue, remodeling and, 557
Ossification of stylohyoid ligament
    clinical features of, 608
    definition of, 608
    differential diagnosis of, 608
    example of, 609f
    localized (traumatic) myositis ossifcans
        and, 610
    management of, 608
    radiographic features of, 608
Ossifying fibromas, 498
    ameloblastoma v., 420
    benign neoplasm v., 412
    craniofacial fibrous dysplasia v., 593
    osteosarcoma v., 469
    radicular cyst v., 387
Ostectomy, crown-root fractures and,
    624
Osteoarthritis, TMJ and, 269
Osteoblastic activity, reactive bone and,
    293
Osteoblastic osteosarcoma, 469
Osteoblastic response, osteomyelitis and,
    380
Osteoblastoma. See Giant osteoid
    osteoma
Osteoblastomas
    benign cementoblastoma v., 435
    benign neoplasm v., 411, 412
    panoramic film of, 453f
    TMJ tumors and, 570
Osteoblasts
    giant osteoid osteoma and, 450
    systemic diseases of bone and, 516
Osteochondroma
    condylar hyperplasia v., 550
    coronoid hyperplasia v., 554
    CT image of, 571f
    degenerative joint disease v., 562
    joint function and, 570
Osteochondromas
    osteomas v., 444
    TMJ tumors and, 570
Osteochondromatosis, 565
    chondrocalcinosis and, 566, 566f
Osteoclastic activity, Paget's disease and,
    509
Osteoclastic bone resorption, periodontitis
    and, 314
Osteoclasts
    resorption, 356
    systemic diseases of bone and, 516
Osteocytes, systemic diseases of bone and,
    516
Osteogenesis imperfecta, overview of,
    347

Osteogenic sarcomas
    bone and, 459
    cementoossifying fibroma v., 501
    fibrous dysplasia and, 489
    hemangioma v., 447f, 448
    odontogenic myxoma v., 434, 435f
    osteoblastomas v., 450
    Paget's disease v., 509
    periosteal reaction and, 293, 293f
    primary intrinsic malignant tumors and,
        571
Osteoid, hypophosphatasia and, 526
Osteoid osteoma
    clinical features of, 452
    overview of, 452
    radiographic features of, 452, 454
Osteoid trabeculae, giant osteoid osteoma
    and, 450
Osteolytic osteosarcoma
    Burkitt's lymphoma v., 480
    non-Hodgkin's lymphoma v., 478
Osteoma cutis
    clinical features of, 609
    definition of, 609
    differential diagnosis of, 610
    management of, 610
    periphery and shape of, 609
    radiographic features of, 609
Osteoma mucosae, osteoma cutis v., 610
Osteomalacia
    clinical features of, 524
    definition of, 524
    radiographic features of, 524
    rickets in adults and, 525
Osteomas
    clinical features of, 443, 586
    coronoid hyperplasia v., 554
    CT scans of, 445f
    definition of, 586
    degenerative joint disease v., 562
    differential diagnosis of, 444
    of frontal sinus, 443, 443f
    Gardner's syndrome and, 445
    overview of, 443
    panoramic radiograph of, 444f
    radiographic features of, 443-444, 586
    rhinoliths v., 608
    three classes of, 443
    TMJ tumors and, 570
    totally radiopaque, 289
Osteomyelitis, 366. See also Acute
        Osteomyelitis
    causes and definition of, 373-374
    cemental dysplasia and, 495
    differential diagnosis for, 375-377
    Ewing's sarcoma v., 474
    fibrous dysplasia and, 489
    florid osseous dysplasia and, 496, 498
    forms of, 374
    fracture and, 636, 636f
    inflammatory lesions and, 367
    management of, 377
    of mandible, 377f
    new bone and, 293, 293f
    osteosarcoma v., 469
    periapical inflammatory lesion v., 367,
        367f, 368, 371
    pericoronitis and, 373
    septic arthritis and, 565
    squamous cell carcinoma v., 461
Osteopathia striata, osteopetrosis v.,
    531

Osteopenia
    juvenile chronic arthritis and, 364
    metastatic tumors v., 467
Osteopetrosis
    clinical features of, 528-529
    definition for, 528
    differential diagnosis of, 531
    osteomyelitis and, 374
    radiographic features of, 529, 531
    synonyms for, 528
    treatment of, 531
Osteophyte formation, rheumatoid
        arthritis v., 563
Osteophytes (spurs), 562f
    condylar hyperplasia v., 551
    condyle and, 539
    degenerative joint disease and, 561,
        562f
    fracture and, 568
    osteomas v., 444
    panoramic projection and, 543, 543f
    remodeling v., 559
Osteoporosis
    clinical features of, 524
    cortical bone and, 203
    Cushing's syndrome and, 523
    definition of, 524
    measurement tools and, 239, 239f
    radiographic features of, 524
    sickle cell anemia and, 533
    treatment of, 524
Osteoradionecrosis
    definition of, 380
    head and neck malignancy and, 482
    irradiation and, 36, 36f
    management of, 382
    radiographic features of, 380, 382, 382f
    squamous cell carcinoma v., 461
Osteosarcoma
    chronic osteomyelitis v., 379
    clinical features of, 469
    definition of, 469
    differential diagnosis of, 469
    Ewing's sarcoma v., 474
    management of, 469, 470
    mandible and, 469, 471f
    osteoblastomas v., 452
    osteomyelitis v., 376
    pericoronitis v., 373
    radiographic features of, 469
    types of, 469
Osteosarcoma of jaws, dentist and, 469
Osteosclerosis
    occult disease and, 268
    osteoid osteoma v., 454
    osteopetrosis v., 531
    periodontal diseases and, 325
Osteotomy, coronoid hyperplasia and, 554
Ostiomatal complex, sinusitis and, 578
Otorhinolaryngologist, rhinoliths and,
    608
Outer cortical plates, aneurysmal bone
    cyst and, 504, 505f, 506f
Overdentures, dentinogenesis imperfecta
    and, 347
Oxalosis, multiple myeloma v., 477
Oxidation, developer and, 102
Oxygen (hypoxia)
    cell survival and, 31-32
    irradiated tissues and, 31
Oxygen enhancement ratio, cell damage
    and

P

Paatero, panoramic radiography principles and, 192
Pagetoid skull bones, Paget's disease and, 508
Paget's disease
    altered trabecular pattern and, 509f
    chronic osteomyelitis v., 379
    craniofacial fibrous dysplasia v., 593
    definition of, 507
    differential diagnosis of, 508-509
    edentulous mandible with, 510f
    florid osseous dysplasia v, 496
    hypercementosis and, 362
    management of, 509
    mandible and, 285
    multiple radiopaque masses in, 510f
    osteosarcoma and, 469
    radiographic features of, 507-508
    three radiographic stages of, 507-508
Pain
    acinic cell carcinoma and, 675
    acute osteomyelitis and, 374
    ameloblastic fibromas and, 428
    aneurysmal bone cyst and, 503
    benign cementoblastoma and, 436
    bifid condyle and, 554
    buccal bifurcation cyst and, 392
    chronic sinusitis and, 579
    dental concussion and, 616
    desmoplastic fibroma of bone and, 454
    diffuse sclerosing osteomyelitis and, 378
    eosinophilic granuloma and, 509
    epithelial papilloma and, 586
    fibrosarcoma and, 474
    giant osteoid osteoma v., 450
    hemangioma and, 445
    inflammation and, 366
    metastatic tumors and, 467
    monostotic fibrous dysplasia and, 485
    nasolabial cyst, 401-402
    neurilemoma and, 439
    neurofibroma and, 441
    neuromas and, 440
    odontogenic keratocyst and, 394
    osteoid osteoma and, 452
    osteoradionecrosis and, 380
    osteosarcoma and, 469
    periapical cemental dysplasia, 492
    periapical inflammatory lesion and, 368
    remodeling and, 559
    rheumatoid arthritis and, 563
    septic arthritis and, 565
    simple bone cyst and, 405
    squamous cell carcinoma and, 461
    squamous cell carcinoma originating in cyst and, 464
    synovial chondromatosis and, 565
    TMJ dysfunction and, 538
    vertical root fractures and, 623
Pain, bone
    acute leukemias and, 481
    multiple myeloma and, 475
    osteomalacia and, 525
    primary hyperparathyroidism and, 517
Pain, low back, multiple myeloma and, 475
Palatal cleft, occlusal radiographs and, 271
Palatal cortex, nasopalatine duct cyst and, 401, 403f
Palatal lesions, 303

Palatal molar roots, 178
Palatal root, 92f
Palate
    film placement and, 126, 130, 134
    gag reflex and, 163
    image field of, 155
    incisive foramen and, 174
    non-Hodgkin's lymphoma and, 477
    occlusal radiography and, 160
    premolar bitewing projection and, 150
    torus mandibularis and, 413
    Treacher Collins syndrome and, 643
Palate bone, mid-facial area and, 204
Palatine torus, 412
Palliation, multiple myeloma v., 477
Pannus, rheumatoid arthritis and, 563
Panoramic, extraoral projections as, 74
Panoramic examination, children and, 267
Panoramic film
    benign tumors and, 410
    buccal bifurcation cyst and, 392, 393f
    cementifying fibroma in, 499f
    condylar hypoplasia in, 552
    darkroom techniques for, 200
    dilated odontome and, 343f
    florid osseous dysplasia and, 496
    simple bone cyst in, 406f
Panoramic image, cropped, large keratocyst in, 397f
Panoramic images
    advantages of, 191
    ameloblastoma and, 420, 424f
    anatomic structures on, 201-209
    CCDs and, 228
    challenges in viewing, 201
    condylar hyperplasia, 551f
    disadvantages of, 191
    extraoral radiography and, 283
    fibrous dysplasia and, 488f
    formation principles of, 192-196
    intellectual segmentation of, 202f
    interpreting, 200-201
    multiple myeloma and, 476f
    odontogenic keratocyst and, 395f
    properly acquired, 201f
    radiolucent airway shadows and, 207
Panoramic machines, 114
    center of rotation and, 193
    exposure factors and, 204
    operation illustrations of, 192, 192f
Panoramic projection
    hard tissue imaging and, 543, 543f
    juvenile arthrosis and, 553, 553f
    transitional dentition and, 273
Panoramic radiographs
    calcified atheromas and, 268
    dental implants and, 677, 678b, 680-681, 680f
    head alignment and, 199f
    implants and, 269
    lesion and, 254f
    multiple myeloma bone destruction in, 477f
    orofacial region and, 271
    periapical cemental dysplasia, 492
    potential implant site and, 680f
    purpose of, 271
    TMJ and, 269
    torus palatinus and, 412
    trauma and, 269
Panoramic tomographic views, coronoid hyperplasia and, 553

Panoramic views
    bifid condyle and, 554
    cemental dysplasia time sequence in, 494f
    mandibular body fractures and, 625
Pansinusitis, overview of, 579
Paper film packets, contamination and, 118
Paper loop, film with, 74f
Paper printers, obstacles to, 235
Papillary crystadenoma lymphomatosum, 672
Papillon-Lefevere syndrome
    aggressive periodontitis v., 324
    periodontal disease and, 327
Paradental cyst of third molar, buccal bifurcation cyst v., 392
Paradental cysts, 392
    buccal bifurcation cyst v., 392
Parafunction
    degenerative joint disease and, 559
    internal derangement and, 555
Parallax unsharpness
    film and, 83f
    results of, 83, 83f
Parallel technique
    bisection technique vs., 62
    maxillary central incisor projection and, 126
    overview of, 123-125, 123f
    periapical radiography and, 121-122
    tooth and, 90, 90f
Paramandibular musculature, fibrosarcoma and, 474
Paranasal sinus mucosa, sinusitis and, 578
Paranasal sinuses, 177, 577
    ameloblastoma and, 419
    cleidocranial dysplasia and, 646, 648
    diseases associated with, 577-578
    epithelial papilloma and, 586
    intrinsic diseases of, 578
    malignant neoplasms of, 586-587
    normal development of, 576-577
    osteomas and, 443, 443f, 444, 586
    overview of, 576
    sinus disease and, 269
    traumatic injuries to, 593
    variations in, 576-577
Parasite lines, linear tomogram and, 247
Parateeth, 330
Parathesia of inferior alveolar nerve, central mucoepidermoid carcinoma and, 465
Parathyroid hormone (PTH)
    functions of, 517
    renal osteodystrophy and, 527
Parenchymal cells, radiation and, 31
Paresthesia
    metastatic tumors and, 467
    neurilemoma and, 439
    neurofibroma and, 441
    pyramidal fracture and, 632
    squamous cell carcinoma and, 461
Paresthesia of cheek, zygomatic arch fractures and, 635
Paresthesia of inferior alveolar nerve, African Burkitt's lymphoma and, 478
Pariapical films, film mount for, 108
Parotid glands
    CT and, 663, 663f
    cystic lesions of, 671
    enlargements of, 658

Parotid glands (Continued)
  malignant tumors of, 673
  radiation and, 33
  sialadenosis and, 670
  sialodochitis and, 668
  stones in, 603
  ultrasonography of, 671f
  Warthin tumor as, 672
Parotid sialoliths, radiography and, 660
Parry-Romberg syndrome, hemifacial
    microsomia and, 643
Parthyroid glands, renal osteodystrophy
    and, 526
Partial image, 125
  faulty radiographs and, 107b
Partial resection, aneurysmal bone cyst
    and, 506
Particulate radiation, overview of, 4-5
Parulis, perapical inflammatory lesions
    and, 371
Pathologic fracture
  fibrosarcoma and, 474
  multiple myeloma and, 476f
  squamous cell carcinoma originating in
    cyst and, 464
Pathologic fracture of jaw, metastatic
    tumors and, 467
Pathology, ghost images and, 208
Patient
  intraoral technique and, 62
  radiographic examination and, 55-56,
    281
  radiographic guidelines and, 272-273
  screen film and, 74
Patient, positioning of, 125
  head alignment and, 197-198
Patient management, children and,
    160-161
Patients, edentulous, radiographic
    examination of, 163
Patients, mentally disabled, radiographic
    examination for, 163
Patients, physically disabled, radiographic
    examination of, 163
PCD. See Peripical cemental dysplasia
    (PCD)
Pcnodysostosis, osteopetrosis v., 531
PDL. See Periodontal ligament (PDL)
    space
Peak kilovoltage (kVp), exposure and, 78
Peg-shaped deformity, microdontia and,
    335f
Penguin gait, osteomalacia and, 525
Penny test, fogging and, 112, 113f
Peptic ulcers, primary
    hyperparathyroidism and, 517
Perapical inflammatory lesions
  clinical features of, 368
  definition of, 367, 367f
  differential diagnosis for, 370
  effects on surrounding structures, 370
  internal structure of, 369, 369f
  management of, 371
  osteomyelitis v., 368
  periphery of, 369, 369f
  radiographic features of, 368, 368f
Perforation
  arthrography v., 548, 549f
  deformed disk and, 559f
Periapical abscess, 367
  perapical inflammatory lesion and, 367,
    367f, 368

Periapical areas, image field and, 126, 128
Periapical cemental dysplasia (PCD)
  benign cementoblastoma v., 436
  clinical features of, 492
  complex odontomas v., 427
  defined periphery of, 492, 495f
  definition of, 492
  differential diagnosis of, 495
  enostoses v., 416
  fibrous dysplasia and, 489
  florid osseous dysplasia v., 496
  internal structure of, 492, 492f
  jaw abnormalities and, 285
  management of, 495
  mature stage of, 495f
  mixed stage of, 492, 494f
  periapical inflammatory lesions v., 370,
    371f
  picture matching and, 283, 284f
  radicular cyst v., 386
  radiographic features of, 492, 495
  synonyms for, 492
Periapical cysts, 385
  primary osseous carcinoma v., 463
Periapical disease
  dental inflammatory lesions and, 588
  mental foramen and, 184, 184f
  mental fossa and, 183, 183f
  occult disease and, 268
  radiographic examination and, 266
Periapical fibroosteoma, 492
Periapical fibrous dysplasia, 492
Periapical films
  buccal bifurcation cyst and, 392, 393f
  dens evaginatus and, 344f
  furcation involvement of mandibular
    molar and, 323f
  image field and, 138
  loose dental implant and, 689
  molar bitewing projection and, 152
  profound radiolucent lesion in, 323f
  radicular cyst and, 386f
  radiolucent-radiopaque internal
    structure in, 486f
  squamous cell carcinoma and, 290f
  torus mandibularis and, 413
Periapical granulomas, 367
  periapical inflammatory lesions v., 367,
    367f, 368, 370
Periapical idiopathic osteosclerosis, 414
Periapical images, 282
Periapical infection, Turner's hypoplasia,
    352
Periapical inflammation, interrelationship
    of results in, 367f
Periapical inflammatory lesions, 167, 366
  acute osteomyelitis v., 375
  dental concussion and, 616
  metastatic tumors v., 467
  pulp and, 366
  synonyms for, 367
Periapical intraoral radiographs, septa
    and, 179
Periapical osteitis, enostoses v., 416
Periapical osteofibrosis, 492
Periapical projections
  lamina dura and, 176
  overview of, 121, 122f
Periapical radiographs
  canine and, 91, 91f
  dental fractures and, 163
  full-mouth examination and, 270

Periapical radiographs (Continued)
  genial tubercles and, 182, 182f
  implants and, 269
  intraoral projection techniques for,
    121-122
  leukemia in, 481f
  occlusal radiographs and, 160, 163
  periapical bone and, 298
  periapical cemental dysplasia, 492
  periodontium and, 316
  purpose of, 270
  torus palatinus and, 412
  trauma and, 269
Periapical radiolucencies, radicular dentin
    dysplasia (type 1) and, 348
Periapical rarifying osteitis
  early cemental dysplasia v., 495
  periapical inflammatory lesions v., 370
Periapical sclerosing osteitis
  benign cementoblastoma v., 436
  bone formation and, 369, 370f
  enostoses v., 416
Periapical surgical defect, radicular cyst v.,
    386
Periapical survey, children and, 160
Periapical views
  children and, 267
  periodontal disease and, 316
  periodontitis and, 267
  purposes for, 73
Pericoronal odontogenic keratocyst,
    adenomaoid odontogenic tumor v.,
    433
Pericoronitis
  clinical features of, 373
  definition of, 371, 373
  differential diagnosis of, 373
  internal structure of, 373, 373f
  management of, 373
  radiographic features of, 373
Peridens, 330
Periodonitis, radiation injury and, 38
Periodontal abscesses
  buccal bifurcation cyst v., 393
  diabetes mellitus and, 327
  maxillary cuspid and, 324f
  overview of, 322
Periodontal bone healing, digital
    subtraction radiography for, 238f
Periodontal disease
  AIDS and, 327
  alveolar bone and, 283
  assessment of, 315
  cancer and, 458
  density of alveolar crest in, 317, 317f
  dental conditions associated with,
    325-326
  dental inflammatory lesions and, 588
  diabetes mellitus and, 327, 523
  differential diagnosis of, 326
  effect of systemic diseases on, 327
  enamel pearl and, 350
  frequency of radiographs in, 316
  gemination and, 338
  indications of, 169
  inflammatory lesions and, 367
  jaws and, 366
  Langerhans' cell histiocytosis v., 513
  limitations of radiographs in, 315
  local irritation factors in, 325-326
  nutrient canals and, 185
  occlusal trauma and, 325

Periodontal disease *(Continued)*
open contacts and, 325
overview of, 267
positioning patient and, 208
radiographic examination and, 266, 274
rotational scenography and, 250
squamous cell carcinoma v., 461
stereoscopy technique and, 249, 249f
tooth mobility and, 325
Periodontal lesions
soft tissue and, 366
vertical root fractures and, 623
Periodontal ligament damage, blood flow and, 617
Periodontal ligament (PDL) space
dental concussion and, 616
dental root fractures and, 621
examination process and, 283
extruded tooth and, 617
fibrous dysplasia and, 489
inflammatory lesions and, 367
luxated tooth and, 617
mandibular canal v., 184
metastatic tumors and, 467
multiple myeloma and, 475
overview of, 170, 170f
periapical cemental dysplasia and, 495
periapical inflammatory lesions and, 370
progressive systemic sclerosis v., 532, 532f
radicular dilaceration and, 340
sarcomas and, 459
vertical osseous defects and, 319
Periodontal membrane
concrescence and, 338
osteosarcoma and, 469, 471f
Periodontal membrane space
abnormalities in, 292
progressive systemic sclerosis and, 532
Periodontal pocket formation, enamel pearl and, 350
Periodontal probe, scout film and, 661
Periodontal therapy
evaluation of, 326-327
periapical film after, 326f
Periodontitis, 267. *See also* Moderate periodontitis
chronic infectious diseases and, 314
etiology of, 314
Periodontium, disorders of, 314
Perioral tissues, *cysticercus cellulosae* and, 601
Periosteal bone formation
Ewing's sarcoma v., 474
periostitis and, 589
Periosteal reaction
mestastic lesions and, 293, 293f
metastatic tumors and, 467
osteomyelitis, 374
Periosteal surfaces, Ewing's sarcoma and, 473
Periosteum
acute osteomyelitis and, 375
inflammatory lesions and, 367
Periostitis
apical inflammatory lesions and, 371f
definition of, 589
radiographic features of, 589, 589f
Periostitis ossificans, 374
Peripheral cortication, central mucoepidermoid carcinoma and, 465

Peripheral invasive squamous cell carcinoma, fibrosarcoma v., 475
Peripheral nerves
fibrosarcoma and, 474
neurilemoma from, 439
neurofibroma and, 440
neuroma and, 440
Peripheral tumors, adenomaoid odontogenic tumor and, 431
Peripheral vascular disease, arteriosclerosis and, 602
Permanent canine, transposition and, 336
Permanent dentitions
fusion of teeth and, 336
hypocalcification/hypocalcification, 345
hypodontia in, 332
taurodontism and, 339
Permanent incisors, congenital syphilis and, 353, 353f
Permanent lateral incisor, fusion of teeth and, 336, 336f
Permanent maxillary lateral incisors, dens in dente and, 342
Permanent molar periapical projection, mixed dentition and, 162
Permanent teeth
crown-root fractures and, 623
dental root fractures and, 620
fractures of dental crown in, 619
hypopituitarism and, 522
odontomas and, 425, 426f
reimplanting, 619
Permeative borders, lesions with, 289
Pernoxyl radicals, biologic molecules and, 26
Personnel, occupational exposure and, 64-65
PET. *See* Positron emission computed tomography (PET)
Petechiae, acute leukemias and, 481
Petrified man condition, progressive myositis ossificans and, 611
Petrotympanic fissure, sagittal plane and, 540
Petrous ridges
panoramic film and, 200, 200f
reverse-Towne projection, 222, 223f
Pharyngeal airway shadow, mandibular ramal area and, 202
Pharynx, ossification of stylohyoid ligament, 609
Phenodin, radiology and, 97
Phleboliths, 597
calcified lymph nodes and, 599
clinical features of, 605
definition of, 605
differential diagnosis of, 605-606
hemangiomas v., 673
radiographic features of, 605, 606f
sialoliths v., 666
Phosphatase, dystrophic calcification and, 598
Phosphate serum, osteomalacia and, 524
Phosphoethanolamine, hypophosphatasia and, 526
Phosphor crystal, intensifying screens and, 83
Phosphor layer, composition of, 76
Phosphor plates, bitewing and, 299f
Phosphorescence. *See* Light (phosphorescence)
Phosphorescent crystals, function of, 76

Phosphors fluorescence, x-ray beam and, 75
Phosphorus, hypophosphatemia and, 527
Photoelectric absorption, 18f
Compton scattering and, 19
diagnostic imaging and, 17
Photomicrograph, of film emulsion, 97, 98f
Photomultiplier tube, photostimulable phosphor plates (PSP), 230f
Photon energies, x-ray machine and, 12, 12f, 13f
Photons, 94, 95f
absorber and, 71
bremsstrahlung interactions and, 12
coherent scattering and, 16-17, 17f
dense objects and, 79
fields associated with, 6f
film density and, 78
focal spot and, 86, 87f
penetration of matter and, 14
quantum theory and, 5-6
radiographic density and, 77
scattered radiation and, 80
Photosensitivity, silver halide grains and, 71
Photostimulable phosphor, radiographic imaging and, 230
Photostimulable phosphor plate (PSP) receptors, comparison of physical properties of, 243t
Photostimulable phosphor plates (PSP)
clinical handling of, 241
exposure latitudes and, 223f
image formation of, 230f
image receptors and, 198
overview of, 230-231, 230f
panoramic machine v, 192
Photostimulable phosphor plates (PSP) images, contralateral treatment with, 242
Photostimulable phosphor plates (PSP) systems
problems with, 242
resolution factors in, 231
Phototiming, radiographic procedures using, 63
PHT. *See* Parathyroid hormone (PTH)
Physically disabled patients. *See* Patients, physically disabled
Physiologic attrition. *See* Attrition
Physiotherapy
degenerative joint disease and, 562
rheumatoid arthritis and, 563
septic arthritis and, 565
Pierre Robin sequence, Treacher Collins syndrome v., 646
Piezoelectric crystal, sonography and, 263
Piezoelectric extracorporeal shock wave lithotripsy, stones and, 605
Pindborg tumor, 422
Pipe stem appearance, arteriosclerosis and, 602
Pituitary adenoma, acromegaly v., 521
Pituitary dwarfism, microdontia in, 335
Pituitary giantism, microdontia and, 335f
Pituitary gland
craniofacial fibrous dysplasia and, 593
hyperpituitarism and, 521
Pituitary tumor, hyperpituitarism and, 521
Pixel matrix, silicon crystals and, 227, 228f

Pixels, 253
    computed tomography (CT) image and,
        251
    digital detector characteristics and, 232
    digital imaging and, 225
    image restoration and, 235
Plain film radiography
    conventional tomography v., 547
    salivary gland disease and, 659
    salivary glands and, 660
Plaque
    aggressive periodontitis and, 324
    inflammatory host response and, 314
Plaque formation, periodontal diseases
    and, 325
Plasma cell granuloma, 588
Plasma cell myeloma, 475
Plasma cells, multiple myeloma and, 475
Plasmacytoma, 475
Plastic barrier sheaths, contamination and,
    118
Plastic surgery, hemifacial microsomia
    and, 643
Pleomorphic adenoma, 672
Pleomorphism of cells, desmoplastic
    fibroma of bone and, 454
Plexiform neurofibromas,
    neurofibromatosis and, 443
Pluripotential lining cells, inflammatory
    lesions and, 367
Pluripotential odontogenic epithelium,
    central mucoepidermoid carcinoma
    from, 465
PM 2002 CC Proline, panoramic machines
    and, 197, 197f
Pocket formation, periodontal diseases
    and, 325
Point of entry
    anterior mandibular occlusal projection
        and, 157
    anterior maxillary occlusal projection
        and, 154
    cross-sectional mandibular occlusal
        projection in, 158
    lateral mandibular occlusal projection
        and, 159
    lateral maxillary occlusal projection and,
        156
    molar bitewing projection and, 153
    occlusal plane and, 153
    paralleling technique and, 127, 129,
        131, 133, 135, 137, 139, 141, 143,
        145, 147
Point of measurement, dental radiography
    and, 52
Polydipsia, diabetes mellitus and, 523
Polymer coat, intensifying screens and,
    77
Polymyositis, autoimmune sialadenitis and,
    669
Polyostotic fibrous dysplasia
    children and, 485
    McCune-Albright syndrome and, 485
Polyposis of sinus mucosa, 582
Polyposis syndromes, enostoses v., 416
Polyps. *See also* Antral polyps
    clinical features of, 582
    definition of, 582
    dystrophic calcification and, 598, 599f
    inflammatory disease and, 578
    radiographic features of, 582, 584
    squamous cell carcinoma and, 587

Polyps, intestinal, Gardner's syndrome
    and, 445
Polytetraflouroethylene implants,
    computed tomography (CT) and, 548
Polyuria, diabetes mellitus and, 523
Porcelain
    metal coping and, 189f
    restorative materials as, 187, 188f
Position and distance rule, occupational
    safety and, 65, 65f
Position artifact, panoramic machines and,
    196f
Positioning, patient, MRI and, 549-550
Positioning indicating device, calibration
    and, 113-114
Positive angulation, projection of central
    ray and, 145
Positron, PET and, 262
Positron emission computed tomography
    (PET)
    classification of salivary tumors and, 665
    diffuse sclerosing osteomyelitis and,
        378
    nuclear medicine and, 262
Postassium hydroxide, developers and, 97
Posterior alveolar process, segmental
    odontomaxillary dysplasia and, 651
Posterior-anterior cephalometric skull
    radiographs, paranasal sinuses and,
    576
Posterior-anterior (PA) skull film,
    panoramic film and, 200, 200f
Posterior attachment (retrodiskal tissues)
    anatomy of, 541
    disk and, 540
    mandibular fossa and, 541
Posterior bitewing films
    children and, 162
    each quadrant with, 149
    mixed dentition and, 162
Posterior cranial occipital condyles,
    submentovertex projection and, 220,
    220f
Posterior dorsum, gag reflex and, 163
Posterior joint space, condyle and, 542,
    5442f
Posterior mandible
    desmoplastic fibromas of bone in, 454
    metastatic tumors and, 459
    neuromas and, 440
    osteomyelitis in, 367
    squamous cell carcinoma and, 461
    trabecular pattern in, 171f
Posterior periapical films
    children and, 162
    external oblique ridge and, 186
    primary dentition and, 161, 161f
Posterior retrodiskal tissues, disk and, 540
Posterior skull radiographs, bony lesions
    and, 660
Posterior skull view, mandibular fracture
    and, 615
Posterior teeth, mylohyoid ridge and, 185,
    185f
Posteroanterior cephalometric projection
    anatomic landmarks in, 216f
    evaluation steps in, 221-222, 222f
    image receptor and, 213
    patient placement and, 213
    resultant image with, 213
Posteroanterior skull radiograph,
    pyramidal fracture and, 631

Posteroanterior skull view
    dystrophic calcification in tonsils and,
        599
    osteoma cutis and, 609
Posteroanterior views, horizontal fracture
    and, 631
Postmenopausal women, osteoporosis and,
    524
Postoperative assessments, radiographs
    and, 687-691
Postradiation dental caries, head and neck
    malignancy and, 482
Posttraumatic myositis ossificans, 610
Potassium bromide
    developing solution and, 97
    restrainers and, 97
Power supply
    functions of, 9
    x-ray machine and, 9-11
Preauricular cyst, parotid and, 658
Preauricular region, joint effusion and,
    567
Precession, magnetic field and, 257
Precision instrument
    dry-heat sterilization for, 117
    film holding and, 124, 124f
    film placement and, 132, 144
    patient examination and, 123
    PID and, 59, 60f
    projection of central ray and, 135
    technique evaluation with, 62
Precision Pedodontic instruments,
    children and, 162
Pregnancy
    fibrous dysplasia and, 491
    ionizing radiation and, 164
    irradiation comparative risk during,
        40t
    Patient Selection Criteria Panel
        regarding, 61
    radiographs, 274-275
Premature craniosynostosis, 640
Premaxilla, 172
Premolar bitewing projection
    central ray projection and, 151
    film placement in, 150
    image field in, 150
Premolar gemination, 338
Premolar projection, 149
    edentulous patients and, 165
Premolar region, torus mandibularis and,
    413
Premolars
    cementoossifying fibroma and, 499
    dental fragments in sinus and, 593
    external resorption and, 358
    film placement and, 132, 138
    image field and, 132, 142
    odontogenic myxoma and, 434
    supplemental teeth and, 332f
    torus mandibularis and, 413
Prenatal irradiation, effects of, 39
Preservatives
    developing solution and, 97
    fixing solution and, 98
Pressure, excessive, resorption and, 356
Primary dentition
    hypopituitarism and, 522
    internal resorption and, 356
    projections used, 161
    taurodontism and, 339
Primary epithelial tumor of jay, 463

Primary hyperparathyroidism
  radiographic manifications of, 518
  teeth v. jaw density in, 518, 519f
Primary intraalveolar epidermoid
  carcinoma, 463
Primary intraosseous carcinoma, 463
  jaw and, 463
  squamous cell carcinoma originating in
    cyst v., 464
Primary lesion, metastatic tumors and, 466
Primary lymphoma, minor salivary glands
  and, 675
Primary malignancy, metastatic tumors
  and, 467, 468f
Primary odontogenic carcinoma, 463
Primary osseous carcinoma
  differential diagnosis of, 463-464
  internal structure of, 463
  management of, 464
  radiographic features of, 463, 463f
Primary teeth
  benign cementoblastoma and, 435
  dentin dysplasia and, 348
  gemination and, 338
  odontomas and, 425
  regional odontodysplasia, 349
Primary tumors, 458
Primordial cysts, 393
  former cysts and, 405
Processing procedures, quality assurance
  program and, 110
Processing room, components for, 99
Processing solutions, 100
  image quality and, 63
  reference film and, 110-111
Processing tanks, 99
Prodromal period, acute radiation
  syndrome and, 37
Progeria, microdontia and, 335
Prognathism, basal cell nevus syndrome
  and, 397
Prognosis
  metastatic tumors and, 467
  radiographic guidelines and, 272
Progressive bone cavity, 405
Progressive myositis ossificans
  definition of, 611
  differential diagnosis of, 611
  management of, 611
  radiographic features of, 611
Progressive osteopenia, osteogenesis
  imperfecta and, 347
Progressive systemic sclerosis (PSS)
  clinical features of, 531
  definition of, 531
  differential diagnosis of, 532
  management of, 532
  radiographic features of, 531-532
Projection geometry, digital subtraction
  radiography (DSR) and, 238-239,
  238f
Projections, 123b
Proliferative periostitis, 374, 377f
  children and, 375
Prophylactic restoration, dens in dente
  and, 343
Proptosis
  craniofacial fibrous dysplasia and, 593
  mucocele and, 585
  polyps and, 582
Prostate metastasis, osteosarcoma v., 469
Prosthesis, imaging stents and, 686

Prosthetic crowns
  dentinogenesis imperfecta and, 347
  dilaceration and, 340
Prosthetic procedures, hypodontia and,
  333
Prosthetic replacement, dentin dysplasia
  and, 349
Prosthetics
  edentulous patients and, 165
  microdontia and, 335
  preoperative planning with, 269
  transposed teeth and, 336
Prosthetics, maxillofacial
  hemifacial microsomia and, 643
  Treacher Collins syndrome and, 646
Protective coat, intensifying screens and,
  77
Protective envelopes, features of, 117
Proteins, irradiation of, 27
Proton-weighted pulse sequences, MRI
  and, 550
Protons, atom structure and, 3, 4
Proximal carious lesions
  bitewing and, 299f
  interproximal radiographs (bitewings)
    and, 271
  susceptible zone in, 304f
Proximal surfaces, fibre-optic
  transillumination (FOTI), 305, 311
Pruritus, non-Hodgkin's lymphoma and,
  477
Pseudarthrosis, ankylosis and, 569
Pseudo-color, digital systems and, 236,
  238
Pseudocysts, 581
  effects on surrounding structures, 582
  internal structure of, 582
  lingual salivary gland depression and,
    651
  periphery and shape of, 582
Pseudogout, 566
  articular loose bodies and, 565
Pseudohypoparathyroidism
  clinical features of, 519-520
  induced dental anomalies in, 521f
  overview of, 519
  radiographic features of, 520
Pseudotrabeculae, localized (traumatic)
  myositis ossificans and, 610
Pseudotumor
  clinical features of, 588
  definition of, 588
  differential diagnosis for, 588
  management of, 588
  radiographic features of, 588
  synonyms for, 588
Pseudotumor of sinuses, 588
Psoriasis, psoriatic arthritis and, 564
Psoriatic arthritis
  overview of, 564
  rheumatoid arthritis v., 563
PSS. *See* Progressive systemic sclerosis
  (PSS)
Psychiatric problems, primary
  hyperparathyroidism and, 517
Psychological distress, missing teeth and,
  333
Pterygoid fovea, condyle and, 539
Pterygoid plates, anatomical overview of,
  181, 181f
Pterygomaxillary fissure, 205, 207f
  CT image and, 205, 207f

Pulp
  calcium hydroxide base and, 187, 188f
  composition of teeth and, 166
  crown-root fractures and, 623
  radiolucent silicate restorations and,
    189f
  tooth crown fractures and, 619
Pulp canal
  antroliths v., 584
  external resorption and, 358, 360
Pulp capping, tooth crown fractures and,
  620
Pulp chamber, 299
  amelogenesis imperfecta and, 346
  attrition and, 354
  coronal dentin dysplasia (type 2), 347,
    348, 348f
  dens in dente and, 342, 342f
  dental concussion and, 616
  dentin dysplasia and, 348
  dentinogenesis imperfecta and, 346
  examination process and, 283
  fusion of teeth and, 336
  gemination and, 338, 338f
  hypophosphatasia and, 526
  hypophosphatemia and, 528
  internal resorption and, 356, 357, 357f
  radicular dentin dysplasia (type 1) and,
    348, 348f
  regional odontodysplasia and, 349, 350f
  secondary dentin and, 360, 360.360f
  segmental odontomaxillary dysplasia
    and, 651
  taurodontism and, 339
Pulp chamber, rectangular, taurodontism
  and, 339, 339f
Pulp channels, composition of teeth and,
  166
Pulp horn
  dens evaginatus, 343
  enamel pearl and, 350
  talon cusp and, 352
Pulp stones
  definition of, 361
  differential diagnosis of, 361
  enamel pearl v., 350
  radiographic features of, 361
  secondary dentin v, 361
Pulpal calcification, pulp stones and, 361
Pulpal disease, dens in dente and, 342
Pulpal infection
  internal resorption and, 357
  regional odontodysplasia and, 349
Pulpal necrosis
  dental concussion and, 616
  dental root fractures and, 622
  periapical inflammatory lesion and, 367,
    367f
  tooth crown fractures and, 620
  traumatized tooth and, 617
Pulpal sclerosis
  definition of, 362
  pulp stones v., 361
  radiographic features of, 362
Pulpectomy, tooth crown fractures and,
  620
Pulpotomy, tooth crown fractures and, 620
Pycnodysostosis
  cleidocranial dysplasia v., 648
  osteopetrosis v., 531
Pyocele, mucocele as, 584, 585
Pyogenic osteomyelitis, 374

Pyramidal fractures, 629
  clinical features of, 631-632
  craniofacial dysfunction v., 633
  definition of, 631
  management of, 632
  radiographic features of, 632
  radiographic position of, 631f

Q

Quality, extraoral images and, 218
Quality assurance
  guide for establishing, 67b
  overview of, 65-66
  radiology and, 110-115
Quantitative computed tomography
  (QCT) programs, osteoporosis and,
  524
Quantum mottle, fast intensifying screens
  and, 82
Quantum theory, overview of, 5-6
Quiescent periods, periodontitis and, 314

R

Rad (radiation absorbed dose), tissue and,
  21
Radiation
  cellular level effects of, 27
  digital detector characteristics and, 233
  digital imaging and, 225
  fibrosarcoma and, 474
  long-term effects of, 31
  nature of, 4-6
  panoramic radiograph, 271
  radiographic guidelines and, 272
  stereoscopy technique and, 249
Radiation beam, horizontal angulation
  and, 148
Radiation biology, overview of, 25
Radiation caries
  dental radiology and, 482
  examples of, 312f
  overview of, 34-36, 36f
  radiation therapy and, 275
  three types of, 35
  tooth destruction of, 305, 312f
Radiation chemistry, overview of, 25
Radiation dose
  CBCT and, 255
  radionuclide-labeled tracers and, 260
Radiation dosimetry report, 66f
Radiation exposure, sources of, 47-51
Radiation genetics, overview of, 42, 42t
Radiation injury, clinical signs after, 37-38
Radiation quantities, summary of, 20t
Radiation therapy
  ameloblastoma and, 422
  central mucoepidermoid carcinoma
    and, 465
  condylar hypoplasia and, 552
  Ewing's sarcoma and, 474
  fibrosarcoma v., 475
  fibrous dysplasia and, 491
  hemifacial microsomia and, 643
  Langerhans' cell histiocytosis and, 514
  malignant lesions and, 32-33
  metastatic tumors and, 467
  multiple myeloma v., 477
  non-Hodgkin's lymphoma v., 478
  osteoradionecrosis and, 380
  osteosarcoma and, 469
  parotid area v., 658
  posterior body of mandible and, 380

Radiation therapy (Continued)
  primary osseous carcinoma and, 464
  radiation-induced xerostomia and, 275
  squamous cell carcinoma and, 461,
    588
  tumors and, 673
  Turner's hypoplasia and, 352
  xerostomia and, 305
Radiation units, summary of, 20t
Radiation weighing factor, 47
Radical neck dissection, malignant tumors
  and, 673
Radicular cysts
  clinical features of, 385
  collapsing of, 387, 387f
  definition of, 385
  differential diagnosis of, 386
  lateral periodontal cyst v., 399
  management of, 387
  nasopalatine duct cyst v., 401
  odontogenic cysts and, 589
  periapical inflammatory lesions v., 370
  periphery and shape of, 385
  radiographic features of, 385, 385f
  retention pseudocysts v., 582
  synonyms for, 385
Radicular dentin dysplasia (type 1)
  dentin dysplasia and, 347, 348
  radiographic features of, 348, 348f
Radioactivity, measurement of, 21
Radiofrequency pulse, angle of rotation
  and, 258
Radiograph
  appearance of lamina dura on, 168
  demineralization process and, 311
  guidelines for ordering, 272
  nutrient canals and, 185f
  overview of, 86
  selection criteria for, 272
  of sinuses, 177, 177f
  thickened mucosa and, 578, 579f
Radiographic appearance, aggressive
  periodontitis and, 324
Radiographic blurring, overview of, 82
Radiographic contrast, overview of, 79
Radiographic cortical boundaries,
  hypophosphatemia and, 527, 529f
Radiographic density, overview of, 77-79
Radiographic examinations
  children and, 160-162
  concrescence and, 337-338
  conduct of, 56
  cost v. benefit of, 266
  criteria of quality for, 121
  dens evaginatus and, 343
  dens in dente and, 342, 342f
  florid osseous dysplasia and, 496
  guidelines for ordering, 265, 266
  of mixed dentition, 162f
  periodontitis and, 267
  properties of, 270t
  taurodontism and, 339, 339f
Radiographic features
  algorithm of diagnostic process in,
    294f
  cherubism and, 507
  primary hyperparathyroidism and,
    518
Radiographic findings, monostotic fibrous
  dysplasia and, 485
Radiographic granular trabecular pattern,
  hypophosphatemia and, 527

Radiographic grids
  composition of, 84-85, 84f
  extraoral radiographic examinations
    and, 210
  function of, 84
  x-ray beam and, 83
Radiographic guidelines
  clinical application of, 275-276
  stage of dental development and, 273
Radiographic image contrast, kilovoltage
  relationship to, 62
Radiographic images
  interpretation steps in, 64, 218, 283
  osteoblastomas and, 450, 451f
Radiographic imaging chain, schematic of,
  227f
Radiographic interpretation
  classification in, 294-295
  developmental v. acquired in, 294
  formulation of, 293
  normal v. abnormal in, 293-294
  steps in, 283
  ways to proceed with, 295
Radiographic joint space, 541, 541f
  overview of, 542
Radiographic mottle, overview of, 81-82,
  82
Radiographic noise, overview of, 81-82
Radiographic procedures, special patient
  considerations in, 162-165
Radiographic report
  clinical information in, 295
  findings and, 295-296
  imaging procedure in, 295
  interpretation (impression) and,
    295-296
  patient and general information in,
    295
Radiographic selection criteria, overview
  of, 56
Radiographic speed, overview of, 81
Radiographic survey, aspects of, 161,
  161f
Radiographic tube housing, occupational
  safety and, 65
Radiography
  categories of, 121
  clinical algorithm for ordering, 268f,
    274
  condyles in children and, 539
  cross-contamination in, 115
  dark, 105b
  dental caries and, 297
  duplicating, 108-109
  exposure and dose in, 51-52
  false-positive carious lesions and, 300
  faulty, common causes of, 105
  guidelines for ordering, 271
  image field and, 126, 128
  luxation and, 617
  periodontal disease and, 315
  potential dental implant sites and, 683
  pregnancy and, 274-275
  previous, uses for, 271
  radiolucent v. radiopaque materials in,
    289
  skull, hyperpituitarism and, 521, 522f
  supplemental teeth and, 331, 332f
  treatment of periodontal disease and,
    326
  viewing conditions in, 282
Radiologists, film printers and, 235

Radiology, dental
   desmoplastic fibromas of bone and, 454
   developing agents in, 97
   fractures and, 615
   monitoring lesions and, 297
   roles in cancer management of, 458
Radiolucency
   acute osteomyelitis and, 375
   calcifying epithelial odontogenic tumors
      and, 423
   chronic osteomyelitis and, 379, 379f
   composite with, 189f
   inflammatory lesions and, 367
   mandibular premolar region of, 399f
   moderate periodontitis and, 318
   periodontal disease and, 322f
   porcelain with, 189f
Radiolucent apical scar, radicular cyst v.,
      386
Radiolucent changes
   occlusal caries with, 302, 307f
   vertical osseous defects and, 320
Radiolucent grid lines, image and, 84
Radiolucent interior, dens in dente and,
      342, 343f
Radiolucent lesions, 384
   examination process and, 283
   metastatic tumors and, 467
Radiolucent object, film and, 79
Radiolucent periphery
   cementoblastoma and, 289
   mature cemental dysplasia and, 495
Radiolucent-radiopaque lesions
   benign cementoblastoma in, 436, 438f
   osteoid osteoma and, 454f
Radiolucent silicate restorations, base and,
      189f
Radiolucent spaces, 82f
Radiolucent structure
   buccal bifurcation cyst with, 392
   eosinophilic granuloma and, 511
   odontogenic keratocyst and, 394, 394f
Radiolucent zone, dental caries and, 297
Radionuclide imaging
   physiologic change and, 260
   uptake of isotope and, 262f
Radionuclide-labeled tracers, radiation
   dose and, 260
Radionuclides, internal radiation and, 49
Radiopacities
   adenomaoid odontogenic tumor and, 431
   calcifying epithelial odontogenic tumor
      and, 424, 425f
Radiopaque (mixed density)
   calcium hydroxide base as, 187, 188f
   dense objects and, 79
   lesion classification as, 289
   restorative materials as, 187-190
   thick trabeculae as, 289f, 290
Radiopaque appearance, orthodontic
   appliances with, 190
Radiopaque areas, washing and, 98
Radiopaque enamel, gemination and, 338
Radiopaque foci
   adenomaoid odontogenic tumor and,
      431, 433f
   osteoid osteoma and, 452
Radiopaque lesions
   corticated periphery and, 288
   enostoses v., 416
   examination process and, 283
   internal structures seen in, 290-291

Radiopaque lines, 82f
Radiopaque mass, periapical film
   revealing, 289f
Radiopaque objects, panoramic machine
   and, 192, 192f
Radiopaque patterns
   cementoossifying fibroma and, 500f
   mucosa thickening and, 579, 579f
Radiopaque regions, florid osseous
   dysplasia and, 496
Radiosensitivity, cell type and, 30
Radiotherapy, malignant tumors and, 572
Radiotracers, radionuclide imaging and,
      260
Radon, 49
Radonuclide uptake, scintigraphy and,
      665, 665f
Rami, anterior mandibular occlusal
   projection and, 157
Rampant caries
   children and, 302, 308f
   mandibular anterior teeth and, 303,
      308f
Ramus
   acromegaly v., 521
   ameloblastic fibromas and, 428, 429f
   arteriovenous (A-V) fistula and, 449
   dentigerous cyst and, 388
   desmoplastic fibromas of bone in, 454
   hemangioma and, 446
   juvenile arthrosis and, 553
   juvenile chronic arthritis and, 364
   neurofibromatosis and, 442, 442f
   osteomas and, 443, 444f
   panoramic image and, 201
Range of motion
   joint effusion and, 567
   synovial chondromatosis and, 565
   TMJ dysfunction and, 538
Ranula, dermoid cysts ., 404
Rapid image acquisition techniques, MRI
   and, 550
Rapid-processing solutions, overview of,
      102
Rare earth filtration, costs of, 61
Rare-earth screens
   calcium tungstate screens *vs.*, 57-58
   speeds of, 77t
   t-grain film and, 58
Rarefaction
   periapical inflammatory lesion and,
      369
   pericoronitis and, 373
Rarefying osteitis
   leukemia v., 481, 482
   radiolucence of, 367
Reabsorption, residual cyst and, 388
Reactive bone, lesion and, 293
Real time imaging, sonography and, 263
Recall visit, radiographs on, 273-274, 274t
Receptor
   image layer and, 194
   panoramic machine and, 192
Receptor selection, ADA and, 56
Recoil electrons (photoelectrons), 17
Rectangular collimation
   benefits of, 59
   E and, 59
Rectangular position-indication device
   (PID), patient skin surface and, 59,
      59f
Rectilinear scanner, tracers and, 262

Recurrance
   aneurysmal bone cyst and, 506
   Langerhans' cell histiocytosis and, 514
   localized (traumatic) myositis ossificans
      and, 611
Red light spectrum, photostimulable
   phosphor plates (PSP) and, 231
Reduced condylar translation, mouth
   opening and, 542
Reducing agents, 96
Reference film, radiographs v., 110, 111f
Reflective layer, 77
Regional lymphadenopathy, squamous cell
   carcinoma originating in cyst and,
      464
Regional mucositis, vertical osseous defects
   and, 320
Regional odontodysplasia
   clinical features of, 349
   definition of, 349
   differential diagnosis of, 349
   management of, 349
   radiographic features of, 349, 350f
   segmental odontomaxillary dysplasia v.,
      651
Reimplantation
   avulsed teeth and, 619
   avulsion v., 619
   external root resorption and, 619
Relative biologic effectiveness (RBE),
   x-rays and, 32
Relative macrodontia, macrodontia v., 334,
      334f
Relative microdontia, microdontia v., 335
Relaxation, resonant RF pulse and, 259
Remineralization
   fluoride use and, 297
   fractures and, 635
   periodontal disease and, 326
Remnant beam
   differential absorption and, 19
   film contrast and, 79
Remodeling
   fibrous ankylosis and, 569
   mandibular condyle fractures and, 627
Remodeling, TMJ, 561f
   clinical features of, 559
   definition of, 557, 559
   differential diagnosis of, 559
   radiographic features of, 559
   treatment of, 559
Renal calculi, primary
   hyperparathyroidism and, 517
Renal disease
   articular loose bodies and, 565
   multiple myeloma and, 476f
Renal osteodystrophy (renal rickets)
   clinical features of, 526
   definition of, 526
   radiographic features of, 526-527
Renal transplant, renal osteodystrophy
   and, 527
Renal tubular disorders,
   hypophosphatemia and, 527
Renulas, cysts and, 671
Replinisher. *See* Developer replenisher
Replinishing solutions, manual tank
   processing and, 101
Resection. *See* Surgery
Resection of jaw
   ameloblastoma and, 422
   central giant cell granuloma v., 503

Residual cyst, 388
  clinical features of, 387
  definition of, 387
  radiographic features of f, 388
Resolution
  digital radiograph, 235
  effect of fast screens on, 77
  radiograph and, 82
Resolving power target, radiograph of, 82f
Resonant RF pulse, relaxation and, 259
Resorption
  benign cementoblastoma and, 436
  dentigerous cyst and, 390f
  inflammatory lesions and, 367
  overview of, 356
  progressive systemic sclerosis and, 532, 532f
Resorption of tooth roots, central giant cell granuloma and, 502
Resource Conservation And Recovery Act of 1976, 104
Respiratory epithelium, epithelial papilloma and, 586
Resportion. See also Bone resorption
Restoration, prophylactic, dens in dente and, 342
Restorations
  congenital syphilis, 353-354
  dental caries and, 266
  examination process and, 283
  subject density and, 78
Restorations, faulty, periodontal diseases and, 325
Restorations,overhanging, periodontal diseases and, 326f
Restorative materials
  overview of, 187-190
  resembling carious lesions, 311f
Restorative procedures
  caries and, 300, 304f
  hypodontia and, 333
  imaging techniques for, 677, 678b
  secondary dentin and, 360
Restorative therapy
  amelogenesis imperfecta, 346
  dentinal lesions and, 301
  microdontia and, 335
Restrainer
  components of, 97
  developing solution and, 97
Retake log
  film errors and, 110
  review of, 111
Retention cyst of maxillary sinus, 581
Retention pseudocysts
  clinical features of, 581-582
  definition of, 581
  differential diagnosis of, 582
  etiology of, 582
  inflammatory disease and, 578
  management of, 582
  odontogenic cysts v., 589
  radiographic features of, 582
  synonyms for, 581
Retinoblastoma, metastatic tumors and, 466
Retrodiskal tissue, MRI and, 550
Retromolar area, image field and, 144, 146
Reverse bias, x-ray and, 11

Reverse-Towne projection (open mouth)
  anatomic landmarks and, 217f
  anatomic landmarks in, 217f
  central x-ray beam in, 218
  evaluation steps for, 222, 223f
  image receptor and, 213
  mandibular condyle fractures and, 626
  patient placement and, 213
  resultant image in, 218
  x-ray beam and, 213
Reverse-Towne view, trauma and, 269
Reversible projection errors, digital subtraction radiography and, 238
Reverting postmitotic cells, radiosensitivity and, 30
Rhabdomyosarcoma, extrinsic malignant tumors and, 571
Rheumatoid arthritis (RA)
  autoimmune sialadenitis and, 669
  clinical features of, 562
  definition of, 562
  degenerative joint disease v., 562
  differential diagnosis of, 563
  juvenile arthrosis v., 553
  progressive myositis ossificans v., 611
  radiographic features of, 563
  treatment of, 563
Rhinoliths
  antroliths v., 584
  clinical features of, 607
  definition of, 607
  differential diagnosis of, 608
  lateral occlusal film of, 607, 607f
  management of, 608
  posterior-anterior skull film of, 607, 607f
  radiographic features of, 607
Rhinorrhea, rhinoliths and, 607
Rhizopus sinusitis, 588
Rickets
  clinical features of, 524
  definition of, 524
  radiographic features of, 524-526
  radiographic features of jaws in, 525
Right angle technique, mandible and, 91
Right-angle views, mandibular body fractures and, 625
Right aveolar process, squamous cell carcinoma and, 462f
Right maxillary canine, adenomaoid odontogenic tumor and, 433f
Right maxillary sinus
  fibrosarcoma and, 474, 474f
  fibrous dysplasia and, 488f
Rinn XCP film-holding instrument, 59f, 60f
  technique evaluation with, 62
Rinsing
  manual tank processing and, 102
  overview of, 97
Roentgen, air kerma vs., 21
Rollers, functions of, 104
Roof of orbit, lateral cephalometric projection and, 218-220, 219f
Root
  chronic osteomyelitis and, 379
  dens in dente involving, 340, 341
  dentinogenesis imperfecta and, 346
  florid osseous dysplasia and, 496
  occlusal radiography and, 160
  periodontitis and, 267
  radicular dilaceration and, 340
  regional odontodysplasia and, 349, 350f

Root absorption, central odontogenic fibroma and, 438
Root apex
  buccal bifurcation cyst and, 392-393
  enostoses v., 416
  external resorption and, 358, 359f
  periodontal lesions and, 367
Root apices, sinus and, 177
Root canal instruments, intraoral periapical examination and, 164
Root canal therapy
  dens in dente and, 342
  fusion of teeth and, 336
  osteomyelitis and, 377
  periapical inflammatory lesions and, 366, 371
  root fragment and, 179
Root canals
  composition of teeth and, 166
  coronal dentin dysplasia (type 2), 347, 348, 348f
  dentinogenesis imperfecta and, 347, 347f
  fused teeth and, 337
  gemination and, 339
  hypophosphatasia and, 526
  hypophosphatemia and, 528, 529f
  incisors with, 167f
  silver points in, 188f
Root caries, 266
Root development
  Burkitt's tumor and, 480
  dens in dente and, 342
Root-form dental implant, 687, 689f
  osseous integration and, 690f
Root fractures
  periodontal diseases and, 325
  trauma and, 269
Root fragments, antroliths v., 584
Root resorption
  ameloblastoma and, 420, 420f
  benign neoplasm v., 411
  dental concussion and, 616
  fibrous dysplasia and, 489
  malignant ameloblastoma and, 466
  nasopalatine duct cyst and, 401, 403f
  neurilemoma and, 439, 439f, 440
  radiolucent ameloblastoma and, 422f
  sarcomas and, 459
Root sheath, dens in dente and, 340
Root structure, periodontal disease and, 315, 315b
Root surface
  composition of teeth and, 166
  external resorption and, 358
  periapical inflammatory lesions and, 366
  toothbrush injury and, 355
Root surface lesions
  cementoenamel junction and, 304
  gingival recession and, 303-304
  radiographic study and, 304, 309f
Root tips
  buccal bifurcation cyst and, 392
  panoramic imaging and, 191
Roots, 167, 167f, 170
  benign cementoblastoma and, 435
  central beam and, 125
  hemangioma and, 448
  hypercementosis and, 362, 363f
  lamina dura and, 168, 169f
  lateral periodontal cyst and, 398
  radicular cyst and, 385

Roots (*Continued*)
    segmental odontomaxillary dysplasia
        and, 651
    stereoscopy technique and, 249, 249f
Roots, lower teeth, mandibular canal v.,
    184, 184f
Rotating anode, dissipating heat and, 8, 9f
Rotating plate scans, PSP systems, 231
Rotational scanography, periodontal
    disease and, 250
Round cell sarcoma, 473
Round position-indication device (PID),
    film holders and, 59
Rubber dam clamp, intraoral periapical
    examination and, 164
RUNX2 gene, cleidocranial dysplasia and,
    646

S

Sacrum, neurilemoma and, 439
Safelight filters, fogging and, 112
Safelighting, equipment for, 98-99, 100f
Sagittal plane
    conventional tomography and, 547
    lateral mandibular occlusal projection
        and, 159
    panoramic imaging and, 208
Sagittal planes, MRI and, 549-550
Sagittal tomogram
    bifid condyle and, 555f
    coronoid hyperplasia and, 554, 554f
    juvenile chronic arthritis and, 364f
Salicylates, giant osteoid osteoma v., 450
Saliva
    dental caries and, 297
    paper film packets and, 118
Saliva, artificial, autoimmune sialadenitis
    and, 670
Salivary duct, 666
Salivary factors, attrition and, 354
Salivary gland disease. *See also* Salivary
    glands
    clinical signs and symptoms of, 658
    definition of, 658
    differential diagnosis in, 658-659, 659b
    image interpretation of, 665-675
Salivary gland parenchyma, MRI and, 260
Salivary gland tumors
    benign mixed tumor v., 672
    salivary glands v., 660
    statistical data on, 671
Salivary glands
    autoimmune sialadenitis, 669
    computed tomography scanners and,
        252
    cystic lesions of, 671
    diagnostic imaging of, 659
        algorithm for, 659, 660
    differential diagnosis of enlargements
        in, 659b
    extraoral radiography of, 660
    extrinsic malignant tumors and, 571
    intraoral radiography of, 660
    malignant ameloblastoma and, 466
    malignant tumors of, 673
    plain film radiography of, 660
    radiation and, 33
    sialodochitis and, 668
    sialography of, 660-663, 662f
    sialoliths in, 603
    tc-pertechnetate and, 664
    therapeutic radiation and, 305

Salivary stimulants
    autoimmune sialadenitis and, 670
    sialadenosis and, 670
Salivary stones, 665
    applied radiology and, 603-604
    sialoliths and, 603
Sarcomas
    mandible and, 459
    posterior jaw region and, 459
Satellite microcysts, odontogenic
    keratocyst and, 394
Scaling
    periodontitis and, 314
    squamous cell carcinoma and, 463
Scanography, overview of, 250, 250f
Scanora integrated imaging system
    mandible and, 683f
    maxilla and, 682f
ScanX system, photostimulable phosphor
    plates and, 231
Scarring, localized (traumatic) myositis
    ossificans and, 610
Scattered radiation, overview of, 80
Schick #2 CMOS sensor, 229f
Schlerotic border, florid osseous dysplasia
    and, 496
Schlerotic metastasis, metastatic tumors
    and, 467
Schwann cells
    neurilemoma from, 439
    neurofibroma and, 440
Schwannomas, 439
    neurofibromatosis and, 441
Scintigraphy
    osteoid osteoma v., 454
    radiopharmaceuticals in glands and, 664
    salivary gland tumors and, 672
    scintillation crystal and, 262
    septic arthritis and, 565
    xerostomia and, 660
Scintillation crystal
    computerized axial transverse scanning
        and, 250
    gamma scintillation camera and, 262
Scleroderma, 531
Sclerosing osteitis
    ill-defined borders in, 288, 289f
    osteoid osteoma v., 454
    radiopaque presentations of, 367
Sclerosis
    fibrosarcoma and, 475
    periapical inflammatory lesion and, 369
    pericoronitis and, 373
    periodontal disease and, 317
Sclerostenosis, osteopetrosis v., 531
Sclerotic bone
    osteoid osteoma and, 452
    periapical cemental dysplasia, 492
    vertical osseous defects and, 320
Sclerotic border, radicular cyst and, 385
Sclerotic margin, periapical cemental
    dysplasia and, 284f, 288
Scout film, infusion of contrast solution
    and, 661
Scout panoramic radiograph, orienting
    subsequent tomograms and, 682f
Screen film, 71
    dentistry and, 74-75
    design of, 74-75
    types of, 74
Screen phosphors, screen structure mottle
    and, 82

Screen structure mottle, fast intensifying
    screens and, 82
Seasoned solution, 97
Second molar
    central ray projection and, 153
    cross-sectional mandibular occlusal
        projection, 158
    dilaceration of root in, 342
Second premolar
    dental anomalies and, 2667
    film placement and, 126, 134, 144
    hypodontia and, 333, 333f
    image field and, 134, 144
    lateral periodontal cyst, 398
    projection of central ray and, 133, 143
Secondary dentin
    clinical features of, 360
    composition of teeth and, 166
    definition of, 360
    differential diagnosis of, 360-361
    management of, 360-361
    radiographic features of, 360-361
Secondary dentition, internal resorption
    and, 356
Secondary electrons, Compton scattering
    and, 19
Secondary hyperparathyroidism
    osteopetrosis v., 531
    overview of, 517
Secondary infections, florid osseous
    dysplasia and, 496
Secondary malignancy, 458, 466
Secondary voltage, 10
Sedation, mentally disabled patients and,
    163
Segmental hemifacial hyperplasia,
    segmental odontomaxillary dysplasia
    v., 651
Segmental neurofibromatosis, 441, 442f
Segmental odontomaxillary dysplasia
    (SOD)
    clinical features of, 651
    definition of, 651
    differential diagnosis of, 651
    hemifacial hyperplasia v., 651
    panoramic view of, 652f
    radiographic features of, 651
Segmentation, image analysis and, 239
Selection criteria, radiographic guidelines
    and, 272
Selective excitation, RF pulse and, 260
Selenium
    flat panel detectors and, 231
    radionuclide-labeled tracers and, 260
Self-rectified, x-ray and, 11
Sella turcica
    hyperpituitarism and, 521, 522f
    lateral cephalometric projection and,
        218-220, 219f
Sensitivity sites, 94
    x-ray film and, 95f
Sensors, contamination and, 118
Septa
    ameloblastoma and, 420, 420f
    aneurysmal bone cyst and, 504
    central giant cell granuloma and, 502,
        503f
    central mucoepidermoid carcinoma
        and, 465
    cysts having, 384
    desmoplastic fibromas of bone in, 454,
        455f

Septa (Continued)
  maxillary sinus and, 179, 179f
  odontogenic keratocyst and, 395f
  odontogenic myxoma and, 434, 435f
Septal bone, periodontal disease and, 321
Septic arthritis
  chronic osteomyelitis and, 379
  clinical features of, 564-565
  definition of, 564-565
  differential diagnosis of, 565
  diffuse sclerosing osteomyelitis and, 378
  joint effusion v., 567
  radiographic features of, 565
  treatment of, 565
Sequestra, osteomyelitis, 374
Sequestrectomy
  osteomyelitis and, 380
  osteoradionecrosis and, 382
Serous nonsecretory retention pseudocyst,
    581
Serum alkaline phosphatase, Paget's
    disease and, 509
Serum alkaline phosphatase level, primary
    hyperparathyroidism and, 518
Severe periodontitis, bone loss and,
    320-321
Shadows, radiolucent airway, soft tissues
    and, 207
Sharpness, 82
  image clarity and, 86
Short reception time (TR), 259
SI system, units of measurement in, 20-21
Sialadenitis
  parotid area and, 658
  salivary glands and, 658
Sialadenosis
  definition of, 670
  radiographic features of, 670
  treatment of, 670
Sialectasia, sialogogue administration and,
    669
Sialectasis, 669, 669f
Sialodochitis
  clinical features of, 668
  definition of, 668
  treatment of, 668
Sialography
  benign tumors presenting on, 672
  cystic lesions and, 671
  lateral view of submandibular gland and,
    668f
  parotid glands, 662f
  salivary gland disease and, 659
  salivary glands and, 658
  sialodochitis v., 668
  staging autoimmune disorders with, 669
  stones and, 604
  submandibular gland and, 663f, 666f,
    667f
Sialolithiasis
  applied radiology and, 603-604
  clinical features of, 603, 665
  definition of, 603, 665
  differential diagnosis and, 604-605
  management of, 605
  radiographic features of, 603, 665
  synonyms for, 665
  treatment of, 666-667
Sialoliths
  calcified lymph nodes v., 599
  cysticercus v., 601
  intraoral radiography and, 660

Sialoliths (Continued)
  occlusal radiographs and, 271
  phleboliths v., 605, 606
  plain film radiography and, 660
  ultrasonography and, 665
Sicca syndrome, 668
Sickle cell anemia
  clinical features of, 533
  definition of, 533
  osteomyelitis and, 374
  radiographic features of, 533
Sickle cell crises, 533
Sievert (Sv), effective dose and, 21
Signal intensity, fourier transform and, 259
Silicates, restorative materials as, 187, 188f
Silicon atom, outer shells of, 228f
Silicon sheet implants, computed
    tomography (CT) and, 548
Silver
  disposing of, 105
  environmental damage and, 104
Silver amalgam, restorative materials and,
    187, 187f
Silver atoms, 96, 96f
Silver bromide crystals, 94, 96, 96f
  developers and, 97
  in emulsion, 95f
Silver halide, 96
Silver halide crystals, 94, 97
  developer and, 97
Silver halide grains
  dental film composition and, 71
  extraoral radiography and, 58
  image sharpness and, 82-83
  x-ray beam and, 77
  x-ray film and, 82
Silver ions, developer and, 96, 96f
Silver points
  endodontic therapy and, 187, 188f
  root canals and, 188f
Silver thiosulfate
  changing solutions and, 102
  washing and, 98
SIMPlant, diagnostic hardware from, 686,
    688f
Simple bone cysts
  clinical features of, 405
  differential diagnosis of, 407
  Langerhans' cell histiocytosis v., 513
  management of, 407-408
  odontogenic myxoma and, 434, 435f
  radiographic features of, 405-406
  shape of, 405, 406f
  synonyms for, 405
Simple odontogenic fibroma, 438
Sinografin, ductal system and, 663
Sinonasal fungal disease, 588
Sinus disease, maxillary teeth pain and,
    269
Sinus floor, sarcomas and, 459, 460f
Sinus mucosa, fractures of alveolar process
    and, 629
Sinus obliteration, craniofacial fibrous
    dysplasia and, 593
Sinus ostium, osteoma and, 586
Sinus polyposis, 584
Sinus polyps, T2-weighted image of, 584f
Sinus tract, endodontics and, 164
Sinuses
  dental structures in, 593
  lateral cephalometric projection and,
    219f, 220

Sinuses (Continued)
  loss of function of
    three sides of, 177
Sinusitis
  clinical features of, 579
  definition of, 578-579
  epithelial papilloma v., 586
  fractured tooth roots and, 593
  management of, 581
  mucosa thickening and, 579f
  odontogenic cysts and, 590
  radiographic features of, 579-581, 581f
  rhinoliths and, 607
  squamous cell carcinoma v., 588
  three subtypes of, 579
Size 2 film
  adults and, 74
  bitewing projection and, 298
Sjögren syndrome, 668
  parotid area v., 658
  submandibular gland and, 659
Skeletal deformities, osteogenesis
    imperfecta and, 347
Skeletal dysplasia, crouzon syndrome and,
    64
Skeletal fractures, panoramic radiographic
    views and, 163
Skin
  cysticercus cellulosae and, 601
  dental radiography and, 52
  hemangioma v., 445
  Langerhans' cell histiocytosis and, 509
  neurofibromatosis and, 441
  progressive systemic sclerosis and, 531
  rectangular position-indication device
    and, 59
Skin lesions, basal cell nevus syndrome
    and, 397
Skull
  ameloblastoma and, 419
  lateral cephalometric projection and,
    218-220, 219f
  ossification of stylohyoid ligament and,
    609
  osteomas and, 443
  Paget's disease in, 507
  submentovertex projection and, 215
  thalassemia and, 534, 534f
  waters projection and, 213
  wide latitude films and, 81
Skull base, submentovertex (SMV)
    projection and, 545
Skull view radiographs, maxillary sinus
    disease and, 577
Skull views, extraoral projections as, 74,
    210
Slice-selecting, MR image and, 260
Slice thickness, frequency range adn, 260
SLOB (same lingual opposite buccal), 91
Slow scan direction, photostimulable
    phosphor plates and, 231
Smoking
  annual E and, 51
  periodontitis and, 314
  prenatal irradiation vs., 39, 40t
SMV projection
  condyle and, 548f
  midsagittal plane and, 548f
Snap-A-Ray, 125
Sodium bicarbonate, developers and, 97
Sodium etidronate, Paget's disease and,
    509

Sodium flouride, radiation caries and, 36
Sodium hypochlorite, film contamination and, 119
Sodium sulfite
    developers and, 97
    developing agents in, 97
Soft mixed odontoma, 428
Soft odontoma, 428
Soft palate, primary carcinomas and, 459
Soft tissue component of TMJ, 540
Soft tissue contrast, MRI and, 260
Soft tissue imaging
    indications for, 542-543
    overview of, 548-550
    trauma and, 615
Soft tissue infections, diagnostic imaging of, 380
Soft tissue injury, craniofacial disjunction and, 633
Soft tissue mass, squamous cell carcinoma and, 461
Soft tissue structures
    dental root fractures v, 622
    MRI and, 664
    overview of, 204f, 207, 208f
    panoramic image and, 204f
Soft tissues
    calcifications and, 597
    coronoid hyperplasia v., 554
    digital detector characteristics and, 232, 233f
    malignant ameloblastoma and, 466
    MRI and, 549-550
Software programs, digital imaging and, 240f
Solitary bone cyst, 405
Solitary intraosseous lesions, Langerhans' cell histiocytosis v., 513
Solitary myositis, 610
Solitary plasmacytoma, osteosarcoma v., 469
Somatic effects
    atomic bomb and, 41
    characteristics of exposure and, 41
    radiation effects and, 39
Sonic energy, sonography and, 263
Soradex Scanora
    facial skeletal images and, 197
    scanography and, 250, 252f
Space-occupying, lesion as, 291
Spatial resolution, digital detector characteristics and, 232
Specific barrier thickness, factors for calculating, 64
SPECT (single photon emission computed tomography)
    Anger camera and, 262
    diffuse sclerosing osteomyelitis and, 378
    nuclear medicine and, 262
Spectrum of photon energies, constant tube voltage (kVp) and, 13, 14f
Sphenoid bones
    fractures and, 629
    Gardner's syndrome and, 445, 446f
    mid-facial area and, 204
Sphenoid sinuses, 205
    development of, 577
    functions of, 577
    lateral cephalometric projection and, 218-220, 219f
    mucocele in, 585

Spiculated bone formation, non-Hodgkin's lymphoma and, 478
Spiculated periosteal response, chronic osteomyelitis and, 380
Spiculation, hemangioma and, 447f
Spin down, MRI and, 256, 257, 258
Spin-spin relaxation time, 259
Spin up, MRI and, 256, 257, 258
Spinal stenosis, 3D CT and, 254, 255f
Spinal structures, panoramic image and, 204f
Spiral scanners, computed tomography (CT) v., 251
Spiral tomography, 246, 246f
Spleen, sickle cell anemia and, 533
Splenomegaly, acute leukemias and, 481
Splint therapy, degenerative joint disease and, 562
Spongiosa. See Cancellous bone
Spontaneous mutations, crouzon syndrome and, 64
Spontaneous rate, cancers and, 41
Spontaneous remission, osteoid osteoma v., 454
Spots, light, faulty radiographs and, 107b
Spots,dark, faulty radiographs and, 107b
Squamotympanic fissure, sagittal plane and, 540
Squamous cell carcinoma
    anterior maxilla and, 290f
    clinical features of, 459, 461, 587
    definition of, 587
    dentigerous cyst and, 392
    differential diagnosis of, 461, 588
    effects on surrounding structures and, 461
    internal structure of, 461
    Langerhans' cell histiocytosis v., 513
    management of, 461, 463, 588
    metastatic lesions of parotid gland and, 675
    metastatic tumors v., 467
    minor salivary glands and, 675
    osteomyelitis v., 376, 377
    osteoradionecrosis v., 382
    overview of, 459
    panoramic image of, 588f
    paranasal sinuses and, 586
    pericoronitis v., 373
    periodontal disease v., 326-327
    periphery and shape of, 461
    radiographic features of, 461, 587-588
Squamous cell carcinoma originating in bone, 463
Squamous cell carcinoma originating in cyst
    clinical features of, 464
    cyst cortex and, 464f
    differential diagnosis of, 464
    effects on surrounding structures and, 464
    internal structure of, 464
    management of, 464
    overview of, 464
    periphery and shape of, 464
    radiographic features of, 464
    synonyms for, 464
Stafne bone cyst, 651
Stafne defect, 651
    residual cyst v., 388
Stainless steel pins
    amalgam restoration and, 188f
    restorative materials as, 187, 188f

Standard conditions of temperature and pressure (STP), exposure and, 20
Standard transmission radiography, scanography v., 250, 252f
Static bone cavity, 651
Stationary anode, 8
Stem cells, gastrointestinal syndrome and, 38-39
Stensen duct, sialoliths and, 660
Step deformity, 202
Step-wedge test
    dosimeter v., 115
    mandibular body fractures and, 625, 626f
    processing system and, 111
Stereoscopy technique, overview of, 248-249
Sterioscopic panoramic plain film projections, sialolith and, 662f
Sternocleidomastoid, localized (traumatic) myositis ossificans and, 610
Steroids, chondrocalcinosis and, 566
Stir solutions, manual tank processing and, 101
Stochastic effect(s), 51
    radiation and, 25
Stones, occlusal radiography and, 160
Storage phosphor plates, bitewings captured on301f
Streak artifacts, MRI and, 664
Streptococci, dental caries and, 297
Stress, periodontal disease and, 327
Strontium-90, Nevada test site and, 51
Sturge-Weber syndrome, arteriosclerosis and, 602
Stylohyoid chain ossification, ossification of stylohyoid ligament, 609
Stylohyoid ligament, ossification of, 609, 609f
Stylohyoid syndrome, ossification of stylohyoid ligament in, 609
Styloid process, ossification of stylohyoid ligament in, 609
Subacute sinusitis, overview of, 579
Subacute suppurative osteomyelitis, 374
Subchondral cyst, rheumatoid arthritis v., 563
Subchondral sclerosis
    degenerative joint disease v., 561, 562f
    remodeling and, 559, 561f
Subcutaneous fibromas, Gardner's syndrome and, 445
Subcutaneous neurofibromas, neurofibromatosis and, 442
Subcutaneous tissues, hemangioma v., 445
Subject contrast, 79
    film contrast and, 79
    film latitude and, 81
    overview of, 79
Subject density, variations in, 78
Subject thickness, image and, 78
Subjective image enhancement, image interpretation and, 235
Sublingual glands
    CT and, 663
    lingual salivary gland depression v., 654
    occlusal radiography and, 160
    stones in, 603
Subluxation of teeth
    overview of, 617
    TMJ dysfunction and, 538
Submandibular duct, sialoliths and, 660

Submandibular fossa, mental fossa and, 183, 183f
Submandibular gland area, enlargements of, 659
Submandibular gland fossa
    anatomical overview of, 185-186, 185f
    lingual salivary gland depression and, 651, 653f
    radiographic image of, 186, 186f
Submandibular glands
    CT and, 663
    malignant tumors of, 673
    occlusal radiography and, 160
    sialodochitis and, 668
    sialoliths and, 603
Submandibular lymph nodes
    calcified lymph nodes and, 599, 600f
    cherubism and, 506
Submandibular salivary glands
    calcified lymph nodes and, 599
    radiation effects on, 34f
Submandibular sialoliths, 605f
Submandibular space infection, submandibular gland and, 659
Submentovertex projection
    anatomic landmarks for, 214f
    central x-ray beam position and, 213
    condyle and, 539
    image receptor and, 213
    interrogating, 220, 220f
    overview of, 545-546
    resultant image in, 213, 215, 217f
    uses for, 546
    zygomatic arch in, 635, 635f
Submentovertex skull view, mandibular fracture and, 615
Subperiosteal implant, denture support and, 678f
Subpixels, 234
Subtraction images
    digital images and, 301
    digital subtraction radiography and, 238, 238f
    radiographs and, 305f
Subtraction radiography, periodontal disease and, 316
Sulfer compounds, 94
Summit of eminence, TMJ and, 540
Superimposed teeth, 207-208
    conrescence and, 337
Superior alveolar nerves, 178
    sinus and, 178
Superior foramina, of nasopalatine canal, 174
Superior foramina of nasopalatine canal, position of, 175f
Superior joint space
    arthrography v., 548
    interarticular disk and, 540, 541f
    radiographic joint space v., 541, 541f
Superior lamina, posterior attachment (retrodiskal tissues) and, 541
Superior sinus wall, 173, 174f
Supernumerary teeth
    clinical features of, 330
    complete twinning and, 338
    dental anomalies and, 2667
    dentigerous cyst and, 388
    differential diagnosis for, 331
    management of, 331-332
    microdontia and, 335
    radiographic features of, 330-331

Supernumerary teeth (Continued)
    synonyms for, 330
    transposition and, 336
Supernumerary teeth, unerupted, cleidocranial dysplasia and, 646, 648, 649f
Supplemental teeth, 330
    deciduous dentition and, 331, 332f
    demographic information on, 330
Sures, Waters projection and, 221
Surface disinfection, 115
Surface exposures, relationship of diagnostic density and, 56f
Surgery. See also Excision, surgical; Orthognathic surgery
    ameloblastoma and, 422
    ankylosis and, 569
    arteriovenous (A-V) fistula and, 449
    benign tumors and, 672
    calcifying epithelial odontogenic tumors and, 423
    carious lesions and, 311
    cemental dysplasia and, 495
    cementoossifying fibroma v., 501
    central mucoepidermoid carcinoma and, 465
    cherubism and, 507
    chondrocalcinosis and, 566
    chrondrosarcoma and, 472, 473
    cleft palate and, 640
    coronoid hyperplasia and, 554
    craniofacial disjunction and, 634
    crouzon syndrome and, 641
    cystic lesions and, 671, 671f
    dentigerous cyst and, 392
    dermoid cysts and, 404
    desmoplastic fibromas of bone v., 454
    Ewing's sarcoma and, 474
    fibrosarcoma v., 475
    fibrous dysplasia and, 489
    fracture and, 568
    hemangioma and, 448
    malignant ameloblastoma and, 466
    malignant tumors and, 572, 673
    metastatic tumors and, 467
    MRI and, 260
    mucocele and, 585
    odontogenic keratocyst and, 396
    odontogenic myxoma v., 434
    osteomyelitis and, 377, 380
    osteosarcoma v., 469
    Paget's disease and, 509
    periodontitis and, 314
    progression of lesion and, 301
    radicular cyst and, 387
    squamous cell carcinoma and, 461, 588
    stones and, 605
    supplemental teeth and, 331
    Treacher Collins syndrome and, 646
Surgery, endoscopic, chronic sinusitis and, 581, 581f
Surgery, joint
    juvenile arthrosis v., 553
    rheumatoid arthritis and, 563
    synovial chondromatosis v., 566
Surgery, orthodontic, juvenile arthrosis v., 553
Surgery, orthognathic
    condylar hyperplasia and, 551
    condylar hypoplasia and, 552
    juvenile arthrosis v., 553
    neonatal fractures and, 569

Surgery, TMJ, fibrous adhesions and, 555-556
Surgical drainage, joint effusion and, 567
Survival curves, irradiation and, 29, 30f, 32f
Sutural synostosis, crouzon syndrome and, 641f
Sutures, posteroanterior cephalometric projection and, 221-222, 222f
Swelling. See also Edema
    ameloblastic fibromas and, 428
    ameloblastoma and, 419
    aneurysmal bone cyst and, 503
    arteriovenous (A-V) fistula and, 449
    calcifying epithelial odontogenic tumor and, 422
    central giant cell granuloma and, 502
    central mucoepidermoid carcinoma and, 465
    cherubism and, 506
    craniofacial disjunction and, 633
    dermoid cysts, 404
    giant osteoid osteoma v., 450
    hemangioma and, 445
    imaging for jaw pathology in, 268
    inflammation and, 366
    jaw lesions and, 469
    neurilemoma and, 439
    neurofibroma and, 441
    osteoid osteoma and, 452
    radicular cyst and, 385
    rheumatoid arthritis and, 563
    salivary glands and, 669
    squamous cell carcinoma originating in cyst and, 464
    synovial chondromatosis and, 565
    TMJ dysfunction and, 538
Swelling, facial
    desmoplastic fibroma of bone and, 454
    monostotic fibrous dysplasia and, 485
Syndromic craniosynostosis, 640
Synodontia, 336
Synovial chondromatosis
    chondrocalcinosis and, 566
    clincal features of, 565
    definition of, 565
    differential diagnosis of, 565-566
    radiographic features of, 565
    synonyms of, 565
    treatment of, 566
Synovial chondrometaplasia, 565
Synovial fluid
    synovial chondromatosis and, 565
    synovial membrane and, 541
Synovial hypertrophy, juvenile chronic arthritis v., 364
Synovial inflammation, juvenile chronic arthritis v., 364
Synovial membrane, synovial fluid and, 541
Synovial membrane inflammation, rheumatoid arthritis and, 563
Synovial osteochondromatosis, 565
    CT image of, 566f
Synovial sarcoma, primary intrinsic malignant tumors and, 571
Synovitis, TMJ and, 269
Synovitis, chronic, chondrocalcinosis and, 566
Synovium, articular loose bodies and, 565
Synthetic phenolic compounds, surface cleaners and, 116

Syphilis, dystrophic calcification in tonsils v., 599

Systematic approach, image analysis with, 282

Systemic diseases
    changes to dental structures in, 516, 518f
    osteomyelitis and, 374
    periodontal disease and, 314, 327
    periodontitis and, 314
    radiographic changes and characteristics in, 516, 517t

Systemic infection, cancer and, 458

Systemic lupus erythematosus, autoimmune sialadenitis and, 669

Systemic steroids, osteopetrosis and, 531

Systems compatibility, digital imaging and, 240-241

T

T2-weighted pulse sequences, MRI and, 550

T-grain film
    extraoral radiography and, 58
    rare earth screens and, 58

T-grains of silver halide, 75f

T-mat films, 74, 75f
    extraoral radiography and, 58
    sensitivity of, 76f

T1 relaxation time, 259

T2 relaxation time, 259

T1-weighted images, 259
    advantages of, 259-260
    hemangiomas and, 673
    TMJ and, 261f

T2-weighted images
    cystic lesions and, 671, 671f
    hemangiomas and, 673
    inflammatory changes and, 260

T1-weighted post contrast, MRI and, 664

T1-weighted pulse sequences, MRI and, 550

Taenia solium (pork tapeworm), cysticercosis and, 601

Talon cusp
    clinical features of, 351-352
    definition of, 351
    differential diagnosis of, 352
    management of, 352
    radiographic features of, 352

Tank, insert, 100

Tank, master, 100

Tank, processing, 100
    diagram of, 101f

Target, purpose of, 8, 9f

Taste buds, radiation and, 33

Taurodontism
    clinical features of, 339
    definition of, 339
    differential diagnosis of, 340
    management of, 340
    radiographic features of, 339, 339f

Tc-pertechnetate, scintigraphy and, 664

TCOF1 gene, Treacher Collins syndrome v., 643

Technetium bone scans
    central giant cell granuloma v., 503
    septic arthritis and, 565

Technetium pertechnetate, radionuclide-labeled tracers and, 260

Teeth. *See* Erupted teeth; Erupted teeth, accelerated; Erupted teeth, delayed; Unerupted teeth
    aging and, 167
    benign neoplasm and, 411
    benign tumors and, 410
    body height and, 333
    central ray and, 127
    cleft palate and, 640
    cleidocranial dysplasia and, 646
    composition of, 166-168
    cysts and, 384
    demineralization progression and, 297
    dental anomalies and, 2667
    dental concussion and, 616
    dental trauma and, 615
    diabetes mellitus and, 523
    disorders of endocrine system and, 516
    fibrosarcoma and, 475
    film holding instruments and, 124-125
    film placement and, 130, 138
    interpretation of images and, 208-209
    irradiation of, 34
    lateral cephalometric projection and, 219f, 220
    leukemia and, 482
    mandibular canal and, 184
    metastatic lesions of, 459, 461f, 467
    non-Hodgkin's lymphoma and, 477
    osseointegrated implants and, 269
    osteomalacia and, 525
    panoramic film and, 200, 200f
    panoramic image and, 201
    premolar bitewing projection and, 150
    projection of central ray and, 143
    rickets and, 525
    segmental odontomaxillary dysplasia and, 651
    sequence of, examination process and, 283
    structure of, attrition and, 354, 354f
    supporting structures of, 168-187
    surface of
        demineralization of, 298
        follow-up radiograph of, 312
        lesion shape and, 299
    traumatic injuries of, 269, 616
    vertical angulation and, 148
    wear patterns of, attrition and, 354, 354f

Teeth, deformed, compound odontomas and, 425

Teeth, developing, lesions in, 292

Teeth, development of, panoramic imaging and, 191

Teeth, displaced
    adjacent teeth to, 617
    odontogenic tumors and, 590

Teeth, embedded, PDL and, 170

Teeth, erupted. *See* Erupted teeth

Teeth, impacted. *See* Impacted teeth

Teeth, loose
    acute leukemias and, 481
    hemangioma and, 446
    osteosarcoma and, 469

Teeth, missing
    aggressive periodontitis and, 324
    maxillary sinus floor and, 178, 178f
    radicular dilaceration and, 340

Teeth, primary, male v. female size of, 334

Teeth, restored, periapical radiographs and, 298

Teeth, subluxated permanent, management of, 618

Teeth, transposed. *See* Transposition

Teeth displacement, cementoossifying fibroma v., 449, 499, 500

Temperature
    film processing and, 102, 104
    processing stations and, 111

Temporal bones
    glenoid fossa, 539, 540f
    hemifacial hyperplasia and, 650
    mid-facial area and, 204
    submentovertex projection and, 220, 220f

Temporal component of TMJ, 540

Temporomandibular joint (TMJ), 205
    anatomy of, 541f
    ankylosing spondylitis and, 564
    computed tomography scanners and, 252, 254f
    coronoid hyperplasia and, 554
    developmental abnormalities of, 550-554
    diagnostic imaging of, 542-565
    disease affecting, 269
    extraoral radiography and, 283
    extrinsic tumors of, 570
    fibrosarcoma and, 474
    film based tomography and, 245
    hemifacial microsomia, 644f
    intrinsic tumors of, 570
    joint effusion and, 567
    juvenile arthrosis and, 553
    juvenile chronic arthritis v., 364
    linear tomogram of, 247f
    MRI and, 260, 261f
    MRI of normal, 549f
    orthophos Plus and, 197
    orthoralix S and, 197
    ossification of stylohyoid ligament and, 609
    osteoblastomas in, 450
    panoramic image and, 201, 202
    PM 2002 CC Proline and, 197, 197f
    psoriatic arthritis and, 564
    radiographic abnormalities of, 550
    rheumatoid arthritis and, 563
    sagittal plane and, 540
    septic arthritis and, 564
    stereoscopy technique and, 249, 249f
    synovial chondromatosis and, 565
    T1-weighted MR image and, 261f
    transorbital projection and, 544-545
    Ultrasound image of, 264f

Temporomandibular joint (TMJ) ankylosis
    bilateral fractures v., 569
    rheumatoid arthritis and, 569

Temporomandibular joint (TMJ) dysfunction
    bifid condyle and, 554
    clinical features of, 538
    condylar hypoplasia and, 552
    diagnostic imaging in, 538-539
    diagnostic imaging of, 542-565
    internal derangement and, 555
    malignancy v., 571
    overview of, 538
    radiographic anatomy of, 539-542
    signs and symptoms of, 538

Temporomandibular joint (TMJ) fractures, condylar neck and, 567

Temporomandibular joint (TMJ) imaging
    goal of, 269
    purposes of, 538-639

Temporomandibular joint (TMJ) pain, soft tissue imaging and, 548
Temporomandibular joint (TMJ) symptoms, panoramic projection and, 543, 543f
Temporoparietal bossing, basal cell nevus syndrome and, 397
Teratomas, 404
Terminal foramina, composition of teeth and, 166, 167f
Terrestrial radiation, overview of, 48-49
Tertiary dentin, 360
Tetany
    hypoparathyroidism and, 519
    pseudohypoparathyroidism and, 519
Thalassemia
    clinical features of, 533
    definition of, 533
    multiple myeloma v., 477
    radiographic features of, 533, 536
    synonyms for, 533
Thermal conductivity, target with, 8
Thermal conductor, target melting and, 8
Thermometer, overview of, 99, 101
Thickened mucous membrane, 578
Thickness of cut, focal plane and, 247
Thin film transistor (TFT)
    computer displays and, 234
    flat panel detectors and, 231
Thiosulfate ions, washing and, 98
Third molar
    ameloblastic fibroma and, 430f
    coronoid process and, 187, 187f
    external oblique ridge v., 186, 186f
    hypodontia and, 333, 333f
    image field and, 134, 144, 146, 156
    lateral mandibular occlusal projection and, 159
    mandibular body fractures and, 625
    microdontia in, 335
    panoramic imaging and, 191
    projection of central ray and, 147
Third molar-retromolar area, reverse-Towne projection and, 218
Third molar buds, hypopituitarism and, 522
3-D Dental software, reformatted CT study using, 684f, 685f
THREE 3D Accuitomo, CBCT and, 255
Three-dimensional reformatting, interpolation and, 252, 253f
Three-walled, vertical osseous defects as, 319
THREE3D CT (three-dimensional images), rotation manipulation of, 254, 255f
(3)D CT (three-dimensional images), 252
Throglossal duct cysts, dermoid cysts v., 404
Thrombi, hemangioma and, 448, 448f
Thrombocytopenia, acute radiation syndrome and, 39
Thymus gland, children and, 41
Thyroid cartilage, lateral cephalometric film of, 606f
Thyroid collar, 62f
    leaded apron with, 61f
Thyroid dose, radiographic examination and, 53
Thyroid exposure, FSFDs and, 59
Thyroid function tests, sialography and, 663

Thyroid glands
    dental radiography and, 52
    hyperthyroidism and, 522
    hypothyroidism and, 519, 522
    Iodine-131 and, 51
    radiation exposure of, 40
    tc-pertechnetate and, 664
Thyroid stimulating hormone (TSH), hypothyroidism and, 522
Thyrotoxicosis, 522
Thyroxin
    hyperthyroidism and, 522
    hypothyroidism and, 522
TIFF (Tagged Image File Format), digital imaging and, 240
Time-termperature processing, film quality and, 63
Timer, x-ray machine and, 11, 114
Timer, interval
    manual tank processing and, 102
    overview of, 99-101
Tinnitus, joint effusion and, 567
Tipped teeth, periodontal diseases and, 325
Tissue, 58
    effect of collimation, 58f
    radiation effects on, 30-32
    radiation-induced cancer and, 40b
    short-term effects of radiation on, 31
Tissue-weighing factor, smoking and, 51
Titanium dioxide, base material and, 76
TMJ remodeling. See Remodeling, TMJ
Tobacco, cancers and, 458
Tomographic angle, focal plane and, 247
Tomographic layer, focal plane and, 247
Tomographic views
    multimodality machines and, 197
    pyramidal fracture in, 632
Tomography, film based
    film radiography and, 245-248
    movements in, 246f
    techniques in, 246f
Tomography, film-based. See also Body section radiograpny; Computed tomography (CT)
Tongue
    anteroposterior position radiograph and, 198
    dystrophic calcification and, 598
    film placement and, 134, 138, 144, 146
    hemifacial hyperplasia and, 650
    lateral cephalometric projection and, 219f, 220
    mandibular ramal area and, 202
    osteoma cutis and, 609
    primary carcinomas and, 459
    squamous cell carcinoma and, 461
Tongue, posterior dorsum, gag reflex and, 163
Tonsil concretions, 599
Tonsillar area
    non-Hodgkin's lymphoma and, 477
    primary carcinomas and, 459
Tonsillar calculi, 599
Tonsilloliths, 599. See also Dystrophic calcification in tonsils
    clinical features of, 599
    radiographic features of, 599
Tools, measurement, digital imaging software and, 239, 239f

Tooth. See Root; Root absorption; Root apex; Root canal therapy
Tooth, crown. See Crown, tooth
Tooth alignment, periodontal diseases and, 325f
Tooth apex, periapical inflammatory lesion and, 370
Tooth avulsion, chest film and, 615
Tooth bud, gemination and, 338
Tooth crown. See Crown, tooth
Tooth displacement
    aneurysmal bone cyst and, 504, 505f, 506f
    central odontogenic fibroma and, 438
    dentigerous cyst and, 390f, 391f
    residual cyst and, 388
Tooth germs
    fusion of teeth and, 336
    missing teeth and, 333
Tooth mobility
    dental root fractures and, 620
    periodontal diseases and, 325
Tooth pulp chamber, remnant beam in, 80
Tooth resorption
    aneurysmal bone cyst and, 504, 505f, 506f
    central giant cell granuloma and, 502
Tooth roots. See Roots
Toothache, periapical inflammatory lesion and, 368
Toothbrush injury
    abrasion and, 355
    clinical features of, 355
    radiographic features of, 355
Torus, osteomas v., 444
Torus mandibularis
    clinical features of, 413-414
    occlusal radiograph of, 416f
    radiographic features of, 414, 415f
Torus palatinus
    clinical features of, 412
    occlusal radiograph of., 414f
    radiographic features of, 412-413
    torus mandibularis v., 413
Total beam exposure, 61
Total E, dental exposure and, 53
Totally radiolucent, lesion classification as, 289
Totally radiopaque, lesion classification as, 289
Towne's projection
    compression fracture in, 568f
    condylar neck fractures and, 545
    dystrophic calcification in tonsils and, 599
Toxic adenoma, hyperthyroidism and, 522
Trabeculae
    ameloblastoma and, 422
    anterior maxilla and, 170
    fibrous dysplasia and, 485
    hemangioma and, 447
    inflammation and, 290
    osteosarcoma and, 469, 470f
    Paget's disease in, 508
    patterns in fibrous dysplasia of, 487
    periapical sclerosing osteitis and, 370
    periodontal diseases and, 325
    remodeling and, 559
    rickets and, 525
Trabecular bone, 282. See also Cancellous bone
    composition of teeth and, 166

Trabecular pattern, 171, 171f
  cementoossifying fibroma and, 500f
  hemangioma and, 447f
Trabecular plates, 170-171, 171f
Trabeculation, alveolar process and, 203
Trachial cartilages, calcification of, 606
Tram-track appearance, arteriosclerosis
  and, 602
Transcranial projections
  conventional tomography v., 547
  hard tissue imaging and, 543, 543f
  left TMJ and, 546f
  transcranial series and, 543, 546f
  transorbital projection v., 545
Transducer, sonography and, 263
Transformer, primary, voltage aat, 10f
Transistor voltage, liquid crystal display
  (LCD) and, 234
Transitional dentition, panoramic
  projection, 273
Transorbital projections
  condylar neck fractures and, 545
  mandibular condyle fractures and, 626
  overview of, 544-545
  TMJ and, 547f
Transorbital view, condyle and, 547f
Transpharyngeal projections
  mandible and, 546f
  overview of, 544
  transorbital projection v., 545
Transport system, automatic film
  processors and, 103
Transposed teeth. See Transposition
Transposition
  clinical features of, 336
  differential diagnosis of, 336
  management of, 336
  radiographic features of, 336, 336f
Transverse fractures, craniofacial
  disjunction and, 634
Trauma, dental
  arteriovenous (A-V) fistula and, 449
  bifid condyle and, 554
  concrescence and, 337
  condylar head fractures and, 625
  condylar hypoplasia and, 552
  condylar neck fractures and, 625
  degenerative joint disease and, 559
  dental crown, 619
  dental root fractures and, 620
  dentin production and, 168
  dislocation and, 567
  effusion and, 566
  fracture and, 567
  intraoral periapical films and, 615
  intruded maxillary central incisor after,
    618f
  lateral incisor after, 618f
  localized (traumatic) myositis ossificans
    and, 610, 611f
  luxation of teeth and, 617
  mandibular, ankylosis and, 569
  mandibular body fractures and, 625
  maxillary sinuses and, 577
  panoramic imaging and, 191
  panoramic radiographs and, 269
  radicular cyst and, 385
  radiographs and, 163
  radiologic examination evaluation for
    secondary dentin and, 360
  submentovertex (SMV) projection and,
    546

Trauma, dental (Continued)
  tooth and, 167-168
  Turner's hypoplasia, 352
  zygomatic arch fractures and, 635
Trauma, facial. See also Trauma, dental
  inflammatory disease and, 578
Traumatic bone cyst, 405
Traumatic neuroma, 440
Treacher Collins syndrome (TCS)
  clinical features of, 643
  definition of, 643
  differential diagnosis of, 643, 646
  radiographic features of, 643
Treatment plan
  radiographic guidelines and, 272
  soft tissue imaging and, 548
Trismus
  fibrosarcoma and, 474
  occlusal radiography and, 160
  osteosarcoma and, 469
  septic arthritis and, 565
  special patient considerations and, 162
  squamous cell carcinoma and, 461
Trisomy 21 syndrome, taurodontism and,
  340
Triticeous, 607
True ankylosis, 569
True cementoma, 434
True concrescence, 337
Tube current (mA)
  filament step-down transformer and, 9
  spectrum of photons and, 13, 14f
Tube head
  angulation of, 125, 148
  disinfection of, 115
  multimodality machines and, 197
  patient procedure using, 122
  stability of, 115
  universal precautions with, 117f
  x-ray machine with, 7f
Tube rating, duty cycle and, 11
Tube shift technique, 91
  spatial position of object and, 91, 91f,
    92f
Tube voltage (kVp)
  changing, 14
  x-rays and, 9-10
Tuberales, 253
  surface formed by, 253
Tubercle, dens evaginates and, 343, 344f
Tuberculosis
  calcified lymph nodes and, 599, 600f
  infection control and, 115
Tuberosity, 282
  image field and, 134
Tumor(s), 428
  ameloblastic fibromas v., 428, 429
  bone-forming, localized (traumatic)
    myositis ossifcans and, 611
  calcifying odontogenic cyst and, 399
  cementoossifying fibroma v., 499
  condylar
    ankylosis v., 569
    TMJ swelling and, 570
  coronoid, benign tumors v., 571
  coronoid hyperplasia v., 554
  dermoid cysts v., 404
  external resorption and, 358
  extrafollicular, 431
  follicular, 431
  high-grade, 673, 675
  intercranial, 3D CT and, 254

Tumor(s) (Continued)
  jaw, characteristics of, 410
  metastatic
    jaws and, 571
    radiographic features of, 571
  neural, anterior loop of mandibular
    canal and, 203
  neurilemoma and, 439
  odontogenic, 418
    overview of, 590, 592
  osteoblastomas and, 452
  overview of, 570
  primary, osteoradionecrosis and, 380
  resorption and, 356
Tumor(s), benign
  adjacent tissues and, 411f
  central mucoepidermoid carcinoma v., 465
  clinical features of, 410, 570
  degenerative joint disease v., 562
  differential diagnosis of, 570-571
  displacement of adjacent teeth and, 412f
  giant osteoid osteoma and, 450
  host bone of, 412f
  of neural origin, 439-456
  overview of, 570, 671
  radiographic features of, 410-411, 570,
    671-672
  treatment of, 571, 672
Tumor cells, fractionation and, 33
Tumor mass, radon and, 33
Tumoral calcinosis, articular loose bodies
  and, 565
Tumors, brown
  cortical expansion of, 519, 520f
  primary hyperparathyroidism and, 518,
    519f
Tumors, malignant. See Malignant tumors
Tumors, metastatic
  definition of, 466
  minor salivary glands and, 674
Tungsten, characteristics of, 8
Tungsten target, 8
Turbinate bone, mid-facial area and, 204
Turner's hypoplasia
  clinical features of, 352
  definition of, 352
  differential diagnosis of, 353
  management of, 353
  radiographic features of, 353, 353f
Turner's tooth, 352
Twinning. See Gemination
Two-walled, vertical osseous defects as, 319
Type 1 collagen, osteogenesis imperfecta
  and, 347

U

Ulcers
  acute leukemias and, 481
  eosinophilic granuloma and, 509
  osteosarcoma and, 469
  radiation injury and, 39
  radiation treatment and, 33
Ultra-speed film, 73f
  characteristic curves and, 81f
  iodide and, 71
Ultra-Vision film, crossover and, 58
Ultrafast computed tomography (CT), CT
  technology and, 255
Ultrasonography
  advanced imaging procedures and, 271
  overview of, 262-263
  solid mass v. cystic and, 665

Ultrasound (US) imaging
   carious lesions and, 311
   cystic lesions and, 671, 671f
   fetus in, 263f
   inflammatory diseases and, 666
   salivary gland disease and, 660
   TMJ in, 263f
   Warthin tumor and, 673
Ultraviolet radiation, intensifying screens
   and, 83
Unerupted teeth
   ameloblastic fibromas and, 428
   ameloblastic fibromas v., 429
   calcifying epithelial odontogenic tumors
     and, 423
   dentigerous cyst and, 388
   Gardner's syndrome and, 445
   occult disease and, 268
   odontogenic keratocyst and, 394
   segmental odontomaxillary dysplasia
     and, 651
Unfavorable fractures, mandibular body
   fractures as, 625
Unicameral bone cysts, 405
Unicystic types, ameloblastoma and, 420,
   420f
Uniform difference image, digital
   subtraction radiography and, 238
Unilateral abnormality, normal anatomy
   and, 283
Unilateral epistaxis, zygomatic arch
   fractures and, 635
Unilateral fibrous dysplasia, 485
Units of measurement, SI system and, 20,
   20t
Universal precautions, cross-contamination
   and, 115
Urine, multiple myeloma and, 475

V

Van der Woude syndrome, facial clefts
   and, 639
Vapor pressure, tungsten and, 8
Variable-intensity light source, image
   density and, 64
Vascular lesions
   hemangioma and, 448
   intrinsic tumors of TMJ, 570
   mandibular canal and, 411
   neurilemoma v., 440
   neurofibroma and, 441
Vascular response, osteoradionecrosis and,
   380
Vascular tissue, jaw abnormalities and,
   285
Vegetative intermitotic cells,
   radiosensitivity and, 30
Vehicle, film and, 71
Vein, arteriovenous (A-V) fistula and, 449
Velocardiofacial syndrome, facial clefts
   and639
Ventilation, darkroom and, 98, 99f
Vertebrae
   lateral cephalometric projection and,
     219f, 220
   Paget's disease in, 507
Vertebral fusion, basal cell nevus syndrome
   and, 397
Vertical angulation
   maxillary anterior occlusal projection
     and, 161
   nasolacrimal canal and, 176

Vertical angulation (Continued)
   projection of central ray and, 127, 143
   tube head and, 125, 148
Vertical bitewing films, overview of, 149,
   149f
Vertical bitewings, periodontium and,
   316
Vertical defects
   moderate periodontitis and, 319-320,
     321f
   periodontal ligament space and, 321f
Vertical root fractures
   clinical features of, 623
   crown-root fractures and, 623
   definition of, 622-623
   management of, 623
   radiographic features of, 623
Videofluoroscopy, arthrography v., 548
Viewboxes, 110, 235
   cleaning of, 112
Villous synovitis, rheumatoid arthritis and,
   563
Vinyl packaging, contamination of film
   and, 119
Viral sialadenitis, submandibular gland
   and, 659
Vitality testing, mandibular canal and,
   184
Vitamin D
   osteomalacia and, 524
   pseudohypoparathyroidism and, 520
Vitamin D metabolite, renal
   osteodystrophy and, 526
Vitamin D-resistant rickets, 527
Voltage, x-rays and, 226
Voltage potential, 10
Vomer bone, 173
   mid-facial area and, 204
   midface fractures and, 629
Vomiting, erosion and, 356
Von Recklinghausen's disease, 441
   neurofibroma v., 440
Von Willebrand disease, pseudotumor and,
   588
Votage, at anode, 10f
Voxel length, computed tomography
   image and, 251
Voxels (volume elements)
   computed tomography image and, 251,
     253f
   Larmor frequency and, 260

W

Warthin tumor
   clinical features of, 672
   definition of, 672
   parotid area v., 658
   radiographic features of, 672
Washing solution
   film, 98
   temperature of, 100
Wastes, hazardous, digital imaging and,
   225
Wastes, radiographic, management of,
   104-105
Water
   radiolysis of, 26
   radionuclides and, 49
Water flouridation, rampant caries and,
   302
Water images, relaxation time and, 260
Water radiolysis, role of, 26

Waters' projection
   anatomic landmarks in, 215f
   central x-ray beam position in, 213
   horizontal fracture and, 631
   image receptor with, 213
   interrogating, 221
   mucosa thickening and, 579-580, 580f
   patient placement with, 213
   pyramidal fracture and, 632
   squamous cell carcinoma and, 587
Waters' skull view, maxillary sinus disease
   and, 578
Waters' tomographic views
   coronoid hyperplasia and, 553
   hypoplasia and, 576
Wavelength, 5
Wear facets, attrition and, 354
Weight loss
   multiple myeloma and, 475
   non-Hodgkin's lymphoma and, 477
Wharton's duct, submandibular stones
   and, 603
Whole blood transfusions, acute radiation
   syndrome and, 39
Whole-body radiation
   effects of, 37-39
   occupational exposure and, 52
Wide-angle tomography, disadvantages v.
   advantages of, 247, 248f
Wide latitude films, films and, 81
Wide uncalcified osteoid seams,
   osteomalacia and, 524
Wilms' tumor, metastatic tumors and, 466
Wire grids, periodontal disease and, 316
Woriman bones
   cleidocranial dysplasia and, 648, 648f
   osteogenesis imperfecta and, 347
World Health Organization (WHO)
   calcifying odontogenic cyst and, 399
   classification of odontogenic tumors by,
     418-419
   odontogenic fibroma and, 438

X

X-ray, medical, annual E of, 50
X-ray beam. *See also* Central x-ray beam
   beam attenuation in, 16
   computerized axial transverse scanning
     and, 250
   coronoid process and, 187
   dental implants and, 687
   double lamina dura nd, 169
   factors controlling, 13-16
   fracture and, 616
   gamma rays *vs.*, 5
   ghost images and, 207
   gold and, 187, 187f
   grid and, 84, 84f
   horizontal bitewing films and, 148
   intermaxillary suture and, 172
   kilovoltage and, 62
   means for limiting size of, 59
   occlusal radiography and, 160
   panoramic machine and, 192, 192f, 193
   photoelectric absorption and, 17
   photons and, 60
   photostimulable phosphor plates and,
     230f
   pixels and, 225
   production of, 12-13
   silver grains and, 77
   subject density and, 78

X-ray beam *(Continued)*
 transorbital projection and, 544-545
 vertical bitewing films, 149, 149f
 vertical root fractures and, 623
X-ray beam alignment, periodontal disease and, 316
X-ray beam collimation, equipment choice of, 56
X-ray examination, stochastic effects from, 54t
X-ray exposure, timer and, 11
X-ray film, 74f
 anterior mandibular occlusal projection and, 157
 composition of, 71-72
 processing of, 77
 radiographic guidelines and, 272, 274t
 timer and, 99-101
X-ray imaging
 morphologic imaging techniques v., 260
 sonography v., 263
X-ray machine, dental
 callibration of, 113-115
 collimators and, 15, 15f
 components of, 7, 7f
 darkroom and, 98, 99f
 disinfection of, 115
 extraoral radiographic examinations and, 210
 federal government designations and, 60
 images from, 11
 overview of, 6, 7
 patient procedure using, 122
 quality assurance program and, 110
 reasons for spectrum of energies in, 12, 13f
 wall chart for, 113f
X-ray photons
 demineralized area and, 297
 scintillating material and, 229f

X-ray receptor, electronic, digital imaging and, 225
X-ray source, movement of, 194f
X-ray tube
 components of, 7-9, 7f
 computed tomography (CT) and, 251
 electrons and, 12
 film based tomography and, 245
 focal spot and, 86
 grids and, 84
 image layer and, 194
 panoramic machine and, 193
 patient examination and, 123
 periodontal disease and, 316
 radiographs and, 121
 Soredex Scanora and, 250, 252f
XCP instruments
 children and, 162
 deciduous maxillary molar periapical projection and, 161
 film holding and, 124, 124f
 film placement in, 152
 horizontal bitewing films and, 148
 patient examination and, 123
 PID and, 59
 sterilizing, 117, 118f
Xerophthalmia, glandular swelling and, 669
Xerostomia
 diabetes mellitus and, 523
 glandular swelling and, 669
 progressive systemic sclerosis and, 531
 radiation and, 33
 radiation caries and, 305
 radiation induced, 36f
 rampant caries and, 303
 sialography and, 660

Z

Zoneography, soft tissue and, 248, 249f
Zygoma bone, midface fractures and, 629

Zygomas
 facial fractures in, 624
 hemifacial hyprplasia and, 650
 horizontal fracture and, 630f
 Treacher Collins syndrome and, 643, 645f
Zygomatic arches, 206, 635
 arch fracture and, 635
 coronoid hyperplasia and, 554, 554f
 panoramic image and, 206
 panoramic projection and, 543, 543f
 submentovertex projection and, 214f
 submentovertex (base) projection and, 213
 transpharyngeal projection, 546f
 Waters projection and, 221
Zygomatic bones
 inferior portion of, 180, 180f
 mid-facial area and, 204
 overview of, 179-180
 zygomatic complex fractures and, 635
Zygomatic bones, missing, Treacher Collins syndrome and, 643
Zygomatic complex fractures, zygomatic bone and, 635
Zygomatic fractures, 629
 clinical features of, 635
 definition of, 634-635
 management of, 635
 radiographic features of, 635
 two types of, 634
Zygomatic process, 205, 282
 film of, 92, 92f
 image field of, 155
 midface and, 206
 odontogenic myxoma and, 434
 overview of, 179-180
 pyramidal fracture and, 632
 radiograph of, 180
Zygomycosis of paranasal sinuses, 588